Allergic Diseases from Infancy to Adulthood

SECOND EDITION

C. WARREN BIERMAN, M.D.

DAVID S. PEARLMAN, M.D.

1988
W. B. SAUNDERS COMPANY
Harcourt Brace Jovanovich, Inc.
Philadelphia ■ London ■ Toronto ■ Montreal ■ Sydney ■ Tokyo

W. B. SAUNDERS COMPANY
Harcourt Brace Jovanovich, Inc.

West Washington Square
Philadelphia, PA 19105

Library of Congress Cataloging-in-Publication Data

Allergic diseases from infancy to adulthood.

  Rev. ed. of: Allergic diseases of infancy,
childhood, and adolescence.
  Includes bibliographies and index.
  1. Allergy. I. Bierman, C. Warren (Charles Warren),
1924–   . II. Pearlman, David S. III. Allergic
diseases of infancy, childhood, and adolescence.
[DNLM: 1. Hypersensitivity. WD 300 A4308]
RC584.A343 1988   616.97   87-26420
ISBN 0-7216-1513-9

Editor: John Dyson
Developmental Editor: Kathleen McCullough
Designer: W. B. Saunders Staff
Production Manager: Bob Butler
Manuscript Editor: Mary Anne Folcher
Illustration Coordinator: Lisa Lambert
Indexer: Lorraine Zawodny

Allergic Diseases from Infancy to Adulthood   ISBN 0–7216–1513–9

Last digit is the print number: 9   8   7   6   5   4   3   2   1

To my late parents, Margery and Linn, my wife Joan, my daughters, Margot, Karen, Charlotte, and Barbara, and my grandchildren, Erin and Cale.

C. Warren Bierman

To my late parents, Benjamin Norman and Sylvia, and to my family, Doris, Michael, Melanie, and Nan.

David S. Pearlman

CONTRIBUTORS

Leonard C. Altman, M.D.
Clinical Professor of Medicine, Oral Biology and Environmental Health; Chief of Allergy, Harborview Medical Center; Staff Physician, University Hospital, Harborview Medical Center, Providence Hospital, Northwest Hospital, Children's Hospital Medical Center, Seattle, Washington.

John A. Anderson, M.D.
Clinical Professor, Department of Pediatrics, University of Michigan, Ann Arbor; Chairman, Department of Pediatrics, Head, Division of Allergy and Clinical Immunology, Henry Ford Hospital, Detroit, Michigan.

Sanford E. Avner, M.D.
Clinical Associate Professor, Department of Pediatrics, University of Colorado Medical School; Senior Staff Physician, National Jewish Center for Immunology and Respiratory Medicine, Denver, Colorado.

H. William Barkman, Jr., M.D.
Professor of Medicine, Department of Medicine, Section of Pulmonary Disease, Tulane University School of Medicine, New Orleans, Louisiana.

C. Warren Bierman, M.D.
Clinical Professor of Pediatrics, University of Washington School of Medicine; Chief, Division of Allergy, Children's Hospital and Medical Center, Seattle, Washington.

Joseph A. Bellanti, M.D.
Professor of Pediatrics and Microbiology, Georgetown University School of Medicine; Director, International Center for Interdisciplinary Studies of Immunology, Georgetown University School of Medicine, Washington, D.C.

Bernard A. Berman, M.D.
Assistant Clinical Professor of Pediatrics, Tufts University School of Medicine; Chief, Pediatric Allergy, St. Elizabeth's Hospital, Boston, Massachusetts.

Hans Bisgaard, M.D.
Senior Registrar, Department of Medicine M, Rigshospitalet, Copenhagen, Denmark.

Charles D. Bluestone, M.D.
Professor of Otolaryngology, University of Pittsburgh School of Medicine; Staff, Children's Hospital of Pittsburgh; Staff, Eye and Ear Hospital of Pittsburgh, Pittsburgh, Pennsylvania.

S. Allan Bock, M.D.
Clinical Associate Professor, Pediatrics, University of Colorado School of Medicine; Senior Staff Physician, National Jewish Center for Immunology and Respiratory Medicine, Denver, Colorado.

Jerome M. Buckley, M.D.
Associate Clinical Professor of Pediatrics, University of Colorado School of Medicine; Senior Clinical Staff, National Jewish Center for Immunology and Respiratory Medicine, Denver, Colorado.

Rebecca H. Buckley, M.D.
J. Buren Sidbury Professor of Pediatrics and Professor of Immunology, Duke University School of Medicine; Chief, Division of Allergy and Immunology, Department of Pediatrics, Duke University Medical Center, Durham, North Carolina.

Robert K. Bush, M.D.
Associate Professor of Medicine, University of Wisconsin; Chief of Allergy, William S. Middleton Memorial Veterans Hospital, Madison, Wisconsin.

William W. Busse, M.D.
Professor of Medicine, University of Wisconsin; Head Allergy Section, Department of Medicine, University Hospital, Madison, Wisconsin.

Hyman Chai, M.D.
Senior Staff Physician, National Jewish Center for Immunology and Respiratory Medicine, Denver, Colorado.

Victor Chernick, M.D.
Professor of Pediatrics, Faculty of Medicine, University of Manitoba; Head, Section of Respirology, Children's Hospital of Winnipeg, Winnipeg, Canada.

Dennis L. Christie, M.D.
Clinical Professor, Department of Pediatrics, University of Washington School of Medicine; Chief, Pediatric Gastroenterology, Children's Hospital and Medical Center; Head, Pediatrics, Virginia Mason Medical Center, Seattle, Washington.

James A. Donaldson, M.D.
Professor of Otolaryngology, University of Washington; Attending, University Hospital; Attending, Children's Hospital, Seattle, Washington.

James G. Easton, M.D.
Clinical Professor of Pediatrics, UCLA; Chief, Department of Allergy and Clinical Immunology, Kaiser Permanente Medical Center, Los Angeles, California.

Peyton A. Eggleston, M.D.
Associate Professor of Pediatrics, The Johns Hopkins University School of Medicine; Attending Physician, Johns Hopkins Hospital, Baltimore, Maryland.

Elliot F. Ellis, M.D.
Professor of Pediatrics, State University of New York at Buffalo; Chief, Division of Allergy/Immunology, Children's Hospital of Buffalo, Buffalo, New York.

Enrique Fernandez, M.D.
Associate Professor of Medicine, University of Colorado Health Sciences Center; Senior Staff Physician, National Jewish Center for Immunology and Respiratory Medicine, Denver, Colorado.

John R. Forehand, M.D.
Instructor in Pediatrics, University of Pennsylvania; Fellow, Children's Hospital of Philadelphia, Philadelphia, Pennsylvania.

S. Lance Forstot, M.D.
Associate Clinical Professor of Ophthalmology, University of Colorado School of Medicine; Ophthalmologist, University Hospital, Veterans Administration Hospital, Denver, Colorado.

Oscar L. Frick, M.D., Ph.D.
Professor of Pediatrics, University of California, San Francisco; Attending physician, University of California, San Francisco, California.

Gilbert A. Friday, M.D.
Professor of Pediatrics, University of Pittsburgh; Chief of Clinical Services, Asthma and Allergic Disease Center, Children's Hospital of Pittsburgh; Children's Hospital of Pittsburgh, Pittsburgh, Pennsylvania.

Vincent A. Fulginiti, M.D.
Professor of Pediatrics, Vice Dean for Academic Affairs, University of Arizona College of Medicine; University Medical Center (active), Tucson Medical Center (consulting), Kino Community Hospital (consulting), Tucson, Arizona.

Dennis L. Fung, M.D.
Professor of Clinical Anesthesia, University of California, Davis; Professor of Clinical Anesthesia, University of California Davis Medical Center, Sacramento, California.

Clifton T. Furukawa, M.D.
Clinical Professor of Pediatrics, University of Washington; Attending Physician, Harborview Hospital; Allergy Education Coordinator, Division of Allergy, Children's Hospital and Medical Center, Seattle, Washington.

Simon Godfrey, M.D., Ph.D.
Professor of Pediatrics, Hadassah-Hebrew University Medical School; Chairman, Department of Pediatrics, Hadassah University Hospital, Mount Scopus, Jerusalem, Israel.

Alan B. Goldsobel, M.D.
Assistant Clinical Professor of Pediatrics, University of California, San Francisco, California.

Anthony R. Hayward, M.D., Ph.D.
Professor of Pediatrics and Microbiology/Immunology, University of Colorado School of Medicine; University Hospital, University of Colorado; National Jewish Center for Immunology and Respiratory Medicine, Denver, Colorado.

Douglas C. Heiner, M.D., Ph.D.
Professor of Pediatrics, UCLA School of Medicine;

Chief, Division of Immunology and Allergy, Department of Pediatrics, Harbor-UCLA Medical Center, Torrance, California.

Leslie Hendeles, Pharm. D.
Professor, Pharmacy and Pediatrics, University of Florida; Clinical Pharmacist, Clinical Pharmacology Division, Pediatrics Department, Shands Hospital of the University of Florida, Gainesville, Florida.

Roger Hollister, M.D.
Associate Professor of Pediatrics, University of Colorado Health Sciences Center; Senior Staff Physician, National Jewish Center for Immunology and Respiratory Medicine, Denver, Colorado.

Alvin H. Jacobs, M.D.
Professor of Dermatology and Pediatrics, Emeritus (Active), Stanford University School of Medicine, Stanford, California.

Richard B. Johnston, Jr., M.D.
Professor of Pediatrics, University of Pennsylvania; Physician-in-Chief and Senior Physician, Children's Hospital of Philadelphia, Philadelphia, Pennsylvania.

Douglas E. Johnstone, M.D.
Clinical Professor of Pediatrics, University of Rochester School of Medicine and Dentistry; Associate Attending Pediatrician, Strong Memorial Hospital, Rochester, New York.

Josef V. Kadlec, S.J., M.D.
Associate Professor of Pediatrics and Microbiology, Georgetown University Medical School; Member, International Center for Interdisciplinary Studies of Immunology, Georgetown University Hospital, Washington, D.C.

Guinter Kahn, M.D.
Director, Pediatric Dermatology Seminars, Miami, Florida.

Michael S. Kaplan, M.D.
Associate Clinical Professor in Pediatrics and Allergy, UCLA; Staff Physician, Kaiser Foundation Hospital, Department of Allergy and Clinical Immunology, Los Angeles, California.

Roger M. Katz, M.D.
Clinical Professor of Pediatrics, UCLA School of Medicine, Director, Allergy Research Foundation, Inc.; UCLA Medical Center; Cedars-Sinai Medical Center, Los Angeles, California.

Robert A. Kinsman, Ph.D.
Clinical Associate Professor, Department of Psychiatry, University of Colorado Medical School, Denver, Colorado.

William T. Kniker, M.D.
Professor of Pediatrics and Microbiology; Chief, Division of Clinical Immunology, University of Texas Health Science Center at San Antonio; Medical Center Hospital, San Antonio; Santa Rosa Medical Center, Texas.

Jane Q. Koenig, Ph.D.
Research Associate Professor, University of Washington, Seattle, Washington.

Gary L. Larsen, M.D.
Associate Professor of Pediatrics, University of Colorado School of Medicine; Head, Section of Pediatric Pulmonary and Critical Care Medicine, University of Colorado Health Sciences Center; Senior Staff Physician, National Jewish Center for Immunology and Respiratory Medicine, Denver, Colorado.

L. Kathleen Mahan, R.D., M.S.
Teaching Associate, Department of Pediatrics, University of Washington; Nutritionist, Pediatric Pulmonary Center, Children's Hospital and Medical Center, Seattle, Washington.

Herbert C. Mansmann, Jr., M.D.
Professor of Pediatrics, Associate Professor of Medicine, Jefferson Medical College of Thomas Jefferson University Hospital; Attending, Thomas Jefferson University Hospital; Attending, Children's Rehabilitation Hospital, Philadelphia, Pennsylvania.

R. Mason, M.D.
Chairman, Department of Medicine, National Jewish Center for Immunology and Respiratory Medicine, Denver, Colorado.

F. Stanford Massie, M.D.
Clinical Professor of Pediatrics, Allergy and Clinical Immunology, Virginia Commonwealth University — Medical College of Virginia; Virginia Commonwealth University — Medical College of Virginia Children's Medical Center; St. Mary's Hospital, Pediatric Allergy and Clinical Immunology, Richmond, Virginia.

Kenneth P. Mathews, M.D.
Professor Emeritus of Internal Medicine, University of Michigan Medical School, Ann Arbor, Michigan;

Adjunct Member, Scripps Clinic and Research Foundation, La Jolla, California.

Timothy P. McBride, M.D.
Assistant Professor, Otolaryngology, University of Pittsburgh School of Medicine; Staff, Children's Hospital of Pittsburgh; Staff, Eye and Ear Hospital of Pittsburgh, Pittsburgh, Pennsylvania.

D. Lee Miller, M.D.
Clinical Associate Professor of Pediatrics, University of Pittsburgh School of Medicine; Chief, Division of Allergy and Immunology, Department of Medicine, The Mercy Hospital of Pittsburgh; Children's Hospital of Pittsburgh, Pittsburgh, Pennsylvania.

Michael E. Miller, M.D.
Professor and Chairman, Department of Pediatrics, University of California, Davis School of Medicine, Davis, California; Professor and Chairman, Department of Pediatrics, University of California, Davis, Medical Center, Sacramento, California.

Niels Mygind, M.D.
Senior Lecturer, Otopathological Laboratory, Department of Otorhinolaryngology, Rigshospitalet, Copenhagen, Denmark.

Harold S. Nelson, M.D.
Clinical Professor of Medicine, University of Colorado Health Sciences Center; Staff Physician, National Jewish Center for Immunology and Respiratory Medicine, Denver, Colorado.

Michael J. Painter, M.D.
Associate Professor, University of Pittsburgh; Children's Hospital of Pittsburgh; Magee-Womens Hospital, Pittsburgh, Pennsylvania.

Frank Parker, M.D.
Professor and Chairman, Department of Dermatology, Oregon Health Sciences University; Oregon Health Sciences University Hospital, Portland, Oregon.

David S. Pearlman, M.D.
Clinical Professor of Pediatrics, University of Colorado School of Medicine; Senior Staff Physician, National Jewish Center for Immunology and Respiratory Medicine, Denver, Colorado.

William E. Pierson, M.D.
Clinical Professor of Pediatrics and Environmental Health, University of Washington School of Medicine; Co-director, Division of Allergy,

Children's Hospital and Medical Center, Seattle, Washington.

Don Warren Printz, M.D.
Former Chief of Operational Research, Venereal Disease Branch, Centers for Disease Control, Atlanta; Dekalb General Hospital, Decatur; Northlake Medical Center, Tucker, Georgia.

Gary S. Rachelefsky, M.D
Clinical Professor, Department of Pediatrics; Director of Allergy Research Foundation; Co-director, Pediatric Allergy Clinic; Associate Director, Allergy, Immunology Training Program, University of California at Los Angeles, Los Angeles, California.

John E. Salvaggio, M.D.
Henderson Professor and Chairman of Medicine, Tulane University School of Medicine, New Orleans, Louisiana.

Michael Schatz, M.D.
Associate Clinical Professor, Department of Medicine and Pediatrics, University of California, San Diego School of Medicine; Active Medical Staff, Kaiser Foundation Hospital; Attending Staff, University Hospital, San Diego, California.

Alan L. Schocket, M.D.
Associate Professor of Medicine, University of Colorado School of Medicine; Associate Director, Department of Medicine, AMI Presbyterian/St. Luke's Medical Center, Denver, Colorado.

Robert H. Schwartz, M.D.
Clinical Professor of Pediatrics, The University of Rochester Medical Center; Pediatrician, Strong Memorial Hospital, Rochester, New York.

Gail G. Shapiro, M.D.
Clinical Professor of Pediatrics, University of Washington School of Medicine; Children's Hospital and Medical Center, Seattle, Washington.

Sheldon C. Siegel, M.D.
Clinical Professor of Pediatrics, UCLA School of Medicine; Co-director of the Pediatric Immunology-Allergy Training Program, UCLA School of Medicine; Cedars-Sinai Hospital, Los Angeles, California; Daniel Freeman Hospital, Centinella Hospital, Inglewood, California.

F. Estelle R. Simons, M.D.
Professor and Deputy Chairman, Department of

Pediatrics and Child Health, University of Manitoba; Head, Section of Allergy and Clinical Immunology, Children's Hospital, Winnipeg, Canada.

Raymond G. Slavin, M.D.
Professor of Internal Medicine and Microbiology, St. Louis University School of Medicine; Attending Physician, St. Louis University Hospital, Cardinal Glennon Children's Hospital and John Cochran Veterans Administration Hospital, St. Louis, Missouri.

R. Michael Sly, M.D.
Professor of Child Health and Development, The George Washington University School of Medicine and Health Sciences; Director of Allergy and Immunology, Children's Hospital National Medical Center, Washington, D.C.

Laurie J. Smith, M.D.
Associate Professor of Uniformed Services, University of Health Sciences in Medicine and Pediatrics; Assistant Chief, Allergy Clinical Immunology Services, Walter Reed Army Medical Center, Washington, D.C.

William R. Solomon, M.D.
Professor of Internal Medicine and Chief, Division of Allergy, University of Michigan Medical School; Attending Physician, University Hospital, Ann Arbor; Consultant, University of Michigan Student Health Service; Consultant, United States Veterans Administration Hospital, Ann Arbor, Michigan.

Sheldon L. Spector, M.D.
Clinical Professor of Medicine, University of California at Los Angeles; Co-director of Allergy Research Foundation; Los Angeles, California.

Jane L. Todaro, M.D.
Clinical Professor of Gastroenterology, Children's Hospital and Medical Center, Seattle, Washington.

James K. Todd, M.D.
Professor of Pediatrics and Microbiology/ Immunology, University of Colorado School of Medicine; Director of Infectious Disease, The Children's Hospital of Denver, Denver, Colorado.

Paul P. VanArsdel, Jr., M.D.
Professor of Medicine and Head, Section of Allergy, University of Washington School of Medicine; Attending Physician, University Hospital; Associate Attending, Harborview Medical Center; Consultant, Children's Orthopedic Hospital and Medical Center, Seattle, Washington.

Stephen I. Wasserman, M.D.
Professor of Medicine and Acting Chairman, Department of Medicine, University of California, San Diego Medical Center; Head, Division of Allergy and Immunology, University of California, San Diego Medical Center, San Diego, California.

Richard W. Weber, M.D.
Training Director, Allergy-Clinical Immunology Training Program, Fitzsimons Army Medical Center; Assistant Clinical Professor of Medicine, University of Colorado School of Medicine; Chief, Allergy-Immunology Service, Fitzsimons Army Medical Center, Aurora, Colorado.

Miles Weinberger, M.D.
Professor of Pediatrics; Chairman, Pediatric Allergy and Pulmonary Division, The University of Iowa, Iowa City, Iowa.

Mark C. Wilson, M.D.
Fellow, Pediatric Allergy and Immunology/ Pulmonary, National Jewish Center for Immunology and Respiratory Medicine and University of Colorado School of Medicine, Denver, Colorado.

James N. Woody, M.D., Ph.D.
Professor of Pediatrics and Microbiology, Georgetown University School of Medicine, Washington, D.C.; Director, Transplantation Research Program Center, Naval Medical Research Institute, Bethesda, Maryland.

John W. Yunginger, M.D.
Professor of Pediatrics, Mayo Medical School; Consultant in Pediatrics and Internal Medicine (Allergy), Mayo Clinic and Foundation, Rochester, Minnesota.

FOREWORD

The new is but the old come true,
Each sunrise sees a new year born.
From *New Year's Morning*
Helen Hunt Jackson (1831–1885)

The disciplines of allergy and immunology are among the most rapidly developing areas in medicine today. Each new idea, each new discovery, each new disclosure, seems to open up a new era in our understanding of the essentials of these specialties. More and more, expansion of our knowledge of immunology is being translated into better understanding of the pathogenesis of the diseases of hypersensitivity and a more rational approach to treatment. As a practical matter, allergy in clinical medicine involves integration of immunology, pathology, physiology, pharmacology, and pulmonology into the whole, and it has become a component part of almost all fields of medicine, cutting across many disciplines and having many similarities in different age groups.

In spite of our increased understanding of these fundamentals, there is a growing body of evidence that suggests that we are not keeping pace with what appears to be a gradual increase in the severity, if not the frequency, of allergic disease, especially in the young. The cause of this phenomenon is not readily apparent, and, regardless of the numerous additions to and improvements in our therapeutic arsenal, asthma is now recognized as the most common medical admission to children's wards. As new and better approaches to treatment are developed, allergic problems seem to increase in severity, so that the newer drugs are required for effective management. We cannot become complacent!

Against this background, the second edition of this text has been designed to increase our understanding of the many facets of allergic disease and to emphasize even more strongly the application of new information in the diagnosis and management of these problems. More stress has been placed on viewing allergy as a continuum, where fundamentals are similar in all age groups, but where tissue responses and clinical manifestations may be modified by age.

The reader will find the new text slightly more constricted, with coverage dealing more directly with clinical allergic disease and with less discussion of tangential material that might more properly relate to fundamental immunologic problems.

The appearance of the second edition of any text is always gratifying, signifying as it does both acceptance of the earlier work and the need for a revision to keep pace with increasing knowledge and changing needs. Future directions in allergy will be based in part on past experience and forward vision. This new text should provide a great deal of both.

William A. Howard, M.D.

PREFACE

Allergy is one of the most common causes of acute and chronic disease. It is a substantial cause of school and work absenteeism for chronic conditions of the respiratory tract and is responsible for a wide range of problems for the patient and family. It may cause physical disability, may interfere with normal psychosocial development of the child and psychosocial relationships of the adult, and often creates severe social and economic difficulties for the family as well. Unfortunately, allergy is a misunderstood and mysterious area of medicine for many physicians. On the one hand, it commonly is invoked as the basis for numerous types of symptoms for which no other explanation is apparent. On the other hand, allergic disease often is not recognized and, even when recognized, is managed inappropriately. This book was first conceived and developed for physicians who provide primary patient care and addresses itself to diagnosis and treatment of those disorders, symptoms, complexes, and signs when the question of "allergy" may arise.

The terminology of allergy suffers from divergent and often vague usage, in itself obstructing recognition and treatment of allergic disease. The term "allergy" was coined in 1906 by von Pirquet following his recognition with Bela Schick that antibodies could cause as well as ameliorate disease. The term, taken from the Greek *allos* ("change in the original state"), referred to the concept that an encounter with a foreign substance induced an alteration in specific responsiveness, so that subsequent contact with that substance was heightened (hypersensitivity) or decreased (hyposensitivity or immunity). Eventually, an association was recognized between immune factors and various clinical syndromes, leading to the idea that these disorders had an immune basis; in this context "allergy" came to refer only to the hypersensitive (adverse) manifestations of the immune response, and the terms "allergic disease" and "allergic disorder" came into use. Current understanding of the pathogenesis of many of these disorders, however, differs from earlier concepts on which the terms were based, and the terms "allergy" or "allergic" often are more confusing than helpful.

Accordingly, we have adopted the following definitions for "allergy" in this book:

An *allergic reaction* is the adverse consequence of a specific immune event, that is, of the interaction between antigen and antibody or sensitized lymphocytes.

An *allergic disorder (disease)* is a complex of symptoms and signs in which immune events are thought frequently to play a major role. It should be recognized that in some individuals with an allergic disease, immune events may not be of major importance or may not participate in the disease at all and, further, that even when "allergy" is an important factor in the disease, it may not be the underlying basis of the disease.

Atopy (from the Greek *atopos* or "strangeness"), another term that requires definition, was first used by Coca and Cooke over 50 years ago with reference to a group of diseases (seasonal rhinitis, perennial rhinitis, asthma) that shared certain clinical features, suggesting a common basis for these disorders. Sulzberger later argued for the inclusion of infantile eczema ("atopic dermatitis") as well. The occurrence of a specific skin-sensitizing substance ("atopic reagin"), now considered to be principally IgE antibody, was recognized in a high proportion of individuals with atopic disorders and was believed to contribute to the pathogenesis of the disorder in such individuals. Though frequently associated, there is considerable evidence that atopic disease can be independent of IgE antibody.

We have chosen, therefore, to consider *atopy* in terms of a constellation of complexes of symptoms and signs that exhibits certain features in common: a familial (and presumably hereditary) basis, an end-organ hypersensitivity to a variety of chemical mediators of inflammation, and a precipitation or an aggravation of the complex by various mechanisms, only one of which may involve IgE antibody. Thus, involvement of IgE antibody is not a required characteristic of an atopic disorder, although the likelihood of an important pathogenetic association with the disorder is considerable. Conversely, the capacity to produce IgE antibody, known to be present in many individuals without any other features of atopy, does not in itself warrant the designation "atopic." Thus, atopic disorders are considered to represent a subgroup of allergic disorders, which include perennial and seasonal allergic rhinitis, asthma, and atopic dermatitis.

This book is for the practicing physician, and its orientation, therefore, is practical. An attempt has been made to reference individual chapters broadly, including review articles and in some cases additional general references on the subject matter covered. We hope that the information and the manner in which it is provided will foster more intelligent diagnosis and therapy of allergy and, in so doing, will encourage the physician to deal more effectively with allergic diseases from childhood through adulthood.

C. Warren Bierman, M.D.
David S. Pearlman, M.D.

INTRODUCTION

VICTOR C. VAUGHAN, III, M.D.

The recorded history of allergic disorders is almost as old as the recorded history of man. Asthma was known to the ancients, as well as the concept that one man's food may be another's poison. The modern perspective with regard to allergy began to be formed early in the 19th century, when Bostock (1819) gave the first modern description of hay fever; a few years later Blackley proved hay fever to be a pollenosis and reported the first confirmatory diagnostic tests, including in 1873 the first skin test. The recognition that asthma and hay fever and certain other clinical syndromes were related to an altered reactivity of the body, often excited by environmental particles, foods, or other conditions, led to a long and exciting period during which the practice of the clinical allergist was dominated by the quest for the identity of those inciting factors.

Immunology is much younger conceptually than allergy. It had its birth in the late 19th century in studies of bacterial infection and resistance, in studies of resistance to snake venom, in the development of antisera against diphtheria and other scourges, and in the description of anaphylaxis. The link between allergy and immunology was forged early in the 20th century by a host of investigators too numerous to list but whose names include Arthus, Calmette, Cooke, Noon, Richet, Schick, Schloss. Theobald Smith, von Behring, and von Pirquet. Richet (1902) described *anaphylaxis* and became the father of modern experimental immunology; von Pirquet (1906) invented the word *allergy* to describe *altered reactivity;* and Leonard Noon (1911) first injected an extract of allergen to treat hay fever by *desensitization* (hyposensitization). The next half century was dominated by a clinical orientation among allergists, based on the concepts developed in these early years. The fundamental notion of allergy was that altered reactivity was based upon prior exposure and that its management was to identify and avoid the inciting factors or to desensitize against those inciting factors when they cannot be avoided altogether and when an effective extract could be prepared.

The romance between allergy and immunology began almost a century ago, and the marriage at its diamond jubilee seems secure, but recent studies have both put the relationship on a more solid conceptual and experimental basis and revealed areas in which appeals to immunology for understanding of allergic problems have failed to find adequate responses. New techniques and new rigors in the scientific study of allergic diseases are changing our perceptions of their natures and are calling upon us to modify or abandon time-honored notions with respect to allergic and related immunologic problems.

The development of sophisticated immunologic tests and their correlation with traditional clinical observation and allergic testing have indicated that some patients with clinical allergy by traditional definitions have no substantial evidence of an immunologic disorder nor any clear-cut sign that traditional measures are likely to be helpful. For such patients, traditional management is to be regarded as unacceptably costly, intrusive, and futile. For them, management with drug therapy may be the only effective present recourse; the same will be true for many other patients who have more traditional forms of allergy. The advances in pharmacologic therapy in the past quarter century have aided in this differentiation and management.

Hyposensitization began to be used in 1911 in the treatment of hay fever. The process was long known as "desensitization" and still may be for some allergists, though it is clear that when wheal and flare reactivity is part of the response to a skin test, this reactivity may not much abate as symptoms are controlled by the injection of extracts. Recent rigorous experimental studies have sharply revised our notions of the effectiveness of this time-honored procedure. The anecdotal evidence of nearly two generations of clinical allergists has supported the procedure with enthusiasm, but studies using modern criteria for statistical reliability and validity were not done until nearly 40 years after desensitization was first introduced. These studies and others that have followed have validated the procedure statistically but have also raised problems as to how the procedure should be properly used in the particular patient. For example, the results of an early study might be interpreted as suggesting that *all* the statistically significantly beneficial effects of desensitization in a study group might have represented major impact on the symptoms of a relatively small subgroup of those who were treated. We are left to wonder how to identify reliably those patients who will and those who will not benefit from or need this form of treatment.

It is clear that attitudes towards allergic diseases are in a state of rather rapid change. Our attitudes towards skin testing and immunization therapy (desensitization or hyposensitization) are more conservative than a decade ago, and with the refined chemical techniques that allow us to accurately measure the levels of drugs (and especially of theophylline) in the blood, we have entered a new era in management of asthma. Cromolyn and corticosteroids also have roles to play in this new development. All of these developments are discussed in detail in the pages that follow, and the contributors to this volume will indicate our present conceptualization of the relationship between the basic sciences and the clinical conundrum known as allergy and will show us where we are sometimes served best by immunology, sometimes best by pharmacology, and sometimes best by an empiric common sense rooted in decades of clinical practice.

Nothing in the foregoing comments should be construed as suggesting that the allergist or any other physician should abandon in any major respect the traditional plan of study of allergic patients, which is to attempt through complete and creative history-taking to identify events or substances precipitating symptoms of allergic disorders. Skin tests have a place in the study of certain patients. Some constraint on exposure to inciting agents is appropriate, and prophylactic constraints often may also be useful. But any of these processes may become cost-ineffective when pushed to the point where the frustration of the physician, the patient, or in the case of a child the patient's parents outweighs relief of tolerable symptoms or to the point where guilt and depression are generated by the failure of intense efforts to abate symptoms that nothing can control. Even though for many years skillful conventional allergic management has brought comfort or relief to millions, we must be ready to test and retest our notions as to what best fits the individual patient and must be ready as soon as possible to identify those patients for whom nonimmunologic therapy is the only kind required or likely to be helpful.

When value systems are in rapid evolution, it is helpful to have substantial reviews such as this volume to bring us to the advancing edge of a changing field and show us where we are, what is going on, and what likely lies ahead. We may guess that what lies ahead for allergic patients and their families is continued progress in clinical immunology, clinical physiology, clinical pharmacology, and clinical psychology. This continuing progress will tell us with ever more confidence what allergic patients need and how to provide it for them.

CONTENTS

Part VIII: Management of Other Allergic Diseases   655

HOST DEFENSE SYSTEMS AND DISORDERS OF HOST DEFENSE

1

The Immune System
MICHAEL E. MILLER, M.D.

Knowledge of the mechanisms of host defense has increased dramatically in recent years. What has emerged is a very complex, yet exciting communications network of cellular and humoral components that interacts to maintain homeostasis and health.

COMPONENTS OF THE IMMUNE-INFLAMMATORY RESPONSE

Cellular Components

Lymphocytes. Lymphocytes are the antigen-specific components of the immune system. They are a highly sophisticated group of cells that act by receptors on their surfaces. Each receptor is highly specific, and different clones of lymphocytes express their own unique specificity. Two major classes of lymphocytes are generally recognized as follows: T lymphocytes and B lymphocytes. (T lymphocytes are so called because of their derivation from or activation by the thymus. B lymphocytes are formed early in the liver of the fetus but subsequently appear to be mainly bone marrow–derived.)

T lymphocytes are required for regulation of immunoglobulin synthesis (in B lymphocytes), mediating delayed hypersensitivity and lysing viral infected and some tumor cells. They can be divided as follows into two major functional subgroups: helper/inducer T cells and cytotoxic/suppressor T cells. The various stages of T cell maturation and the ultimate development into helper/inducer or cytotoxic/suppressor subgroups are correlated with the expression of

specific surface molecules (Reinherz et al., 1980). These molecules are designated by the letter T followed by a number (currently 1 through 11). The OK series of hybridoma antibodies are monoclonal antibodies that react against determinants of human T cells. Detection of the specific surface marker can be made by the use of highly specific monoclonal antibodies such as the OK series. Table 1–1 lists the characteristics and distribution of the various T cell markers and monoclonal antibodies. Helper/inducer T cells are identified by T4 antibodies, and cytotoxic/suppressor T cells by T8 monoclonal antibodies.

B lymphocytes play a primary role in immunoglobulin production and secretion (Inglis, 1982). They display immunoglobulins as integral proteins on their surface membranes. The actual secreted immunoglobulins differ somewhat from those expressed on the B cell surface. Membrane immunoglobulins, for example, contain an additional, hydrophobic peptide at their carboxy terminus and have one less site for glycosylation on their heavy chains (see subsequent discussion of immunoglobulins) (Waldmann and Broder, 1982).

As is the case with T cells, B cells display numerous receptors that also can be identified by monoclonal antibodies. Receptors for IgG, IgA, IgM, IgE, or IgD are found on individual B cells. In addition to the immunoglobulin receptors, B cells have receptors for multiple other antigens, including Epstein-Barr virus (EBV); complement components (C3d, C3b, C4); histocompatibility antigens (HLA-B, HLA-C, HLA-A, and HLA-D); pokeweed mitogen: lipoprotein polysaccharide; and hormones, such as insulin. It is obvious that the B cell may be activated under many different circumstances and by multiple agents (Waldmann and Broder, 1982). Activated B cells either differentiate into immunoglobulin secreting plasma cells or divide and return to a resting state. Such cells are called "memory cells" because they rapidly differentiate into plasma cells when exposed again to the same antigen. Plasma cells represent the

TABLE 1-1. T Cell Markers

Surface Molecule	Molecular Weight (Daltons)	Present on Thymocytes (%)	Present on Peripheral T Cells (%)
OKT1	67,000	95	100
OKT3	20,000-26,000	20	100
OKT4	60,000	75	65
OKT6	44,000	70	0
OKT8	32,000-43,000	80	35
OKT9	190,000	10	0
OKT10	37,000	95	5
OKT11	55,000	95	100

final differentiation of mature B cells. A single plasma cell can release thousands of antibody molecules per second. Unlike the B cell, a plasma cell contains few membrane receptors and has a very short life span of less than 4 days. Most plasma cells are found in the lymphoid tissues and not in the circulation.

Macrophages. The term macrophage was first coined by Metchnikoff at the turn of the century; this term referred to cells that were fixed tissue phagocytes. Over the years, such cells have been identified as histiocytes, alveolar macrophages, Kupffer cells, pleural and peritoneal macrophages, osteoclasts, microglial cells, and synovial type A cells. In recent years, a new classification of macrophages — monocytes and their precursor cells — has been recognized. The common origin of all of these cells from a specific hematopoietic stem cell, along with their common morphology and observed functions, has led to grouping these cells together as the mononuclear phagocyte system. The first identifiable precursor of this system is the monoblast, which matures into a promonocyte and then into a monocyte in the bone marrow. Tissue macrophages arise by maturation of monocytes that have migrated from blood and also by proliferation of local, immature macrophages. The relative contribution of each source to the mature tissue macrophage pool is controversial.

Macrophages play two prominent roles (Nathan, 1980; Shevach, 1984; Parker, 1984). The first is their long recognized role as phagocytes; macrophages are able to recognize and attack foreign or damaged materials. The second, and more recently recognized role, involves their participation in the immune response. Although they are not thought to be specific for any particular antigen, macro-phages are crucial in concentrating and presenting antigens to lymphocytes. The macrophage probably determines which population of T cells will be preferentially activated by various antigens. Macrophages also secrete several biologically active mediators (see subsequent discussion), which regulate the type and degree of response of T and B cells following antigen exposure (Karnovsky and Lazdins, 1978).

In order to accomplish these diverse and sophisticated roles, mononuclear phagocytes display numerous receptors on their cell surfaces, including a number of "nonspecific" receptors for products of other phagocytic and T and B cells (Parker, 1984). Table 1-2 lists some of the receptors of mononuclear phagocytes. The complexity of macrophages is further demonstrated by observing the huge number of substances secreted by activated macrophages. These substances include protein and nonprotein materials, the effects of which influence multiple immune and inflammatory events (Table 1-3).

Finally, it is now recognized that macrophages influence T cell function by an intricate, genetically determined mechanism. An important component of this mechanism is the requirement that the T cell and macrophage that interact display the same histocompatibility-encoded determinants. These are the so-called Ia antigens (see Chapter 2). Only a percentage of mononuclear phagocytes from an activated population express this marker.

Polymorphonuclear Leukocytes (PMNs). PMNs (the "macrophages" of Metchnikoff)

TABLE 1-2. Some Surface Receptors of Mononuclear Phagocytes

Immunoglobulins — Fc domain
  IgG (monomeric and polymeric)
  IgE
Complement
  C3b
  C3d
Macrophage activation factor (MAF)
Macrophage migration inhibition factor (MIF)
Hormone receptors
  Insulin
  Colony stimulating factor (CSF)
Complex carbohydrates
Fucosyl and mannosyl terminal glycoproteins
α 2-Macroglobulin proteinase complexes
Lactoferrin
Transferrin
Fibronectin
Fibrin/fibrinogen
Lipoproteins

TABLE 1-3. Secreted Products of Macrophages*

Enzymes
  Neutral proteinases
    Plasminogen activator
    Metal-dependent elastase
    Collagenase, specific for interstitial collagens (types I, II, III)
    Collagenase, specific for basement membrane collagen (type IV)
    Collagenase, specific for pericellular collagen (type V)
    Cytolytic proteinase
  Arginase
  Lysozyme
  Lipoprotein lipase
  Angiotensin-converting enzyme
  Acid hydrolases
    Proteinases and peptidases
    Glycosidases
    Phosphatases
    Lipases
    Others
Plasma Proteins
  α_2-Macroglobulin
  Fibronectin
  Transcobalamin II
  Apolipoprotein E
  Coagulation proteins
    Tissue thromboplastin
    Factor V
    Factor VII
    Factor IX
    Factor X
  Complement components
    C1
    C2
    C3
    C4
    C5
    Properdin
    Factor B
    Factor D

Plasma Proteins (cont'd)
  Factor I
    (C3b inactivator)
  Factor H
    (β_1H, C3b inactivator accelerator)
Reactive Metabolites of Oxygen
  Superoxide anion
  Hydrogen peroxide
  Others
Bioactive Lipids
  Prostaglandin E_2
  6-Ketoprostaglandin $F_{1\alpha}$
  Thromboxane B_2
  Leukotriene C (slow reacting substance of anaphylaxis)
  12-Hydroxyeicosatetraenoic acid
  Others
Nucleotide Metabolites
  cAMP
  Thymidine
  Uracil
  Uric acid
Factors Regulating Cellular Functions
  Interleukin-1 (endogenous pyrogen)
  Angiogenesis factor
  Interferon
  Factors promoting proliferation of —
    Fibroblasts
    Endothelial cells
    T cells
    B cells
    Myeloid cell precursors (colony-stimulating factor)
  Factors inhibiting proliferation of —
    Tumor cells
    Listeria monocytogenes
  Erythropoietin

* Reproduced, with permission, from Stites DP et al. (eds.): Basic and Clinical Immunology, 5th ed. Copyright 1984 by Lange Medical Publications, Los Altos, California.

serve as a first line of defense against invading microorganisms. It has become evident that these "professional phagocytes" accomplish this function through a set of highly complex and coordinated mechanisms (Cline, 1975). Mobilization of PMNs to the site of infection is initiated in the circulation. The process involves adherence to endothelium, followed by extravascular emigration. Once outside the vessel, PMNs migrate directly towards the foreign particle (chemotaxis). Once the PMN is in the inflammatory arena, membrane recognition and attachment to the particle take place, followed by ingestion (phagocytosis). Within the PMN, fusion of the phagocytic vacuole (containing the organism) with lysosomes takes place, followed by discharge of lysosomal products into the vacuole (degranulation). Membrane attachment and the subsequent steps are accompanied by a burst of oxidative metabolism with generation of oxygen-derived free radicals and hydrogen peroxide. These metabolites, along with the lysosomal bactericidal products, participate in killing the ingested bacteria. Deficiencies in any of the above steps result in impaired host defenses and predictable clinical abnormalities. The disorders of phagocyte function are described in Chapter 4.

PMNs are end stage cells that have a half-life of 6 to 7 hours once released from the bone marrow. Differentiation of committed granulocyte precursors *in vitro* is induced by a glycoprotein substance known as colony-stimulating factor or activity (CSA). Major generation of

CSA occurs following the interaction of monocytes and T lymphocytes. A number of potential feedback regulators of granulopoiesis have been identified, including lactoferrin (see subsequent discussion), endotoxin, and neutrophil breakdown products. Approximately 10^{11} PMNs enter and leave the circulation daily. The total neutrophil pool in the body is approximately, equally divided between circulating and marginated cells. In acute infections, both populations are called into play. Available data suggest that there may be functional heterogeneity among circulating PMN populations.

In view of the complexity of PMN mechanisms it is not surprising that these cells also have a number of identifiable surface receptors similar to lymphocyte and mononuclear phagocytes (Snyderman and Goetzl, 1981). For example, structurally specific receptors for C5a, N-formyl methionyl peptides, leukotrienes, and leukocyte-derived chemotactic factors, have been demonstrated on human PMN membranes.

Basophils, Mast Cells, and Eosinophils. While these cells participate in the immune-inflammatory response, their primary roles appear to lie within the areas of immediate and delayed hypersensitivity. It should be noted, however, that various products of activated basophils, mast cells, and eosinophils may activate cells described previously and humoral systems, such as complement (see following section). These cells are discussed in detail in the appropriate sections of the text.

Humoral Components

Immunoglobulins. The secretory products of mature plasma cells, the immunoglobulins, are the protein molecules that carry antibody activities (Wasserman and Capra, 1977; Jeske and Capra, 1984). These proteins compose approximately 20 percent of the total serum protein pool. Immunoglobulins are found within the circulation, the extravascular fluids, the exocrine secretions, and on the surface of some lymphocytes. Immunoglobulins are composed of approximately 82 to 96 percent polypeptide and 4 to 18 percent carbohydrate. They constitute an extremely heterogeneous group of proteins, among which the five following major subgroups have been recognized: IgG, IgA, IgM, IgD, and IgE. These immunoglobulins are defined by antigenic differences in the C regions of the H chains as now described.

The basic general structure of immunoglobulin molecules is shown in Figure 1–1. Each subgroup contains at least one basic unit or monomer of four polypeptide chains. One pair of polypeptide chains is designated as light (L) chains, and the other pair as heavy (H) chains. The designation is based upon molecular weight, the H chains' containing approximately twice the number of amino acids and twice the molecular weight as the L chains. The heterogeneity of immunoglobulins results from a variable (V) region of each polypeptide chain (amino terminal). Each chain also contains a constant (C) portion at its carboxy terminal portion.

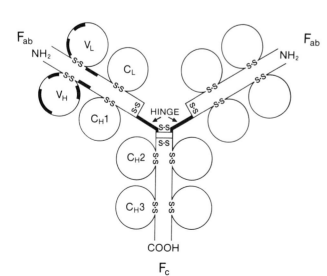

FIGURE 1–1. Multichain structure of human IgG, showing both inter- and intra-chains disulfide bridges, homology regions, and complementarity determining (antigen-binding) regions, located on the variable portions of the H (V_H) and the L (V_l) chains (thick lines). The hinge region is denoted by the heavy solid bars.

Understanding of the molecular structure of immunoglobulins has evolved to the point where an entire text could be devoted to this subject. One of the most important evolutionary concepts involves the new field of immunogenetics. The discovery of the human major histocompatibility complex (MHC) dates from the mid 1950's, and subsequent work has led to the recognition of an elaborate and intricately controlled immunogenetic response, which is discussed in Chapter 2.

FUNCTIONAL ACTIVITIES OF
IMMUNOGLOBULIN SUBGROUPS

Activities of all immunoglobulin subgroups can be divided into two basic functions as follows: (1) binding of antigens and (2) triggering of a spectrum of biologic activities, such as complement fixation and histamine release by mast cells. Antigen binding is localized to the combined action of the V regions of the H and L chains, and the triggering of biologic activities to the C regions of the H chains (Jeske and Capra, 1984).

IgG. IgG makes up approximately 75 percent of the total pool of immunoglobulins in normal adults (Table 1–4) and has a molecular weight of about 180,000 daltons. Four subclasses of IgG have been recognized, and their production is under genetic control. Of the four IgG subclasses, IgG1 makes up 60 to 70 percent of the total IgG pool; IgG2, 14 to 20 percent; IgG3, 4 to 8 percent; and IgG4, 2 to 6 percent.

IgG is the only immunoglobulin class that crosses the placenta. This transport is an active process involving the specific configuration of the Fc portion of the IgG molecule (see Fig. 1–1). The IgG subclasses differ somewhat in their efficiency of placental transport, with IgG2 being the most slowly transported. The biologic significance of these differences, if any, is unknown.

IgG contains multiple antibodies against a wide variety of bacterial and viral antigens and is capable of fixing and activating serum complement. IgG subclasses vary considerably in their ability to fix complement, as follows: IgG3 > IgG1 > IgG2. IgG4 has little, if any, ability to activate complement by the classic pathway (binding of C1q) but may activate the alternative pathway (see following discussion). Interaction between IgG molecules and macrophages is facilitated by the presence of surface receptors on macrophages for the Fc portion of IgG1 and IgG3. Macrophages that have bound IgG1 or IgG3 are activated to exert cytotoxic activities against appropriate target cells or particles.

IgA. IgA is the major constituent of mucosa-produced or secretory immunoglobulins. In addition to two molecules of the basic four-chain polypeptide units, IgA contains one molecule of secretory component and one of J chain (Fig. 1–2). The secretory component is a single polypeptide chain of 70,000 daltons mol wt. Based upon its amino acid composition, secretory component appears to be structurally unrelated

TABLE 1–4. Levels of Immunoglobulins in Sera of Normal Subjects by Age*

Age	IgG		IgM		IgA		Total Immune Globulin	
	MG/DL	PERCENT OF ADULT LEVEL	MG/DL	PERCENT OF ADULT LEVEL	MG/DL	PERCENT OF ADULT LEVEL	MG/DL	PERCENT OF ADULT LEVEL
Newborn	1031 ± 200†	89 ± 17	11 ± 5	11 ± 5	2 ± 3	1 ± 2	1044 ± 201	67 ± 13
1 to 3 mo	430 ± 119	37 ± 10	30 ± 11	30 ± 11	21 ± 13	11 ± 7	481 ± 127	31 ± 9
4 to 6 mo	427 ± 186	37 ± 16	43 ± 17	43 ± 17	28 ± 18	14 ± 9	498 ± 204	32 ± 13
7 to 12 mo	661 ± 219	58 ± 19	54 ± 23	55 ± 23	37 ± 18	19 ± 9	752 ± 242	48 ± 15
13 to 24 mo	762 ± 209	66 ± 18	58 ± 23	59 ± 23	50 ± 24	25 ± 12	870 ± 258	56 ± 16
25 to 36 mo	892 ± 183	77 ± 16	61 ± 19	62 ± 19	71 ± 37	36 ± 19	1024 ± 205	65 ± 14
3 to 5 yr	929 ± 228	80 ± 20	56 ± 18	57 ± 18	93 ± 27	47 ± 14	1078 ± 245	69 ± 17
6 to 8 yr	923 ± 256	80 ± 22	65 ± 25	66 ± 25	124 ± 45	62 ± 23	1112 ± 293	71 ± 20
9 to 11 yr	1124 ± 235	97 ± 20	79 ± 33	80 ± 33	131 ± 60	66 ± 30	1134 ± 254	85 ± 17
12 to 16 yr	946 ± 124	82 ± 11	59 ± 20	60 ± 20	148 ± 63	74 ± 32	1153 ± 169	74 ± 12
Adults	1158 ± 305	100 ± 26	99 ± 27	100 ± 27	200 ± 61	100 ± 31	1457 ± 353	100 ± 24

* From Stiehm, E.R., Fudenberg, H.H.: Serum levels of immune globulins in health and disease. Reproduced by permission of Pediatrics 37:715, 1966.
† One standard deviation.
   Values shown were derived from measurements made in 296 normal children and 30 adults. Levels were determined by the radial diffusion plate method using specific rabbit antisera to human immunoglobulins.

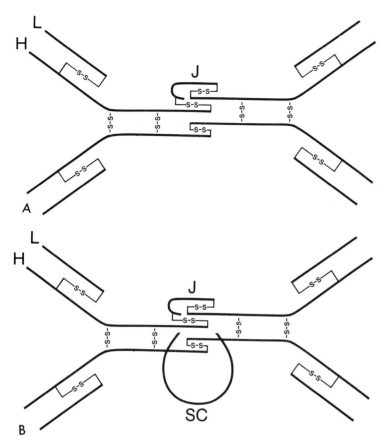

FIGURE 1–2. *A,* Schematic diagram of human serum IgA dimer. The model utilizes the clasp configuration proposed by Koshland (1975, Advan. Immunol. 22:232). *B,* Secretory IgA dimer. The location of the secretory component (SC) is hypothetic.

to other immunoglobulin chains, including J chain. Secretory component is synthesized by epithelial cells at the mucosal surface where actual immunoglobulin secretion occurs. It may be found free in the secretions of individuals with serum or secretory IgA deficiencies. It is considered by many to be a transport protein that enables IgA molecules to reach the secretions from mucosal tissues. J chain is a low molecular weight (15,000 daltons) glycopeptide, which is associated with all multipolymeric forms of immunoglobulins, i.e., two or more basic four-chain units. Although the role of the J chain is controversial, it appears to facilitate polymerization of basic units of IgA and IgM.

IgA may exist in multiple polymeric forms, giving mixtures of disulfide bonded polymers with eight-chain, twelve-chain, or larger multiples of the basic four-chain structure. It is found in high concentrations in saliva, tears, bronchial mucosa, nasal mucosa, prostatic secretions, mucous secretions of the small intestine, and breast milk. It functions at these sites as an initial primary defense mechanism against bacteria and viruses, as well as a deterrent to passage

of antigens across mucosal surfaces where they otherwise would gain exposure to the immune system.

IgM. IgM usually circulates as a pentamer, containing five basic four-chain units with a resultant molecular weight of 900,000 daltons (Fig. 1–3). IgM is not transported across the placenta and is an early antibody formed in response to antigenic challenge (see subsequent discussion of the ontogeny of the immune response in this chapter). IgM has antibody activity particularly against a number of gram-negative organisms. It is a highly efficient activator of complement through the classic pathway (C1q binding) and, along with IgD, is the major immunoglobulin expressed on the B cell surface.

IgD. Despite much effort to characterize the function of IgD, its role in the body remains unknown. Earlier studies suggested a role for IgD in initiating the IgM response, but more recent studies have disproved this hypothesis (see discussion of ontogeny). IgD's predominance, along with IgM, on the surface of B cells continues to suggest a role in differentiation of these cells, but no convincing data have been produced in support of this speculation. The IgD molecule is a monomer, with a molecular weight of approximately 180,000 daltons.

IgE. IgE antibodies have been well characterized as atopic reagins (skin-sensitizing antibodies), and their major role lies in the mediation of the allergic response. As such, they are discussed in considerable detail elsewhere (see Chapter 6). Their major functional activity results from their extraordinarily efficient ability to attach with high affinity to effector cells, such as mast cells, via a site on their Fc region. Following fixation to mast cells, the latter release a panoply of pharmacologic mediators (see Chapter 5), resulting in the characteristic wheal and flare response seen in atopic individuals following a skin test to a particular allergen. Mast cell activation occurs following combination of IgE antibodies by their Fab portion with specific antigens or allergens. A measure of the extreme efficiency of IgE antibodies is provided by the recognition that they make up only 0.004 percent of the total serum immunoglobulins.

Individuals with atopic allergies, in general, have higher levels of IgE than do nonatopic individuals, but this correlation is imperfect. IgE is not passed into the breast milk or across the placenta.

Lymphokines and Cytokines. The mechanisms by which cells of the immune-inflammatory response communicate with one another

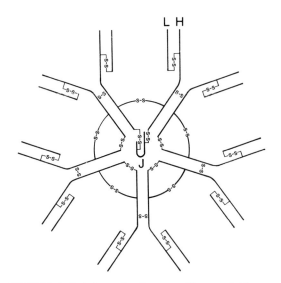

FIGURE 1–3. Schematic diagram of human IgM pentamer, showing inter-subunits, disulfide bridges, and the possible location of the J-piece.

and coordinate their responses involve the production and secretion of effector molecules. Lymphokines are genetically unrestricted, lymphocyte-derived peptides that modulate a wide spectrum of inflammatory and immune responses. The various lymphokines have activities affecting all of the cell types previously described. A similar group of effector molecules is produced by a variety of other cell types. Together with lymphokines, these molecules are collectively known as cytokines (Cohen et al., 1979). We will consider here the most pivotal cytokines and lymphokines, which modulate the immune-inflammatory response.

The major cytokines that amplify both the afferent and efferent limbs of the immune response are the interleukins and interferons. These molecules exert effects upon macrophages, lymphocytes, PMNs, and other cell types, and they may be considered as "second messengers," which amplify the initial response to antigen exposure.

Three *interleukins* have been clearly identified, as follows: interleukin-1 (IL-1), interleukin-2 (IL-2), and interleukin-3 (IL-3) (Dinarello and Mier, 1986; Spivak et al., 1985). *IL-1 is secreted primarily by activated macrophages and monocytes, although a variety of other cells also can participate, including dendritic cells, Langerhans cells, B cells, endothelial cells, melanoma cells, mesangial cells, astrocytes, glioma cells, PMNs, fibroblasts, keratinocytes, corneal cells, and sperm cells. Many antigens and foreign particles can stimulate IL-1 production. The nature of the stimulating particle determines which IL-1 is produced and, if so, whether it remains in the intracellular environment or is secreted into the extracellular environment. A few agents have inhibitory effects upon IL-1 production, including hydrocortisone and products of the cyclooxygenase pathway, such as prostaglandin E_2. Several cultured B cell lines also have produced inhibitors of IL-1.

IL-1 has a number of diverse effects upon the cells of the immune-inflammatory response. IL-1 is effective at augmenting antigen-induced or lectin-induced proliferation of some T cells; it is particularly active towards thymocytes in the thymic medulla and much less so towards peripheral T lymphocytes. More immature subsets of T lymphocytes do not respond to IL-1. Thus, it appears to augment responses of T cells, which have reached a certain developmental stage. Full activation of susceptible T cells requires contact between a lymphocyte and a histocompatible macrophage and IL-1. Depletion of macrophages prevents lymphocyte activation even in the presence of IL-1. IL-1 also can directly augment lymphoproliferative and antibody-producing responses of B cells.

IL-1 also increases and promotes expression of B cell immunoglobulin receptors and T cell differentiation markers, including receptors for responsiveness to IL-2. Other lymphocytes are stimulated by IL-1 to produce IL-2, that, in turn, acts upon lymphocytes bearing IL-2 receptors. In addition, IL-1 also enhances specific cytotoxic effector functions of lymphocytes. In conjunction with IL-2 or interferon (or both), it also can enhance nonspecific natural killer (NK) cells. IL-2 also has been shown to promote the growth and functional activities of a wide variety of nonlymphoid cells involved in inflammatory responses, including fever, increased erythrocyte sedimentation rate, acute phase protein production, and fibrosis. Finally, IL-1 is believed to be the same molecule previously characterized as endogenous pyrogen. Its fever-producing effects are modulated by stimulation of arachidonic acid and prostaglandin production.

The total effects of IL-1, therefore, suggest that it plays a critical role in host defenses against infections. Purification of IL-1 and development of monoclonal antibodies against this molecule promise to initiate an exciting new phase in our understanding of the immune-inflammatory response.

IL-2 is produced by mature T cells. In humans, it appears that both helper and suppressor T cells can produce IL-2 upon appropriate stimulation. IL-2 release from producer cells requires interaction of lectin or antigen with cell membrane, Ir gene products, and IL-1. An indication of the importance of the role of IL-2 in augmentation of immune response is provided by the observation that several immunosuppressive agents, such as glucocorticoids, cyclosporine, and prostaglandin E_2, probably exert their effects by inhibiting its production. Augmentation of IL-2 production results from IL-1 stimulation. In addition, a number of other agents increase IL-2 production, including phorbol myristate acetate, vasopressin and other neurohormones, sodium azide, and a number of cell surface–active compounds.

The development of responsiveness of a cell to IL-2 production requires the development of a specific receptor on that cell surface. Expression of this receptor, known as Tac, is increased following antigen presentation and activation involving IL-1 as discussed previously. An additional factor, known as receptor inducing factor (RIF), also is involved. RIF has not yet been fully characterized. A monoclonal antibody (anti-Tac) has been developed that will block IL-2 production of previously activated T cells. This antibody also has been used to partially characterize the IL-2 receptor. Ontogeny of Tac is discussed subsequently in this chapter.

IL-3 is produced by various cells, including T lymphocytes following exposure to mitogens (Ihle et al., 1981). Currently available data suggest that IL-3 promotes the proliferation of erythroid (BFU-E), megakaryocytic (CFU-Meg), and granulocyte-macrophage (CFU-GM) progenitors and mast cells (Spivak et al., 1985). It also may enhance the proliferation of pluripotent hematopoietic stem cells, i.e., spleen colony-forming units (CFU-S). Since IL-3 increases the number of stem cells in the cell cycle, it may be useful in enhancing the incorporation of new genetic material into these cells as well (Williams et al., 1984). Preliminary evidence for a fourth interleukin *(IL-4)*, and even IL-5 and IL-6, awaits more definitive characterization before they can be accepted as identified factors, however.

Interferons have been recognized as important, nonspecific inhibitors of viral replication. It is known that they also exert important immunoregulatory effects. Three major types of interferons have been recognized as follows: alpha (IFNα), beta (IFNβ), and gamma (IFNγ) (Stewart, 1982).

IFNα is produced by viral or polyribonucleotide-stimulated leukocytes, primarily lymphocytes. This type was previously known as leukocyte or type 1 interferon. Fourteen or more distinct IFNα genes have been cloned. *IFNβ* is produced primarily by viral- or polyribonucleotide-stimulated fibroblasts, epithelial cells, and macrophages. Previous designations were fibroblast interferon and type 1 interferon. IFNβ differs antigenically from IFNα. *IFNγ* was previously called type 2 or immune interferon. It is primarily produced by stimulation of T lymphocytes with antigens, or mitogens.

A wide spectrum of immunoregulatory effects has been attributed to the interferons. It is not yet clear what the specific roles are for each type. Their production can result from stimulation of any of the various cell types indicated. Although the predominant cell types in which each is produced are identifiable, in fact various cell types in combination generally are activated in immune-inflammatory response. The interferons modulate a wide variety of nonspecific inflammatory functions, which is similar to

IL-1. For example, they have profound effects upon activation of phagocytosis, enzyme production, mediator production, and antigen presentation by macrophages. In addition, they exert direct effects on T cells and B cells. The nature of these interactions and the precise ways in which the interferons interact with IL-1 and IL-2 are not yet known. They all are produced following stimulation of cells of the immune system and consequently have been considered "immunohormones." They appear and act in the following sequence: production of IL-1 leading to production of IL-2, leading to production of interferons.

Reactivity of T cells is enhanced by the release of numerous lymphokines, which in turn act as antigen-nonspecific modulators of other cells of the immune-inflammatory response. Not only do they act upon effector cells, but they also can act upon other T and B cell populations. Many lymphokines have been identified, but the clinical relevance of some is conjectural. Among those that are believed to play a role in host defenses are migration inhibition factor (MIF), macrophage activation factor (MAF), leukocyte inhibition factor (LIF), colony stimulating factor (CSF), fibroblast activation factor, B cell growth factor (BCGF), and B cell differentiation factors (BCDF).

Complement. Complement consists of a system of interacting proteins that yields biologic activities upon activation (Brown et al., 1984). Over 20 proteins have been identified, and a number of these have been characterized. The proteins interact in an orderly sequence or "cascade," much like the coagulation system. There are two recognized pathways of complement activation, the classic pathway and the alternative (old name, properdin) pathway (see Chapter 4).

Following activation of various complement components, three major types of biologic activities may result. The first type of activities is cytotoxic reactions. These result from interaction of multiple components upon a given cell surface or membrane. The best known example is hemolysis of antibody-sensitized sheep erythrocytes, in which complement damages the membrane and permits osmotic lysis of the cell. The second type of reactions involves changes that occur on the surface of antigen-antibody particles, as the individual complement components sequentially fix to the complex. For example, a pneumococcus with antibody fixed to its surface will activate complement. Once activation reaches the stage in which active C3 is fixed to the surface of the particle, PMNs in the area avidly attack and phagocytize the pneumococcus. PMNs would not attack the pneumococcus in the absence of complement participation.

Finally, complement may influence the immune-inflammatory response by liberating "split products," of low molecular weights, which are broken off the intact molecules during the process of surface activation. Unlike the native molecules that circulate in a biologically inactive state, the split products possess potent activities, such as histamine release (anaphylatoxins) and attraction of leukocytes (chemotactic factors). Such activities have wide potential in the modulation of numerous steps of the inflammatory response. Normal and abnormal functions of the complement system are discussed further in Chapter 4.

Other Mediators. In addition to complement and the cell-derived mediators described, the roles of a number of other substances found in the circulation in association with the immune-inflammatory response are being investigated. Two of these, lactoferrin and fibronectin, have been implicated as important participants.

Lactoferrin is an iron-binding protein found in the secondary, or specific, granules of PMNs. This protein has been implicated as having an important role in bacteriostasis and in enhancement of PMN functions, such as movement and ingestion. An important role for lactoferrin in PMN adhesiveness has been suggested, as based upon the identification of patients with genetic deficiencies of lactoferrin and impaired PMN adhesiveness (see Chapter 4).

Fibronectin is a high molecular weight glycoprotein that is present in soluble and insoluble forms. The soluble form (plasma fibronectin) is found in blood, lymph, and other tissue fluids. The insoluble form (tissue fibronectin) is found primarily in connective tissue and in association with basement membranes. Plasma fibronectin opsonizes numerous antigenic and nonantigenic particles and increases phagocytosis *in vitro*. Tissue fibronectin may be involved in cell-cell interactions and adherence to substratum. It may play a significant role in wound healing.

Chemical mediators of the allergic inflammatory response are considered in detail in Chapter 5.

DEVELOPMENTAL IMMUNOLOGY

The remainder of this chapter considers the development of the various components and functions of the immune-inflammatory response from fetal life to early childhood. Such information is important for three reasons. First, data on this period of life have contributed significantly to our understanding of the interrelationships of the various components of host defenses and their genetically determined control mechanisms. Second, understanding of the ontogeny of the immune-inflammatory response has markedly increased our knowledge of the large group of immune-deficiency and inflammatory-deficiency disorders identified in this text. Finally, information gained from studies of ontogeny of host defenses has played a major role in the understanding of and designing of therapeutic strategies for the continuing problem of neonatal sepsis.

Cell mediated immunity (CMI) is important for protection against infections with viruses, fungi, and protozoa. It also plays a pivotal role in the host's ability to recognize and react against allogeneic histoincompatible cells. Cell mediated immune reactions take place through specifically modified, or "sensitized," T cells. The early fetal development of immunocompetent T cells prevents fetal infections and protects the fetus against destruction by immunocompetent, histoincompatible, maternal T cells.

Ontogeny of T Cell Immunity

T Lymphocyte Subpopulations. The use of monoclonal antibodies for the identification and characterization of surface receptors on various types of T cells has been described. This technique also has been used to investigate the maturation of the T cell system in the fetus and neonate. Three maturational stages of differentiation have been described (Reinherz et al., 1980). In stage 1, early thymocytes show OKT9+ and OKT10+ surface markers (see Table 1–1). In stage 2, common thymocytes are detected in the thymic cortex. These cells are OKT4, 6, 8, and 10+. Two subsets also are found within this population, precursors of helper/inducer T cells (OKT4 + 8−) and precursors of suppressor/cytotoxic T cells (OKT4 − 8+). In stage 3, mature thymocytes are found in the thymic medulla (OKT3+, OKT10+). Of the thymocytes eventually released into peripheral blood, fewer than 5 percent retain the OKT10+ marker.

As detected by monoclonal antibodies, cord blood ratios of helper : suppressor T cells are greater than ratios of adult peripheral blood

(1 : 2 vs. 1 : 3) (Griffiths-Chu et al., 1984). The absolute number of T cells in newborns, however, actually is greater than in adults. A significant proportion of T cells in cord blood shows immature T cell markers. These are primarily suppressor cells which are OKT3−.

Antigen Recognition and Binding. Recognition and binding of antigen are among the earliest steps in the immune response. Several techniques have been utilized to measure these functions in fetal life. Fetal thymocytes acquire these abilities early during gestation. By the technique of binding of radiolabeled antigen, fetal thymocytes were observed with bound antigens by 10 to 13 weeks' gestation (Dwyer et al., 1972). When measured by mixed lymphocyte reactions, responses were seen as early as 10 weeks' gestation. Human splenic lymphocytes develop graft versus host (GVH) reactivity as early as 13 weeks' gestation (Stites et al., 1974). This finding indicates that fetal thymus or lymphoid tissues given to reconstitute immune function in children with T cell deficiencies probably should be obtained from fetuses of no more than 10 to 14 weeks' gestation in order to avoid inducing GVH reactions in the recipients.

Cytotoxic Activities of Lymphocytes. Antigen-activated lymphocytes destroy or lyse appropriate target cells *in vitro*. This activity, known as cell-mediated lympholysis (CML), appears to develop during intrauterine life, although it has been demonstrated less consistently with neonatal than with adult lymphocytes in various studies (Granberg et al., 1976).

Response to T Lymphocyte Mitogens and Antigens. Extensive data have been obtained on the response of fetal and neonatal T cells to nonspecific mitogens (Miller, 1978). Fetal lymphocytes respond to mitogens, such as phytohemagglutinin (PHA), as early as 10 weeks of gestation. Responsive cells can be identified first in the thymus and in the peripheral blood and spleen 3 to 4 weeks later. Data on response of cord blood lymphocytes to PHA are conflicting. Depending upon study design, PHA responsiveness of cord blood lymphocytes has been found to be equal to, greater than, or less than that of adult lymphocytes. Some of the contradictory findings probably stem from the failure to obtain highly purified populations of nonactivated cord blood lymphocytes. Also, when interpreting cell responsiveness to mitogens, it is important to recognize that PHA may not be a suitable prototype for all other mitogens (Alford et al., 1976). For example, responsiveness to PHA appears to develop earlier and more vigorously than does responsiveness of fetal lymphocytes to another mitogen, ConA (Leino et al., 1980). This finding suggests the possibility that the PHA and ConA responsive lymphocytes may come from different subpopulations.

Fetal and cord blood responses to specific antigens have been studied less well than has mitogen-induced blastogenesis. The few studies available indicate that lymphocytes of some newborn infants can respond to stimulation by *Salmonella* or *Candida in vitro*, following prior exposure (Leiken and Oppenheim, 1971; Alford et al., 1976).

Suppressor Activity. Studies of suppressor activity of neonatal lymphocytes suggest a relative increase compared with maternal or adult lymphocytes (Altman et al., 1984; Jacoby et al., 1984). It is unclear whether this increased suppressor activity is due to cellular or humoral factors or to a combination of both, as will be reviewed.

Neonatal Suppressor Cell Activity. Studies that have demonstrated increased neonatal T cell suppression, for the most part, have examined inhibition of mitogen responses of adult lymphocytes by neonatal lymphocytes (Hayward, 1981). Data have been obtained using a variety of mitogens, including PHA, pokeweed mitogen (PWM), and mixed lymphocyte cultures. Suppression by a given neonate's lymphocytes is specific for its mother's cells (Olding and Oldstone, 1974 and 1976). Fetal studies have demonstrated that proliferation of maternal lymphocytes may be decreased by fetal lymphoid cells from liver at 8 weeks of gestation and by fetal blood lymphocytes at 14 weeks or later of gestation (Unander and Olding, 1981). This suppressor activity towards maternal lymphocytes has been found in lymphocytes as late as 11 months after birth. Identification of the subset of T cells responsible for the suppressor activity of newborn cells suggests that it is an OKT8+ lymphocyte. In virtually all of the studies published to date, the possible role of other cell types in the cultures has not been fully evaluated, however. The precise nature of suppressor cell activity in the fetus and neonate, therefore, remains to be determined.

Soluble Suppressor Factors. Soluble factors that cause suppression have been demonstrated by several investigators. The suppressor activity of newborn lymphocytes can be inhibited completely, for example, by prior irradia-

tion with 6000 rads. This finding suggests that cell division may be required for the development of the suppressor effect of neonatal cells upon maternal cells *in vitro* (Olding et al., 1977). In several studies, the cell-free supernates generated by stimulation of lymphocytes with antigens or mitogens have shown suppression of *in vitro* antibody responses.

Preliminary characterization of a humoral neonatal suppressor factor has been carried out. The factor is dialyzable, stable at 56°C for 30 minutes but inactivated by heating at 80°C for 10 minutes. This factor has been named "cord T cell–derived suppressor factor (CTSF)" (Miyawaki et al., 1979). It has been suggested that CTSF may work in concert with monocytes. CTSF has a molecular weight of less than 500 daltons (Johnsen and Olding, 1983). It also has been suggested that prostaglandins (PG) are the probable effector molecules. Suppression can be blocked, for example, with the use of either indomethacin or anti-PGE_2 antibodies (Durandy et al., 1982). PGE_1 and PGE_2 appear to be the major immunosuppressive species. The difference in sensitivity between neonatal and maternal lymphocytes to prostaglandin E may in part reflect fewer high-affinity receptors on the surface of cord blood lymphocytes.

Activity of Natural Killer and Killer Cells. Two types of effector cells have been identified within the lymphocyte population that have the capability of causing death or lysis to appropriate target cells. Natural killer (NK) cells are lymphocytes that are spontaneously cytolytic for certain tumor cell lines and viral infected cells. Killer (K) cells are a different population of effector cells that mediate antibody dependent cellular cytotoxicity (ADCC). NK cells appear to be a subpopulation of peripheral blood mononuclear cells, which morphologically are large granular lymphocytes. Utilizing a monoclonal antibody that identifies NK cells, the ontogeny of appearance has been evaluated (Abo et al., 1982). The number of NK cells progressively increases from a very low level during the newborn period to normal adult level by the age of 30 years. Numbers increase in rough correlation with age between the newborn and adult periods. Of the few studies on NK function in newborn infants, results are highly variable, and information is insufficient to correlate functional activity with cell number. Data on K cell activity are too limited at present to permit even speculative comments.

A possible role for hormonal regulation in the development of NK cells in humans has been suggested. Males show slight but significantly greater NK activity than females (Abo et al., 1982). Administration of estrogen in mice blocks maturation of NK cells in bone marrow (Seaman et al., 1979). Dosages of hormones used in the experimental studies, however, were much greater than physiologic, and the significance of the findings mentioned is unclear.

Ontogeny of B Cell Immunity

Through the use of monoclonal antibodies much information also is available about the fetal and neonatal development of B cell function. Maturation of B cells during fetal life involves two distinct stages (Lawton and Cooper, 1977; Raff et al., 1976). The first stage consists of the development of lymphoid cells containing intracellular (cytoplasmic) IgM. In the human fetus, these first appear from 7.5 to 10 weeks of gestation. The next stage of development is the ability to express IgM on the surface of the cells. Such cells are first detected in fetal liver commencing at approximately 10 weeks' gestation. IgD does not precede but rather follows expression of IgM. This fact is of interest as it was thought for some time that IgD was the first immunoglobulin expressed and that it was a necessary precedent to the development of normal B cell function. B lymphocytes emerge sequentially, in a specific chronology, by an antigen independent process. The order of development in studies to date is IgM, IgD, IgG, and IgA. Although the precise sites of B cell development in humans have not yet been positively identified, most evidence favors fetal liver and then bone marrow, as serving sequentially in this capacity (Lawton and Cooper, 1977).

Most of the B cells in the fetus are found in blood (30 percent), spleen (35 percent), and lymph nodes (13 percent) (Gathings et al., 1976). The relative proportion of each isotype appears to be antigen independent and genetically predetermined.

Fetal Immunoglobulin Production. Intrauterine infection from organisms such as rubella virus, cytomegalovirus, *Treponema pallidum*, and *Toxoplasma gondii* leads to increased production of IgM antibody by the fetus (Alford, 1970). In addition, an infection acquired at or shortly after birth stimulates IgM synthesis. However, the post-natal IgM level must be significantly greater than the expected physiologic level to be considered a reliable indicator of intrauterine infection, since IgM levels rise rapidly after birth (probably as a result of bacterial colonization of the gastrointestinal tract).

Antibody Responses. Studies on the antibody response in fetal lambs produced a major contribution in this area (Sterzl and Silverstein, 1967). Indwelling catheters were placed into the large vessels in the neck of fetal lambs, thereby permitting injection of antigens into the fetal circulation and periodic withdrawal of blood samples for antibody measurements without further surgical intervention. A variety of antigens were administered, including bacteriophage ϕX 174, ferritin, egg albumin, and salmonella. These studies revealed that the fetal lamb was able to produce antibodies against most of the antigens long before birth and that there was a stepwise maturation or "hierarchy" of antigen responsiveness. In other words, the fetal lambs developed the ability to respond to each of the antigens at different stages of gestation. Thus, antibodies to phage were observed at days 34 to 41 of gestation, antibodies to ferritin were first observed at day 55, and antibodies to egg albumin were observed at day 125. Anti-salmonella antibody had not appeared in fetuses by term (150 days). More recent studies have demonstrated a similar stepwise maturation in the opossum and the rat.

This hierarchy of antigen responsiveness has major implications in the understanding of mechanisms of the fetal immune response. The initial explanation, that the stepwise development of antibody responses to various antigens reflected the development of separate clones of antibody-producing cells, has little evidence to support it. An alternative hypothesis for which there are supportive data relates to stepwise maturation of antigen-processing cells, such as macrophages. Various antigens, for example, may not stimulate antibody production until development of mechanisms for their degradation by macrophages and subsequent presentation to the antibody-producing B cells. Antibody responses in newborn sheep, mice, and rats are increased by the addition of adult macrophages but not by adult lymphocytes (Blaese et al., 1970; Argyris, 1968).

Immunoglobulins. The human fetus produces little IgG. Serum levels remain below 100 mg/dl until approximately 17 weeks of gestation, at which time a gradual and steady increase occurs. By term the fetal IgG level usually exceeds the maternal level by 5 to 10 percent. IgA has been detected in 30-week-old human fetuses. Only limited synthesis occurs, so serum levels seldom are in excess of 5 mg/dl. Little, if any, IgA is transferred across the placenta. Most newborns beyond 30 weeks of gestation have low but detectable and measurable IgM in cord serum. Buckley and coworkers (1969) reviewed the results of seven studies of cord blood IgM levels and found that mean levels varied from 5.8 to 15.8 mg/dl; levels at two standard deviations varied from 1 to 10 mg/dl (lower limit) to 12.9 to 27.4 mg/dl (upper limit). In premature infants, IgM levels usually are slightly lower than in term infants but not in a predictable fashion. The proportion of infants without detectable cord IgM increases with decreasing gestational age. There is no known clinical significance to the absence of cord IgM. In contrast, as discussed, an elevated cord IgM level indicates intrauterine antigenic stimulation, often the result of intrauterine infection. IgD also does not cross the placenta and usually is not detectable in cord blood. When present, IgD levels are 5 to 30 percent of the normal adult level of 3 mg/dl. Maternal IgD levels tend to increase in pregnancy. IgE does not cross the placenta (Bazaral et al., 1971). Synthesis of IgE has been detected by week 11 *in utero* in fetal lung and by week 21 in liver (Miller et al., 1973). Rate of synthesis is usually low, as suggested by the low mean cord serum IgE concentrations of approximately 2 IU/ml (see also Chapter 6.).

The Antibody Response of the Neonate. A number of circulating factors may inhibit or suppress the neonatal antibody response. Transplacentally acquired maternal antibody inhibits active antibody formation in the newborn period. For example, infants with passively acquired diphtheria antitoxins or poliomyelitis antibodies have decidedly diminished responses when given diphtheria toxoid or inactivated poliomyelitis vaccine. Inhibition can be overcome at least for certain potent antigens (e.g., tetanus) by employing larger antigen doses, more frequent immunizations, or adjuvants. Other humoral factors may exert an immunosuppressive effect upon neonatal antibody production. Bilirubin, for instance, can suppress antibody responses to pertussis, diphtheria, tetanus, and *Escherichia coli* until 1 year of age (Nejedla, 1970).

The studies by Smith et al. (1964) of antibody responses to *Salmonella* flagellar (H) antigens and somatic (O) antigens illustrate the antibody response of the human newborn. Passively acquired maternal antibody influenced immune responsiveness; only those newborns without detectable maternal antibody or with titers (< 1:20) exhibited antibody responses. Most premature and term neonates with passively acquired *Salmonella* agglutinins were able to produce antibodies to flagellar (H) antigens when immunized with *Salmonella* vaccine, but older infants (> 13 days) were more responsive than newborn infants. The response was not related to maturity since over 50 percent of the premature infants (< 2500 gm birth weight) produced flagellar agglutinins in titers of at least 1:10 by day 7 following immunization; more than 80 percent had responded by day 14. In many instances, the titers of flagellar agglutinins were comparable with those found in adults. Dancis and coworkers (1953), utilizing diphtheria toxoid, found that a small proportion of full-term and premature neonates immunized with toxoid during the first week of life developed diphtheria antitoxin within 1 month. All premature infants responded when immunized with diphtheria toxoid at their estimated birth dates. The antigenic stimulus supplied by the bacterial flora acquired at birth seems to play a major role in the development of the antibody response.

Smith et al. (1964) also found that premature or full-term neonates rarely developed agglutinins to the somatic O antigen, in contrast to H agglutinins, whereas immunized older children and adults developed O agglutinins by day 14. The capacity to produce agglutinins to O antigens developed between 3 and 9 months of age. Even though the assay technique used in measuring O agglutinins is less sensitive than that used in measuring H agglutinins, it is evident that a significant difference exists in the ability of neonates to respond to those two antigens. Whether immune or nonimmune (processing) maturational factors are responsible for the different reactions to these antigens is not clear, however.

The antibody response to H antigen also followed a sequential development similar to that seen in the adult. The first antibody activity to appear in the neonate was found in the macroglobulin fraction, probably IgM, followed by activity in the IgG fraction. Although the heterogeneity of response was similar to that seen in adults, the newborns differed in the timing of the appearance of activity in the IgG fraction. IgM was present exclusively in the neonates for prolonged periods, up to 20 to 30 days following immunization. Adults showed IgG-antibody activity at 5 to 15 days. The prolonged transition from IgM to IgG antibody in neonates has been found to last from 1 to 6 months of age.

Passive Immunity in the Newborn. The fetus receives IgG antibodies passively via the placenta; the breast-fed infant additionally receives secretory antibodies (which are not absorbed) via the oral route. Passively acquired maternal IgG antibodies confer the neonate with protection against certain disorders, such as measles, rubella, meningococcal infections, streptococcal disease, and *Haemophilus influenzae* infection. Some protection against certain other infections (such as vaccinia, varicella, pertussis, tetanus, and diphtheria) also may result. However, since protective IgG antibodies to these agents do not persist in high titers, only recently infected or immunized mothers tend to provide protective IgG antibodies to their infants. Certain maternal antibodies to antigens of gram-negative organisms, such as *Escherichia coli* and Salmonelleae, reside chiefly within the IgM class and do not cross the placenta; consequently, the infant does not receive all of the mother's antibodies to these organisms. Gitlin and coworkers (1963) postulated that this deficiency of IgM may be responsible, at least in part, for the unusual susceptibility of newborns to infections with gram-negative organisms. However, IgG antibodies to somatic antigens of gram-negative organisms do cross the placenta and can provide protection for most infants.

It should be recognized that lack of placental transfer of certain maternal IgM antibodies is advantageous to the neonate. For example, the presence of maternal IgM isoagglutinins (natural anti-A and anti-B) in the infant would result in ABO hemolytic disease in every ABO incompatible maternal-newborn pair.

Skin Reactivity and Inflammatory Response

Since many assays of inflammatory immune function depend upon some form of skin response, it must be recognized that an abnormal response can be due to abnormal skin reactivity as well as to defective inflammatory or immune function. Gaisford (1955) found that infants immunized with BCG (bacille Calmette-Guérin vaccine) developed positive Mantoux test reactions in 14 to 21 days as in the adult, but the intensity of the reactions was diminished by comparison. Also infants under 1 year of age were found to develop less contact sensitivity to a *Rhus* allergen, pentadecylcatechol, than adults.

Uhr et al. (1960) studied the development of delayed type (contact) hypersensitivity in premature and term neonates exposed to 2,4-dinitrochlorobenzene. Reactions developed in all of the control subjects and in two of five term neonates and three of ten premature infants studied. Reactions in the neonates were less intense than those in the older infants, but the histology of the lesions was qualitatively similar to that seen in contact-type hypersensitivity in the adult. Responses to sensitization did not correlate with the weight of the premature infants or the full-term neonates. The investigators concluded that a newborn has the capacity to develop cell-mediated immunity at or shortly after birth but that the response is uneven, partly due to a diminished ability to maintain an inflammatory response at this age.

Many newborn animals exhibit poor inflammatory responses to dermal infections and have reduced capacities to localize such infections. They also demonstrate delayed migration of neutrophils and mononuclear cells. The skin of human newborns responds poorly to irritation and fails to localize inflammation when compared with the skin of older children (Eitzman and Smith, 1959). Studies of cutaneous inflammation in neonates by the Rebuck-Crowley skin window method also have demonstrated a relatively delayed and less intense shift from the predominantly polymorphonuclear to the mononuclear phase than in adults (Eitzman and Smith, 1959; Bullock et al., 1969). Skin homografts applied to human infants at birth are rejected, although more slowly than in adults (Fowler et al., 1960).

Sterzl and Hrubesova (1959) demonstrated passive transfer of tuberculin skin test reactivity from skin test–negative piglets to adult pigs by sensitizing newborn leukocytes. Salvin et al. (1962) immunized guinea pigs during the first 2 weeks of life with diphtheria toxoid. Although the newborn guinea pigs failed to show cutaneous reactivity to toxoid, their leukocytes were able to passively transfer cutaneous reactivity to toxoid to adult guinea pigs. In most studies of humans, newborns fail to accept sensitized cells or manifest a delayed allergic skin test reaction after receiving sensitized cells. Fireman et al. (1970) studied purified protein derivative (PPD) reactivity in infants between 1 and 2 days of age born of mothers with positive tuberculin test results. No reactivity to PPD by skin test or in lymphocyte culture was found in any infant. Passive transfer of PPD reactivity with leukocytes or leukocyte transfer factor from PPD-positive mothers was studied in neonates of both PPD-positive and PPD-negative mothers. Infants who received either intact leukocytes or transfer factor from PPD-positive donors showed increased activity to PPD in lymphocyte cultures *in vitro*, as assessed by blast transformation or incorporation of ³H-thymidine into nucleoprotein. By contrast, these infants showed no *in vivo* response to PPD skin testing. When leukocytes from three infants who had failed to develop a delayed skin test reaction after passive sensitization were injected into PPD-negative adult recipients, two of three of the latter became PPD-positive. The investigators then administered BCG to the passively sensitized infants as well as to a group of normal nonsensitized infants. *In vivo* skin and *in vitro* leukocyte responses to PPD were not different in the two groups. The development of the *in vitro* leukocyte response to PPD preceded the development of the *in vivo* skin reactivity by 1 to 3 weeks. These studies demonstrate that the neonatal lymphocyte is capable of responding immunologically to antigen, despite the absence of a skin test response.

In addition to the decreased cutaneous responsiveness of newborn skin, defects have been observed in the phagocyte and complement systems of neonates (Miller, 1979a and 1979b). Although the degree to which these individual deficiencies contribute to the overall diminished skin response is unclear, it is highly probable that some (or all) of them play a role. (These areas are covered in detail elsewhere in this text, and only information relevant to the newborn period is summarized here.)

Ontogeny and Function of Phagocytic Cells

Polymorphonuclear Leukocytes. Neonatal PMNs show decreased movement compared with adult PMNs (Miller, 1971). Pahwa et al. (1977) compared movement of cord blood PMNs with that of PMNs from healthy adults towards two stimuli, as follows: endotoxin-activated serum and lymphocyte-derived chemotactic factor (LDCF). Cord blood PMNs moved significantly less rapidly than did adult PMNs. Klein et al. (1977) utilized an agarose technique and also found deficient movement in neonatal PMNs.

Miller (1975) adapted the assay of cell elastimetry to the study of neonatal PMNs. Neonatal PMNs were markedly less deformable than adult PMNs. In other words, significantly greater negative pressures were required to aspirate neonatal PMNs than adult PMNs into equal sized micropipettes. This increased rigidity of the neonatal PMNs was hypothesized to play a significant role in the impaired movement of these cells. Kawaoka and coworkers (1981) compared the effects of the synthetic chemotactic peptide, N formyl leucyl phenylalanine (f-Met-Leu-Phe), upon the deformability and filter movement of PMNs. Alterations in PMN deformability occurred as a natural consequence of chemotactic factor stimulation. It was concluded that increased deformability might be a prerequisite to efficient PMN movement. If so, the decreased deformability found in neonatal PMNs might be responsible for compromised movement and function.

Miller and Cheung (1980 and 1982) utilized videotape and multiple speed cinemicrographic analysis to further examine these relationships. Newborn PMNs failed to adhere and deform properly; therefore, these cells are at a mechanical disadvantage when compared with adult PMNs or their more distant ancestors, the amoebae. These mechanical limitations result in an inability of the newborn PMNs to obtain leverage for directed migration and effective translocation.

A variety of studies implicate modulation through the cell membrane as the level responsible for the decreased deformability of neonatal PMNs. Mease et al. (1980) found phytohemagglutinin-induced (PHA-induced) aggregation and chemotactic response of cord PMNs to be selectively decreased. The chemotactic response of neonatal PMNs showed a positive correlation with PHA-induced aggregation. Chemokinesis of newborn PMNs was the same as adult PMNs. These investigators suggested that the decreased chemotactic response of newborn PMNs might be due to developmental membrane differences that adversely affect the membrane or the availability of C5a receptors (or both).

Kimura et al. (1981) investigated the phenomenon of concanavalin A–induced (ConA–induced) capping in cord blood PMNs. The phenomenon reflects membrane fluidity, which in turn reflects submembranous cellular events, including the functional state and activity of the cytoskeletal component of the PMNs. In normal human adult PMNs, ConA capping is significantly increased following incubation of the cells with an agent such as colchicine, a microtubule disruptor. Prior to incubation with colchicine, adult and cord blood PMNs showed a comparable proportion of spontaneously capped cells. Upon preincubation with colchicine, a significant increase from 16 percent to 48 percent capped cells occurred with adult PMNs. In contrast, the colchicine-treated cord PMNs failed to show any increase in capping over spontaneous levels. The mean value of spontaneous capping in cord PMNs was 18 percent, and colchicine preincubated cord PMNs increased to only 22 percent.

Cheung et al. (1985) utilized the tritonation (demembranation)/reactivation technique to study the functional compromises of cord blood PMNs. Normal adult PMNs demonstrated random movement and pseudopodial formation that were lost during tritonation. Reactivation by ATP helped to restore these activities. Such reactivated models, however, did not regain their chemotactic responsiveness. Thus, the tritonation process left the cytoskeletal structures functionally intact, but the same process partially and selectively destroyed the cell membrane enough to eradicate its chemotactic sensation/integration function. Cord blood PMNs also demonstrated random movement and pseudopodial formation under normal conditions but lacked chemotactic responsiveness. As with adult PMNs, tritonated cord blood PMNs lost their movement characteristics and regained them with addition of ATP.

Monocyte/Macrophage Activity. Immune reactivity of neonatal macrophages may be somewhat less developed than adult macrophages. Braun and Lasky (1967) were able to increase the antibody response to sheep erythrocytes in 2-day-old C47B1 mice by the addition of adult macrophages. Argyris (1968) obtained similar results in C3H/He mice. Blaese (1970) studied the role of macrophages in the antibody response in newborn rats. Administration of adult macrophages, but not adult lymphocytes, enhanced antibody response of newborn rate to antigen challenge.

Fetal macrophages appear to have relatively little capacity to suppress immunoglobulin synthesis in mitogen-stimulated cultures (Jacoby et al., 1984; Olding and Oldstone, 1976). Cord blood macrophages had no effect upon normal mitogen-driven responses of adult lymphocytes (Durandy et al., 1982). Rodriguez et al. (1981) showed that selection with the monoclonal antibody OKM1 (which selects for monocytes) did exert significant suppression in such cultures.

Expression of Ia on the surface of macrophages is important for the processing of certain antigens, such as polysaccharides. Prostaglandins, such as PGE_2, can suppress Ia expression. Snyder and coworkers (1982) found that concentrations of PGE_2 found in fetal circulation decreased the expression of Ia on macrophages *in vitro* to below detectable levels. This finding may be implicated in the poor response of the newborn to certain polysaccharide antigens.

Limited data are available on secretory products of macrophages. Gerdes et al. (1984) studied the production of fibronectin and the second component of complement (C2) in cultured monocyte-macrophages from cord and adult blood. Cord and adult cells synthesized equal amounts of C2, but cord cells synthesized significantly less fibronectin than adult cells. The researchers suggested that this observation may explain, in part, the reduced plasma fibronectin concentration and reticuloendothelial system hypofunction found in the newborn infant.

Functional activity of neonatal macrophages compared with that of adult macrophages is not well understood. Wilson and Haas (1984) found that newborn macrophages activated by adult ConA stimulated–lymphocyte supernatants killed *Toxoplasma gondii* as well as similarly activated adult macrophages (see also section on Cytokines and Lymphokines). Data on neonatal macrophage movement, ingestion, and killing are limited and somewhat contradictory.

Complement Ontogeny and Activation

Ontogeny of complement in neonates has been studied by the three following basic techniques: (1) synthesis of individual components by isolation of fetal tissues and study *in vitro* (Colten, 1977); (2) in the case of genetic polymorphism, demonstration of different maternal-fetal genetic type; and (3) demonstration of a specific complement component in fetal or neonatal serum that the mother lacks as the result of a genetic deficiency, thereby implying fetal synthesis of that component. Immunochemical demonstration of C3 synthesis by fetal tissues has been demonstrated as early as 5.5 weeks of gestation. Little, if any, placental transfer of maternal complement to fetal circulation occurs.

Numerous measurements of complement components and activities of classic and alternative pathways in the fetus and neonate have been reported (Miller, 1978). In general, both classic and alternative pathway activities have been relatively deficient in neonates, as compared with adults. Previous studies that have examined low birth weight infants have found that the defects in alternative and classic pathway activities are relatively greater than in normal birth weight infants. It was not clear from these studies, however, whether the relatively greater defect in low birth weight infants was the result of premature birth or of intrauterine growth retardation. Recent data of Notarangelo et al. (1984) suggest that in infants of comparable birth weights, complement activity is significantly influenced by differences in gestational age. Shapiro and coworkers (1981) also found no differences between complement levels in AGA (appropriate for gestational age) and SGA (small for gestational age) term infants (i.e., of different birth weights but of comparable gestational ages). In summary, complement factors increased gradually during gestation, and intrauterine growth retardation did not affect development of complement factors.

Studies of complement component levels and hemolytic activities may not reflect functional activity of the complement system (Miller, 1978). Thus such activities as opsonic and chemotactic functions may require separate measurements to assess actual level of functional development.

Cytokines and Lymphokines

The assessment of functional activity of the various cytokines and lymphokines is difficult, as the assay systems are complex and involve cells as well as humoral factors. For example, newborn leukocytes synthesize similar amounts to adult leukocytes. The addition of alpha-interferon to newborn cells, however, increased NK cell activity against herpes simplex–infected targets less than its addition to adult cells. Addition of alpha-interferon or gamma-interferon to newborn leukocytes induces less antiviral activity than addition to adult leukocytes.

Few data are available on the relative production and functional activity of lymphokines in the fetal and neonatal periods. Eife and coworkers (1974) measured lymphotoxin production by neonatal lymphocytes, as compared with production by adult lymphocytes. Lymphotoxin is a lymphokine that is cytotoxic for a variety of target cells and is produced by lymphocytes exposed to PHA, ConA, a variety of antigens, or allogeneic cells. Newborn lymphocytes produced only 25 percent as much lymphotoxin as did adult lymphocytes.

Macrophage migration inhibitory factor (MIF) production has been compared between newborn and adult mononuclear cells. As with lymphotoxin, newborn cells produced significantly less MIF. Lymphocyte derived chemotactic factor (LDCF) production by neonatal cells also is relatively decreased.

Macrophage activation is dependent in adults on a series of lymphokine signals, including macrophage activating factor (MAF). Wilson and Hass (1984) compared MAF production and response to MAF in newborns with that in adults. Both of these functions were decreased in the newborn macrophages. These workers and others have suggested that gamma-interferon may be the major MAF in the newborn. Cord blood MAF producing lymphocytes may be deficient in number, MAF-producing capacity, or interleukin-2 (gamma-interferon) producing capacity.

Other Mediators

Yoder and coworkers (1983) studied plasma fibronectin levels in healthy term and premature newborn infants and compared them with those of normal adults. The term and premature groups had significantly lower plasma fibronectin levels. In infants suffering from perinatal asphyxia or respiratory distress syndrome, the levels were even lower. Comparable data of fibronectin levels are reported by McCafferty and coworkers (1983).

Synthesis of fibronectin by cultured monocyte/macrophage preparations was studied by Gerdes and coworkers (1984). Cultured monocytes from cord blood synthesized far less fibronectin than comparable cells from adult blood. By contrast, synthesis of another macrophage product, C2, was the same for both cultures thereby suggesting that the fibronectin synthetic defect was selective. Both cord and adult cells showed similar functional morphologic properties on long-term culture.

REFERENCES

Abo, T., Cooper, M.D., Balch, C.M.: Postnatal expansion of the natural killer and killer cell population in humans identified by the monoclonal HNK 1 antibody. J. Exp. Med. 155:321–326, 1982.

Alford, C.A.: Immunologic status of the newborn. Hosp. Pract. 5:88–94, 1970.

Alford, R.H., Cartwright, B.B., Sell, S.H.: Ontogeny of human cell-mediated immunity: Age-related variation of *in vitro* infantile lymphocyte transformation. Infect. Immun. 13:1170–1175, 1976.

Altman, Y., Handzel, Z.T., Levin, S.: Suppressor T-cell activity in newborns and mothers. Pediatr. Res. 18:123–126, 1984.

Argyris, B.F.: Role of macrophages in immunological maturation. J. Exp. Med. 128:459–467, 1968.

Bazaral, M., Orget, H.A., Hamberger, R.N.: IgE levels in normal infants and mothers and an inheritance hypothesis. J. Immunol. 107:794–801, 1971.

Blaese, R.M., Henrichon, M., Waldmann, T.A.: Ontogeny of the immune response: The afferent limb (abstract). Fed. Proc. 29:699, 1970.

Braun, W., Lasky, L.F.: Antibody formation in newborn mice initiated through adult macrophages (Abstract). Fed. Proc. 26:642, 1967.

Brown, E.J., Joiner, K.A., Frank, M.M.: Complement. *In* W. E. Paul (ed.); Fundamental Immunology. Raven Press, New York, 645–668, 1984.

Buckley, R.H., Younger, J.B., Brumley, G.W.: Evaluation of serum immunoglobulin concentrations in the perinatal period by use of a standardized method of measurement. J. Pediatr. 75:1143–1148, 1969.

Bullock, J.D., Robertson, A.F., Bodenbender, M.T., Kontras, S.B., Miller, C.E.: Inflammatory response in the neonate re-examined. Pediatrics 44:58–61, 1969.

Cheung, A.T.W., Miller, M.E., Donovan, R.M., Goldstein, E., Kimura, G.M.: Reactivation of tritonated models of human polymorphonuclear leukocytes (PMNs): A computer-assisted analysis. J. Leuk. Biol. 38:203–211, 1985.

Cline, M.J.: The White Cell. Harvard University Press, Cambridge, 1975.

Cohen, S., Pick, E., Oppenheim, J.J.: Biology of the Lymphokines. Academic Press, Orlando, 1979.

Colten, H.R.: Development of host defenses: The complement and properdin systems. *In* M.D. Cooper, D.H. Dayton (eds.); Development of Host Defenses. Raven Press, New York, 165–173, 1977.

Dancis, J., Osborn, J.J., Kunz, H.W.: Studies of immunology of the newborn infant. IV. Antibody formation in the premature infant. Pediatrics 12:151–156, 1953.

Dinarello, C.A., Mier, J.W.: Interleukins. Ann. Rev. Med. 37:173–178, 1986.

Durandy, A., Fischer, A., Griscelli, G.: Inability of newborns' or pregnant women's monocytes to suppress pokeweed mitogen-induced responses. J. Immunol. 128:525–529, 1982.

Dwyer, J., Warner, N.L., McKay, I.R.: Specificity and nature of the antigen-combining sites on fetal and mature thymus lymphocytes. J. Immunol. 108:1439–1446, 1972.

Eife, R.F., Eife, G., August, C.S., Kuhre, W.L., Staehr-Johansen, K.: Lymphotoxin production and blast cell transformation by cord blood lymphocytes: Dissociated lymphocyte function in newborn infants. Cell Immunol. 14:435–442, 1974.

Eitzman, D.V., Smith, R.T.: The non-specific inflammatory cycle in the neonatal infant. Am. J. Dis. Child, 97:326–334, 1959.

Fireman, P., Kumate, J., Gitlin, D.: Development of delayed hypersensitivity in neonates (abstract). Excerpta Med. (Amst.), Sect. VII. International Congress of Allergology, No. 211, 1970.

Fowler, R., Jr., Schubert, W.K., West, C.D.: Acquired partial tolerance to homologous skin grafts in the human infant at birth. Ann. N.Y. Acad. Sci. 87:403–428, 1960.

Gaisford, W.: Protection of infants against tuberculosis. Br. Med. J. 2:1164–1171, 1955.

Gathings, W.E., Cooper, M.D., Lawton, A.R., Alford, C.A.: B cell ontogeny in humans. Fed. Proc. 35:276a, 1976.

Gerdes, J.S., Douglas, S.D., Kolski, G.B., Yoder, M.C., Polin, R.A.: Decreased fibronectin biosynthesis by human cord blood mononuclear phagocytes *in vitro*. J. Leuk. Biol. 35:91–99, 1984.

Gitlin, D., Rosen, F.S., Michael, J.G.: Transient 19S gamma-deficiency in the newborn infant and its significance. Pediatrics 31:197–208, 1963.

Granberg, C., Manninen, K., Toivanen, P.: Cell-mediated lympholysis by human neonatal lymphocytes. Clin. Immunol. Immunopath. 6:256–263, 1976.

Griffiths-Chu, S., Patterson, J.A.K., Berger, C.L., Edelson, R.L., Chu, A.C.: Characterization of innovative T cell subpopulations in neonatal blood. Blood 64:296–300, 1984.

Hayward, A.R.: Development of lymphocyte responses and interactions in the human fetus and newborn. Immunol. Rev. 57:39–60, 1981.

Ihle, J.N., Pepersack, L., Rebar, L.: Regulation of T cell differentiation: *in vitro* induction of 20 α-hydroxysteroid dehydrogenase in splenic lymphocytes is mediated by a unique lymphokine. J. Immunol. 126:184–189, 1981.

Inglis, J.R., (ed.): B Lymphocytes Today. Elsevier Science Publishing Co., Inc., New York, 1982.

Jacoby, D.R., Olding, L.B., Oldstone, M.B. A.: Immunologic regulation of fetal-maternal balance. Adv. Immunol. 35:157–208, 1984.

Jeske, D.J., Capra, J.D.: Immunoglobulins: Structure and function. *In* W.E. Paul (ed.); Fundamental Immunology. Raven Press, New York, 131–165, 1984.

Johnsen, S.A., Olding, L.B.: Differences in binding sites for prostaglandin E2 on mononuclear leukocytes from human newborns and from their mothers. Scand. J. Immunol. 17:389–394, 1983.

Karnovsky, M.L., Lazdins, J.K.: Biochemical criteria for activated macrophages. J. Immunol. 121:809–813, 1978.

Kawaoka, E.J., Miller, M.E., Cheung, A.T.W.: Chemotactic factor induced effects upon deformability of human polymorphonuclear leukocytes. J. Clin. Immunol. 1:41–45, 1981.

Kimura, G.M., Miller, M.E., Leake, R.D., Raghunathan, R., Cheung, A.T.W.: Reduced concanavalin-A capping of neonatal polymorphonuclear leukocytes (PMNs). Pediatr. Res. 14:1271–1273, 1981.

Klein, R.B., Fischer, T.J., Gard, S.E., Biberstein, M., Rich, K.C., Stiehm, E.R.: Decreased mononuclear and polymorphonuclear chemotaxis in newborns. Pediatrics 60:467–472, 1977.

Lawton, A.R., Cooper, M.D.: Two new stages of antigen-independent B cell development in mice and humans. *In* M.D. Cooper, D.H. Dayton (eds.); Development of Host Defenses. Raven Press, New York, 43–54, 1977.

Leiken, S., Oppenheim, J.J.: Differences in transformation of adult and newborn lymphocytes stimulated by antigen, antibody and antigen-antibody complexes. Cell Immunol. 1:468–475, 1971.

Leino, A., Hirvonen, T., Soppi, T.: Ontogeny of phytohemagglutinin and concanavalin A responses in the human fetus: Effect of thymosin. Clin. Immunol. Immunopathol. 17:547–555, 1980.

McCafferty, M.H., Lepow, M., Saba, T.M., Cho, E., Meuwissen, H., White, J., Zuckerbrod, S.F.: Normal fibronectin levels as a function of age in the pediatric population. Pediatr. Res. 17:482–485, 1983.

Mease, A.D., Fischer, G.W., Hunter, K.W., Roymann, F.B.: Decreased phytohemagglutinin-induced aggregation and C5a-induced chemotaxis of human newborn neutrophils. Pediatr. Res. 14:142–146, 1980.

Miller, D.L., Hirvonin, T., Gitlin, D.: Synthesis of IgE by the human conceptus. J. Allergy Clin. Immunol. 52:182, 1973.

Miller, M.E.: Chemotactic function in the human neonate: Humoral and cellular aspects. Pediatr. Res. 5:487–492, 1971.

Miller, M.E.: Developmental maturation of human neutrophil motility and its relationship to membrane deformability. In J.A. Bellanti, D.H. Dayton (eds.); The Phagocytic Cell in Host Resistance. Raven Press, New York, 295–307, 1975.

Miller, M.E.: Host Defenses in the Human Neonate. Grune and Stratton, New York, 1978.

Miller, M.E.: The immunodeficiencies of immaturity. In E.R. Stiehm, V.A. Fulginiti (eds.); Immunologic Disorders in Infants and Children, 2nd ed. W.B. Saunders Co., Philadelphia, 219–238, 1979a.

Miller, M.E.: The inflammatory and natural defense systems. In E.R. Stiehm, V.A. Fulginiti (eds.); Immunologic Disorders in Infants and Children, 2nd ed. W.B. Saunders Co., Philadelphia, 165–180, 1979b.

Miller, M.E., Cheung, A.T.W.: Characterization of the movement defect of human neonatal polymorphonuclear leukocytes (PMNs). Pediatr. Res. 14:549a, 1980.

Miller, M.E., Cheung, A.T.W.: Functional alterations in the membrane of motile polymorphonuclear leukocytes. Am. J. Pediatr. Hem. Oncol. 4:77–82, 1982.

Miyawaki, T., Seki, H., Kubo, M., Taniguchi, N.: Suppressor activity of T lymphocytes from infants assessed by coculture with unfractionated adult lymphocytes in the pokeweed mitogen system. J. Immunol. 123:1092–1096, 1979.

Nathan, C.F., Murray, H.W., Cohn, Z.A.: The macrophage as an effector cell. N. Engl. J. Med. 303:622–626, 1980.

Nejedla, A.: The development of immunological factors in infants with hyperbilirubinemia. Pediatrics 45:102–104, 1970.

Notarangelo, L.D., Chirico, G., Chiara, A., Columbo, A., Rondini, G., Plebani, A., Martini, A., Ugazio, A.G.: Activity of classical and alternative pathways of complement in preterm and small for gestational age infants. Pediatr. Res. 18:281–285, 1984.

Olding, L.B., Murgita, R.A., Wigzell, H.: Mitogen-stimulated lymphoid cells from human newborns suppress the proliferation of maternal lymphocytes across a cell-impermeable membrane. J. Immunol. 119:1109–1114, 1977.

Olding, L.B., Oldstone, M.B.A.: Lymphocytes from human newborns abrogate mitosis of their mother's lymphocytes. Nature 249:161–162, 1974.

Olding, L.B., Oldstone, M.B.A.: Thymus derived peripheral lymphocytes from human newborns inhibit division of their mothers lymphocytes. J. Immunol. 116:682–686, 1976.

Pahwa, S., Pahwa, R., Grimes, E., Smithwick, E.: Cellular and humoral components of monocyte and neutrophil chemotaxis in cord blood. Pediatr. Res. 11:677–680, 1977.

Parker, C.W.: Mediators. In W.E. Paul (ed.); Fundamental Immunology. Raven Press, New York, 703–707, 1984.

Raff, M.C., Jegson, M., Owen, J.J.T., Cooper, M.D.: Early production of intracellular IgM by B-lymphocyte precursors in mouse. Nature 259:224–226, 1976.

Reinherz, E.L., Kung, P.C., Goldstein, G., Levey, R.H.,

Schlossman, S.F.: Discreet stages of human intrathymic differentiation: Analysis of normal thymocytes and leukemic lymphoblasts of T cell lineage. Proc. Natl. Acad. Sci. (U.S.A.) 77:1588–1592, 1980.

Rodriguez, M.A., Bankhurst, A.D., Ceuppens, J.L., Williams, R.C.: Characterization of the suppressor cell activity in human cord blood lymphocytes. J. Clin. Invest. 68:1577–1585, 1981.

Salvin, S.B., Gregg, M.B., Smith, R.F.: Hypersensitivity in newborn guinea pigs. J. Exp. Med. 115:707–722, 1962.

Seaman, W.E., Merigan, T.C., Talal, N.: Natural killing in estrogen-treated mice responds poorly to poly IC despite normal stimulation of circulating interferon. J. Immunol. 123:2903–2905, 1979.

Shapiro, R., Beatty, D.W., Woods, D.L., Malan, A.F.: Serum complement and immunoglobulin values in small-for-gestational-age infants. J. Pediatr. 99:139–141, 1981.

Shevach, E.M.: Macrophages and other accessory cells. In W.E. Paul (ed.); Fundamental Immunology. Raven Press, New York, 71–107, 1984.

Smith, R.T., Eitzman, D.V., Catlin, M.E., Wrirz, E.O., Miller, B.E.: Development of the immune response: Response of newborn and mature humans to salmonella vaccines. Pediatrics 33:163–183, 1964.

Snyder, D.S., Beller, D.I., Unanue, E.R.: Prostaglandins modulate macrophage Ia expression. Nature 299:163–165, 1982.

Snyderman, R., Goetzl, E.J.: Molecular and cellular mechanisms of leukocyte chemotaxis. Science 213:830, 1981.

Spivak, J.L., Smith, R.R.L., Ihle, J.M.: Interleukin 3 promotes the in vitro proliferation of murine pluripotent hematopoietic stem cells. J. Clin. Invest. 76:1613–1621, 1985.

Sterzl, J., Hrubesova, M.: Attempts to transfer tuberculin hypersensitivity to young rabbits. Folia Microbiol. (Praha) 4:60–61, 1959.

Sterzl, J., Silverstein, A.M.: Developmental aspects of immunity. Adv. Immunol. 6:337–359, 1967.

Stewart, W.E., II: The Interferon System, 2nd ed. Springer-Verlag, New York, 1982.

Stites, D.P., Carr, M.C., Fudenberg, H.H.: Ontogeny of cellular immunity in the human fetus: Development of responses to phytohemagglutinin and to allogeneic cells. Cell Immunol. 11:257–271, 1974.

Uhr, J.W., Dancis, J., Neumann, C.G.: Delayed-type hypersensitivity in premature neonatal humans. Nature 187:1130–1131, 1960.

Unander, A.M., Olding, L.B.: Ontogeny and postnatal persistence of a strong suppressor activity in man. J. Immunol. 127:1182–1186, 1981.

Waldmann, T.A., Broder, S.: Polyclonal B cell activators in the study of the regulation of immunoglobulin synthesis in the human system. Adv. Immunol. 32:1–63, 1982.

Wasserman, R.L., Capra, J.D.: Immunoglobulins. In M.I. Horowitz, W. Pigman (eds.); The Glycoconjugates. Academic Press, New York, 323–348, 1977.

Williams, D.A., Lemischka, I.R., Nathan, D.G., Mulligan, R.C.: Introduction of new genetic material into pluripotent haematopoietic stem cells of the mouse. Nature 310:476–480, 1984.

Wilson, C.B., Haas, J.E.: Cellular defenses against Toxoplasma gondii in newborns. J. Clin. Invest. 73:1606–1616, 1984.

Yoder, M.C., Douglas, S.D., Gerdes, J., Kline, J., Polin, R.A.: Plasma fibronectin in healthy newborn infants: Respiratory distress syndrome and perinatal asphyxia. J. Pediatr. 102:777–780, 1983.

2

Immunogenetics

JOSEPH A. BELLANTI, M. D.
JOSEF V. KADLEC, S. J., M. D.
JAMES N. WOODY, M. D., PH.D.

Immunogenetics is the study of processes involved in the immune response that may have a *genetic* basis. It includes all factors that control immune responsiveness as well as transmission of antigenic specificities from generation to generation.

Immune responses are carried out by a highly sophisticated multicompartmental system of cells and cell products that respond in a coordinated fashion to the presence of antigen. The integration of major opposing functions, i.e., regulation of helper and suppressor function and maintenance of some immune balance, is under strict genetic control. Polymorphic genetic systems encode for the various immunoglobulins, major histocompatibility (MHC) antigens, and T-cell receptors. There are also genes that code for other mediators and components of immune reactions. All interact in generating, regulating, and fostering an effective immune response.

CLINICAL IMPORTANCE OF IMMUNOGENETICS

An understanding of immunogenetics is assuming increased clinical importance because the genetic variability from individual to individual appears to form the basis for determining susceptibility to infection and predisposition to many of the allergic (atopic) and other hypersensitivity diseases, autoimmune diseases, and malignant diseases. Immune imbalance may be an important factor in the pathogenesis of disease entities such as systemic lupus erythematosus (SLE), rheumatoid arthritis, multiple sclerosis, Kaposi sarcoma, and Addison disease, all of which have demonstrable immune abnormalities and often exhibit an association with the genetically determined major histocompatibility complex (MHC) antigens. Knowledge of immunogenetics also provides tools for the diagnosis, treatment, and prevention of disease. The recent development of highly specific monoclonal antibodies has fostered research in basic and clinical disciplines within and outside immunology.

A knowledge of the genetic factors controlling the antigenic specificities of the ABO, Rh, and human leukocyte antigen (HLA) systems is of clinical importance. In addition to forming the basis for understanding of hemolytic diseases of the newborn, transfusion reactions, and factors involved in transplantation of tissues and organs, associations between histocompatibility types and rheumatoid, malignant, immune, atopic, and other diseases have been identified that present new and exciting diagnostic possibilities. For example, there is evidence for an association among ragweed hayfever, production of IgE antibody to ragweed, and markers for immune response genes closely linked to the histocompatibility system.

GENETICS OF IMMUNE REGULATION

A large number of genes (collectively called immune response or IR genes) code for regulatory molecules or components of the immune network. It was originally thought that the genes controlling the immune response were located within the genetic segment coding for histocompatibility antigens. Although the histocompatibility-linked IR genes certainly play an important role in immune responses, only part of the system is histocompatibility linked. Certain IR genes may code for cellular receptors for antigen, for instance, immunoglobulin molecules that act also as surface receptors on B cells. Another group of recently identified genes code for receptors on T cells. There is reason to believe that other genes exist that control mediator secretions or cellular receptors. Thus, there appears to be a multigenic system that exists on several levels, which controls the capacity to respond to antigens and regulates the type and duration of the immune response.

Disorders of this complex and multigenic immunoregulatory network, whether genetic or environmental, can lead to serious consequences, which range from an inability to respond to antigenic exposure *(hyporesponsiveness)*, as seen in patients with acquired immunodeficiency syndrome (AIDS), to autoimmune disorders, as seen in SLE *(hyperresponsiveness)*, or to allergic diseases.

The three best studied polymorphic systems in humans that form the genetic basis of immune responsiveness include the major histocompatibility complex (MHC), the genes that code for immunoglobulins and for IgE antibody production, and the recently discovered genes responsible for polymorphism of the T-cell receptor.

THE MAJOR HISTOCOMPATIBILITY COMPLEX (MHC) OF HUMANS—HLA

The human MHC is called the human leukocyte antigen (HLA) system and is located within a chromosomal region on the short arm of chromosome 6. The MHC consists of a series of genes that code for the expression on cell surfaces of strong transplantation antigens. These antigens are present on the surface of most nucleated cells and, generally, are glycoprotein in composition. The MHC in mammals also is the region where the histocompatibility-linked IR genes are located. This chromosomal HLA segment has many functions, as follows: it controls the synthesis of transplantation antigens responsible for graft rejection and influences immune responses to infectious agents as well as susceptibility to development of immunologically mediated diseases.

Several major genetic loci have been established within the HLA complex (Fig. 2–1). The A, B, and C functional loci code for Class I anti-

gens, whereas the D subregion with functional loci DP (SB), DQ (MB=DC), and DR/Dw codes for Class II molecules. Some of the complement components also are coded within the HLA region, and their products sometimes have been referred to as Class III antigens.

Each of the HLA genes has many alleles (i.e., alternative forms) that represent small variations in the nucleotide sequence of the gene. These small changes in the gene result in small variations in cell surface glycoproteins, perhaps a change of one or two amino acids, or in a small difference in molecular stereoconfiguration. These variations in HLA antigen structure are called "specificities" and can be detected either by specific HLA typing antisera (Class I) or by certain typing cells specific for Class II molecules (Fig. 2–2). The HLA genes are inherited in a codominant fashion as a group, in accordance with mendelian principles. Individuals receive one set of "haplotype" genes from each parent.

Structure and Function of Human Class I Antigens

In humans, three structural genes (HLA-A,-B,-C) on chromosome 6 code for Class I antigens. Each Class I antigen consists of a large transmembrane glycoprotein heavy chain (of about 350 amino acids, 44K mol wt) noncovalently associated with beta-2 microglobulin (a 100 amino acid, 12K mol wt protein). Beta-2 microglobulin is coded for by genes on a separate chromosome from those coding for the Class I heavy chain. The arrangement of these molecules on the cell surface is shown schematically in Figure 2–3. Each of the HLA-A, -B, or -C genes has multiple alleles at each locus. The HLA-B gene has the largest number of detect-

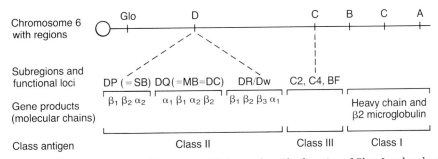

FIGURE 2–1. Schematic representation of the human HLA complex. The function of Class I molecules is to serve as target antigens for immune recognition and killing. The function of Class II antigens is to serve as restricting molecules in cellular regulation. Class III antigens are the components of the complement system. Both new and old (in parentheses) nomenclature for the subregions (functional loci) are given.

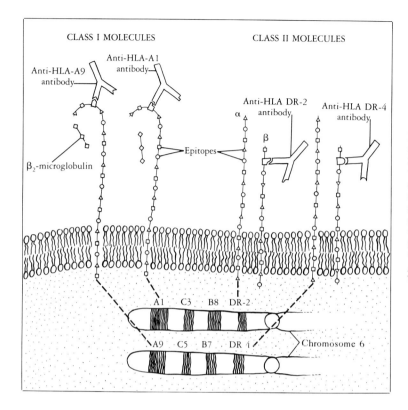

FIGURE 2–2. Schematic representation of HLA antibodies showing how serologic (allelic) specificities are detected. The small symbols in the schematic molecules represent areas with amino acid variations that can be recognized by specific antibodies. These variations recognized by antibodies are known as "epitopes" or "specificities." (From Bellanti, J. A.: Immunology III, Philadelphia, W.B. Saunders Co., 1985.)

able alleles (specificities) with 32 and is said to be the most polymorphic. The HLA-A genes have 17 alleles or specificities, which have been detected. The currently accepted list of alleles is shown in Table 2–1. Each of the alleles has been numerically designated. For example,

HLA-A1 and HLA-Aw30 represent alleles of the HLA-A gene. For a tentative assignment of a new specificity, the prefix "w" (workshop) has been assigned by the International Workshop for HLA Genetics to indicate that it is under consideration for acceptance as a formal

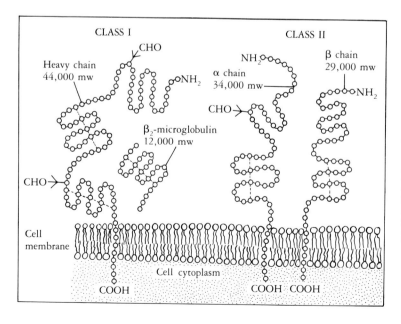

FIGURE 2–3. Schematic representation of Class I and Class II histocompatibility antigens within the cell membrane. Class I type glycoprotein antigens are coded for by HLA-A, B, and C genes in humans, and by H-2 K, D, L, Qa, and TLa genes in mice. Class II antigens are coded for by HLA-DR, DC, and SB genes in humans, and by IA and IE genes in mice. (From Bellanti, J.A.: Immunology III, Philadelphia, W.B. Saunders Co., 1985.)

TABLE 2–1. HLA Alleles Identified as Serum Specificities*

A HLA-A	B HLA-B	C HLA-C	D HLA-D	DR HLA-DR
A1	B7	Cw1	Dw1	DR1
A2	B8	Cw2	Dw2	DR2
A3	B13	Cw3	Dw3	DR3
A11	B14	Cw4	Dw4	DR4
Aw23 (A9)	B18	Cw5	Dw5	DR5
Aw24 (A9)	B27	CW6	Dw6	DRw6
A25 (A10)	Bw35	CW7	Dw7	DR7
A26 (A10)	B37	CW8	Dw8	DRw8
A28	BW38 (B16)		Dw9	DRw9
A29	Bw39 (B16)		Dw10	DRw10
Aw30 (Aw19)	Bw41		Dw11	
Aw31 (Aw19)	Bw42		Dw12	
Aw32 (Aw19)	Bw44 (B12)			
Aw33 (Aw19)	Bw45 (B12)			
Aw34	Bw46			
Aw36	Bw47			
Aw43	Bw48			
	Bw49 (B21)			
	Bw50 (B21)			
	Bw51 (B5)			
	Bw52 (B5)			
	Bw53			
	Bw54 (Bw22)			
	Bw55 (Bw22)			
	Bw56 (Bw22)			
	Bw57 (B17)			
	Bw58 (B17)			
	Bw59			
	Bw60 (Bw40)			
	Bw61 (Bw40)			
	Bw62 (B15)			
	Bw63 (B15)			

* Some of the early antisera contained antibodies that detected several alleles or specificities. In some instances, the original allele was "split" into several. A good example is Bw22, which is now known to contain three alleles; Bw54, Bw55, and Bw56. Alleles in parentheses represent the original allele that has now been split. The letter w indicates a workshop or temporary designation. (From Bellanti, J.A.: Immunology III, Philadelphia, W.B. Saunders Co., 1985.)

allele (e.g., HLA-Bw47). The allelic Class I products are found on most nucleated cells, exceptions being sperm and trophoblastic cells, and are generally detected by using human or mouse alloantisera that bind to the cell surface molecules, bearing the particular specificity determinant (see Fig. 2–2). Lymphocytes of the patient are commonly used for the HLA typing because they are easily obtainable. Antibodies against the HLA-A, -B, and -C specificities are commonly found in the sera of multigravida or individuals who have received numerous transfusions.

Class I molecules in humans are thought to serve as determinants necessary for immune recognition and for elimination of viral infected cells. It is thought that the T8+ killer cell uses the T8 molecule to recognize self-MHC antigen,

and the T3-associated T-cell-"idiotype" region to recognize and bind to foreign antigen (associative or dual recognition). In addition, Class I antigens may serve as targets in graft rejection, which can be mediated both by antibody and sensitized cells. For this reason, donor's tissues must be carefully "matched" to the recipient for Class I antigens prior to transplantation.

Structure and Function of Human Class II Antigens

Class II antigens consist of two noncovalently associated glycoproteins (alpha and beta chains) of about 34 and 29K mol wt, respectively (see Fig. 2–3). In humans, at least three genes have been identified that code for Class II antigens, although several more candidates currently exist. The three functional loci have been designated DR/Dw, DP(SB), and DQ(MB=DC). The Class II cell surface glycoprotein molecules, also collectively referred to as Ia (immune-associated) antigens, also are involved in the control of the immune response. In humans, they are coded in the HLA-D region within the short arm of chromosome 6 and therefore are called HLA-DR (HLA-D related) antigens.

Since the Class II antigens are made up of two chains, alpha and beta, two genes are necessary to code for a single Class II antigen. Several types of alpha chains may combine with various beta chains to make cell surface "hybrid" molecules. Using standard tests, some of the Class II antigens can be serologically detected (HLA-DR antigens). Others (DW and DP antigens) are recognized only through T lymphocytes, which proliferate (in a one-way, mixed lymphocyte culture), in response to foreign Class II determinants. The DW and DP type antigens have been termed lymphocyte defined or LD antigens (in contrast to the former Class I

antigens, termed SD or serologically defined) to designate the need for cellular recognition for their detection. However, in many cases, antibodies also have been found that bind to the same or similar determinants (epitopes) on the same molecule. Because of differences in detection of similar determinants by various methods, the correlation between serologic and cellular HLA-D typing has proved difficult.

Class II antigens are involved at many levels in immune interactions. There is a need for sharing of certain Class II molecules (HLA-DR or DP) between macrophages and T cells for effective induction of T-helper cells. In some cases of kidney graft rejection, killer cells specific for HLA-D/DR antigens have been identified. They also play a major role in graft versus host disease (e.g., in bone marrow transplantation). The early events in allograft rejection include the production of T cells that recognize foreign HLA antigens. These cells may kill cells bearing foreign Class I or Class II antigens or release mediators (lymphokines) that induce macrophages and neutrophils to enter the graft site, leading to graft destruction. Shortly after

TABLE 2–2. HLA and Disease Associations*

Disease Type	HLA Allele	Relative Risk
RHEUMATOLOGIC DISEASES		
Ankylosing spondylitis	B27	88
Reiter's syndrome	B27	37
Acute anterior uveitis	B27	10
Juvenile arthritis	B27, Dw5, or Dw8	4
Rheumatoid arthritis	Dw4(DR4)	4
AUTOIMMUNE/ENDOCRINE DISEASES		
Chronic hepatitis	Dw3(DR3)	14
" "	B8	9
Celiac disease	Dw3(DR3)	11
Graves disease	Dw3(DR3)	4
Hashimoto thyroiditis	Dw5(DR5)	3
Idiopathic Addison disease	Dw3(DR3)	6
Juvenile-onset diabetes mellitus	Dw4(DR4)	6
" " " "	Dw3(DR3)	3
Congenital adrenal hyperplasia (21-hydroxylase deficiency)	B47	15
" " "	B5	4
Myasthemia gravis	B8	4
" "	Dw3(DR3)	3
Multiple sclerosis	Dw2(DR2)	4
Systemic lupus erythematosus	Dw3(DR3)	6
MALIGNANT DISORDERS		
Chronic myelocytic leukemia	A2	39
Chronic lymphocytic leukemia	B18	5
Acute lymphoblastic leukemia	A2	1
Hodgkin disease	A1, A11, B8, B15	1–8

* From Bellanti, J.A.: Immunology III, Philadelphia, W.B. Saunders Co., 1985.

initiation of cellular immune response, antibodies to Class I and Class II antigens can be detected, which also play a role in destruction.

HLA and Disease Association

Associations between various diseases and HLA antigens are primarily statistical in nature, and the significance of these associations is often not known. However, it is generally agreed that these associations are likely to have great relevance. The most common approach for investigating a possible association between a particular disease state and HLA involves determining the HLA types of a group of patients with the particular disease and comparing types with HLA types of a random panel of unaffected individuals from the same ethnic group and geographic area. The general statistical approach for evaluation of this data is by a 2×2 contingency table. Dr. Arne Svejgaard, in Copenhagen, has established an international registry to evaluate HLA and disease associations. The results are periodically updated and published. A few of the more interesting examples are given in Table 2–2. It also is possible to perform formal linkage analysis between a genetic disease and an HLA allele. This analysis requires large families in which several members may have the disease. The information gained, however, is more conclusive and may allow investigators to formally map disease-linked genes.

A number of the rheumatologic, autoimmune, and endocrine disorders show an association with HLA alleles of the D/DR region. In many of these disorders, antibodies are found that have specificity for the target organ. One could postulate that the MHC-linked "immune response" alleles in these individuals permit an elevated or exaggerated response to cross reactive exogenous antigens or to endogenous antigens per se, which results in the production of autoantibodies. To account for some of the observations, one might anticipate that individuals who are homozygous for a particular allele may be more affected than individuals who are heterozygous. However, this is not the case, and environmental factors also appear to be important to the initiation of the disease process. Although a strong association between HLA antigens and susceptibility to infectious diseases has been anticipated to date, such an association has been found only for tuberculoid leprosy. There has been speculation that MHC genes may influence susceptibility to infection by various direct or indirect mechanisms, such as through an influence on receptor binding for toxins, oncogenic viruses, bacteria, or other pathogenic materials. Alternatively, they may not be responsible for disease susceptibility but rather are linked with others as yet undefined genes, which play more important roles in disease susceptibility.

IMMUNOGLOBULIN GENETICS

The germ line of an individual contains genes that code for the constant regions of immunoglobulins and others that code for the variable segments. In humans, studies of B cell malignancies and advances in recombinant DNA technology allowed investigators to identify and study the immunoglobulin (Ig) genes. There are three chromosomes that bear human Ig genes. Chromosome 14 contains a gene that encodes for heavy chains; chromosome 2, a gene that encodes for κ light chain; and chromosome 22, a gene that encodes for λ light chain. Three distinct gene families that are involved in generating the variable region of heavy chains exist side by side. These gene families, variable (V_H), diversity (D), and joining (J_H), together generate the unique specificity of an antibody. During B cell differentiation, V_H, D, and J_H segments physically move closer together through a loss of the intervening sequences, using a process termed rearrangement. This results in the formation of a V-D-J gene. Subsequently, the V-D-J gene and one constant region gene are transcribed, and the derived messenger RNA encodes for the complete immunoglobulin heavy chain (Fig. 2–4), deleting the introns (intravening noncoding sequences).

The temporal sequence in which the various immunoglobulins are expressed (μ, δ, γ, ε, α) follows the order of heavy chain, constant region genes. Following gene arrangement, a given heavy chain, constant region gene is expressed and is transcribed with the variable region gene. When a "switch" in Ig classes occurs, the previously expressed constant gene appears to be deleted, and a subsequent constant gene is activated and transcribed. In this fashion, a single cell can produce sequentially several different classes of immunoglobulin with the same antibody specificity. A similar process occurs with the assembly of the messenger for light chains, except that D genes do not exist in the

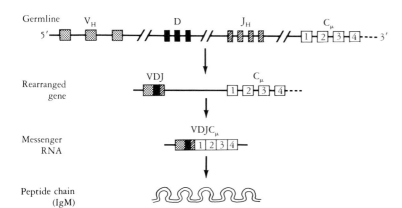

FIGURE 2–4. Schematic representation of the process whereby gene segments are linked and transcribed. One of many V_H region genes, one of several D genes, and one of several J_H genes are linked through rearrangement with loss of the other V_H, D, and J_H genes. This complex, which now codes the variable regions of the antibody, is transcribed along with the C region genes of the appropriate class into messenger RNA. (From Bellanti, J.A.: *Immunology III*, Philadelphia, W.B. Saunders Co., 1985.)

repertoire; there are only V, J, and constant region genes. In the final assembly of antibodies, the heavy and light chains are themselves linked through disulfide bonds and secreted by the antibody forming cell.

In addition, during the life of the cell, it appears that a significant degree of somatic mutation occurs, which further defines and refines antibody specificity. (Thus, elements of both germ line and mutational theories, which sought to account for the basis of antibody diversity, have been shown to be correct.)

THE T CELL ANTIGEN RECEPTOR

T cells, like B cells, interact with antigen via cell surface receptors. However, unlike the B cells, the T cells must in addition recognize the "self"—MHC determinants together with the antigen on the surface of the antigen-presenting cell (APC). This phenomenon, called MHC-restricted antigen recognition, is a key feature of T cell responses. The nature of the T-cell receptor eluded investigators until recently when a two-chain polypeptide "heterodimer" was found to be associated with the T3 molecule (Meuer et al., 1983). The putative T-cell receptor chains were named alpha and beta. A short time later, Mak and colleagues (Yanagi et al., 1984) were able to clone the genes for the beta chain and demonstrated that it had 50 to 60 percent homology with immunoglobulin. Recently, a third T cell specific gene, designated gamma, has been isolated and has been shown to be another component of the T-cell receptor complex (Saito et al., 1984). The T-cell receptor chains, which are disulfide linked on the cell surface, have corresponding gene structures very similar to those for immunoglobulin. Specifically, they have variable (V), diversity (D),

and joining (J) segments that rearrange with a constant segment to generate a complete gene in a fashion identical to that of the immunoglobulin genes shown in Figure 2–4. Despite the similarities to the immunoglobulin molecule, the T-cell receptor alpha chain genes are located on chromosome 14 (Croce et al., 1985; Isobe et al., 1985), whereas beta and gamma chain genes are located on chromosome 7 (Morton et al., 1985; Murre et al., 1985), all being unassociated with the immunoglobulin genes.

It is clear that at least alpha and beta polypeptide chains are associated with T3 on the cell surface and that this complex forms the T-cell receptor for antigen. It is still uncertain where exactly the specificities for the antigen and MHCs are located in the primary structure of the T-cell receptor polypeptide chains. It is generally accepted, however, that the T-cell receptor consists of a heterodimer that forms a single receptor complex, similar to the Ig heavy and light chains, that binds to the appropriate MHC antigen configuration (Brenner et al., 1986). There is evidence from animal models to indicate that T helper cells, killer cells, and suppressor cells use slightly different alpha, beta, and gamma genes for assembling their receptors (Kronenberg et al., 1985; Brenner et al., 1986).

In summary, three separate polymorphic systems exist that compose the "IR gene family," including the MHC, immunoglobulin, and T-cell receptor genes.

GENETIC CONTROL OF IgE PRODUCTION AND IgE ANTIBODY FORMATION

Any description of immunogenetics and allergic diseases must of necessity include discussion of genetic control of total IgE levels as well as factors controlling specific IgE antibody formation. There appear to be a number of factors influencing IgE levels, some of which are genetic but others of which are environmentally influenced. For example, elevated IgE levels are seen in cigarette smokers and in patients with bacterial infections (e.g., pertussis) and viral infections (e.g., respiratory syncytial virus).

IgE antibody production in the human appears to be under genetic control. Conflicting data exist concerning whether genetic transmission of IgE production is recessive or dominant. Most recent studies by Blumenthal and Bach (1983) suggest a polygenic mode of inheritance that is not associated with the HLA system.

In contrast to total IgE production, which is not HLA related, there appears to be an HLA association with specific IgE antibody responses to allergens. For example, reactivity to ragweed antigen, Ra5, appears to be associated with HLA-B7. An Ir Ra3 locus for another ragweed antigen, Ra3, may be associated with HLA-A3 and HLA-B12 (Blumenthal and Bach, 1983). The gene for ragweed sensitivity appears in some families to map on chromosome 6.

Despite numerous problems in studying the immunogenetics of atopic disease (e.g., limitations to population studies to establish the genetics of a disease or immune response), there is information for at least two genetic mechanisms in humans. The first relates to specific Ir gene associations with MHC chromosome 6 and disease (e.g., ragweed hay fever). However, the association of any specific immune response to a specific HLA antigen has not been firmly established. A second genetic control, postulated for the regulation of levels of IgE, does not appear to be associated or linked with HLA. Further studies are needed to establish the linkage between a major locus and polymorphic marker locus to establish the mode of inheritance of serum IgE levels.

REFERENCES

Acuto, O., Reinherz, E.L.: The human T cell receptor, structure and function. N. Engl. J. Med. 312:1100, 1985.

Bellanti, J.A.: Immunology III. W.B. Saunders Co., Philadelphia, 1985.

Blumenthal, M.N., Bach, F.H.: Immunogenetics of atopic disease. *In* Allergy, Principles and Practice, 2nd ed., vol. 1. Middleton, E., Jr., Reed, C.E., Ellis, E.F. (eds.), C.V. Mosby Co., St. Louis, 1983.

Brenner, M.B., et al.: Identification of a putative second T cell receptor. Nature 322:145–149, 1986.

Croce, C.M., et al.: Gene for alpha chain of human T-cell receptor: Location on chromosome 14 region involved in T-cell neoplasms. Science 227:1044, 1985.

Dausset, J., Svejgaard, A.: HLA and Disease. Williams & Wilkins, Baltimore, 1977.

Isobe, M., et al.: Location of gene for beta subunit of human T-cell receptor and band 7q 35, a region prone to rearrangements in T cells. Science 228:580, 1985.

Johnson, R.H., Hartzman, R.J., Robinson, M.A.: HLA: The Major Histocompatibility Complex. *In* Clinical Diagnosis and Management by Laboratory Methods. Henry, J. (ed.), W.B. Saunders Co., Philadelphia, 1984.

Kronenberg, M., et al.: Rearrangement and transcription of the beta-chain genes of the T-cell antigen receptor in different types of murine lymphocytes. Nature 313:647, 1985.

Meuer, S.C., et al.: Evidence for the T3-associated 90K heterodimer as the T-cell antigen receptor. Nature 303:808, 1983.

Morton, C., et al.: Genes for beta chain of human T-cell antigen receptor map to regions of chromosomal rearrangement in T cells. Science 228:582, 1985.

Murre, C., et al.: Human gamma chain genes are rearranged in leukaemic T cells and map to the short arm of chromosome 7. Nature 316:549–552, 1985.

Saito, H., et al.: Complete primary structure of a heterodimeric T cell receptor deduced from cDNA sequences. Nature 309:757–762, 1984.

Schaller, J., Hansen, J.: HLA relationship to disease. Hosp. Prac. 41, 1983.

Siu, G. et al.: The human T-cell antigen receptor is encoded by variable, diversity, and joining gene segments that rearrange to generate a complete V gene. Cell 37:393, 1984.

Yanagi, Y., et al.: A human T cell–specific cDNA clone encodes a protein having extensive homology to immunoglobulin chains. Nature 308:145, 1984.

Zaleski, M.B., et al.: Immunogenetics. Boston, Pitman, 1983.

3

Immune Deficiency Disease

Anthony R. Hayward, M.D., Ph.D.

Immunodeficiency syndromes were originally recognized as consequences of otherwise unexplained recurrent infections. The association of different types of infection with different patterns of inheritance led to the characterization of the commonest primary immunodeficiencies and the recognition that other immunologic abnormalities, particularly autoimmunity and allergy, could still occur despite the lack of useful immunity. Specific and nonspecific factors contribute to protection from infection. Some nonspecific factors, such as lactoferrin, can act on their own, while the function of others (complement and neutrophils) is much more efficient in the presence of specific factors, such as antibody. This chapter deals exclusively with defects of specific immunity (the production of antibodies and of cell mediated immunity); primary defects are covered in more detail than are secondary defects. Understanding of the etiology of most primary immunodeficiency syndromes is incomplete, so classification systems are still being evolved. Definitive classification will have to await the elucidation of the biochemical mechanisms involved. Until that time, the most coherent approaches to classification are based on the supposed pathogenetic mechanisms; therefore, these are discussed first, and a description of the more common syndromes follows.

CLASSIFICATION AND PATHOGENESIS

Defects of specific immunity are associated with a range of lymphocyte abnormalities in which there is either a failure of development or a lack of function (Fig. 3–1). Classification of immunodeficiency on the basis of which lymphocyte populations are present or absent is at best a temporary measure. The approach is of help for some severe, combined immunodeficiency syndromes (which are discussed first), but it is of limited help in understanding most cases of antibody deficiency, in which lymphocytes are present in normal numbers.

Lack of Stem Cell Development and Severe Combined Immunodeficiency

Complete failure of lymphoid stem cell and granulocyte development is rare, and so-affected infants generally have died early before the mechanism of the defect could be determined. The immune consequences of the defect are antibody deficiency and absence of cell mediated immunity (a combination described as severe combined immunodeficiency), with the addition of neutropenia. Occurrence of the syndrome in siblings of different sex suggests an autosomal recessive inheritance, with a single gene defect.

T cells and B cells are absent in about a third of infants with severe combined immunodeficiency syndromes. Arrest in the differentiation of a lymphoid precursor cell seems a likely cellular mechanism for this phenotype (Neudorf et al., 1985); when inheritance can be established it usually is autosomal recessive. Whereas the number of small lymphocytes in the blood of these patients is greatly reduced, monocytes and large granular lymphocytes may be present in normal or increased number. Granular lymphocytes lack surface CD 3 antigens of T cells and immunoglobulins of B cells. When granular lymphocytes are expanded in number by culture with interleukin-2 (IL-2), they generally are found to have surface characteristics of natural killer (NK) cells.

Lack of T and B Lymphocyte Function

Most infants with severe combined immunodeficiency (SCID) have some B lymphocytes in the blood or bone marrow but lack T cells. These patients lack B cell function, as judged by the absence of antibody responses to injected antigen, although their B cells can be stimulated to make IgM in tissue cultures to which normal T cells are added. Since help from T cells is required for antibody responses by B cells, the

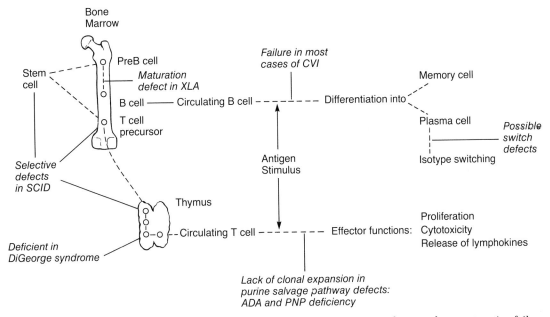

FIGURE 3–1. Diagram indicating points in normal lymphocyte differentiation pathways where maturation failures may be associated with primary specific immunodeficiency syndromes.

lack of T cells is an adequate explanation for the deficiency of both antibody and cell mediated immunity in these cases of SCID. Whether the primary defect in these patients is of T cell differentiation in the thymus (Pyke et al., 1975), or whether an earlier stage of differentiation may be blocked, is unknown.

A rarer form of SCID is characterized by a selective lack of CD 4 cells, with normal numbers of CD 8 cells. The CD 8 cells of two boys with this phenotype had an XX karyotype (Conley et al., 1984), suggesting that they were maternal in origin and presumably had crossed the placenta before delivery. Engraftment by maternal lymphocytes of infants with SCID is increasingly recognized (by HLA typing cells grown in tissue culture), and it seems likely to contribute to the heterogeneity of the clinical picture. The infant possesses histocompatibility (HLA) antigens derived from the father which maternal T lymphocytes would be expected to recognize as foreign. Persistence of maternal cells in the infant without causing graft versus host disease suggests that either they are nonspecific effectors (such as NK cells) or they do not include T cells, with specificity for paternally derived HLA antigens. The potential occurrence of colonization by maternal cells makes the classification of SCID syndromes on the basis of blood or bone marrow lymphocyte findings unsatisfactory and underlines the need

for biochemical classification. The simple inheritance pattern of most SCID syndromes suggests that only a single gene is responsible for the immunodeficiency. However, adenosine deaminase (ADA) deficiency is the only example of SCID syndrome in which there is a plausible biochemical explanation for the functional defects of lymphocytes.

ADA is a polymorphic enzyme in which the gene locus is on chromosome 20. It catalyzes the conversion of adenosine and deoxyadenosine to inosine and deoxyinosine, respectively. When the enzyme is deficient, the level of deoxyadenosine increases sufficiently to drive the phosphorylation pathway to ATP and dATP (Fig. 3–2). There are at least three adverse consequences of raised intracellular dATP levels. One is a fall in intracellular nicotinamide adenine dinucleotide (NAD) levels which, when experimentally induced, leads to the death of both resting and dividing T cells after about 8 hours (Seto et al., 1985). An additional and independent action is the inhibition of ribonucleotide reductase and limitation in production of other deoxynucleoside diphosphates for DNA synthesis. T cells are, as a result, unable to divide. Lack of ADA also may allow adenosine to rise to levels that inhibit the recycling of S-adenosyl homocysteine and S-adenosylmethionine, with consequent inhibition of methylation reactions. The proliferation

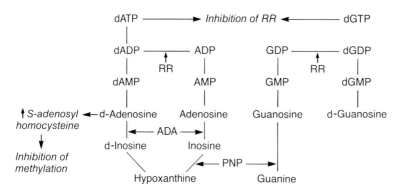

FIGURE 3–2. Purine salvage pathways involved in the pathogenesis of immunodeficiency. ADA = adenosine deaminase, PNP = purine nucleoside phosphorylase, RR = ribonucleotide reductase. Adverse consequences of excess purine metabolite levels are shown in italics.

of T cells is more severely impaired in ADA deficiency than that of other somatic cells. This may be because T cells remain in G_0 for long periods until antigen stimulation normally triggers rapid proliferation. The special susceptibility of T cells also may reflect their lack of an endo-5'-nucleotidase, which allows other cells to eliminate excess dATP. ADA deficiency accounts for about 25 percent of cases of SCID in which the inheritance is autosomal recessive.

SCID with X-linked inheritance often is different from other forms in that patients may produce serum IgM and may have high (60 percent or more) proportions of circulating B lymphocytes. These B cells are not of maternal origin, and they sometimes can be induced to differentiate into immunoglobulin secreting cells by mitogen or Epstein-Barr virus (EBV) stimulation. Patients with this form of SCID nevertheless remain antibody deficient until they are effectively engrafted. These observations suggest that some forms of SCID may result from a lack of T lymphocytes alone. The underlying defect could be at the level of T cell differentiation in the thymus or at a post-thymic level.

Selective Deficiency of T Cell Function

It is unusual for defects of T cell function to affect only cell mediated immunity and to leave antibody production intact. Indeed, the maintenance of antibody production suggests that sufficient T cells are present to provide soluble, B cell growth and differentiation factors. Immunodeficiency as a consequence of thymic defects is rare, and in the best characterized example (Di George syndrome) T cell production usually is delayed rather than absent.

Many infants with the typical features of Di George syndrome possess at least small numbers of T cells in their blood in the first weeks of life, and the numbers of these cells tend to increase in the ensuing months. These infants make normal amounts of immunoglobulin, while those with the lowest number of blood T cells are antibody deficient. The variability of the immune features in this condition most probably reflects the different degrees of thymic defect and hence the number of T cells available to provide help for B cells to produce antibody.

The most selective defect of T cell function occurs in purine nucleoside phosphorylase (PNP) deficiency. The enzyme catalyzes the conversion of inosine to hypoxanthine (see Fig. 3–2). PNP-deficient patients excrete increased amounts of inosine, guanosine, and deoxyguanosine in their urine. Deoxyguanosine is thought to be the most detrimental to T cell function, acting primarily by inhibiting ribonucleotide reductase and hence T cell division. The conservation of antibody production is intriguing and suggests that T cells remain capable of releasing soluble helper factors after antigen stimulation.

Defects of Antibody Production

Although a lack of T cells severely compromises antibody production, the reverse does not appear to hold true in that cell mediated immunity is normal in patients with congenital X-linked agammaglobulinemia (XLA), the most selective form of immunoglobulin deficiency. XLA patients have few if any B cells in their blood, although they have normal numbers of B cell precursors (preB cells characterized by cytoplasmic μ chain but lack of surface IgM) in their bone marrow (Pearl et al., 1978). Following transformation by EBV, cell lines expressing immunoglobulin genes can be grown from the patient's marrow. Abnormality of the μ heavy chain (a lack of regions encoded by V, D, and J) is reported from one laboratory (Schwaber et al., 1983), but too few patients have been studied to conclude that this is the primary mechanism. Gene mapping studies now suggest that the defective gene is on the proximal part of the long arm of the X chromosome, between the phosphoglycerate kinase (PGK) and hypoxanthine guanine phosphoribosyl transferase (HGPRT) loci.

Most patients with antibody deficiency syndromes have low to normal numbers of B cells in their blood, but these cells do not differentiate normally into immunoglobulin secreting cells following mitogen or antigen stimulation. Some patients with acquired hypogammaglobulinemia syndromes possess circulating T cells, which suppress responses by B cells in tissue culture. However, it appears that this is a rare mechanism in the pathogenesis of antibody deficiency and that most patients' T cells make differentiation factors for B cells normally, following nonspecific stimulation in tissue culture (Platts-Mills et al., 1981). It seems likely, therefore, that the differentiation failure resides in the B cell. The genes for immunoglobulin heavy chains are normal, so the defect appears to be at the level of the cellular response to activation by antigen. Patients with hypogammaglobulinemia associated with thymoma are exceptions in that they often possess T cells with strong suppressor activity in their blood. Patients with selective immunoglobulin production defects generally have B cells with the surface isotype of the deficient class in their circulation; why these cells fail to differentiate and function normally is not known. In selective IgA deficiency, for example, B cells with surface alpha chains are present in the blood, but the cells are immature as shown by their coexpression of surface μ chains and their limited differentiation into IgA-secreting plasma cells, following mitogen stimulation (Conley and Cooper, 1981). IgG2 and IgG4 deficiencies often occur in association with selective IgA deficiency. Since the genes for $\gamma 2$, $\gamma 4$, and α chains are all in the second group on chromosome 14, the primary defect may be one of heavy chain gene rearrangement during isotype switching.

PRIMARY IMMUNODEFICIENCIES —ANTIBODY DEFICIENCY SYNDROMES

Congenital X-Linked Agammaglobulinemia (XLA)

XLA occurs exclusively in boys. Affected infants usually are protected from infection for the first 3 to 6 months of life by maternal immunoglobulin acquired before birth. Symptoms, when they arise, usually result from infection by encapsulated pyogenic bacteria, particularly streptococci, meningococci, and *Haemophilus* species. The respiratory tract most often is involved along with otitis media, sinusitis, or pneumonia, but spread via the blood to the brain, bone, or joints is common. The skin is another important site for infection; gram-positive cocci are the predominant organisms and recurrence, with scarring, occurs. Untreated patients sometimes develop arthritis affecting the knee or ankle. The etiology of this arthritis is not understood; pyogenic organisms usually are not recovered by culture of joint aspirates, though in one case mycoplasma was cultured. The joint itself is swollen, and movement is restricted.

Lack of tonsillar lymphoid tissue is an important physical sign, which may suggest the diagnosis during the first infection. Often the child is treated effectively with a course of antibiotics only to relapse when the course is completed. A patient in whom the diagnosis of the underlying immunodeficiency is delayed tends to have multiple and chronic infections, which damage the respiratory mucosa and lead ultimately to bronchiectasis.

Diagnosis is based primarily on the presence of low or undetectable levels of serum IgM and IgA. The IgG level is normal at birth but falls to values between 100 and 200 mg/dl by 6 months of age. The test results for cell mediated immunity and the number of T cells in the blood are normal unless the patient is malnourished or has an active virus infection. B cells usually are absent; their presence in normal numbers should raise the suspicion that the patient has another type of antibody deficiency. A more specific diagnosis likely will become possible when probes for the defective gene become available.

Treatment of the agammaglobulinemia is by IgG replacement, in the form of either intramuscular injection or intravenous infusion. The various protocols for giving the IgG are described under Treatment of Antibody Deficiency. The minimum dosage to provide protection from infection is about 25 mg/kg/wk.

Complications. The following problems arise only in a minority of antibody deficient patients. Although they are not complications in the strict sense, they are discussed separately, since they require different treatments.

Diarrhea is common in patients with antibody deficiency (Asherson and Webster, 1980). The etiologic agent sometimes is a rotavirus or *Giardia lamblia,* in which case the clinical response to metronidazole is good. A minority of patients has a more chronic diarrhea associated with malabsorption and failure to thrive. The changes observed radiographically in the small intestine may resemble those of Crohn disease, and usually no organism can be clearly incriminated. Appropriate management includes studies for less common pathogens, such as *Cryptosporidium* and *Campylobacter,* since infections caused by these pathogens are treatable.

A dermatomyositis-like syndrome occurs in 5 to 10 percent of patients in association with encephalitis. The skin rash is variable, but most of these patients develop thickening of the skin and subcutaneous tissues of the legs, cyanosis of the fingers and toes and, if they survive, flexion deformities of the knees and elbows. The encephalitis may initially be experienced as impaired vision due to optic atrophy, convulsions, or slowly progressive intellectual impairment. Many of these patients have had echovirus cultured from brain and cerebrospinal fluid. Successful treatment with infusions of high titered, anti-echovirus antibody is reported, but not all patients respond well (Mease et al., 1981).

Immunoglobulin Deficiency with Normal or Increased IgM

Children with this syndrome have a more diverse clinical spectrum than those with XLA. In particular, they may present with *Pneumocystis carinii* pneumonia or severe diarrhea, as do infants with combined immunodeficiency. Sometimes there is a history of affected male relatives, suggesting an X-linked transmission, but sporadic cases occur in females. The usual immunoglobulin findings include very low IgG and IgA levels with raised IgM. Similar findings would be expected to result from persistent EBV infection in patients with the common, variable

forms of antibody deficiency, so the heterogeneity of the syndrome is not surprising. When the IgM levels are high, they sometimes fall to normal levels after treatment with IgG replacement. It is important to test cell mediated immunity of infants suspected of having this syndrome to rule out SCID.

One reason for classifying these patients apart from patients with congenital XLA and those with more common varied immunodeficiency is that they tend to be more difficult to treat. Problems include the occurrence of intermittent or continuous neutropenia or thrombocytopenia and of lymphadenopathy, with or without splenomegaly. Some of the patients retain the ability to make IgM antibodies. This can be troublesome, since it can include the production of autoantibodies or antibodies to IgA present in immunoglobulin preparations used in replacement therapy.

Common Variable Immunodeficiency (CVI) Affecting Predominantly Antibody Formation

Most adults and children with congenital or acquired failures of antibody production do not "fit" into any of the aforementioned syndromes and, pending the evolution of a better classification, are described as having common variable immunodeficiency. Subcategorization of these patients on the basis of the age of onset of infections or the levels of individual immunoglobulin classes is not very useful, since there often are differences among affected relatives. The occurrence of immunodeficiency, arthritis, and allergy in different members of the same family suggests that an underlying immunoregulatory disorder exists but may be variously expressed.

Respiratory Tract Symptoms. Symptoms in CVI result mainly from recurrent respiratory tract infection. Pathogens are the same as those found in XLA. A small number of patients develop lymphoid infiltrates in their lungs, and these infiltrates can progress to reduce lung compliance and cause respiratory failure. Histologically, the lesions resemble nodular lymphoid hyperplasia of the bowel (see next section). Steroid treatment sometimes is useful for preserving lung function in these patients.

Gastrointestinal Symptoms. About 50 percent of adults with CVI have reduced gastric acidity even after gastrin stimulation, and in some the production of intrinsic factor is impaired so that megaloblastic anemia develops. Test results for parietal cell antibodies are negative, and it may be chronic infection rather than autoimmunity that is responsible for gastritis and achlorhydria. The incidence of gastric carcinoma appears to be increased in CVI (Asherson and Webster, 1980).

Diarrhea and malabsorption are common in antibody deficient patients; giardiasis is the leading cause, with occasional cases of gluten sensitive enteropathy or colonization of the small intestine by bile salt–splitting bacteria. Lymphoid nodules in the wall of the small or large intestine are often visualized as small filling defects on radiographs with barium meal or enemas. This condition is called "nodular lymphoid hyperplasia." Histologically, the nodules are composed of small lymphocytes with a central area of larger, pale staining cells that includes a few macrophages. Although the nodules can become very large in the colon, there is no evidence to indicate that they become malignant.

Selective Defects of Immunoglobulin Production

IgG Subclass Deficiencies

IgG1 normally accounts for about 60 percent of serum IgG, IgG2 for 25 percent, and IgG3 and IgG4 combined account for the remainder. There is considerable difference in the distribution of antibodies in the various subclasses; most antitetanus toxoid activity is in IgG1, herpesvirus antibodies are equally distributed between IgG1 and IgG3, and bacterial polysaccharide antibodies are almost entirely IgG2. The best recognized forms of IgG subclass deficiency occur with low overall levels of serum IgG (Yount et al., 1970). Such patients are best regarded as having common variable antibody deficiency syndromes. Recently, a small population of children with normal serum IgG levels but selective deficiencies of IgG2 or IgG3 and recurrent respiratory tract infections has been recognized (Smith et al., 1984; Umetsu et al., 1985). The types of respiratory tract infections experienced by these patients seem no different from those in other types of antibody deficiencies; therefore, the diagnosis can be made only by subclass measurement. A low titer of antibodies to bacterial capsular polysaccharide, with little response to immunization, would be suggestive of IgG2 subclass deficiency. There is

a clinical impression of benefit from replacement of IgG, but this benefit has not been formally evaluated.

IgG4 deficiency may occur alone, with or without recurrent infections (Beck and Heiner, 1981), or with deficiencies of IgA (Oxelius et al., 1981) or IgG2 (Oxelius, 1974). Infections are predominantly of the respiratory tract (see Chapter 7 for additional discussion of IgG subclasses and subclass deficiency).

Selective IgA Deficiency

This condition is defined as a serum IgA level below 5 mg/dl, with normal levels of IgG and IgM. Infants normally have low IgA levels, so the condition cannot be diagnosed with confidence before the age of 3 years. About 1 in 700 blood donors has selective IgA deficiency; most of these individuals are healthy, and any discussion of symptoms associated with selective IgA deficiency is clouded by the fact that some IgA deficient individuals otherwise appear to be perfectly normal. In immunodeficiency clinics, patients diagnosed as IgA deficient are referred most often because of frequent upper respiratory tract infections. However, studies of patients with chronic lung disease show little if any excess of patients with IgA deficiency. There does appear to be an association between low serum IgA levels and recurrent pharyngitis or tonsillitis (Ostergaard, 1977). The other principal disorders associated with IgA deficiency are allergic or autoimmune (Ammann and Hong, 1971). The degree of association with these phenomena also is not clearly established.

Confusion probably arises in part from the heterogeneity of selective IgA deficiency. Some patients have chromosomal abnormalities, some patients have relatives with common variable immunodeficiency, other patients have ataxia telangiectasia, and some patients have cases that arise secondarily from taking drugs (principally anticonvulsants), which lower serum IgA levels. IgA deficient patients with symptoms of infection or immune complex disease often fail to make IgG2 antibodies (Oxelius et al., 1982). Occasionally, patients who present with recurrent infections and are found to lack only IgA subsequently develop low levels of all immunoglobulin classes. The major symptoms ascribed to IgA deficiency are summarized in the following sections.

Diarrhea. There are two associations with selective IgA deficiency, as follows: (1) affected children have an excess of celiac disease (Asquith, 1974) and (2) adults, an excess of post-vagotomy diarrhea (McLoughlin et al., 1976). The clinical features in each resemble those of patients who do not have IgA deficiency, and some with celiac disease have been reported to respond to a gluten free diet.

Autoimmunity. Up to 60 percent of symptomatic IgA deficient patients have auto-antibodies; these include antinuclear and, in some studies, anti-DNA antibodies. Up to 33 percent of IgA deficient patients have rheumatoid arthritis. Systemic lupus, thyroiditis, pernicious anemia, Sjögren syndrome, Addison disease, hemolytic anemia, and thrombocytopenia (in approximate order of frequency) all are recognized associations. Anti-IgA antibodies are rare but important because they can cause transfusion reactions or, rarely, reactions to replacement IgG preparations, since these preparations contain small amounts of IgA.

Allergy. There is an association between asthma precipitated by infection and reduced (but not absent) serum IgA levels. In some uncontrolled studies, an increased incidence of low levels of serum IgA have been reported in atopic subjects. Lack of secretory antibodies is a possible contributory factor, though this is not established. One potentially important correlation exists among the presence of circulating immune complexes, milk precipitins, arthritis, and IgA deficiency (Cunningham-Rundles et al., 1981). Overall, the importance of IgA deficiency in the pathogenesis of atopic disease remains controversial.

Treatment. Asymptomatic patients require no treatment. Those who have recurrent upper respiratory tract infections should be tested for IgG subclass deficiency and, if possible, antibody responses to pneumococcal polysaccharides. Those patients who lack an IgG2 antibody response may benefit from IgG replacement, though this remains to be established. An alternative approach is to give long-term treatment with an antibiotic such as trimethoprim-sulfa. Patients with IgA deficiency should be warned that there is a small possibility of reaction to transfused blood or plasma and to gamma globulin because of the IgA content. This is particularly true for patients who have no IgA whatsoever and who, therefore, may develop antibodies to IgA so infused.

SELECTIVE IgM DEFICIENCY

This syndrome is rare. Some of the few patients reported have had severe viral infections in addition to bacterial meningitis or respiratory tract infections (Faulk et al., 1971). IgM deficiency without an excess of infections also is reported (Ross and Thompson, 1976). The diversity of the infecting microorganisms in symptomatic individuals suggests that patients may have a failure of IgG antibody and cell mediated immunity in addition to the selective IgM deficiency. The diagnosis is made from immunoglobulin measurements (IgM levels < 10 mg/dl); isohemagglutinins and pneumococcal polysaccharide antibodies usually are low. Replacement of IgG in symptomatic patients is rational; IgM has too short a half-life for it to be replaced. Long-term antibiotic treatment is a possible alternative. Significant complications include thrombocytopenia, splenomegaly, and hemolytic anemia. EBV infection may be an etiologic factor in some of these complications.

LIGHT CHAIN DEFICIENCIES

These deficiencies are rare and mostly the subject of single case reports. One female patient reported by Zegers and coworkers (1976) lacked kappa chains and IgA and also had cystic fibrosis. Her kappa chain locus on chromosome 2 has been cloned, and it appears that there is a single point mutation that prevents the formation of the intrachain disulfide bond (Stavnezer-Nordgren et al., 1985). Lambda chain deficiencies also occur, usually with abnormal levels of serum IgG. It is reasonable to regard the light chain deficiencies as variable immunodeficiency syndromes and to treat them with IgG replacement if they are associated with antibody deficiency.

TRANSIENT HYPOGAMMAGLOBULINEMIA

This is a diagnosis that can be applied retrospectively to infants who had low levels of immunoglobulins in the first year of life that subsequently returned to normal. Serum IgG levels normally dip to a mean of 520 mg/dl (with 240 mg/dl 2 SD below the mean) between 4 and 6 months of age as maternally derived IgG is diluted and catabolized and before endogenous synthesis has matured. Transient hypogammaglobulinemia in many infants is most likely an accentuation of this normal trough, and its recognition depends on the symptoms of these infants' being severe enough for the immunoglobulin levels to be measured. Since the disorder by definition resolves spontaneously, the frequency with which it is diagnosed depends on the readiness of pediatricians to measure immunoglobulin levels in infants with frequent infections. Some centers have found transient hypogammaglobulinemia in the siblings of infants with severe combined immunodeficiency; the possibility that it may result from heterozygosity for a more severe immunodeficiency also exists. In our own experience and that of Tiller and Buckley (1978), transient hypogammaglobulinemia is rare. Rather, most patients whose immunoglobulin levels in infancy were low continue to have low levels in later childhood.

Clinical Features. Recurrent upper respiratory tract infections or episodes of bronchitis with wheezing are the usual indications for measuring serum immunoglobulin levels, which lead to the diagnosis. Occasional infants have had pneumonia, meningitis, or even paralytic poliomyelitis following routine immunization with attenuated poliovirus.

Diagnosis and Treatment. Usual criteria are normal serum levels of one immunoglobulin class (in practice this usually is IgM), with low levels of one or both other classes, and spontaneous return to normal in 2 to 3 years. Test results of nonspecific and cell mediated immunity are normal. These patients usually have benign courses, so the therapeutic dilemma is whether to start them on replacement immunoglobulin. Our own practice is to test all infants with low immunoglobulin levels for antibody production (see Tests). Patients with poor or absent antibody responses are started on IgG replacement, which is continued until immunoglobulin levels are reached that are within the normal range for age. Those with normal responses are given immunoglobulin only if they have had infections with systemic spread. Routine immunizations with live viruses should be delayed while IgG replacement is being given and if the final diagnosis is not established.

Treatment of Antibody Deficiency

IgG replacement confers substantial protection from infection on patients with congenital and acquired hypogammaglobulinemia syndromes (Buckley, 1985). Conventional immune serum immunoglobulin preparations for intramuscular injection have about 150 mg/ml of IgG, with trace amounts of IgA. Some of the IgG aggregates during preparation and storage; these aggregates activate complement. Consequently, this material is not safe for intravenous administration. Several aggregate-free preparations for intravenous use are now marketed.

The first requirement in treating antibody deficient patients is to give enough replacement as follows: 25 mg/kg/wk of IgG is an approximate minimum dosage and will raise the serum IgG level of an agammaglobulinemic patient to the 200 to 300 mg/dl range. When given as an intramuscular injection, this dosage, for a 70 kg adult, corresponds to 12 ml/wk (or 24 ml every 2 weeks) of concentrate. This amount should be sufficient to protect a patient from septicemia and pneumonia, but it may not prevent sinusitis, particularly when there is a long history of recurrent sinusitis. Clinical indications that the IgG dosage should be increased include persistence or recurrence of arthritis or mild conjunctivitis (with matting of the eyelashes on awakening). The discomfort and frequency of injection prompts many patients to change to intravenous treatment in which the discomfort is much less (much larger amounts of IgG can be given), but cost is about 50 times greater. Unusual circumstances, such as lack of muscle bulk, may dictate the use of intravenous IgG. Comparisons of the intravenous and intramuscular preparations given at equivalent dosage show no significant differences in efficacy. The intramuscular preparations of IgG can be given by slow subcutaneous infusion (Berger et al., 1980). The anterior abdominal wall usually is the most satisfactory site, and flow rates of 1 to 2 ml/hr are tolerable. Motivated patients may be able to infuse themselves at home with 12 ml three times weekly and achieve serum IgG levels of 400 mg/dl or greater. Subcutaneous infusions generally are tolerated poorly by children.

Currently available preparations of IgG for intravenous use have aggregates removed either by physical or mild chemical means, and they are then stabilized by adding 5 to 10 percent of various sugars to the solution. There are no trials available comparing the clinical efficacy of the different preparations. Those made by mild alkylation and reduction are thought to have lower proportions of the IgG3 subclass and to be rather less active in tests of bacterial opsonizing activity (van Furth et al., 1984).

Reactions characterized by anxiety, back pain, chills, tachycardia, bronchospasm, and cyanosis are the main hazards of IgG replacement. These reactions usually occur 2 to 20 minutes following intramuscular injections and are thought to be due to rapid entry of aggregates into the circulation. Overall, about 10 percent of patients have reactions. However, they occur intermittently, so the risk with any one injection is less than 1 percent. A small number of patients have reactions following each injection. In many instances the response is to the IgA in the concentrates (Buckley, 1985), and IgE antibodies may be responsible (Burks et al., 1986). Sometimes a change to another batch of intramuscular IgG or an intravenous preparation may be of benefit. Reactions that are not due to IgA and persist may be due to B lipoprotein. Mild reactions require only reassurance; when severe they are treated with oxygen and epinephrine. In general, patients who do not have anti-IgA antibodies should be encouraged to continue with IgG replacement treatment despite the occasional reaction. Patients who may have allergic reactions to IgA could be treated with antibiotics until antibody tests have been completed. One of the subjects reported by Burks and coworkers (1986) tolerated an intravenous IgG preparation that contained only 1.6 μg/ml of IgA.

Many antibody deficient patients continue to have sinusitis and chronic productive cough after IgG replacement treatment is started. Permanent damage to the ciliary epithelium from previous infections seems the most likely explanation for persistence of symptoms. It is probably unwise to abandon IgG replacement under these circumstances, as the patient would be vulnerable to septicemia. Long-term antibiotic treatment sometimes is helpful; trimethoprim-sulfa preparations have the advantage of sufficient once-a-day medication, but many patients develop neutropenias or skin rashes. Additional lines of treatment include nasal steroid sprays, in the hope of reducing congestion and improving drainage, and nasal irrigation with warmed water.

COMBINED IMMUNODEFICIENCY DISORDERS

"Combined" in this context indicates a deficiency of antibody and cell mediated immunity. This group of disorders is heterogeneous and their classifications are likely to be revised as their etiologies are defined. The following descriptions are predominantly clinical, as considerable potential for confusion with allergic symptoms (e.g., diarrhea, skin rash, and cough) exists in infants.

Congenital Severe Combined Immunodeficiency (SCID)

Common presenting symptoms are diarrhea, vomiting, and cough with onset between 1 and 3 months of age. This is earlier than usual in antibody deficiency syndromes. A subgroup of patients presents with seborrheic dermatitis (see Combined Immunodeficiency with Reticuloendotheliosis). Diarrhea often is treated by changes in formula, which may result in temporary improvement. If the underlying immunodeficiency is not recognized, the infant suffers increasingly severe failure to thrive, weight loss, and death from infection. Fatal graft versus host disease is another common event, secondary to the transfusion of blood given for anemia. Candidiasis, particularly of the diaper area and the mouth, often is severe and should alert the physician to the possibility of an immunodeficiency, as should the development of a bilateral interstitial pneumonia caused by *Pneumocystis carinii.* Many other rare or exotic infections by opportunists are described, including *Mycobacterium Kansasii,* bacille Calmette-Guérin (BCG), and vaccinia (when vaccination was still routinely practiced). Without treatment, most affected infants die before the first year of age.

The most useful physical sign is a lack of palpable lymph nodes. Cervical nodes normally are detectable by 1 month of age, and inguinal nodes usually are palpable by 3 months, particularly in infants with diaper dermatitis. The thymus is not visible on chest radiographs, but this finding is too nonspecific to be of use in differential diagnosis. Lymphopenia is the most common abnormality in routine blood counts, but the presence of a normal differential blood count does not exclude SCID; the numbers of monocytes and large granular lymphocytes are often increased as a result of infection and may be counted as lymphocytes.

The diagnosis of SCID requires the demonstration of deficiencies of both antibody and cell mediated immunity. Lack of detectable serum IgM over 1 month of age generally is considered adequate evidence for antibody deficiency. The subset of patients who make IgM should be immunized with DPT (diphtheria, pertussis, tetanus) or, if available, with bacteriophage ϕ X174 and retested 7 to 10 days later to determine whether they have made any antibody. A lack of cell mediated immunity is inferred from a lack of T cells in blood, and, as might be expected, many patients are lymphopenic. The presence of normal numbers of lymphocytes in conventionally stained blood films does not exclude the diagnosis, as functional T cells are sometimes replaced by NK cells. Lack of proliferative responses by blood mononuclear cells in cultures stimulated with mitogens or with unrelated histocompatibility antigens (mixed lymphocyte culture) is the most useful functional test. In practice, increasing reliance is being placed on phenotyping of blood lymphocytes; when a diagnosis is made *in utero*, this usually is the only evidence available.

Variants of Severe Combined Immunodeficiency Syndromes

COMBINED IMMUNODEFICIENCY WITH NEUTROPENIA (RETICULAR DYSGENESIS)

Neutropenia greatly increases the susceptibility of newborns with combined immunodeficiency to infection. Consequently, most affected infants have survived for only a few weeks. This short time span has hindered full characterization of the syndrome, and it is uncertain whether the neutropenia is secondary (e.g., to infection) or whether it is primary, resulting from failure of development of a common stem cell. The presence of neutrophil precursors in the marrow of several affected infants, and variation in neutrophil count between affected siblings, argues against the failure of a common stem cell in many cases. Two affected infants have been successfully treated through the transplantation of bone marrow and subsequent reconstitution.

COMBINED IMMUNODEFICIENCY WITH THE PRESENCE OF IMMUNOGLOBULINS (NEZELOF SYNDROME)

Some infants with the clinical features of SCID have severely impaired or absent cell mediated immunity, but they do make some immunoglobulins (usually IgM). Agammaglobulinemia was at one time regarded as essential to the diagnosis of SCID syndrome; therefore, infants with some Ig were classified separately. This approach may be helpful in understanding the pathogenesis of SCID but has been of little help clinically. The immunoglobulin that is made usually does not include antibody to antigens used for immunization; conceivably, it may be made by B cells that are triggered nonspecifically by mitogens in the gut. The occurrence of monoclonal immunoglobulin "spikes"

in some patients could be secondary to EBV infection of B cells. Even without bone marrow transplantation some affected infants have survived 2 to 3 years, a little longer than the SCID infants who do not make immunoglobulin.

COMBINED IMMUNODEFICIENCY WITH RETICULOENDOTHELIOSIS

This is a descriptive term applied to infants with hypogammaglobulinemia and absent cell mediated immunity who have erythematous scaly skin rash, lymphadenopathy, and hepatosplenomegaly in addition to diarrhea and failure to thrive usually found in SCID. T cell numbers are uniformly reduced, but there is considerable heterogeneity in the extent of depression of individual subsets and the individual immunoglobulin classes among the cases reported (Fischer et al., 1983). The existence of one large family with multiple affected infants suggests that sometimes there may be genetic predisposition to this syndrome rather than classic SCID (Karol et al., 1983). Varying levels of maternal T cell engraftment and consequent graft versus host disease in infants with SCID are plausible explanations for the characteristic histiocytic infiltrates of the skin rash and the lymph nodes.

The SCID with reticuloendotheliosis syndrome is important principally because of the potential for misdiagnosis as Letterer-Siwe syndrome, Leiner disease, or even severe eczema. The presence of immunoglobulins or even low numbers of T cells in the circulation is not sufficient to exclude the diagnosis of SCID in an infant with a severe seborrheic skin rash with intractable diarrhea, and tests of immune function should be performed.

Defective Expression of Histocompatibility Antigens (Bare Lymphocyte Syndrome)

The patients originally described as having the bare lymphocyte syndrome had reduced expression of HLA-A, -B, -C, and β_2 microglobulin on the surface of their lymphocytes (Touraine and Betuel, 1983). The clinical findings were heterogeneous but included opportunistic infections and failure to thrive. More recently, the syndrome has been divided to separate those with defective expressions of Class I and Class II major histocompatibility (MHC) antigens.

Defective expression of Class II (HLA-DP, -DQ, -DR) antigens was first recognized in children whose clinical findings were those of SCID but who had lymphocytes in normal numbers and normal responses to mitogens in the blood (Griscelli et al., 1984). Expression of Class I antigens (HLA-A, -B, -C) is reduced but not absent in these patients. Genes for the Class II HLA-DR antigens are present in the patients' DNA, but there is no production of mRNA for these molecules (Lisowska-Grospierre et al., 1985). The primary defect, therefore, is thought to affect HLA-DR gene transcription; it is not reversed by gamma-interferon treatment of the patient's cells. The other group of patients with bare lymphocyte syndrome has defective Class I (HLA-A, -B, -C) antigen expression but makes normal amounts of Class II antigens. Blood mononuclear cells from these patients have low amounts of mRNA for Class I antigens, but cell lines derived from them express normal amounts of Class I antigens in long-term culture. The clinical features of these patients are dominated by intractable diarrhea and respiratory tract infections.

Treatment of SCID

The treatment of choice remains bone marrow transplantation. When a sibling is available as a donor, who is HLA matched with the recipient by both serologic and mixed lymphocyte culture nonreactivity, the chances of success are over 70 percent. Special facilities are not usually needed. The patient normally is started on IgG replacement (intravenous often is indicated because of poor muscle mass) and, as prophylaxis against *Pneumocystis* pneumonia, trimethoprim-sulfa. Infants who have been symptomatic for more than 3 months usually are wasted and are more easily managed with the placement of a Broviac line and with intravenous hyperalimentation.

Bone marrow is aspirated under sterile conditions from the iliac crests of the donor and transferred, anticoagulated with heparin, to a blood donation bag. Sufficient marrow is required to give a dose of about 4×10^8 nucleated cells for each kilogram of recipient weight, and this dose is infused over 1 to 2 hours to avoid causing respiratory embarrassment due to pulmonary microembolization. Mild fever and mild erythematous rash are common in the first week after the transfusion; more severe disturbance is suggestive of infection or, if there has been an error in matching, of graft versus host disease. In the absence of these complications the blood lymphocyte count usually starts to rise after about 7 days, and T cells are detected in tests of proliferation shortly afterwards. Diarrhea usually is the first symptom to improve, followed by candidal skin rash. Serum immunoglobulins do not usually start to rise for 3 to 4 weeks, and during the first 3 months monoclonal proteins may be made transiently.

The majority of SCID patients do not have matched siblings as potential donors. Incompletely matched (e.g., parental) marrow is dangerous for these subjects because of the mature T cells it contains. It is only in the past 5 years that reasonably reliable means have been evolved to prepare T cell–depleted marrow preparations. The greatest clinical experience is currently with a method using a soybean differential agglutination step followed by a rosetting and a density gradient centrifugation (Reisner et al., 1983). Much larger amounts of marrow are required from the donor, and engraftment of the recipient may be achieved only following a course of cytotoxic drugs. Three months or more may be required to achieve engraftment (judged either by the appearance of donor type cells or by clinical improvement), much longer than is the case with unseparated grafts. Nevertheless, 80 percent or more of patients grafted by these techniques at centers with experienced staffs are reconstituted for T cell immunity. Reconstitution for antibody production is significantly less reliable and was achieved in only 35 percent of one recent series (O'Reilly et al., 1986).

SELECTIVE DEFECTS OF CELL MEDIATED IMMUNITY

Purine Nucleoside Phosphorylase (PNP) Deficiency

This is a very rare syndrome characterized immunologically by severely impaired cell mediated immunity associated with normal antibody production. Most of the patients described have lacked PNP activity in their erythrocytes and are assumed to have a defective structural gene for the enzyme on chromosome 14. One family had a functionally abnormal PNP. Patients recognized to date have had recurrent respiratory tract infections and severe infections with herpesviruses, especially varicella-zoster virus. There are no characteristic physical findings, and diagnosis depends on laboratory test results. These generally show low numbers of circulating T cells, low lymphocyte count, and little proliferative response to phytohemagglutinin (PHA). The serum immunoglobulins are normal, as are antibody responses to both primary and secondary immunization. The diagnosis is suggested by the increased excretion of inosine and deoxyinosine in the urine; it is confirmed by direct assay of the enzyme in red blood cells. There is no simple, established treatment. Transfusion of red blood cells for enzyme replacement has been tried without clear clinical benefit (Staal et al., 1980) and may result only in the production of anti-red blood cell antibodies. Bone marrow transplantation may have a place in treatment, but most probably requires that the recipient be heavily immunosuppressed.

Complications of PNP deficiency include megaloblastic changes in the bone marrow, mild orotic acidemia, neurologic spasticity, and autoimmune hemolytic anemia. The metabolic changes and spasticity arise from the purine and secondary pyrimidine pathway abnormalities, while the autoimmunity may result from failure of normal immunoregulation. There is no established treatment for these complications.

Thymic Hypoplasia (Di George Syndrome)

Infants with the most complete forms of this syndrome lack parathyroid and thymus glands, and they have abnormal development of the aortic arch. Additional features include low set ears, mid-line facial defects, and small jaws. Most cases are sporadic, and it is assumed that they result from interrupted differentiation of the endodermal epithelium before the twelfth week of gestation. The degree of cardiac, parathyroid, and thymic impairment varies independently, and this makes it difficult to compare the effects of one treatment with another.

The most serious symptoms result from the cardiac defects, particularly when there is truncus arteriosus or total anomalous pulmonary venous drainage. Infants who survive surgery or do not require surgery develop hypocalcemia, which responds only to calcium and vitamin D supplements. Immune problems develop later or not at all. Potentially, the most serious problem is graft versus host disease fol-

lowing the transfusion of unirradiated blood during corrective surgery, but this outcome seems very rare. Almost all affected infants make some immunoglobulin, though it may not include antibody to antigens, such as tetanus toxoid, which have been used for immunization. Less severely affected infants have normal antibody production and only moderately depressed numbers of circulating T cells.

Treatment by grafts of fetal thymus is followed by increased cell mediated immunity (August et al., 1970). Grafts of immunocompetent cells carry a risk of causing graft versus host disease; therefore, very young fetal thymus (less than 12 weeks' gestation) is preferred. The immune basis for the response to fetal thymus is unclear, and thymus graft treatment has not been compared with no treatment. There is a spontaneous though slow increase in the number of circulating T cells in infants who are not grafted. Injection of thymic humoral factors is a potential line of treatment. Susceptibility to severe bacterial infections is reduced by giving replacement IgG; this may be the initial approach of choice while spontaneous improvement is awaited.

Common Variable Immunodeficiency Affecting Predominantly Cell Mediated Immunity

This encompasses children and adults with unclassified congenital or acquired primary defects of cell mediated immunity but intact or relatively unimpaired antibody responses. This is a much rarer combination than hypogammaglobulinemia. The patients are heterogeneous and commonly present with severe or progressive virus infections. When herpesviruses are involved, infection may take the form of recurrent zoster, prominent hepatosplenomegaly with cytomegalovirus (CMV) infection, or chronic EBV infection. Individuals with more severely depressed cell mediated immunity may develop disseminated herpes simplex virus (HSV) infection, Pneumocystis carinii lung infection, and mucosal candidiasis. Positive family histories for similar infections in some patients suggest that selective defects of cell mediated immunity can be genetically determined. With the recent advances in characterizing the in vitro responses of lymphocytes, it may be possible to define the defects in some of these individuals in the future and plan some rational treatment. Previous empirical approaches to treatment have included injections of thymic extracts or synthetic polypeptides with putative thymic humoral factor activities. Transfer factor, which is prepared as a dialyzable extract of blood lymphocytes from healthy donors, also has been used. Both of these approaches remain experimental. There are numerous reports of benefits in individual patients (Hobbs et al., 1984), but difficulties in standardizing and assaying the preparations have hindered useful controlled studies. Treatment with putative immunostimulatory drugs such as levamisole also has had little success.

OTHER DISORDERS WITH ASSOCIATED DEFECTS OF SPECIFIC IMMUNITY

Ataxia Telangiectasia (AT)

This is a complex multisystem disorder characterized by cerebellar ataxia, telangiectases in the conjunctivae and facial skin, and a variable degree of immunodeficiency. The disorder has an autosomal recessive inheritance and an incidence of about 1 in 40,000 live births. The biochemical basis for the symptoms is not understood; the most characteristic metabolic defect is of DNA repair, following ionizing radiation (Paterson and Smith, 1979). The abnormal DNA repair seems likely to contribute to the high frequency of chromosome abnormalities in AT patients and their increased susceptibility to lymphoid and epithelial malignances. The lymphomas often are T cell in origin (Stevens and Golde, 1979), and in about 50 percent of cases translocations involve the 14q32 band. This finding is of interest because the immunoglobulin heavy chain genes are at 14q32, and the gene for the alpha chain of the T cell receptor is at 14q11. Break and translocation points in the patients' lymphomas, therefore, commonly involve recognized rearrangement points.

Clinical presentation usually begins with ataxia between 3 and 6 years of age; telangiectasia may not become noticeable for several more years. The ataxia progresses so that patients lose the ability to walk and feed themselves, but intellectual function is less obviously impaired. Associated abnormalities include gonadal dysgenesis and biochemical changes, such as raised alpha-fetoprotein levels, glucose intolerance, and low serum IgA and IgE levels. Total IgG levels usually are normal, though the IgG2 subclass is low or absent (Oxelius et al.,

1982). IgM levels are normal, but the proportion with low molecular weight is increased. Cell mediated immunity commonly is normal at diagnosis but becomes progressively impaired, as judged by responses to PHA and delayed hypersensitivity skin test reactions. Recurrent sinusitis and chronic lung disease are common, and pneumonia is a cause of death. Immunoglobulin deficiencies and failure of antigen-specific T cell responses (Nelson et al., 1983) are likely contributing factors.

Wiskott-Aldrich Syndrome

This syndrome is characterized by eczema, thrombocytopenia, and immunodeficiency. It has an X-linked recessive inheritance with a minimum incidence (calculated from retrospective surveys) of about 5/million live male births (Perry et al., 1980). The separate components of the syndrome are variable in severity, and since splenectomized patients have platelets of normal size and function it seems likely that the platelet defect is secondary. The nature of the primary defect is obscure, but it appears to result in abnormal expression of a glycoprotein (gpL115) on the surface of the patient's lymphocytes (Remold-O'Donnell et al., 1984). The most common immune abnormality is a lack of serum antibodies to carbohydrate antigens, including isohemagglutinins, and patients respond poorly or not at all to immunization with pneumococcal polysaccharide. The serum IgG and IgA levels are mostly normal or raised, whereas mean IgM levels are about half normal (50 to 60 mg/dl). Many patients have high IgE levels, findings consistent with apparent, atopic eczema.

Clinical presentation of Wiskott-Aldrich syndrome usually is in childhood, with eczema typical of atopic dermatitis in appearance and distribution. As the child's activity increases, bruising following even mild trauma becomes more marked. A small number of patients have more acute onsets, either with intracerebral bleeding or with bloody diarrhea. The diagnosis is suspected from the association of bruising and eczema in a boy, especially when there is a family history of affected male relatives on the mother's side.

Complete correction of the condition is possible with transplantation of matched sibling bone marrow, following immunosuppression of the recipient with cyclophosphamide and busulfan (Kapoor et al., 1981). Grafting of patients who lack matched siblings with T cell depleted marrow is difficult to achieve, but there is little experience with this treatment at present. Until biochemical correction of the underlying metabolic defect is possible, bone marrow grafting is likely to remain the treatment of choice. Although splenectomy does not correct the immunodeficiency, it does protect the patient from the risk of intracerebral and other bleeding and so substantially prolongs the time before grafting needs to be attempted. Following splenectomy, susceptibility to severe septicemia is increased so that continuous antibiotic treatment with a broad spectrum agent, such as trimethoprim-sulfa, is recommended (Lum et al., 1980). Intravenous IgG can be given to patients with histories of septicemia, but it is probably better to rely on antibiotics. Benefit from injections of Transfer Factor has been reported, but problems of preparation and uncertainty over the chances of success have limited the popularity of this approach.

Immunodeficiency with Transcobalamin II Deficiency

Transcobalamin II is a transport protein for vitamin B_{12} in blood and tissues. Deficiency of this transport protein is rare, and in the case of a Moroccan boy was accompanied by severe megaloblastic anemia and hypogammaglobulinemia. Immunoglobulin production increased following treatment with B_{12}, but the patient subsequently developed a neutrophil bactericidal defect. The defect responded to large doses of formyl tetrahydrofolic acid (Seger et al., 1980).

Immunodeficiency with Thymoma

Patients with thymomas develop a range of autoimmune disorders of which the most common is myasthenia gravis, affecting about 40 percent; red blood cell aplasia or aplastic anemia, 20 percent; and hypogammaglobinemia, only about 5 percent. Clinical presentation is rare before the age of 40 years. Symptoms arise either from thymoma (which is usually of the spindle cell type and benign) or from recurrent infection due to antibody deficiency. These patients have few if any B cells in their blood, and their bone marrows lack preB cells. Many patients have circulating T cells, which express suppressor activity in tissue culture (Brenner et

al., 1984); it is possible that suppressor T cells are responsible for the interference with B cell precursor function in the marrow. Other cell lines also are affected as follows: (1) eosinophils are rare or absent in thymoma patients, and (2) anemia, leukopenia, and thrombocytopenia are common. Serum immunoglobulins usually are very low, although secretory IgA tends to be preserved. Blood lymphocyte counts generally are normal, but patients may have abnormal T cell function as judged by negative and delayed hypersensitivity skin test results or depressed proliferative responses to mitogens. Removal of the thymoma does not reverse the hypogammaglobulinemia, and treatment is by IgG replacement.

Immunodeficiencies Associated with Short Stature

These associations may occur in at least two ways. The first is the impaired growth seen in children with chronic infection, secondary to the immunodeficiency. A second possibility is that a single metabolic defect has adverse effects on the proliferation of both cartilage and lymphocytes. The achondroplasia-like syndrome, which occurs in infants with SCID due to adenosine deaminase (ADA) deficiency, appears to be an example of the first, while cartilage hair hypoplasia (CHH) may be an example of the second.

Cartilage Hair Hypoplasia (CHH)

This is a rare condition characterized by proportional but short stature, thin and sparse hair, and severe reactions to virus infections. The inheritance is autosomal recessive, and some of the original patients, amongst the Amish, died of severe varicella infections (McKusick and Cross, 1966). Subsequent experience indicated that the degree of immunodeficiency is variable both between patients and in a single patient, over the course of time. Immunoglobulins generally are normal, as are antibody responses, but there may be lymphopenia, reduced numbers of T cells (both CD 4 and CD 8 subsets are affected) in the blood, and reduced proliferative responses to mitogens and antigens.

Clinically, the concern with these patients remains their susceptibility to severe herpesvirus, particularly varicella-zoster, infections. Until the safety of the Oka herpesvirus vaccine strain is established, and prophylaxis becomes possible, it is probably advisable to offer zoster immune globulin protection to immunodeficient CHH patients following varicella exposure. Acyclovir treatment would be expected to help those who do develop severe herpes simplex or varicella infections.

Chronic Mucocutaneous Candidiasis

This disorder is characterized by chronic infection of the skin, nails, and mouth with *Candida*. Some patients have no further problems, whereas others have associated endocrine deficiencies, granulomas, or recurrent infections. The occurrence of familial cases sharing the same associations is the basis for their separate classification (Wells et al., 1972). Although the chronicity and severity of the infections are evidence for immunodeficiency, the pathogenesis of the disorder is obscure. Immunoglobulin levels and antibody responses usually remain normal even when the candidiasis is severe. T lymphocyte responses (delayed hypersensitivity skin test results, proliferation to mitogens and *Candida* antigens) are low in some patients but not in others. T cell responses tend to return to normal following treatment of the candidiasis; therefore, it is likely that many of the abnormalities reported in the medical literature are secondary to immunosuppression by *Candida* polysaccharides (Fischer et al., 1978).

The clinical onset usually is in childhood, with presentation as severe diaper dermatitis or oral candidiasis. The nails are usually involved within a year or two. The diagnosis should be based on detection of *Candida* hyphae in a potassium hydroxide preparation. The skin rash can be confused with atopic eczema. Local treatment with miconazole usually reduces scaling, but relapse is common when application is discontinued. Oral ketoconazole usually is sufficient to suppress the *Candida*, but continuous treatment is necessary. Injections of lymphocyte extracts (Transfer Factor) have been tried without clear evidence of benefit. If it is to be tried, it should be given with antifungal drugs (Kirkpatrick and Smith, 1974).

Three of the conditions associated with chronic mucocutaneous candidiasis deserve special mention. The endocrinopathy typically involves the parathyroids, the adrenals, and occasionally the thyroid or pituitary glands (Blizzard and Gibbs, 1968). Granulomas can be particularly disfiguring; in one study, they oc-

curred in patients who retained delayed cutaneous hypersensitivity to *Candida* antigen. Recurrent infections may be due to herpesviruses or, in others, to staphylococci, in which cases they take the form of recurrent abscesses.

Lymphopenia with Lymphocytotoxins

Antilymphocyte antibodies are found in patients with a range of autoimmune disorders and in others with different virus infections, including acquired immune deficiency syndrome (AIDS). In most cases, the antibodies are IgM class and fix complement. A few patients have been reported with severe, episodic lymphopenias and recurrent, lower respiratory tract infections; an affected boy subsequently died, with a reticulum cell sarcoma (Gelfand et al., 1975).

SECONDARY IMMUNODEFICIENCIES

Secondary immunodeficiencies occur far more commonly than do primary syndromes. The diversity of mechanisms that interfere with normal immunity is so great that only a general survey is given here. Major causes are summarized in Table 3–1. Loss of immunoglobulins with or without cells is described first because it is the simplest mechanism by which immunodeficiency occurs.

TABLE 3–1. Major Causes of Secondary Immunodeficiency

Nutritional defects
    Malnutrition
    Loss of protein or cells from gut or kidney

Infections

    Human immunodeficiency viruses (HIV)
    Other viruses, especially CMV, EBV, rubella, measles
    Malaria

Malignancies
    Lymphoid, especially leukemias, Hodgkin disease, myeloma
    Other

Drugs

Extremes of age

Surgery
    Splenectomy

Loss of Immunoglobulin
from the Kidney

Kidney diseases that result in nonselective proteinuria can result in the loss of large amounts of immunoglobulin each day. IgG levels are lowered most, because of molecular size and the fact that this isotype has the highest serum levels and the longest half-life. All immunoglobulin classes are lost in patients with nonselective proteinuria syndromes. Infections in patients with hypoproteinemia secondary to renal loss are common and occur particularly at sites exposed to bacterial colonization (such as the peritoneal cavity during dialysis). The recognition of protein loss syndromes is facilitated when proteinuria is detected or hypoproteinemia is severe enough to cause edema. Laboratory confirmation comes from the demonstration of a low serum albumin level and raised 24-hour urinary protein loss. Treatment of renal loss needs to be directed to the primary cause. Replacement of IgG is of little use in the face of continued protein loss.

Gut Loss

Protein losing enteropathy has several causes, but in most instances the loss is not severe enough to cause clinically significant immunodeficiency on its own. Losses in severe Crohn disease and in hypertrophic eosinophilic gastritis are principally of protein; cell mediated immunity is preserved unless there is significant malnutrition or steroid treatment. In the rare condition of intestinal lymphangiectasia, the primary defect is part of a generalized disorder of the lymphatic system that results in dilatation of the lymphatic channels and leakage into the gut lumen of plasma proteins and lymphocytes (Vardy et al., 1975). Symptoms, which may not appear until the second year of life, usually include diarrhea and edema with failure to thrive. Laboratory results that are useful diagnostically include low serum albumin and IgG levels together with lymphopenia and evidence for reduced T cell responses by delayed skin hypersensitivity reactions and *in vitro* testing. Problems with infections are variable, and some infants have serum IgG levels below 200 mg/dl without respiratory tract involvement. The high rate of IgG synthesis and the persistence of NK cell activity may account for the relative rarity of severe infections in this disorder. Replacement of IgG is difficult in the presence of continued severe gut loss.

Malnutrition

Worldwide, this is by far the most common cause of secondary immunodeficiency. The adverse effects of malnutrition on the immune system are reviewed in detail by Chandra (1980) and are only summarized here. In general, antibody responses to new antigens are impaired well before serum immunoglobulin levels fall; cell mediated immune responses are impaired early in the course of the deficiency. By affecting immunity, malnutrition increases infection that in turn interferes with nutrition. The effects of malnutrition are complicated by possible deficiencies of defined essential dietary factors, such as vitamin B_{12}, folic acid, and zinc. Zinc is selectively deficient in a rare disorder, acrodermatitis enteropathica, which has an autosomal recessive inheritance. Early symptoms are dermatitis, affecting particularly the face and perianal area, and diarrhea. The number of circulating T cells is low; *in vitro* T cell responses are usually abnormal, and a minority of patients has antibody deficiency. Treatment with zinc supplements usually is effective.

Virus Infections

Acquired Immunodeficiency Syndrome (AIDS). AIDS results from the infection of a subset of T lymphocytes with a retrovirus named human immunodeficiency virus (HIV). Unique features of all the lymphotropic retroviruses include the binding to the T cell through the CD 4 antigen and the ability to cause either a transformation (leading to leukemia) or a cytopathic effect (leading to immunodeficiency) (Wong-Staal and Gallo, 1985). The infection is mostly acquired through sexual contact, but transmission also is through blood transfusion and contact with blood products, including Factor VIII concentrates, and occasional perinatal transmission from mother to child. Following infection the virus has been recovered from blood, lymphoid tissues, plasma, semen, saliva, and tears, whether or not the subject has serum antibody to the virus. The extent to which the disease progresses following exposure is variable and, because of the slow course of the infection, not yet fully defined. More people have antibody to the virus than have experienced symptoms, which are due clearly to HIV infections. The antibodies can neutralize the infectivity of the virus *in vitro*, so there is a clear potential for immunity.

The rate of AIDS diagnosis continues to be highest amongst homosexuals, followed by drug abusers, blood transfusion and Factor VIII recipients, and heterosexual contacts. The mildest clinical manifestation of the infection is often called either pre-AIDS or AIDS-related complex (ARC). This is manifest as lymphadenopathy with varying degrees of fever, malaise, and weight loss. At the other end of the spectrum are patients with opportunistic infections (e.g., *Pneumocystis carinii, Candida,* herpesviruses, and fungi) and AIDS-associated neoplasms, particularly Kaposi sarcoma and B cell lymphoma. Presenting symptoms in infants and children are mostly infections due to encapsulated bacteria, and the early course resembles that of boys with agammaglobulinemia. With progression of the infection, affected children develop interstitial pneumonia, thrush, and enlargement of the salivary glands.

The diagnosis may be suspected in a patient with persistent lymphadenopathy and a known risk factor. It usually can be confirmed by the presence of serum antibody to HIV and evidence for immunodeficiency. Laboratory test result abnormalities typical for these patients include selctive loss of CD 4 positive lymphocytes, reduced proliferative responses to T cell mitogens, reduced production of IL-2 by T cells, and often raised serum IgG levels (Rosen, 1985). Antibody responses to recall antigens (e.g., tetanus toxoid) usually are normal, whereas the ability to make antibody to new antigens is impaired.

Although the rate of replication of HIV in tissue culture can be slowed by drugs, it has not yet been possible to reverse the course of clinical infection. Some relief of symptoms in affected infants is provided by immunoglobulin replacement. Since the patients tend to have high IgG levels, the half-life of IgG administered to the recipients is reduced; more than the basic maintenance dose for antibody deficiency should be given. Approximately 150 mg/kg/wk is recommended. Interstitial pneumonia may require oxygen supplementation.

Epstein-Barr Virus (EBV) Infections and X-linked Lymphoproliferative Syndrome. This syndrome describes a range of adverse consequences of Epstein-Barr virus (EBV) infections in individuals with preexisting genetic susceptibility (Hamilton et al., 1980). The disorder was first recognized in a large kindred with six affected males, and their inheritance of the susceptibility was X-linked and recessive. Affected males have been in good health until infected with EBV. The outcome of infection is of two main types, those with and those without lymphoproliferation. The most common clinical phenotype is fatal infectious mononucleosis (with lymphoproliferation); other phenotypes in this group include immunoblastic sarcoma, Burkitt lymphoma, and immunodeficiency with hyper-IgM. The aproliferative phenotypes include agranulocytosis, aplastic anemia, and hypogammaglobulinemia. The etiology of the condition remains obscure, though a failure of T cell recognition and NK cell activation seems likely. Prospects for treatment may depend on the development of more effective anti-EBV drugs.

Infectious Mononucleosis. Acute infectious mononucleosis is accompanied by increases in the number of CD 8 cells, and reduced percentages of CD 4 cells, in the circulation. Circulating T cells obtained during the acute stage of infection suppress mitogen stimulated B cell responses, and they also display nonspecific cytotoxicity to cell lines (Svedmyr et al., 1984). Most patients make uneventful recoveries, but a minority develops a syndrome suggestive of persistent infection (Rumke et al., 1984).

Measles. Delayed hypersensitivity skin responses are suppressed during and shortly after acute measles infections. A transient increase in circulating activated T cells may contribute to this effect.

Rubella. Congenital rubella infections are associated with an increased incidence of immunoglobulin deficiency, mostly IgA and IgG (South et al., 1975), and of autoimmune disorders, particularly juvenile onset diabetes mellitus. Since autoimmunity also is independently associated with immunodeficiency, a single mechanism may account for these various effects.

Drugs. The immunosuppressive effects of drugs that interfere with cell division, and so prevent clonal expansion of antigen stimulated cells, are familiar and to be expected. Corticosteroids act variously by (1) interfering with mediator release from monocytes, (2) altering the circulation of lymphocytes so that T cells accumulate in the marrow, and (3) interfering with T cell effector functions such as NK cell activation and cytotoxicity (Claman, 1984). Interference with mediator release has proved to be an effective means to suppress both new and established immune responses; cyclosporin A is an example of this type of drug. Other drugs have immunosuppressive effects that might not be expected based on their routine clinical uses. These include phenytoin, which usually lowers serum IgA levels and in some subjects interferes with IgG and IgM syntheses. Low immunoglobulin levels sometimes are seen with other anticonvulsants, though it is unclear whether this is a primary or secondary effect.

Tumors. Common tumors, such as those of the lung, often are observed with pneumonia following interference with local immunity. Impairment of specific immunity can follow as a result of anorexia, leading to malnutrition, or treatment with cytotoxic drugs or with irradiation. Malignancy of the lymphoid system itself can cause a more severe defect of specific immunity earlier in the course of the disease. Patients with chronic lymphocytic leukemia most often have reduced IgM levels, followed by reduced IgG levels. The reduction is due to reduced synthesis and may result from the large numbers of circulating leukemia cells and the secondary interference with efficient cell cooperation. Leukemia cells themselves are unresponsive to mitogen stimulation except in a minority of patients whose cells have some capacity for further differentiation. Patients with antibody deficiency and recurrent bacterial infections may be helped by IgG replacement.

Multiple myeloma patients have monoclonal bands and high levels of the corresponding immunoglobulin class. The levels of polyclonal immunoglobulin can be very low, and the susceptibility to bacterial infection increased. Suppression of normal immunoglobulin production appears to play a role in immunodeficiency in addition to hypercatabolism of immunoglobulins.

Hodgkin disease patients differ from those with lymphoid malignancies in that cell mediated immunity is affected more than antibody responsiveness. A clinical correlate of the abnormalities of T cell function is an increased frequency of fungal and mycobacterial infections, together with reactivation of varicella-zoster virus to give herpes zoster.

THE PATIENT WITH RECURRENT INFECTION

The commonest cause for referral to an immunodeficiency clinic is recurrent upper respiratory tract infection. Most of the children investigated have normal specific and nonspecific immune responses by currently available tests. Often, environmental factors such as exposure in preschool groups appear to be the most likely cause; in a minority, allergy is a major etiologic factor. Most adults who have clear histories for increases in infections have secondary immunodeficiencies. Attention should be directed, therefore, at all ages, to exclude common secondary causes. In children, this list of causes includes cystic fibrosis, inhaled foreign bodies, and anatomic abnormalities; in adults, malignancies and AIDS should be considered. The following sections summarize points in the history, examination, and laboratory tests that help in the recognition of primary immunodeficiency syndromes.

History

Only a few clinical conditions are strongly suggestive of particular immunodeficiency syndromes. These include recurrent staphylococcal abscesses, involving groups of lymph nodes in chronic granulomatous disease (CGD); progressive BCG infection in SCID; and recurrent *Candida* infections in chronic mucocutaneous candidiasis. Table 3–2 lists the organisms to which susceptibility is enhanced, according to the kind of immune deficit. In CGD and SCID, infections start in the first 4 months of age, while antibody deficiency syndromes do not usually appear before 6 months of age. This difference in age of onset reflects the protection provided by maternal IgG antibody for the first months of life.

The family history is useful when it is positive for a defined immunodeficiency. When this history provides no more than an account of unexplained early deaths in childhood, it is important to consider the socioeconomic conditions prevailing at the time.

Examination

This usually is more helpful in defining the degree of structural damage caused by infections than in characterizing the underlying immunodeficiency. Exceptions, which sometimes are clinically useful, include the absence of tonsils in patients with congenital agammaglobulinemia or SCID. Characteristic physical signs are the hallmarks of rare conditions, such as ataxia telangiectasia and CHH. Bruising due to thrombocytopenia is seen with Wiskott-Aldrich syndrome.

TABLE 3–2. Infectious Agents Characteristically Associated with Immunodeficiency Syndromes

Organism	Antibody*	Complement C3	Complement C5-9	Neutrophil	T cell	Combined
Bacteria						
Streptococcus pneumoniae	+	+	−	−	−	+
Haemophilus influenzae	+	+	−	−	−	+
Staphylococcus aureus (skin)	+	+	−	+	−	+
Disseminated *Neisseria*	−	−	+	−	−	−
Protozoa						
Pneumocystis carinii	+/−	−	−	−	+	+
Giardia (gut)	+	−	−	−	−	+/−
Cryptosporidium (gut)	+	−	−	−	−	+/−
Viruses						
Poliovirus	+	−	−	−	−	+/−
Echovirus	+	−	−	−	−	−
Herpes zoster	+	−	−	−	+	+

*The + signifies that the agent is a common or significant pathogen in the condition indicated; the +/− indicates that the agent is a relatively uncommon pathogen.

Tests

The range of tests continues to increase faster than does expertise in interpreting the results. A selection that will help screen for the more common immunodeficiencies is ranked in Table 3–3 in approximate order of diagnostic yield. Where tests cover similar responses, it is best to choose one with which the laboratory staff is familiar. Points that bear on interpretation are summarized next.

Serum Immunoglobulins. These usually need to be measured, if only to exclude deficiency. For children, it is essential to use pediatric control standards for interpretation of results. Patients, including children, with recurrent viral upper respiratory tract infections but no allergy tend to have higher serum IgG levels than do healthy controls; these patients also produce brisk increases in secretory IgA during infections (Isaacs et al., 1984). Selective IgA deficiency is easily recognized, but low IgA levels may also be important, as in children whose upper respiratory tract infections are accompanied by asthma or recurrent tonsillitis (Donovan and Soothill, 1973).

Patients with recurrent respiratory tract infections but normal total serum IgG levels may need to have IgG subclasses measured. This usually requires sending the sample to an established referral laboratory. Measurement of antibody responses to a polysaccharide (pneumococcal or *Haemophilus* polysaccharide) and a protein (tetanus toxoid) antigen also is useful to the diagnosis in the rare patient with antibody deficiency and normal IgG levels.

Counts of B cell numbers in the blood are of clinical value in the diagnosis of suspected hypogammaglobulinemia due to thymoma or possible X-linked agammaglobulinemia; in

TABLE 3–3. Screening Tests for Immunodeficiency

First level screening tests

Blood count to exclude neutropenia, thrombocytopenia, anemia
Serum immunoglobulins to exclude hypogammaglobulinemia
HIV antibodies, T cell count or response when AIDS is considered
Nitroblue tetrazolium dye (NBT) test in recurrent staphylococcal abscesses

Second level tests for antibody response

Pre- and post-immunization antibody titers to pneumococcus and tetanus toxoid
Serum IgG subclasses

Second level tests for complement function

Total hemolytic complement titer—if low, measure individual components.

Second level tests for neutrophil function

Bacterial killing test

Second level tests for cell mediated immunity

Delayed hypersensitivity skin tests
T cell subset counts
T cell proliferative response to mitogens or antigens

both instances, they are markedly reduced or absent. In the more common acquired antibody deficiency syndromes B cells are present in normal or moderately reduced numbers, but this information has no useful prognostic value. Bone marrow examinations are useful when there is a possibility of malignancy.

Cell Mediated Immunity. The simplest tests of cell mediated immunity are delayed hypersensitivity skin tests. When done to demonstrate normal responses, it is important to select antigens to which the subject is likely to be responsive (see Chapter 17, Table 17–4). For adults, *Candida*, measles, mumps, and tetanus toxoid antigens are suitable. For infants whose sensitization is uncertain, tetanus toxoid is often the best choice provided that routine immunizations have been given. A normal response (induration as well as erythema) indicates that the antigen was processed and presented to T cells and that inflammatory cells were recruited into the response following lymphokine release. If skin test results are negative, the separate components of the response need to be tested in other ways. This step entails measuring an antibody response to tetanus toxoid or another antigen that normally requires processing. T cells should be counted in the blood after a blood count and differential have been obtained so that the proportions of CD 3, CD 4, and CD 8 cells can be expressed as absolute numbers. *In vitro* responses of T cells to antigen or mitogen are measurable as cell proliferation and IL-2 release. The frequency of T cells with specificity for single antigens is difficult to quantify, unless a laborious limiting dilution approach is used; IL-2 assays may be increasingly used. Tests for specialized mediator release (migration inhibition factors, macrophage activating factors) are less used than formerly, though this trend may be reversed with the introduction of simple kits for mediators such as gamma interferon.

REFERENCES

Ammann, A.J., Hong, R.: Selective IgA deficiency: Presentation of 30 cases and a review of the literature. Medicine 50:223, 1971.

Ammann, A.J., Wara, D.W., Pillarisetty, R.J., Talal, N.: The prevalence of autoantibodies in T-cell, B-cell and phagocytic immunodeficiency disorders. Clin. Immunol. Immunopathol. 14:456, 1979.

Asherson, G.L., Webster, A.D.B.: Diagnosis and Treatment of Immunodeficiency Diseases. Blackwell Scientific Publications, Inc., Oxford, 1980.

Asquith, P.: Immunology of celiac disease. Clin. Gastroent. 3:213, 1974.

August, C.S., Berkel, A.L., Levey, R.H., Rosen, F.S.: Establishment of immunological competence in a child with congenital thymic aplasia by a graft of fetal thymus. Lancet 1:1080, 1970.

Beck, C.S., Heiner, D.C.: Selective immunoglobulin G$_4$ deficiency and recurrent infections of the respiratory tract. Am. Rev. Respir. Dis. 124:94, 1981.

Berger, M., Cupps, T.R., Fauci, A.S.: Immunoglobulin replacement therapy by slow subcutaneous infusion. Ann. Int. Med. 93:55, 1980.

Blizzard, R.M., Gibbs, J.H.: Candidiasis: Studies pertaining to its association with the endocrinopathies. Pediatrics 42:231, 1968.

Brenner, M.K., Reittie, J.G.E., Chadda, H.R., Pollock, A., Asherson, G.L.: Thymoma and hypogammaglobulinemia with and without T suppressor cells. Clin. Exp. Immunol. 58:619, 1984.

Buckley, R.H.: Gamma-globulin replacement. Clin. Immunol. Allerg. 5:141, 1985.

Burks, A.W., Sampson, H.A., Buckley, R.H.: Anaphylactic reactions after gammaglobulin administration in patients with hypogammaglobulinemia. N. Engl. J. Med. 314:560, 1986.

Chandra, R.K.: Immunology of Nutritional Disorders. Edward Arnold, London, 1980.

Claman, H.N.: Anti-inflammatory effects of corticosteroids. Clin. Immunol. Allerg. 4:317, 1984.

Conley, M.E., Cooper, M.D.: Immature IgA B cells in IgA deficient patients. N. Engl. J. Med. 305:495, 1981.

Conley, M.E., Nowell, P.C., Henle, G., Douglas, S. XX T cells and XY B cells in two patients with severe combined immune deficiency. Clin. Immunol. Immunopathol. 31:87, 1984.

Cunningham-Rundles, C., Brandeis, W.E., Pudifin, D.J., Day, N.K., Good, R.A.: Autoimmunity in selective IgA deficiency: Relationship to anti-bovine protein antibodies, circulating immune complexes and clinical disease. Clin. Exp. Immunol. 45:299, 1981.

Donovan, R., Soothill, J.F.: Immunological studies in children undergoing tonsillectomy. Clin. Exp. Immunol. 14:347, 1973.

Faulk, W.P., Kiyasu, W.S., Cooper, M.D., Fudenberg, H.H.: Deficiency of IgM. Pediatrics 47:399, 1971.

Fischer, A., Ballet, J.J., Griscelli, C.: Specific inhibitor of *in vitro* candida-induced lymphocyte proliferation by polysaccharide antigens present in the serum of patients with chronic mucocutaneous candidiasis. J. Clin. Invest. 62:1005, 1978.

Fischer, A., Ledeist, F., Durandy, A., Hamet, M., Arnaud-Battandier, F., Griscelli, C.: Heterogeneity of immunologic and enzymatic deficiencies in the familial reticuloendotheliosis syndrome. *In* Primary Immunodeficiency Diseases, Wedgwood, R.J., Rosen, F.S., Paul, N.W. (eds.). A. R. Liss, New York, 1983.

Gelfand, E.W., Parkman, R., Rosen, F.S.: Lymphocytotoxins and immunological unresponsiveness. *In* Immunodeficiency in Man and Animals, Bergsma, D., et al. (eds.), Sinauer Press, Sunderland, Massachusetts, 1975.

Griscelli, C., Fischer, A., Grospierre, B., Durandy, A., Bremard, C., Charron, D., Vilmer, E., Virelizier, J-L.: Clinical and immunologic aspects of combined immunodeficiency with defective expression of HLA antigens. Prog. Immunodef. Res. Therap. 1:19, 1984.

Hamilton, J.K., Paquin, L.A., Sullivan, J.L., et al.: X-linked lymphoproliferative syndrome registry report. J. Pediatr. 96:669, 1980.

Hobbs, J.R., Byrom, N., Nagvekar, N., Rowland-Payne, C.M.E., Oates, J.K.: Post-viral T cell deficiencies and their treatment. *In* Progress in Immunodeficiency Research and Therapy I, Griscelli, C., Vossen, J. (eds.), Excerpta Medica Press, Elsevier, Amsterdam, 1984.

Isaacs, D., Webster, A.D.B., Valman, H.B.: Immunoglobulin levels and function in pre-school children with recurrent respiratory tract infections. Clin. Exp. Immunol. 58:335, 1984.

Kapoor, N., Kirkpatrick, D., Blaese, R.M., Oleske, J., Hilgartner, M.H., Chaganti, R.S.K., Good, R.A., O'Reilly, R.J. Reconstitution of normal megakaryopoiesis and immunologic functions in Wiskott-Aldrich syndrome by marrow transplantation following myeloablation and immunosuppression with busulfan and cyclophosphamide. Blood 57:692, 1981.

Karol, R.A., Eng, J., Cooper, J.B., Dennison, D.K., Sawyer, M.K., Lawrence, E.C., Marcus, D.M., Shearer, W.T.: Imbalances in subsets of T lymphocytes in an inbred pedigree with Omenn's syndrome. Clin. Immunol. Immunopathol. 27:412, 1983.

Kirkpatrick, C.H., Smith, T.K.: Chronic mucocutaneous candidiasis: Immunologic and antibiotic therapy. Ann. Int. Med. 80:310, 1974.

Lisowska-Grospierre, B., Charron, D.J., dePreval, C., Durandy, A., Griscelli, C., Mach, B.: A defect in the regulation of major histocompatibility complex class II gene expression in human HLA-DR negative lymphocytes from patients with combined immunodeficiency syndrome. J. Clin. Invest. 76:381, 1985.

Lum, L.G., Tubergen, D.G., Corsah, L., Blaese, R.M.: Splenectomy in the management of the thrombocytopenia of Wiskott-Aldrich syndrome. N. Engl. J. Med. 289:921, 1980.

McKusick, V.A., Cross, H.E.: Ataxia telangiectasia and swiss type agammaglobulinemia: Two genetic disorders of the immune system in related Amish sibships. J. Am. Med. Assn. 195:739, 1966.

McLoughlin, G.A., Bradley, J., Chapman, D.M., Temple, J.G., Hede, J.E., McFarland, J.: IgA deficiency and severe post vagotomy diarrhoea. Lancet 1:168, 1976.

Mease, P.J., Ochs, H.D., Wedgwood, R.J.: Successful treatment of echovirus meningoencephalitis and myositis-fasciitis with intravenous immunoglobulin therapy in a patient with X-linked agammaglobulinemia. N. Engl. J. Med. 304:1278, 1981.

Nelson, D.L., Biddison, W.E., Shaw, S.: Defective *in vitro* production of influenza virus specific cytotoxic T lymphocytes in ataxia telangiectasia. J. Immunol. 130:2629, 1983.

Neudorf, S., Kersey, J., Filipovich, A.: Lymphoid progenitor cells in severe combined immunodeficiency. J. Clin. Immunol. 5:26, 1985.

O'Reilly, R. J., Brochstein, J., Collins, N., Keever, C., Kapor, N., Kirkpatrick, D., Kernan, N., Dupont, B., Burns, J., Reisner, Y.: Evaluation of HLA-haplotype disparate parental marrow grafts depleted of T lymphocytes by differential agglutination with a soybean lectin and E-rosette depletion for the treatment of severe combined immunodeficiency. Vox. Sang. 51 (Suppl. 2):81, 1986.

Ostergaard, P.A.: IgA levels and carrier rate of pathogenic bacteria in 27 children previously tonsillectomized. Acta Path. Microbiol. Scand. 85:178, 1977.

Oxelius, V.A.: Chronic infections in a family with hereditary deficiency of IgG2 and IgG4. Clin. Exp. Immunol. 17:19, 1974.

Oxelius, V-A., Berkel, I., Hanson, L.A.: IgG2 deficiency in ataxia telangiectasia. N. Engl. J. Med. 306:515, 1982.

Oxelius, V-A., Laurell, A-B., Lindquist, B., Golbiowska, H., Axelsson, U., Bjorkander, J., Hanson, L.A.: IgG subclasses in selective IgA deficiency. N. Engl. J. Med. 304:1476, 1981.

Paterson, M.C., Smith, P.J.: Ataxia telangiectasia: An inherited human disorder involving hypersensitivity to ionizing radiation and related DNA damaging chemicals. Ann. Rev. Genet. 13:291, 1979.

Pearl, E.R., Vogler, L.B., Okos, A.J., Christ, W.M., Lawton, A.R., Cooper, M.D.: B lymphocyte precursors in human bone marrow: An analysis of normal individuals and patients with antibody deficiency states. J. Immunol. 120:1169, 1978.

Perry, G.S., Spector, B.D., Schuman, L.M., Mandel, J.S., Anderson, E., McHugh, R.B., Hanson, M.R., Fahlstrom, S.M., Krivit, W., Kersey, J.H.: The Wiskott-Aldrich syndrome in the United States and Canada (1892-1979). J. Pediatr. 97:72, 1980.

Platts-Mills, T.A.E., De Gast, G.C., Pereira, R.S., Webster, A.D.B., Asherson, G.L., Wilkins, S.R.: Two immunologically distinct forms of late onset hypogammaglobulinemia. Clin. Exp. Immunol. 44:383, 1981.

Pyke, K., Dosch, H-M., Ipp, M., Gelfand, E.R.: Demonstration of an intrathymic defect in a case of severe combined immunodeficiency disease. N. Engl. J. Med. 293:424, 1975.

Reisner, Y., Kapoor, N., Kirkpatrick, D., Pollack, M.S., Cunningham-Rundles, S., Dupont, B., Hodes, M.Z., Good, R.A., O'Reilly, R.J.: Transplantation for severe combined immunodeficiency with HLA-A,B,D,DR incompatible parental marrow cells fractionated by soybean agglutinin and sheep red cells. Blood 61:341, 1983.

Remold-O'Donnell, E., Kenney, D., Parkman, R., Cairns, L., Savage, B., Rosen, F.S.: Characterization of a human lymphocyte surface sialoglycoprotein that is defective in Wiskott-Aldrich syndrome. J. Exp. Med. 159:1705, 1984.

Rosen, F.S.: The acquired immunodeficiency syndrome. J. Clin. Invest. 75:1, 1985.

Ross, I.N., Thompson, R.A.: Severe selective IgM deficiency. J. Clin. Path. 29:773, 1976.

Rumke, H.C., Terpstra, F.G., Weening, R.S., Zeijlmaker, W.P., Vossen, J.M.: B and T cell functions in children with persistent EBV infection tested in a PWM-driven system. Prog. Immunodef. Res. Therap. 1:297, 1984.

Schwaber, J., Molgaard, H., Orkin, S.H., Gould, H.J., Rosen, F.S.: Early pre B cells from normal and X-linked agammaglobulinemia produce Cu without an attached V_H region. Nature 304:355, 1983.

Seger, R., FraterSchroder, M., Hitzig, W.H., Wildfeuer, A., Linnell, J.C.: Granulocyte dysfunction in transcobalamin II deficiency responding to leukovorin or hydroxycobalaminplasma transfusion. J. Inher. Metab. Dis. 3:9, 1980.

Seto, S., Carrera, C.J., Kubota, M., Wasson, D.B., Carson, D.A.: Mechanism of deoxyadenosine and 2-chlorodeoxyadenosine toxicity to nondividing human lymphocytes. J. Clin. Invest. 75:377, 1985.

Smith, T.F., Morris, E.C., Bain, R.P.: IgG subclasses in non-allergic children with chronic chest symptoms. J. Pediatr. 105:896, 1984.

South, M.A., Montgomery, J.R., Rawls, W.E.: Immunodeficiency in congenital rubella and other viral infection. *In* Immunodeficiency in Man and Animals. Bergsma, D. (ed.), Sinauer Press, Sunderland, Massachusetts, 1975.

Staal, G.E., Stoop, J.W., Zegers, B.J., Henkelom, L.H., van der Vlist, M. J., Wadman, S.K., Martin, D.W.: Erythrocyte metabolism in purine nucleoside phosphorylase deficiency after enzyme replacement therapy by infusion of erythrocytes. J. Clin. Invest. 65:103, 1980.

Stavnezer-Nordgren, J., Kekish, O., Zegers, B. J.: Molecular defects in a human immunoglobulin kappa chain deficiency. Science 230:458, 1985.

Stevens, R.H., Golde, D.W.: Helper and suppressor T lymphocyte leukemia in ataxia telangiectasia. N. Engl. J. Med. 300:700, 1979.

Svedmyr, E., Ernberg, I., Seeley, J., et al.: Virologic, immunologic and clinical observations on a patient during the incubation, acute and convalescent phases of infectious mononucleosis. Clin. Immunol. Immunopathol. 30:437, 1984.

Tiller, E.L., Buckley, R.H.: Transient hypogammaglobulinemia of infancy: Review of the literature, clinical and immunologic features of 11 new cases and long-term follow-up. J. Pediatr. 92:347, 1978.

Touraine, J-L., Betuel, H.: The bare lymphocyte syndrome: Immunodeficiency resulting from the lack of expression of HLA antigens. *In* Primary Immunodeficiency Disorders, Wedgwood, R.J., Rosen, F.S., Paul, N.W. (eds.), Birth Def. Orig. Art. Series 19:83, 1983.

Umetsu, D.T., Ambrosino, D.M., Quinti, I., Siber, G., Geha, R.S.: Recurrent sinopulmonary infection and impaired antibody response to bacterial polysaccharide antigen in children with selective IgG-subclass deficiency. N. Engl. J. Med. 313:1247, 1985.

van Furth, R., Leijh, P.C.J., Klein, F.: Correlation between opsonic activity for various microorganisms and composition of gammaglobulin preparations for intravenous use. J. Inf. Dis. 149:511, 1984.

Vardy, P.A., Lebenthal, E., Shwachman, H.: Intestinal lymphangiectasia: A reappraisal. Pediatrics 55:842, 1975.

Wells, R.S., Higgs, J.M., Macdonald, A., Valdimarsson, H., Holt, P.J.L.: Familial chronic mucocutaneous candidiasis. J. Med. Genet. 9:302, 1972.

Wong-Staal, F., Gallo, R.C.: Human T-lymphotropic retroviruses. Nature 317:395, 1985.

Yount, W.J., Hong, R., Seligmann, M., Good, R.A., Kunkel, H.G.: Imbalances of gammaglobulin subgroups and gene defects in patients with primary hypogammaglobulinemia. J. Clin. Invest. 49:1957, 1970.

Zegers, B.J.M., Maertzdorf, W.J., van Loghem, E., et al.: Kappa chain deficiency. N. Eng. J. Med. 294:1026, 1976.

4

Complement and Phagocyte Function in Health and Disease

JOHN R. FOREHAND, M.D.
RICHARD B. JOHNSTON, JR., M.D.

The complement system, circulating and tissue sequestered phagocytes, and physical and anatomic barriers provide the host with "nonspecific" protection against microorganisms. These factors do not require prior exposure to provide protective capabilities and exist with more or less the same potential activity in all normal individuals. The "immune response" in host defense acts as an integrated system, involving humoral and cellular components. The important initial event in the specific response is the formation of specific antibody and sensitized T cells. However, complement and phagocytic cells are required to remove the infectious agent and may be effective in some cases even in the absence of specific antibody. That antibody and cell mediated immunity alone are ineffective in host protection is evidenced by the various clinical problems that arise when defects occur in a nonspecific host defense mechanism, particularly in the complement or phagocytic system.

PHYSICAL AND ANATOMIC BARRIERS

Defects in the normal physical and anatomic barriers to microbial invasion, as a group, are the most common causes of recurrent infection. A break in the integument; an obstruction to the outflow of mucus, air, or urine; an attenuation of normal microbial flora by antibiotic usage; a compromised vascular perfusion, as seen in diabetes mellitus or sickle cell disease; and fluid retention (edema) associated with the nephrotic syndrome are all examples of conditions that predispose the host to recurrent bacterial (and sometimes fungal) infection (Johnston, 1984).

As a group, infections due to defective barriers are characterized by recurrence in the same locations.

COMPLEMENT

The complement system is comprised of 19 serum proteins (Table 4–1). This system provides the host with nonspecific protection, primarily through the following activities (Muller-Eberhard, 1985; Johnston, 1986): (1) release of mediators of inflammation (anaphylatoxins); (2) enhancement of phagocytosis of foreign materials; and (3) mediation of direct cytotoxicity against various cells and microorganisms.

These host defense mechanisms are the product of activation of the complement system by one or both pathways (the classical and alternative pathways). Agents that initiate activation of the classical pathway or permit propagation of the alternative pathway are reviewed in Table 4–2. Activation leads to the sequential enzymatic cleavage of component proteins, with eventual formation of the membrane attack complex and subsequent cell death (Fig. 4–1). The molecular fragments that are generated possess significant biologic properties, as follows: C5a, C3a, and C4a interact with mast cells to release histamine; C5a is a potent chemotactic factor; C5a has enhancing activity on antibody synthesis; and C3a has suppressive action on antibody synthesis.

The clinical manifestations of various deficiency states attest to the importance of the complement system in host defense against infection and the importance of understanding the complement system in the practice of medicine. Defects in the complement system can be inherited or acquired and can involve either the classical or alternative complement pathways.

Hereditary Defects of the Complement System

Complete or almost complete deficiencies of each of the components of the classical pathway have been described as hereditary disorders (Ross and Densen, 1984; Guenther, 1983; Alper and Rosen, 1984; and Johnston, 1986) (Table 4–3). C2 deficiency has been re-

TABLE 4–1. Complement Components

Complement Proteins	Serum Concentration (μg/ml)	Molecular Weight (daltons)
CLASSICAL PATHWAY		
C1q	70	400,000
C1r	34	190,000
C̄1s	31	87,000
C4	600	206,000
C2	25	117,000
C3	1,200	185,000
ALTERNATIVE PATHWAY		
Properdin	25	224,000
Factor B	200	95,000
Factor D	1	25,000
MEMBRANE ATTACK COMPLEX		
C5	85	180,000
C6	75	128,000
C7	55	121,000
C8	55	153,000
C9	60	72,000
CONTROL PROTEINS		
C1 INA	180	105,000
C4bp	—	560,000
Factor H	500	150,000
Factor I	34	86,000
S protein	300	80,000

TABLE 4–2. Activators of Complement Pathways

Classical pathway

Immunoglobulins (IgM, IgG subclasses 1, 2, and 3)
Bacterial lipopolysaccharides
C-reactive protein
Proteases (plasmin)
Urate crystals
Polyanions (heparin)
Nephritic factor
Certain viruses

Alternative pathway

Polysaccharides
Bacterial or yeast cell walls
Viruses, fungi, and parasites
Tumor cells
Nephritic factor
X-ray contrast agents
Dialysis membranes
Erythrocytes from patients with paroxysmal nocturnal hemoglobinuria

ported in more than 100 individuals, whereas congenital deficiencies of the other components are less commonly reported. However, these reports have appeared only in recent years, and the true incidence of these defects remains to be determined.

THE COMPLEMENT SYSTEM

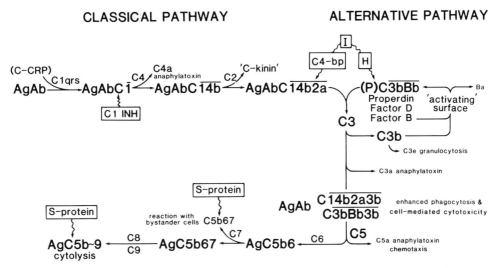

FIGURE 4–1. Sequence of activation of the components of the classical pathway of complement and interaction with the alternative pathway. Ag = antigen (bacterium, virus, tumor cell, or erythrocyte); Ab = antibody (IgG or IgM classes only); C-CRP = C carbohydrate–C reactive protein; C1 INH = C1 inhibitor; C3b INA = C3b inactivator; C4-bp = C4-binding protein. Regulator proteins are each enclosed in a box. (From Johnston, R.B., Jr.: Complement. *In* Nelson's Textbook of Pediatrics, 13th ed., Behrman, R.E., Vaughan, V.C., III, (eds.). Philadelphia, W.B. Saunders Co., 1987.)

TABLE 4–3. Genetic Deficiencies of Complement Components

Deficient Protein	APPARENT INHERITANCE	Associated Clinical Findings*	
		COLLAGEN-VASCULAR DISEASE	INFECTIONS
COMPONENT			
C1q	?	SLE, dermal vasculitis, MPGN, DLE	Recurrent bacterial, fungal; dermatitis, meningitis
C1q dysfunction	ACD	SLE	
C1r	ACD	CGN, SLE, dermal vasculitis	Pneumonia,[†] meningitis[†]
C1s	?	SLE	
C4	ACD	SLE, H-A purpura,[†] Sjögren syndrome[†]	Bacteremia,[†] meningitis[†]
C2	ACD	SLE, DLE, CGN, MPGN, H-S purpura, dermal vasculitis, dermatomyositis,[†] ITP[†]	Recurrent septicemia, especially pneumococcal; meningitis, pneumonia
C3	ACD	MPGN, SLE, dermal vasculitis	Severe, generalized bacterial
C5	ACD	SLE[†]	Disseminated gonococcal or meningococcal; pyoderma[†]; meningitis[†]
C5 (dysfunction)	?AD		Pyoderma, septicemia
C6	ACD	SLE,[†] DLE,[†] MPGN,[†] Sjögren syndrome[†]	Disseminated gonococcal or meningococcal
C7	ACD	SLE,[†] scleroderma,[†] ankylosing spondylitis,[†] RA	Disseminated gonococcal or meningococcal, or both
C8	ACD	SLE[†]	Disseminated gonococcal or meningococcal
C9	ACD		Meningococcal meningitis[†]
Factor D	?		Recurrent sinusitis, bronchitis; bronchiectasis
Factor B	ACD		
CONTROL PROTEINS			
Factor I	ACD		Severe pyogenic
Factor H	ACD		
Properdin	XLR		Meningococcal meningitis
C3b receptor (CR1)	ACD	SLE	

*Key: CGN = chronic glomerulonephritis; DLE = discoid lupus erythematosus; H-S = Henoch-Schönlein; ITP = idiopathic thrombocytopenic purpura; MPGN = membranoproliferative glomerulonephritis; RA = rheumatoid arthritis; SLE = systemic lupus erythematosus; XLR = X-linked recessive; ACD = autosomal codominant; AD = autosomal dominant; ? = mode of inheritance unproved in most.
[†]Finding reported uncommonly in patients with this deficiency.
Modified from Johnston, 1986, with permission of the publisher.

Deficiency of each C1 subcomponent has been described. C1q deficiency has been reported in association with collagen-vascular disorders, glomerulonephritis, recurrent infections, and as a partial deficiency with hypogammaglobulinemia and severe combined immunodeficiency disease. Restoration of C1q levels occurred in four patients with combined immunodeficiency following bone marrow transplantation for restoration of lymphocyte function (Ballow et al., 1973). Patients with nonfunctional C1q protein (C1q dysfunction) have had systemic lupus erythematosus (SLE). C1r deficiency has been reported in association with autoimmune diseases, including SLE, an SLE-like syndrome, and chronic nephritis. C1s deficiency has been described in association with low C1r levels and as an isolated defect. Some patients have been normal, and others have had an antinuclear antibody-positive lupus-like illness.

Among complement deficient patients, patients with C4 deficiency have the highest risk of developing SLE. Inheritance has conformed to an autosomal recessive pattern, with heterozygous family members having approximately half the normal C4 levels, a pattern referred to as autosomal codominant. This same inheritance pattern is seen with most of the complement proteins (see Table 4–3). In one individual, genetic studies showed that the C4 gene was located on chromosome 6, which also carries the genes that code for antigens of the major histocompatibility complex (MHC), factor B, and C2. Certain MHC antigens in this family were inherited with the C4 gene, indicating linkage between the C4 gene (MHC class III) and genes for histocompatibility antigens (MHC class I).

C2 deficiency is the most commonly reported hereditary complement deficiency. The first two cases described were in healthy immunologists (Alper and Rosen, 1984). Some patients have had increased incidences of autoimmune diseases, including anaphylactoid purpura, dermatomyositis, discoid lupus, SLE, inflammatory bowel disease, cold urticaria, common variable immunodeficiency, and glomerulonephritis (Ross and Densen, 1984). Heterozygous family members, who have half the normal C2 levels, may have an increased incidence of SLE or juvenile rheumatoid arthritis (JRA) (Glass et al., 1976). These patients are the exceptions to the general finding that patients heterozygous for a deficient complement protein are healthy. Half the normal level of a complement component in heterozygous individuals usually allows completely normal complement functions, as studied *in vitro*.

Some patients with homozygous C2 deficiency have had recurrent infections, including pneumococcal bacteremia (Newman et al., 1978). Freedom from infection in most patients with C2 deficiency is presumed to be due to a normally functioning alternative pathway. However, many C2 deficient patients have had approximately half the normal levels of factor B. Thus, the alternative pathway may not serve to fully protect these individuals from infections.

The reason for an association between complement deficiencies and autoimmune disease is unclear. Various (not mutually exclusive) explanations have been hypothesized, but they remain speculative. For example, there may be an increased incidence of clinically inapparent viral infections in complement deficient patients due to defective virus neutralization, with a resultant increased incidence of autoimmune disease. It also is possible that reduced systemic clearance of immune complexes, a process that requires complement, may predispose patients to development of autoimmune disease. Finally, immune response genes have been suggested as important in permitting autoimmune disease to occur. If the defective complement genes are closely linked to these immune response genes, there may be a linked genetic transmission of complement deficiencies and abnormal immune functions that predisposes an individual to autoimmune disease.

C3 is the major component responsible for effective enhancement of phagocytosis (opsonization) of infectious agents. Fixation of C3b to the microorganism through either the classical or the alternative pathway results in binding and subsequent ingestion of the microorganism. Since fixation of C3b is crucial for enhancement of phagocytosis of most bacteria, it is not surprising that patients with absent C3 have recurrent infections. Most of the individuals described with C3 deficiency have had severe recurrent infections with extracellular pyogenic bacteria, manifested as meningitis, pneumonia, or septicemia (Alper et al., 1972). The exceptional C3 deficient individuals who have not had serious infections have had symptoms of collagen-vascular disorders. The heterozygotes have not demonstrated abnormalities in handling infectious agents.

The absence of C5 was first described in two half sisters; one had SLE and superficial infections, and the other was healthy (Rosenfeld, 1976). Patients have been reported subsequently and have had predisposition to neisserial infections — gonococcal arthritis or meningococcal meningitis.

Several infants have been described with a syndrome similar to Leiner disease, including severe seborrheic dermatitis, diarrhea, and recurrent infections with gram-negative organisms and *Staphylococcus aureus* (Miller et al., 1968). Despite normal levels of C5 protein and normal hemolytic activity of the complement system in these patients, the C5 present in their sera appears to function abnormally. This finding is manifested as defective enhancement of phagocytosis of yeast and defective generation of chemotactic activity. Their clinical symptoms are improved with infusion of normal plasma. The structure of dysfunctional C5 appears to be normal, but its activity declines more rapidly on storage when compared with normal C5.

Patients with C6 deficiency also have had neisserial infections; some have had disseminated gonococcal infections, and others have had recurrent meningococcal meningitis or meningococcemia. Their sera lacked bactericidal activity against several bacteria, including *Neisseria.* However, opsonization of these same bacteria was normal. Preparing bacteria for effective phagocytosis is the most important function of the complement system in response to infection and undoubtedly protects against most organisms. Killing of organisms by the complement system is evidently not as important in bacterial defense. *Neisseria* may represent an important exception to this rule.

C7 deficiency has been reported in patients with autoimmune diseases (including SLE, scleroderma, ankylosing spondylitis, and JRA) or severe neisserial infections. Some individuals with C7 deficiency are reported to be healthy. C8 deficiency can be divided according to which of the two major subunits is missing (beta or alpha-gamma chain). Individuals with the C8 beta chain deficiency have been white and as a rule have neisserial infections, whereas those without the C8 alpha-gamma chain have been black or Hispanic and have disseminated gonococcal infections.

A familial pattern of C9 deficiency has been reported in several families who had no associated rheumatic disorders or increased susceptibility to infections. Serum from C9 deficient individuals is capable of immune hemolysis, albeit at a much slower rate. More recently, a previously healthy 17-year-old female with C9 deficiency developed meningococcal meningitis. Her hemolytic complement titer was less than half the lower limit of normal, which has been true of the other reported individuals with C9 deficiency (Ross and Densen, 1984).

Patients with genetically determined defects in the alternative pathway have been reported. Individuals with a deficiency of factor I (C3b/C4b inactivator) have experienced recurrent pyogenic infections, similar to individuals with a C3 deficiency (Alper et al., 1970; Ross and Densen, 1984). The function of factor I is to remove C3b attached to any surface. Without removal of C3b, the enzyme responsible for activating C3 through the alternative pathway, C3bBb, continues to destroy C3. This results in a deficiency of C3 and an extreme susceptibility to bacterial infections, including pneumonia, septicemia, and recurrent meningitis. Infusions of plasma or purified factor I can restore serum C3 levels and opsonization of bacteria.

An HLA-A11B27–linked partial deficiency of factor B has been described in six healthy individuals through three generations (Guenther, 1983). Identical twin sisters had a functional deficiency of factor D (Kluin-Nelemans, 1984). Both sisters had recurrent infections of the upper and lower respiratory tracts. Their serum hemolytic complement activity was normal, but alternative pathway activity ranged from 6 to 12 percent of normal. Three males in an extended family had a selected deficiency of properdin (Sjoholm, 1982). One died from meningococcal septicemia and meningitis. Further history disclosed three additional male relatives with similar fatal infections. In another family, factor H (beta 1H globulin) deficiency has been reported in two brothers ages 6 and 7 years (Thompson and Winterborn, 1981). The younger brother had hemolytic uremic syndrome at 8 months of age. His hemolytic complement titer was 13 μ/ml (normal, 25 to 45), his serum C3 level was 12 mg/dl (normal, 75 to 175), and his serum C4 level was normal. Factor H activity was 6 percent and 7 percent of normal in the two brothers; their parents had factor H activity of approximately 50 percent of normal. Miyakawa et al. (1981) found the C3b receptor missing on the erythrocytes in 37 of 56 patients with SLE; only 1 of 51 normal controls lacked the glycoprotein. Although there was no increased incidence of infections, the defect was persistent even during remission of their disease. Pedigree analysis disclosed an autosomal codominant mode of inheritance (Wilson et al., 1982).

Acquired Defects of the Complement System

Numerous disease states are associated with a partial decrease in one or more complement components (Table 4–4). C1 inactivator (C1 INA) deficiency, which results in hereditary angioedema, occurs on a genetic basis. An acquired deficiency of C1 INA has been described in several patients with lymphoproliferative diseases. Episodic angioedema was present in all.

The serum concentration of the early acting components of the classical pathway (C1, C4, C2, and C3) frequently are decreased in SLE, as a consequence of activation of C1q by immune complexes. Treatment restores component levels to normal, and serum C3 concentrations serve as sensitive means of following the activity of the disease. An interesting SLE-like syndrome with recurrent urticaria, angioedema with laryngeal edema, and arthralgia, but with negative antinuclear antibody titers, has been described in several individuals. Unlike those with typical SLE, these individuals have had persistently decreased C1q and C3.

TABLE 4-4. Acquired Defects of the Complement System

Deficient Component	Underlying Mechanism	Associated Clinical Findings[*]
C4, C2	C1 INA deficiency	Lymphoproliferative diseases,
C1, C4, C2, C3	Immune complexes	SLE, leprosy, SBE, VJS, mononucleosis, dengue fever, hepatitis, AGN, dermatitis herpetiformis, celiac disease
C3	Decreased synthesis	Malnutrition
C3	Accelerated consumption	Burns, post-perfusion syndrome, nephritic factor (MPGN, SLE)
Any	None	Normal physiologic state of neonates
Alternative pathway function	Not known	Sickle cell anemia, beta thalassemia, splenectomy, hypogammaglobulinemia

[*]Key: SLE = systemic lupus erythematosus; SBE = subacute bacterial endocarditis; VJS = ventricular jugular shunt; AGN = acute glomerulonephritis; MPGN = membranoproliferative glomerulonephritis.

Adults with paroxysmal nocturnal hemoglobinuria lack a 70,000 mol wt protein on their erythrocyte membranes (Nicholson-Weller et al., 1985). This protein (decay accelerating factor, DAF) suppresses complement activation by inhibiting the assembly of the C3 convertase, C3bBb. Patients whose erythrocytes lack DAF suffer bouts of hemolytic anemia, resulting from the effects of the uninhibited activation of the complement cascade and membrane lysis. This condition is acquired in adulthood for reasons that are not understood. Early erythrocyte precursors in the bone marrow express DAF activity and are resistant to complement-mediated lysis. During erythropoiesis this activity is lost, and erythrocytes become complement sensitive (Moore et al., 1985).

Hypocomplementemia involving the early reacting components has been described in cases of leprosy, subacute bacterial endocarditis, ventriculojugular shunts, malaria, infectious mononucleosis, dengue hemorrhagic fever, viral hepatitis, acute glomerulonephritis, dermatitis herpetiformis, and celiac disease. All of these disorders involve immune complexes, which activate the classical pathway, with the reduction in C1, C4, C2, and C3. Schwartz et al. (1982) reported 16 patients with hypocomplementemic urticarial vasculitis. All patients had decreased total complement activity, 15 had low levels of C4, and 12 had low levels of C3. Levels of other components (C1q, C2, and C3-C9) were measured in a few patients and were usually below normal limits. The mechanism of complement consumption is unknown. Both malnutrition and burns can result in hypocomplementemia, as reflected in low C3 levels. The mechanism is not known but may involve excessive loss or decreased synthesis.

Patients with membranoproliferative glomerulonephritis have long been known to have depressed levels of C3. These patients have been found to have a serum protein termed "C3 nephritic factor," which promotes the cleavage of C3 (Spitzer et al., 1969). The cleavage takes place through the alternative pathway; the alternative pathway C3-cleaving enzyme (C3bBb) is protected from inactivation by the C3 nephritic factor, which is an autoantibody to the C3bBb complex. An analagous classical pathway C3 nephritic factor, an autoantibody to the C42 enzyme, can occur in SLE. Two reports of transplacental transport of nephritic factor have appeared in which the infants had transient hypocomplementemia. Many patients with nephritic factor and hypocomplementemia also have partial lipodystrophy. These patients sometimes develop renal disease, and at least one patient had recurrent bacterial infections. The relationship of hypocomplementemia to glomerulonephritis is unclear. A recent hypothesis suggests that hypocomplementemia predisposes the patient to increased infections, which result in glomerulonephritis.

Abnormal opsonization of pneumococci, described in sickle cell anemia, appears to involve the alternative pathway. Other assays of alternative pathway activity also have been abnormal in some patients with sickle cell disease (Johnston et al., 1973), apparently because of low grade activation and consumption of complement (Chudwin et al., 1985). Such a defect may help explain these patients' known susceptibility to pneumococcal disease.

Neonates have long been noted to have increased susceptibility to infections. Along with other defects in their immune system, cord blood levels of C3, factor B, and early components of the classical pathway are reduced to about two thirds of adult levels.

Adverse reactions to radiocontrast agents have been shown to be mediated through the alternative pathway. The dyes directly activate C3 and C5 through the alternative pathway, resulting in production of the anaphylatoxins C3a and C5a. Binding of these peptides to mast cells results in degranulation and symptoms of anaphylaxis in susceptible individuals.

When to Suspect Defects in the Complement System

Defects in the complement system should be suspected in several clinical situations.

Autoimmune diseases, such as SLE, anaphylactoid purpura, dermatomyositis, chronic nephritis, and other vasculitis syndromes, are most suspicious, particularly if the clinical and laboratory findings are not completely typical. These diseases occur most frequently with congenital deficiencies of C1q, C1r, C1s, C4, C2, and C3. It is important to make the diagnosis of a complement deficiency since the prognosis, associated problems, and risk to other family members may differ from those of other patients.

Recurrent severe infections with extracellular pyogenic organisms occur with C3 or factor I deficiency. These infections resemble those in hypogammaglobulinemia. Meningitis and septicemia are particularly common. Recurrent pneumococcal septicemia should support the suspicion of C2 deficiency.

Recurrent gonococcal or meningococcal infections, even those beginning in adulthood, should raise the possibility of deficiency of a late-acting component (C5, C6, C7, C8, or C9) or of properdin.

Evaluation of Complement System

Whole Complement Titer (CH50). When there is a suspicion that a patient with "collagen disease" or recurrent infections has a complement deficiency, blood should be drawn for determination of the whole complement titer (CH50). The blood must be carefully handled by separating the serum from the clot and freezing the serum at $-70°C$ *within 1 hour.* The assay (available in most hospital laboratories) tests the capacity of serum to lyse antibody-coated sheep erythrocytes; this reaction requires all nine components of the classic pathway. The assay easily identifies all homozygous complement deficient patients, since the hemolytic capacity of their serum invariably is zero. Therefore, a normal CH50 eliminates the possibility of a deficiency of the classical pathway as a cause of recurrent infections. Once a patient is identified as having a zero CH50, family members also should be investigated. Heterozygous family members (with half the normal levels of the defective component) will have normal or slightly subnormal CH50. To pinpoint the exact component defect, the individual complement components in the patient's serum should be determined. Certain medical centers and some commercial laboratories can perform these determinations; serum should be prepared as for CH50 testing. Patient and family members also will require genetic counseling. It should be remembered that an individual heterozygous for C2 deficiency may have a clinical disease (JRA or SLE) and a normal CH50. The level of C2 in the serum must be measured to make this diagnosis.

Alternative Pathway Function. Patients with recurrent infections who have normal CH50s do not have abnormalities of the classical pathway of complement that can explain their problem. However, if a cause for the patient's infections cannot be found and the clinician remains suspicious, an abnormality of the alternative pathway should be considered. Determinations of alternative pathway function are not commercially available but can be performed at many medical centers.

Concentrations of Individual Components

As mentioned, complement abnormalities occur as secondary phenomena in many disease states. Determination of the individual component values listed in Table 4–1 may be of value in diagnosis of these diseases, as well as in pinpointing deficiencies. This can be done in many hospital laboratories using radial immunodiffusion. Low levels of the early components, C4, C2, and C3, may be due to activation by immune complexes; a low C3 level in a patient with chronic renal disease suggests membranoproliferative glomerulonephritis in association with a C3 nephritic factor.

PHAGOCYTE FUNCTION

Effective phagocytic function involves an orderly sequence of events, resulting in destruction of the invading microorganism. The initial step by the phagocytes is *adherence* to blood vessel walls adjacent to the site of invasion, followed by *chemotaxis*, which leads to contact with the organism. Upon contact, if the organism has been properly opsonized, *phagocytosis* occurs, moving the organism into the cell's interior. During ingestion, the phagocyte undergoes a burst of metabolic activity in which oxygen is consumed and reduced to toxic by-products required for killing most microorganisms. Simultaneously, intracellular granules fuse with the phagocytic vacuole as it forms, and intracellular *killing* begins. Any break in this sequence — adherence, chemotaxis, ingestion, and killing — impairs the host's ability to resist infection.

Defects of Adherence

Neutrophils that lack critical surface glycoproteins fail to spread on glass or plastic surfaces, move poorly in response to a chemotactic gradient, and demonstrate minimal phagocytosis of particles opsonized with antibody and complement (Anderson et al., 1985). The absent major surface membrane glycoproteins (gp) share a common beta chain of approximately 95,000 daltons. The best studied of these is the gp termed Mo1, which serves as the receptor for cleaved C3b (i.e., C3bi). Affected individuals have delayed separation of the umbilical cord, recurrent infections of the skin and respiratory tract, severe periodontal disease, and diminished migration of cells into areas of inflammation. The mode of inheritance appears to be autosomal recessive, with parents having lower levels of the Mo1 glycoprotein but normally functioning neutrophils.

Primary Cellular Defects of Chemotaxis

Several defects of chemotaxis result from primary abnormalities of the phagocyte itself (Table 4–5). The *Chédiak-Higashi syndrome* (CHS) is a genetically determined, probably autosomal recessive, disease characterized by recurrent infections; partial loss of pigment of the

skin, iris, and retina; photophobia; nystagmus; and giant granules in most granule-containing cells (Blume and Wolff, 1972). Most patients develop a "malignant phase," with a lymphoma-like illness consisting of pancytopenia, lymphadenopathy, and hepatosplenomegaly. The majority of patients die of infection or hemorrhage in childhood. An analogous syndrome occurs in several animal species.

The loss of pigmentation ("partial albinism") is among the most constant features of the disease and may be present at birth. The depigmentation may be subtle and appears only as a silver hue of the hair. Melanin is not lost but is aggregated in large granules rather than distributed homogeneously in the cell. Abnormally

TABLE 4–5. Defects of Chemotaxis[*]

Primary cellular abnormalities

Plasma membrane glycoprotein deficiency
Chédiak-Higashi syndrome
Increased microtubule assembly and elevated GMP
Kartagener syndrome
Glycogenesis type Ib
Specific granule deficiency
Lazy leukocyte syndrome

Secondary cellular abnormalities

Burns
The neonatal state
Hyperimmunoglobulinemia E syndrome
Diabetes mellitus
Acrodermatitis enteropathica
Hypophosphatemia
Ethanol intoxication
Influenza A viral infection
Artificial blood substitutes
Periodontal disease
Rheumatoid arthritis
Mannosidosis
Down syndrome
Cancer
Malnutrition
Therapy with corticosteroids or immunosuppressive agents
Bone marrow transplantation

Humoral deficiencies

Abnormality of chemotactic factor production (C3 or C5 deficiency)
Absence of antagonist of chemotaxis inhibitor

Humoral inhibitors

Chemotactic factor inhibitors; cancer, cirrhosis, sarcoidosis, leprosy, chronic granulomatous disease
Elevated IgA level
Circulating chemotactic factors; Wiskott-Aldrich syndrome, nephritis

[*]From Forehand and Johnston, 1985.

large granules are present in many other cells, including all neutrophils, eosinophils, and basophils, and a variable number of lymphocytes, but the granules do not appear in platelets or erythrocytes. Recognition of depigmentation and abnormal granules in patients with frequent infections leads to the diagnosis.

Information on infections associated with the defect is scant. However, in four carefully studied patients, 29 pyogenic infections were documented. *Staphylococcus aureus*, group A beta-hemolytic streptococci, and *Haemophilus influenzae* organisms were the most common pathogens. Sites of infection included the lungs, skin, subcutaneous tissue, and upper respiratory tract (along with otitis media and sinusitis). All infections responded appropriately to antibiotics.

The predisposition to recurrent bacterial infections is, at least in part, the result of multiple phagocytic defects. Neutropenia may be profound. The granulocytes have impaired chemotactic ability and move sluggishly to the site of infection. Characteristically, peripheral leukocytosis fails to occur even with severe infections. Once granulocytes are at the site of infection, ingestion of the organisms appears normal. Degranulation of lysosomes into the phagocytic vacuole is impaired, however. The levels of lysosomal enzymes are normal, as is phagocytosis-associated oxidative metabolism. There is a mild defect in phagocytic killing of bacteria, similar to the defect found in carriers of chronic granulomatous disease (CGD), who rarely have increased infections. This bactericidal defect most likely results from the slow release of lysosomal enzymes into the phagocytic vacuoles containing bacteria. Recurrent infections appear to be due to the neutropenia and the chemotactic defect.

Recent evidence indicates that the impaired chemotaxis and degranulation of leukocytes in CHS may be due to a defect in function of cellular microtubules. The function of microtubules, which serve as a cell skeleton, is regulated by the cyclic nucleotides cAMP and cGMP. The *in vitro* addition of cGMP, or of cholinergic agents that increase cGMP, to leukocytes from CHS patients improves chemotaxis, degranulation, and bactericidal activity of the cells. Oral administration of ascorbate — known to increase intracellular cGMP levels — resulted in normalization of *in vitro* chemotaxis, degranulation, and bactericidal activity, and in freedom from infection for a year in one patient. The neutro-

penia and abnormal granules were unchanged, however (Boxer et al., 1976).

The *congenital absence of neutrophil specific granules* is associated with diminished *in vitro* chemotaxis and recurrent pyogenic infections. Three possible explanations for the chemotactic defect have been proposed, as follows: (1) a deficiency of lactoferrin (LF), a principal constituent of specific granules that is capable of inducing adherence (Boxer et al., 1982); (2) an inability of the cell to replenish its chemotactic factor receptors, which may be derived from specific granule membrane (Gallin and Seligmann, 1984); and (3) an absence of the membrane glycoprotein Mo1 whose alpha chain is translocated from the specific granule to the plasma membrane during neutrophil stimulation (Todd et al., 1984).

The *lazy leukocyte syndrome* involves the combination of severe neutropenia with normal numbers and types of cells in the marrow, abnormal neutrophil chemotaxis into "skin windows," and defective neutrophil chemotaxis *in vitro* (Miller et al., 1971). The clinical findings consist of recurrent gingivitis, stomatitis, otitis media, furunculosis, and pneumonia. Phagocytosis and bactericidal activity are normal. The ability of neutrophils to deform in order to squeeze through narrow spaces is decreased, which is a possible explanation for the functional abnormalities. Other syndromes of defective chemotaxis, some of which are familial, have been reported (see Table 4–5) (Gallin, 1981; Forehand and Johnston, 1985).

Secondary Cellular Defects of Chemotaxis

Another group of chemotactic disorders consists of conditions in which the cellular abnormality results from a primary underlying disease state.

A number of patients have been reported who have shown decreased neutrophil chemotaxis and hyperimmunoglobulinemia E (HIE) in association with a variety of clinical syndromes and increased susceptibility to infection. These patients include several with mucocutaneous candidiasis. A combination of chronic dermatitis, usually eczematous, and recurrent staphylococcal abscesses has been associated with elevated IgE level and depressed chemotaxis (Hill and Quie, 1974). These patients include those with Job syndrome. The same syndrome with ichthyosis rather than eczema has been described. Several patients have had urticaria or allergic rhinitis. Other infections have included furunculosis, cellulitis, pneumonia, empyema, otitis media, and occasionally a deep abscess or septicemia. *S. aureus* has been the most common pathogen. Some patients have had this clinical syndrome with HIE and defective cell mediated immunity but transient or no defects in chemotaxis (Buckley et al., 1972). The chemotactic defect in any of these HIE syndromes may not be persistent. In addition, patients with atopic dermatitis without elevated IgE levels have been reported to have chemotactic defects.

In these syndromes it is unlikely that the defect in chemotaxis is directly due to the hyperimmunoglobulinemia E. Donabedian (1985) and Chikazawa and coworkers (1984) have identified inhibitors of neutrophil chemotaxis produced by mononuclear cells from patients with HIE. As a second possibility, histamine release from IgE-coated basophils could be responsible. Histamine inhibits chemotaxis of normal neutrophils *in vitro*, perhaps because it elevates intracellular cAMP. Treatment of some of these patients' neutrophils with the blocker of the H_2 histamine receptor, burimamide, produced significant improvement in chemotaxis.

Patients with diabetes mellitus have been reported to have abnormal chemotaxis and ingestion. The chemotactic defect can be corrected *in vitro* by the addition of insulin (Mowat and Baum, 1971; and Hill et al., 1974). Insulin deficiency theoretically could result in defective neutrophil function through potassium or glucose deficiency. The significance of the relationship between phagocyte dysfunction and infection in diabetes is unclear.

Chemotactic Defects Attributable to Humoral Abnormality

Defective chemotaxis can be due to an abnormality of plasma either from a deficiency of factors necessary for the process to occur or from inhibitory activity (see Table 4–5). Direct inhibitors of chemotactic factors have been found in the sera of patients with a variety of chronic inflammatory disorders. Similar inhibitors are present in normal sera but at much lower levels. Thus, chronic inflammation may stimulate increased production of what may be a normal control mechanism.

Defects of Ingestion

Defects of ingestion by neutrophils also result in recurrent infections (Table 4–6); these have been reviewed elsewhere in detail (Stossel, 1978; Horowitz, 1982). A striking abnormality in ingestion occurs when serum opsonization is defective owing to reduced concentrations of antibody or C3. Neutropenia is a well known cause of recurrent infections (Howard et al., 1977). Since the extent of phagocytosis is decreased, the basic defect might be considered one of ingestion. *S. aureus* is the most common pathogen involved, but *Pseudomonas* organisms and *Escherichia coli* are involved almost as frequently. The most common types of infections are pneumonitis, otitis media, and abscesses. Neither meningitis nor serious viral or fungal infections have been reported in patients with isolated neutropenia.

Splenic hypofunction, whether due to congenital asplenia, surgical removal of the spleen, or the sludging of erythrocytes in sickle cell disease, can be considered a defect of ingestion, since a large mass of phagocytic cells is actually or functionally absent. The clinical picture contrasts with that of neutropenia in that superficial infections are rare, since neutrophil function at the periphery is normal. However, septicemia and meningitis are relatively common, since blood stream filtering by splenic macrophages does not occur. Pyogenic bacteria, especially the pneumococci, are the usual infecting organisms (Singer, 1973).

TABLE 4–6. Defects of Ingestion*

Deficit opsonization
  Antibody deficiency
  C3 deficiency

Neutropenia

Hyposplenia

Primary cellular abnormality
  Membrane glycoprotein (Mo1) deficiency

Secondary cellular abnormalities
  Hypophosphatemia
  Diabetes mellitus
  Viral infection
  Corticosteroid therapy
  Galactosemia
  Circulating immune complexes
  Macrophage "blockade" (e.g., with damaged erythrocytes)

---

*From Forehand and Johnston, 1985.

Intrinsic cellular abnormalities also can result in ingestion abnormalities. Deficiency of Mo1 leads to a defect in phagocytosis of C3-opsonized particles. Incubation of normal neutrophils with monoclonal antibodies directed against the Mo1 antigen (C3bi receptor) mimics the abnormalities of Mo1 deficient cells (Arnaout et al., 1983; Dana et al., 1984).

Defects of Microbicidal Activity

Killing of the intracellular organisms after normal chemotaxis and ingestion is the final step in phagocytic function. Defects in the microbicidal activity can have profound effects on health. Defects of microbicidal activity are listed in Table 4–7 and reviewed in Babior (1978), Johnston (1980), and Forehand and Johnston (1985).

The term chronic granulomatous disease (CGD) has been applied to a syndrome of recurrent purulent infections of the skin, lymph nodes, liver, and lungs, associated with an inability of phagocytes to kill fungi and bacteria that do not produce hydrogen peroxide (H_2O_2). Recent evidence suggests that the syndrome can be caused by various molecular defects (Tauber et al., 1983; Forehand and Johnston, 1985).

X-linked and autosomal recessive modes of inheritance of CGD have been demonstrated. The existence of different "varieties" of CGD in addition to those represented by different modes of inheritance seems likely.

The most characteristic clinical abnormalities reflect the involvement of the reticuloendothelial system. Lymphadenopathy has been described in all but a few infants and children with a milder form of the disease. Hepatomegaly,

TABLE 4–7. Defects of Microbicidal Activity[*]

Chronic granulomatous disease
G-6-PD deficiency
Myeloperoxidase deficiency
Alkaline phosphatase deficiency
Pyruvate kinase deficiency
Malakoplakia
Granule defects
   Chédiak-Higashi syndrome
   Absence of specific granules
   Myelogenous or histiocytic leukemia
Felty syndrome
Leukemia
Viral infections

[*]From Forehand and Johnston, 1985.

splenomegaly, and hepatic or perihepatic abscesses are common. All of these findings reflect the accumulation of bacteria or fungi by phagocytic cells that cannot kill them (Johnston and Newman, 1977). The second major group of signs reflects the inability of circulating phagocytes to kill invading bacteria at the site of penetration. These include pneumonitis, subcutaneous abscesses, furunculosis, osteomyelitis, perianal abscess, conjunctivitis, and ulcerative stomatitis. These serious infections are generally localized, but septicemia or meningitis may occur if defenses are overwhelmed. Other features, which are less easily explained, include eczematoid or seborrheic dermatitis, often present on eyelids, external nares, or around the mouth; persistent diarrhea; and rhinitis.

The majority of patients manifest the disease in the first year of life—some in the first week. Many children die before the age of 10 years. With milder forms of disease, survival of some patients into the sixth decade has been reported. Pulmonary disease has been the cause of death in the majority, although septicema and meningitis have been lethal in several patients.

Staphylococci and enteric bacteria are the predominant infecting organisms. *Aspergillus* and *Candida* also have been common pathogens. *Salmonella* is the most common cause of septicemia or meningitis. The rarity of *H. influenzae*, pneumococci, and streptococci correlates with the ability of CGD phagocytes to kill these catalase-negative, peroxide-producing organisms *in vitro*. Tuberculosis and disseminated BCG infection have occurred.

Cells from patients with CGD do not undergo the normal phagocytosis associated increase in oxygen consumption and conversion to microbicidal metabolites, including superoxide anion and H_2O_2. Presumably, the basic molecular defect of CGD is deficient activity of an enzyme (or enzyme system) responsible for conversion of oxygen to bactericidal species.

Deficiency of glucose-6-phosphate dehydrogenase (G-6-PD) involving leukocytes as well as erythrocytes could be considered a variant of CGD; at least it represents the first enzyme defect shown clearly to cause the CGD syndrome. When G-6-PD levels are less than 1 percent of normal, the patient suffers a clinical syndrome that mimics CGD but is milder (Baehner, 1972).

In *primary myeloperoxidase (MPO) deficiency*, peroxidase activity is absent in both neutrophils and monocytes but normal in erythrocytes.

MPO deficiency is the most common abnormality of the neutrophil with an associated dysfunction. Both partial and complete MPO deficiency have been described with an estimated incidence of one in 2100. The routine use of MPO staining to perform blood leukocyte differential counts has revealed that partial deficiency occurs commonly in otherwise apparently normal individuals. Patients are generally not abnormally susceptible to disease (Kitahara et al., 1981; Parry et al., 1981; Larrocha et al., 1982). However, one patient with disseminated candidiasis and one with fatal candidal pneumonia, and both with diabetes mellitus, have been reported. MPO deficiency also may occur as a secondary phenomenon in association with leukemia, anemia, psoriasis, and neuronal storage disease. Functionally, the MPO deficient leukocytes have impaired microbicidal activity that is not as severe as that in CGD. Microbicidal mechanisms independent of MPO appear to protect effectively against infections.

Impaired bactericidal activity has been associated in a few instances with an abnormality of neutrophil granules. Bactericidal defects also have been reported in Felty syndrome, leukocyte alkaline phosphatase deficiency, neutrophil pyruvate kinase deficiency, and leukemia (see Table 4–7). The biochemical basis for the killing defects associated with these disorders is not known.

When to Suspect a Defect of Phagocyte Function

Infections in patients with defects of chemotaxis characteristically occur at the interface between the host's and microbe's worlds, where a small inoculum can become significant if the neutrophil response is delayed or absent. Thus, patients should be investigated for abnormalities of chemotaxis if recurrent infections of the skin, subcutaneous tissue, or respiratory tract are present. Recurrent furunculosis, subcutaneous abscesses, sinusitis, otitis media, and pneumonia are the most common clinical manifestations, with deep abscesses or septicemia being unusual (Johnston, 1984). Particular attention should be given to patients who exhibit these infections and have hyperimmunoglobulinemia E, eczema, or elevated IgA levels.

Neutropenia predisposes patients to a pattern of infections similar to that seen with chemotactic defects. Patients with overwhelming septicemia, especially with the pneumococcus, may have actual asplenia or functional asplenia (e.g., the asplenia in sickle cell disease).

Marked lymphadenopathy with suppuration, dermatitis, hepatic abscesses, perianal abscesses, and recurrent pneumonia suggests an ability of phagocytes to ingest but not to kill microorganisms. The prototypic disorder with these clinical findings is chronic granulomatous disease. The other defects of microbicidal activity, e.g., glucose-6-phosphate dehydrogenase deficiency, have a similar clinical pattern, but infections are less severe.

Evaluation of Phagocyte Function

When the history and physical examination suggest a disorder of phagocyte function, evaluation should begin with total and differential leukocyte counts, hematocrit values, and red and white blood cell morphology (Hill, 1980; Bloch and Salvaggio, 1982; Johnson et al., 1984; and Johnston, 1984). Neutropenia and Chédiak-Higashi syndrome, in which granulocytes and monocytes contain abnormal granules, can be diagnosed by these simple procedures. The presence of abnormal erythrocyte morphology or Howell-Jolly bodies in erythrocytes suggests the presence of splenic hypofunction. A sickle cell preparation should be ordered for patients with anemia and recurrent pneumococcal infections.

A Rebuck skin window test provides a screening test for chemotactic disorders that can be performed in the physician's office (Rebuck and Crowley, 1955). A patient suspected of having a defect in chemotaxis should be referred to a facility where chemotaxis can be evaluated in a standardized *in vitro* assay.

A patient suspected of a disorder of microbicidal activity should be tested; a nitroblue tetrazolium (NBT) test should be performed on the leukocytes (Johnston et al., 1985). This test is available at many hospitals and serves as an effective screening test for chronic granulomatous disease and G-6-PD deficiency. A normal reaction requires the neutrophils to reduce oxygen to superoxide anion and other microbicidal products. Testing for MPO is done in hematology-oncology laboratories as a means of differentiating certain leukemias, and this is a suitable screening test for MPO deficiency.

If results of any screening procedures are abnormal, further studies to define the defects, e.g., phagocytic killing, chemotaxis, and ingestion, should be performed at immunology centers where the required laboratory procedures are available. In most cases, curative therapy is not available, but supportive therapy can be effective in reducing the frequency of infections. Since these disorders are often inherited, genetic counseling is important.

REFERENCES

Alper, C.A., Abramson, N., Johnston, R.B., Jr., Jandl, J.H., Rosen, F.S.: Increased susceptibility to infection associated with abnormalities of complement-mediated functions and of the third component of complement (C3). N. Engl. J. Med. 292:349–354, 1970.

Alper, C.A., Colten, H.R., Rosen, F.S., Rabson, A.R., Macnab, G.M., Gear, J.S.S.: Homozygous deficiency of C3 in a patient with repeated infection. Lancet 2:1179-1181, 1972.

Alper, C.A., Rosen, F.S.: Inherited deficiencies of complement proteins in man. Springer Semin. Immunopathol. 7:251-261, 1984.

Anderson, D.C., Schmalsteig, F.C., Finegold, M.J., Hughes, B.J., Rothlein, P., Miller, L.J., Kohl, S., Tosi, M.F., Jacobs, R.L., Waldrop, T.C., Goldman, A.S., Shearer, W.T., Springer, T.A.: The severe and moderate phenotypes of heritable Mac-1, LFA-1, deficiency: Their quantitative definition and relation to leukocyte dysfunction and clinical features. J. Inf. Dis. 152:668–689, 1985.

Arnaout, M.A., Todd, R.F. III., Dana, N., Melamed, J., Schlossman, S.F., Colten, H.R.: Inhibition of phagocytosis of complement C3- or immunoglobulin G-coated particles and C3bi binding by monoclonal antibodies to a monocyte granulocyte membrane glycoprotein (Mol). J. Clin. Invest. 72:171–179, 1983.

Babior, B.M.: Oxygen-dependent microbial killing by phagocytes. N. Engl. J. Med. 298:659–668, 721–725, 1978.

Baehner, R.L., Johnston, R.B., Jr., Nathan, D.G.: Comparative study of the metabolic and bactericidal characteristics of severely glucose-6-phosphate dehydrogenase deficient polymorphonuclear leukocytes and leukocytes from children with chronic granulomatous disease. J. Reticuloendotheliol. Soc. 12:150–169, 1972.

Ballow, M., Day, N.K., Biggar, W.D., Park, B.H., Yount, W.J., Good, R.A.: Reconstitution of C1q after bone marrow transplantation in patients with severe combined immunodeficiency. Clin. Immunol. Immunopathol. 2:28–35, 1973.

Bloch, K.J., Salvaggio, J.E.: Use and interpretation of diagnostic immunologic laboratory tests. J.A.M.A. 248:1734–1758, 1982.

Blume, R.S., Wolff, S.M.: The Chédiak-Higashi syndrome: Studies in four patients and a review of the literature. Medicine 51:247–280, 1972.

Boxer, L.A., Haak, R.A., Yang, H., Wolach, J.B., Whitcomb, J.A., Butterick, C.J., Baehner, R.L.: Membrane-bound lactoferrin alters the surface properties of polymorphonuclear leukocytes. J. Clin. Invest. 70:1049–1057, 1982.

Boxer, L.A., Satanabe, A.M., Rister, M., Besch, H.R., Allen, J., Baehner, R.L.: Correction of leukocyte function in Chédiak-Higashi syndrome by ascorbate. N. Engl. J. Med. 295:1041–1045, 1976.

Buckley, R.H., Wray, B.B., Belmaker, E.Z.: Extreme hyper-

immunoglobulinemia E and undue susceptibility to infection. Pediatrics 49:59–70, 1972.

Chikazawa, S., Nunoi, H., Endo, F., Matsuda, I., Honda, M.: Hyperimmunoglobulin-E associated recurrent infection syndrome accompanied by chemotactic inhibition of polymorphonuclear leukocytes and monocytes. Pediatr. Res. 18:365–369, 1984.

Chudwin, D.S., Korenblit, A.D., Kingzette, M., Artrip, S., Rao, S.: Increased activation of the alternative complement pathway in sickle cell disease. Clin. Immunol. Immunopathol. 37:93–97, 1985.

Dana, N., Todd, R.F. III., Pitt, J., Springer, T.A., Arnaout, M.A.: Deficiency of a surface membrane glycoprotein (Mo1) in man. J. Clin. Invest. 73:153–159, 1984.

Donabedian, H.: Human mononuclear cells exposed to staphylococci rapidly produce an inhibitor of neutrophil chemotaxis. J. Inf. Dis. 152:24–32, 1985.

Forehand, J.R., Johnston, R.B., Jr.: Phagocytic defects. Clin. Immunol. Allerg. 5:351–369, 1985.

Gallin, J.I.: Abnormal phagocyte chemotaxis: Pathophysiology, clinical manifestations and management of patients. Rev. Inf. Dis. 3:1196–1220, 1981.

Gallin, J.L., Seligmann, B.E.: Mobilization and adaptation of human neutrophil chemoattractant fMet-Leu-Phe receptors. Fed. Proc. 43:2732–2736, 1984.

Glass, D., Gibson, D.J., Carpenter, C.B., Schur, P.H.: Hereditary C2 deficiency: HLA gene complex associations with recombinant events. J. Immunol. 116:1065–1070, 1976.

Guenther, L.C.: Inherited disorders of complement. J. Am. Acad. Dermatol. 9:815–839, 1983.

Hill, H.R.: Laboratory aspects of immune deficiency in children. Pediatr. Clin. N. Am. 27:805–830, 1980.

Hill, H.R., Quie, P.G.: Raised serum IgE levels and defective neutrophil chemotaxis in three children with eczema and recurrent bacterial infections. Lancet 1:183–187, 1974.

Hill, H.R., Sauls, H.S., Dettloff, J.L., Quie, P.G.: Impaired leukotactic responsiveness in patients with juvenile diabetes mellitus. Clin. Immunol. Immunopathol. 2:395–403, 1974.

Horowitz, M.A.: Phagocytosis of microorganisms. Rev. Inf. Dis. 4:104–135, 1982.

Howard, M.W., Strauss, R.G., Johnston, R.B., Jr.: Infections in patients with neutropenia. Am. J. Dis. Child. 131:788–790, 1977.

Johnson, C.M., Rhoades, K.H., Katzmann, J.A.: Neutrophil function tests. Mayo Clin. Proc. 59:431–433, 1984.

Johnston, R.B., Jr.: Biochemical defects of polymorphonuclear and mononuclear phagocytes associated with disease. In The Reticuloendothelial System, Sbarra, S.I., Strauss, R. (eds.), Plenum Publishing Corp., New York, 1980.

Johnston, R.B., Jr.: Recurrent bacterial infections in children. N. Engl. J. Med. 319:1237–1243, 1984.

Johnston, R.B., Jr.: Complement. In Nelson Textbook of Pediatrics, 12th edition, Behrman, R.E., Vaughan, V.C. (eds.), W.B. Saunders Co., Philadelphia, 1986.

Johnston, R.B., Jr., Newman, S.L.: Chronic granulomatous disease. Pediatr. Clin. N. Am. 24:365–376, 1977.

Johnston, R.B., Jr., Newman, S.L., Struth, A.G.: An abnormality of the alternative pathway of complement activation in sickle cell disease. N. Engl. J. Med. 288:803–808, 1973.

Johnston, R.B., III., Harbeck, R.J., Johnston, R.B., Jr.: Recurrent severe infections in a girl with apparently variable expression of mosaicism for chronic granulomatous disease. J. Pediatr. 106:50–57, 1985.

Kitahara, M., Eyre, H.J., Simonian, Y., Atkin, C.L., Hasstedt, S.J.: Hereditary myeloperoxidase deficiency. Blood 57:888–893, 1981.

Kluin-Nelemans, H.C., van Velzen-Blad, H., vanHelden, H.P.T., Daha, M.R.: Functional deficiency of complement factor D in a monozygous twin. Clin. Exp. Immunol. 58:724–730, 1984.

Larrocha, C., de Castro, M.F., Fontan, G., Vilaria, A., Fernandez-Chacon, J.L., Jimenez, C.: Hereditary myeloperoxidase deficiency: Study of 12 cases. Scand. J. Haematol. 29:389–397, 1982.

Miller, M.E., Oski, F.A., Harris, M.B.: Lazy leukocyte syndrome: A new disorder of neutrophil function. Lancet 1:665–669, 1971.

Miller, M.E., Seals, J., Kaye, R., Levinsky, L.C.: A familial, plasma associated defect of phagocytosis: A new cause of recurrent bacterial infection. Lancet 2:60–63, 1968.

Miyakawa, Y., Yamoda, A., Kosaka, K., Tsuda, F., Kosugi, E., Mayumi, M.: Defective immune adherence (C3b) receptor on erythrocytes from patients with systemic lupus erythematosus. Lancet 2:493–497, 1981.

Moore, J.G., Frank, N.M., Muller-Eberhard, H.J., Young, N.S.: Decay-accelerating factor is present on paroxysmal nocturnal hemoglobinuria erythroid progenitors and lost during erythropoiesis *in vitro*. J. Exp. Med. 162:1182–1192, 1985.

Mowat, A.G., Baum, J.: Chemotaxis of polymorphonuclear leukocytes from patients with diabetes mellitus. N. Engl. J. Med. 284:621–627, 1971.

Muller-Eberhard, H.J., Miescher, P.A.: Complement. Springer-Verlag, Berlin, 1985.

Newman, S.L., Vogler, L.B., Feigin, R.D., Johnston, R.B., Jr.: Recurrent septicemia associated with congenital deficiency of C2 and partial deficiency of factor B and the alternative complement pathway. N. Engl. J. Med. 299:290–292, 1978.

Nicholson-Weller, A., Spicer, D.B., Austen, K.F.: Deficiency of the complement regulatory protein: "Decay-accelerating factor" on membranes of granulocytes, monocytes and platelets in paroxysmal nocturnal hemoglobinuria. N. Engl. J. Med. 312:1091–1096, 1985.

Parry, M.F., Root, R.K., Metcalf, J.A., et al.: Myeloperoxidase deficiency prevalence and clinical significance. Ann. Int. Med. 95:293–301, 1981.

Rebuck, J.W., Crowley, J.H.: A method of studying leukocyte functions *in vitro*. Ann. N.Y. Acad. Sci. 59:757–805, 1955.

Rosenfeld, S.I., Kelly, M.E., Leddy, J.P.: Hereditary deficiency of the fifth component of complement in man. J. Clin. Invest. 57:1626–1634, 1976.

Ross, S.C., Densen, P.: Complement deficiency states and infection. Medicine 63:243–273, 1984.

Schwartz, H.R., McDuffie, F.C., Black, L.E., Schroeter, A.L., Conn, D.L.: Hypocomplementemic urticarial vasculitis. Mayo Clin. Proc. 57:231–238, 1982.

Singer, D.B.: Postsplenectomy sepsis. Perspect. Pediatr. Pathol. 1:285–311, 1973.

Sjoholm, A.G., Bracenier, J.H., Szderstrom, C.: Properdin deficiency in a family with fulminant meningococcal infections. Clin. Exp. Immunol. 50:291–297, 1982.

Spitzer, R.E.: The complement system. Pediatr. Clin. N. Am. 24:341–364, 1977.

Spitzer, R.E., Vallota, E.H., Forristal, J., Sudora, E., Stitzel, A., Davis, N.C., West, C.D.: Serum C3 lytic system in patients with glomerulonephritis. Science 164:436–437, 1969.

Stossel, T.P.: How do phagocytes eat? Ann. Int. Med. 84:398–402, 1978.

Tauber, A.I., Borregaard, N., Simons, E., Wright, J.: Chronic granulomatous disease: A syndrome of phagocyte oxidase deficiencies. Medicine 62:286–309, 1983.

Thompson, R.A., Winterborn, M.H.: Hypocomplementemia due to a genetic deficiency of beta 1H globulin. Clin. Exp. Immunol. 46:110–119, 1981.

Todd, R.F. III., Armaout, M.A., Rosin, R.E., Crowley, C.A., Peters, W.A., Babior, B.M.: Subcellular localization of the large subunit of Mo1 (Mo1: formerly gp 110), a surface glycoprotein associated with neutrophil adhesion. J. Clin. Invest. 74: 1280–1290, 1984.

Wilson, J.G., Wong, W.W., Schur, P.H., Fearon, D.T.: Mode of inheritance of decreased C3b receptors on erythrocytes of patients with systemic lupus erythematosus. N. Engl. J. Med. 307:981–986, 1982.

5
Chemical Mediators of Inflammation
STEPHEN I. WASSERMAN, M.D.

An important increase in our understanding of the mediators of inflammation and the cells responsible for generating them has developed during the last decade. A number of new mediators have been identified and several have been characterized structurally, synthesized, and elucidated in regard to their functional properties. A previous unappreciated heterogeneity of cells that generate mediators has been demonstrated, and the growth, differentiation, and localization of these cells have been defined. These advances have permitted construction of cogent new theories of the roles of inflammatory mediators and cells in the genesis and expression of allergic disorders as well as in various phases of other non-IgE mediated disorders. It is the purpose of this chapter to delineate these advances and to provide a framework for the new concepts of the roles of mediators and cells in allergy.

MAST CELLS AND BASOPHILS

Characterization

Three different cells are known to possess both high affinity receptors for the Fc portion of IgE and the metachromatic granules that contain histamine. Although basophils have long been differentiated from mast cells by morphology, site or origin, and tissue distribution, only recently has it been appreciated that two classes of mast cells exist (Metcalfe, 1983). These mast cell subtypes are most clearly recognized in rodents but are represented in humans as well. One, the "typical" or connective tissue type, is prominent in loose connective tissue, on serosal surfaces, and in skin. The other, the "atypical" or mucosal mast cell, is richly represented in gastrointestinal mucosa and perhaps in other mucosal and epithelial locations as well. The connective tissue mast cell is large, contains nu-

merous small (0.1 to 0.4 μ) granules, which stain intensely with metachromatic dyes owing to their content of heparin. The growth and development of this mast cell type is uncertain but does not appear to be regulated solely by T lymphocytes. The mucosal mast cell, as does its connective tissue counterpart, possesses a mononuclear nucleus and numerous small granules that, because they lack heparin at least in the rodent, stain less intensely with metachromatic dyes (Razin et al., 1982). Precursors for this mast cell type arise in the bone marrow and then populate various target tissues; they subsequently differentiate into mast cells under the influence of the T lymphocyte–derived lymphokine, interleukin-3 (Ihle et al., 1983).

Although typical connective tissue mast cells and atypical mucosal mast cells can be differentiated by microscopic and biochemical techniques, their relationship is unknown. It is possible that these are merely different forms of a single cell type expressed at different times in cell maturation, although current opinion favors the concept that these cells differ either in their progenitor cell or in specific growth and differentiation factors that lead to their final expression. These factors may be tissue specific.

Mast cells occur throughout the body, and they are especially prominent in the skin (Mikhail and Muller-Milinska, 1964), the upper and lower respiratory tract (Paterson et al., 1976), and the gastrointestinal tract mucosa (Enerbach, 1981). They also exist free in the bronchial lumen and in the loose connective tissue around small blood vessels and nerves. Mast cell numbers are increased in bone marrow in association with malignant disorders (Yoo et al., 1979), in the gut with inflammatory and parasitic diseases, and in the lung with asthma and fibrotic diseases.

Basophils arise in the bone marrow from precursors in the polymorphonuclear leukocyte series and are most closely related to eosinophilic polymorphonuclear leukocytes. Basophils, similar to mast cells, possess on their surfaces 50,000 to 100,000 receptors for the Fc portion of IgE. They have larger but fewer non-heparin containing metachromatic granules (Metcalfe, 1984). Basophil growth regulation has not been elucidated, but the production of basophils occurs normally only in the bone marrow. The cells generally are found only in the marrow or peripheral blood (0.1 to 2 percent) but can be identified in tissue in various inflammatory situations, most particularly in contact dermatitis (Dvorak and Dvorak, 1975).

Activation

Numerous agents have been demonstrated to induce mast cells and basophils to generate and secrete mediators. This process is noncytolytic and, in the case of IgE mediated signals, is due to cross linking of cell surface–bound IgE molecules. In addition to antigens recognized by cell surface–bound IgE, activators of mast cells include highly charged molecules; peptides, such as opiates, neurotensin, and substance P; ATP; divalent cation ionophores; anaphylatoxins C3a and C5a; and many drugs and complex carbohydrates. Even hyperosmolar solutions and physical stimuli can activate these cells (Wasserman, 1983). The mechanisms by which these processes induce activation are extraordinarily complex and include the following: (1) alterations in intracellular calcium concentrations, (2) changes in transmembrane calcium flux, (3) metabolism of phospholipids to generate inositol polyphosphates and diacylglycerol, (4) increases in cAMP, (5) utilization of several protein kinases, (6) phosphorylation of cellular proteins, (7) solubilization and swelling of granules, (8) fusion of granules with cell membranes, and (9) eventual liberation of granule contents. These processes essentially occur simultaneously, and their inter-relationships, sequence, and in fact true relevance to mediator generation and secretion remain to be fully elucidated.

Whatever the precise biochemical processes might be, their successful completion is accompanied by the release of the constituent amines, peptides, proteins, and proteoglycans of the granules and by the generation of purine nucleosides, prostanoids, and complex lipids. These generated and released materials have been termed mediators, as they possess a variety of biologic activities best categorized as vasoactive-spasmogenic, chemotactic, enzymatic, and structural proteoglycans.

MEDIATORS

Vasoactive-Spasmogenic Mediators (Table 5–1)

Histamine is the only preformed, granule associated mediator in this class. It is formed by the decarboxylation of histidine and is stored bound to the protein-proteoglycan backbone of mast cell and basophil granules (5 and 1 $\mu g/10^6$ cells, respectively). Histamine is released when granules are exposed to cations and circulates in blood at concentrations of 100 to 300 pg/ml (Dyer et al., 1982), which are maximal in the early morning (Barnes et al., 1980). Histamine and its metabolic products are excreted in large amounts in the urine primarily as imidazole acetic acid or methylated histamine. The biologic activities of histamine are a consequence of its interaction with H_1 and H_2 receptors (Black et al., 1972). H_1 receptors predominate in the skin and smooth muscle and are inhibited by classic antihistamines. H_2 receptors are found in the skin, the lungs, the stomach, and a variety of leukocytes, and are selectively inhibited by cimetidine and ranitidine. The biologic response to histamine reflects the ratio of these receptors activated by histamine in a given tissue. By its action upon H_1 receptors, histamine induces contraction of respiratory and intestinal musculature, enhances vascular permeability by means of endothelial disconnections, causes pulmonary vasoconstriction, and stimulates nasal mucus production. Indirect effects of the H_1 action of histamine also occur and are thought to be a consequence of its ability to induce production of prostaglandins (PGE_2, $PGF_2\alpha$, PGI_2, and thromboxane) from local tissue (Platshon and Kaliner, 1978). Conversely, relaxation of respiratory smooth muscle, increased airway mucus production, suppression of lymphocytotoxicity, and increased suppressor T cell function are mediated by histamine action on H_2 receptors. Together, H_1 and H_2 receptor activation are responsible for cutaneous vasodilation, cardiac irregularities, and pruritus (Marquardt, 1983).

Increases in blood levels of histamine occur in physical urticaria, asthma, anaphylaxis, and systemic mastocytosis. Such increases in histamine are small, and only recent improvements in technique have permitted accurate assessment of these small changes (Brown et al., 1982).

Platelet activating factor (PAF) is an unstored lipid, the structure of which is 1-O-alkyl-2-acetyl-sn-glyceryl-3-phosphorylcholine (Demopoulos et al., 1979). It is generated by human mast cells after IgE-dependent activation by the addition of an acetate group to the sn-2 position of the lyso-alkyl moiety. Degradation of PAF occurs by the action of acetyl hydrolase, which removes the acetate. This enzyme is very active

TABLE 5–1. Vasoactive-Spasmogenic Mediators

Mediator	Preformed or Generated	Function	Therapeutic Inhibitor	Human Disease Association
Histamine	Preformed	H_1: Contract smooth muscle Increase vascular permeability Generate prostaglandins Induce pulmonary vasoconstriction Increase nasal mucus production	Classic antihistamines	Asthma Anaphylaxis Urticaria Rhinitis
		H_2: Increase vascular permeability Increase gastric acid secretion Increase airway mucus production Stimulate suppressor lymphocytes Inhibit skin and basophil histamine release Cause bronchodilatation Induce idioventricular responses	Cimetidine Ranitidine	
		H_1 and H_2: Pruritus Induce vasodilatation Reduce threshold for ventricular fibrillation		
PAF	Generated	Aggregate and activate platelets and neutrophils Sequester platelets in tissue Induce vascular permeability Induce vasodepression Induce bronchoconstriction		
Arachidonic acid metabolites LTC_4, LTD_4, LTE_4 Slow reacting substance of anaphylaxis (SRS-A)	Generated	Constrict smooth muscle Increase vascular permeability Decrease peripheral blood flow Increase airway mucus production Induce cardiac depression Induce coronary vasoconstriction Inhibit lymphocyte response to mitogen	Glucocorticoids may prevent generation	Anaphylaxis ?Asthma Rhinitis
PGD_2	Generated	Contract smooth muscle Increase vascular permeability	Aspirin and nonsteroidal antiinflammatory agents block generation	Mastocytosis Rhinitis
Prostaglandin-generating factor	?Preformed	Induce production of prostaglandins		
Adenosine	Generated	Augment mast cell degranulation Contract asthmatic airways Increase airway mucus Induce coronary vasodilation	Methylxanthines	Asthma

in human plasma (Farr et al., 1983). In addition, removal of the polar head group by phospholipase C or D can occur. Whenever the parent compound is altered, biologic activity is lost.

Initially PAF was identified as a molecule capable of aggregating and degranulating platelets after IgE mediated, basophil-dependent reactions, and it is the most potent compound known in causing aggregation of human platelets (Mc Manus et al., 1980). PAF also causes a wheal and flare permeability response (Pinkard et al., 1980) that can be associated with local leukocyte infiltration (Humphrey et al., 1982). It directly contracts pulmonary and intestinal musculature and induces vasoconstriction. PAF is a marked hypotensive agent capable of causing cardiovascular collapse and death; it may alter coronary blood flow and lead to cardiac dysrhythmia (Halonen et al., 1980). PAF also can cause pulmonary artery hypertension, pulmonary edema, rapid shallow breathing, increase in total pulmonary resistance, and decrease in dynamic compliance. The factor causes rapid sequestration of platelets in the lung accompanied by release of platelet factor 4 and thromboxane. Of these PAF mediated responses, only the changes in pulmonary resistance and compliance are platelet dependent (Halonen et al., 1981).

Several mediators in this class are *products of arachidonic acid metabolism.* Arachidonic acid is a 20-carbon fatty acid with four double bonds present in all mammalian cells, as one of the fatty acid constituents of membrane phospholipids. It is liberated from membrane phospholipids in activated cells by the action of phospholipase A_2 or by the concerted action of phospholipase C and diacylglycerol lipase. The metabolic fate of liberated arachidonic acid is quite varied. At least 20 potential end products can be generated from this substrate, but no one cell type generates them all. Two enzymes, lipoxygenase and cyclooxygenase, regulate the pattern of metabolites generated from arachidonic acid. Mast cells generate a restricted pattern of arachidonic acid metabolites, representing products of each of these enzymes.

Human mast cells preferentially generate prostaglandin D_2 along with lesser amounts of thromboxane (Lewis et al., 1982), as products of cyclo-oxygenase action. Connective tissue mast cells of rodents also generate PGD_2 in large amounts, whereas mucosal-type mast cells generate only small quantities of this metabolite. Generation of PGD_2 by mast cells can be inhibited by agents that can inhibit cyclo-oxygenase, including aspirin and other nonsteroidal anti-inflammatory drugs as well as dapsone (Ruzicka et al., 1983). PGD_2 is a potent inducer of wheal and flare responses, which are more persistent than those caused by histamine and which may be accompanied by perivascular neutrophil accumulation (Flower et al., 1976). This prostaglandin is thought to be responsible for attacks of flushing and hypotension seen in some patients with mastocytosis (Roberts et al., 1980). In addition, PGD_2 is a potent bronchoconstrictive agent.

An indirect pathway for mast cell dependent generation of prostaglandins also has been identified. Both a peptide, termed prostaglandin generating factor, and histamine are capable of inducing generation of a diverse group of prostaglandins, including $PGF_2\alpha$, PGE_2, and thromboxane (Steel and Kaliner, 1981).

The substitution of hydroperoxy groups to arachidonic acid is catalyzed by a family of enzymes termed lipoxygenases. Each lipoxygenase adds the hydroperoxy group to a specific position on the arachidonic acid molecule; in the mast cell, it is the 5-lipoxygenase enzyme that is most active. The action of this enzyme produces an unstable intermediate, 5-HPETE (hydroperoxy-eicosatetraenoic acid), which can be further metabolized to 5-HETE (hydroxy-eicosatetraenoic acid) or, as in the mast cell, to leukotriene A. This last product is then further metabolized by the addition of the tripeptide glutathione (cys-gly-glu) to generate the sulfidopeptide leukotriene C_4 (LTCA) (Samuelsson et al., 1979 and 1980). Removal of the terminal glutamic acid generates LTD_4, and removal of the glycine residue from LTD_4 generates LTE_4. These three products *(LTC_4, LTD_4, and LTE_4)* compose what was once termed the slow reacting substance of anaphylaxis.

IgE mediated activation of human mast cells leads to generation of substantial quantities of LTC_4 (MacGlashan et al., 1982). Rodent mucosal but not connective tissue mast cells also generate large amounts of this leukotriene (Razin et al., 1982). The sulfidopeptide leukotrienes are potent inducers of wheal and flare responses accompanied by local discomfort (Sotor et al., 1983). They also induce constriction of gastrointestinal and respiratory smooth muscle, induce hypotension directly and through cardiodepression, and may inhibit lymphocyte function. In most systems, LTD_4 is most potent and LTE_4 is least active (Lewis and Austen, 1981).

The action of leukotrienes is mediated through action on specific receptors for each, and binding appears to depend on both sulfidopeptide and hydrophobic portions of the molecule. Degradation of these molecules occurs via transformation of the peptide portion (LTC_4 to LTE_4) and oxidation. This latter reaction can proceed by specific enzymes or by the action of H_2O_2, hypochlorous acid, and other oxygen radicals (Henderson and Klebanoff, 1983).

Activation of mast cells consumes ATP and thereby generates *adenosine.* This purine nucleoside is released parallel with histamine from activated mast cells (Marquardt et al., 1984). Upon its release, adenosine is metabolized via adenosine deaminase to inosine and hypoxanthine or may be taken up into cells and phosphorylated to AMP. Circulating levels of adenosine approximate 0.3 μM (Mills et al., 1976) and may rise ten-fold upon induction of asthma or hypoxia (Mentzer et al., 1975). Adenosine is a potent vasodilator and causes bronchoconstriction in asthmatics but not in healthy subjects (Holgate et al., 1984). Adenosine is unique in its ability to enhance mast cell mediator release through its action on a mast cell receptor specific for this nucleoside (Marquardt et al., 1985). Adenosine action upon the mast cell receptor and its ability to induce bronchospasm can be inhibited by therapeutic concentrations of theophylline, a known adenosine receptor blocker.

Chemotactic Mediators (Table 5 – 2)

Neutrophil Directed Activities. Several molecules generated during mast cell activation are capable of altering neutrophil migration. Some, including PGD_2, leukotriene B_4, several monohydroxy fatty acids, and platelet activating factor, are not specific for neutrophils and rather are broadly chemotactic or chemokinetic acting upon a variety of migratory cell types.

A high molecular weight (660 Kd), neutral isolectric point protein (HMW-NCF) has been identified in blood of patients with antigen or exercise-induced bronchospasm (Atkins et al., 1976) or experimentally induced physical urticaria (Wasserman et al., 1977). In subjects developing a second, late bronchospastic response to antigen, a second peak of HMW-NCF has been noted (Nagy et al., 1982). This factor is specific for neutrophils, and after its appearance in serum, a transient inhibition of neutrophil chemotactic responsiveness termed deactivation occurs (Center et al, 1979). Other specific neutrophil directed chemotactic activities, termed inflammatory factors of anaphylaxis, have been partially isolated from the granules of rodent mast cells (Oertel and Kaliner, 1981).

Eosinophil Directed Activities. Factors capable of attracting the directed migration of eosinophils have been identified in human lung mast cells (Paterson et al., 1976) and isolated from the blood of those experiencing antigen-induced bronchospasm and experimentally induced physical urticaria (Wasserman et al., 1982). At least three such factors exist separable by their molecular weight, charge, and hydrophobicity. Other factors, including LTB_4, PAF, monohydroxy fatty acids, PGD_2, and histamine, also can modulate eosinophil responsiveness but are not selectively active on this cell type.

Other Chemotactic Activities. Factors capable of attracting lymphocytes, mononuclear leukocytes, and basophils have been found to be released after IgE mediated activation of mast cells in various model systems. The presence of these activities in humans remains to be investigated.

Enzymatic Mediators (Table 5 – 3)

Several enzymes have been identified in isolated human or rodent mast cells by their extraction from isolated populations of these cell types or by their identification in supernatant fluids after IgE mediated cell activation.

Neutral Proteases. The most abundant human mast cell granular protein is the tetrameric, 144,000 daltons mol wt enzyme tryptase (Schwartz et al., 1981). This enzyme is tightly bound to heparin and constitutes nearly half of the mast cell granular protein content. It is released from the mast cell upon IgE dependent activation. Mast cells located in both connective tissue and mucosal sites possess this enzyme. Tryptase has a tryptic specificity; its function is enhanced and its stability is improved by its interaction with heparin. The enzyme is capable of cleaving kininogen and C3 (Schwartz et al., 1982) and also is thought capable of liberating bradykinin from kininogen. Tryptase is not known to be inhibited by plasma antiproteases.

A second neutral protease, with chymotryptic specificity, has also been identified in a subset of human mast cells. This enzyme was first noted in human skin, and its mast cell origin was surmised from the fact that its content was greatly increased in the lesions of mastocytosis (Schechter et al., 1983). It is prominent in mast cells of the skin and those present in loose connective tissue (Irani et al., 1986). This enzyme is thought capable of cleaving angiotensinogen. Other activities attributed to mast cell proteases include cleavage of plasminogen and activation of Hageman factor and prekallikrein.

Acid Hydrolases. The enzymes beta hexosaminidase, arylsulfatase, beta glucuronidase myeloperoxidase, superoxide dismutase, and carboxypeptidase all have been noted in mast cells from rodents or humans. Some of these enzymes are released upon IgE mediated mast cell activation, but their persistence or role outside the cell remains speculative (Schwartz, 1983).

TABLE 5-2. Chemotactic Mediators

Mediator	Preformed or Generated	Function	Therapeutic Inhibitor	Human Disease Association
Eosinophil chemotactic factor of anaphylaxis (ECF-A)	Preformed MW ~500	Attract and deactivate eosinophils Increase eosinophil complement receptors	Glucocorticoids block effect	Physical urticaria Asthma
ECF oligopeptides	Preformed MW ~2000	Attract and deactivate eosinophils and mononuclear leukocytes (more acidic peptides)	Glucocorticoids block effect	Physical urticaria Asthma
HMW-NCF	?Preformed MW ~60,000	Attract and deactivate neutrophils	Glucocorticoids block effect Xanthines, β-agonists, and cromolyn inhibit release	Physical urticaria Asthma
T lymphocyte chemotactic factor	MW ~14,000	Activate T lymphocyte directed migration	?	
B lymphocyte chemotactic factor	MW ~500	Activate B lymphocyte directed migration	?	
Lymphocyte chemokinetic factor	MW ~300	Activate T and B lymphocyte random migration	?	
Inflammatory factors of anaphylaxis (mast cells)	Preformed MW ~1400 and 4000	Induce cutaneous neutrophil (early) and mononuclear (late) cellular infiltrate	?	
Histamine	Preformed	Activate (H_1) or inhibit (H_2) directed and random migration of eosinophils and neutrophils	Classic antihistamines Cimetidine Ranitidine	Asthma Anaphylaxis Urticaria
Arachidonic acid metabolites Cyclooxygenase products PGD$_2$	Generated	Augment neutrophil and eosinophil migration	Aspirin and nonsteroidal anti-inflammatory agents prevent generation	
Lipoxygenase products LTB$_4$	Generated	Augment random and directed migration of neutrophils and eosinophils Increase neutrophil granule release and oxidative metabolism	? Glucocorticoids prevent generation	
PAF	Generated	Augment neutrophil directed migration, enzyme release, and oxidative metabolism		

TABLE 5-3. Enzymatic Mediators

Mediator and Source	Preformed or Generated	Function	Human Disease Association
Tryptase	Preformed MW ~140,000	Generates C3a Generates bradykinin Proteolysis Cleaves fibrinogen Degrades kininogen	Mastocytosis Rhinitis
Chymotryptic protease		Cleaves angiotensinogen	Mastocytosis
Hageman factor activator	MW ~13,000	Activates Hageman factor	
Prekallikrein activator	MW ~80,000	Activates prekallikrein	
Myeloperoxidase	Preformed	Degrades peroxide	
Superoxide dismutase	Preformed	Degrades superoxide	
Lysosomal hydrolases			
Beta glucuronidase	Preformed	Cleaves glucuronide residues	
Beta hexosaminidase	Preformed	Cleaves hexosamines	
Arylsulfatase	Preformed	Cleaves sulfate esters	

Proteoglycans (Table 5–4)

The major proteoglycan of the human mast cell (Metcalfe et al., 1979), and the constituent that confers metachromasia to this cell type, is heparin. This molecule is released on cell activation, promotes anticoagulation, angiogenesis, and bone remodeling, and inhibits complement activation.

Other chondroitin sulfates, including over-sulfated ones, have been found in rodent mast cells. Their presence in human mast cells remains to be unequivocally demonstrated.

MEDIATOR INTERACTIONS

The mediators generated and released after mast cell activation have been isolated, identified, and characterized as individual factors, whereas physiologic and pathologic events reflect their combined interactions. Given the number of mediators; the knowledge that many mediators have yet to be purified (or even identified); the lack of understanding of appropriate ratios of mediators generated or released *in vivo*; and their varying solubilities, kinetics of action, and degradation; it is not surprising that there is very little reliable data regarding these interactions. The smooth muscle effects of histamine and leukotrienes are synergistic *in vitro*, and both are known to cause prostaglandin generation. This property is shared by $PGF_{2\alpha}$. PGD_2, whether generated primarily by the mast cell or secondarily by the action of mast cell mediators on other cell types, may augment chemotactic factor action; other prostaglandins may affect leukotriene-induced cutaneous responses. Heparin can enhance tryptase function, whereas histamine may potentiate or inhibit leukocyte migration. The ability of histamine and other mast cell–dependent factors (e.g., chemotactic factors, inflammatory factor of anaphylaxis, arachidonate metabolites) to attract circulating leukocytes, to modulate their metabolic activity, and to induce superoxide generation and the production of inflammatory lipids suggests further potential interactions for mast cell mediators. Taken together, it is apparent that the number and type of mast cell mediator interactions are potentially enormous; their pathobiologic consequences are relevant to a variety of homeostatic and disease processes. These interactions remain largely unexplored.

EOSINOPHILS

The association of eosinophils with allergic diseases has been long noted. Recent evidence indicates that this association, in addition to providing diagnostic information, also has pathogenetic implications.

Growth and Differentiation. Eosinophils develop in the bone marrow from precursors that have common lineage with neutrophils and basophils (Fishkoff et al., 1984). Eosinophil production is regulated by T lymphocyte factors (Griffin et al., 1984). Eosinophils mature in the marrow and circulate for only a few hours before appearing at the tissue sites to which they have been directed. The vast majority of eosinophils are in the tissue or bone marrow; less than 1 in 200 are in the circulation.

Eosinophil Constituents. Eosinophils contain granules with a unique crystalline core structure, as viewed under the electron microscope. The granules are composed of a variety of enzymes and some novel peptides and proteins. It is this combination of factors, together with the specificity of eosinophil chemotactic responses, that is believed to give this cell its special functions.

Of the enzymes present in the eosinophil granules, peroxidase, arylsulfatase B, phospho-

TABLE 5–4. Proteoglycans

Mediator and Source	Preformed or Generated	Function	Inhibitor	Human Disease Association
Heparin	Preformed MW ~60,000	Bind histamine Anticoagulant inhibit complement activation Bind platelet factor 4 Bind and activate tryptase	Protamine	Mastocytosis
Oversulfated Chondroitin sulfate	Preformed	? Bind histamine		

lipase D, and histaminase are the ones that distinguish this cell from other granulocytes. The peroxidase is distinguishable immunologically and functionally from myeloperoxidase and is capable of inducing mast cell degranulation when H_2O_2 and halide anion are present (Henderson et al., 1980). Arylsulfatase B can bind sulfidopeptide leukotrienes; phospholipase D is capable of inactivating platelet activating factor; and, of course, histaminase can degrade histamine. The relevance of these functions to allergic disease, however, has been questioned since prominent eosinophilia is associated with more severe disease rather than with its amelioration. Conversely, corticosteroids that depress eosinophil levels are generally beneficial in therapy of allergic disorders.

Several peptides and proteins unique to the eosinophil have been characterized and are now thought to be responsible for the adverse effects of this cell type. The major basic protein of eosinophils (MBP) is a peptide of approximately 11,000 daltons, with an isoelectric point of 10. It constitutes nearly half of the granule protein (Gleich et al., 1976). This peptide is toxic to tracheal epithelium, is a cause of mast cell and basophil degranulation, and is thought to be important in killing parasites. A functionally related molecule, eosinophil cationic peptide (Olsson and Venge, 1974), is somewhat larger (~17,000 daltons) than MBP, but it too is toxic to parasites; it has potent actions upon the lymphocytes and upon the proteins in the clotting and fibrinolytic cascades. Another peptide, termed eosinophil derived neurotoxin (Durach et al., 1981) of ~18,000 daltons has been shown capable of damaging the neurons of the central nervous system. Its role in disease, however, is speculative. Finally, an eosinophil membrane associated enzyme with lysophospholipase activity has been identified (Weller et al., 1980). Aggregates of this protein compose the Charcot-Leyden crystals, which are so characteristic of eosinophilic inflammatory processes. Both Charcot-Leyden crystal protein and MBP are present, albeit in much reduced amounts, in basophils. In addition to these preformed constituents, activation of eosinophils by immune complexes or by divalent cation ionophores can lead to the production of the sulfidopeptide leukotriene LTC_4 (Weller et al., 1983), whereas chemotactic factors cause this cell to generate platelet activating factor (Lee et al., 1984).

The mechanism of release of eosinophil granular constituents was long debated, but it now appears to be a noncytolytic process that is enhanced in states of eosinophil activation. Such granule release is associated with the presence of eosinophils with reduced bouyant density in the circulation (Prin et al., 1984). These bear new antigenic determinants, which are metabolically activated (Bass et al., 1980).

Eosinophil Localization in Allergic Disease

The blood and tissue association of eosinophils with allergic disorders implies a mechanism by which IgE mediated mast cell activation can be communicated to this cell type. Several factors that specifically regulate eosinophil migratory responses have been identified in mast cells or in blood or tissue after mast cell activation. A tetrapeptide termed ECF-A, or eosinophil chemotactic factor of anaphylaxis (Goetzl and Austen, 1975), has been identified in human lung; a similar activity, in a preformed state, in rodent mast cell granules (Wasserman et al., 1974) and in isolated human mast cells (Paterson et al., 1976), has been reported. In the blood of individuals experiencing antigen induced bronchospasm or experimentally induced mast cell–dependent physical urticaria, several eosinophil directed chemotactic activities have been identified. These molecules are of low molecular weight and differ in their charge and hydrophobicity (see previous discussion). Additionally, histamine at low concentrations enhances and at higher concentrations inhibits eosinophil migratory responses to a variety of attractants. Thus, the generation of a family of specific eosinophil directed chemoattractants upon mast cell activation (directly from mast cells or indirectly from the action of mast cell mediators on other cells or on plasma proteins) is thought to be the mechanism by which allergic disorders and eosinophils are so tightly associated.

Other Cells in Allergy. Chemoattractants for neutrophils, lymphocytes, basophils, and mononuclear leukocytes have been identified in various models of mast cell activation (see previous section). The association of tissue neutrophils with the acquisition of bronchial hyperreactivity and its prevention in animal models by maneuvers that deplete neutrophils suggest that these cells also may play an important role in human allergic diseases. It is, however, beyond the scope of this chapter to delineate the many functions of this important cell. Similarly, the complex functions of mononuclear leukocytes and lymphocytes is dealt with in Chapters 1 and 4.

THE ROLE OF CELLS AND MEDIATORS IN ALLERGIC DISEASE

The most complete evidence for the role of mast cells and mediators in allergic disease is derived from experiments in which IgE dependent mast cell activation in skin tissue is caused by specific antigen (or by antibody to IgE). The participation of other immunoglobulin classes, and thus other inflammatory pathways, has been excluded in such studies by using purified IgE to sensitize nonimmune individuals. Activation of mast cells by antigen results initially in a pruritic wheal and flare reaction, which begins in minutes and persists for 1 hour to 2 hours, followed in 6 to 12 hours by a large, poorly demarcated, erythematous, tender, and indurated lesion (Dolovitch et al., 1973; Solley et al., 1976). The initial response, as assessed by light microscopy, is accompanied by mast cell degranulation, dermal edema, and endothelial cell activation. The later reaction is characterized by infiltration of the dermis by neutrophils, eosinophils, basophils, lymphocytes, and mononuclear leukocytes; in some instances, it is characterized by hemorrhage, blood vessel wall damage, and fibrin deposition of sufficient severity to warrant the diagnosis of vasculitis. A similar dual phase reaction is experienced by allergic subjects undergoing antigen bronchoprovocation. Such challenges result in an immediate bronchospastic response followed by recovery and, 6 to 24 hours later, by recurrence of asthmatic signs and symptoms. Although biopsy proven correlates of this pulmonary response are lacking, direct bronchoalveolar examination and lavage results reveal an early edematous, hyperemic phase associated with neutrophils in the airway followed by a later influx of eosinophils. The mediators responsible for these pathophysiologic manifestations have not yet been delineated fully, but clues to their identity can be derived from knowledge of the effects of pharmacologic manipulation, by the identification of mediators in blood or tissue fluid obtained when the inflammatory response occurs, and by the known effects of isolated mediators.

Pharmacologic intervention suggests that the initial phase is mast cell–dependent in both skin and lung tissues. The initial response in the skin may be inhibited by antihistamines and in the lungs by cromolyn. In both tissues, glucocorticoids effectively inhibit only the late response, reflecting its inflammatory nature. Studies of skin blisters have identified histamine and an eosinophil chemotactic factor (Ting et al., 1981), as well as metabolites of arachidonic acid early in the lesion. These mediators also are identified in blister fluids obtained later in the course of the reaction. In antigen challenges of allergic asthmatics, early increases in the plasma content of histamine, eosinophil and neutrophil chemotactic factors, and platelet activating factor 4 have been identified coincident with the initial response, whereas another peak of histamine and the chemotactic factors occurs during the late response. In nasal mucosa a similar dual response pattern is noted with histamine, LTC_4, esterase, and kinin. Such activities are identified in nasal washings both early and late, whereas PGD_2, a mast cell but not a basophil mediator, is present during the initial phase only. This finding has been taken to imply early mast cell activation and later basophil response.

The exact pathophysiology of the dual phase responses is uncertain. It seems likely that histamine, PGD_2, leukotrienes, platelet activating factor, and adenosine are sufficient to cause the early or immediate clinical responses to mast cell activation. As leukocyte accumulation is not prominent during the early response, this construct seems plausible. However, it is possible that resident leukocytes, antigen responsive T lymphocytes, and mononuclear leukocytes also can produce mediators capable of inducing early changes. Moreover, in response to newly generated or released mediators, it is likely that endothelial cells, fibroblasts, and other connective tissue cells also contribute biologically active products capable of modulating the early response.

The late phase in skin, nasal mucosa, and lung reflects the extent and persistence of the early phase as well as the effects of newly arrived leukocytes (responding to chemotactic factors) and the action of enzymes upon tissue and plasma protein substrates. Most important in this regard appears to be the marked influx of eosinophils beginning within hours of mast cell activation, which persists for many hours to days. This influx has been documented in skin and nasal epithelium and is manifest in bronchial alveolar washings. The potent inflammatory constituents of the eosinophil and its ability to generate inflammatory lipids and toxic oxygen species suggest this cell is important in extending mast cell events beyond immediate responses. The beneficial effects of glucocorticoids on late responses to mast cell activation in association with their potent eosinopenic effects further strengthen this hypothesis. By whatever mechanism it is engendered, the late response carries implications beyond its clinical expression. Thus, asthmatic patients' experiencing such reactions manifest, as a consequence, heightened nonspecific bronchial hyperreactivity, a response not noted to occur after isolated early responses (Cockcroft et al., 1977). This heightened reactivity due to mast cell initiated inflammation then is capable of causing prolonged (and less obviously allergen associated) clinical changes.

Although these relationships are tenuously drawn and somewhat speculative at present, the rapid advances occurring in this area make it certain that our understanding of mast cell mediated inflammation will continue to sharpen in focus, enabling better approaches to diagnosis and therapy of allergic disorders.

REFERENCES

Atkins, P.C., Norman, M., Werner, H., et al.: Release of neutrophil chemotactic activity during immediate hypersensitivity reactions in humans. Ann. Intern. Med. 86:415, 1976.

Barnes, P., et al.: Nocturnal asthma and changes in circulating epinephrine, histamine, and cortisol. N. Engl. J. Med. 303:263, 1980.

Bass, D.A., Grover, W.H., Lewis, J.: Comparison of human eosinophils from normals and patients with eosinophilia. J. Clin. Invest. 66:1265, 1980.

Black, J.W., et al.: Definition and antagonism of histamine H₂ receptors. Nature 236:385, 1972.

Brown, M.J., et al.: A novel double isotope technique for the enzymatic assay of plasma histamine: Application to estimation of mast cell activation assessed by antigen challenge in asthmatics. J. Allergy Clin. Immunol. 69:20, 1982.

Center, D.M., Soter N.A., Wasserman S.I., Austen, K.F.: Inhibition of neutrophil chemotaxis in association with experimental angioedema in patients with cold urticaria: A model of chemotactic deactivation *in vivo*. Clin. Exp. Immunol. 35:112, 1979.

Cockcroft, D.W., Ruffin, R.E., Dolovich, J., et al.: Allergen-induced increase in nonallergic bronchial hyperreactivity. Clin. Allergy 7:503, 1977.

Demopoulos, C.A., Pinkard, R.N., Hanahan, D.J.: Platelet-activating factor. Evidence for 1-O-alkyl-2-acetyl-sn-glyceryl-3-phosphorylcholine as the active component. J. Biol. Chem. 254:935, 1979.

Dolovitch, J., et al.: Late cutaneous allergic response in isolated IgE-dependent reactions. J. Allergy Clin. Immunol. 52:38, 1973.

Durach, D.T., Ackerman, S.J., Loegering, D.A., et al.: Purification of human eosinophil–derived neurotoxin. Proc. Natl. Acad. Sci. (USA) 78:5165, 1981.

Dvorak, H.F., Dvorak, A.M.: Basophilic leukocytes: Structure, function, and role in disease. Clin. Haematol. 4:651, 1975.

Dyer, J., et al.: Measurement of plasma histamine: Description of an improved method and normal values. J. Allergy Clin. Immunol. 70:82, 1982.

Enerbach, L.: The gut mucosal mast cell. Monogr. Allergy 17:222, 1981.

Farr, R.S., et al.: Human serum acid-labile factor is an acyl-hydrolase that inactivates platelet-activating factor. Fed. Proc. 42:3120, 1983.

Fishkoff, S.A., Pollak, A., Gleich, G.J., et al.: Eosinophilic differentiation of the human promyelocytic leukemia cell line HL-60. J. Exp. Med. 160:179, 1984.

Flower, R.J., Harvey, E.A., Kingston, W.P.: Inflammatory effects of prostaglandin D₂ in rat and human skin. Br. J. Pharmacol. 56:229, 1976.

Gleich, G.J., Loegering, D.A., Mann, K.G., et al.: Comparative properties of the Charcot-Leyden crystal protein and the major basic protein from human eosinophils. J. Clin. Invest. 57:633, 1976.

Goetzl, E.J., Austen, K.F.: Purification and synthesis of eosinophilotactic tetrapeptides of human lung tissue: Identification as eosinophilotactic factor of anaphylaxis (ECF-A). Proc. Natl. Acad. Sci. (USA) 72:4123, 1975.

Griffin, J.D., Meuer, S.C., Schlossman, S.F., et al.: T cell regulation of myelopoiesis: An analysis at a clonal level. J. Immunol. 133:1863, 1984.

Halonen, M., Palmer, J.D., Lohman, I.C., et al.: Respiratory and circulatory alterations induced by acetylglyceryl ether phosphorylcholine, a mediator of IgE anaphylaxis in the rabbit. Am. Rev. Resp. Dis. 122:915, 1980.

Halonen, M., Palmer, J.D., Lohman, I.C., et al.: Differential effects of platelet depletion in the cardiovascular and pulmonary alterations of IgE anaphylaxis and AGEPC infusion in the rabbit. Am. Rev. Resp. Dis. 124:416, 1981.

Henderson, W.R., Chi, E.Y., Klebanoff, S.J.: Eosinophil peroxidase–induced mast cell secretion. J. Exp. Med. 152:265, 1980.

Henderson, W.R., Klebanoff, S.J.: Leukotriene B4, C4, D4, and E4 inactivation by hydroxyl radicals. Biochem. Biophys. Res. Commun. 110:266, 1983.

Holgate, S.T., et al.: Pharmacological modulation of airway caliber and mediator release in human models of bronchial asthma. *In* Asthma: Physiology, Immunopharmacology and Treatment, Austen, K.F., Lichenstein, L.M., and Kay, A.B. (eds.), London, Academic Press, 1984.

Humphrey, D.M., Hanahan, D.J., Pinkard, R.N.: Induction of leukocytic infiltrates in rabbit skin by acetylglyceryl ether phosphorylcholine. Lab. Invest. 47:227, 1982.

Ihle, J.N., et al.: Biologic properties of homogeneous interleukin 3. I. Demonstration of WEHI-3 growth factor activity, mast cell growth factor activity, P cell-stimulating factor activity, colony-stimulating factor activity, and histamine-producing cell-stimulating factor activity. J. Immunol. 131:282, 1983.

Irani, A.A., Schechter, N.M., Craig, S.S., DeBlois, G., Schwartz, L.B.: Two types of human mast cells that have distinct neutral protease composition. Proc. Natl. Acad. Sci. (USA) 83:4464, 1986.

Lee, T.C., Lenihan, D.J., Malone, B., et al.: Increased biosynthesis of platelet-activating factor in activated human eosinophils. J. Biol. Chem. 259:5526, 1984.

Lewis, R.A., Austen, K.F.: Mediation of local homeostasis

and inflammation by leukotrienes and other mast cell–dependent compounds. Nature 293:103, 1981.

Lewis, R.A., et al.: Prostaglandin D_2 generation after activation of rat and human mast cells with anti-IgE. J. Immunol. 129:1627, 1982.

MacGlashan, D.W., Jr., Schleimer, R.P., Peters, S.P., et al.: Generation of leukotrienes by purified human lung mast cells. J. Clin. Invest. 70:747, 1982.

Marquardt, D.L.: Histamine. Clin. Rev. Allergy 1:343, 1983.

Marquardt, D.L., Gruber, H.E., Wasserman, S.I.: Adenosine release from stimulated mast cells. Proc. Natl. Acad. Sci. (USA) 81:6192, 1984.

Marquardt, D.L., Wasserman, S.I.: Adenosine binding to rat mast cells—pharmacologic and functional characterization. Agents Actions 16:453, 1985.

McManus, L.M., Hanahan, D.J., Pinkard, R.N.: Human platelet stimulation by acetylglyceryl ether phosphorylcholine. J. Clin. Invest. 67:903, 1980.

Mentzer, R.M., Rubio, R., Berne, R.M.: Release of adenosine by hypoxic canine lung tissue and its possible role in pulmonary circulation. Am. J. Physiol. 229:1625, 1975.

Metcalfe, D.D.: Effector cell heterogeneity in immediate hypersensitivity reactions. Clin. Rev. Allergy 1:311, 1983.

Metcalfe, D.D., Bland, C.E., Wasserman, S.I.: Biochemical and functional characterization of proteoglycans isolated from basophils of patients with chronic myelogenous leukemia. J. Immunol. 132:1943, 1984.

Metcalfe, D.D., Lewis, R.A., Silbert, J.E., et al.: Isolation and characterization of heparin from human lung. J. Clin. Invest. 64:1537, 1979.

Mikhail, G.R., Miller-Milinska, A.: Mast cell population in human skin. J. Invest. Dermatol. 43:249, 1964.

Mills, G.C., et al.: Purine metabolism in adenosine deaminase deficiency. Proc. Natl. Acad. Sci. (USA) 73:2867, 1976.

Nagy, L., Lee, T.H., Kay, A.B.: Neutrophil chemotactic activity in antigen-induced late asthmatic reaction. N. Engl. J. Med. 306:497, 1982.

Oertel, H., Kaliner, M.: The biologic activity of mast cell granules. III. Purification of inflammatory factors of anaphylaxis (IF-A) responsible for causing late-phase reactions. J. Immunol. 127:1398, 1981.

Olsson, I., Venge, P.: Cationic proteins of human granulocytes. Blood 44:235, 1974.

Paterson, N.A.M., et al.: Release of chemical mediators from partially purified human lung cells. J. Immunol. 117:1356, 1976.

Pinkard, R.N., Knicker, W.T., Lee, L., et al.: Vasoactive effects of 1-O-alkyl-2-acetyl-sn-glyceryl-phosphorylcholine in human skin. J. Allergy Clin. Immunol. 65:196, 1980.

Platshon, L.F., Kaliner, M.: The effects of the immunologic release of histamine upon human lung cyclic nucleotide levels and prostaglandin generation. J. Clin. Invest. 62:1113, 1978.

Prin, L., Charon, J., Capron, M., et al.: Heterogeneity of human eosinophils. Clin. Exp. Immunol. 57:735, 1984.

Razin, E., et al.: Culture from mouse bone marrow of a subclass of mast cells possessing a distinct chondroitin sulfate proteoglycan with glycosaminoglycan rich in N-acetylgalactosamine-4,6 disulfate. J. Biol. Chem. 257:7229, 1982.

Roberts, L.J., Sweetman, B.J., Lewis, R.A., et al.: Increased production of prostaglandin D_2 in patients with systemic mastocytosis. N. Engl. J. Med. 303:1400, 1980.

Ruzicka, T., et al.: Inhibition of rat mast cell arachidonic acid cyclooxygenase by dapsone. J. Allergy Clin. Immunol. 72:365, 1983.

Samuelsson, B., et al.: Introduction of a nomenclature: Leukotrienes. Prostaglandins 17:785, 1979.

Samuelsson, B., et al.: Leukotrienes and slow-reacting substance of anaphylaxis. Allergy 35:375, 1980.

Schechter, N.M., et al.: Human skin chymotryptic proteinase: Isolation and relation to cathepsin g and rat mast cell proteinase I. J. Biol. Chem. 258:2973, 1983.

Schwartz, L.B.: Enzyme mediators of mast cells and basophils. Clin. Rev. Allergy 1:397, 1983.

Schwartz, L.B., Lewis, R.A., Austen, K.F.: Tryptase from human pulmonary mast cells: Purification and characterization. J. Biol. Chem. 256:11939, 1981.

Schwartz, L.B., Schratz, J.J., Vik, D., et al.: Metabolism of human C3 by human mast cell tryptase. J. Allergy Clin. Immunol. 69:94S, 1982.

Solley, G.O., et al.: The late phase of the immediate wheal-and-flare skin reaction: Its dependence upon IgE antibodies. J. Clin. Invest. 58:408, 1976.

Soter, N.A., et al.: Local effects of synthetic leukotrienes (LTC_4, LTD_4, LTE_4, and LTB_4) in human skin. J. Invest. Dermatol. 80:115, 1983.

Steel, L., Kaliner, M.A.: Prostaglandin-generating factor of anaphylaxis: Identification and isolation. J. Biol. Chem. 256:12692, 1981.

Ting, S., Zweiman, B., Lavker, R.M., et al.: In vivo release of eosinophil chemoattractant activity in human allergic skin reactions. J. Immunol. 127:557, 1981.

Wasserman, S.I.: Mediators of immediate hypersensitivity. J. Allergy Clin. Immunol. 72:101, 1983.

Wasserman, S.I., Austen, K.F., Soter, N.A.: The function and physiochemical characterization of three eosinophilotactic activities released into the circulation by cold challenge of patients with cold urticaria. Clin. Exp. Immunol. 47:570, 1982.

Wasserman, S.I., Goetzl, E.J., Austen, K.F.: Preformed eosinophil chemotactic factor of anaphylaxis. J. Immunol. 112:351, 1974.

Wasserman, S.I., Soter, N.A., Center, D.M., et al.: Cold urticaria: Recognition and characterization of a neutrophil chemotactic factor which appears in serum during experimental cold challenge. J. Clin. Invest. 60:189, 1977.

Weller, P.A., Goetzl, E.J., Austen, K.F.: Identification of human eosinophil lipophospholipase as the constituent of Charcot-Leyden crystals. Proc. Natl. Acad. Sci. (USA) 77:7440, 1980.

Weller, P.A., Lee, C.W., Foster, D.W., et al.: Generation and metabolism of 5-lipoxygenase pathway leukotrienes by human eosinophils: Predominant production of leukotriene C_4. Proc. Natl. Acad. Sci. (USA) 80:7626, 1983.

Yoo, D., Lessin, L.S., Jensen, W.: Bone-marrow mast cells in lymphoproliferative disorders. In The Mast Cell: Its Role in Health and Disease, Pepys, J., Edwards, A.M. (eds.), Kent, England, Pitman Medical Publ. Co., 1979.

6

IgE Antibody in Health and Disease

REBECCA H. BUCKLEY, M.D.

As recently as 1963, Stanworth wrote that skin sensitizing antibodies represented a nebulous concept to most immunologists. Many crucial discoveries since then not only have firmly established that the substances responsible for skin sensitizing activity are "true" antibodies but also have documented that most skin sensitizing antibodies belong to a single immunoglobulin class.

DEFINITIONS AND SYNONYMS

Skin sensitizing antibodies are defined as antibodies that exhibit a high affinity for membrane receptors on the basophils and mast cells of members of the same or closely related species. Although it is clear that a majority of such molecules belong to the IgE class, there also is some evidence in animals and humans to suggest that some skin sensitizing antibodies may belong to the IgG class. Whether these antibodies are of clinical significance is as yet unknown. The interaction of antigen with two or more basophil or mast cell bound antibodies results in the release of chemical mediators that cause a variety of biologic effects. When antigen is injected into the skin, the mediators released from dermal mast cells cause vasodilatation, pruritus, and increased capillary permeability — resulting in an immediate wheal and flare reaction. Synonyms for skin sensitizing antibodies include reaginic antibodies, atopic reagin, anaphylactic antibodies, and homocytotropic antibodies; the names reflect the various levels of understanding of the functions of these antibodies at the times the terms came into use.

HISTORICAL BACKGROUND

Prausnitz in 1921 demonstrated the feasibility of transferring immediate wheal and flare skin test reactivity to himself by the intracutaneous injection of serum from his fish sensitive patient, Küstner. In spite of that demonstration, scientists were puzzled for the next four decades over the fact that sera from allergic subjects lacked activity in the classic *in vitro* immunologic reactions of precipitation, agglutination, complement fixation, and guinea pig passive cutaneous anaphylaxis (PCA). This peculiar reactivity in the sera of patients with hay fever and asthma was termed "atopic reagin" by Coca and Grove in 1925 (Stanworth, 1963).

Not until the early 1960's did the notion evolve that antibodies of different immunoglobulin classes might have different biologic properties. In 1963, Ovary et al. demonstrated that the fraction of 7S antibody protein in immune guinea pig serum capable of passively transferring both cutaneous and systemic anaphylaxis to normal guinea pigs was of $\gamma 1$ electrophoretic mobility, whereas the fraction causing complement fixation was of $\gamma 2$ mobility. Similarly, although it had been shown repeatedly that sera from allergic individuals did not give positive PCA reactions in guinea pigs challenged with allergen, such sera were found to give strongly positive reactions in monkey PCA experiments (Buckley and Metzgar, 1965). From these experiments, the terms homocytotropic and heterocytotropic came into usage; the former referred to antibodies capable of transferring skin sensitization or anaphylaxis to members of the same or closely related species, and the latter to those capable of transferring similar reactivity across species to lower animals.

In 1966, Ishizaka and Ishizaka isolated a fraction from allergic human serum that did not contain detectable amounts of any of the then known immunoglobulin classes, yet contained reaginic activity that could be removed by absorption of the fraction with antibodies to human immunoglobulin light chains (Ishizaka and Ishizaka, 1975). Immunization of rabbits with this fraction (which contained only minute amounts of protein) yielded an antiserum that, when absorbed with immunoglobulins of the other known classes, could remove all reaginic activity from the original fraction. By chance a year later, Johansson and his coworkers identified a myeloma protein, which they termed ND (IgND), that had antigenic characteristics different from any of the four known immunoglobulin classes (Bennich et al., 1976). This protein subsequently was shown to have antigenic identity with the protein found by Ishizaka and Ishizaka to carry reaginic activity. The World Health Organization officially designated this unique immunoglobulin class "IgE."

IgE SKIN SENSITIZING ANTIBODIES

Sites of IgE Production

IgE producing plasma cells are found predominantly in paragut and pararespiratory lymphoid tissues and in regional lymph nodes (Table 6–1). In addition, germinal centers of tonsils, adenoids, and bronchial and mesenteric lymph nodes contain IgE producing cells. By contrast, few plasma cells containing IgE are found in the spleen or in subcutaneous lymph nodes. Thus, the distribution of IgE producing plasma cells is similar to the distribution of plasma cells that produce IgA (Bloch, 1976). This fact and the fact that many allergens that cause allergic symptoms are inhaled or ingested have raised the question whether IgE producing lymphoid tissue may represent a distinct local immune system. Although this possibility remains, since IgE has been detected in nasal washings, colostrum, and saliva, no conclusive evidence for selective local production has been presented thus far. In addition, a structure analogous to secretory piece has not been found on IgE molecules in external secretions.

Peculiarities of Antigens that Induce IgE Formation

Antigens that induce most IgE antibody responses are widespread in nature and innocuous to most nonallergic subjects. The major categories of antigens include pollen, food, mold, insect, animal, and parasitic antigens; these are discussed in detail in Chapters 10 to 12. Many other antigens are known to elicit vigorous immune responses of other types but do not selectively stimulate IgE production. Antigens that stimulate IgE antibody production usually are protein in nature and are of medium size, most ranging from approximately 20,000 to 40,000 daltons mol wt (King, 1976). Major antigenic components have been purified from a few of these agents, including ragweed, rye and timothy grasses, cat dander, house dust mite, codfish, and *Ascaris,* but thus far no common or unique structures have been identified to account for their tendency to stimulate IgE antibody synthesis. Certain types of adjuvants, such as aluminum hydroxide gel or killed *Bordetella pertussis* organisms, also facilitate an IgE antibody response (Tada, 1975; Ishizaka, 1984).

Physicochemical Characteristics of IgE

The availability of myeloma proteins of the IgE class enabled extensive characterization of the physicochemical properties of IgE (Bennich et al., 1976). IgE myeloma proteins consist of

TABLE 6–1. Distribution of IgE Forming Cells in Lymphoid Tissues*

Lymphoid Tissues	Human		Monkey	
	PLASMA CELLS	GERMINAL CENTER	PLASMA CELLS	GERMINAL CENTER
Tonsil	+~+++	+~++	+	++
Adenoid	+~+++	+~++		
Bronchial and peritoneal	++	(+)†	++	(+)
Subcutaneous lymph nodes	±~+	−	±	−
Spleen	±~+	−	+~++	±
Respiratory mucosa	+	−	+	−
Gastrointestinal mucosa	+~++	−	+~++	(+)‡
Lung	−	−	−	−
Blood	−	−	ND§	
Bone marrow	−	−	ND	

* From Ishizaka, T., Ishizaka, K.: Biology of immunoglobulin E. Progr. Allergy 19:60–121, 1975; used with permission.
† Results in parentheses were negative in some cases.
‡ 1+ in Peyer's patches.
§ ND = not done.

four polypeptide chains, two identical heavy (epsilon) chains and two identical light chains, which may be of either the kappa or lambda type (Fig. 6–1). IgE antibodies are considerably heavier than IgG antibodies, having a molecular weight of approximately 190,000 daltons and a sedimentation coefficient of 8.0S. The molecule also differs from IgG in the content of carbohydrate, which represents 12 percent of IgE's total weight. The estimated molecular weight of each heavy chain is 72,300 daltons and of each light chain, 22,500 daltons.

When IgE is treated with enzymes such as papain and pepsin, it can be cleaved into smaller fragments the same way molecules of the other immunoglobulin classes can be (see Fig. 6–1) (Bennich et al., 1976). If papain is used, three fragments result, one termed Fc (or crystallizable fragment) and the other two, Fab (or antigen binding fragments). Pepsin digestion, on the other hand, results in destruction of the carboxyl terminal two thirds of the Fc portion, yielding one large fragment called F(ab')2. Use of these enzymatic probes has allowed analysis of the antigenic characteristics of various segments of the molecule. From such studies it has been learned that the Fc fragment has two different immunoglobulin class specific antigenic determinants. These are termed E1 and E2, with E2 residing on the carboxyl terminal ends of the epsilon chains and E1 on the adjacent heavy chain segment in the amino terminal third of the Fc fragment, designated Fc' (see Fig. 6–1). In addition, a third determinant is present in the Fab fragment on the Fd portion of the epsilon chain, the EO antigenic determinant. The EO, or idiotypic determinant, differs in the hypervariable portion for all IgE molecules having different antigenic specificities.

The remainder of the Fab fragment is composed of a light chain.

Each IgE molecule contains 40 half-cysteine residues or 20 disulfide bonds (Bennich et al., 1976). Sixteen of these are intrachain bonds, 12 on the epsilon chains and four on the light chains. Two others link the epsilon chains within the Fc' region, and the remaining two connect the light chains to the Fc portions of the heavy chains at the hinge region. The amino acid sequence of the epsilon chains as well as the locations of the intrachain disulfide bonds have been determined, and five domains on the epsilon chain, two in the Fd portion, and three in the Fc portion have been defined (Bennich et al., 1976). By using varying concentrations of sulfhydryl bond reducing agents, such as dithiothreitol, it has been possible to cleave selectively certain disulfide bonds and study the effects of disruption of these bonds on the biologic activity of the molecule.

Biologic Properties of IgE

IgE exists in serum and other body fluids in minute concentrations that are significantly lower than those of the other four immunoglobulin classes (Johansson and Bennich, 1982). Reported geometric mean serum IgE concentrations have ranged from 11.8 to 74.6 IU/ml (28.3 to 179 ng/ml) in studies of different normal populations (Homberger, 1986). Metabolic studies done by Waldmann et al. (1976) demonstrated the low concentration to be due to both a low total body synthetic rate and a very short serum half-life (2.7 days). As discussed subsequently, however, other biologic characteristics of IgE more than compensate for its low avail-

FIGURE 6–1. Structure of immunoglobulin IgE and sites of action of enzymes, as drawn by Ishizaka and Ishizaka (Progr. Allerg. *19*:60, 1975) from the data of Bennich and von Bahr-Lindstrom (Progress in Immunology, Amsterdam, North Holland, 1974; used with permission.) There are three major antigenic determinants on each of the epsilon chains. Proceeding from right to left, the class specific E2 determinant is associated with the carboxy terminal portion of the Fc fragment and not included in the F (ab')₂ fragment; the E1 determinant is present on the FC' segment; and the EO (or idiotypic) determinant is in the Fd or N terminal segment.

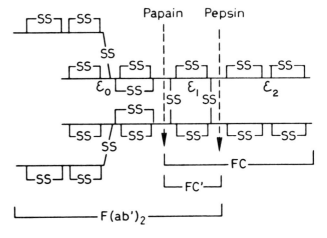

TABLE 6–2. Properties of Homocytotropic Antibodies*

Properties	IgG Type				IgE Type						
	HUMAN	GUINEA PIG†	MOUSE	RAT	HUMAN	MONKEY	DOG	RABBIT	GUINEA PIG	RAT	MOUSE
Sedimentation coefficient	6.5	6.5	6.5	6.5	8.0	8.0	8.0	8.0	8.0	8.0	8.0
Heat lability	−	±	±	−	+	+	+	±	+	+	+
Sulfhydryl lability	−	±	±	−	+	+	+	+	+	+	+
Optimal latent period	4 to 6 h	3 to 6 h	1 to 2 h	3 h	1 day	1 to 2 days	2 days	3 days	6 days	3 days	3 days

* From Ishizaka, T., Ishizaka, K.: Biology of immunoglobulin E. Progr. Allergy 19:60–121, 1975; used with permission.

† Properties of guinea pig antibody in this table are IgG 1a antibody. Guinea pig has IgG 1b antibody in which the optimal latent period is 16 h. The IgG 1b antibody is heat stable but susceptible to reduction-alkylation treatment.

ability, since devastating effects on human health can result upon interaction of antigen with just a few strategically located IgE molecules.

General Characteristics. Before discussing its high affinity for basophil and mast cell membrane receptors—the most prominent biologic characteristic of IgE—it is important to note the similarities and dissimilarities of IgE to other immunoglobulin classes (Ishizaka and Ishizaka, 1975). IgE antibodies in serum are unique in their heat lability, losing their capacity to sensitize normal skin, blood basophils, or lung mast cells passively, following heating at 56°C for 2 to 4 hours (Table 6–2). Treatment of IgE molecules with sulfhydryl bond reducing agents, such as 2-mercaptoethanol and dithiothreitol, similarly will affect their ability to sensitize. In addition, IgE antibodies, similar to antibodies of the IgA, IgM, and IgD classes, fail to cross the placenta from the mother to the fetus. They are incapable of mediating guinea pig PCA even when concentrated many times more than *in vivo* (Table 6–3) (Ishizaka and

Ishizaka, 1975). Although highly concentrated preparations are able to agglutinate erythrocytes coated with ragweed antigen, it is doubtful that agglutination is an important biologic function of IgE antibodies, since concentrations of the magnitude required to demonstrate this effect are not achieved in the natural state. The ability of IgE molecules to fix complement was investigated by using nonspecifically aggregated IgE myeloma protein and its enzymatically produced fragments. High concentrations of aggregated IgE do not activate the complement system by the classic pathway but can do so by the alternative pathway. Aggregated Fc fragments also are capable of activating the alternative pathway, whereas F(ab')2 fragments do not (see Table 6–3).

Cell Membrane Affinity. The most important biologic property of IgE antibody molecules is their extremely high binding affinity for membrane receptors on homologous basophils and mast cells (Ishizaka and Ishizaka, 1975 and 1984). Using ^{125}I-labeled anti-IgE and ^{125}I-labeled IgE myeloma proteins, Ishizaka and his

TABLE 6–3. Immunologic Properties of IgE*

Reactions	Minimum Concentration of Antibody; μg N/ml	Activity
In vitro		
Agglutination	10^{-2}	+
C fixation (classic)	>800†	−
C fixation (alternative)	80†	+
In vivo		
PK in human	4×10^{-5}	+
PCA in monkey	10^{-3}	+
PCA in guinea pig	>100	−

* From Ishizaka, T., Ishizaka, K.: Biology of immunoglobulin E. Progr. Allergy 19:60–121, 1975; used with permission.

† Aggregated IgE.

coworkers were able to show that IgE binds preferentially to primate basophils and mast cells. In contrast, similar studies with radiolabeled human IgG or anti-IgG showed that IgG molecules attach predominantly to membrane receptors on primate monocytes and neutrophils. Equilibrium constants of the binding affinities of these two types of immunoglobulins for their respective preferred cell receptors were found to be $10^{-9}/M$ for IgE and $10^{-5}/M$ for IgG (Ishizaka and Ishizaka, 1975). Despite the high avidity of IgE for basophil and mast cell receptors, it is well known that there is a minimum latent period of about 4 hours before skin sensitization can be detected in passive transfer experiments, and full sensitization is not accomplished until approximately 24 hours. The extremely high avidity of IgE for basophils and mast cells allows these molecules to persist in tissues far longer than in serum. Although there are reports that passively transferred IgE antibodies may persist for weeks or even months, the half-life of radiolabeled IgE injected into human skin is between 12.5 and 18 days (Ishizaka and Ishizaka, 1975).

The structural portion of IgE that binds to basophil and mast cell membrane receptors has been identified through experimental attempts to block passive sensitization by pretreatment with fragments of the molecule (Ishizaka and Ishizaka, 1975). These studies have shown that only Fc fragments are capable of such binding. Moreover, failure of Fc' fragments to block indicates that the carboxyl terminal two thirds of the Fc fragment contains the structures essential for binding to these receptors. Further evidence in support of the last conclusion was obtained by Bennich and Dorrington (Bennich et al., 1976), who demonstrated that the long recognized heat lability of IgE is due to irreversible conformational changes in the Fc fragment, resulting in loss of its affinity for mast cell and basophil receptors. No such conformational changes were seen with the Fc' or F(ab')2 fragments. Finally, reduction and alkylation studies, using dithiothreitol, showed that cleavage of intra-epsilon chain disulfide bonds located at the junction of the hinge and Fc portions also resulted in loss of affinity of IgE molecules for their natural cell receptors (Ishizaka and Ishizaka, 1975). Since these bonds are remote from the carboxyl terminal two thirds of the Fc portion, it is postulated that their cleavage must have a secondary effect on the conformation of the Fc portion.

Role in Allergic Reactions. It is entirely possible that IgE antibodies would be essentially functionless molecules if they did not have the capacity to bind to homologous basophils or mast cells. With this capacity, they are able to trigger one of the body's most potent biologic amplification systems upon interaction with antigen to cause "explosive" reactions. These reactions are caused by the sudden release of a variety of chemical mediators from blood basophils or tissue mast cells or both subsequent to interaction of antigen with very few molecules of cell bound IgE. These cells are major sources of blood and tissue histamine and produce many other substances that mediate IgE associated hypersensitivity reactions (Wasserman, 1983). The latter include vasoactive substances, such as histamine, platelet activity factor (PAF), prostaglandin D_2 (PGD$_2$), thromboxanes, and leukotrienes C, D, and E; chemotactic factors for neutrophils, eosinophils, and other cell types; enzymes, including neutral proteases and acid hydrolases; and proteoglycans, such as heparin and chondroitin sulfates (see Chapter 5). These substances, depending upon the extent and sites of their release, may produce a wide variety of allergic reactions clinically and experimentally. They include active and passive systemic anaphylaxis, active and passive local anaphylaxis (as in the direct immediate skin test, the Prausnitz-Küstner reaction, and the homologous PCA reactions), asthma, allergic rhinitis, urticaria, and angioedema.

The events that initiate generation or release (or both) of these chemical mediators take place on and in the basophil and mast cell membranes. In the usual situation in which IgE antibodies are involved, bridging of two membrane attached antibody molecules appears to be required in order to initiate the series of biochemical events that leads to basophil or mast cell degranulation and mediator release (Ishizaka and Ishizaka, 1984). Conroy et al. (1977) have reported that the number of IgE molecules bound to the surfaces of blood basophils ranged from 4000 to 100,000 per cell for normal individuals and from 100,000 to 500,000 per cell for allergic individuals. Since these molecules most likely have many diverse specificities, the chance is remote that two IgE molecules having the same antigenic specificity would occupy adjacent Fc receptors on the cell membrane. It is known, however, that minute amounts of allergen (10^{-8} to 10^{-10}M) can trigger histamine release or induce wheal and flare skin reactions in sensitive individuals. These considerations are difficult to reconcile with the bridging hypothesis, unless one assumes that IgE molecules bound to cell surface Fc receptors are constantly moving and that antigen may bind to one IgE molecule and be carried with it by normal receptor movement until another IgE molecule with the same antigenic specificity is encountered, at which time the bridging would occur. Until recently, little was known about the molecular events that occur subsequent to IgE or IgE receptor bridging that lead to the release of histamine and other mediators. It is now known that a series of enzymatic reactions occur within the plasma membrane to provide the mechanism for signal transmission (Ishizaka and Ishizaka, 1984). Phospholipids are distributed asymmetrically throughout the plasma membrane; phosphatidyl ethanolamine (PE) is oriented toward the inner side, whereas phosphatidyl choline (PC) is oriented toward the outside (Fig. 6–2). The relative concentrations of PE and PC are regulated by the activity of two different phospholipid methyl transferase enzymes (PMT I and PMT II), which catalyze the sequential methylation of PE to form phosphatidyl-N-monomethylethanolamine (PME) and of PME to form PC. In mast cell membranes, IgE receptor bridging stimulates the activity of PMT I and PMT II. The resulting cascade of enzymatic reactions favors the formation of PC in that segment of the membrane. The PC formation causes decreased membrane viscosity and promotes the influx of Ca^{++} ions and the release of histamine. Ca^{++} ions also promote increased activity of phospholipase A_2, which catalyzes the hydrolysis of PC to form lysophosphatidyl choline. Lysophosphatidyl choline, through its detergent-like activity, promotes the fusion of plasma membranes which likely contributes to exocytosis of histamine rich granules from mast cells. IgE receptor cross-linking also causes localized activation of adenylate cyclase, which promotes the formation of cyclic AMP and the activation of cyclic AMP–dependent protein kinase, leading to the release of histamine (see Fig. 6–2).

Possible Beneficial Roles. Augmented IgE biosynthesis is associated with the atopic diseases; certain bacterial, fungal, and parasitic diseases; and a number of the primary immunodeficiency diseases (Buckley, 1987). Studies in rats experimentally infested with *Nippostrongylus braziliensis* or *Schistosoma mansoni* have implicated important roles for IgE antibodies in host defense against these parasites. It is well known that IgE antibody-antigen reactions result in the influx of eosinophils into the local site. Butterworth et al. (1977) demonstrated antibody-dependent eosinophil cytotoxicity against[51]Cr-labeled schistosomula that appears to be mediated by IgG antibody and is inhibited by antigen-antibody complexes. These workers also have demonstrated that eosinophil major basic protein can damage such larvae directly (Butterworth et al., 1979). In addition, there is evidence that IgE antibodies can interact with membrane Fc epsilon receptors on macrophages to increase the binding of these cells to *Schistosoma mansoni* schistosomula and enhance the lethal effect of IgG antibody dependent, macrophage mediated cytotoxicity (Capron et al., 1977). The predominant production of both IgA and IgE immunoglobulins by plasma cells in lymphoid tissues adjacent to mucosal surfaces suggests that, if IgE antibodies do have a protective role, it would be as mediators of local immunity (Bloch, 1976). Although there is no firm evidence either for a local protective action of IgE antibodies or for a collaborative interaction between IgA and IgE antibodies in humans, it does not seem likely from a

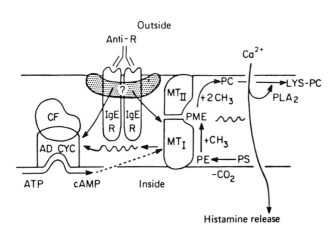

FIGURE 6–2. Schematic model for the relationship among IgE receptors (IgE R), methyltransferases (MT_I and MT_{II}), and adenylate cyclase (AD CYC) in rat mast cell membrane. Anti-R = antireceptor antibody; CF = coupling factor; PS = phosphatidylserine; PE = phosphatidylethanolamine; PME = phosphatidyl-N-monomethylethanolamine; PC = phosphatidylcholine; LYS-PC = lysophosphatidylcholine; PLA_2 = phospholipase A_2; ? = putative proteolytic enzymes. (From Ishizaka and Ishizaka, Progr. Allerg. 34:188, 1984; used with permission.)

teleologic standpoint that IgE would have survived in evolution on the basis of its harmful properties. In addition to the aforementioned roles, it also has been postulated that vasoactive substances released following the interaction of antigen with mast cell – fixed or basophil-fixed IgE antibodies may alter vascular permeability to facilitate the passage of other components of the immune system into sites where they are needed.

IgG SKIN SENSITIZING ANTIBODIES

Although IgG skin sensitizing antibodies exist in several lower species, including guinea pigs, mice, and rats (Bloch and Ohman, 1971), such antibodies have been difficult to demonstrate in humans. Investigations in the early 1970's provided some evidence for the existence of IgG homocytotropic antibodies in humans (Parish, 1973; Bryant et al., 1975). It is not likely that such antibodies cause frequent clinical problems, however, since this type of skin sensitizing activity could not be found in any of the sera obtained from 149 patients highly sensitive to a variety of allergens (Nelson and Branch, 1977). All such sera did contain IgE antibody to appropriate antigens.

Physicochemical Characteristics of IgG

IgG homocytotropic antibodies identified in all species have had molecular weights of approximately 150,000 daltons and sedimentation coefficients of 6.5S, both of which are lower than the values for IgE (see Table 6 – 2). IgG antibodies are four-chain monomers, with both inter- and intra-chain disulfide bonds, as are IgE antibodies. The IgG skin sensitizing antibodies of several lower species have been characterized as follows: (1) in the guinea pig they have been found in the IgG1a and IgG1b classes; (2) in the mouse they are IgG1; and (3) in the rat they are IgGa (Bloch and Ohman, 1971). Parish (1973) coined the term "short-term sensitizing" antibody, or IgG S-T S, for human IgG skin sensitizing antibodies. There has been considerable interest in the possibility that human IgG skin sensitizing antibodies might belong to a particular IgG subclass. Vijay and Perelmutter (1977) found that IgG4 (but no other IgG subclass) myeloma protein was capa-

ble of blocking passive sensitization of monkey skin and human basophils by IgE antibody, evidence which strongly supports such a hypothesis. Moreover, anti-IgG4 antiserum caused histamine release from human basophils sensitized by IgG4.

Biologic Properties of IgG

In order for IgG antibodies to function as skin sensitizing antibodies, they must have the capacity to bind to basophils and mast cells. Direct evidence that some IgG molecules possess this property was obtained from autoradiographic studies of basophils and from demonstration of histamine release upon treatment with anti-IgG or anti-IgG4 (Vijay and Perelmutter, 1977). As noted previously, the equilibrium constant for the binding affinity of IgG to neutrophils and monocytes has been estimated at 10^{-5}/M. Since so few IgG molecules have the capacity to bind to basophils and mast cells, IgG's binding affinity for these cell types has not been determined. Nevertheless, it is likely that the affinity is far lower than that of IgE antibodies; studies of the disappearance rate of radiolabeled IgG injected into human skin have estimated a half-life of only 2 days, in contrast to the much longer tissue half-life of IgE (Ishizaka and Ishizaka, 1975). The optimal sensitization (or latent) period for all IgG homocytotropic antibodies studied thus far has been much shorter than that for IgE, with the times ranging from 1 to 2 hours in mice and from 4 to 6 hours in humans (see Table 6 – 2) (Bloch and Ohman, 1971; Parish, 1973).

Other biologic properties that distinguish IgG skin sensitizing antibodies from those of the IgE class include the failure of reduction and alkylation or of heating at 56°C for 2 to 4 hours to affect the binding of IgG homocytotropic antibodies to basophils and mast cells in all species except the guinea pig (see Table 6 – 2) (Bloch and Ohman, 1971).

Parish (1973) used these observations to establish the IgG nature of skin sensitizing antibodies present in sera from persons who had immediate wheal and flare skin reactions to milk proteins or to bacterial antigens but who did not have demonstrable IgE antibodies to these antigens. The skin sensitizing activity was demonstrated by passive sensitization of monkey skin with both heated (56°C for up to 6 hours) and unheated sera, injecting the sera 24, 4, and 1.5 hours prior to antigen challenge. Sera from these patients showed greater reactions at the sites sensitized for 4 hours and none at those sensitized for 24 hours. Moreover, there was no difference between the sites injected with heated and unheated sera and with sera reduced with 2-mercaptoethanol.

Parish (1973) also reported that many of the sera with S-T S antibody contained precipitins. Reactions observed after 1.5 to 2.5 hours appeared to be distinguishable from Arthus reactions by virtue of the fact that no latent period is required for passive Arthus reactions. Moreover, S-T S activity was demonstrable in monkeys depleted of neutrophils and in those with greatly reduced levels of serum complement, both of which are needed for Arthus reactions.

The antigens to which IgG homocytotropic antibodies are directed appear to be more restricted than those that induce IgE antibody responses, since there have been few documented examples of IgG S-T S antibodies against pollen allergens. Parish (1973) found IgG homocytotropic antibodies in sera from patients with serum sickness due to horse globulin, from those with severe local reactions due to tetanus toxoid, from some with cutaneous vasculitis due to streptococcal infection, and from some patients with pulmonary disorders. Finally, Bryant et al. (1975) found serum IgG skin sensitizing antibodies that were neither removed by anti-IgE antibodies nor inactivated by heating or reduction and alkylation in asthmatic patients with positive bronchial provocation test results to antigens from the house dust mite, *Dermatophagoides pteronyssimus.*

METHODS OF MEASURING SKIN SENSITIZING ANTIBODIES

Skin sensitizing antibodies may be detected by immediate skin testing procedures, which involve mediator release *in vivo*, histamine release *in vitro* from peripheral leukocytes, and radioimmunoassays. Details of skin testing and indications for the various tests are given in Chapter 17; only general principles are described here.

Immediate Skin Testing

Direct Testing. This test for skin sensitizing antibodies is both the oldest and the most sensitive technique available (Stanworth, 1963; Ishizaka and Ishizaka, 1975). Allergen injected into the epidermis or placed on the abraded skin

of an allergic patient interacts with IgE molecules attached to skin mast cells and induces release of histamine, which causes a wheal and flare reaction within 5 to 15 minutes. This test detects skin sensitizing antibodies on tissue mast cells that may be relevant to the patient's allergy. The major limitation of this test is that it provides only a rough estimate of the amount of the particular IgE antibody detected for two reasons as follows: (1) it is not a primary binding assay; therefore, results are dependent on releasability of mediators from recipient mast cells and (2) the amount of IgE detected is quantifiable only in terms of the least amount of antigen required to elicit a wheal and flare reaction.

Passive Transfer Tests. Most commonly these studies have been done by injecting a 1:10 or higher dilution of serum from an allergic individual into the skin of a nonsensitized individual, as described originally by Prausnitz and Küstner in 1921 (Stanworth, 1963). This procedure thus is usually referred to as the "P-K test." After allowing time for donor IgE to bind optimally to the recipient's skin mast cells (usually 24 hours), antigen is injected into the site sensitized earlier by serum, as well as into an unsensitized site as a control. Buffer alone is injected into another sensitized site as an additional control. A wheal and flare reaction developing within 5 to 15 minutes only at the antigen injected sensitized site indicates that IgE antibodies to that antigen were present in the donor serum. In the past, this procedure was used to test for IgE antibodies in sera from patients with generalized dermatitis, dermatographia, or histories of anaphylactic reactions to drugs or insect stings, and to quantify serum IgE antibodies by sensitizing with varying dilutions of donor serum. Since the procedure carries the risk of transmitting hepatitis and other viral agents, however, it has been replaced by radioimmunoassays described subsequently.

Nonhuman primates also can be used as recipients of IgE passive transfer tests (Buckley and Metzgar, 1965). Skin sensitization of anesthetized monkeys is done in exactly the same manner as the P-K test, and a similar latent period of 24 to 48 hours is allowed to elapse before antigen challenge is given. The procedure differs from the P-K test, however, in that antigen is usually given intravenously, along with a colloidal blue dye. When antigen reacts with IgE molecules on mast cells at the previously sensitized skin site, mediators are released, resulting in increased vascular permeability; bluing occurs at the sites due to leakage of the dye from the intravascular space. This procedure is called passive cutaneous anaphylaxis (PCA), since a local anaphylactic reaction occurs at the passively sensitized skin site.

Mediator Release Procedures

Leukocyte Mediator Release. This assay detects IgE antibodies on peripheral blood basophils of allergic subjects by quantifying the amount of one or more of the primary chemical mediators released as a consequence of antigen and basophil-fixed IgE antibody interaction. It also can be used to detect IgE antibodies in the sera of allergic donors by preincubating those sera with basophils from nonsensitized subjects. The test is performed by separating leukocytes from heparinized blood by dextran sedimentation and suspending them in a buffer containing Ca^{++} and Mg^{++}. Varying quantities of allergen are added to tubes containing fixed numbers of cells, and the tubes are incubated at 37°C for 1 hour. The mediators released into the supernatants can be quantified by a variety of methods (see Chapter 5). The assay also can be used to detect serum blocking antibodies by adding sera inactivated for IgE binding by heating at 56°C for 4 hours to a parallel set of test tubes. In most studies designed to detect IgE, histamine has been measured (Brown et al., 1982). The quantity of histamine released per tube is expressed as a percentage of the total histamine available in the cells and as a function of the dose of allergen added. The amount of allergen needed to cause 50 percent histamine release usually is between 10^{-4} and 10^{-6} μg/ml (King, 1976). Histamine release assays define not only the specificity of cell bound IgE antibodies but also assess the functional integrity of mediator releasing mechanisms. However, the same following limitations apply to this method that apply to skin testing: (1) it does not measure primary binding of antigen to antibody, (2) the results in the direct assay are dependent upon the releasability of the chemical mediators from the subject's basophils (approximately 15 percent of subjects have basophils that do not release histamine *in vitro*), and (3) the amount of IgE detected in the direct assay is quantifiable only in terms of the least amount of antigen needed for 50 percent histamine (or other mediator) release. Results of leukocyte histamine release assays generally have correlated with results of skin tests, although the skin

tests are more sensitive. Because of the technical difficulty in performing mediator release tests, they are used primarily for investigational purposes. They have been particularly well suited for this, since they provide more quantifiable data than skin testing does. This type of assay also can be used to quantify IgG blocking antibody titers in patients undergoing immunotherapy. It may also be used to identify loss of cell sensitivity during immunotherapy and to study pharmacologic modulation of mediator release.

Mediator Release from Tissues. The same methods for detecting mediator release may be employed to determine mast cell–fixed IgE present in small tissue fragments or in skin *in vivo* by creating small artificial blisters. Tests have been performed with chopped human or monkey lung, with skin slices or blister fluids, and with nasal polyps. These procedures, which are used strictly as investigational tools, have the same limitations as basophil assays.

Radioimmunoassays

Radioimmunoassays have advantages over skin tests or mediator release tests in that they are performed *in vitro* and do not require either sensitized cells or tissues. The assays measure binding of antigen and IgE antibody directly rather than indirectly through mediator release. In general, however, these tests are less sensitive than skin tests because they lack the amplified read-out provided by mast cell and basophil mediator release. The types of radioimmunoassays employed in IgE measurements can be divided into those that involve competitive displacement of radiolabeled IgE (Wide, 1971) and those that involve solid phase antigen or anti-IgE and radiolabeled anti-IgE, the so-called two site or immunoradiometric assays (IRMA) (Homberger, 1986).

Competitive Displacement Assays. In these assays, antibody to IgE is allowed to react with radiolabeled purified IgE protein in antigen excess (Wide, 1971; Gleich et al., 1971). Known quantities of unlabeled IgE or unknown quantities in test samples are added to the mixtures; these molecules displace radiolabeled IgE from its binding with antibody so that less labeled IgE is bound. In solid phase assays, which employ Sephadex, microcrystalline cellulose, or filter paper discs, antibody bound IgE is separated from nonbound IgE by washing the solid phase material to remove nonspecifically

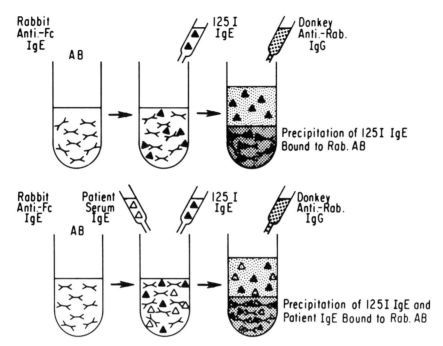

FIGURE 6–3. Principle of the double antibody radioimmunoassay for IgE, as used in my laboratory (Buckley and Fiscus, J. Clin. Invest. 55:157, 1975). This is a competitive displacement assay, i.e., the more cold IgE in the test sample, the fewer counts detected in the precipitate.

bound IgE. In double antibody radioimmunoassays, anti-IgE in solution reacts with radiolabeled and unlabeled IgE in the same manner as in the solid phase assay (Fig. 6–3). By employing a second antibody directed against the anti-IgE antibody, bound IgE is precipitated from solution and is removed by centrifugation. The quantity of bound IgE in unknown samples is determined by reading from a calibration curve established by plotting known concentrations of unlabeled IgE added against the percentage of counts per minute detected in the solid phase material or precipitate, as compared with the counts per minute in the tubes containing no unlabeled IgE. The best known version of this test is the sensitive double antibody radioimmunoassay (Gleich et al., 1971), which has been used to measure IgE concentrations in serum, body fluids, and supernatants of cultured blood mononuclear cells at concentrations as low as 0.2 ng/ml (Fiser and Buckley, 1979; Sampson and Buckley, 1981).

Two Site or Immunoradiometric Assays (IRMA). In these procedures, analogous in principle to the indirect Coombs test, either antigen or anti-IgE antibody is covalently coupled to a solid material. Either cellulose or other types of particles (Fig. 6–4), filter paper discs (Fig. 6–5), or plastic tubes or cuvettes may be used as the solid phase material. Antigen is allowed to interact with antibodies to it, or anti-IgE is permitted to react with known or unknown quantities of IgE (Wide, 1971). After 4 to 24 hours' incubation, the solid phase is washed, and radiolabeled immunospecifically purified anti-IgE is added. After a second wash, the solid phase is analyzed for radioactivity. If antigen is used for coupling, the more antigen specific IgE antibody present in the standard or test sample, the greater the radioactivity finally associated with the solid material. The most widely known version of this test is the radioallergosorbent test or RAST (see Fig. 6–4 and Fig. 6–5), but variations of this test employing other solid phase carriers of antigen are becoming legion (MAST, FAST, and so forth). RAST results usually are expressed in terms of percent of total counts of radiolabeled anti-IgE antibody added bound or in units of an arbitrary scoring system based on the counts per minute bound by a known, high titered positive serum. Jacob and Homberger (1982) found the cutoff between positive and negative scoring to be most reliably selected by defining the test result in terms of multiples of negative control counts per minute (cpm) as follows: <150 percent = negative; 150 to 250 percent = borderline, and >250 percent = positive. False negative results may be

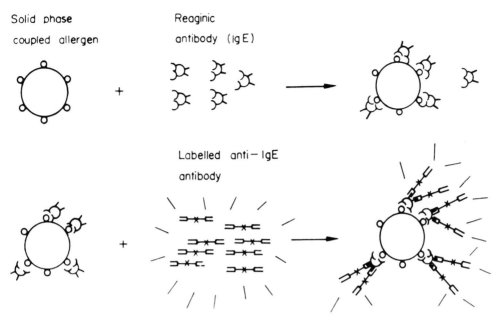

FIGURE 6–4. Principle of the radioallergosorbent test (RAST) for detecting and quantifying IgE antibodies to allergens. In this example of a two-site IRMA, the solid phase material is anti-IgE coupled to cyanagen bromide–activated cellulose particles. (From Wide, Solid Phase Antigen-Antibody Systems. *In* Kirkham and Hunter (eds.), Radioimmunoassay Methods. Edinburgh, Churchill Livingstone, Inc., 1971; used with permission.)

caused by inhibition of binding of IgE antibodies by IgG antibodies, commonly found in the sera of patients receiving allergen immunotherapy. Serial RASTs, therefore, are not helpful in monitoring IgE antibody levels in patients on allergy vaccines. The assay is most useful for detecting and semiquantifying (the actual concentrations are not determined) IgE antibodies to various allergens and for measuring the potency of various allergenic extracts. Allergen

potency can be measured by varying the amounts of standard and test allergen extracts coupled to the solid phase material (referred to as the direct RAST) or by measuring the degree that the allergen inhibits the binding of IgE antibodies in a known allergic serum to solid phase antigen (RAST inhibition).

In the situation where anti-IgE is coupled to the solid phase, the more IgE present in the standard or test sample, the greater the radioac-

FIGURE 6–5. The RAST assay using allergen coupled to a filter paper disc as the solid phase material. If anti-IgE had been coupled to the disc instead of allergen, the schematic would illustrate the paper radioimmunosorbent or PRIST test for total IgE.

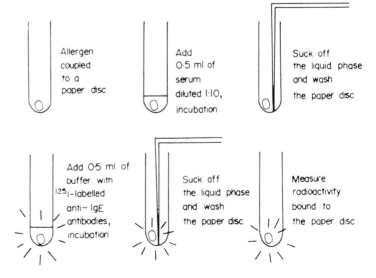

tivity ultimately associated with the solid phase. A standard curve can be constructed by plotting the counts bound against known quantities of IgE added. This method forms the basis for the well-known paper disc radioimmunosorbent (PRIST), a sensitive, accurate, and easily performed method for measuring total IgE in sera or other body fluids. Maximum precision is achieved at concentrations of IgE ranging from 7.5 to 50 IU/ml (18 to 120 ng/ml), but concentrations as low as 0.5 IU/ml (1.2 ng/ml) can be measured.

Enzyme-Linked Immunoassays (ELISA)

These assays are similar in principle and application to the two site IRMA except that the anti-IgE antibody used in the final phase is coupled to an enzyme rather than being radiolabeled. The amount of enzyme-linked anti-IgE antibody reacting with the solid phase material is detected and quantified by measuring the intensity of color that results from adding the enzyme's substrate. This technique has obvious advantages over radioimmunoassays, it is safer because it does not involve radioactivity and it does not require an expensive gamma counter.

ONTOGENY OF IgE BIOSYNTHESIS

Fetal IgE Synthesis. Miller et al. (1973) demonstrated that the human fetus is capable of synthesizing IgE as early as 11 weeks of gestation *in utero*. Synthesis of IgE may occur by 11 weeks in fetal lung and liver and by 21 weeks in fetal spleen. Even though the capacity for IgE synthesis develops very early, the fetal synthesizing rate is low in most instances, as evidenced by the low cord serum IgE concentrations (<1.0 IU/ml) and the fact that injection of anti-IgE antibody into the skin of neonates does not cause an immediate wheal and flare reaction. The latter is not due to a paucity of skin mast cells, however, since both premature and full-term newborns have been shown to be capable of developing wheal and flare reactions when they served as recipients in P-K tests (Orgel, 1975). The low rate of IgE synthesis in fetal and neonatal life correlates well with the known freedom of infants from IgE-mediated diseases up to 2 to 3 months of age.

IgE in Normal Individuals. In 114 apparently nonallergic, healthy infants, the serum IgE concentration 2 S.D. above the geometric mean was 1.5 IU/ml at birth but increased to 20 IU/ml by 1 year of age (Kjellman, 1976). In 93 nonallergic children, it was 40 IU/ml at age 2 years and peaked at 140 IU/ml at age 10 years, gradually declining thereafter. IgE concentrations reported in this study were lower overall than those in a study by Gerrard et al. (1974), possibly because the patients in the latter study were unselected and because Kjellman employed the two site IRMA PRIST assay, which generally gives lower IgE values. Nevertheless, a similar trend was seen in both studies. Geometric mean serum IgE concentrations reached adult levels by 4 years of age and then increased gradually until a maximum level was reached between 10 and 12 years of age. They then dropped sharply, to reach adult levels again by age 14 years (Fig. 6–6). Adult normal values have varied widely between laboratories because of different methods, standards, nomenclature, sample sizes, and statistical analyses employed in deriving the normative data. Published mean IgE values for normal adults have ranged from 11.8 to 74.6 IU/ml. In my laboratory, in which a double antibody radioimmunoassay is employed (Gleich et al., 1971), the normal geometric mean is 55 IU/ml, and the 95 percent confidence interval is 5 to 621 IU/ml. The latter very wide normal range is due to the fact that serum IgE concentrations in normal populations do not follow an arithmetic Gaussian distribution. For proper statistical analysis, logarithmic transformation of the data is neces-

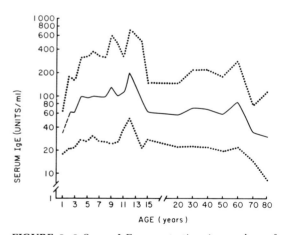

FIGURE 6–6. Serum IgE concentrations in members of 80 families. The solid line represents the geometric mean and the dotted line the anti-log of the mean log ± 1 S.D. of the logarithms of the data. (From Gerrard et al., J. Pediatr. *85*:660, 1974, as modified by Orgel, Pediatr. Clin. North Am. *22*:17, 1975; used with permission.)

sary, resulting in very broad normal ranges. This fact also means that many allergic adults have serum IgE concentrations within the normal range. The usefulness of IgE measurement in older children and adults is, therefore, not as great as in infants (see next section).

IgE and IgA in Atopic Infants and Children. In 34 infants whose IgE concentrations were followed serially throughout the first year of life, every one who developed a serum IgE concentration greater than 20 IU/ml by 1 year of age had evidence of atopic disease by 2 years of age (Table 6–4) (Orgel, 1975). An initial IgE level 1 S.D. above the mean in the first year of life in 114 infants appeared predictive of allergy in that 75 percent of those with elevated IgE levels had developed atopic or probable atopic disease 18 months later, as compared with only 6.4 percent of those with normal serum IgE levels (Kjellman, 1976). A similar trend occurred in 93 children from 2 to 14 years of age, in whom 41.7 percent of those with elevated IgE values (> 1 S.D. above mean) had obvious or probable atopy 18 months later, compared with only 5 percent of those with normal initial IgE values. Thus, serum IgE concentrations appear useful in predicting future atopy in infants and may be especially useful in evaluating the likelihood of atopy in offspring of atopic parents (Michel et al., 1980). Nevertheless, a normal serum IgE concentration at birth or during infancy does not exclude the development of atopy later.

Since both IgA and IgE are produced predominantly in paragut and pararespiratory lymphoid tissues (Ishizaka and Ishizaka, 1975; Bloch, 1976), it has been suggested that IgA deficiency may contribute to increased mucous membrane permeability to antigens, leading to stimulation of increased IgE production and consequently a greater likelihood of developing the atopic state. Evidence by Platts-Mills et al.

(1976), however, suggests that the opposite is true in atopic patients, i.e., individuals predisposed to make increased IgE antibodies have a normal or even an increased ability to produce allergen specific IgA antibodies.

GENETIC CONTROL OF IgE BIOSYNTHESIS

Since the diseases with which increased IgE production are associated have long been recognized for their heritable nature, there is reason to believe that genetic factors regulate IgE biosynthesis. As with the mode of inheritance of the atopic diseases (Lebowitz et al., 1984), however, studies done in animals and humans to date indicate that control of IgE biosynthesis appears to be multifactorial, with at least two genetic loci implicated (Levine, 1974; Orgel, 1975; Tada, 1975; Watanabe et al., 1976). One of these controls the level of IgE antibody production and appears to be unassociated with the major histocompatibility complex (MHC) (Levine, 1974; Watanabe, 1976). The other controls immune recognition of allergens and may be linked to the MHC (Levine, 1974).

Genetic Influence on Overall Level of IgE Production

IgE Production in Mice. When various strains of mice were immunized with multiple antigens, all were found to produce IgE antibodies to one or more antigens, but only certain strains exhibited high or moderate reaginic antibody responses (Levine, 1974). The differences noted in these studies pertained only to the IgE response, regardless of the antigen or dose administered. Breeding experiments dem-

TABLE 6–4. Correlation Between Serum IgE Level at 1 Year of Age and Symptoms and Signs of Atopic Disease Manifested by 2 Years of Age*

Serum IgE U/ml by 1 Year of Age	n	Symptoms or Signs of Atopic Disease by 2 Years of Age		
		DEFINITE	POSSIBLE	DEFINITE AND POSSIBLE
<10	17	2 (12 percent)	4	6 (35 percent)
10 to 20	5	1 (20 percent)	1	2 (40 percent)
20.1 to 100	6	5 (83 percent)	1	6 (100 percent)
>100	6	3 (50 percent)	3	6 (100 percent)
Total	34	11	9	20

* From Orgel, H.A.: Genetic and developmental aspects of IgE. Pediatri. Clin. N. Am. 22:17–32, 1975; used with permission.

onstrated that the genetic control for high or low IgE response in these strains was not linked to the MHC. Studies by Watanabe et al. (1976) and Chiorazzi et al. (1977) in IgE "non-responder" mice of the SJL strain and "low responder" mice of the AKR strain revealed that such animals are converted to IgE "responders" by elimination of suppressor T cell activity through irradiation or the use of cyclophosphamide. The augmented IgE production in such mice also is terminated by the transfer of syngeneic normal thymocytes or spleen cells. These findings demonstrate that poor IgE antibody formation in untreated SJL and AKR strains of mice is not based on a genetically determined inability to develop IgE responses but rather on an inherited capacity to inhibit IgE antibody formation. It is possible that high IgE "responder" humans also inherit an insufficient IgE regulatory capacity.

Human IgE Production. In several studies of serum IgE concentrations in unselected populations of adults, the distribution of values appears to be multimodal. The explanation for this distribution is not clear, but the multimodality likely is due to a combination of genetic and environmental influences. Twin studies provide strong evidence for an appreciable genetic effect on basal serum IgE concentrations (Orgel, 1975). The effect appears greater in monozygous twin adults. Those studies also demonstrated that nongenetic factors also may contribute to variability in IgE levels, making it more difficult to analyze the genetic mechanisms. Three separate population studies suggest that serum levels of IgE in humans are controlled by two alleles at a single locus (Gerrard et al., 1978). Marsh et al. (1981) hypothesized from their data that high levels of IgE are inherited as a recessive trait. Gerrard et al. (1978) presented evidence for a single major regulatory locus for serum IgE concentration, the locus having two alleles, a dominant allele designated RE and a recessive allele, re. Persons who are re/re homozygotes maintain persistently high levels of IgE, whereas persons who are heterozygotes or RE/RE homozygotes have normal or low levels. The gene frequency of re was found to be 0.489 by Gerrard et al. (1978), and the displacement was 1.67 S.D. Whether this locus is analogous to that described previously for mice, determining "high" and "low" IgE responder types, and whether the genetic control is by suppressor T cells remain to be demonstrated.

Immune Response (Ir) Genes that Control IgE Antibody Synthesis

Ir Genes in Mice. It is well established that genes controlling immune responsiveness to synthetic branched polypeptides in mice are linked to the H 2 complex (Orgel, 1975). In studies designed to investigate whether reaginic antibody responses are regulated by genes within the MHC, Levine and Vaz found clear-cut differences among inbred strains of mice in reaginic antibody responsiveness to repeated minute (0.1 μg) doses of benzylpenicilloyl-bovine γ globulin. This difference in responsiveness correlated with the H 2 genotype of the strain (Levine, 1974). It should be noted, however, that the differences among strains were demonstrable only with repeated, low dose immunization. In addition, the differences extended to general immune responsiveness to the particular antigen, rather than being unique to reagin production, in contrast to the strain differences in overall IgE responsiveness previously discussed.

Ir Genes in Humans. A number of studies have sought evidence in humans for genes analogous to Ir genes in mice (Levine, 1974; Orgel, 1975). Levine (1974) and his coworkers examined seven families with a high familial incidence of ragweed hay fever and showed that the occurrence of hay fever and intense immediate skin sensitivity to ragweed antigen E were highly correlated with a particular HLA haplotype in successive generations of allergic families. The associated haplotype varied from family to family, however, and differed for each of the seven families studied. Studies of IgE antibodies to antigen E revealed that the presence of these antibodies also correlated in most cases with the presence of hay fever. However, since some family members with the haplotype in question failed to manifest either hay fever or skin reactivity to ragweed antigen E, whereas none of those lacking the haplotype had hay fever or antigen E reactivity, Levine and his associates concluded that the presence of an Ir gene linked to a particular HLA A and B locus haplotype within a family is necessary but not sufficient for the development of an intense IgE immune response to antigen E and clinical hay fever (Levine, 1974). Similar findings were reported by Blumenthal et al. (Orgel, 1975), who studied a very large family through three generations and found that sensitivity to ragweed antigen E was associated with the HLA

A2, B12 haplotype. In contrast to these studies, Marsh et al. (1981) were unable to confirm a within family haplotype association for ragweed hay fever and skin sensitivity to antigen E. However, in populations of unrelated, highly allergic individuals, Marsh and his coworkers did report a significant correlation between skin sensitivity to the ragweed antigen Ra5 and the presence of the HLA B7 cross-reacting group of antigens. As in the studies of Levine (1974), the presence of IgG antibodies to Ra5 was found only in those able to produce IgE antibodies to Ra5. It seems probable that multiple genetic factors interact to influence the expression of IgE mediated disease in a given individual (Levine, 1974; Orgel, 1975).

T CELL REGULATION OF IgE BIOSYNTHESIS

Rodent Studies

Important observations bearing on mechanisms of IgE immunoregulation were made by Tada and his associates in 1971 when they demonstrated enhancement of ongoing IgE antibody production in the rat by treating the animals with small doses of antithymocyte serum, whole body irradiation, and adult thymectomy and splenectomy, or by administering various immunosuppressive drugs before or shortly after immunization (Tada, 1975). Further studies revealed that administration of carrier specific T lymphocytes inhibited ongoing hapten specific homocytotropic antibody formation. The augmentation of ongoing homocytotropic antibody production by immunosuppressive manipulations was surprising and paradoxical, since those workers had shown earlier that

priming of carrier specific T helper cells was necessary for production of homocytotropic antibody by hapten specific antibody forming B cells. IgE synthesis thus appeared to require T helper cells for initiation but also to be under active T suppressor cell control. Since those initial studies, the mechanisms of T cell regulation of IgE formation have been investigated extensively by various workers (Tada, 1975; Ishizaka, 1984). Information as to how thymocytes could be both inhibiting and facilitating came from further work by Tada and his coworkers (1975), who found an antigen specific T cell factor derived from mechanically disrupted rat thymocytes that had a negative regulatory effect on IgE antibody synthesis.

More recent studies of IgE immunoregulation have focused on nonantigen specific but IgE isotype specific regulatory cells and factors (Ishizaka, 1984). Working with *Nippostrongylus braziliensis* infested rats, Ishizaka et al. (1984) were able to demonstrate that mesenteric lymph node cells produced factors that had the capacity to bind IgE. If the cells were obtained 2 weeks after infestation, they produced a factor that caused enhanced IgE production; if they were obtained 1 week after infestation, they produced a factor that suppressed IgE synthesis. Both factors are produced by rat T helper cells, have molecular weights of 13,000 to 15,000 daltons and bind IgE, but there is a mannose-rich oligosaccharide on the enhancing factor (Table 6–5). Studies with complete Freund adjuvant treated rats demonstrated that T cells (having a phenotype corresponding to suppressor T cells in humans) produce a glycosylation inhibiting factor, which appears to be a fragment of lipomodulin. It inhibits phospholipase activity, thereby inhibiting glycosylation of the binding factors produced by the helper T

TABLE 6–5. Comparisons Between IgE-Potentiating Factor and IgE-Suppressive Factor*

Properties	IgE-Potentiating Factor	IgE-Suppressive Factor
Source	Fc R + W 3/25 + T cells†	W 3/25 + T cells†
Molecular weight	13,000 to 15,000	13,000 to 15,000
Affinity for IgE	+	+
Affinity for		
Lentil lectin	+	−
Concanavalin A	+	−
Peanut agglutinin	−	+

* Modified from Ishizaka, K.: Ann. Rev. Immunol. 2:159, 1984.
† W 3/25 + T cells are rat T helper cells.

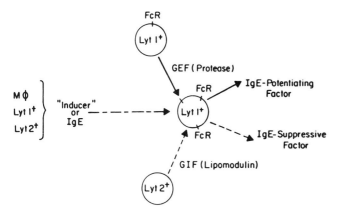

FIGURE 6-7. Schematic model for the selective formation of rat IgE-potentiating factor or IgE-suppressive factor. FcR$^+$ Lyt 1$^+$ T helper cells form IgE-potentiating factor in the presence of GEF, produced by a different T helper cell, but the same T helper cells form IgE-suppressive factor in the presence of GIF, produced by a T suppressor cell. (From Ishizaka, Ann. Rev. Immunol. 2:159, 1984; used with permission.)

cells, so that IgE suppressor factors are formed (Fig. 6-7). In contrast, rats given *Bordetella pertussis* were found to have Fc receptor positive helper T cells that produced a glycosylation enhancing factor. This factor has kallikrein-like activity and is postulated to enhance the glycosylation of IgE binding factors through the activation of phospholipase, so that IgE potentiating factors are formed (see Fig. 6-7). Ishizaka, Huff, and coworkers have now developed rat-mouse (Huff et al., 1982) and human (Huff and Ishizaka, 1984) T cell hybridomas that produce IgE binding factors; Kishimoto, Sugimura, and coworkers (Sugimura et al., 1982) have murine hybridomas producing IgE suppressor molecules. Huff et al. (1984) have demonstrated the presence of an antigenic determinant common to rat IgE potentiating factor, IgE suppressive factor, and FcεR on T and B lymphocytes. However, a curious finding concerning cDNA clones isolated from such rat-mouse hybridomas and encoding these rodent IgE binding factors is their remarkable homology to gag and DNA endonuclease coding sequences of the endogenous, retrovirus-like, intracisternal A particle gene families of the Syrian hamster and mouse (Toh et al., 1985; Moore et al., 1986). Recently, an IgE potentiating activity was found in the supernatants of concanavalin A stimulated murine T helper cell clones, which appears to be identical with B cell differentiation factor (Coffman and Carty, 1986). It remains to be shown whether this activity has any structural similarity to the rat IgE potentiating factor described by Ishizaka (1984). In 1981, Ishizaka and Sandberg reported the detection of IgE binding factors in supernatants of cultured blood lymphocytes from allergic humans. However, little progress had been made until recently on the functional characterization of human IgE binding factors (see subsequent discussion).

Cells Bearing Fc Epsilon Receptors

In addition to high affinity Fc epsilon receptors (Fcε R) on basophils and mast cells, other types of cells also have been found to have lower affinity Fcε R, including lymphocytes, monocytes, and eosinophils (Spiegelberg, 1984). Fcε R+ cells have been detected in normal human peripheral blood and in increased numbers in atopic subjects; these were initially described primarily among the B cell population (Spiegelberg, 1984). However, there have been reports of Fcε R detection on human T cells (Yodoi and Ishizaka, 1979 and 1980; Ishizaka and Sandberg, 1981). Similar to the situation with lymph node cells from *Nippostrongylus braziliensis* infested rats, incubation of human mononuclear blood cells (MNC) with IgE and antigen or addition of IgE to mixed leukocyte cultures reportedly increase the proportion of Fcε R+ cells (Yodoi and Ishizaka, 1980; Ishizaka and Sandberg, 1981). Soluble IgE binding factors (BFs) were also detected in the supernatants (1) of blood mononuclear cells from ragweed sensitive patients when incubated with antigen E plus IgE; (2) of two way, mixed leukocyte culture of cells from two normal individuals followed by incubation with IgE; and (3) of normal blood T cells cultured in the presence of interleukin-2 (IL-2) then incubated with IgE (Ishizaka and Sandberg, 1981). However, Thompson, Spiegelberg, and I (1985) enumerated T cells bearing Fcε R in patients with the hyper IgE syndrome and found few if any Fcε R+ T cells. Thompson et al. (1983) had had similar findings in patients with atopic eczema and elevated serum IgE concentrations. These observations are consistent with recent findings by Suemara, Kishimoto, and coworkers (1986), using monoclonal antibodies to lymphocyte Fcε Rs, that (1) such receptors are present only on a subset of B lymphocytes (IgM+, IgD+), (2) they could not be induced on T lymphocytes even after incubation with IgE and IL-2, and (3) they are not present on T lymphocytes from patients with the hyper IgE syndrome. Indeed, recent studies by that group have shown that the Fcε R on B lymphocytes is antigenically identical to the B cell surface antigen CD23 (Owaki et al., 1987). It has been postulated that the Fcε R is transiently expressed on mature B cells prior to isotype switching.

Immunodeficiency Disorders Characterized by Excessive IgE Production

The most convincing evidence to date suggesting an association between impaired thymus dependent immunity and excessive IgE production in humans derives primarily from associations found in patients with certain types of immunodeficiency diseases (Buckley and Fiscus, 1975). Patients with partial deficiencies in thymus dependent immunity may have sufficient numbers of T helper cells for initiation of IgE antibody formation but an inadequate number of T suppressor cells, resulting in augmented IgE biosynthesis. The regular association of increased IgE biosynthesis with a particular immunodeficiency disorder was first noted in patients with the Wiskott-Aldrich syndrome (Buckley, 1987). Later, my associates and I described two adolescent boys with lifelong histories of severe recurrent staphylococcal abscesses involving the skin, lungs, and joints, who had exceptionally high serum IgE concentrations but normal concentrations of other immunoglobulins (Buckley and Sampson, 1981; Buckley, 1987). In 1972, Polmar et al. reported that an infant with DiGeorge syndrome consistently had an elevated serum IgE concentration, and in 1973 Kikkawa et al. first described a high serum IgE concentration in an infant with a variant of thymic alymphoplasia (the so-called Nezelof syndrome) (see Buckley, 1987). In other studies in my laboratory (Buckley and Fiscus, 1975), concentrations of IgE were measured in sera from 165 patients with a variety of well-defined primary immunodeficiency disorders. IgE concentrations were significantly lower than normal in patients who had marked deficiencies in all three major immunoglobulin classes, such as those with severe combined immunodeficiency and X-linked and non-X-linked agammaglobulinemia. In ad-

dition, IgE concentrations were depressed in patients with X-linked immunodeficiency with hyper IgM and in those with ataxia telangiectasia. In contrast, IgE values were significantly elevated in patients with the Wiskott-Aldrich and Nezelof syndromes, with the selective IgA deficiency, and with the hyper IgE syndrome. Except for the patients with selective IgA deficiency, all immunodeficiency patients with excessive IgE production have had impaired but not absent cell mediated immunity (Buckley, 1987). The fact that elevated IgE production also has been associated with graft versus host disease following bone marrow transplantation (when there are T cell subset imbalances) is further evidence for an important role for T cell regulation of human IgE synthesis (Ringden et al., 1983; Sindel et al., 1984).

Studies of Human IgE Biosynthesis

Direct examination of cellular regulatory events in human IgE antibody synthesis has not been possible due to an inability to conduct experiments with cells from lymphoid organs *in vitro* or in human subjects *in vivo*, as has been done in rodents. Thus, efforts in the study of human IgE regulation have involved mainly the only readily accessible tissue, i.e., venous blood (Fiser and Buckley, 1979; Sampson and Buckley, 1981). However, study of IgE production *in vitro* has been difficult, owing to the very small quantities of IgE made by blood lymphocytes even in disease states characterized by extremely elevated serum IgE concentrations (Massicott and Ishizaka, 1986). An additional limitation is that, unlike blood B cell production of IgG, IgA, and IgM, these lymphocytes fail to respond with augmented IgE production upon stimulation with polyclonal B cell activators, such as pokeweed mitogen, *Staphylococcus aureus* Cowan I, and Epstein-Barr virus. While low nanogram quantities of IgE have been detected in supernatants of cultured mononuclear blood cells from patients with elevated serum IgE concentrations, it still is not clear in most cases how much of this was actually synthesized by the cultured cells or how much was preformed *in vivo* and merely released into the supernatant during incubation. Though much has been published about *in vitro* IgE synthesis in humans over the past 8 years, most findings, interpretations, and conclusions are suspect because of two major technical problems. The first of these is the failure to appreciate that, because of the very small quantities of IgE being detected, all preformed IgE must be accounted for before one can actually say that "synthesis" has occurred. A variety of means has been used in attempts to do this, including the addition of protein synthesis inhibitors (puromycin, cyclohexamide) to parallel cultures of control cells, freezing and thawing control cells on day zero, and the addition of 1 N HCl to control cells on day zero and to experimental cells at the time of harvest (Turner et al., 1983). The last method results in release of more than twice as much preformed IgE as any other (Table 6–6). Few published studies have employed that method in controlling for preformed IgE. In my laboratory, donors whose cells had been considered to be good producers of IgE were found to actually synthesize no IgE *in vitro* when all of the preformed IgE was accounted for by the 1 N HCl method (see Table 6–6). However, a few atopic or hyper IgE syndrome donors' cells have been found to synthesize more than two-fold the preformed amount, albeit very low nanogram quantities. A second major technical problem in many published studies has been falsely high supernatant IgE measurements due to the detection of IgG molecules because of contaminating antibodies in the anti-IgE reagent that recognize a cross-reactive idiotype on IgG molecules (Spiegelberg et al., 1983). When both of

these sources of technical artifact are eliminated from *in vitro* studies, there are few donors whose B cells truly synthesize IgE, and the amounts produced rarely exceed 1 to 2 ng/ml. In a recent multicenter (22) study evaluating the sensitivity, specificity, and precision of different methods of measuring IgE in culture supernatant, wide variability was found in all of these parameters; moreover, only 13 of the 22 laboratories could detect any IgE in a sample containing 500 pg/ml (Helm et al., 1986). These problems point out the limited usefulness of mononuclear blood cell cultures in studies of human IgE regulation (Massicot and Ishizaka, 1986).

Without a reproducibly positive system of *in vitro* human IgE production, it has been impossible to evaluate the effects of regulatory cells and factors on that production, as has been done in rodent studies (Ishizaka, 1984). The most promising evidence to suggest that human blood lymphocytes can be used for the study of IgE immunoregulation comes from the work of Lanzavecchia and Parodi (1984) who reported the induction of synthesis of nanogram quantities of IgE by normal B lymphocytes by culturing them with alloreactive T helper cell clones, having specificity for HLA Class II antigens on their surfaces. Using this technique, these workers estimated that from 1 in 2200 to 1 in 6000 B cells in the blood of normal donors can be activated to produce measurable amounts of IgE. This effect is not isotype specific, however, as such alloreactive T cell clones trigger B cell synthesis of all isotypes. Cloned human antigen specific T helper cells also were shown to be capable of triggering antigen specific B cells to produce antibody, and it has been estimated that a single B cell so activated is capable of producing 10 ng of antibody (Lanzavecchia et al., 1983). Thus, if these approaches can be applied reproducibly for the stimulation of IgE-producing B cells, it seems likely that the quantities of IgE (and even of allergen specific IgE) synthesized *in vitro* should be well within the sensitivity of immunoassays and that such systems could lend themselves to studies of cellular and molecular regulation of IgE. Because of a lack of such a system thus far, recent studies of the activities of human IgE binding factors had to be performed on rat mesenteric lymph node cells (Huff et al., 1986). The fact that human molecules with the same physicochemical characteristics as rat IgE suppressive and potentiating factors exhibited the same immunoregulatory activities strongly suggests that

TABLE 6–6. Evaluation of Methods to Determine Preformed IgE*

Treatment	Number of Days Incubation	IgE (pg/ml) DONOR NO. 1	IgE (pg/ml) DONOR NO. 2
Freeze-thaw four times day 0	0	380	<200
	2	490	<200
	4	620	<200
	6	1030	<200
	8	1190	<200
	10	1320	<200
	12	1240	<200
Freeze-thaw four times day 0 plus 1 N HCl	0	2250	410
1 N HCl only	0	2480	380
Culture cells 12 days and then freeze-thaw four times	12	2930	<200
Culture cells 12 days and then freeze-thaw four times plus 1 N HCl	12	2250	320
Culture cells 12 days and then 1 N HCl only	12	2080	—

*Data from Buckley, R.H. In Massicot, J.G., Ishizaka, K.: J. Allergy Clin. Immunol. 77:544, 1986; used with permission.

human IgE synthesis is controlled by mechanisms similar to those in the rat.

REFERENCES

Bennich, H., Johansson, S.G.O., Bahr-Lindstrom, H., and Karlsson, T.: Function and structure of immunoglobulin E (IgE). *In* Johansson, S.G.O., Strandberg, K., and Uvnas, B. (eds.): *Molecular and Biological Aspects of the Acute Allergic Reaction.* New York, Plenum Press, 1976.

Bloch, K.J.: The special relationship of IgA and IgE antibodies to mucosal surfaces. *In* Bouheys, A. (ed.): *Lung Cells in Disease.* Amsterdam, North-Holland, 1976.

Bloch, K.J., and Ohman, J.L.: The stable homocytotropic antibodies of guinea pig, mouse and rat. Some indirect evidence for the *in vitro* interaction of homocytotropic antibodies of two different rat immunoglobulin classes at a common receptor on target cells. *In* Austen, K.F., and Becker, E.L. (eds.): *Biochemistry of the Acute Allergic Reaction.* Oxford, Blackwell Scientific Publications, Ltd., 1971.

Brown, M.J., Ind, P.W., Causon, R., and Lee, T.H.: A novel double isotope technique for enzymatic assay of plasma histamine — application to estimation of mast cell activation assessed by antigen challenge in asthmatics. J. Allerg. Clin. Immunol. 69:20, 1982.

Bryant, D.H., Burns, M.W., and Lazarus, L.: Identification of IgG antibody as a carrier of reaginic activity in asthmatic patients. J Allergy Clin. Immunol. 56:417, 1975.

Buckley, R.H.: Disorders of the IgE system. *In* Stiehm, E.R. (ed.): *Immunologic Disorders of Infancy and Childhood,* 3rd ed. Philadelphia, W.B. Saunders Co., 1987.

Buckley, R.H., and Fiscus, S.A.: Serum IgD and IgE concentrations in immunodeficiency diseases. J. Clin. Invest. 55:157, 1975.

Buckley, R.H., and Metzgar, R.S.: The use of nonhuman primates for studies of reagin. J. Allergy Clin. Immunol. 36:382, 1965.

Buckley, R.H., and Sampson, H.A.: The hyperimmunoglobulinemia E syndrome. *In* Franklin E.C. (ed.): *Clinical Immunology Update.* New York, Elsevier Science Publishing Co., 1981.

Butterworth, A.E., Remold, H.G., Houba, U., David, J.R., Franks, D., David, P.H., and Sturrock, R.F.: Antibody-dependent eosinophil-mediated damage to ^{51}Cr-labelled schistosomula of *Schistosoma mansoni:* Mediation by IgG and inhibition by antigen-antibody complexes. J. Immunol. 118:2230, 1977.

Butterworth, A.E., Wassom, D.L., Gleich, G.J., Loegering, D.A., and David, J.R.: Damage to schistosomula of *Schistosoma mansoni* induced directly by eosinophil major basic protein. J. Immunol. 122:221, 1979.

Capron, A., Dessaint, J.P., Joseph, M., Torpier, G., Capron, M., Rousseaux, R., Santoro, F., and Bazin, H.: IgE and cells in schistosomiasis. Am. J. Trop. Med. Hyg. 26:39, 1977.

Chiorazzi, N., Fox, D.A., and Katz, D.H.: Hapten-specific IgE antibodies in mice. VII. Conversion of IgE "non-responder" strains to IgE "responders" by elimination of suppressor T cell activity. J. Immunol. 118:48, 1977.

Coffman, R.L., and Carty, J.: A T cell activity that enhances polyclonal IgE production and its inhibition by interferon-γ. J. Immunol. 136:949, 1986.

Conroy, M.C., Adkinson, N.F., Jr., and Lichtenstein, L.M.: Measurement of IgE on human basophils: Relation to serum IgE and anti-IgE–induced histamine release. J. Immunol. 118:1317, 1977.

Fiser, P.M., and Buckley, R.H.: Human IgE biosynthesis *in vitro:* Studies with atopic and normal blood mononuclear cells and subpopulations. J. Immunol. 123:1788, 1979.

Gerrard, J.W., Horne, S., Vickers, P., Mackenzie, J.W.A., Goluboff, N., Garson, J.Z., and Maningas, C.S.: Serum IgE levels in parents and children. J. Pediatr. 85:660, 1974.

Gerrard, J.W., Rao, D.C., and Morton, N.E.: A genetic study of immunoglobulin E. Am. J. Hum. Genet. 30:46, 1978.

Gleich, G.J., Averbeck, A.K., and Swedlund, H.A.: Measurement of IgE in normal and allergic serum by radioimmunoassay. J. Lab. Clin. Med. 77:690, 1971.

Helm, R.M., Buckley, R.H., Adkinson, N.F., Squillace, D.L., Gleich, G.J., and Yunginger, J.W.: Variability of IgE protein measurement in cell culture supernatants: Results from a multicenter collaborative study. J. Allerg. Clin. Immunol. 77:880, 1986.

Homberger, H.A.: Diagnosis of allergy: *In vitro* testing. CRC Crit. Rev. Clin. Lab. Sci. 23:279, 1986.

Huff, T.F., and Ishizaka, K.: Formation of IgE binding factors by human T cell hybridomas. Proc. Natl. Acad. Sci. (USA) 81:1514, 1984.

Huff, T.F., Jardieu, P., and Ishizaka, K: Regulatory effects of human IgE-binding factors on the IgE response of rat lymphocytes. J. Immunol. 136:955, 1986.

Huff, T.F., Uede, T., and Ishizaka, K.: Formation of rat IgE-binding factors by rat-mouse T cell hybridomas. J. Immunol. 129:509, 1982.

Huff, T.F., Yodoi, J., Uede, T., and Ishizaka, K.: Presence of an antigenic determinant common to rat IgE-potentiating factor, IgE-suppressive factor, and Fcε R receptors on T and B lymphocytes. J. Immunol. 132:406, 1984.

Ishizaka, K.: Regulation of IgE synthesis. Ann. Rev. Immunol. 2:159, 1984.

Ishizaka, K., and Sandberg, K.: Formation of IgE binding factors by human T lymphocytes. J. Immunol. 126:1692, 1981.

Ishizaka, T., and Ishizaka, K.: Biology of immunoglobulin E. Progr. Allergy 19:60, 1975.

Ishizaka, T., and Ishizaka, K.: Activation of mast cells for mediator release through IgE receptors. Prog. Allergy 34:188, 1984.

Jacob, G.L., and Homberger, H.A.: The analytical accuracy of specific IgE antibody results determined by a blind proficiency survey. J. Allergy Clin. Immunol. 69:110, 1982.

Johansson, S.G.O., and Bennich, H.H.: The clinical impact of the discovery of IgE. Ann. Allergy 48:325, 1982.

King, T.P.: Chemical and biologic properties of some atopic allergens. Adv. Immunol. 23:77, 1976.

Kjellman, N.-I.M.: Predictive value of high IgE levels in children. Acta Paediatr. Scand. 65:465, 1976.

Lanzavecchia, A., and Parodi, B.: *In vitro* stimulation of IgE production at a single precursor level by human alloreactive T helper clones. Clin. Exp. Immunol. 55:197, 1984.

Lanzavecchia, A., Parodi, B., and Celada, F.: Activation of human B lymphocytes: Frequency of antigen-specific B cells triggered by alloreactive or by antigen-specific T cell clones. Eur. J. Immunol. 13:733, 1983.

Lebowitz, M.D., Barbee, R., and Burows, B.: Family concordance of IgE, atopy and disease. J. Allergy Clin. Immunol. 73:259, 1984.

Levine, B.B.: Genetics of atopic allergy and reagin production. *In* Brostoff, J. (ed.): *Clinical Immunology-Allergy in Paediatric Medicine.* Oxford, Blackwell Scientific Publications, Ltd., 1974.

Marsh, D.G., Meyers, D.A., and Bias, W.B.: The epidemiology and genetics of atopic allergy. N. Engl. J. Med. 305:1551, 1981.

Massicot, J.G., and Ishizaka, K.: Workshop on measurement of *in vitro* IgE synthesis and regulation of IgE synthesis. J. Allergy Clin. Immunol. 77:544, 1986.

Michel, F.B., Bousquet, J., Greiller, P., Robinet-Levy, M., and Coulomb, Y.: Comparison of cord blood immunoglobulin E concentrations and maternal allergy for the prediction of atopic diseases in infancy. J. Allergy Clin. Immunol. 65:422, 1980.

Miller, D.L., Hirvonin, T., and Gitlin, D.: Synthesis of IgE by the human conceptus. J. Allergy Clin. Immunol. 52:182, 1973.

Moore, K.W., Jardieu, P., Miety, J.A., Trounstine, M.L., Kuff, E.L., Ishizaka, K., and Martens, C.L.: Rodent IgE-binding factor genes are members of an endogenous, retrovirus-like gene family. J. Immunol. 136:4283, 1986.

Nelson, H.S., and Branch, L.B.: Incidence of IgG short-term sensitizing antibodies in an allergic population. J. Allergy Clin. Immunol. 60:266, 1977.

Orgel, H.A.: Genetic and developmental aspects of IgE. Pediatr. Clin. North Am. 22:17, 1975.

Ovary, Z., Benacerraf, B., and Bloch, K.J.: Properties of guinea pig 7S antibodies. II. Identification of antibodies involved in passive cutaneous and systemic anaphylaxis. J. Exp. Med. 117:951, 1963.

Owaki, H., Kikutani, H., Suemura, M., Yamasaki, K., Yukawa, K., Yokota, A., Nakamura, H., Barsumean, E.L., Hardy, R.R., and Kishimoto, T.: A B cell specific differentiation antigen, CD23, is a receptor for IgE (Fcε R) on lymphocytes. J. Immunol. (in press), 1987.

Parish, W.E.: Reaginic and non-reaginic reactions on anaphylactic participating cells. *In* Goodfriend, L., Sehon, A.H., and Orange, R.P. (eds.): *Mechanisms of Allergy: Reagin-mediated Hypersensitivity.* New York, Marcel Dekker, Inc., 1973.

Platts-Mills, T.A.E., Von Maur, R.K., Ishizaka, K., Norman, P.S., and Lichtenstein, L.M.: IgA and IgG anti-ragweed antibodies in nasal secretions: Quantitative measurements of antibodies and correlation with inhibition of histamine release. J. Clin. Invest. 57:1041, 1976.

Ringden, O., Persson, U., and Johansson, S.G.O.: Are increased IgE levels a signal of an acute graft-versus-host reaction? Immunol. Rev. 71:57, 1983.

Sampson, H.A., and Buckley, R.H.: Human IgE synthesis *in vitro*: A reassessment. J. Immunol. 127:829, 1981.

Sindel, L.J., Buckley, R.H., Schiff, S.E., Ward, F.E., Mickey, G.H., Huang, A.T., Naspitz, C., and Koren, H.: Severe combined immunodeficiency with natural killer cell predominance: Abrogation of graft-versus-host disease and immunologic reconstitution with HLA identical bone marrow cells. J. Allergy Clin. Immunol. 73:829, 1984.

Spiegelberg, H.L.: Structure and function of Fc receptor for IgE on lymphocytes, monocytes and macrophages. Adv. Immunol. 35:61, 1984.

Spiegelberg, H.L., Plummer, J.M., Ruedi, J., Thompson, L.F., Mellon, M.H., and Zeiger, R.S.: Lack of pokeweed mitogen induced IgE formation *in vitro* by human peripheral blood mononuclear cells: Detection of cross-reacting idiotypic determinants on polyclonal Ig by antibodies to a single IgE myeloma protein. J. Immunol. 131:3001, 1983.

Stanworth, D.R.: Reaginic antibodies. Adv. Immunol. 3:181, 1963.

Suemura, M., Kikutani, H., Barsumian, E.L., Hattori, Y., Kishimoto, S., Sato, R., Maeda, A., Nakamura, H., Owaki, H., Hardy, R.R., and Kishimoto, T.: Monoclonal anti-Fcε receptor antibodies with different specificities and studies on the expression of Fcε receptors on human B and T cells. J. Immunol. 137:1214, 1986.

Sugimura, K., Nakanishi, K., Maeda, K., Kashiwamura, S-I., Suemura, M., Shiko, O., Yamamura, Y., and Kishimoto, T.: The involvement of two distinct subsets of T cells for the expression of the IgE class-specific suppression: Establishment and characterization of PC-specific, T 15 idiotype positive T hybridomas and IgE class-specific, antigen-nonspecific T hybridomas. J. Immunol. 128:1637, 1982.

Tada, T.: Regulation of reaginic antibody formation in animals. Progr. Allergy 19:122, 1975.

Thompson, L.F., Mellon, M.H., Zeiger, R.S., and Spiegelberg, H.L.: Characterization with monoclonal antibodies of T lymphocytes bearing Fc receptors for IgE (Tε cells) and IgG (Tγ cells) in atopic patients. J. Immunol. 131:2772, 1983.

Thompson, L.F., Spiegelberg, H.L., and Buckley, R.H.: IgE Fc receptor positive T and B lymphocytes in patients with the hyper IgE syndrome. Clin. Exp. Immunol. 59:77, 1985.

Toh, H., Ono, M., and Miyata, T.: Retroviral gag and DNA endonuclease coding sequences in IgE-binding factor gene. Nature 318:388, 1985.

Turner, K.J., Holt, P.G., Holt, B.J., and Cameron, K.J.: *In vitro* synthesis of IgE by human peripheral blood leukocytes. III. Release of preformed antibody. Clin. Exp. Immunol. 51:387, 1983.

Vijay, H.M., and Perelmutter, L.: Inhibition of reagin-mediated PCA reactions in monkeys and histamine release from human leukocytes by human IgG4 subclass. Int. Arch. Allergy Appl. Immunol. 53:78, 1977.

Waldmann, T.A., Iio, A., Ogawa, M., McIntyre, O.R., and Strober, W.: The metabolism of IgE: Studies in normal individuals and in a patient with IgE myeloma. J. Immunol. 117:1139, 1976.

Wasserman, S.I.: Mediators of hypersensitivity. J. Allergy Clin. Immunol. 72:101, 1983.

Watanabe, N., Kojima, S., and Ovary, Z.: Suppression of IgE antibody production in SJL mice. I. Nonspecific suppressor T cells. J. Exp. Med. 143:833, 1976.

Wide, L.: Solid phase antigen-antibody systems. *In* Kirkham, K.E., and Hunter, W.M. (eds.): *Radioimmunoassay Methods.* Edinburgh, Churchill Livingstone, Inc., 1971.

Wide, L.: Clinical significance of measurement of reaginic (IgE) antibody by RAST. *In* Brostoff, J. (ed.): *Clinical Immunology-Allergy in Paediatric Medicine.* Oxford, Blackwell Scientific Publications, Ltd., 1974.

Yodoi, J., and Ishizaka, K.: Lymphocytes bearing Fc receptors for IgE. 1. Presence of human and rat lymphocytes with Fcε receptors. J. Immunol. 122:2577, 1979.

Yodoi, J., and Ishizaka, K.: Induction of Fcε receptor bearing cells *in vitro* in human peripheral lymphocytes. J. Immunol. 124:934, 1980.

7

Non-IgE Antibody in Allergic Disease

DOUGLAS C. HEINER, M.D.

Von Pirquet initially used the word *allergy* to describe an altered immune responsiveness to a foreign substance. Common usage has since restricted the term largely to unusual responses not seen in the majority of individuals exposed to comparable amounts of a particular foreign substance. A few authors of medical literature and some physicians restrict the term to indicate only those conditions that are IgE mediated. This is an arbitrary restriction that eliminates from consideration certain instances of hypersensitivity, including many that have delayed type onsets. Even if excessive responses other than IgE were not considered to be allergic, it would be essential to understand the interrelationships between different immunoglobulin classes and the roles played by both humoral and cellular components of immune responses. Non-IgE antibody responses as well as cell-mediated immune responses may occur alone or may accompany IgE-mediated responses, modifying their intensity and duration and contributing to clinical manifestations of disease. Thus, the importance of recognizing non-IgE antibodies and of understanding how they participate in clinical responses is evident.

Since the first edition of this book was published, much has been learned about the genetic mechanisms of antibody production and the importance of IgG subclasses. We now know that there is not a single gene for IgG heavy chains but separate genes directing the synthesis of each of four IgG subclasses, IgG1–4, and two genes for IgA1–2. Subclass responses thus will be considered in this chapter. Different kinds of humoral immune responses that occur, with or without concomitant involvement of IgE, also are reviewed as are certain immunoregulatory mechanisms.

The classification of allergic responses by Gell and Coombs into four major categories has been helpful over the years in the study and understanding of hypersensitivity disorders. As originally stated, it is an oversimplification of the situation actually encountered in the laboratory or observed in the patient. Nevertheless, there is utility for this classification. Briefly, tissue damage is considered in the following four general categories (Coombs and Gell, 1975):

Type I or *Anaphylactic Reactions.* IgE antibodies attached to specific receptors on basophils or mast cells are the classic examples. Antibody that, on contact with antigen, triggers the release of chemical mediators from the cells, results in a local or systemic anaphylactic response. It is now recognized that IgE-mediated reactions may manifest themselves rapidly or evolve over a few hours. Considerations involving non-IgE antibodies are discussed in subsequent sections.

Type II or *Cytotoxic Reactions.* These involve antibody directed towards a cell component or an antigen affixed to the cell. Damage to the cell can then result from the action of complement or mononuclear cells that are focused onto the cell surface by the antibody.

Type III or *Antigen-Antibody Complex Induced Tissue Injury.* This usually is due to microprecipitates in or around small blood vessels or basement membranes. The greatest damage is caused by immune complexes of 1 million daltons or more molecular weight formed at equivalence or slight antigen excess which are capable of activating complement.

Type IV or *Delayed Type (Cell-Mediated) Tissue Damage.* This classically is due to the triggering of sensitized T lymphocytes (bearing antigen specific receptors on the cell surface) which, on contact with antigen, release lymphokines. Cell-mediated cytotoxicity ensues.

HOMOCYTOTROPIC IgG ANTIBODY

It has long been known that there are two distinct types of cytotropic antibody response in rodents involving antibodies with an affinity for mediator releasing cells (Becker, 1971). Homocytotropic antibodies adhere to specific cells in animals of the same species. The cells that possess receptors for the immunoglobulin are considered to be sensitized when a critical density of specific antibody has accumulated on the cell surface, so that on exposure to small or moderate amounts of antigen, chemical mediators are released and an allergic response ensues.

IgE antibodies are the classic homocytotropic antibodies (see Chapter 6). They are denatured by heating at 56°C, after which they no longer bind to cellular receptors; they require a latent period of several hours or days following injection into a recipient's skin before maximal passive cutaneous anaphylactic (PCA) responses occur; they persist at the local site for several days or weeks; and the PCA response (Prausnitz-Küstner response in humans) can be blocked by prior exposure of the involved basophils or mast cells to an excess of purified E myeloma protein or can be abrogated by specific removal of IgE from the donor serum before passive transfer. A second type of homocytotropic antibody also passively sensitizes recipient skin for PCA reactions. These antibodies, however, are heat stable at 56°C; they do not require a prolonged latent period for maximal expression; and passive sensitization usually lasts less than 36 hours. Maximal responses can be obtained within a few hours or less of passive sensitization. Sensitizing activity of rodent serum is abrogated by specific removal of IgG1 before it is used for passive transfer.

Several investigators have performed experiments that suggest human IgG antibodies also may be homocytotropic and contribute to allergic responses. In these instances, the characteristics of the IgG antibody were similar to those of rodent IgG1.

The majority of these investigators considered IgG4 to be the most likely candidate for non-IgE homocytotropic antibodies. IgG4 levels are elevated in subjects with atopic dermatitis and asthma, particularly in those with positive delayed onset bronchial challenges. However, a number of workers have found no evidence that IgG4 acts as a homocytotropic antibody to cause histamine release from human basophils. Van der Giessen et al. (1976) were the first to suggest that IgG4 antibodies may have a "blocking" function, since they increase dramatically following hyposensitization with pollen antigens. Many studies have shown that IgG4 antibodies are markedly elevated in beekeepers who have frequent stings yet show no evidence of hypersensitivity. Thus, if IgG4 antibodies are involved in the production of allergic symptoms, this must occur only under special circumstances such as might exist if antigen-antibody complexes had a pathogenic role in a narrowly defined range of antibody content. Receptors for IgG are present on human basophils, and these bind aggregated IgG much more avidly than uncomplexed IgG.

Studies in our laboratory and others suggest that IgG4 antibodies generally are present in higher concentrations in untreated allergic patients than in nonallergic subjects exposed to a similar amount of a given allergen. Although there is little evidence that IgG4 antibodies contribute significantly to allergic responses when elevated above the normal range, they may provide a clue that a subject is allergic to a specific allergen. The problem lies in defining ranges of normal. This should involve the study of 50 or more nonallergic subjects of a given sex and age for each antigen and for each technique used. At the present time, only a few laboratories have determined the normal ranges of serum IgG4 antibody concentrations to any antigens. Until such ranges are determined, utilization of IgG or IgG4 antibodies in the diagnostic evaluation of allergic diseases is unwarranted. Another important factor is the degree of patient exposure to the allergen under study. Healthy subjects with high degrees of exposure have higher IgG and IgG4 antibody levels than healthy subjects with lesser degrees of exposure.

ANTITISSUE OR ANTICELL ANTIBODIES

Antibodies reactive with a number of different cell types or tissues have been associated with tissue damage. A classic example is Coombs positive hemolytic anemia, in which antibody coated red blood cells have a markedly shortened life span. In an analogous manner, anti-platelet antibodies may cause thrombocytopenia and purpura, and antibodies to polymorphonuclear leukocytes can result in neutropenia. Anti-basement membrane antibodies are important in both the renal and pulmonary manifestations of Goodpasture syndrome. Anti-skin antibodies probably participate in the production of dermatitis herpetiformis, pemphigus, and bullous pemphigoid. Antibodies to gastric parietal cells are common in pernicious anemia. Antinuclear and anti-DNA antibodies are prevalent in disseminated lupus erythematosus. Many other examples have been cited. Not all antitissue antibodies have been shown convincingly to be tissue damaging, but some, particularly those involving cells of the hematologic system, have been shown to possess this capability.

ANTIGEN-ANTIBODY COMPLEXES

Disseminated lupus erythematosus is one disease that has long been known to be associated with the presence of antigen–non-IgE–antibody complexes, both in the serum and in deposits in the renal glomeruli. Serum sickness is another example of a disease in which antigen-antibody complexes of non-IgE type appear to play a central pathogenetic role. In this instance, a single dose of antigen produces a series of immunologic changes that result in vasculitis and multisystem disease. Symptoms accompany the antibody production and the accumulation of circulating antigen-antibody complexes. After the complexes have been eliminated, symptoms decline and pathologic lesions regress. It is of interest that an IgE response frequently precedes or accompanies the appearance of antigen-antibody complexes and may contribute to the clinical manifestations of the disease process. Indeed, it may well be that an IgE-mediated increase in vascular permeability contributes to the actual deposition of antigen-antibody complexes in vessel walls and the subsequent production of vasculitis (Benveniste et al., 1976).

It appears that IgE responses may constitute an integral part of many antigen-antibody complex diseases, examples of which are hepatitis B infection and allergic bronchopulmonary aspergillosis. Circulating immune complexes that contain IgE are more common in food allergic than in nonallergic subjects. However, the presence of immune complexes in serum per se should not be construed to be pathologic. Circulating immune complexes have been reported to occur regularly in normal infants following ingestion of cow milk (Delire et al., 1978). It is likely that formation of immune complexes is a common, perhaps daily, occurrence in the blood and interstitial fluids of most humans. This underscores the need for laboratory tests that can discriminate between pathologic and innocuous immune complexes.

The nature of antigen-antibody complexes and the way in which the body handles them are probably critical determinants in whether or not manifestations of disease result. Benveniste et al. (1976) suggest that the development of glomerular lesions in acute serum sickness depends on the simultaneous presence of circulating immune complexes of a particular size and a critical degree of IgE-induced basophil degranulation with mediator release. Scherzer and Ward (1978) have shown that pulmonary damage from immune complexes administered intratracheally to rats depends on a critical ratio of antigen to antibody in the complexes, those preformed at antigen-antibody equivalence being most injurious. Other studies suggest that immune complex binding to lymphocyte receptors for Fc and complement can modulate lymphocyte proliferation and function. For example, altering the ratio of antigen to antibody in complexes can either stimulate or depress antigen-induced lymphocyte reactivity (Eisen and Karush, 1964; Banks, 1973; Kontiainen and Mitchison, 1975; Askonas, 1976).

Antigen-antibody complexes also may play an important role in immunoregulatory mechanisms in that they can suppress *in vitro* antibody production by spleen cells, possibly by acting on antigen receptors (Diener and Feldmann, 1972).

COMPLEMENT-FIXING ANTIBODIES

Non-IgE antigen-antibody reactions that activate complement may induce allergic symptoms through release of chemical mediators (see Chapter 4). Antitissue antibodies, anti-blood cell antibodies, antigen-antibody complexes (whether circulating or deposited in blood vessels or glomeruli), and many autoantibodies are capable of activating complement. Although complement is principally activated by IgG and IgM antibodies, complexes containing antibodies of other classes, or substances that are not antibody-dependent such as endotoxin, yeasts, polysaccharides, and radiopaque contrast material, may activate complement by the alternative pathway (see Chapter 4).

INTERRELATIONS BETWEEN ANTIBODIES OF DIFFERENT IMMUNOGLOBULIN CLASSES

The usual immune response to an antigen involves antibodies of several, and frequently of all, immunoglobulin classes. Interrelationships between different types of antibodies, and between antibodies and cells, may be important in tissue injury. Research has only begun to unravel these interactions. Some antibodies may be additive in causing tissue damage, whereas some directed at the same antigen may have opposing actions and modify the reaction. Antibodies may act to inhibit or to enhance further antibody synthesis. Antibodies of all immunoglobulin classes probably play important interrelated roles in a vast immunoregulatory network (Jerne, 1974).

An example of additive antibody effects is seen in the activation of complement by both IgG and IgM antibodies. Under most circumstances, IgM antibodies appear earlier in immune responses and persist for a shorter time. Both, however, activate the classic complement pathway following reaction with antigen, assisting in the neutralization or killing and removal of microorganisms and macromolecules. IgG ordinarily has a higher affinity for monovalent haptens than does IgM. However, at a molecular level, IgM activates complement more efficiently than does IgG. IgM also is more effective as a hemagglutinin or bacterial agglutinin. IgM is larger and can form more bonds with multivalent antigens than IgG. Thus, IgM and IgG reinforce each other, and the two acting together may be much more effective than either alone. It is likely that the tissue damaging effects of IgG and IgM antibodies also are additive. Examples include the anti-DNA antibodies that may participate in the pathogenesis of disseminated lupus erythematosus, IgG and IgM rheumatoid factors in the joints of patients with rheumatoid arthritis, and mixed IgM-IgG cryoglobulins in some forms of cryoglobulinemia.

There is evidence, on the other hand, that the presence of IgG antibodies under certain circumstances may ameliorate or block the tissue injuring effects of other immunoglobulins, such as IgE. For example, allergy injection therapy for IgE-mediated disease, such as hay fever, stimulates the production of IgG "blocking" antibodies which may combine with antigen, restricting its access to the circulation and mast cells. It also may inhibit IgE antibody synthesis.

CONSIDERATIONS CONCERNING IgG SUBCLASSES

It is likely that each IgG subclass is important in resistance to infections. Isolated absences of one or more subclass are associated usually with frequent recurrent infections, although instances of very low or absent levels of certain subclasses have been found in apparently healthy subjects (Van Loghem et al., 1980; Lefranc et al., 1979). It would appear that subjects with marked deficiency or absence of a particular IgG subclass are near the "cutting edge" between effective and ineffective resistance to bacterial and fungal infections. Some are able to compensate better than others. Of those who exhibit frequent infections, most improve dramatically when replacement therapy is instituted. Some children have a transient deficiency of one or more subclasses during the first few years of life, during which time they have recurrent or severe infections. They may subsequently develop normal immunoglobulin levels at which time there is an improvement in, or a disappearance of, the recurrent infections. Other subjects have a persistent subclass deficiency and a persistently increased susceptibility to infections. It is our current practice to treat children under six years of age with gamma globulin or single donor plasma therapy only during times of infection and not when symptom free. Our presumption is that they may synthesize normal amounts of the deficient subclass at an earlier age if not given continual replacement therapy. This, however, remains to be proved.

Each IgG subclass has distinctive immunochemical and biologic properties. Some of these are summarized in Table 7–1. The majority of antipolysaccharide antibodies probably belong to the IgG2 subclass of immunoglobulins, and

TABLE 7–1. Properties of IgG Subclasses

Property	G1	G2	G3	G4
Mean percent of serum IgG	65	25	6	3
Half-life (days)	23	23	11	22
Complement fixation	4+	2+	4+	0
Binding to staphylococcal protein A	+	+	−	+
Sensitizes basophils	−	−	−	±
Net molecular charge	Pos	Pos	Pos	Neg
Antibody to foods in normal subjects	2+	±	1+	3+
Antibody to foods in allergic patients	3+	1+	2+	4+

there may be selective deficiencies of antibodies to specific organisms (Umetsu, 1985). There is evidence, however, that antipolysaccharide antibodies also are found in the three other subclasses of IgG. There may be a difference in subclass response to various polysaccharide antigens. Hammarstrom et al. (1985) found that many IgA deficient subjects preferentially produced IgG1 and IgG3 anti-dextran antibodies even though their total levels of IgG2 were normal. There is evidence that antipneumococcal polysaccharide and antistaphylococcal teichoic acid antibodies in children are largely of the IgG1 subclass, whereas antibodies to these polysaccharides in adults are largely of the IgG2 subclass. We have evidence that IgG4 antibodies to the polyribose phosphate antigen of *Haemophilus influenzae* predominate in the responses of Alaskan Eskimo children who have invasive *H. influenzae* disease (Ramadas et al., 1986). It also is known that antibodies to protein antigens can be found in each of the subclasses of IgG (Seppala et al., 1984; Mohammad et al., 1983; Dengrove et al., 1986). Autoantibodies to clotting factors often are preferentially IgG4 (Andersen et al., 1968; Coots et al., 1979; Allain et al., 1981). The data available at present suggest that IgG1 antibodies compose the majority of those directed towards most protein antigens and that IgG4 antibodies may be the next most active, at least with regard to antibodies to tetanus toxoid. IgG2 appears to be the least likely, and the slowest, to respond to tetanus immunization. It is likely that antibodies to certain protein antigens are preferentially of a specific subclass, whereas antibodies to other protein antigens may belong largely to other subclasses (Husby et al., 1985). The subclass distribution of antibodies to specific viruses also may have unique characteristics (Sarnesto et al., 1985).

There is evidence that certain IgG subclasses tend to be deficient in association with other deficiencies. Thus, IgG2 and IgG4 deficiencies commonly coexist, and each is present more frequently when there is a low or absent level of IgA. IgG4 levels frequently are elevated in the same patients that have high levels of IgE, and low levels of IgG4 are commonly associated with low levels of IgE. These relationships appear to have some connection to the linear arrangement of heavy genes for these subclasses on chromosome 14. They suggest that some of the factors that enhance or suppress the rate of synthesis of the various subclass antibodies act at the DNA or RNA level.

Because they are negatively charged, IgG4 molecules may have a particular affinity for renal glomerular basement membranes (Melvin et al., 1984) and are prominent in the immune deposits of certain forms of renal disease (Doi et al., 1984). Devey et al. (1985) suggested that IgG4 antibodies may be of low avidity in relation to antibodies of other subclasses. This suggests a specialization of function, which is yet to be elucidated. The work of Mayumi et al. (1984) suggests that mitogens can differentially stimulate subclass antibody production by plasma cells; synthesis of one subclass is favored by T cell factors and pokeweed mitogen, whereas other subclasses are favored by stimulation with phytohemagglutinin.

IMMUNOREGULATORY EFFECTS OF ANTIBODY

The ability of specific antibodies to regulate the synthesis of tissue damaging antibodies is used clinically to prevent Rh sensitization of D-negative mothers. Anti-D antibody (Rho-GAM) administered during late pregnancy or at delivery binds to D-positive infant cells, facilitating their removal and preventing maternal sensitization (Freda et al., 1964). A small amount of passively administered antibody given at the proper time inhibits the formation of maternal anti-D antibody, permitting subsequent pregnancies to proceed to term without the development of erythroblastosis.

As the concentration of serum IgG increases, so does its catabolic rate (Morell et al., 1970). This is an autoregulatory mechanism by which antibody influences its own concentration.

Jerne (1974) proposed a provocative theory of immune regulation involving a network of antibody molecules in which each specific antibody has a unique antigenic structure or idiotype specificity, which itself elicits and reacts with anti-idiotype antibodies within the system. When a critical concentration of anti-idiotype antibodies is reached, antigen-specific humoral and cellular immune responses are turned off. Anti-allotypic antibodies, on the other hand, may turn off class-specific immune responses. Antibodies of high affinity are more immunosuppressive than antibodies of low affinity. In general, IgG antibodies are more suppressive than IgM antibodies. Passively administered antibodies, and presumably naturally occurring antibodies, have less inhibitory effect on secondary immune responses than on primary responses.

It has been demonstrated that identical idiotype specificities exist on B and T lymphocytes of the same individual, suggesting that both of these cell types participate in the network. Both T and B lymphocyte responses have been demonstrated to be directed toward idiotypes present on an animal's own immunoglobulin molecule. Anti-idiotypic antibodies passively administered will suppress T and B lymphocyte function when the lymphocyte possesses the corresponding idiotype. Anti-idiotype T cells also can suppress the production of antibodies carrying the corresponding idiotype just as can auto-anti–idiotypic antibodies. Mixed lymphocyte, graft versus host, and lymphocyte cytotoxicity reactions—all of which can cause tissue damage—are inhibited either by anti-idiotypic antibodies directed towards antibody and lymphocyte idiotypes or by anti-allotypic antibodies directed towards histocompatibility antigens. Thus, anti-idiotype antibodies are now known to play an important regulatory role in the immune system. A possible result of their deficiency could be the overproduction of specific antibodies seen in certain immunodeficiency disorders with immunoglobulins of restricted heterogenicity, also the oligoclonal cerebrospinal fluid (CSF) gammopathies seen in multiple sclerosis and subacute sclerosing panencephalitis (SSPE), and the benign and malignant gammopathies of old age, including myelomas and lymphomas.

INTERRELATIONSHIPS BETWEEN ANTIBODIES AND LYMPHOCYTES THAT MAY CONTRIBUTE TO TISSUE DAMAGE

There are many ways in which antibodies and lymphocytes cooperate to produce a particular immune response. For example, in kidney graft rejection, antibodies may act with lymphocytes to destroy histoincompatible donor kidney cells. The reaction has been termed antibody-dependent, cell-mediated cytotoxicity (ADCC), and the antibodies have been called lymphocyte dependent antibodies (LDA). Such antibodies can also sensitize mononuclear cells (K or killer cells) from unimmunized subjects and cause them to destroy target cells. Complement is not required, the antibodies are not cytophilic, and their action can be inhibited by immune complexes. These antibodies usually are of the IgG variety and only low concentrations are needed. Antibody-dependent lymphocyte cytotoxicity may be particularly important in immune defenses against malignant cells that arise as the result of cellular mutation or transformation.

INTERRELATIONSHIPS BETWEEN NON-IgE ANTIBODIES AND NONLYMPHOID CELLS

IgG or IgM antibody, acting with complement, may cause cell lysis by a mechanism independent of lymphocytes. These "cytotoxic" antibodies often are important in hyperacute renal graft rejection. Such tissue damage requires a higher level of antibody than that of ADCC. Cytotoxic antibodies may play a role in other hypersensitivity phenomena. For instance, antiplatelet antibody plays an important pathogenetic role in many cases of thrombocytopenia in newborn infants. In these cases, maternal IgG antiplatelet antibody induces the disease, which clears spontaneously as the maternal antibodies disappear from the infants' circulation. Antibodies to polymorphonuclear leukocytes, produced after many blood transfusions, may cause neutropenia in some subjects. Antineutrophil antibodies also are seen in systemic lupus erythematosus and other autoimmune disorders, in which they may contribute to neutropenia. Anti-red blood cell antibodies are a common cause of hemolytic anemia. Such reactions may be drug-induced (Ackroyd, 1975) or idiopathic. A wide variety of tissue damaging autoantibodies to nonhematologic tissues are noted in Table 7–2.

Antibodies, particularly those of the IgG class, may affix to nonlymphoid cells by means of Fc receptors and impart to these cells such properties as antigen recognition, complement-related chemotaxis, and opsonic activity, leading to enhanced phagocytosis. Both polymorphonuclear leukocytes and monocytes possess surface membrane IgG receptors and may be passively sensitized to specific soluble or cellular antigens. Fc-receptor bearing leukocytes thus can be involved in antibody-dependent, tissue damaging reactions.

NON-IgE ANTIBODIES IN TISSUE DAMAGE

One method of implicating antibodies in the pathogenesis of tissue damage is to demonstrate antigen-induced tissue damage following passive transfer of antibodies to an otherwise unaffected recipient. Nature performs this experiment in newborn infants who receive transplacental IgG anti-red blood cell antibodies from the mother. Unfortunately, in most situations, such a clear-cut cause and effect cannot be demonstrated because of the complexity of immune responses that ordinarily follow contact with antigen.

Celiac Disease. A disease of interest is gliadin-induced celiac disease. There is little or no evidence that a deficiency in intestinal mucosal peptidase is primarily responsible for this disease, as was once thought. There is, however, an array of immune and genetic associations that suggests the importance of immune mechanisms in its genesis. Non-IgE antibodies to gliadin are much more prominent than in control populations (Taylor et al., 1961; Heiner et al., 1962; Bertele et al., 1985). *In vitro* lymphokine production upon exposure of peripheral blood lymphocytes to gluten is increased, as are delayed skin responses to gliadin. These observations suggest a role for cell-mediated hypersensitivity. An increase in circulating immune complexes during active disease also has been reported, as has a high incidence of autoantibodies to reticulin, a tissue protein that cross-reacts with wheat gliadin (Seah et al., 1973). Fifteen subjects with biopsy confirmed, gluten-related celiac disease were studied with a sensitive radioimmunoassay for specific IgE antibodies to wheat gliadin in my laboratory. None had high levels of specific IgE antibody, and, perhaps more importantly, none had absent IgE antibodies as was found in 20 percent of healthy subjects. High levels of specific IgE antibodies would favor an immediate type reaction that might preclude sufficient wheat ingestion to cause celiac disease. Perhaps the development of celiac disease requires low levels of IgE antibody to increase gastrointestinal permeability and facilitate the deposition of antigen-antibody complexes or to activate other immune mechanisms in a host genetically programmed for hyperreactivity to gliadin.

The HLA antigens D8 and Dw3 are found with increased frequency in celiac disease (Falchuk et al., 1972). An inherited B cell surface antigen called GSE Ag also occurs together with HLA D8 or Dw3 much more frequently in subjects with celiac disease than in controls (Mann et al., 1976). These findings indicate a strong genetic influence in the pathogenesis of celiac disease and suggest that specific immune re-

sponses may play a major role in the disease. It is probable that several immune mechanisms participate in causing the jejunal mucosal damage in celiac disease, although the relative importance of each is unclear at present.

Other Disorders of Immune Response. A similar discussion is pertinent to many disorders that are associated with aberrant immune responses. Since responses to provoking antigens are complex and include the development of various kinds of antibodies, investigators and practitioners alike should observe caution in ascribing the etiology or pathogenesis of a hypersensitivity disorder to a single mechanism simply because of the presence of a particular antibody. Even allergic reactions that appear clinically to be solely IgE-mediated usually occur in the presence of antibodies of various immunoglobulin classes as well as sensitized lymphocytes, all of which may play important pathogenetic roles in specific instances.

Tests to Identify Non-IgE-Mediated Tissue Damage. A thorough discussion of laboratory procedures designed to identify non-IgE-mediated tissue damage and follow its progress is beyond the scope of this chapter. Such procedures, in fact, are multiplying at such a rapid pace that what is optimal this year may be out of date next year. One must utilize wisely the facilities and personnel available, relying largely on laboratories where there is experience and skill in performing particular procedures and knowledge concerning interpretation of results. A partial listing of procedures that may be of assistance in the diagnosis and management of selected disorders is given in Table 7–2. A brief general description of some of these procedures follows.

Fluorescence microscopy is used to identify antibodies directed towards specific autologous antigens. Antinuclear antibodies are identified routinely by fluorescence microscopy, as are linear and lumpy deposits of immunoglobulin and complement, for example, in renal glomeruli in Goodpasture syndrome and lupus erythematosus, respectively.

Fluorescence microscopy helps considerably in studying specific antibody responses in subjects with a variety of dermatologic diseases, e.g., complement fixing IgG antibodies to epithelial intercellular cement in pemphigus vulgaris; linear deposits of IgG antibodies to epithelial basement membrane in bullous pemphigoid; and granular accumulations of IgA and C3 along dermal-epidermal junctions in dermatitis herpetiformis. It also has facilitated

TABLE 7-2. Non-IgE Antibodies and Related Immunologic Findings that May Help in Diagnosis and Management of Selected Diseases

Disease	Findings
Non-IgE allergic bronchial asthma	Negative scratch and prick skin test reactions Positive intradermal skin test reactions Heat-stable, short-term sensitizing antibody Positive bronchial challenge Negative results in IgE studies
Extrinsic allergic alveolitis	Serum precipitins to offending antigen, e.g., to *Micropolyspora faeni* in farmer's lung and to pigeon serum or droppings in pigeon-breeder's lung. Cell-mediated immunity to offending antigen.
Allergic bronchopulmonary aspergillosis	Dual skin reactions (15 minute and 8 hour) Precipitins to one or several *Aspergillus fumigatus* antigens in low to moderate titer. Elevated total IgE, IgE antibodies.
Aspergilloma	Serum precipitins to multiple *A. fumigatus* antigens in relatively high titer. Normal total and antibody IgE.
Systemic lupus erythematosus	LE cell formation Antinuclear antibodies in serum including anti-DNA, anti-Sm, anti-DNP, anti-histone, anti-Ro, anti-La Serum DNA-anti-DNA immune complexes Decreased serum C3, C4, CH50 levels Granular deposits of Ig, C, sometimes DNA in glomerular basement membrane (GBM) False positive reaction for syphilis Anti-histone antibodies in drug-induced lupus
Post-streptococcal glomerulonephritis	Elevated serum ASO titer Decreased serum C3, C4, CH50 levels
Hypocomplementemic membranoproliferative nephritis	Decreased serum C3, not C4 level Alpha$_2$D and C3 NeF in serum Granular C3 deposits in GBM
Subacute bacterial endocarditis	Serum immune complexes Decreased serum C3, CH50 levels Positive blood culture results Decreased antibody response to new antigens
Rheumatoid arthritis	Rheumatoid factor in serum, joint fluid Anti-RANA antibodies Complexes of IgG and rheumatoid factor in synovium, joint fluid
Rheumatic fever	Anti-myocardial sarcolemmal antibodies Elevated antistreptolysin, antistreptokinase, and antihyaluronidase titers
Sjögren syndrome	Antibodies to Ro and La antigens Positive rheumatoid factor Antithyroglobulin and antinuclear antibodies

greater understanding of gastrointestinal disturbances such as celiac disease, milk-induced enteropathy, Crohn disease, and ulcerative colitis. The technique is widely used in detecting autoantibodies in disorders such as Hashimoto thyroiditis, hyperthyroidism, Addison disease, and certain types of diabetes. In spite of its limitations, which include the need for subjective interpretation and the lack of precise quantitation, this technique will continue to be used in the foreseeable future to detect non-IgE tissue reactive antibodies.

Immune electron microscopy is a specialized technique which, like fluorescence microscopy, will permit identification of tissue binding antibodies according to specific immunoglobulin class. Its greater resolving power will permit localization of antibodies not only to specific cell types but also to certain organelles, providing a more detailed picture of their potential pathogenetic role than would be otherwise possible. This procedure is too specialized and expensive to be used for routine investigative studies in more than a few medical centers or in any but the most provocative circumstances. Electron microscopy also is of value in searching for viruses which, if found, might be implicated in tissue damage, either directly or in consort with antibodies.

Cell and organ cultures offer promise of insight into the nature of immunologic responses at the cellular and tissue levels. Cultures of lym-

Table 7-2 *(Continued)*

Disease	Findings
Goodpasture syndrome	Linear deposits of immunoglobulin on renal GBM, pulmonary epithelial basement membranes Serum antibodies to glomerular and pulmonary basement membranes
Celiac disease	Chronic jejunal inflammatory changes clear on gluten-free diet, reappear on challenge. High titer of non-IgE serum antibodies to alpha gliadin Arthus-like skin responses to gluten *In vitro* induction of leukocyte inhibitory factor (LIF) lymphokine by gliadin
Milk-induced enteropathy	Jejunal inflammatory changes clear on milk-free diet, reappear on challenge. Excessive loss of ^{51}Cr-tagged red blood cells, or albumin clears with milk-free diet, returns on challenge.
Mixed connective tissue disease	Antibodies to ribonucleoprotein
Milk-induced pulmonary hemosiderosis in children	Serum precipitins in high titer to cow milk antigens Positive intradermal skin tests with cow milk antigens
Autoimmune hemolytic anemia	Positive direct Coombs test (IgG, IgM antibody and/or complement on red blood cell) Positive indirect Coombs test (serum antibody to autologous red blood cells)
Erythroblastosis fetalis	Positive direct Coombs test on cord or neonatal cells Positive indirect Coombs test using mother's serum, infant's red blood cells
Dermatitis herpetiformis	Granular IgA and C3 along dermal-epidermal junctions
Pemphigus vulgaris	IgG antibodies to epithelial intercellular cement Complement (C3) deposition along with the antibodies
Bullous pemphigoid	Linear deposits IgG on epithelial basement membranes
Pernicious anemia	Antibodies to intrinsic factor Antibodies to gastric parietal cells
Hashimoto thyroiditis	Antibodies to thyroglobulin in high titer Antibodies to thyroid microsomes
Graves disease	Long-acting thyroid stimulator antibodies Low levels of antithyroglobulin
Addison disease	Anti-adrenal mitochondrial antibodies Anti-thyroglobulin, anti-gastric parietal cell, and anti-intrinsic factor antibodies
Acquired immunodeficiency syndrome (AIDS) in adults	Antibodies to HTLV III (HIV) Elevated serum immunoglobulins Inability to make antibodies to new antigens Elevated serum immune complexes Reduced T4 lymphocytes Diminished delayed skin responses Decreased *in vitro* lymphocyte responses
AIDS in children	Same as in adults plus IgG subclass deficiencies Recurrent pyogenic respiratory tract infections

phocytes and of jejunal mucosal biopsies are examples. It is possible to quantitate intrinsic antibody production according to immunoglobulin class, to observe and test for tissue binding antibodies produced elsewhere, and to observe the effects of added antigen, antibody, lymphoid cells, lymphokines, other chemical mediators, and hormones on *in vitro* enzyme production and on antibody synthesis and tissue integrity.

Tests for complement activation or depletion have provided presumptive evidence for the involvement of non-IgE antibodies in many instances of tissue injury. The lowering of serum C3 and C4, which accompanies disease activity in disseminated lupus erythematosus, is an ex-

ample. Oral administration of cow milk to milk sensitive children and of wheat gluten to celiac disease patients has been reported to cause activation of complement and to decrease levels of serum complement components. Most such studies do not provide proof of pathogenetic involvement of complement fixing antibodies, but they suggest a possible role.

Tests for circulating antigen-antibody complexes are developing at a rapid pace. At present, however, it may be advantageous to study patients by at least two different techniques as a check on both the sensitivity and reproducibility of the tests being used. The C1q binding and Raji cell tests commonly are employed. Each depends on complexes that activate the complement system, and each has the potential drawback of false positive results, if there is nonspecific aggregation of immunoglobulins or generation of C3b by improper serum handling. Searches for cryoprecipitins; lowered total complement (CH50), C3, or C4; and presence of rheumatoid factor are other techniques of value. These and other procedures and their clinical applications have been ably summarized by Kohler (1983) and by Zubler and Lambert (1978).

Radioimmunoassays and enzyme linked immunosorbent assays (ELISA) provide sensitive techniques for measuring specific antibodies of each immunoglobulin class and subclass as well as for measurements of specific antigen, antigen-antibody complexes, chemical mediators of allergic responses, and thymic hormones. Allergists and pediatricians are perhaps most aware of the availability of tests to measure specific antibodies of the IgE class. Modifications have been used to measure antibodies of other immunoglobulin classes, and it is possible to measure specific antibodies of any of the five immunoglobulin classes or of their subclasses by appropriate radioimmunoassay procedures.

Radioimmunoassays have the decided advantage of providing a sensitive quantitative measurement of antibodies when low concentrations are present. They also permit quantitative studies concerning the timing and magnitude of humoral immune responses following specific antigen challenge or during the course of specific diseases. Like most other tests, they do not in themselves prove that the antibody identified is responsible for a specific symptom or tissue injury.

Immunodiffusion in gel permits simple demonstration and identification of precipitating antibodies. Radial immunodiffusion provides the simplest quantitation of total IgG, IgA, and IgM concentrations. Serum levels of IgG1, IgG2, and IgG3 also can be determined by immunodiffusion. When precipitating antibodies are observed by double immunodiffusion, one can be certain that a high concentration of antibody is present, usually of the IgG class, but IgA or IgM also may contribute. Neither radial nor double immunodiffusion is sufficiently sensitive to reflect accurately total or antigen-specific IgD, IgE, or IgG4. Caution must be exercised to prove that observed precipitates are indeed antigen-antibody reactions rather than nonspecific protein or polysaccharide aggregates. The experienced worker can do this through ensuring the quality of reagents and the proper use of standards and controls. One should also remember that many subjects have antibodies of the IgG, IgM, or IgA variety that are demonstrable by other techniques but are not detected by the relatively insensitive precipitin technique.

Radioimmunodiffusion and crossed radioimmunoelectrophoresis (CRIE) add sensitivity and specificity to the versatility of double immunodiffusion. These permit identification of minute amounts of specific antigen or of specific antibody according to immunoglobulin class. However, such procedures still lack the quantitative precision and reproducibility of properly performed radioimmunoassays.

Passive transfer tests. Human IgG heat stable antibodies that cause passive cutaneous anaphylactic (PCA) reactions have been demonstrated by tests both in experimental animals and in humans. Positive immediate skin tests in humans ordinarily indicate that IgE antibodies are present, but in some instances IgG antibodies have been incriminated. Preheating serum to 56°C for one half hour abrogates IgE but not IgG responses. Because of the possibility of passive transfer of hepatitis or HTLV-III viruses during passive transfer tests between human subjects, passive sensitization tests should be done on monkeys. Perhaps the most convincing method of proving the immunoglobulin class of an antibody involved in PCA or other physiologic responses involves the removal of individual immunoglobulins, using specific anti-heavy chain antisera and then demonstrating that removal of only the incriminated immunoglobulin abrogates the untoward response.

Additional tests to detect non-IgE antibodies have been used, with varying degrees of success, in relating the findings to clinical symptoms and tissue injury. Many of these are discussed in other chapters of this book. Immunoassays of lymphokines, of complement components and derivatives, of circulating immune complexes, and of chemical mediators of inflammation hold considerable promise in providing much-needed simple tests to quantitate the various types of immune responses which occur in patients.

REFERENCES

Ackroyd, J.F.: Immunological mechanisms in drug hypersensitivity. *In* Gell, P.G.H., Coombs, R.R.H., and Lachmann, P.G. (eds.): *Clinical Aspects of Immunology,* 3rd ed. Oxford, Blackwell Scientific Publications, Ltd., 1975.

Allain, J.P., Gaillandre, A., Lee, H.: Immunochemical characterization of antibodies to factor VIII in hemophilic and nonhemophilic patients. J. Lab. Clin. Med. 97:791–800, 1981.

Andersen, B.R., Terry, W.D.: Gamma G_4-globulin antibody causing inhibition of clotting factor VIII. Nature 217:175–176, 1968.

Ashkenazi, A., Idar, D., Handzel, Z.T., Ofarim, M., Levin, S.: An *in vitro* immunological assay for diagnosis of coeliac disease. Lancet 1:627–629, 1978.

Askonas, B.A., McMichael, A.J., Roux, M.E.: Clonal dominance and the preservation of clonal memory cells mediated by antigen-antibody. Immunology 31:541–550, 1976.

Banks, K.L.: The effect of antibody on antigen-induced lymphocyte transformation. J. Immunol. 110:709–716, 1973.

Becker, E.L.: Nature and classification of immediate-type allergic reactions. Adv. Immunol. 13:267–308, 1971.

Benveniste, J., Egido, J., Gutierrez-Millet, V.: Evidence for the involvement of the IgE-basophil system in acute serum sickness. Clin. Exp. Immunol. 26:449–456, 1976.

Bertele, R.M., Burgin-Wolff, A., Berger, R., Gorny, R.M., Harms, H.K.: The fluorescent immunosorbent test for IgG gliadin antibodies and the leucocyte migration inhibition test in coeliac disease; comparison of diagnostic value. Eur. J. Pediatr. 144:58–62, 1985.

Coombs, R.R.A., Gell, P.G.H.: Classification of allergic reactions responsible for clinical hypersensitivity and disease. *In* Gell, P.G.H., Coombs, R.R.A., Lackmann, P.G. (eds.): *Clinical Aspects of Immunology,* 3rd ed. Oxford, Blackwell Scientific Publications, Ltd. 1975.

Coots, M.C., Muhleman, A.F., Glueck, H.I.: A factor V inhibitor: *In vitro* interference by calcium. Am. J. Hematol. 7:178–180, 1979.

Delire, M., Cambiaso, C.L., Misson, P.L.: Circulating immune complexes in infants fed on cow's milk. Nature 272:632, 1978.

Dengrove, J., Lee, E.J., Heiner, D.C., St. Geme, Jr, J.W., Leake, R., Baraff, J., and Ward, J.J.: IgG and IgG subclass specific antibody responses to diphtheria and tetanus toxoids in newborns and infants given DTP immunization. Ped. Res. 20:735–739, 1986.

Devey, M.E., Bleasdale, K.M., French, M.A., Harrison, G.: The IgG4 subclass is associated with a low affinity antibody response to tetanus toxoid in man. Immunology 55:565–567, 1985.

Diener, E., Feldmann, M.: Relationship between antigen and antibody induced suppression of immunity. Transplant. Rev. 8:76–103, 1972.

Doi, T., Mayumi, M., Kanatsu, K., Suehiro, F., Hamashima, Y.: Distribution of IgG subclasses in membranous nephropathy. Clin. Exp. Immunol. 58:57–62, 1984.

Eisen, H.N., Karush, F.: Immune tolerance and an extracellular regulatory role for bivalent antibody. Nature 202:677–682, 1964.

Falchuk, Z.M., Rogentine, G.N., Strober, W.: Predominance of histocompatibility antigen HL-A8 in patients with gluten-sensitive enteropathy. J. Clin. Invest. 51:1602–1605, 1972.

Freda, V.J., Gorman, J.G., Pollack, W.: Successful prevention of experimental sensitization in man with an anti-Rh gamma globulin antibody preparation. Transfusion 4:26–32, 1964.

Gwynn, C.M., Morrison-Smith, J., Leon, G.L., Stanworth, D.R.: Role of IgG4 subclass in childhood allergy. Lancet 1:910–911, 1978.

Hammarstrom, L., Persson, M.A.A., Smith, C.I.E.: Immunoglobulin subclass distribution of human anti-carbohydrate antibodies; aberrant pattern in IgA-deficient donors. Immunology 54:821–826, 1985.

Heiner, D.C., Lahey, M.E., Wilson, J.F., Gerrard, J.W., Shwachman, H., Khaw, K.T.: Precipitins to antigens of wheat and cow's milk in celiac disease. J. Pediatr. 61:813–830, 1962.

Husby, S., Oxelius, V.A., Teisner, B., Jensenius, J.C., Svehag, S.E.: Humoral immunity to dietary antigens in healthy adults. Occurrence, isotype and IgG subclass distribution of serum antibodies to protein antigens. Int. Arch. Allergy Appl. Immunol. 77:416–422, 1985.

Jerne, N.K.: Towards a network theory of the immune system. Ann. Immunol. Inst. Pasteur 125:373–389, 1974.

Kohler, P.F.: Immune complexes and allergic disease. *In* Middleton, E., Jr., et al. (eds.): *Allergy Principles and Practice,* vol. I, 2nd ed. St. Louis, C.V. Mosby Co., 1983.

Kontiainen, S., Mitchison, N.A.: Blocking antigen-antibody complexes on the T-lymphocyte activation during *in vitro* incubation before adoptive transfer. Immunology 28:523–533, 1975.

Lafranc, G., Dumitresco, S.M., Salier, J.P., et al.: Familial lack of the IgG3 subclass. Gene elimination or turning off expression and neutral evolution in the immune system. J. Immunogenet. 6:215–221, 1979.

Mann, D.L., Katz, S.I., Nelson, D.L., Abelson, L.D., Strober, W.: Specific B-cell antigen associated with gluten sensitive enteropathy and dermatitis herpetiformis. Lancet 1:110–111, 1976.

Mayumi, M., Kuritani, T., Cooper, M.D.: T-cell regulation of IgG subclass expression by mitogen-induced plasma cells: Soluble factors versus the T cells. J. Clin. Immunol. 4:287–293, 1984.

Melvin, T., Kim, Y., Michael, A.F.: Selective binding of IgG4 and other negatively charged plasma proteins in normal and diabetic human kidneys. Am. J. Pathol. 115:443–446, 1984.

Mohammad, I., Ogunmekan, D., Heiner, D.: IgG subclass antibody responses to diphtheria and tetanus immunizations. Abstracts of American Academy of Pediatrics Section on Allergy and Immunology, San Francisco, October 23, 1983.

Morell, A., Terry, W.D., Waldmann, T.A.: Metabolic properties of IgG subclasses in man. J. Clin. Invest. 49:673–680, 1970.

Parish, W.E.: Short-term anaphylactic IgG antibodies in human sera. Lancet 2:591–592, 1970.

Ramadas, K., Petersen, G.M., Heiner, D.C., Ward, J.I.: Class and subclass antibodies to *Haemophilus influenzae* type b capsule: Comparison of invasive disease and natural exposure. Infect. Immun. 53:486–490, 1986.

Sarnesto, A., Julkenen, I., Makela, O.: Proportions of Ig classes and subclasses in mumps antibodies. Scand. J. Immunol. 22:345–350, 1985.

Scherzer, H., Ward, P.A.: Lung injury produced by immune complexes of varying composition. J. Immunol. 121:947–957, 1978.

Seah, P.P., Fry, L., Holborow, E.J., Rossiter, M.A., Doe, W.F., Magalhaes, A.F., Hoffbrand, A.V.: Antireticulin antibody: Incidence and diagnostic significance. Gut 14:311–315, 1973.

Seppala, I.J.T., Routonen, N., Sarnesto, A., Mattila, P.A., Makela, O.: The percentages of six immunoglobulin isotypes in human antibodies to tetanus toxoid: Standardization of isotype-specific second antibodies in solid-phase assay. Eur. J. Immunol. 14:868–875, 1984.

Taylor, K.B., Truelove, S.C., Thompson, D.L., et al.: An

immunological study of coeliac disease and idiopathic steatorrhea: Serological reactions to gluten and milk proteins. Brit. Med. J. 2:1727–1729, 1961.

Umetsu, D.T., Ambrosino, D.M., Quinti, I., Siber, G.R., Geha, R.: Recurrent sinopulmonary infection and impaired antibody response to bacterial capsular polysaccharide antigen in children with selective IgG-subclass deficiency. N. Engl. J. Med. 313:1247–1251, 1985.

Van der Giessen, M., Homan, W.L., Van Kernebeek, G., Aalberse, R.C., Dieges, P.H.: Subclass typing of IgG antibodies formed by grass pollen allergic patients during immunotherapy. Int. Arch. Allergy Appl. Immunol. 50:625–639, 1976.

Van Loghem, E., Sukernik, R.I., Osipova, L.P., et al.: Gene deletion and gene duplication within the cluster of human heavy-chain genes. Immunogenetics 7:285–299, 1980.

Zubler, R.H., Lambert, P.H.: Detection of immune complexes in human diseases. Prog. Allergy 24:1–48, 1978.

8

Immunizations and Adverse Reactions to Vaccines

VINCENT A. FULGINITI, M.D.

The use of bacterial and viral vaccines has changed the face of childhood permanently. Smallpox is gone, measles, mumps, and rubella are reduced to minor occurrences in the United States, and natural polio is virtually nonexistent. Pertussis still occurs but at rate magnitudes below that of the early part of this century. Diphtheria is almost gone, and tetanus and rabies are rare. Thus, despite the fact that this chapter is devoted, in fact dwells on, the adverse effects of immunization, the reader is advised to remember that the enormous benefits of vaccines far outweigh the few instances of reactions and adverse events that will be documented.

All vaccines are not alike; therefore, as might be expected, reactions to individual vaccines are related to the properties of the specific biological. However, some generalizations are possible from analysis of all reported reactions; some properties are common, many are not.

A vaccine is intended to provide the host with an immunizing experience that simulates natural immunity, with minimal or no undesirable side effects (Fulginiti, 1982). No vaccine achieves this ideal perfectly. All vaccines have predictable consequences; some are trivial and temporary, some severe and long lasting. A few may very rarely cause the death of the recipient. However, all adverse events must be taken in the context of the benefits of the vaccine for the recipient and the risk of acquiring a given disease for the unvaccinated, with that disease's attendant morbidity and mortality. Undesirable and unwanted as are the side effects, in this context they are infinitesimal when compared with the risks of the corresponding diseases and their consequences.

Reactions may be divided into categories, as follows:

1. *Injury* that results from *improper use*, such as injection by an inappropriate route, use of too large a dose, or use of an outdated product.
2. *Intrinsic biologic properties* of a constituent of the vaccine that result in an adverse reaction, such as the potential infectivity of the central nervous system of live, attenuated poliovirus vaccine.
3. *Hypersensitivity* to some component of the vaccine, which can produce any of a variety of adverse immune (allergic) reactions (types I, II, III, IV of Gell and Coombs, 1968). Examples include mercury sensitivity, antibiotic hypersensitivity, egg allergy, and cell mediated reactions to tetanus toxoid.
4. *Idiosyncratic reactions* for which no biologic explanation exists or has been discovered, such as the pertussis "collapse syndrome," in which an infant may become hyporesponsive and hypotonic shortly after receipt of diphtheria, tetanus, and pertussis (DTP) vaccine (Cody et al., 1981).

The ingredients of various vaccines in common use are listed in Table 8–1, with the potential consequences for the recipient. It is emphasized that the listed consequences are, in fact, potential complications which may have been recorded only rarely.

IMPROPER USE OF VACCINES

This category of reactions may be further subdivided into errors in administration as follows: (1) contamination of the vaccine, of the site of injection, or of the apparatus used for injection; (2) administration of the vaccine to an inappropriate age group; and (3) failure to heed precautions and contraindications for a specific vaccine (Fulginiti, 1982; Centers for Disease Control (CDC), 1983).

Errors in administration encompass all uses of the vaccine for which no standard exists or for which prior experience has demonstrated an adverse consequence. Most vaccines have been field tested within limited bounds and released with stringent guidelines for their administration in order to achieve the desired immune response and avoid or minimize side effects. For example, DTP, the vaccines diphtheria, tetanus

TABLE 8–1. Vaccine Constituents and Potential Reactions (for Commonly Administered Vaccines)

Vaccine	Primary Constituent	Other Constituents	Potential Reactions
DPT (diphtheria, pertussis, tetanus)	Diphtheria toxoid		Hypersensitivity
			Toxicity
	Tetanus toxoid		Arthus
			? Peripheral neuropathy
	Pertussis bacilli		? Hypersensitivity
			Local irritation
			Mild systemic toxicity
			Pyrogenicity
			Collapse syndrome
			Seizures
			Encephalopathy
		Aluminum Salts	"Sterile" abscess
			Granuloma
Live poliovirus	Polioviruses 1,2,3		Paralytic disease
		Streptomycin	? Hypersensitivity
		Neomycin	? Hypersensitivity
MMR (measles, mumps, rubella)	Live measles virus		Fever, rash
			Atypical measles*
	Live rubella virus		Fever, rash
			Lymphadenopathy
			Arthritis, arthralgia
			Peripheral neuritis
	Live mumps virus		Parotitis (rare)
		Neomycin	Hypersensitivity
		Ovalbumin	Anaphylaxis
Influenza	Killed influenza Virus or portions		Fever
			Toxicity
		Egg antigens	Anaphylaxis
Pneumococcal	Polysaccharide		Local irritation
			Systemic toxicity
			Rare anaphylaxis
Killed poliovirus (rarely used)	Inactivated polioviruses 1,2,3		Local reactions
			? Others

* For description of atypical measles, see text.

(DT) and adult tetanus, diphtheria (Td) should always be administered into an adequate muscle mass employing a technique that avoids insertion or leakage of the biological into the subcutaneous or intradermal areas. If these products are injected into an inappropriate site, a mild to severe inflammatory reaction may occur in some individuals, with local heat, erythema, and induration. In a few individuals, a so-called sterile abscess may follow the injection of the vaccine and its aluminum adjuvant into the subcutaneous tissues. Inadvertent intravenous administration may have disastrous consequences, since these products have toxic properties and sudden high toxic blood levels can produce shock and other severe reactions.

Inadvertent intradermal administration, particularly in an individual who has previously been sensitized by one or more doses of the vaccine in the past, can result in either an immediate or a delayed type hypersensitivity response.

There have been some reports of oral poliovirus vaccine being given by injection, rather than by the standard oral route. I am unaware of any serious consequences of such administration, but the potential for bypassing the regional lymphoid tissue of the gut and the intestinal mucosa may predispose the recipient to central nervous system localization.

INTRINSIC BIOLOGIC HAZARDS

Almost all vaccines pose a potential threat to some individuals. The reasons for this are not clear but may be related, in some instances, to genetic receptivity to the undesired effect of the vaccine (Jones and Fulginiti, 1982). For example, live, attenuated poliovirus vaccine very rarely produces paralysis in some recipients or in a susceptible contact of a recipient (Schonberger et al., 1976). Types III and I poliovirus, attenuated for vaccine use, have been shown to undergo reversion to neurovirulence by passage in laboratory animals or in humans (Melnick, 1984; Vallancourt, 1984). Several lines of evidence suggest that the rare occurrence of paralytic disease after oral poliovirus vaccine (OPV) is not by chance but may be related to the immunogenetic composition of host cells. Cells, grown *in vitro*, from some individuals will support invasion by poliovirus, whereas others will not (Green, 1974). In other studies, certain haplotypes at the MLC locus on chromosome 6 appear more frequently among paralytic poliovirus–infected individuals than would be expected by chance (Van Eden et al., 1983). Abundant, increasing animal and human experience suggests that genetic predisposition to both infection and severity of disease for some pathogens resides in the MLC region of chromosome 6 in the human and comparable loci in experimental animals. One can speculate that each of us has a fixed capacity to respond to specific antigens, including those possessed by infectious agents (Brinton and Nathanson, 1981). This capacity may be sufficient to ensure both intact survival and immunity after contact with the agent. Further, the individual's inherent responsiveness may determine the severity of disease. This may range from inapparent infection to mild or moderate with good immune response to severe or lethal with little or no immune response. Additionally, a population group may be identified for some infectious agents that is midway between these two extremes, with adequate immune responsiveness but also moderately severe disease.

Another type of intrinsic hazard is only manifest in an individual whose response is congenitally absent or abridged by either acquired disease or therapy, which results in immunosuppression (Fulginiti, 1971). For example, live attenuated measles virus appears incapable of producing more than very mild disease in normal recipients; this occurs in fact in only 5 to 15 percent of normal individuals, and the remainder experience no symptoms at all. However, if the vaccine virus is administered to a child whose immune response is blunted or absent, disseminated, severe, and even lethal infection may result (Lipsey et al., 1967; Nahmias et al., 1967).

Yet another intrinsic property of some vaccines is a toxic effect due to toxins of the agent included in the vaccine. For example, pertussis vaccine contains endotoxin in variable amounts from lot to lot; the endotoxin can induce severe reactions in the infant or child who receives the vaccine (Hooker, 1981; Mortimer, 1980). This is a direct effect of one of the unavoidable constituents of the vaccine and is not a hypersensitivity or idiosyncratic reaction.

HYPERSENSITIVITY REACTIONS

The modified Gell and Coombs classification will be used to discuss the possible "allergic" or, more properly termed, hypersensitivity reactions to vaccine constituents. Type I reactions are immediate hypersensitivity responses, usually mediated by IgE-specific antibody. Anaphylactic reactions, severe forms of type I or IgE-antibody mediated reactions, can result from prior sensitization to a constituent of the vaccine used. For example, influenza vaccine is produced in fertilized hens' eggs and despite purification, trace amounts of ovalbumin and other egg-derived antigens persist in the final product (Isaacson, 1971). An individual highly sensitive to egg antigens (e.g., ovalbumin) may experience anaphylactic shock or lesser anaphylactoid reactions upon receipt of the vaccine. Recently, the same phenomenon has been demonstrated for live measles virus vaccine that is produced in chick embryo tissue culture but contains nanogram amounts of ovalbumin (Hermann et al., 1983). In several children who had IgE-specific anti-ovalbumin antibody, administration of live measles virus vaccine resulted in anaphylaxis.

Examples of type II mechanisms among vaccine reactions are rare and poorly studied, for the most part. One possible example may be the post-virus vaccine thrombocytopenia that has been reported occasionally (Kelton, 1981). It is assumed that the viral antigen in the vaccine (e.g., rubella virus) attaches to the platelet and produces a combined antigen against which an immune reaction develops. Cytotoxic antibodies directed either against the combination or against a platelet component then destroy the cell (either platelet or megakaryocyte). Peripheral thrombocytopenia can occur and, in extreme instances, petechial and other forms of bleeding result.

Type III hypersensitivity results from immune complex formation between the vaccine antigen and antibody directed against it. The atypical measles syndrome seen in recipients of killed measles virus vaccine (KMV) may represent a type III reaction (Bellanti et al., 1969). In the case of wild virus exposure, the killed measles virus vaccine recipient may experience the atypical onset, course, and manifestations of measles. The rash has a different appearance, distribution, and evolution from those observed in unimmunized individuals. It is more petechial and urticarial than that of natural measles. The disease may affect joint, pleural, peritoneal, and other tissues. Bellanti and coworkers (1969) demonstrated the presence of IgG-specific antibody and complement components in the skin lesions of such patients and an inflammatory cellular response more typical of type III reactions than any other immune type. Other investigators, including us, contend that a different mechanism is responsible for the observed disease or that a type III reaction is only one component of a complex immune response to the killed antigen (Fulginiti et al., 1967 and 1968).

If the person who received the KMV vaccine is subsequently given live measles virus vaccine (LMV), a local reaction at the site of injection may occur, and systemic symptoms appear that differ from those seen in unimmunized individuals given LMV. Bellanti and coworkers also have demonstrated histopathologic and immunopathologic changes at least consistent with a type III mechanism in the lesions associated with this response.

Type IV reactions have been documented infrequently after vaccines, in part because many of the observations were made at a time when relatively unsophisticated tests for cell-mediated immunity (CMI) were available. Atypical reactions related to the use of killed measles virus cited previously have been hypothesized to be due to type IV reactivity, specifically because of a disparity between a positive and persistent CMI response and lack of protective antibody in the recipient of killed vaccine (Fulginiti et al., 1967 and 1969). This disparity was believed to allow expression of CMI (type IV) immune reactions and to account for the unusual vasculitis-like manifestations observed.

Another atypical reaction to an experimental, killed virus vaccine produced similar heightened disease on natural exposure. Some infants immunized with killed respiratory syncytial virus vaccine had more severe manifestations of bronchiolitis when infected with wild virus

(Fulginiti et al., 1969). These manifestations occurred despite the demonstration of some antibody response to the vaccine. These infants were proved to have in vitro CMI responses that did not occur in naturally infected individuals, suggesting that type IV hypersensitivity was the predominant cause of the atypical bronchiolitis (Fulginiti et al., 1968).

SPECIFIC VACCINES

The usual schedule for commonly administered vaccines is indicated in Table 8–2.

DIPHTHERIA

Immunity and the Vaccine

Diphtheria is primarily a toxic disease, resulting from the absorption of a potent exotoxin from the local site of infection, most commonly the upper respiratory tract. Immunity against disease, and to some extent against infection, is related to the presence of circulating antitoxin. Hence, the immunization procedure consists of injections of diphtheria toxoid, diphtheria toxin that has been altered chemically to render it nontoxic without destroying its immunogenicity, and that evokes antitoxin in the recipient. The vaccine is administered by intramuscular injection deep into a large enough muscle to contain the full dose (CDC, 1983). Vaccine

TABLE 8–2. Usual Schedule for Commonly Administered Vaccines

Age	Vaccine*	Comments
2 months	DTP	0.5 ml I.M.
	OPV	Oral
4 months	DTP	
	OPV	
6 months	DTP (OPV)	Optional; in high risk areas
12 months	PPD	Test for tuberculosis
15 months	MMR	0.5 ml subcutaneous
18 months	DTP	
	OPV	
2 years	HIB	Subcutaneous, intramuscular
4 to 6 years	DTP	At or before entry into school
	OPV	
14 to 16 years	Td	Repeat every 10 years

* DTP = Diphtheria and tetanus toxoids; pertussis vaccine
OPV = Attenuated, live poliovirus vaccine
MMR = Live, attenuated measles, mumps, and rubella viruses
HIB = *Haemophilus influenzae*, type b, killed vaccine
PPD = Purified protein derivative (tuberculin)
Td = Tetanus and diphtheria toxoid, adult type

preparations include diphtheria toxoid alone (D), in combination with tetanus toxoid at full strength (DT, pediatric type), in combination with tetanus toxoid at reduced concentration (Td, adult type, containing approximately one twentieth the amount of diphtheria toxoid as is contained in DT or DPT), and in combination with tetanus toxoid and pertussis vaccine (DTP).

Adverse Reactions

Reactions to diphtheria toxoid are difficult to separate from those to other antigens contained in the combined vaccines (DT, DTP, and Td). That is, in most reports, they are usually considered together. The CDC maintains a passive surveillance system for reactions to vaccines that is totally voluntary, which reports "adverse events" occurring within 30 days after immunization. Table 8–3 displays the major reactions reported in this CDC surveillance system for vaccines containing diphtheria toxoids (CDC, 1984).

Local reactions are common when pertussis vaccine is included with diphtheria toxoid. The reduction in rates associated with lesser doses of diphtheria toxoid (Td) suggests that diphtheria toxoid may contribute somewhat to the local reaction. On the other hand, allergic reactions appear to be equivalent between DT and Td, suggesting the possibility that this is a dose-independent phenomenon. Unfortunately, rates for tetanus toxoid alone or diphtheria toxoid alone are not available in the CDC system, and one cannot argue from subtractive logic as to the contribution of each of these reactions.

There appears to be no age relationship to diphtheria toxoid reactions in these data, whereas the DTP reactions do diminish with increasing age, suggesting that the pertussis component is largely responsible for age-related reactions. One study demonstrated a significantly higher frequency of wheal and flare reactions to intradermal testing with diphtheria toxoid in atopic individuals compared with nonatopic individuals. Acute anaphylaxis also has been described in the older literature with the use of alum-precipitated diphtheria toxoid alone. Acute reactions of the anaphylactic type have been reported after Schick testing, consisting of swelling and wheals at the site of injection, puffiness of the face, generalized urticarial or scarlatiniform rash, faintness, cyanosis, and dyspnea; all patients recovered. This reaction has been attributed to the peptone used in preparing the Schick test material.

Reactions to full strength diphtheria toxoid in immune individuals appear to be more prevalent after age seven. Accordingly, only the lower doses of diphtheria toxoid should be used as Td, which contains one twentieth the concentration used in DTP and DT, and should be administered to individuals 7 years and older.

A recent investigation of DT in children suggests that the rate of local reactions is only 11.9 percent; fever occurred in only 19 percent, none higher than 39.0°C (Barkin et al., 1985). In 587 children examined after either DT or DTP, fever occurred more frequently after receipt of plain vaccines (without adjuvant) than after receipt of alum-adsorbed preparations (Waight et al., 1983). DT produced fewer fever episodes than did DTP, either plain or adsorbed. In the largest recent study, investigators at University of California at Los Angeles (UCLA) found significant differences between DTP and DT recipients for almost all reactions (Cody et al., 1981). In this study, 784 DT injections were compared with 15,752 DTP injections given to children from early infancy to 6 years of age. Table 8–4 sum-

TABLE 8–3. Reactions to DT, DTP, and Td within 30 Days of Receipt of Vaccine as Reported to the CDC for 1979–1982*

	DTP		DT		Td	
	NUMBER	RATE†	NUMBER	RATE†	NUMBER	RATE†
Local reactions	885	30.4	5	10.7	250	20.1
Fever	1334	45.8	11	23.5	145	11.7
Rash	259	8.9	2	4.3	33	2.7
Febrile convulsions	219	7.5	1	2.1	6	1.3
Allergic reactions	146	5.0	1	2.1	32	2.6

* (Modified from *Adverse Events Following Immunization-Surveillance.* USDHHS, PHS, CDC, Report No. 1, 1979–1982, Issued August 1984.)

† = Rates are calculated per million doses administered. Because of nature of reporting, these rates should be interpreted as indexes of the true rates.

TABLE 8-4. Reactions to DTP and DT in the UCLA Study*

	DT Recipients		DTP Receipients	
	NUMBER	RATE	NUMBER	RATE
LOCAL				
Redness	60	7.6	5891	37.4
Swelling	60	7.6	6411	40.7
Pain	78	9.9	8018	50.9
SYSTEMIC				
Fever > 38°C	27	9.3	3605	46.5
Drowsiness	117	14.9	4962	31.5
Fretfulness	177	22.6	8412	53.4
Vomiting	20	2.6	977	6.2
Anorexia	55	7.0	3292	20.9
Persistent crying	5	0.7	488	3.1
High pitched cry	0		17	0.1

* Adapted from Cody, C.L. et al.: Nature and rates of adverse reactions associated with DTP and DT immunizations in infants and children. Pediatrics 68:650, 1981.

marizes the results of this study. As can be seen, by subtractive reasoning the pertussis component appears to be responsible for the majority of reactions to DTP. A residual rate of reactions is apparent for DT, but which of the two components is responsible for this is unknown. Moreover, how much of this residual rate would be greater than that in nonimmunized children in the same time span of observation is unclear.

TETANUS TOXOID

Immunity and the Vaccine

Tetanus toxoid is one of the most effective vaccines currently available. Prolonged immunity, perhaps for a lifetime, follows full primary immunization with adequate booster doses at 10-year intervals thereafter. Immunity is antitoxic in nature; vaccinees can acquire infection with *Clostridium tetani* but are immune to the toxic effects of the infection (CDC, 1983).

Adverse Reactions

Tetanus toxoid shares with diphtheria toxoid the capacity to produce local irritation. Tables 8-3 and 8-4 list the rates of some reactions reported for combinations of the two toxoids. It is not possible to differentiate between the two vaccines as to cause of the reactions. Tetanus toxoid alone is administered to some individuals, and reactions to it have been catalogued. There is an anecdotal report of a large overdose of tetanus toxoid (3.8 ml in contrast to the usual 0.5 ml) that resulted in a local reaction of mild erythema, heat induration, tenderness, and pain at the injection sites, peaking at 48 hours after injection (Lerner, 1974). The reaction gradually resolved within 5 days, with no systemic symptoms and no residuae. The physician interpreted this as a delayed reaction without serum sickness, probably of the CMI type.

Tetanus toxoid alum-adsorbed vaccine is associated with more adverse reactions than the fluid preparation. In one study involving 9703 injections of alum-precipitated vaccine, severe local reactions were noted in 19 instances (White, 1980). Twelve occurred after booster doses administered to individuals who had received the full primary series. Moderate reactions occurred 74 times, again with a predominance among booster dose recipients. In another study involving 220 adults given booster doses 25 to 30 years after primary immunization, reactions were without serious side effects and were observed in 39.5 percent (Simonsen et al., 1984). Fever and malaise were reported in only two individuals (1 percent).

Few studies have attempted to investigate responses to tetanus toxoid other than antitoxic antibody levels. In one group of infants aged 1 to 2 years, DTP immunization resulted in elevation of IgE antibody to tetanus toxin. In three infants, the DTP injection was associated with local erythema, swelling, and tenderness, and all had markedly elevated levels of toxin specific–IgE antibody (700 to 4000 units/ml) (Matuhasi and Ikegami, 1982).

Tetanus toxoid is known to induce CMI responses in recipients. Several investigators have shown that it is a useful test for delayed cutaneous hypersensitivity (or CMI), in the assessment of possible immune deficiency (Delafuente et al., 1983). From 60 to 100 percent of prior recipients of tetanus toxoid have been reported to have positive delayed skin test reactions. The extent to which CMI plays a role in adverse reactions has not been investigated systematically. One group investigated the ratio of T-helper to T-suppressor cells before and after immunization with tetanus toxoid. In 11 healthy adults, a significant decrease in the helper/suppressor ratio was noted; in four of the 11, the ratio dropped to one or less, a value considered abnormal and often associated with early stages of acquired immune deficiency syndrome (AIDS) (Eibl et al., 1984). The clinical relevance of these changes in T-cell populations, however, is unknown.

Most investigators have attributed the severe local reactions to tetanus toxoid to a type III (Arthus) reaction, resulting from excessive levels of preformed antibody to tetanus toxin interacting with the locally injected booster dose to produce vascular inflammation with necrosis (Edsall, 1971). Reaction "proneness" has been related to titers of tetanus antitoxin in the serum of greater than or equal to 5 units/ml. The reaction-prone group is a small minority of those with similarly high titers, therefore, other factors also are operative. In any event, an individual with a history of previous reaction to tetanus toxoid appears more likely to fall into this small group of individuals susceptible to further reactions, which may be severe. Such persons should not receive subsequent doses of tetanus toxoid.

PERTUSSIS

Immunity and the Vaccine

Precise identification of that part of the immune response that accounts for the observed 85 to 95 percent protection among recipients of pertussis vaccine has not been achieved (Mortimer, 1980). A variety of serum antibodies have been identified, but only loose correlation with protection has been found. At this point, it appears that at least two of the identifiable pertussis antigens may be related to induction of immunity to infection, as follows: the (1) fimbria antigen and the (2) lymphocytosis-promoting factor. A vaccine containing these antigens currently is being evaluated in Japan and the United States (Sato et al., 1984). Preliminary results suggest that it is both effective and relatively safe, with fewer side effects locally and systemically, than whole bacterial vaccine in wide use.

Adverse Reactions

Whole bacterial vaccine consists of billions of pertussis organisms, some of which are fragmented and contain a variety of components of the bacilli, including endotoxin. It is not surprising that a large number of local reactions occur after injection of this product. Tables 8-3 and 8-4 indicate the high frequency of local reactions attributable to the pertussis component of DTP (Cody et al., 1981).

Most of the local reactions appear to be due to physical irritation at the site of injection with attendant inflammation, although there is little or no objective evidence to substantiate this idea. Local reactions can develop into so-called sterile abscesses (Church et al., 1985). Some investigators believe that these are secondary to the leakage or direct injection of vaccine into the subcutaneous tissues or to hypersensitivity to one or more components. Bacterial infections may also occur at the site of injection (CDC, 1984; Stetler et al., 1985; Kassanoff et al., 1971). Usually these infections are caused by the pyogenic cocci, occasionally by anaerobic organisms. Clusters of patients with this complication can be related to contamination of a multiple dose vial, with subsequent inoculation of the organisms into additional vaccinees. Individual instances of pyogenic abscesses may be related to improper sterilization of the vial cap, the syringe, or the site of injection.

Generalized reactions are believed secondary to any of a number of "toxins" of pertussis (Mortimer, 1980). Systemic reactions range from fever to central nervous system (CNS) irritability. The most serious consequence, postpertussis vaccine encephalopathy, appears with a frequency estimated at one per 310,000 inoculations (Miller et al., 1981). The cause of the encephalopathy is uncertain. Fenichel (1982) disclaims an association of pertussis vaccine with any definable CNS disorder. Most workers accept the concept that an encephalopathy rarely can be caused by the vaccine, but as there are no definitive tests and no characteristic pathologic findings even at autopsy, proof of causation is not possible. In addition, the occurrence of other CNS diseases in the same age group as that during which pertussis vaccine is administered complicates the assessment of cause. For example, viral meningoencephalitis can occur and coincidentally follow pertussis vaccine administration. Even more dramatic are infantile spasms (infantile myoclonic seizures), an illness shown to be independent of pertussis vaccine but having its onset in the 2- to 6-month-old infant. Several studies have shown that infantile spasms are seen with the same frequency in unimmunized and immunized infants, and the frequency does not change even if the first dose of vaccine is delayed until 6 months of age (Melchior, 1977; Bellman, 1983). It is clear that the onset of infantile spasms appears to cluster within 1 week of receipt of vaccine; but the frequency is no different overall than that of nonrecipients of vaccine, for a 30 day period following the time of vaccination.

Allergic reactions to the pertussis component are difficult to sort out, since pertussis almost always is used in one form of DTP vaccine. Thus, if an urticarial reaction develops within hours of receipt of DTP, it is uncertain which component the child is reacting to. Shira (1985) tested a small group of children who had urticaria after injections of one of the vaccines (DTP, DT, or Td). Only one of seven children had a positive (actually marginal) immediate skin test reaction to the corresponding vaccine. He administered the next due dose of the vaccine to the six children with negative skin test results in full dose, without reactions. In the seventh child, he gave fractional doses until the full 0.5 ml dose was reached, again without adverse reaction. This small, informal experience does not provide sufficient guidelines to indicate that this is the correct procedure; it is reassuring enough to imply that such testing and cautious administration of the needed next dose of vaccine are acceptable procedures until additional information is forthcoming.

POLIOVIRUS VACCINES

Immunity and the Vaccines

Two types of poliovirus vaccine are available, as follows: Sabin live, attenuated, oral vaccine (OPV) and Salk inactivated, killed vaccine (IPV) (Ray, 1982). Both stimulate systemic IgG antibody to all three types of poliovirus. After a full vaccination series, more than 95 percent of recipients are antibody positive to all three types of poliovirus. OPV also stimulates IgA-specific antibody in the gastrointestinal and upper respiratory tract, which IPV does not. Such topical antibody prevents infection by wild-type viruses in OPV recipients. In contrast, IPV vaccinees, despite systemic antibody, can be infected with wild polioviruses of the same type.

Currently, OPV is recommended for routine use in infants and children and in persons at high risk of contracting wild poliovirus at any age (American Academy of Pediatrics (AAP), 1986). However, IPV is recommended for individuals at greater risk of paralytic diseases from OPV, such as those immunosuppressed by disease or treatment, those over the age of 18 years, and those who may contact and therefore transmit the vaccine viruses to others who are immunosuppressed.

Adverse Events

OPV has one serious adverse consequence, i.e., the development of paralytic disease caused by one of the three types of poliovirus in the vaccine (Schonberger, et al., 1976). Paralytic disease occurs rarely; the rate for primary recipients of the vaccine has been estimated over the years as approximately one instance in 3 to 5 million doses of vaccine distributed. It is uncertain why normal individuals develop paralysis, although there is a strong suspicion that genetic predisposition, perhaps linked to immune response genes in the major histocompatibility locus of chromosome 6, may play a critical role (Van Eden et al., 1983). Adult contacts of immunized infants and children also are more susceptible to the rare event of paralysis after OPV. Such persons may not have encountered wild virus nor have received poliovirus vaccines, or having received poliovirus vaccines may be among those who did not respond to the vaccine. Thus, they are fully susceptible to the particular type of poliovirus that is excreted by the primary vaccinee, and after oral or pharyngeal contact may develop paralysis. The rate of paralytic disease is higher than for primary vaccinees, approximately one per 3 to 4 million doses distributed, possibly because the virus reverts to neurovirulence upon passage and growth in the gastrointestinal tract. A genetic predisposition to disease, previously alluded to, also may be operative in these individuals (Green, 1974; Van Eden et al., 1983).

Immunosuppressed persons experience a 10,000-fold greater risk of paralysis than do normal persons. Such immunosuppression may be congenital or acquired. Acquired causes include lymphatic malignancies and other tumors associated with reduction in host defense mechanisms. In addition, persons receiving immunosuppressive therapy may be susceptible to paralysis upon contact with vaccine viruses.

There are no other known adverse consequences of oral poliovirus vaccines. Apart from local irritation in a minority of IPV recipients, it is generally believed that serious side effects do not occur in recipients of this vaccine.

MEASLES VIRUS VACCINE

Immunity and the Vaccine

Live, attenuated measles virus provides children over the age of 15 months with more than

95 percent assurance that they will be immune to the natural disease after receipt of a single dose of the vaccine (AAP, 1986). The vaccine is effective in any individual at any age older than 15 months who neither has had the natural disease nor has been immunized previously. However, for infants under the age of 15 months, residual maternal antibody prevents successful multiplication of the vaccine virus in some. This effect is most pronounced in the early months of life and gradually diminishes at 13 to 14 months of age because of the waning of maternal antibody. At 6 months of age, as few as 50 percent of infants are capable of responding to vaccine; at 9 months of age, approximately 65 percent respond; and at 13 to 14 months of age, more than 95 percent respond with production of neutralizing antibody. Efficacy against disease on exposure to the wild virus is directly correlated with the presence of any detectable serum antibody.

Prior to 1965 in the United States and to 1970 in Canada, killed or inactivated measles virus vaccine was used for some children (Fulginiti et al., 1967 and 1968). It has been estimated that 600,000 individuals were immunized in the United States. This vaccine appeared to be effective, as judged by serum antibody levels and resistance to infection, for variable periods after immunization. However, protection eventually waned, and an atypical, often severe, form of measles occurred upon exposure to natural virus. Consequently, the vaccine was removed from the market and has not been in use since.

Adverse Effects

Live measles virus (LMV) vaccine produces fever and rash within 5 to 14 days after receipt of the vaccine in fewer than 15 percent of children immunized. This "illness" is mild and often unnoticed, usually producing no impairment of function or sense of well-being. No other serious side effects have been noted in healthy individuals. Although CNS disease has been noted after receipt of vaccine, the frequency is no different in vaccinees than in unvaccinated individuals of the same age (CDC, 1984). Specifically no increase in subacute sclerosing panencephalitis has been observed after LMV. In fact, there has been a marked reduction in the frequency of this disorder, suggesting that elimination of the measles in much of the population has reduced the "hidden" infection of the CNS previously associated with natural infection.

LMV vaccine has produced systemic dissemination and death in individuals severely compromised immunologically by virtue of hematologic malignancies, congenital immunodeficiencies, and immunosuppressive therapy (Lipsey et al., 1967; Nahmias et al., 1967).

In atopic children, LMV was originally thought to be harmless, despite the theoretical possibility that egg antigens from the chicken might be present in the chick embryo tissue culture in which the live virus was grown to prepare the vaccine. In fact, several studies supported the safety of the vaccine for egg-sensitive children. More recently, Hermann and coworkers (1983) reported anaphylactic reactions in extremely egg-sensitive children given the LMV vaccine. Investigation showed both the presence of nanogram amounts of ovalbumin in the vaccine and IgE anti-ovalbumin antibody in egg-sensitive children who reacted to the vaccine. These investigators concluded that any child with a history of anaphylactic reactions to egg should first undergo skin-testing with vaccines containing LMV, which are to be administered. If the test result is negative, the vaccine can be given in full dosage under closely supervised circumstances, with the administrator prepared and capable of responding to an anaphylactic reaction. In skin test–positive potential recipients, it is suggested that an elaborate scheme of small incremental doses be administered (see Fig. 8–1). Using this technique, Hermann noted that 20 nonallergic children had negative prick test results and tolerated the vaccine without any immediate reactions; of 21 children without a history of egg white sensitivity, none had positive prick or intradermal test results, and none reacted adversely to the vaccine. In six children who had positive histories of generalized urticaria, angioedema, wheezing, or laryngeal edema after exposure to egg white, four had positive prick skin test results, two had positive intradermal test results, and all were immunized with the incremental series (outlined in Fig. 8–1) without adverse consequences.

RUBELLA VIRUS VACCINE

Immunity and the Vaccine

Administration of live rubella virus vaccine (LRuVV) is followed by development of serum antibody in more than 95 percent of recipients (Alexander, 1982). In contrast to measles vaccination, immunity wanes sufficiently that a

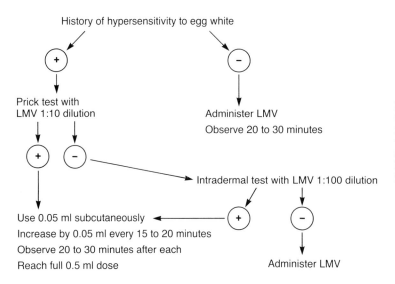

FIGURE 8–1. Schema for administration of vaccines containing live measles virus (LMV) to children who have histories of anaphylactic reactions to eggs. (Adapted from Hermann, J.J. et al., J. Pediatr. *102*:196, 1983.)

fairly large proportion of these vaccinees can be infected by natural virus, albeit without disease and without detectable viremia. In fact, the reinfection by wild virus produces a boost in antibody titer. In some individuals, serum antibody appears to wane over a period of years to undetectable levels (Orenstein et al., 1984), raising the question of whether reimmunization may be necessary in order to ensure lifelong protection. However, when such individuals, originally immunized with demonstrable positive antibody response but now without detectable antibody, are given a second dose of LRuVV, they respond rapidly with an increase in IgG antibody, indicative of an immune or a secondary response (Balfour, 1981). Thus, they appear to be protected despite the seeming lack of antibody. In some instances, serum antibody that is undetectable by standard testing in fact is present when more sensitive tests are used.

It now appears that a single immunization with live virus vaccine suffices to provide very long-term immunity, probably for a lifetime, although definitive proof of this immunity will be provided only with continued measurement and observation of those vaccinated over their lifetimes (Hermann et al., 1982). An additional feature of LRuVV immunization is the fact that virus can be recovered in low titer from a vaccinee's upper respiratory tract. This finding led to the speculation that vaccine virus might be transmissible to others and that, in women, the virus might also be present in the blood at or near the time of conception and, thus, be transmitted to the fetus. No convincing evidence for transmissibility has been shown. Even bed-

mates in a residential institution for the mentally retarded failed to seroconvert when exposed intimately to a recent vaccinee. Alleged instances of transmission are clouded by the finding that wild virus was present in the same population that received vaccine. Thus, the infected person may have acquired the infection naturally instead of through contact with vaccine-related virus.

The possibility that vaccine virus could infect the fetus appears to be adequately refuted by the experience of a large number of pregnant women who were inadvertently immunized shortly before conception to 3 months after conception (CDC, 1983). In individuals in this group who were known to be serologically negative, hence susceptible, and who seroconverted with vaccine infection, congenital rubella syndrome has not been observed. In a few instances, there has been serologic evidence of infection in a normal offspring, but in none of these patients has abnormalities attributable to vaccine virus infection been noted. Many of the children born to the mothers who were inadvertently immunized have been followed for as long as 7 years without observable adverse effects from possible exposure to the vaccine virus *in utero.*

Adverse Effects

LRuVV has predictable side effects including mild disease-like symptoms, arthritis/arthralgia, rarely peripheral neuropathy, and possibly thrombocytopenia (CDC, 1983). Mild rubella-like symptoms occur in <10 percent of vaccinees; symptoms are transient and without serious manifestations or sequelae. Arthritis/arthralgia is more frequent in recipients, occurring in an estimated 8 percent of children and in as many as 40 percent of adult females. Occasionally, the painful joints may last for a week or more. No proven instance of rheumatoid arthritis–like disease, persisting beyond the immediate post-vaccine period, has been identified; although there are isolated reports of the arthritic syndrome after immunization but without obvious causal link to the vaccine. Peripheral neuropathy is a rare event, with two distinct syndromes identified; one involves the lower extremity, and the other involves the upper extremity. Pain can be severe and may last for long periods, although permanent effects have not been described.

In recent years, only a human diploid cell line has been used to prepare the vaccine. Thus, egg sensitivity is not a concern with this product.

LIVE MUMPS VIRUS VACCINE

Immunity and the Vaccine

More than 95 percent of individuals who receive LMuVV respond with antibody and are protected against natural exposure (CDC, 1983). Despite apparent breakthroughs, true mumps virus infection (parotitis) has not been demonstrated in an immune vaccinee (AAP, 1986). Other infections that cause parotitis may occur in vaccinated individuals and may be mistakenly considered to be vaccine failures. These instances will be more apparent in a population that is largely immune to mumps by virtue of immunization, with the residual instances of parotitis occurring in the unvaccinated or in the population as a whole from other infectious agents. Some primary failures are inevitable, however. Thus, some individuals with histories of mumps vaccinations will contract the disease. Nevertheless, careful studies that compare rates between unimmunized and immunized individuals demonstrate more than 85 to 95 percent protection afforded recipients of the vaccine.

Adverse Events

Parotitis has been reported rarely. Presumably, egg allergy could be a problem (see

Measles Virus Vaccine) although reports have *not* been recorded. Similarly, allergy to neomycin in the vaccine is a potential problem.

INFLUENZA VACCINE

Influenza vaccine is effective in preventing disease in immunized persons, and side effects with the use of recently developed vaccines are fairly minimal (Alexander, 1982). In the past, when purification processes were less satisfactory than at the present, considerable toxicity was associated with the vaccine. By techniques such as zonal centrifugation, the current inactivated influenza vaccines produce few reactions that are severe. Self-limited local and mild systemic reactions are infrequent. Egg allergy remains a potential problem for the egg-sensitive patient; the vaccine is still produced by growth of the virus in fertilized hens' eggs prior to inactivation. Small amounts of egg antigens are carried over into the final product, with the result that anaphylactic reactions have been recorded among individuals known to be highly egg-sensitive. Influenza vaccine should not be administered to patients with histories of anaphylactic reactions to egg white, unless skin test results to the vaccine are negative (Bierman et al., 1977).

RABIES VACCINE

The older rabies vaccines derived from animal nervous tissue were often associated with severe CNS reactions. Duck embryo vaccine had fewer CNS reactions, but local and systemic allergic reactions were common (Harrison, 1982). The only vaccine recommended today is grown in human diploid cell culture and is devoid of serious reactions of any type, although a number of irritating symptoms have been recorded after its administration (CDC, 1984).

HAEMOPHILUS INFLUENZAE VACCINE

The newest entry into immunization practice is a polysaccharide vaccine prepared from capsular material of the organism, *H. influenzae*, type b (AAP, 1986). It is a highly purified and concentrated product and has had only one serious reaction (in Finland) associated with its administration. One child among 50,000 who received the vaccine developed an acute anaphylactic reaction, which responded promptly and fully, without recurrence, to epinephrine. Other reactions include fever (1 percent) and local heat, redness, and tenderness (25 percent).

In summary, vaccines are among the most effective preventive measures that we have in medicine. They are not perfect, however, and reactions ranging from annoying to lethal are associated with some. Virtually every vaccine consists of a biologic product, derived from the natural organism, that is either inactivated or attenuated. As a result, the injection of these antigens produces undesired, but intrinsically predictable, reactions in the host. Efforts to reduce reactivity in the future include the following: (1) improvement of purification steps; (2) removal of unwanted and unnecessary antigens from the vaccine; (3) preparation of narrow spectrum vaccines from concentrated antigens of specific type known to induce the desired immune response; (4) recognition of host factors that enhance adverse effects either to administer the vaccine in a different way than is usual (such as occurs in the egg-sensitive individual with live measles virus vaccine) or to avoid the vaccine; and (5) synthetic preparation of vaccine antigens using DNA cloning techniques and genetic manipulation, resulting in highly specific antigens only of the type desired.

REFERENCES

AAP (American Academy of Pediatrics): *Report of the Committee on Infectious Diseases,* 20th ed. Evanston, Illinois, 1986.

Alexander, E.R.: Influenza. *In* Fulginiti V.A. (ed.), *Immunization in Clinical Practice,* Philadelphia, J.B. Lippincott Co., 1982.

Alexander, E.R.: Rubella. *In* Fulginiti, V.A. (ed.), *Immunization in Clinical Practice,* Philadelphia, J.B. Lippincott Co., 1982.

Balfour, H.H., Groth, E., Edelman, C.K., Best, J., Banatuala, J.E.: Rubella viremia and antibody responses after rubella vaccination and revaccination. Lancet 1:1078–1080, 1981.

Barkin, R.M., Pichichero, M.E., Samuelson, J.S., Barkin, S.Z.: Pediatric diphtheria and tetanus toxoids vaccine: Clinical and immunologic response when administered as the primary series. J. Pediatr. 106:779–781, 1985.

Bellanti, J.A., Sanga, R.L., Klutinis, B., Brandt, B., Artenstein, M.S.: Antibody responses in serum and nasal secretions of children immunized with inactivated and attenuated measles virus vaccines. N. Engl. J. Med. 280:628–633, 1969.

Bellman, M.H., Ross, E.M., Miller, D.L.: Infantile spasms

and pertussis immunization. Lancet 1:1031–1032, 1983.

Bierman, C.W., Shapiro, G.G., Pierson, W.E., Taylor, J.W., Foy, H.M., Fox, J.P.: Safety of influenza vaccination in allergic children. J. Infect. Dis. 136:652–655, 1977.

Brinton, M.A., Nathanson, N.: Genetic determinants of virus susceptibility. Epidemiol. Rev. 3:115–139, 1981.

CDC (Centers for Disease Control): M.M.W.R. 32:1–17, 1983.

CDC: Adverse Events Following Immunization; surveillance. USDHHS, PHS, Document 00–4405, Report 1, August, 1984.

CDC: Rubella vaccination during pregnancy, United States, 1971–1982. M.M.W.R. 32:429–432, 437, 1983.

CDC: Rabies prevention and control. M.M.W.R. 33:393–402, 1984.

Church, J.A., Richards, W.: Recurrent abscess formation following DTP immunization. Pediatrics 75:899–900, 1985.

Cody, C.L., Baraff, L.J., Cherry, J.D., Marcy, S.M., Manclark, C.R.: The nature and rate of adverse reactions associated with DTP and DT immunization in infants and children. Pediatrics 68:650–660, 1981.

Delafuente, J.C., Eisenberg, J.D., Hoelzer, D.R., Slavan, R.G.: Tetanus toxoid as an antigen for delayed cutaneous hypersensitivity. J.A.M.A. 249:3209–3211, 1983.

Edsall, G.: The current status of tetanus immunization. Hosp. Pract. 6:57–66, 1971.

Eibl, M.M., Mannhalter, J.W., Zlabinger, G.: Abnormal T-lymphocyte subpopulations in healthy subjects after tetanus booster immunization. N. Engl. J. Med. 310:198–199, 1984.

Fenichel, G.: Neurological complications of immunization. Ann. Neur. 12:119–128, 1982.

Fulginiti, V.A.: Abnormalities in Vaccine Responsiveness. *In* Kagan, B., Stiehm, E.R. (eds.), *Immunologic Incompetence,* Chicago, Year Book Medical Publishers, Inc., 1971.

Fulginiti, V.A.: Practical Aspects of Immunization. *In* Fulginiti, V.A. (ed.), *Immunization in Clinical Practice,* Philadelphia, J.B. Lippincott Co., 1982.

Fulginiti, V.A., Arthur, J.H., Pearlman, D.S., Kempe, C.H.: Altered reactivity to measles virus, local reactions following measles virus immunization in children who previously received a combination of inactivated and attenuated vaccines, Am. J. Dis. Childh. 115:671–677, 1968.

Fulginiti, V.A., Eller, J.J., Downie, A.W., Arthur, J.H., Pearlman, D.S.: Altered reactivity to measles virus. J.A.M.A. 202:1078–1080, 1967.

Fulginiti, V.A., Eller, J.T., Sieber, O.F., Joyner, J.W., Minimitani, M.: Respiratory virus immunization. Am. J. Epidemiol. 89:435–448, 1969.

Gell, P.G.H., Coombs, R.R.A.: *Clinical Aspects of Immunology.* Oxford, Blackwell Scientific Publications Ltd., 1968.

Green, H.: The gene for the poliovirus receptor, N. Engl. J. Med. 290:303, 1974.

Harrison, H.R.: Rabies, *In* Fulginiti, V.A. (ed.), *Immunization in Clinical Practice,* Philadelphia, J.B. Lippincott Co., 1982.

Hermann, J.T., Schneiderman, R.: Allergic reactions to measles (rubeola) vaccine in patients hypersensitive to egg protein. J. Pediatr. 102:196–200, 1983.

Hermann, K.L., Halstead, S.B., Wiebanga, N.H.: Rubella antibody persistence after immunization. J.A.M.A. 247:193–196, 1982.

Hooker, J.M.: A laboratory study of the toxicity of some

diphtheria-tetanus-pertussis vaccines. J. Biol. Stand. 9:493–506, 1981.

Issacson, P., Stone, A.: Allergic reactions associated with viral vaccines. Prog. Med. Virol. 13:239–247, 1971.

Jones, J., Fulginiti, V.A.: Immunology of Immunization. *In* Fulginiti, V.A. (ed.), *Immunization in Clinical Practice,* Philadelphia, J. B. Lippincott Co., 1982.

Kassanoff, I., Nahmias, A.J., Abrutyn, E.: Fatal staphylococcal septicemia associated with use of jet injector for measles vaccination. Pediatrics 47:135 137, 1971.

Kelton, J.G.: Vaccination-associated relapse of immune thrombocytopenia. J.A.M.A. 245:369–371, 1981.

Lerner, S.: Overdose of tetanus toxoid (letter). J.A.M.A. 228:159, 1974.

Lipsey, A.I., Kahn, M.J., Bolande, R.P.: Pathologic variants of congenital hypogammaglobulinemia: An analysis of 3 patients dying of measles. Pediatrics 39:659–661, 1967.

Matuhasi, T., Ikegami, H.: Elevation of levels of IgE antibody to tetanus toxin in individuals vaccinated with DTP vaccine. J. Infect. Dis. 146:290, 1982.

Melchior, J.C.: Infantile spasms and early immunization against whooping coughs: Danish survey from 1970 to 1975. Arch. Dis. Child. 52:134–138, 1977.

Melnick, J.L.: Live attenuated oral poliovirus vaccine. Rev. Infect. Dis. 6:323–327, 1984.

Miller, D.L., Ross, E.M., Alderslade, R., Bellman, M.H., Rawson, N.S.B.: Pertussis immunization and serious neurological illness in children. Brit. Med. J. 282:1595–1599, 1981.

Mortimer, E.A., Jr.: Pertussis immunization: Problems, perspectives, prospects. Hosp. Pract. 15:103–118, 1980.

Nahmias, A., Griffith, D., Salsbury, C., Yoshida, K.: Thymic aplasia with lymphopenia, plasma cells and normal immunoglobulins in relation to measles virus infection. J.A.M.A. 201:103–108, 1967.

Orenstein, W.A., Bart, K.J., Hinman, A.R., Preblud, S.R., Greaves, W.L., Doster, S.W., Stetler, H.C., Sirotkin, B.: The opportunity and obligation to eliminate rubella from the United States. J.A.M.A. 251:1988–1994, 1984.

Ray, C.G.: Poliomyelitis. *In* Fulginiti, V.A. (ed.), *Immunization in Clinical Practice,* Philadelphia, J.B. Lippincott Co., 1982.

Sato, Y., Kimura, M., Fukimi, H.: Development of a pertussis component vaccine in Japan. Lancet 1:122–126, 1984.

Schonberger, L.B., McGousan, J.E., Gregg, M.B.: Vaccine-associated poliomyelitis in the United States, 1961–1972. Am. J. Epidemiol. 104:202–211, 1976.

Shira, J.: Personal communication, 1985.

Simonsen O., Kjeldsen, K., Heron, J.: Immunity against tetanus and effect of revaccination 25–30 years after primary vaccination. Lancet 1:1240–1244, 1984.

Stetler, H.C., Garbe, P.L., Dwyer, D.M., Facklam, R.R., Orenstein, W.A., West, G.R., Dudly, K.J., Bloch, A.B.: Outbreaks of group-A streptococcal abscesses following Diptheria-Tetanus-Pertussis Vaccination. Pediatrics 75:299–303, 1985.

Vallancourt, R.J.: Current poliovirus vaccines. Rev. Infect. Dis. 6:328–333, 1984.

Van Eden, W., Persijn, G.G., Bijkerk, H., deVries, R.R.P., Schuurman, R.K.B., van Rood, J.J., Persijn, G.G.: Differential resistance to paralytic poliomyelitis controlled by histocompatibility leucocyte antigens. J. Infect. Dis. 147:422–426, 1983.

Waight, P.A., Pollock, T.M., Miller, E., Coleman, E.M.: Pyrexia after diphtheria/tetanus/pertussis and diphtheria/tetanus vaccines. Arch. Dis. Child. 58:921–933, 1983.

White, W.G.: Reactions after plain and adsorbed tetanus vaccines. Lancet 1:42, 1980.

ETIOLOGIC AND PATHOGENETIC FACTORS IN ALLERGIC DISEASES

9

Epidemiologic Considerations in Atopic Disease

LAURIE J. SMITH, M.D.
RAYMOND G. SLAVIN, M.D.

As defined in the first preface to this book, an allergic disease is considered to be "a complex of symptoms and signs in which immune events are thought frequently to play a major role." Atopic disorders represent a group of so-called allergic diseases in which there is a familial tendency, and which often coexist in the same individual. Epidemiologic and clinical studies support an association between the propensity to produce IgE antibody and the atopic diseases, such as asthma, seasonal and perennial allergic rhinitis, and atopic dermatitis. Although IgE antibody frequently is found in these diseases, its involvement is not universal. Even when present, its role in the pathogenesis of a particular atopic disease often is unclear. Thus, while there is an association between IgE antibody and the atopic diseases, the heritability of the atopic diseases and the genetics of IgE production appear to be separate.

EPIDEMIOLOGIC STUDIES

Epidemiologic studies intend to characterize certain facets of disease, as follows: *cumulative prevalence* — the proportion of the general population that currently has a particular disease or has had it previously; *point prevalence* — the proportion of the population that has a disease currently or at a given time; *incidence* — the number of new cases of a particular disease identified during a specified observation period. Epidemiologic studies also cover mortality rates, hospital admission rates, and economic impact of a disease, including days lost from school and work, cost of medicines and medical care, and lost revenues. These studies are subject to a large number of variables, which may affect interpretation of results. Identification of a disease, such as asthma or allergic rhinitis, may be made from medical records, verbal reports, questionnaires, or actual physical examination and physiologic studies. Atopy may be inferred merely by the finding of allergic antibody in an individual in some studies; in others, establishment of an association between positive allergy test results and symptoms, or a positive family history may be required. How stringently one defines a disease, such as asthma, may affect data results. A question such as "Have you ever wheezed?" will generate a different prevalence rate than "Has a physician ever diagnosed or treated you for asthma?" When different methodologies are applied to the study of the same disease, therefore, enormous variations occur in the estimates of prevalence of a disease, such as asthma (Table 9–1). Some variations may reflect true differences in disease prevalence, whereas others may merely reflect sampling and methodologic differences.

GENERAL EPIDEMIOLOGIC CONSIDERATIONS

Despite enormous problems encountered in assessing epidemiologic aspects of atopic disease, it is possible to make certain observations. Each disease is considered separately later in this chapter, but a few general comments concerning several epidemiologic factors are warranted first.

Prevalence and Incidence. The prevalence and incidence of atopic respiratory disease vary considerably in different parts of the world (Table 9–1 and Table 9–2). There is evidence that asthma is increasing in prevalence both in

121

TABLE 9–1. Prevalence of Asthma
(Percent Population)

<1.5	1.5 to 6	>6
Sweden	France	Denmark
Finland	Britain	Australia
Germany	United States	New Zealand
Switzerland	Tanzania	United States
Gambia	South Africa	Maldive Islands
Japan	Sweden	
India	Israel	
Norway	Canada	

the United States and other areas of the world. This increase appears to transcend differences in study methodologies and most likely represents a true increase in disease rate and morbidity and mortality rates of asthma.

Genetic Factors. Atopic allergic diseases are reported to be clustered in families. Studies performed in Iowa by Smith (1975) revealed that 87 percent of children who developed an atopic disorder before 10 years of age had a close relative with an atopic disorder. It was found that 16 percent of girls and 28 percent of boys born into households in which someone already had an atopic respiratory disorder had developed asthma or allergic rhinitis by age 20 years, compared with 0.08 percent of girls and 1.5 percent of boys born into households in which no atopic respiratory disorder was present.

This familial occurrence of atopic disorders suggests a genetic basis for their appearance. Some investigators have reported an increased incidence of HLA-B8 and HLA-Dw3 and HLA-Dw2 associated with allergic diseases (Smith, 1983). This association is weak, and most in-

vestigators feel a polygenic type of inheritance is involved in atopic diseases (see also Chapter 2). There is a familial concordance of IgE levels reported both in identical twins and in families (Lebowitz et al., 1984). Even identical twins, however, do not demonstrate complete concordance with atopic disorders. This concordance is higher for monozygotic than dizygotic twins but neither exceeds 50 percent (Lubs, 1971). It has been suggested that the presence of atopic diseases in the mother may be of more importance than that in the father in predisposing a child to an atopic disease (Smith, 1983).

It has also been shown convincingly that atopy, defined as producing allergic antibody, is inherited separately from bronchial hyperreactivity. Sibbald et al. (1980) demonstrated an increased prevalence of asthma in relatives of both atopic (i.e., allergic) and nonatopic asthmatics, as compared with nonasthmatic individuals. Also, the prevalence of atopic asthma was higher in relatives of both atopic and nonatopic probands, suggesting that asthma is inherited separately from allergic reactivity. Sibbald and coworkers suggest that an increased prevalence of asthma in relatives of atopic asthmatics arises from an increased susceptibility for asthma in individuals who inherit separately a predisposition to both asthma and atopy. In another study, Sibbald and Turner-Warwick (1979) found that hay fever and eczema were more common among relatives of atopic asthmatics than of nonatopic asthmatics, again emphasizing the separate pattern of inheritance of asthma per se and atopic diseases.

Atopic dermatitis or infantile eczema has been characterized as a disease with hyperreactive skin. Although 80 to 90 percent of cases are

TABLE 9–2. Prevalence of Allergic Rhinitis (Percent Population)*

	Boys	Girls	Both	Adults
Sweden		1.5		14.8
Finland	14	8	2.7	10
United States	4.9–9	3.6–8	3.1	9.7–10.6
Switzerland			0.5–4.4	
Puerto Rico			11	
Maldive Islands			20.4	
Belgium				0.5
New Zealand				6.2–10.4
Wales (over 70)				7.9
Canada				9.1
Tokelau (on the island)			14	
(in New Zealand)			28	

* Derived from data in Smith, 1983. The varying percent prevalance rates in the same countries come from studies performed by different researchers at different times.

associated with increased serum levels of IgE (Rasmussen and Provost, 1983), IgE antibody cannot be implicated in the pathogenesis of the disease in most cases. Nevertheless, atopic dermatitis is found frequently in association with other atopic diseases, both in individuals with other disorders and in families of such individuals. In fact, when the group of asthmatics reported by McNicol and Williams in 1973 was followed to age 21, 50 percent of the milder asthmatics and 75 percent of the more severe asthmatics were found to have had allergic rhinitis; 35 percent of the most severe asthmatics were found to have had atopic dermatitis persisting into adult life (Martin et al., 1981). Others have also demonstrated an association between atopic dermatitis and the occurrence and persistence of asthma (Blair, 1977; Horwood et al., 1985). However, a recent study from New Zealand demonstrated that, although parental asthma and eczema and childhood asthma and eczema were related, there was a specific inheritance pattern in which parents with eczema tended to have children with eczema, with no association with childhood asthma, and parents with asthma tended to have children with asthma (Fergusson et al., 1983). It is interesting that hyperreactive skin (decreased threshold for itching) can occur in the absence of IgE antibody production, which suggests some parallel in the case with asthma and indicates further the complexity of the genetic scheme of atopic inheritance.

Environmental Versus Genetic Factors. A major influence on the prevalence of allergic disease may be the amount and nature of allergens in different environments. Some apparent racial differences, in fact, may be due to differences in environmental influences. The prevalence of asthma in Asian and West Indian children born in England has been found to be similar to that of English children, whereas children born in Asia and the West Indies who then moved to England had a lower prevalence than their counterparts born in England. Also the prevalence rates found in immigrant children born in the Indian subcontinent and the West Indies were higher than those found in India or the West Indies, suggesting the importance of environmental factors for differences in prevalence rates. Tokelauan children migrating to New Zealand had a cumulative prevalence of asthma (25.3 percent) far higher than that found in Tokelau (11 percent). These children who migrated to New Zealand also had a higher prevalence of rhinitis (28.3 percent

versus 13.7 percent) and eczema (8.5 percent versus 0.1 percent) (Gregg, 1983).

Age. The atopic diseases generally begin in early childhood, but they can arise at any age. The majority of patients with allergic asthma develop symptoms before 20 years of age and most before age 10. In an Iowa study (Smith, 1965), 80 percent of patients had developed allergic symptoms by age 20. However, in some geographic locations, asthma in childhood is rare; in Sweden, only 20 percent of asthma cases occurred before age 18. In the New Guinea Highlands, even though most asthmatics had positive skin test results, it was rare to find asthmatics under age 30 (Anderson, 1974).

Atopic dermatitis begins most commonly in infancy or early childhood, whereas seasonal allergic rhinitis tends to begin somewhat later. Perennial allergic rhinitis may develop earlier than seasonal rhinitis, perhaps as a result of earlier exposure to perennial allergens.

Sex. In most studies, boys have twice the prevalence of asthma in childhood as do girls. Boys also have a higher rate of atopic dermatitis. Although it is often stated that girls achieve near equality in asthma prevalence with boys during their teen years and throughout middle age and may actually exceed the prevalence rate of that for boys, current statistics concerning prevalence of asthma by sex in the United States do not reflect this trend. Prevalence rates for males can be seen to be higher at all ages (Table 9–3). A population survey in Wales found a prevalence for asthma in those over 70 years of age of 6.5 percent, with 5.1 percent in males and 1.8 percent in females (Burr et al., 1979). Asthma was carefully distinguished from other chronic obstructive pulmonary diseases in this study.

Race. It would appear that asthma is rarer in some races, including American Indians, Eskimos, and the natives of the New Guinea Highlands. There is evidence, however, for increasing prevalence in some of these races. A recent study in the Papua New Guinea highlands in 1985 suggests an increase in asthma prevalence to as much as 39 times as great as that found in 1972 (Dowse et al., 1985). This finding has been attributed in part to the introduction of more "civilized" customs. In particular, cotton blankets were introduced into the country several years ago. Dowse and co-workers identified extremely high quantities of dust mites in the cotton bedding of the Papuan subjects, and over 90 percent of those with

TABLE 9-3. Cumulative Prevalence of Asthma*

	Age				
	All Ages	3-11	12-44	45-64	65-74
Total	10.6†	10.2	9.9	11.8	12.4
Male	11.4	12.0	10.2	12.9	15.5
Female	9.7	8.3	9.7	10.8	9.9
White	10.4	9.7	9.7	11.8	12.4
Black	12.2	13.4	12.0	11.5	11.8

* United States population age 3 to 74 years, from the National Health
and Nutrition Examination Survey, 1976–1980.
† Rates per 100 persons

asthma had positive skin test results to mite allergen. It is of interest that, despite equal exposure rates, Papuan children had lower total IgE levels to mites and virtually no asthma. Recent data suggest an overall increase in the prevalence of asthma in the United States, with the greatest increase being in hospitalization rates for asthma in young black males (Evans et al., 1985).

Other Risk Factors in Developing Atopic Diseases. Other factors often cited in association with risk for developing atopic diseases include elevated neonatal or cord blood IgE levels, early infant feeding practices, maternal smoking, and viral infections (also see Chapters 6, 14 and 21).

Several studies have suggested that elevated levels of IgE precede the manifestation of atopic symptoms (Orgel et al., 1975; Kjellman, 1976). A recent consecutive study of 1701 infants studied at birth and at 18 months of age found that 8.3 percent had some manifestation of atopy (Croner et al., 1982). Of those infants, 73 percent with a family history for atopy and an elevated IgE level developed atopic disease; only 3 percent with no family history for atopy and normal IgE levels developed atopic disease.

Numerous studies have evaluated the impact of breast-feeding on the subsequent development of allergy. This literature has been critically reviewed by Burr (1983) who found that the risk of developing allergic disease was positively associated with cow's milk or mixed feeding in early infancy in 13 of 24 studies. One study showed a positive association between breast-feeding and allergy, and ten studies showed no convincing association between development of allergic diseases and infant feeding practices. Burr concluded that although this issue is not settled, the balance of evidence appears to favor the hypothesis that early feeding

with cow's milk or solids increased the risk of developing atopic allergic disease (see also Chapter 21).

Cigarette smokers have been shown to have higher IgE levels (Burrows et al., 1981), and they are more likely to have positive skin test results than nonsmokers (Welty et al., 1984). A recent study by Weiss et al. (1985) indicates that maternal smoking leads to an increased risk of atopy in nonsmoking children. The etiology for the increase in atopic disease in children of mothers who smoke is not known. This phenomenon was independent of any effect of a possible increased incidence of respiratory infections in children of smoking parents, although an increased incidence of respiratory infections in children of parents who smoke has been demonstrated (Fergusson et al., 1980). Weiss and coworkers did not find an increased incidence of bronchial responsiveness in children of smokers.

Many studies have purported to demonstrate a relationship between early viral respiratory infections and later development of asthma. A history of bronchiolitis or recurrent croup in early childhood appears to be associated with a marked increase in bronchial hyperreactivity later in life. Frick et al. (1979) found a temporal relationship between the development of atopic disease and viral infections. The relationship between the frequency of respiratory infections and the development of allergy is not clear. Cogswell et al. (1982) followed 92 infants prospectively from birth to 3 years of age. Each infant had one parent with asthma or hay fever. Respiratory infections were not more common in those children later shown to be atopic than in those who were not. Weiss et al. (1985) found an increased prevalence of atopic allergy in children of mothers who smoked but not an increased incidence of atopic allergy in children who had respiratory infections in early life. However, children who had acute respiratory illnesses in early life had increased airway hyperresponsiveness in later life. These studies underline the discordance between the development of asthma and atopic allergic reactivity.

EPIDEMIOLOGIC CONSIDERATIONS IN ALLERGIC RHINITIS

Seasonal allergic rhinitis lends itself easily to characterization and study. A history of seasonal nasal symptoms with demonstration of IgE antibody to allergens appropriate to the seasonal symptoms are characteristics that can be obtained without difficulty. Perennial allergic rhinitis is more difficult to study. Evidence of IgE antibody in these so-affected patients often less clearly can be related to causation of the disease. Up to 39 percent of asymptomatic normal subjects have been shown to have positive skin test results to at least one allergen on intradermal screening (Haahtela et al., 1980). An assessment by history of a causal relationship between perennial symptoms and evidence of allergic antibody is difficult to achieve in studies utilizing questionnaires and interviews by relatively unskilled persons.

The frequency of allergic rhinitis in childhood is not known with certainty; reports range from a prevalence rate of 0.5 percent to over 20 percent (see Table 9–2). The prevalence is lower in the very young and increases progressively with age. Fewer than 2.9 percent of children age 4 years or younger are reported to have allergic rhinitis (Broder et al., 1974). For all age groups, the prevalence of allergic rhinitis in the United States usually is cited as 8 to 10 percent. Most studies of university student populations provide figures higher than that, however, ranging from 12 to 20 percent (Smith, 1983). A study of twelfth graders revealed a prevalence of 21 percent for seasonal allergic rhinitis and approximately 9 percent for perennial symptoms (Freeman and Johnson, 1964). Hagy and Settipane (1969) found a prevalence in college students of 21.1 percent seasonal allergic rhinitis and 5.2 percent perennial rhinitis.

Males and females appear to have equal prevalence of allergic rhinitis at any age. Racial factors contributing to prevalence of allergic rhinitis in varying populations are difficult to interpret, as lower reported prevalences in European, African, and Asian populations may be attributable to differences in study design. Foreign students attending an American university had a prevalence of allergic rhinitis comparable to that of American students (Maternowski and Mathews, 1962). This finding might indicate that the prevalence of allergic rhinitis in a foreign student population was higher in the United States than in the native country because more sensitive criteria were employed. Alternatively, it could also mean that environmental allergens, such as ragweed pollen, were more likely to induce allergic rhinitis in students who were atopic in the United States, which might have been avoided if they had remained in their native country. An increased prevalence of IgE antibodies and symptoms of allergic rhinitis have been reported in higher socioeconomic groups (Lebowitz, 1977) but whether changes in socioeconomic status or other phenomena are responsible is not clear.

Family histories of atopic disease in patients with allergic rhinitis range as high as 87 percent. In general, the risk for a child developing allergic rhinitis increases when one parent has atopic disease and is even greater when both parents have atopic disease.

Allergic rhinitis tends to develop in childhood, persists into adulthood, and declines in old age. However, Burr et al. (1979) reported a prevalence of allergic rhinitis in a population over age 70 of 7.9 percent. Spontaneous remission occurs possibly in 15 to 25 percent cases when followed over 5 to 7 years. Perennial rhinitis is less likely to remit than seasonal rhinitis, and both are less likely to remit than asthma.

Treatment success, i.e., amelioration of symptoms, has been reported in 43 to 100 percent of patients who are treated with immunotherapy compared with similar improvement in 10 to 56 percent treated with placebo. It is evident that immunotherapy has an impact on the morbidity of allergic rhinitis; there is reason to believe it has a significant effect on the ultimate course as well. It has been suggested that immunotherapy for allergic rhinitis is indicated to prevent the development of asthma. However, there is little evidence to support or refute this, and the onset of asthma more often precedes the onset of allergic rhinitis. Less than 10 percent of children were reported to have allergic rhinitis for more than 1 year before asthma began (Freeman and Johnson, 1964).

EPIDEMIOLOGIC CONSIDERATIONS IN ASTHMA

Asthma is a particularly difficult disease to study epidemiologically because of varying criteria employed. If one requires wheezing, a diagnosis by a physician, and 15 percent reversibility of airflow limitation by a bronchodilator drug, epidemiologic information will be far different than that obtained simply from historical reports of episodic wheezing, cough, and dyspnea. Further, if bronchial hyperreactivity to stimuli, such as histamine, methacholine, and exercise, is evaluated as indicators of asthma without requiring symptoms of airways disease, the prevalence of asthma will be considered to be very high indeed. Now that reversible airways obstruction with symptoms of cough or dyspnea without wheezing (or both) has been identified and considered to be the same disease as asthma with wheezing (Corrao et al., 1979), it is evident that many surveys have underestimated the prevalence of asthma in the past. In a recent examination of third grade schoolchildren, Speight et al. (1983) found 179 children who had wheezed since entering school. Of that group, only 11.7 percent had been diagnosed as having asthma, although nearly all of them had seen a physician for respiratory symptoms. A total of 87 of these undiagnosed children had more than four episodes of wheezing each year, and about half had missed more than 50 days of school each year because of their respiratory disease. School absenteeism fell ten-fold when the diagnosis was made and continued prophylactic treatment for asthma was offered. This study emphasizes the high rate of asthma underdiagnosis and also underlines the importance of recognizing asthma, in order to offer proper treatment of this respiratory disease.

Although asthma occurs in patients with allergic rhinitis and atopic dermatitis, it seems to have a separate pattern in inheritance from these disorders, as previously indicated. Nonallergic and allergic asthmatics have similar family histories for asthma, although relatives of allergic asthmatics have a higher incidence of allergic rhinitis. In various surveys, the incidence of allergic rhinitis in patients with asthma is as high as 67 percent; generally, allergic rhinitis is far more common in those asthmatics with positive than those with negative allergy skin test results. In addition, from 6 to 63 percent of asthmatic patients have been reported to have eczema. McNicol and Williams (1973) found that children with wheezy bronchitis and children with moderate to severe asthma had similar incidences of allergic rhinitis and of positive skin test results to allergens, both higher than in control subjects. In addition, the investigators found eczema to be more common in those with more severe asthma.

The reported prevalence of asthma varies from less than 3 percent to more than 20 percent of the population. An 11 percent prevalence reported by McNicol and Williams (1973) includes children who had unequivocal diagnoses of repeated wheezing and continued to have wheezing at age 10 years (3.7 percent) together with children who had more than five episodes of wheezing, but whose asthma had ceased by age 10 years (7.7 percent). The report excluded an additional group of schoolchildren with histories of fewer than five episodes of wheezing associated with infection, however. (These children were mentioned previously as being indistinguishable by allergic parameters from the asthmatic group.) Had these children been included, there would be an overall prevalence of 18 to 19 percent.

Broder et al. (1974) reported similar figures in children under age 15 in Tecumseh, Michigan, with a cumulative prevalence of 8 percent in boys and 4.8 percent in girls. Note the current United States prevalence figures listed by age, sex, and race in Table 9–3. The cumulative prevalence rate for all ages is 10.6 percent.

Asthma tends to develop (or at least to be diagnosed) at an earlier age than does allergic rhinitis. In a group of asthmatics studied by Blair (1977) and followed for 20 years, 39 percent had onset of symptoms within the first year of life; 57 percent had signs of asthma by 2 years; and 84 percent by 5 years. There is a tendency for asthma to begin at an earlier age in patients prone to develop IgE antibody. Rackemann and Edwards (1952) reported that 74 percent of patients with asthma whose disease began prior to age 15 years were allergic, whereas, of those in whom it began after age 45 years, only 32 percent were allergic. There often is a feeling that the asthmatic who does not have positive allergy test results has a worse prognosis than the asthmatic who does have positive allergy test results. A recent analysis of a clinic population of asthmatics did indeed indicate that those with negative allergy skin test results had more severe disease than those with positive allergy skin test results. However, when a subpopulation was matched for age and duration of asthma there was no significant difference in the severity of asthma between the patients with skin test positive results and those with negative results (Inouye et al., 1985). Thus, factors of age and duration of asthma may have more prognostic significance than do allergy skin test results or, in other words, allergic reactivity.

In nearly every study of the natural history of asthma, significant spontaneous improvement in asthma has been reported by 10 to 14 years of age, with improvement rates ranging from 26 to 78 percent. One of the problems encountered in analyzing the results of these childhood asthma studies has been the difference in duration of follow-up. Clearly, in many studies, children were not followed long enough. The original group of children studied by McNicol and Williams was recently followed to age 21 years (Martin et al., 1980a). Most of the subjects improved during adolescence, and 55 percent of those whose wheezing had started before age 7 and stopped during adolescence remained wheeze free. However, 45 percent of those who had stopped wheezing by age 14 subsequently had minor recurrences between 14 and 21 years. Fewer than 20 percent of those with persistent wheezing in childhood stopped wheezing by age 21. Surprisingly, 21 percent of the original nonasthmatic control group who could be followed to age 21 had to be dropped from the study because of wheezing episodes that occurred during adolescence!

Most of the subjects who were still wheezing by age 21 had abnormal pulmonary function test results, although many of those with episodic wheezing exhibited normal function test results (Martin et al., 1980b). It was estimated that 60 percent of those who had ceased wheezing had abnormal bronchial responsiveness to histamine. This study did not find that an early age of onset of asthma was associated with a worse prognosis. The follow-up study of the population at age 21 found a higher prevalence of persistent and recurrent wheezing than did the study of the same population at age 14. It is apparent that when asthmatic children are followed through adolescence into early adulthood, there is considerable recurrence of symptoms and persistence of airways hyperreactivity.

A recent survey of the available statistics concerning asthma found a marked increase in the hospitalization rate for asthma in the United States, a moderate increase in the death rate, and a smaller increase in the overall prevalence of asthma (Table 9–4) (Evans et al., 1985).

TABLE 9–4. Hospital Discharge Rates and Deaths from Asthma in the United States*

Year			
1973	1978	1980	1982
Deaths (actual number)			
1912	1872	2891	3154
Hospital discharges (in thousands)			
161	201	408(257)†	434(273)

* This data is from the Hospital Discharge Survey, 1965–1983, and Vital Statistics of the US, Mortality vol. 2 (Evans, 1985).

† Numbers in parentheses represent recalculation of actual numbers to account for terminology change in 1979.

Rates of hospitalization for asthma in the United States between 1965 and 1983 have increased by 50 percent for adults and over 200 percent for children. In many pediatric hospitals, asthma has become the most common reason for admission. There has been a substantial increase in deaths from asthma, especially among the older age group. The death rate for asthma in children has risen less strikingly. Reasons for these apparent changes are unclear.

Because of the heterogeneous nature of asthma and the multiple factors capable of precipitating an attack, the role of immunotherapy in altering the course and prognosis of asthma is difficult to assess. The related literature reveals nearly equal numbers of reports either supporting or denying efficacy of immunotherapy in asthma. Assessment of severity of asthma and perception of need for medication are subjective criteria in a disease noted for discrepancies between objective pulmonary abnormalities and patient (and often physician) assessment of degree of obstruction. However, these criteria were most often used to grade response to immunotherapy in asthma. A scientifically valid conclusion concerning overall efficacy of immunotherapy in asthma and its influence on the natural history of the disease, therefore, is difficult to reach at this time.

EPIDEMIOLOGIC CONSIDERATIONS IN ATOPIC DERMATITIS

The prevalence of atopic dermatitis as judged by patient history is difficult to assess. In the mild form, atopic dermatitis may be forgotten or ignored. In older children, other skin conditions may be confused with it. The prevalence of atopic dermatitis is estimated to be 1 to 3 percent of the general population. In populations in which asthma is uncommon, eczema also is uncommon. The sex distribution is approximately the same as in asthma, i.e., twice as common early in life in boys as in girls. The proportion of patients with atopic dermatitis who subsequently develop asthma ranges from 20 to 60 percent, with the onset of asthma being significantly earlier in children affected with atopic dermatitis. Figures for subsequent development of allergic rhinitis range from 30 to 45 percent. Thus, in a patient with atopic dermatitis the risk of developing atopic disease of the upper or lower respiratory tract or both is five to ten times greater than in the population at large.

Atopic dermatitis generally begins in infancy or early childhood, but rarely before 5 weeks of age. Cutaneous autonomic dysfunction in the form of increased vasoconstriction and xerosis generally is found. Serum IgE levels frequently are elevated, and IgE antibodies to foods are present in 43 to 72 percent of patients.

Spontaneous resolution of the condition occurs in about two thirds of patients by the age of 6 years. Unfavorable prognostic factors for resolution have been reported to be, in order of importance, severe (widespread) dermatitis in childhood, family history of atopic dermatitis, associated allergic rhinitis or asthma or both, female sex, and early age of onset (Rystedt, 1985). Persistence of dry itchy skin in adulthood also is associated with persistent or recurring atopic dermatitis to a significantly higher degree than if the skin is otherwise normal.

Although anti-allergic therapy in some cases may modify the disease, and avoidance of certain foods may lessen symptoms, there is no evidence that symptomatic treatment or specific anti-allergic therapy shortens the duration of the disease.

OTHER ALLERGIC DISEASE STATES

Whereas there is firm support for a familial association among asthma, allergic rhinitis, and atopic dermatitis, the evidence for an association with other allergic conditions is vague. Urticaria varies in frequency from 2.9 to 14 percent in patients with atopic diseases; in the general population, it varies from 3.2 to 12.8 percent.

Hymenoptera sensitivity and some drug sensitivities, such as penicillin allergy, are mediated by IgE antibody. However, the prevalence of atopic disease (e.g., atopic dermatitis, allergic rhinitis, and asthma) is not increased in subjects with Hymenoptera sensitivity or penicillin allergy. Prevalence of Hymenoptera sensitivity is generally cited at 0.4 to 0.8 percent of the population. However, a recent questionnaire-type survey at a plant found 4 percent of workers reporting histories of systemic reactions to insect stings (Valentine, 1984). Estimates of prevalence of penicillin allergy have ranged from 0.7 to 8 percent with approximately 10 percent of these reactions being life threatening (Sullivan et al., 1981).

It is evident from this review that although much information is accumulating regarding the etiology and pathogenesis of atopic disease, much work remains to be done. The basic question, why an individual develops a particular disease at a particular time in life, remains unanswered. Whatever the reason, once developed, these diseases tend to persist. There is a critical need for studies that lead to a better understanding of the prevalence and impact of allergic diseases on the individual, his or her family, and society in general. Atopic diseases constitute a public health problem, involving millions of patients and hundreds of millions of dollars in health care costs. Evidence points to an increase in the number of patients affected and in the complexity of diseases associated with a technologically advanced society.

REFERENCES

Anderson, H.R.: The epidemiological and allergic features of asthma in the New Guinea Highlands. Clin. Allergy 4:171, 1974.

Blair, H.: Natural history of childhood asthma. Arch. Dis. Child. 52:613, 1977.

Broder, I., Barlow, P.P., Horton, R.J.M.: Epidemiology of asthma and allergic rhinitis in a total community: Tecumseh, Michigan. J. Allergy Clin. Immunol. 54:100, 1974.

Burr, M.L.: Does infant feeding affect the risk of allergy? Arch. Dis. Child. 58:561, 1983.

Burr, M.L., Charles, T.J., Roy, K., Seaton, A.: Asthma in the Elderly: An epidemiological survey. Brit. Med. J. 1:1041, 1979.

Burrows, B., Halonen, M., Barbee, R.A., Lebowitz, M.D.: The relationship of serum immunoglobulin E to cigarette smoking. Am. Rev. Respir. Dis. 124:523, 1981.

Cogswell, J.J., Halliday, D.F., Alexander, J.R.: Respiratory infections in the first year of life in children at risk of developing atopy. Brit. Med. J. 284:1011, 1982.

Corrao, W.M., Bramen, S.S., Irwin, R.S.: Chronic cough as the sole presenting manifestation of bronchial asthma. N. Engl. J. Med. 300:633, 1979.

Croner, S., Kjellman, N-I.M., Ericsson, B., Roth, A.: IgE screening in 1701 newborn infants and the development of atopic disease during infancy. Arch. Dis. Child. 57:364, 1982.

Dowse, G.K., Turner, K.J., Stewart, G.A., Alpers, M.P., Woolcock, A.J.: The association between *Dermatophagoides* mites and the increasing prevalence of asthma in village communities within the Papua New Guinea Highlands. J. Allergy Clin. Immunol. 75:75, 1985.

Evans, R., Mullaly, D., Wilson, R., Gergen, P., Rosenberg, H., Grauman, J., Edmonds, F., Feinleib, M.: Present evidence on mortality and morbidity of asthma. Transcript of proceedings, NIH, International Workshop on the Etiology of Asthma, June 25–27, 1985, Bethesda, Md.

Fergusson, D.M., Horwood, L.J., Shannon, F.T.: Parental smoking and respiratory illness in infancy. Arch. Dis. Child. 55:358, 1980.

Fergusson, D.M., Horwood, L.J., Shannon, F.T.: Parental asthma, parental eczema and asthma, and eczema in early childhood. J. Chron. Dis. 36:517, 1983.

Freeman, G.L., Johnson, S.: Allergic diseases in adolescents. II. Changes in allergic manifestations during adolescence. Am. J. Dis. Child. 107:560, 1964.

Frick, O.L., German, D.F., Mills, J.: Development of allergy in children. I. Association with virus infections. J. Allergy Clin. Immunol. 63:228, 1979.

Gregg, I.: Epidemiological Aspects. *In* Clark, T.J.H., Godfrey, S. (eds.), Asthma, 2nd ed. London, Chapman & Hall, 1983.

Haahtela, T., Heiskala, M., Suoniemi, I.: Allergic disorders and immediate skin test reactivity in Finnish adolescents. Allergy 35:433, 1980.

Hagy, G.W., Settipane, G.A.: Bronchial asthma, allergic rhinitis, and allergy skin tests among college students. J. Allergy 44:323, 1969.

Horwood, L.J., Fergusson, D.M., Shannon, F.T.: Social and familial factors in the development of early childhood asthma. Pediatrics 75:859, 1985.

Inouye, T., Tarlo, S., Broder, I., Corey, P., Davies, G., Leznoff, A., Mintz, S., Thomas, P.: Severity of asthma in skin test-negative and skin test-positive patients. J. Allergy Clin. Immunol. 75:313, 1985.

Kjellman, N-I.M.: Predictive value of high IgE levels in children. Acta. Paediatr. Scand. 65:465, 1976.

Lebowitz, M.D.: The relationship of socio-environmental factors to the prevalence of obstructive lung diseases and other chronic conditions. J. Chron. Dis. 30:599, 1977.

Lebowitz, M.D., Barbee, R., Burrows, B.: Family concordance of IgE, atopy, and disease. J. Allergy Clin. Immunol. 73:259, 1984.

Lubs, M.L.: Allergy in 7000 twin pairs. Acta Allergol. 26:249, 1971.

Martin, A.J., Landau, J.I., Phelan, P.D.: Natural history of allergy in asthmatic children followed to adult life. Med. J. Aust. 2:470, 1981.

Martin, A.J., McLennan, L.A., Landau, L.I., Phelan, P.D.: The natural history of childhood asthma to adult life. Brit. Med. J. 280:1397, 1980a.

Martin, A.J., Landau, L.I., Phelan, P.D.: Lung function in young adults who had asthma in childhood. Am. Rev. Resp. Dis. 122:609, 1980b.

Maternowski, C.J., Mathews, K.P.: The prevalence of ragweed pollinosis in foreign and native students at a midwestern university and its implications concerning methods for determining the inheritance of atopy. J. Allergy 33:130, 1962.

McNicol, K.N., Williams, H.B.: Spectrum of asthma in childhood. I. Clinical and physiological components. II. Allergic components. Brit. Med. J. 4:7, 12, 1973.

Orgel, H.A., Hamburger, R.N., Bazaral, M., Gorrin, H., Groshong, T., Lenoir, M., Miller, J.R., Wallace, W.: Development of IgE and allergy in infancy. J. Allergy Clin. Immunol. 56:296, 1975.

Rackemann, F.M., Edwards, M.C.: Asthma in children. N. Engl. J. Med. 246:815, 1952.

Rasmussen, J.E., Provost, T.: Atopic Dermatitis. *In* Middleton, E., Reed, C.E., Ellis, E.F. (eds.), Allergy: Principles and Practice, 2nd ed. St. Louis, C.V. Mosby, 1983.

Rystedt, I.: Long-term follow-up in atopic dermatitis. Acta. Derm. Venereol. 114:117, 1985.

Sibbald, B., Horn, M.E.C., Brain, E.A., Gregg, I.: Genetic factors in childhood asthma. Thorax 356:71, 1980.

Sibbald, B., Turner-Warwick, M.: Factors influencing the prevalence of asthma among first degree relatives of extrinsic and intrinsic asthmatics. Thorax 34:332, 1979.

Smith, J.M.: Studies of the prevalence of asthma in childhood. Allergol. Immunopathol. 3:127, 1975.

Smith, J.M.: Epidemiology and natural history of asthma, allergic rhinitis, and atopic dermatitis. *In* Middleton, E., Reed, C.E., Ellis, E.F. (eds.), Allergy: Principles and Practice, 2nd ed. St. Louis, C.V. Mosby, 1983.

Smith, J.M., Knowler, L.: Epidemiology of asthma and allergic rhinitis. I. In a rural area. II. In a university centered community. Am. Rev. Respir. Dis. 92:16, 1965.

Speight, A.N.P., Lee, D.A., Hey, E.N.: Underdiagnosis and undertreatment of asthma in childhood. Brit. Med. J. 286:1253, 1983.

Sullivan, T.J., Wedner, H.J., Shatz, G., Yecies, L.D., Parker, C.W.: Skin testing to detect penicillin allergy. J. Allergy Clin. Immunol. 68:171, 1981.

Valentine, M.D.: Insect venom allergy: Diagnosis and treatment. J. Allergy Clin. Immunol. 73:299, 1984.

Weiss, S.T., Tager, I.B., Munoz, A., Speizer, F.: The relationship of respiratory infections in early childhood to the occurrence of increased levels of bronchial responsiveness and atopy. Am. Rev. Respir. Dis. 131:573, 1985.

Welty, C., Weiss, S.T., Tager, I.B., Munoz, A., Becker, C., Speizer, F.E., Ingram, R.H.: The relationship of airways responsiveness to cold air, cigarette smoking, and atopy to respiratory symptoms and pulmonary functions in adults. Am. Rev. Respir. Dis. 130:198, 1984.

10

Adverse Reactions to Foods

JOHN A. ANDERSON, M.D.

Adverse reactions to foods represent an important aspect of allergic or allergic-like diseases. Surveys involving parents indicate that as many as 20 percent of infants in the first year of life have had adverse reactions (5 percent probable incidence of significant reactions) to something in the diet (Foucard, 1984). Food-induced adverse reactions may be broadly classified on the basis of the mechanism of the reaction. *Allergic or food hypersensitivity* reactions are those that result from an immune event involving the exposure to a food or a food additive (Anderson and Sogn, 1984). The classic example of such reactions is food anaphylaxis. This type of reaction usually involves IgE antibody with the release of chemical mediators. All other nonimmune adverse reactions to food can be classified as *food intolerance.* An anaphylactoid reaction is an example of food intolerance; the reaction is anaphylaxis-like in clinical appearance but results from nonimmune release of chemical mediators. Other food intolerances include pharmacologic and metabolic reactions, food toxicity, and food idiosyncrasy.

Drug-like or pharmacologic food reactions can be caused by natural chemicals present in some foods (e.g., amines and caffeine). Some toxic reactions to ingredients of foods may have the appearance of an allergic reaction — especially those due to histamine "poisoning" from contaminated fish. Metabolic food reactions usually are the result of enzymatic deficiencies, for example, primary lactose intolerance. An *idiosyncratic reaction* is an abnormal response to a substance in the diet that differs from its physiologic or pharmacologic effect; it may resemble an allergic or a hypersensitivity reaction. Reactions to food additives, such as tartrazine, sulfites, and monosodium-L-glutamate, are examples of such reactions.

FOOD ALLERGENS

Raw Foods

Food is a composite mixture of many different molecules, including nutrients as well as potential antigens (allergens). These allergens are proteins, glycoproteins, or polypeptides (Aas, 1984). A given allergen, and different types of allergens, present in a single food can induce a variety of immune responses affecting various components of the immune system simultaneously. For the most part, the allergist is concerned most commonly with those allergens that induce the production of IgE antibodies and with those reactions that occur on reexposure to those allergens.

Foods are derived from animal and vegetable sources. Foods can be classified according to similar biologic relationships (Table 10–1). In some food groups, allergy to one member of the group may result, to a variable degree, in allergy to other members of the same food group because of common cross-reacting allergens. The clinical importance of such interrelationships may not be so common as previously believed, however. Of particular importance to the allergist are the legumes (soybean, bean, pea, and peanut); fish; mollusks (clam, oyster, scallop); and crustaceans (shrimp, lobster, crab, crayfish).

Although anaphylaxis to peanuts is more common than anaphylaxis to other legumes, a person allergic to peanuts may be at some risk when exposed to other members of the legume family (probably uncommon). In an individual allergic to peanuts, however, the risk of sensitivity to individual tree nuts (e.g., cashews and walnuts), which bear no botanic relationship to peanuts, also may be increased. An individual allergic to fish of one species is at risk when eating fish of other species. However, an individual allergic to seafood may be allergic to only one family type, either crustaceans (most likely) or mollusks; this sensitivity generally does not imply sensitivity to fish. It is of interest that, within a given animal species, various components of the animal are not necessarily cross reactive enough to evoke a clinical problem. Patients allergic to milk usually can tolerate beef; patients allergic to eggs usually have no diffi-

TABLE 10–1. Biologic Relationships of Foods Important in Food Allergy*

Animal Groups

Birds
  Chicken, duck, turkey
Eggs (Bird)
  Ovomucoid, ovovitellin, white, yoke
Fish
  Freshwater and saltwater
Meats
  Red
Milk (Cow, Goat)
  Butter, buttermilk, casein, cheese, cream, ice cream, lactalbumin, milk (condensed, evaporated, homogenized, powdered, raw, skimmed), most infant formulas, yogurt
Seafoods
  Crustaceans
    Crab, crayfish, lobster, prawn, shrimp
  Mollusks
    Abalone, clam, cockle, mussel, octopus, oyster, scallop, snail (escargot), squid

Plant Groups

Apple
  Apple (cider, vinegar), crabapple, pear
Banana
Buckwheat
  Buckwheat, rhubarb
Cashew
  Cashew nuts, mango, pistachio nuts
Citrus
  Grapefruit, kumquat, lemon, lime, orange, tangelo, tangerine
Cola
  Chocolate (cocoa), cola (kola) nut
Fungi
  Mushroom, yeast
Gourd (Melon)
  Cantaloupe, cucumber, honeydew melon, pumpkin, summer squash, watermelon

Plant Groups (*Continued*)

Grape
  Champagne, grape, raisin, vinegar (wine), wine
Grass
  Barley, corn, popcorn, oats, rice, rye, sorghum, sugar cane, wheat
Lecythis
  Brazil nut
Lily
  Asparagus, chives, garlic, leek, onion
Madder (Coffee)
Mallow (Marshmallow)
Morning Glory
  Sweet potato, yam
Mustard
  Broccoli, brussel sprouts, cabbage, cauliflower, collards, horseradish, mustard, radish, rutabaga, turnip, watercress
Nightshade
  Bell pepper, chick pepper, eggplant, white potato, tomato, tobacco
Parsley
  Carrot, celery, dill, fennel, parsley, parsnip
Pea (Legume)
  Peas, beans, chick pea, lentil, licorice, soybean, peanut
Pepper
  Black
Pineapple
Plum
  Almond, apricot, cherry, peach, nectarine, plum, prune
Rose
  Blackberry, raspberry, strawberry
Sunflower (Composite, Aster)
  Artichoke, dandelion, lettuce, sunflower seeds (cross-reactivity with ragweed, melon, banana)
Tea
Walnut
  Walnut, pecans

* Adapted from Anderson, J., Sogn, D. (eds.): Adverse Reactions to Foods, AAAI and NIAID, NIH Pub. No. 84–2442, pp. 21–25, July, 1984.

culty eating chicken or inhaling materials associated with chicken feathers.

There is a reported relationship between inhaled pollen sensitivity in certain patients and localized oral or pharyngeal reactions to ingested fresh fruits and vegetables. In the United States, patients allergic to ragweed pollen have reported oral pruritus and swelling after ingestion of melons and bananas (Anderson et al., 1970). Similarly, patients allergic to birch pollen may react to the ingestion of apples, pears, carrots, parsnips, potatoes, and hazelnuts (Lahti et al., 1980).

Most studies of food allergy involve raw food allergens. Double-blind, placebo-controlled food challenges of children with atopic dermatitis indicate that the five most common foods causing sensitization in the United States are cow's milk, egg, peanut, wheat, and soy raw food allergens (Sampson and Albergo, 1984). In older children as well as in adults, food-induced anaphylactic sensitivity most commonly involves fish, crustacean-type shellfish, and nuts. However, it is important to recognize that severe reactions can occur to almost any food.

Partially Purified and Purified Food Allergens

In studies of foods in which either partially purified or purified food allergens have been examined, the physical and chemical properties of these allergens have been found to be similar to those of the major allergens of ragweed pollen (Bleumink, 1970) (Table 10–2).

TABLE 10-2. Purified and Partially Purified Food Allergens*

	Cow's Milk	Egg White	Codfish	Food Peanut	Soybean	Shrimp	Wheat	Tomato
Allergen	Beta-lactoglobulin	Ovomucoid	Allergen M	Peanut I	Soybean trypsin inhibitor	Allergen II	Gluten derivatives	Tomato
Active component	GP†	GP	GP	GP	GP	GP	GP	
Molecular weight (daltons)	36,000	31,500	12,328	180,000 (approx)	20,000	38,000	Unknown	20,000
Heat stability	+	+	+	+	+	+	+	+

* Adapted from Anderson, J., Sogn, D. (eds.): Adverse Reactions to Foods, AAAI and NIAID, NIH Pub No. 84–2442, pp. 7–16, July, 1984.
† Glycoprotein.

Purified food allergens have been identified as glycoproteins with small molecular weights (18,000 to 38,000 daltons) and represent only a small fraction of the parent food. Since purified food allergens tend to resist protein denaturation, their antigenicity probably depends more on their primary sequence than their confirmational structure (Aas, 1984). Foods that have been best studied include cow's milk, egg white, codfish, soybean, peanut, tomato, wheat, shrimp, and cottonseed.

Cow's Milk

Cow's milk contains several proteins that have been shown to produce allergic sensitivity (Bahna and Heiner, 1980). Casein constitutes approximately 80 percent of the milk proteins; whey proteins account for the remaining 20 percent. In purified form, four major caseins have been identified. These have molecular weights ranging from 18,000 to 24,000 daltons. The major whey protein and most important milk allergen is beta-lactoglobulin. This protein contains two polypeptide chains, each with a molecular weight of 18,000. Alpha-lactalbumin and bovine serum albumin and globulin also are well-known milk allergens.

Most milk allergens, with the exception of some casein allergens, are heat resistant. Thus, almost all milk products and cow's milk protein formulations (such as infant formula) are potentially capable both of sensitizing humans and precipitating an allergic reaction in those already sensitized. Though most clinical studies of milk allergy have employed whole cow's milk, results of studies that have used purified milk allergens are similar to those that have used whole milk (Anderson et al., 1974).

Children commonly react allergically to cow's milk in a variety of ways, and reactions typical of types I, III, and IV (Gell and Coombs classification) may be seen (Kletter et al., 1971). Of particular importance are reactions that result in anaphylaxis, rhinitis, and asthma in early infancy, atopic dermatitis, milk-induced enteritis, and milk-induced gastrointestinal bleeding, all of which are considered to be primarily type I reactions. In milk-induced chronic pulmonary disease (Heiner syndrome), a type III antigen-antibody complex/complement–mediated and a type IV cell-mediated immune injury probably are involved.

Chicken Eggs

Patients allergic to eggs usually react only to egg white. Egg white is known to contain six major proteins, as follows: ovalbumin, ovomucoid (trypsin inhibitor), conalbumin (ovotransferrin), ovomacroglobulin, ovomucin, and lysozyme (Hoffman, 1983). Most of the egg white is composed of ovalbumin, which is easily denatured on heating. Lysozyme accounts for 11 percent and ovomucoid for 4 percent of the egg proteins. In clinical studies involving purified protein from fresh eggs, hard boiled eggs (cooked at 100°C for 20 minutes) and soft boiled eggs (cooked at 100°C for 3 minutes), both ovalbumin and ovomucoid were found to retain strong allergenicity in egg-allergic individuals. Conalbumin was less potent, and lysozyme was found to be a weak allergen. Despite denaturation, in other words, both ovalbumin and ovomucoid are present in an immunologically recognizable form in both hard and soft boiled eggs. As with cow's milk allergens, clinical reactions to egg proteins involve IgE (type I) responses. Individuals allergic to egg may have anaphylaxis, urticaria, atopic dermatitis, or acute gastrointestinal reactions.

Fish

Fish allergy plays a classic role in the history of allergy and immunology. In experiments involving passive transfer, the serum of Dr. Küstner, who was allergic to boiled haddock, was transferred to the skin of Dr. Prausnitz, who was nonallergic. A positive skin test result to fish was subsequently observed at the site of the passive serum transfer and established a biologic basis for reagin (Prausnitz, 1921). In recent years, this transferable serum factor has been found to be IgE antibody.

Codfish muscle protein (allergen M) is the most purified food allergen and has been well studied (Aas, 1984). Codfish extracts contain more than 20 antigenic components. Purification has been performed to produce a crystalline form. This allergen is an acidic protein (isoelectric point of 4.75) and has a molecular weight of 12,328 daltons; it is composed of 113 amino acids and one glucose residue. The amino acid sequence of the molecule has been defined. Allergen M is derived from a large class of vertebrate muscle proteins known as parvalbumins, which are characterized by low molecular weight, high solubility in water, and ability to chelate calcium. Parvalbumins are present in fish and amphibian muscle but not in mammalian muscle. Thus, this allergen is present in all saltwater and freshwater fish probably worldwide (Anderson and Sogn, 1984).

The biologic relevance of codfish allergen M in stimulating an IgE allergic response has been established in fish allergic individuals. Clinical sensitivity has been demonstrated by double-blind placebo-controlled food challenge (anaphylactic, dermatologic, respiratory, and gastrointestinal symptomatology). Almost perfect correlation has been found with positive oral challenge and prick skin test, double-blind passive transfer or Praunitz-Küstner (PK) test, *in vitro* release of histamine from chopped human lung sensitized with appropriate antisera, and *in vitro* allergen-specific IgE radioallergosorbent test (RAST) (Aas, 1984).

Peanuts

Allergic reactions to peanuts, particularly in children, are becoming recognized with increasing frequency. This fact is especially important, since peanuts and other legumes are being used more often as protein sources in the average American diet. The isolation and partial characterization of major peanut allergen, designated as Peanut-I, recently has been described by Sachs et al. (1981).

In 1916, the two major proteins of peanuts were identified and named arachin and conarachin. Arachin has a molecular weight of 330,000 daltons, and its monomeric form, 180,000 daltons. Conarachin is a high molecular weight heterogeneous protein complex with several subfractions. It is the most important of the two storage peanut proteins. The molecular weight ranges from 140,000 to 295,000 daltons.

Peanut-I allergen is an acidic glycoprotein (pH 8.9) and probably constitutes one of the subfractions of the large storage peanut proteins. The molecular weight of Peanut-I has been estimated to be approximately 180,000 daltons. The allergen contains 11 percent nitrogen and 8.7 percent carbohydrate. In a small number of peanut allergic patients, concordant results were found between double-blind placebo-challenge, positive prick skin test, *in vitro* Peanut I–induced histamine release from human leukocytes, and Peanut-I, IgE RAST. In addition, RAST has demonstrated that, although Peanut-I may be the most potent allergen, it is not the only allergen that can be isolated from peanut.

In other clinical studies of peanut allergy in children, partially purified peanut allergens were not inactivated by heating to 145°C for 1 hour to simulate commercial roasting (Kemp, 1985). However, commercial peanut oil has been found to be free of peanut allergens (Taylor et al., 1981). Allergic reactions to peanuts include anaphylaxis, atopic dermatitis, and gastrointestinal reactions (vomiting, pain, diarrhea) in particular.

Soybean

Similar to peanuts, soybeans have been used worldwide with increasing frequency in recent years as protein extenders or food supplements. Soy allergy also has been recognized with increasing frequency in the United States and Europe.

Soybean protein can be divided into globulin and whey fractions. The globulin, which constitutes 85 percent of the total soy protein, consists of four subcomponents. One subcomponent, 2S globulin, contains two molecules with molecular weights of 18,000 and 32,000 daltons. The most biologically active of the soy proteins in soy allergic patients reside in these two molecules of 2S globulin. These are the most heat stable of the soy proteins analogous to what has been found with other important food allergens (Shibasaki et al., 1980).

In the whey fraction of soy protein, one enzyme, Kuni soybean trypsin inhibitor, caused anaphylaxis in a research worker using this protein (Moroy et al., 1980). This protein (20,000 daltons) was the sole soybean allergen to which this person was allergic. The patient had several episodes of anaphylaxis on eating soybean containing foods, and had positive skin test results, positive passive transfer (PK), and positive RAST results to this soy protein. This allergen is acid resistant, suggesting that the allergen can retain allergenicity in the gastrointestinal tract.

As in the case of peanut oil, commercial soybean oils are free of soy allergens and should be considered safe for soy allergic patients (Bush et al., 1985). Clinical studies have shown that soy sensitivity may result in anaphylactic, respiratory, dermatologic, and gastrointestinal reactions. Of concern is the fact that children who have milk-induced chronic gastrointestinal disease have an increased likelihood of becoming allergic also to soy formulas, which are the main type of substitute infant formula available in the United States.

Shrimp

Shrimp is a member of the crustacean family of seafood. This food frequently produces reactions such as hives or systemic anaphylaxis or both in sensitive individuals. Hoffman (1981) was able to identify two purified allergens (I and II) from raw shrimp. Allergen-I was found (1) to be a dimer of two polypeptide chains with a molecular weight of 21,000 daltons, (2) to have a carbohydrate content of 0.5 percent, and (3) to be heat sensitive. Allergen II, a heat stable allergen, could be identified in cooked shrimp and had a molecular weight of over 200,000 daltons (probably due to heat aggregation). The most probable size of this allergen is estimated to be 38,000 daltons. The carbohydrate content was found to be 4 percent. The amino acid sequences of both allergen I and II have been defined. In patients known to be allergic to shrimp (reactions include urticaria, systemic anaphylaxis, and contact urticaria), antibody to allergen II has been identified by RAST.

Wheat

Wheat proteins can be divided into six major fractions as follows: gluten, albumin, starch, euglobulins, pseudoglobulins, and gliadin. In patients with gluten-sensitive enteropathy (celiac disease), a component of gluten has been identified that causes damage of the jejunal mucosa. Peptic-tryptic digests of this gluten (fraction III) have been further divided into fractions B (B_1, B_2, B_3) and C. The toxic fractions seem to be B_2 and B_3 (Anand, 1977).

RAST tests of sera of patients allergic to wheat have implicated the major allergens as wheat albumin, euglobulins, and pseudoglobulins (Hoffman, 1975). However, some patients have been found to have allergen-specific IgE antibodies directed against gliadin (Goldstein et al., 1969) and against gluten and gliadin (Scudomore, 1982). In one study of patients with celiac disease, no specific IgE antibody response to gluten fraction B was identified in vitro, but a short-term sensitizing IgG anaphylactic antibody (IgG-STS of Parish) could be demonstrated by monkey passive cutaneous anaphylaxis test in 33 percent of the patients studied (Rawcliffe, 1985). Recently, studies of bakers who are allergic to inhaled wheat flour have indicated that they are allergic to a wide variety of insoluble wheat proteins, as well as to the water soluble albumin. Using a modified IgE RAST technique, employing nitrocellulous sheets and 1-percent potassium hydroxide solvent, reactions were found to globulin, gliadin, gluten, and wheat allergens (Walsh et al., 1985).

Most allergic reactions to wheat allergen involve type I (IgE) reactions. In celiac syndrome, however, increasing evidence suggests that it is a type IV cell-mediated reaction to wheat. Regardless of the type of reaction, intestinal reactions are the most common adverse manifestations of sensitivity to wheat proteins. Exceptions include the atopic dermatitis of wheat allergic children and the asthma induced upon wheat flour inhalation ("baker's asthma") but not upon cooked bakery product ingestion.

FACTORS THAT MAY INFLUENCE THE PATIENT'S POTENTIAL TO REACT TO FOOD

Denaturation of Food Allergen

The most important food allergens studied are heat resistant. Thus, in most cases, heating or cooking food neither changes nor decreases its allergenicity. However, food allergens can be heat sensitive, such as some milk allergens (Bahna and Heiner, 1980) or some shrimp allergens (Hoffman et al., 1981). Dr. Küstner was allergic to cooked fish and not to raw fish (Prausnitz and Küstner, 1921). Mild heating of milk in the presence of lactose can produce a "browning reaction": beta-lactoglobulin increases N-glycoside bound carbohydrates and is rendered more allergenic. Similarly, ripened tomatoes are more allergenic than green (unripened) tomatoes (Anderson and Sogn, 1984).

Gastrointestinal digestion of food can affect allergenicity, not only by degradation and rendering the food nonallergenic, but also by increasing allergenicity. Spies and his colleagues (1970) showed that new antigenic determinants could be demonstrated when cow's milk was exposed to a short course of pepsin or trypsin digestion. Although initially it was thought that it was possible to find IgE antibodies in humans directed solely to the protein digest of cow's milk, later studies showed that all patients studied who were allergic to the protein digest of cow's milk were also allergic to whole milk (Schwartz et al., 1980).

Heredity and the Risk of Food Allergy

Familial factors greatly influence the risk of development of food allergy. In two recent studies in Sweden involving 528 children, the risk of food allergy ranged from 9 to 13 percent if neither parent was allergic; 17 to 29 percent if one parent was allergic; and 53 to 58 percent if both parents were allergic (Foucard, 1984).

Rarely, food sensitization may occur *in utero* or may be the result of transfer of small amounts of foreign food protein ingested by the mother to the infant via breast milk. Infants sensitized in this way may be considered "high IgE-antibody responders" to antigenic stimulation. These infants are at increased risk when the food is first introduced directly into their diet. It has been shown that normal children may make small amounts of IgE food-specific antibodies transiently without demonstrating clinical signs and symptoms of allergy. In contrast, the IgE response in atopic children to a potent allergen such as cow's milk or eggs is more prolonged and intense. The main defect in an atopic child may be a reduced capacity to turn off a naturally induced IgE antibody response (Foucard, 1985).

Age of the Child and Food Exposure

Using cow's milk allergy as a model, the risk of developing allergy is greater when cow's milk is introduced at an early age (Foucard, 1985). Early introduction of solid foods probably induces a similar risk of allergy. On reviewing the many studies concerning breast-feeding, the following facts are apparent: (1) if the parents are allergic or have other food allergic children, the mother should reduce her intake of potentially allergenic foods, such as milk or eggs, during pregnancy and nursing (Anderson and Sogn, 1984; Foucard, 1985); (2) rapid weaning of the child to solids after the age of 6 months probably is preferable to slow weaning particularly before this age; and (3) delayed introduction of solid foods until 5 to 6 months is preferable to early introduction (Foucard, 1985).

Natural History of Food Allergy

In general, those foods that cause an allergic reaction during early childhood are less likely to be a problem as the child grows than are those food sensitivities that are acquired later in life. Thus, individuals with reactions to cow's milk, egg, soy, and peanut have good prognoses (Foucard, 1985; Kemp et al., 1985). Food reactions to allergens such as fish and nuts that develop later in life are likely to persist (Johansson et al., 1984). The patient's prognosis with cow's milk allergy that develops early in life is favorable, with 60 to 90 percent of children able to tolerate cow's milk clinically by 2 to 3 years of age. This tolerance may occur in spite of a persistence of positive prick test results or positive RAST results to milk. Hamburger (1974) has found in a prospective study that a positive IgE skin test result and a positive IgE RAST result to food allergens may precede the development of clinical symptoms. Therefore, the younger the child with a positive food skin test result or food IgE RAST result, the more likely these test results indicate a causal relationship to clinical illness.

The Influence of Food Allergen Absorption

The potential for an allergic reaction to food is influenced by the rate and by the type of macromolecular food particles that are normally absorbed across the intestinal mucosa (Anderson and Sogn, 1984). During early infancy, the absorption of food macromolecules is greater than during later childhood. Evidence for an immune response to these foods is demonstrated by the abundance of circulating serum antibodies to commonly ingested proteins, such as cow's milk and eggs, which occur more commonly in infants than in adults. Most normal infants fed a cow's milk formula show increasing IgG and IgA anti-milk antibodies up to 3 to 9 months of age and, thereafter, a gradual decline (Foucard, 1984). This natural increase in food macromolecular absorption places atopic infants at particular risk of developing an IgE-mediated response to these foods.

Macromolecular food particle absorption may be increased because of a number of acquired factors (Bienenstock, 1984). Malnutrition, vitamin A deficiency, decreased gastric acidity, and absence of digestive enzymes can result in increased food particle absorption. In patients with immunodeficiency disease, particularly IgA deficiency, increased macromolecular food particle absorption is common. Bacterial, viral, parasitic, and toxic enteritis cause damage to the intestinal mucosa and permit the passage of partially digested food allergens (Anderson and Sogn, 1984). It is not uncommon that urticaria to a wide variety of foods may occur in patients during or immediately following an episode of diarrhea. In atopic states, such as atopic dermatitis, increased macromolecular food particle absorption, even in those individuals who do not have food allergy, is apparent compared with nonallergic individuals.

FOOD INTOLERANCE (NONIMMUNOLOGICALLY MEDIATED ADVERSE FOOD REACTIONS)

The true incidence of adverse reactions to food is unknown. Most reactions to foods actually are nonimmune in nature. Table 10–3 lists nonimmune reactions to foods that commonly are confused with allergic reactions as well as the foods that are usually associated with these conditions.

Pharmacologic Reactions to Foods

Pharmacologic adverse reactions to foods are due to chemicals naturally present in foods or to chemicals added to foods that exert a drug-like effect on the individual. Adverse effects to the methylxanthines, including caffeine, may be one of the most frequent nonimmunologically mediated food reactions at all ages. The methylxanthines as well as vasoactive amines, such as tryptophane, tyramine, dopamine, phenylethylamine, norepinephrine, serotonin, and histamine, can cause a wide variety of common symptoms, especially in the central nervous system and the gastrointestinal tract (Anderson, 1984). These chemicals are present in many foods (see Table 10–3). Methylxanthines and vasoactive amines found in common foods, such as cola drinks, chocolate, cocoa, and cheese, can induce headaches.

The most allergic-like reaction due to a nonimmune mechanism is the *anaphylactoid reaction.* This type of adverse food reaction can occur for several reasons (see Table 10–3). It is often confused with allergic reactions to food when the reaction is due either to the direct release of histamine and other mediators from food interacting with mast cells and basophils or to the ingestion of food that contains large amounts of histamine. Strawberries, shellfish, egg whites, wine, and Swiss cheese are of particular importance as potent histamine-releasing foods. Histamine intoxication can occur after the ingestion of fish that contains large amounts of histamine. Scombroid fish (tuna and mackerel) and mahi-mahi (dolphin) can become spoiled and contaminated with *Proteus morganii* or *Klebsiella pneumoniae,* which results in microbial decarboxylation of histidine, yielding histamine (Anderson, 1984).

The possible relationship between the attention deficit disorder of childhood (with or without hyperkinesis) and natural salicylates and food additives, particularly colors, was first presented by Dr. Benjamin Feingold in 1973 (Ribon, 1982). Dr. Feingold claimed that a special diet would produce improvement in 50 percent of children with hyperkinesis. A consensus development conference convened by the National Institutes of Health (NIH) evaluated the information on this subject in 1982 and concluded that only a small number of patients could be helped by a diet devoid of added colors. Swanson and Kinsbourne (1980) found that, with a high dose challenge of food color mixture (particularly tartrazine or yellow no. 5), children with attention deficit syndrome made progressively more mistakes on a learning test than with a challenge of placebo; the food colors mixture appeared to act like a drug. Animal studies have shown that erythosine (FD&C red dye no. 3) also may affect behavior. However, these effects, if consistent, appear to be unusual (also see Chapters 27 and 57).

Metabolic Reactions to Food

Metabolic reactions to food usually affect a susceptible subpopulation of patients. Intestinal oligosaccharide deficiency, an inborn error of metabolism, is the most important cause of carbohydrate malabsorption worldwide. The most frequent problem is lactose intolerance. The intestinal wall enzyme, lactase, is necessary for the metabolism of lactose found in cow's milk. A lack of this enzyme results in the fermentation of the lactose to lactic acid and in an osmotic diarrhea as well as signs of food malabsorption.

Primary lactose intolerance varies dramatically among population groups, with an incidence among North American blacks, Mexicans, and Asiatics of 70 to 80 percent and in whites of 5 to 20 percent (Gray, 1980). Intermediate ranges are found among Puerto Ricans (21 percent). The problem with lactose sugar metabolism usually becomes manifested between the ages of 3 and 15 years. However, viral or bacterial gastroenteritis at a younger age may initiate the signs of this problem earlier. Transient, secondary lactose intolerance is a common problem following infectious enteritis regardless of racial background.

The effects of high sugar intake on behavior have been widely debated. High sugar intake has been correlated with low academic achievement in children; aggressive and restless behavior has been demonstrated in children with hyperkinesis, and increased activity has been demonstrated in normal children (Prinz et al., 1980). Other workers have been unable to demonstrate such effects. Rapoport (1982 to 1983), using double-blind food glucose, sucrose, or saccharin placebo challenge, in fact, demonstrated a calming effect by the sugar on motor and behavioral activity. Recently, Conner (1985) has shown that the background dietary intake, particularly the carbohydrate to protein ratio, is an important factor in modulating the effect of simple sugar intake. Pure carbohydrate appears to degrade attentional efficiency in children, but this effect is offset by a normal background diet of protein (Conner, 1985) (see also Chapter 27).

Adverse metabolic reactions that may be

TABLE 10–3. Food Intolerance— Nonimmunologically Mediated Adverse Food Reactions and Commonly Associated Foods

Pharmacologic Adverse Food Reactions

Caffeine
  Coffee, tea, cola, soft drink, cocoa
Theobromine
  Chocolate, tea
Histamine*
  Toxicity or poisoning (contaminated tuna or mackerel)
  Histamine-releasing foods (strawberry, shellfish, egg white, Swiss cheese)
Tyramine
  Cheese
Serotonin, tyramine, dopamine, phenylethylamine (in chocolate), *norepinephrine*
Food colors
  Particularly tartrazine (yellow dye no. 5) in commercial foods

Metabolic Food Reactions

Disaccharidase deficiency
  Bowel wall lactase—"lactose intolerance"; sucrase, isomaltase) (cow's milk, milk products, fruits)
Gluten sensitivity
  Celiac syndrome (wheat, rye)
Sugar and protein diet content
  Normal diet
Phenylketonuria
Glucose-6-phosphate dehydrogenase deficiency
Ceruloplasmin deficiency
  Wilson disease
Hypoglycemia
  Particularly diabetes mellitus

Food Idiosyncratic Reactions

Reactions to food colors (dyes)*
  Tartrazine (yellow dye no. 5)
  In commercial foods
Reactions to food preservatives*
  Sulfites and SO_2 (particularly in restaurant foods, such as fresh salads, fruits and seafood; commercial foods, such as dried fruits, potato chips, vinegar, cider, baked products, shrimp, beer, wine, and some fruit drinks).
  Sodium benzoate, butylated hydroxyanisole (BHA), and butylated hydroxytoluene (BHT) (in commercial foods).
Reactions to flavor enhancers*
  Monosodium-L-glutamate (MSG) (Chinese restaurant syndrome or shock; restaurant and home-cooked foods).
Reactions to exercise
  Following a meal or ingestion of a specific food (particularly shrimp and celery).†

* Anaphylactoid reactions (mediator release, anaphylaxis-like reactions).
† May be anaphylactoid or anaphylactic (see text).

confused with allergic reactions also may be observed in children with glucose-6-phosphate dehydrogenase deficiency and with ceruloplasmin deficiency (Wilson disease), and in diabetics suffering from hypoglycemic reactions.

Food-Induced Idiosyncratic Reactions

Food-induced, allergic-like idiosyncratic reactions usually are recognized in adults rather than in children. Aspirin and nonsteroidal antiinflammatory drugs (but not natural dietary salicylates) have been shown to induce asthma, rhinitis, urticaria and angioedema, and anaphylactoid-type reactions. Similar reactions may occur with tartrazine; food preservatives, such as sulfites and sulfur dioxide; and food flavor enhancers, such as monosodium L-glutamate.

Tartrazine (Yellow Dye No. 5). The coal tar-derived (azo-) dye tartrazine has been reported to be responsible for asthma and for urticaria and angioedema (Lockey, 1977). In most cases of tartrazine-induced asthma, the patient also is sensitive to aspirin and cross-reactivity is suspected. However, intolerance to tartrazine may exist without intolerance to aspirin (Genton et al., 1985). Recent controlled studies would indicate that tartrazine-induced asthma is unusual (Simon, 1984).

Tartrazine has been reported to be responsible for chronic urticaria in a substantial number of patients, especially by European investigators (Genton et al., 1985). This finding appears to be rare in North America.

Sulfites, Sulfur Dioxide, and other Food Preservatives. Adverse reactions to foods that contain sulfite preservatives have been recognized only since 1976, despite the use of these chemicals in food and drink for over 2500 years (Stevenson and Simon, 1984). Ingestion of food containing sulfites may cause exacerbations of asthma or anaphylactoid, "shock-like" reactions. Anecdotal reports of sulfite-induced acute urticaria also have surfaced. The exact mechanisms of this reaction are unknown. Although asthmatics in general are hyperreactive to SO_2, probably through stimulation of irritant cholinergic receptors, some sulfite-sensitive individuals are exquisitely sensitive to SO_2 inhalation. The food preservative salts, potassium metabisulfite ($K_2S_2O_2$) and sodium sulfite (Na_2SO_3), when added to water will form the sulfite radical (HSO_3^-). At the air fluid interface, H_2SO_3 and SO_2 are in equilibrium (Simon, 1984). One explanation of the sulfite reaction is that in the process of food sulfite mastication, or after swallowing, eructation occurs, so that the prime route of stimulation of the respiratory irritant receptor is by SO_2 inhalation. Another explanation favors travel of the HSO_3^- radical in plasma from the gut to the bronchial mucosa. Some sulfite-sensitive asthmatics may lack sulfite oxidase in their cells, so that they cannot properly metabolize and eliminate this chemical (Jacobson et al., 1984).

The exact incidence of this condition is unknown, but careful epidemiologic studies in adults estimate that 5 percent of asthmatics are at risk (Buckley et al., 1985). Other investigators were not able to identify sulfite-sensitive individuals in a group of adults who presented with a history of "idiopathic anaphylaxis" after a restaurant meal (Sonin and Patterson, 1985).

Sulfites have been used extensively in the restaurant industry as "stay fresh" agents; they are frequently sprayed on salad and fresh fruits. They also are found in soft drinks, wine, beer, vegetables sealed in cellophane, dried fruits (e.g., apricots), avocados, potato chips, French fries, bakery products, and on shrimp.

The condition was recognized as early as 1977 when Freedman, in England, reported reactions to SO_2 released from sulfite preservatives in orange drinks ingested by adults and children with asthma. A study in Australia reported a high incidence (66 percent) in a group of asthmatic children who experienced decreased pulmonary function after oral challenge with an acidic solution of sulfite (Towns and Mellis, 1984). In the United States, Friedman and Easton (1985) reported that 7 of 17 unselected asthmatics (39 percent), ages 5 to 16 years, had significant drops in FEV_1 following challenge with potassium metabisulfite in lemonade (pH 2.4).

Sodium benzoate, butylated hydroxyanisol (BHA), and butylated hydroxytoluene (BHT), all food preservatives, have been reported to cause allergic-like reactions in a few patients (Ribon et al., 1982; Genton et al., 1985). Most of these reactions have been in adults and have not been confirmed (Simon, 1984).

Monosodium L-Glutamate (MSG). MSG is a nonessential dicarboxylic amino acid that constitutes about 20 percent of our normal dietary protein. For example, Camembert cheese naturally contains about 1 percent glutamic acid. MSG is added to foods by cooks in restaurants and homes and to some commercially prepared foods to enhance flavor. MSG has been reported to cause the "Chinese restaurant syndrome," which includes headache, myalgias, backache, neck pain, chest tightness, diaphoresis, and nausea. The incidence of this syndrome is unknown but probably is less than originally reported (Kerr et al., 1979). Although it affects adults for the most part, it has been reported in a child (Asnes, 1980).

MSG has been claimed to cause urticaria (Genton, 1985); other investigators have failed to identify any cases of urticaria induced by MSG (Simon, 1984). One case of MSG-induced "asthma," a late phase reaction similar to some of the reported sulfite-induced reactions, has been published (Allen and Baker, 1981).

Exercise-Induced Anaphylaxis Following a Meal. A newly recognized syndrome of exercise-induced anaphylaxis, following food ingestion, has been described (see also Chapter 31). This syndrome differs from other exercise-induced "physical allergy" syndromes in that the predominant manifestation is shock and, on occasion, urticaria and angioedema. Exercise-induced asthma and cholinergic urticaria do not occur.

Study of a patient reported to have developed exercise-induced anaphylaxis 1 to 2 hours after ingesting a meal found no elevation of plasma histamine level in contrast to other patients with exercise-induced anaphylaxis whose reactions were unrelated to meals (Novey et al., 1983). The mechanism for the resulting shock and urticaria and angioedema is unknown in this patient, but the meal may have amplified tendencies for blood volume redistribution to the abdominal vessels, postexercise hypotension, and mediator release.

Specific food ingestion, particularly to shrimp and celery, also has been associated with the triggering of exercise-induced anaphylactic episodes (Kidd et al., 1983). These events may represent the combination of both immune (IgE allergen-specific antibody) and nonimmune mechanisms.

REFERENCES

Aas, K.: Antigens in food. Nutri. Rev. 42:85, 1984.

Allen, D.H., Baker, G.J.: Chinese-restaurant asthma. N. Engl. J. Med. 305:1154, 1981.

Anand, B.S., Truelove, S.C., Offord, R.E.: Skin test for coeliac disease using a subfraction of gluten. Lancet 1:118, 1977.

Anderson, J., Sogn, D. (ed.): Adverse Reactions to Foods, AAAI Committee on Adverse Reactions to Foods and NIAID. NIH Publication no. 84–2442, July 1984.

Anderson, J.A.: Non-immunologically mediated food sensitivity. Nutri. Rev. 42:109, 1984.

Anderson, J.A., Weiss, L., Rebuck, J.W., Cabal, L.A., Sweet, L.C.: Hyperreactivity to cow's milk in an infant with LE and tart cell phenomenon. J. Pediatr. 84:59, 1974.

Anderson, L.B.J., Dreyfuss, E.M., Logan, J., Johnstone, D.E., Glaser, J.: Melon and banana sensitivity coincident with ragweed pollinosis. J. Allergy Clin. Immunol. 45:310, 1970.

Asnes, R.S.: Chinese-restaurant syndrome in an infant. Clin. Pediatr. 19:705, 1980.

Bahna, S.L., Heiner, D.C.: Allergies to Milk. New York, Grune and Stratton, 1980.

Bienenstock, J.: Mucosal barrier functions. Nutri. Rev. 42:105, 1984.

Bleumink, E.: Food allergy: The chemical nature of the substance eliciting symptoms. World Rev. Nutri. Diet 12:505, 1970.

Buckley, C.E. III, Saltzman, H.A., Sieker, H.O.: The prevalence and degree of sensitivity to ingested sulfites. (Abstract.) J. Allergy Clin. Immunol. 75:144, 1985.

Bush, R.K., Taylor, S.L., Nordlee, J.A., Busse, W.W.: Soybean oil is not allergenic to soybean-sensitive individuals. J. Allergy Clin. Immunol. 76:242, 1985.

Conner, C.K.: National Children's Hospital and Medical Center, Washington, D.C. Personal communication, 1985.

Egger, J., Wilson, J., Carter, C., Turner, M., Soothill, J.: Is migraine food allergy?—A double-blind, controlled trial of oligoantigenic diet X? Lancet 2:865, 1983.

Ferguson, A., Ziegler, K., Strobel, S.: Gluten intolerance (coeliac disease). Ann. Allergy 53:637, 1984.

Foucard, T.: Developmental aspects of food sensitivity in children. Nutri. Rev. 42:98, 1984.

Foucard, T.: Development of food allergies with special reference to cow's milk allergy. Pediatrics 75:177, 1985.

Freedman, B.J.: Asthma induced by sulphur dioxide, benzoate and tartrazine contained in orange drinks. Clin. Allergy 7:407, 1977.

Friedman, M., Easton, J.: Oral metabisulfite (MBS) challenges in children with asthma. Presented at American Academy of Pediatrics, San Antonio, Texas, October 20, 1985.

Genton, C., Frei, P.C., Pecoud, A.: Value of oral provocation tests to aspirin and food additives in the routine investigation of asthma and chronic urticaria. J. Allergy Clin. Immunol. 76:40, 1985.

Goldstein, G.B., Heiner, D.C., Rose, B.: Studies of reagins to γ gliadin in a patient with wheat hypersensitivity. J. Allergy 44:37, 1969.

Gray, G.M.: Absorption and malabsorption of dietary carbohydrate. In Winick, M. (ed.): Nutrition and Gastroenterology. New York, John Wiley & Sons Inc., 1980.

Hamburger, R.N.: Diagnosis of food allergies and intolerance in the study of prophylaxis and control groups in infants. Ann. Allergy 53:673, 1974.

Hoffman, D.R.: The specificities of human IgE antibodies combining with cereal grains. Immunochemistry 12:535, 1975.

Hoffman, D.R.: Immunochemical identification of the allergens in egg white. J. Allergy Clin. Immunol. 71:481, 1983.

Hoffman, D.R., Day, E.D., Miller, J.S.: The major heat state allergen of shrimp. Ann. Allergy 47:17, 1981.

Jacobson, D.W., Simon, R.A., Singh, M.: Sulfite oxidase deficiency and cobalamine protection in sulfite-sensitive asthma. J. Allergy Clin. Immunol. 73:135, 1984.

Johansson, S.G.O., Dannaeus, A., Lilja, G.: The relevance of anti-food antibodies for the diagnosis of food allergy. Ann. Allergy 53:665, 1984.

Kemp, A.S., Mellis, C.M., Barnett, D., Sharota, E., Simpson,

J.: Skin test, RAST, and clinical reaction to peanut allergens in children. Clin. Allergy 15:73, 1985.

Kerr, G.R., Wu-Lee, M., Ed-Lozy, M., McGandy, R., Stare, F.J.: Prevalence of the "Chinese Restaurant Syndrome." J. Am. Diet Assoc. 75:29, 1979.

Kidd, J.M., III, Cohen, S.H., Sosman, A.J., Fink, J.N.: Food dependent exercise-induced anaphylaxis. J. Allergy Clin. Immunol. 71:407, 1983.

Kletter, B., Gray, L., Freier, S., et al.: Immune response in normal infants to cow's milk. Int. Arch. Allergy Appl. Immunol. 40:656, 1971.

Lahti, A., Bjorksten, F., Hannuksela, M.: Allergy to birch pollen and apple. Cross-reactivity of the allergen studies with the RAST. Allergy 35:297, 1980.

Lockey, S.D., Sr.: Hypersensitivity to tartrazine (FD&C yellow no. 5) and other dyes and additives present in foods and pharmaceutical products. Ann. Allergy 38:206, 1977.

Matthews, T., Soothill, J.: Complement activation after milk feeding in children with cow's milk allergy. Lancet 2:893, 1970.

Minor, J.D., Tolber, S.G., Frick, O.L.: Leukocyte inhibition factor in delayed onset of food allergy. J. Allergy Clin. Immunol. 66:314, 1980.

Moroy, L.A., Young, W., Kunitz, H.: Soybean trypsin inhibitor — A specific allergen in food anaphylaxis. N. Engl. J. Med. 302:1126, 1980.

National Institutes of Health (NIH) Consensus Development Panel 2062: Defined Diets in Childhood Hyperactivity. Bethesda, Maryland, Office for Medical Applications of Research, 1982.

Novey, H.S., Fairshter, R.D., Salness, K., Simon, R.A., Curd, J.G.: Post-prandial exercise-induced anaphylaxis. J. Allergy Clin. Immunol. 71:498, 1983.

Parish, W.E.: Short-term anaphylactic IgE antibodies in human serum. Lancet 2:591, 1970.

Prausnitz, C., Küstner, H.: Studien uber Ubernempfindlichkeit, Centralbl. f. Bakteriol. I, Abt. Orig. 86:160–169, 1921. Translated from German by Carl Prausnitz in "Clinical Aspects of Immunology," Gell, P.G.H., Coombs, R.R.A. (eds.) Oxford, Blackwell Scientific Publications, Inc. 1962.

Prinz, R.J., Roberts, W.A., Hoatuum, E.: Dietary correlates of hyperactive behavior in children. J. Consult. Clin. Psychol. 48:760, 1980.

Rapoport, J.L.: Effects of dietary substance in children. J. Psychiatri. Res. 17:187, 1982–1983.

Rawcliffe, P.M., Jewell, D.P., Faux, J.A.: Specific IgG subclass antibodies, IgE and IgG S-Ts antibodies to wheat gluten fraction B in patients with coeliac disease. Clin. Allergy 15:155, 1985.

Ribon, A., Joshi, S.: Is there any relationship between food additives and hyperkinesis? Ann. Allergy 48:275, 1982.

Sachs, M.I., Jones, R.T., Yunginger, J.W.: Isolation and partial characterization of a major peanut allergen. J. Allergy Clin. Immunol. 67:27, 1981.

Sampson, H.A.: Role of immediate food hypersensitivity in the pathogenesis of atopic dermatitis. J. Allergy Clin. Immunol. 71:473, 1983.

Sampson, H.A., Albergo, R.: Comparison of the results of skin tests, RAST, and double-blind, placebo-controlled food challenges in children with atopic dermatitis. J. Allergy Clin. Immunol. 74:26, 1984.

Schwartz, H.R., Nerarkar, L.S., Spies, J.R., Scanlan, R.T., Bellanti, J.A.: Milk hypersensitivity: RAST studies using new antigen generated by pepsin hydrolysis of beta-lactoglobulin. Ann. Allergy 45:242, 1980.

Scudomore, H.H., Phillips, S.F., Swedlund, H.A., Gleich, G.J.: Food allergy manifested by eosinophilia, elevated immunoglobulin E level, and protein-losing enteropathy: The syndrome of allergic gastroenteropathy. J. Allergy Clin. Immunol. 70:129, 1984.

Shibaski, M., Suzuki, S., Tajima, S., Nemoto, H., Kuroune, T.: Allergenicity of major component proteins of soybean. Int. Arch. Allergy. Appl. Immunol. 61:441, 1980.

Simon, R.A.: Adverse reactions to drug additives. J. Allergy Clin. Immunol. 74:623, 1984.

Sonin. L., Patterson, R.: Metabisulfite challenge in patients with idiopathic anaphylaxis. J. Allergy Clin. Immunol. 75:67, 1985.

Spies, J.R., Steven, M.A., Stein, W.J., Conkon, E.J.: The chemistry of allergens XX: New antigens generated by pepsin hydrolysis of bovine milk proteins. J. Allergy 45:200, 1970.

Stevenson, D.D., Simon, R.A.: Sulfites and asthma (editorial). J. Allergy Clin. Immunol. 74:469, 1984.

Swanson, J.M., Kinsbourne, M.: Food dyes impair performance of hyperactive children on a laboratory learning test. Science 207:1485, 1980.

Taylor, S.L., Busse, W.W., Sachs, M.I., Parker, J.A., Yunginger, J.W.: Peanut oil is not allergenic to peanut-sensitive individuals. J. Allergy Clin. Immunol. 68:372, 1981.

Towns, S.J., Mellis, C.M.: Role of acetyl salicylic acid and sodium metabisulfite in chronic childhood asthma. Pediatrics 73:631, 1984.

Walsh, B.J., Wrighley, S.W., Musk, A.W., Baldo, B.A.: A comparison of the binding of IgE in the sera of patients with Baker's asthma to soluble and insoluble wheat-grain proteins. J. Allergy Clin. Immunol. 76:23, 1985.

11

Common Pollen and Fungus Allergens

WILLIAM R. SOLOMON, M.D.

FUNGI

Allergy to inhaled fungal allergens is a common factor in allergic rhinitis and asthma. The clinical impact on respiratory allergy of many widespread, potential offenders still must be determined, however. The overall role of fungus materials in urticaria and eczema is speculative.

Basic Characteristics of Fungi

Fungi compose a unique group of organisms, which differ fundamentally from plants, animals, actinomycetes, and slime molds (Myxomycetes). Fungi have true nuclei and cell walls of chitin or cellulose. Except for unicellular forms, fungi are composed of microscopic strands or "hyphae"; these (Fig. 11–1) proliferate simply, as in "molds," or form specialized fleshy structures, as in mushrooms and sac fungi. In most forms, well-defined septa divide the hyphal strands, and metabolic debris tends to occupy older, more central segments as growth proceeds peripherally.

Most allergenic fungi can grow on nonliving organic matter, while other types, i.e., obligate parasites, require a living host. Both groups need moisture, oxygen, preformed carbohydrate, and occasionally additional growth factors.

Many familiar fungi grow actively at 20°C and may flourish well above or below this temperature; others require low temperatures, proliferating even under refrigeration. A small group of "thermophilic" fungi grow *only* at temperatures of 50°C or higher, while certain types (e.g., *Aspergillus fumigatus*) tolerate these temperatures but also grow well below 50°C. With adequate moisture, many fungi grow actively at 20°C on nutritionally barren substrates (Fig. 11–2) in homes and work environments.

Fungal vegetative strands may be ingestant allergens; however, inhaled spores are the major source of exposure. Spores are specialized reproductive structures that usually are resistant to harsh environmental conditions. Depending upon the fungus (or even upon a particular growth phase), spores may be asexual (diploid) or sexual (haploid) with dissimilar "mating types." Many fungi may produce sexual and asexual spores at different phases of their life cycles. Since these stages may occur separately, they often have been described and named as if they were individual organisms.

Those types that generate asexual spores (i.e., imperfect fungi) are classified according to the form of their spore-producing organs. However, it is now clear that biologically dissimilar fungi may have imperfect (asexual) stages, which are morphologically almost alike. Since the arrangement of the imperfect fungi does not necessarily reflect natural affinities, its taxa are termed *"form* species," and these are grouped in *"form* genera." While the concept of *form* taxa imparts some order to a large and difficult group, it is clear that members of *form* genera cannot be expected automatically to contain identical allergens. This limitation often has been overlooked in the past, both by physicians and pharmaceutical suppliers, in labelling fungus extracts with "generic" names only.

Classes of Fungi

The taxonomy of fungi is based largely upon the morphology and mode of development of their spores. Although many species exist, including many that are wholly aquatic, air-borne molds constitute the most important source of allergens. They can be classified into the five following principal groups.

Fungi Imperfecti (Deuteromycetes). This class of fungi that reproduce asexually includes most of the currently recognized fungal allergens. With a few exceptions, these form taxa are saprophytic, and spores ("conidia") develop on more or less specialized hyphal structures. In one subclass (Sphaeropsidales), spores arise in flask-shaped organs and are extruded in slimy masses, which are dispersed by dew and rain-

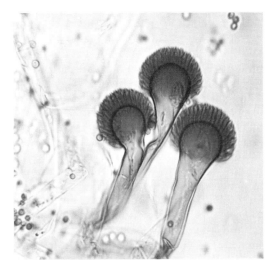

FIGURE 11–1. Photomicrograph of *Aspergillus fumigatus*, a typical filamentous imperfect fungus. Hyphal strands (left) are the basic structural units of these organisms. Spores (conidia) are characteristically borne on specialized hyphae (conidiophores), which, in *Aspergillus* form species, are terminally expanded; three such "vesicles" are shown at the right.

drops; *Phoma* exemplifies this group. Another distinctive subclass (Melanconiales) has spore-forming hyphae in cushion-like masses; some members are plant pathogens, but apparently none serve as important allergens. The imperfect fungi bear spores, singly or multiply on exposed hyphae except for a tiny group (Mycelia Sterilia), which appears to multiply by vegetative appendages alone. Tenuous attachments permit spores of many taxa to be scoured and dispersed readily by air currents; such "dry

spore" dispersal is typical of such common genera as *Alternaria* (Fig. 11–3), *Cladosporium* (formerly *Hormodendrum*), and *Penicillium* species. Out of doors, these types are most prevalent on hot, dry, windy days. By contrast, many fungi (e.g., species of *Phoma*, *Fusarium*, and *Cephalosporium*) produce mucinous masses of "slime" spores dispersed during rainy and humid periods.

Although allergists are most familiar with imperfect fungi, there remains substantial uncertainty concerning their clinical role for a variety of reasons; gaps in knowledge of their prevalence in many areas of the country and of the amount of exposure in specific environments or with specific activities, a dearth of information on the intensity of exposure necessary to induce symptoms, and unclear antigenic relationships between biologically related genera.

Table 11–1 is an annotated list of imperfect fungi of acknowledged or widely suspected clinical importance.

Downy Mildews (Oömycetes). These relatively primitive fungi include economically important parasites of plants and certain insects. Agricultural exposure to heavily infected crops occasionally provokes allergic respiratory responses.

Sugar and Bread Molds (Zygomycetes). The allergic impact of this class is due largely to members of the order Mucorales, including species of *Rhizopus*, *Mucor*, and *Absidia*. These fungi are prominent saprophytes of biologic debris, including food residues and leaf litter. While ubiquitous in soil, their level in air usually is low. However, with seepage of

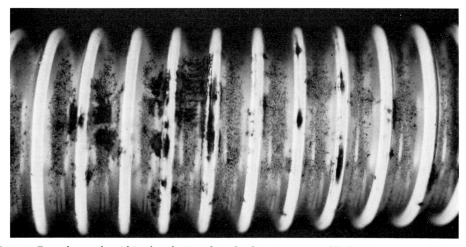

FIGURE 11–2. Fungal growth within the plastic tubing leading to a water-filled spirometer used for ventilatory testing. Airborne dust and droplets of saliva provide the only nutrient source for these organisms. An ample supply of moisture permits fungi to colonize such marginal sites.

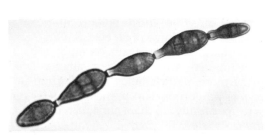

FIGURE 11-3. *Alternaria alternata* spores borne in characteristic chains. These brown, multiseptate particles are widely abundant in outdoor air and are among the most clinically important fungus allergens.

ground water or soiling of furnishings with food, these organisms may flourish indoors. Close inspection of infected substrates may disclose the dark globular reproductive structures (sporangia), each containing myriad spores (sporangiospores). Members of the order Mucorales typically have comparatively broad hyphae with few septa.

Ascomycetes (Sac Fungi). These fungi produce sexual spores (ascospores) in a sac-like cell (or "ascus"). Ascospores often are actively launched into air by processes requiring moisture reaching greatest abundance in humid or rainy weather. Many familiar imperfect fungi, including *Aspergillus*, *Fusarium*, and *Helminthosporium* form species, are asexual states of ascomycetes. Brewer's (baker's) yeast is an additional member of this class. The few ascospore types evaluated as allergens have induced moderate rates of reactivity in exposed atopic subjects (Bruce, 1963).

Basidiomycetes (Mushrooms, Puffballs, Rusts, and Smuts). These fungi resemble asco-

TABLE 11-1. Imperfect Fungi of Special Interest to Allergists

Form Genus and Major Form Species*	SRR†	Noteworthy Characteristics D = dark gray or black colonies ("Dematiaceous")
Alternaria—*A. alternata* = *A. tenuis*	++++	Widespread on vegetation: probably most clinically reactive airborne fungus allergen (D)
Cladosporium (formerly Hormodendrum)—*C. cladosporioides, C. herbarum*	++	Highest outdoor spore levels in most regions. Form species' allergens may differ (D)
Epicoccum—*E. purpurascens*	++	Especially on grains, grasses: produces orange pigments but sporulates poorly on many agar media
Stemphylium—*S. botryosum*	+++	Imperfect form of *Pleospora herbarum*, an ascomycete (D)
Curvularia—*C. lunata*	+++	Especially in warmer areas (D)
Helminthosporium—*H. solani*	+++	Agriculturally centered, epidemic at times (D) (*Drechslera* and *Bipolaris* are similar form genera)
Fusarium—*F. roseum, F. nivale*	++	Imperfect forms of several ascomycete genera: colonies produce slime spores and prominent pigments. Ascospores may produce much *Fusarium* growth
Phoma—*P. herbarum*	+++	Sphaeropsid: slime-spored: reactivity said to parallel that to *Alternaria* form species and both may be asexual forms of certain ascomycete species
Penicillium (more than a dozen common types)	+	Often perennially present *indoors* and outdoors: *unrelated* to sensitivity to penicillin
Aspergillus—*A. flavus, A. fumigatus, A. amstelodami, A. glaucus*, others	++	Indoor and occupational exposures common: *A. fumigatus, A. flavus* also produce allergic aspergillosis
A. niger	(±)	Prominent on wood and paper
Candida—*C. albicans, C. tropicalis*	++	*C. albicans* is a common human gut and orificial saprophyte; uncommon in air
Rhodotorula—*R. glutinis*	+	Prominent during wet weather; acid-tolerant red yeast: grows well in indoor fluid reservoirs
Aureobasidium—*A. pullulans*	++	Formerly termed "Pullularia"; common soil, leaf saprophyte. Pleomorphic on agar media (D)
Monilia sitophila	+	Prominently associated with milling and bakery trades: extremely rapid grower
Botrytis—*B. cinerea*	++	Prevalence regionally variable; prominent plant pathogen
Geotrichum—*G. candidum*	+	Vaguely defined form genus; probably asexual forms of basidiomycetes
Sporobolomyces—*S. roseum*	++	Yeast, usually pink, actively discharging spores; suspected autumn allergen in Great Britain
Gliocladium—*G. roseum*	++	Slime-spored; young growth *Penicillium*-like
Trichoderma—*T. viride*	+	Prominent in soil; rapid grower

* Note that additional form genera including *Cephalosporium, Verticillium, Sporothrix, Pithomyces*, and numerous yeasts are widely encountered but have received little or no clinical evaluation.

† SRR = Estimated relative Skin Reactivity Rate among exposed atopic subjects in North America using available materials.

mycetes in producing sexual spores (among other types), which are shot from their points of origin, given adequate moisture, and are abundant at night and during rainy periods. Characteristic spores, "basidiospores," are formed — most commonly in tetrads — on specialized cells or "basidia." In addition, many parasitic forms (e.g., smuts, bunts, and rusts) produce additional spores during stages of development, often on a succession of hosts. Heavy agricultural exposures to spores of rusts and grain smuts have produced allergic symptoms, but it is not known whether lesser exposures are harmful. Asthma has been associated with homes containing spores of the dry rot fungus (*Merulius lacrymans*), and skin sensitivity to other basidiospores has been described (Gold, 1984; Santilli, 1981).

Concepts of Fungus Prevalence and Their Limitations

Unlike pollens and animal allergens, which come from obvious sources, airborne fungi originate largely from inapparent microscopic growth. Consequently, insight into exposure necessitates direct air sampling. Collection techniques must be carefully chosen to give a true picture of prevalence. Total reliance upon molds that grow on exposed agar media, for example, has limited data to *viable* particles and excluded possibly significant allergens that fail to grow recognizably. Selective recovery is a property of all known media, although some, e.g., malt extract agar and Sabouraud glucose agar, are less restrictive than others. Prevalence data also are readily biased by collecting particles on greased slides or on open plates of growth media by fallout. Since the variations in

air speed, direction, and turbulence affect deposition and the volume of air contributing particles is unknown, data obtained cannot be readily compared sequentially or among sites. Furthermore, particle fallout on collection surfaces is proportional to particle diameter (or, more specifically, to diameter squared) so that larger particles will predominate in collections (Fig. 11–4). Recent applications of techniques, accurate for particles of all sizes, have emphasized the true abundance of many ascospores and basidiospores as well as of small imperfect fungus spores, which previously were unnoticed (see Ogden et al., 1974, for additional details).

Many airborne fungi possess distinctive morphology that enables identification microscopically. Identification by microscopic examination is applicable especially to the dark-spored imperfect fungi (see Table 11–1), to many sexual spores of fleshy fungi, and to rust and smut spores. Though there is no comprehensive guide available, illustrations of selected particles have been published (Gregory, 1973). An extensive set of ascospore drawings (Dennis, 1978) and monographs depicting the spores of imperfect fungus taxa also can be found (Barron, 1977; Barnett, 1972; Ellis, 1971; Ellis and Ellis, 1985).

The growth of fungi on semisolid media is essential for numerous taxa (e.g., form species of *Penicillium* and *Aspergillus*, yeasts and zygomycetes) with minute, nondescript, spheroidal spores. The interested reader is referred to the publication by Arx (1981), which describes generic identification, also to Barron (1968), Barnett, 1972), Ellis (1971), and Onions (1982) for technical advice in identifying fungi.

Recoveries in culture considerably underestimate prevalence, as judged by spores in micro-

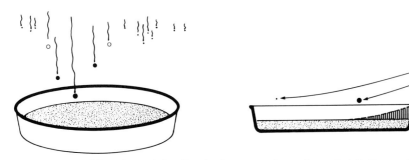

FIGURE 11–4. Problems in particle collection by open culture plates. At left, the markedly greater fallout of larger (than smaller) particles is emphasized using the (unnatural) example of still air. A similar effect is easily observed with normal atmospheric motion (right). Here again, recovery varies with particle size, and in rapidly moving air, deposition may be hindered by the protruding lip of the culture dish.

scopic deposits. In addition, it is clear that many airborne spore types — especially sexual spores of certain fleshy fungi — cannot be identified because they are neither distinctive in form nor capable of growing on available media.

Fungi Outdoors. Since fungi grow principally on leaf surfaces and in plant litter and soil, spore concentrations vary with local cycles of plant growth and are decreased by snow cover. Airborne fungi are prominent throughout the growing season in temperate areas, but peak spore levels are in late summer and autumn, particularly during hot, breezy periods when "dry-spore" forms abound. Recoveries at these times are dominated by spores of *Alternaria* and *Cladosporium* species, which seem to achieve their highest levels in grassland and cultivated (especially, grain-growing) areas. At night and on rainy days, ascospores and basidiospores reach maximum prevalence along with splash-dispersed spores of imperfect taxa. Whether respiratory symptoms that worsen during humid and rainy weather reflect exposure to these little studied particles is unknown. Symptoms are induced in fungus-sensitive subjects by many situations and activities that accentuate exposure. Spore levels are higher close to the ground in natural areas than at rooftop sites. Substantial airborne dispersion of fungus particles occurs when plant growth is disturbed (e.g., by traversing vegetated areas). Exposure peaks also may occur with mowing lawns or harvesting grains. Composting of plant materials poses special hazards for mold-sensitive patients because fungi flourish in composts. Fungus-sensitive persons commonly develop symptoms after exposure to hay, ensilage, mulches, dry soil, commercial peat moss, compost piles, and leaf litter. Yet, there is little objective support for the belief that spore levels are specifically increased in the vicinity of lakes and other surface waters.

Fungi Indoors. Occupational contact with plant or animal products — especially in humid interiors — is associated with heavy exposure to air-borne fungal antigens, and perennial symptoms may result. When spores are numerous out of doors, they will dominate recoveries made in normally ventilated interiors; fungi originating indoors are more likely to be evident when buildings are closed (e.g., in winter or with central air conditioning in summer) and especially when outdoor fungi levels are low. At these times, *Penicillium, Aspergillus,* and *Fusarium* form species and occasionally *Rhodotorula* and other yeasts may predominate. This

contrasts sharply with the "*Cladosporium-Alternaria*" pattern so typical of outdoor air in northern states in summer (Solomon, 1975).

In winter, the correlation between relative humidity and indoor fungus level has been strong. This association probably reflects both moisture promoted fungus growth and colonization of humidifying devices by fungi. "Coolmist" vaporizers are frequently contaminated and emit fungus-laden aerosols (Solomon, 1974); presumably, furnace humidifiers may do so also. Pets and active small children foster increased indoor fungus levels by soiling surfaces with food residues and outside dust. It is possible that houseplants may promote mold exposure, but current information does not justify total elimination of houseplants.

Reduction of indoor mold spore exposure depends upon meticulous general hygiene, with either eliminating or encasing in plastic both fiber and foam-filled furnishings. Central air conditioning will permit window closure during warm periods, thus excluding outdoor particles and reducing relative humidity. At other times, supplementary humidification should be restrained, with levels of 20 to 25 percent relative humidity viewed as adequate. Shower curtains, refrigerator drip trays, and window moldings as well as cold basements and outside walls where water condenses or seeps deserve special concern. If these areas are cleaned with solutions of sodium hypochlorite, Lysol, or other commercial products, such as zephiran (available as Roccal, and used 1 ounce in 1 gallon of tap water), mold growth is inhibited, although microbial regrowth occurs all too quickly. Specific indoor antifungal agents have not yet been proved safe and effective. Small moldy objects may be decontaminated by placing them in a plastic bag for 12 to 24 hours with a small amount of paraformaldehyde or propylene oxide. Fungus growth in limited spaces also may be attacked by volatilizing paraformaldehyde. These fumes are toxic, however, and treated areas must be completely ventilated before use.

Sampling indoor air by use of open culture dishes ("settling plates") has dubious value in evaluating obscure symptoms. If this method is used, the physician must beware of the serious limitation of preferential recovery of large particles, with exclusion of smaller particles (Solomon, 1975). This fact is especially important since small-spored fungi often predominate in indoor air.

Fungi in Foods. Fungi are important in the

production of many foods and industrial chemicals (Onions, 1982). Various yeasts *(Saccharomyces cerevisiae)* are employed in preparation of baked goods, beer, wines, and some liquors as well as vinegar and vinegar products—especially processed meats. Most cheeses result from bacterial fermentations but are readily contaminated in storage; in addition, Camembert and blue-veined cheeses (e.g., Roquefort) utilize specific *Penicillium* species. Commercial mushrooms, the spore-producing organs of basidiomycetes *(Agaricus bisporis)*, are rarely ingestant allergens. Soy and steak sauces are produced using *Aspergillus oryzae.* Fungi are employed in the early stages of chocolate production. In addition, fungi commonly contaminate stored foodstuffs, even at refrigeration temperatures.

Although massive ingestion of yeast-containing foods (e.g., a wine, cheese, and pizza feast) will, at times, provoke respiratory symptoms in young adults, ingested fungi probably are an infrequent cause of prolonged allergic problems. Highly allergic patients occasionally may benefit from a trial withdrawal of dietary fungi followed by a diagnostic challenge. The "mold-free diet" eliminates fresh rolls, coffee cakes, pizza dough, dried yeast, and foods refrigerated over 72 hours as well as fermented beverages and foods. Fresh fruits and vegetables should be peeled or scrubbed before consumption. Products such as jellies and preserves are acceptable, as are commercial breads. Duration should be tailored to individual clinical needs. Often, avoidance of a few foods can provide a major decrease in ingested fungus materials.

Significance of Fungus Sensitivity. Evaluation of sensitivity to fungi is difficult because of their diversity, their uncertain regional distribution, and often prolonged periods of exposure. Clinical allergy to fungal allergens *alone* is uncommon. However, there is little doubt that IgE-mediated allergy to fungi is widespread, especially to species of *Alternaria* and other dark-spored imperfect genera. These may be responsible for symptoms throughout most of a local growing season or, at least, at times different from major pollen peaks. Although many additional molds produce positive skin test reactions, their clinical importance and allergenic similarities, if any, are yet to be fully defined. Determining fungus prevalence in air remains a key to estimating exposure and to setting priorities for clinical evaluation.

POLLENS

Pollen allergy (pollinosis) is the most frequently recognized allergic syndrome. Symptoms are caused by exposure to wind-borne pollens of subjects allergic to them. Manifestations induced are seasonal allergic rhinitis (hay fever), asthma, and may include conjunctivitis. Atopic dermatitis occasionally flares during pollen seasons while pollen-provoked urticaria is usually related to running through fields of pollinating tall grass or ragweed.

Pollen in Reproductive Biology

Pollen grains—common to all flowering plants—serve as vectors for male gametes or reproductive cells. Pollens develop in distinctive floral structures (Fig. 11–5), the *anther sacs,* which are lined by a specialized tissue, the *tapetum.* One or more anther sacs with suitable protective coverings, i.e., the anthers, are usually borne on stalks or *filaments* and termed *stamens.* The total developmental process that provides mature pollen grains for dispersal is termed *anthesis.*

In most flowering plants, *pollination* (i.e., the transport of mature pollen) is effected by one or more animal vectors—generally insects. However, all of the grasses, many of the trees of temperate regions, and a minority of broad-leafed herbs (or "forbs") have developed adaptations for wind dispersal of pollen (and are termed "anemophilous"). The goal of pollen transport, in either case, is deposition of viable grains on a receptive *stigma,* the terminal and most exposed part of the female floral organ (or "pistil"), as shown in Figure 11–5. After this is accomplished, both grain and stigmatic surface release one or more poorly characterized "recognition substances." Aside from their fundamental biologic importance to the plant, many of these substances (e.g., antigen E of short ragweed) appear to be important as clinical allergens. When an exchange of chemical signals occurs between a compatible grain and stigma, it may be followed by *pollen germination.* In this process, a tubular structure emerges from the grain, penetrates the stigma, and grows down through the subjacent *style,* finally reaching the *ovary,* the reproductive nexus of the pistil. Gametes are formed during pollen tube development and effect fertilization, producing both an

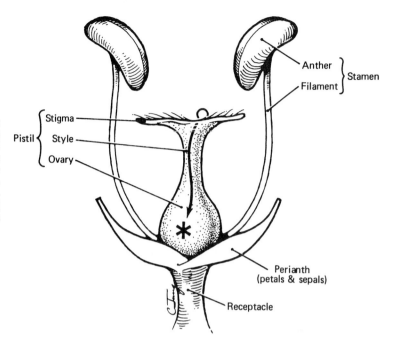

FIGURE 11-5. Structure of a wind-pollinated flower. Note the relatively large anthers, broad stigma, and reduced perianth; no nectaries are present. The arrow indicates the general path of pollen tube growth to effect fertilization (*). Having both male and female organs, this flower is "perfect."

embryo and nutritive *endosperm*, the components of the future seed.

Sources of Wind-borne Pollen

Floral Similarities Among Wind-pollinated Plants. Since anemophilous plants rely upon random transport of pollen, increasing the number of pollen grains dispersed optimizes fertilization rates. To increase this number, similarities in floral pattern (Fig. 11-6) have evolved in all wind-pollinated species. Modifications include production of numerous, minute, grouped flowers; increased output of pollen per stamen; and reduction or absence of brightly colored parts and of scent (which attract insects). In addition, anemophilous flowers commonly have relatively expanded stigmas, long anther filaments, and may be *imperfect,* i.e., of two types—with only male or only female parts in a single floret. Most windborne grains are relatively smooth surfaced and are among the smaller pollens, with diameters of 15 to 60 microns.

Tree, Grass, and Weed Sources. Plants associated with pollinosis often are subclassified colloquially into trees, grasses, and weeds—useful terms which, however, deserve qualification. Trees are woody plants capable of reaching heights of 20 feet or more at maturity.

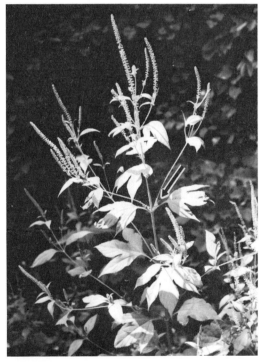

FIGURE 11-6. Giant ragweed, a highly successful wind-pollinated species. Male flowers are produced in crowded terminal spikes, whereas female flowers (arrow) are fewer and occupy the bases of the leaves. The three-lobed leaves are the basis of the Latin name of this plant, *Ambrosia trifida.*

Members of many plant families share this growth form, leaving no reason to expect allergenic similarities among diverse tree pollens. Pollination by tree species usually occurs early in the local growing season and often before leaf expansion is complete. While this schedule probably aids pollen penetration of forest canopies, it means flower buds must form in the autumn and are subject to losses due to winter. For this reason and because of the unpredictable weather of early spring in colder regions, the period and intensity of airborne pollens of trees vary widely from year to year.

All grasses are wind-pollinated; yet, only a few shed sufficient pollen to serve as *clinically* important sources. Pollens from certain grasses are antigenically similar. Peaks of grass pollen prevalence generally occur in the early to mid-summer period but may extend throughout a prolonged growing season in warmer regions.

"Weed" pollens generally are those derived from any sources besides trees and grasses. While many such broad-leafed herbs are horticultural pests (i.e., "weeds" in the strict sense), they represent numerous plant families and allergenic specificities. Furthermore, many grasses and trees also display "weediness," i.e., growth where they are unwanted.

Bases of Pollen Recognition

Pollens and Plant Taxonomy. Morphologic characteristics, evident on light microscopy, suffice to distinguish airborne pollens of most major plant groups. In some cases, the source of pollen grains may be identified only to the level of an *order* (e.g., Graminales, the grass order) while, rarely, individual species may produce distinctive particles or only a single local source may be implicated. Relationships among anemophilous plants and pollens are best examined beginning with the order level. Each order comprises several related *families*, each composed of (one or more) *genera*, sharing closer similarities. Each *genus* contains one or more *species*, the narrowest classification level with circumscribed structural traits and mating affinities.

Fundamentals of Pollen Structure. Typical wind-borne pollen grains are spherical or ovoid structures (Fig. 11–7), often of a faintly yellow hue. An outermost layer, the *exine*, is notable for its rigidity, resistance to chemical degradation, and capacity to be stained with certain dyes (e.g., basic fuchsin). The exine may show shallow sculpturing (e.g., spines and undulations) or may be essentially smooth. In addition,

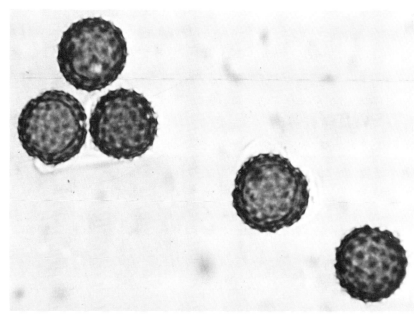

FIGURE 11–7. Photomicrograph of short ragweed pollen stained with fuchsin. Spiny grains, each with three pores, are typical of ragweed and of many additional species of the family Compositae. Several grains show intramural air spaces between the pores.

most pollen types have apertures in the exine that are round ("pores") or elongate ("furrows"). Within the exine is a continuous wall layer, the *intine,* composed largely of cellulose and enclosing the *protoplast,* with its nuclear material and subcellular organelles.

Criteria for pollen identification center largely on grain size and shape (in aqueous mounting media) as well as on ornamentation and apertural characteristics of the exine. However, the overall width of the transparent intine (as in yews, junipers, and their allies) or discrete thickenings in this layer (as in birches) may create distinctive appearances. Even protoplast structures may aid identification, as with the easily observed starch granules of dock and sorrel pollens. Additional features give a distinctive appearance to certain pollen types, such as those airborne as tetrads (e.g., broad-leafed cattail) or larger aggregates *(Mimosa).* Grains of pines, spruces, and firs are noteworthy for their two lateral air-filled bladders, which add to the buoyancy of these large (> 50 microns) particles. Although salient features of major airborne pollens will be noted, the reader is referred to several illustrated references for a systematic approach to identification (Ogden et al., 1974; Kapp, 1969; Hyde and Adams, 1958; Charpin et al, 1975).

Ecology of Airborne Pollen Prevalence

The prevalence of pollen grains depends upon the number produced by each plant, the number of plants, and the efficiency of airborne transport; the effect on the individual reflects also that person's activities as well as the degree of allergy to the pollen.

In general, pollen emission is fostered by relatively warm, dry conditions. Ragweed pollen shedding, for example, falls off sharply or ceases when the temperature is below 10°C or relative humidity is above 70 percent at "anther" level. Requirements for warm, dry air may explain the tendency for most pollens to be released during daylight hours. Ragweed can shed in complete darkness, however, and certain grasses may show peak anthesis at night.

The process of pollen release often is complex, although only a few types (e.g., mulberries) actively expel grains from the anthers. In short ragweed, it is a multistage process in which anther protrusion by individual florets is followed by drying, plication, and ultimate cracking of the anther wall and spillage of moist pollen onto leaf surfaces (Bianchi et al., 1959). The sequence begins before dawn and is abetted by solar warming (and lowered humidity) after sunrise. Deposited grains dry, separate, and become airborne as heat-induced air movement stirs the foliage. Close to source plants, airborne levels are maximal 2 to 3 hours after sunrise, whereas at greater distances, diurnal peaks are delayed, reflecting transport time.

It is difficult to characterize the effects of weather on pollen transport. Rain washes pollen from the air, and particle removal varies principally with the duration rather than intensity of precipitation. This scouring process, however, may be offset by associated air turbulence and impacting raindrops, which refloat particles. Rainfall also is accompanied frequently by atmospheric temperature inversions, which tend to concentrate particles close to the ground.

Brisk winds promote pollen transport, but active atmospheric mixing also carries pollen aloft, thereby diluting levels, to which humans are exposed, near the ground. During evening hours, atmospheric stability often is restored, and particle-bearing air from higher altitudes moves downward toward the surface.

Determining Pollen and Spore Prevalence

"Gravity" Slides and Plates. Atmospheric variables that affect particle prevalence also can modify the behavior of pollen and spores with respect to sampling devices. These effects are most troublesome with traditional "fallout" techniques using greased microslides (Ogden et al., 1974) or open plates of culture medium. Horizontal surfaces will collect particles, and pollen data have been gathered in this way for decades. In practice, an adhesive-coated, 1-in by 3-in glass slide is exposed for 24 hours in a housing of standard design (Durham, 1946). Particles are deposited from turbulent air flow, and, following exposure, are identified microscopically by transmitted light. Data are expressed as "particles per unit area" (usually per cm^2) of slide surface. Viable recoveries have also been studied by substituting plates of nutrient agar in the standard housing (or Durham sampler) for 12- to 60-minute periods. Colonies are identified after incubation of the culture plate for 1 to 7 days.

Sampling by fallout is simple and requires inexpensive, readily available materials. Unfortunately, with gravitational techniques, the volume of air from which particles are recovered cannot be determined, adding uncertainty to comparisons of particle prevalence from different dates or locations. Recoveries by gravity slides (and plates) vary with wind speed, wind direction, and turbulence levels. Furthermore, collections are sparse for all but the most abundant pollens and spores, and larger particles are more likely to accumulate than smaller ones. For these reasons, "gravitational" techniques are useful in identifying prominent pollens "qualitatively" but do not yield reliable "quantitative" pollen concentrations.

Volumetric Samplers. "Volumetric" denotes the ability to relate recoveries to unit volumes of air. Recently, two types of mechanical samplers have been introduced that provide particle data in relation to unit volumes of air (Fig. 11–8). These are (1) impactors, in which an adhesive-coated sampling surface is whirled in a circular path through particle-bearing air, and (2) suction samplers (spore traps), which aspirate air at fixed rates into flow channels with sharp bends. Particles with too much momentum to follow the angular path strike the walls at predictable points where sampling surfaces are positioned. Both types of devices provide quantitative data on the concentration of particles per unit volume of air. Popular impactors include the rotorod sampler, while the drum (Burkard) version of the Hirst spore trap is widely used. Suction devices that provide volume-related recoveries on agar media include several slit samplers and the Andersen sampler. Further information about these devices is available in Ogden et al., 1974; Solomon and Mathews, 1983; and Solomon, 1984.

Use and Abuses of Atmospheric Data

Although it is generally assumed that there is a direct relationship between pollen exposure and allergic symptoms, neither threshold levels nor dose-response effects have been explored. British workers have observed that grass pollen-sensitive patients, with few exceptions, develop symptoms when mean (24 hour, integrated) levels reach 20 grains/m³. Comparable data for ragweed are not available, although a modal value of about 100 grains with considerable intersubject variation in threshold, might be anticipated. In addition, the nasal response appears to be related to recent exposure to other allergens as well as to the intensity of pollen

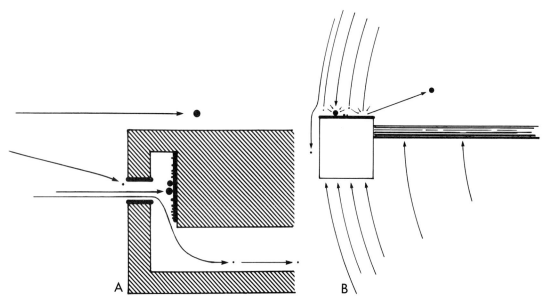

FIGURE 11–8. Collection principles employed by volumetric samplers. *A*, Suction traps (impingers) deposit particles at bends in their internal flow systems. These devices have especially high efficiency for small particles, which readily enter the traps from a moving air stream. *B*, Rotating arm impactors employ rapidly rotated, adhesive-coated, narrow surfaces to intercept particles. The efficiency of impaction varies predictably with increasing particle size. "Bounce-off" can occur, and its frequency defines the "adhesive efficiency" of the collecting surface.

exposure. Previous exposure to sensitizers appears to "prime" the nasal mucosa to react at lower levels of the same or an unrelated pollen allergen (Connell, 1969). For these reasons, the value of "pollen counts" in predicting severity of pollen symptoms is limited, especially when counts are derived from gravity samplers. Further, there are differences between pollen counts done at rooftop level and ground level and from place to place within a community. Optimally performed "background" samples reveal major pollens in the air at a given time, but they will not reflect true personal levels of exposure.

Despite these reservations, aeroallergen data provide, at the least, a qualitative view of exposure for correlation retrospectively with clinical events. Annual dates of pollen and mold appearance and disappearance may be estimated, and peak periods identified. For relatively abundant pollens and larger fungus spores, even gravity slides allow prevalence trends to be identified, although their correlative value is limited.

In areas where ragweed is prevalent, pollen counts based on gravity slide data often are announced by news media to an eager public. Unfortunately, the limitations of these data are mentioned only rarely, and patients often are perplexed by apparent discrepancies between their symptoms and published exposure levels. In general, such reports, describing periods one or more days previously, are no more informative than trends derived from several previous pollen seasons. Moreover, patients often are needlessly distressed by minor day-to-day variation in published data, viewing these as predictors of serious discomfort. Physicians should recognize these misunderstandings about the significance of pollen counts and should try to educate their patients accordingly.

MAJOR POLLEN ALLERGENS AND THEIR SOURCES

Grasses

The grasses (Family Gramineae) are the most successful and widely distributed natural grouping of wind-pollinated plants. Grass pollinosis is recognized on all major land masses and is the principal form of pollen allergy in Great Britain, central Europe, and much of Asia. Symptoms provoked by exposure to (flowering) hay fields long ago prompted the term "hay

fever," which has now been broadened to connote all forms of seasonal allergic rhinitis.

Despite a profusion of grass species, only a limited number shed sufficient pollen to deserve clinical interest. In North America, Bermuda grass (*Cynodon dactylon*), timothy (*Phleum pratense*), and orchard grass (*Dactylis glomerata*) are probably the most copious pollen producers, although over a dozen species play noteworthy secondary roles. Grass pollen grains are subspherical bodies with finely pitted surfaces and single pores (Fig. 11–9). Emanations of most species average 28 to 35 microns; however, some are larger (e.g., rye, 60 microns, and corn, over 100 microns). Typically, pores are closed by a membrane derived from the intine, which bears a single fleck of exine substance (the "operculum").

Several characterizable antigens (groups I, II, and III), described from rye grass (*Lolium perenne*) pollen, have been identified also in certain other temperate zone grass pollens but *not* in that of Bermuda grass, which has its own unique sensitizers. A molecular weight of 27,000 daltons has been estimated for rye grass group I, which constitutes approximately one third of the extractable pollen protein.

The sedges (Cyperaceae), rushes (Juncaceae), and cattails (Typhaceae) are families of grass-like plants that shed wind-borne pollens in moderate amounts. Their allergens appear to differ from those of the grasses, but their clinical impact is not clear.

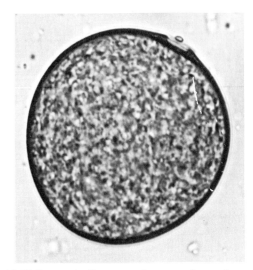

FIGURE 11–9. Pollen grain of a grass. The single pore, with its "operculum" of exine substance, is seen in side view and optical section.

Weeds (Broad-leafed Herbs or "Forbs")

Ragweeds. Members of the ragweed genus *(Ambrosia)* are confined largely to the Western Hemisphere. Within this range, however, they are the most important source of pollinosis, annually affecting over 5 million persons. Of approximately 40 American ragweeds, less than a dozen are substantial local pollen sources, with "common" or "dwarf" ragweed *(A. artemisiifolia)* and giant ragweed *(A. trifida)* the most widely abundant offenders. Ragweed pollinosis in eastern North America involves these species exclusively, except for contributions from southern ragweed *(A. bidentata)* present in Missouri and surrounding states. To the west, perennial ragweed *(A. psilostachya)* and additional species, including perennial slender ragweed *(A. confertiflora)* and annual bur ragweed *(A. acanthocarpa),* are prominent in the Great Plains and Great Basin areas, while canyon ragweed *(A. ambrosioides),* rabbit bush *(A. deltoidea),* and burroweed *(A. dumosa)* are prominent in southwestern deserts. Several of these species previously were classified in the genus *Franseria* (as "false ragweeds"); however, they appear to be valid ambrosias with respect to both form and pollen allergens. Floral development in most ragweeds is stimulated by increasing periods of darkness (longer nights), a response that determines their late summer period of anthesis. Where killing frost ($\sim -3\,^\circ$C at night) occurs, its advent terminates pollen dispersion by ragweeds, although anthesis usually has declined to low levels weeks before. (Several exceptional ragweed species, e.g., burroweed *(A. dumosa)* and rabbit bush *(A. deltoidea),* shed pollen during late spring in arid portions of the southwest and may elicit symptoms at that time.)

Although some ragweeds are confined to remote areas, the more familiar species (e.g., short ragweed) are truly "weedy," serving as prominent pests of cultivated sites. Despite their success, the persistence of these types requires disturbance of competing perennial species, and ragweeds can be crowded out over several years by grasses and perennial herbs. Ragweeds readily utilize soils "disturbed" by flowing water, cultivation, and winter salting of roads, and, in Michigan, peak (short) ragweed abundance has been identified with cultivated grain fields (Fig. 11–10). Ragweeds obtain competitive advantages also by their rapid seedling growth in spring and by seed longevity, which may exceed 60 years.

Pollen grains of common ragweed species are relatively small (18 to 23 microns) and are covered with short conical spines. Typically, three equally spaced pores are discernible, lying in a single (equatorial) plane. Between the pores, the outer wall layers separate to form shallow air spaces, which increase buoyancy and give a mildly trilobate outline to the grains.

Of several defined ragweed allergens, principal interest has centered on antigen E, a two-chain, linear protein of 37,800 daltons mol wt that appears to carry over 90 percent of the allergenic potency of whole pollen eluate. Yet, antigen E constitutes less than 0.5 percent of the solid and less than 6 percent of the protein extractable from short ragweed pollen. Trace amounts of antigen E may be detectable in vegetative organs of short ragweed (e.g., stems and leaves); however, this material is confined essentially to pollen, where it appears to function as a recognition factor during pollination. Other described allergens include antigens K (38,200 daltons), Ra3 (ca 15,000 daltons), and Ra5 (ca 5000 daltons), all of which appear to sensitize fewer persons than antigen E; additional components probably remain to be identified.

Ragweeds are members of the large composite family (Compositae), characterized by many small specialized flowers ("florets") borne in tight aggregates. While few of the composites are anemophilous, many species have pollens that resemble those of ragweeds morphologi-

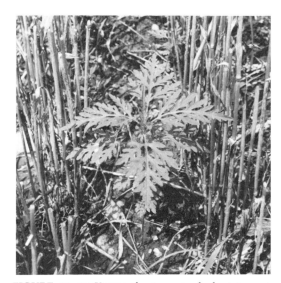

FIGURE 11–10. Young short ragweed plant in grain stubble of a Michigan oatfield. In many areas, agricultural disturbance makes cultivated fields dominant sources of ragweeds and their pollens.

cally and may cross-react antigenically, although human exposure to them may be sporadic. Such cross-reactivity seems to depend on components besides antigen E in most cases (Yunginger and Gleich, 1972). Clinically prominent ragweed relatives include the wind-pollinated marsh elders (*Iva*), especially burweed marsh elder or "prairie ragweed" (*I. xanthifolia*) and rough marsh elder (*I. ciliata*) of the south-central and Gulf states. Additional *Iva* species —including poverty weed (*I. axillaris*) of the far West and *I. frutescens* of eastern salt marshes— appear to shed relatively little pollen. A similar verdict seems justified in the case of the abundant cockleburs (*Xanthium* species), in which doubt is cast on the importance traditionally assigned to these plants as allergen sources.

The sages, sagebrushes, wormwoods, and mugworts of the genus *Artemisia* constitute a second group of clinically important, anemophilous plants within the Compositae. Although herbs of this group are widespread, substantial pollen levels are confined to western regions, where common sagebrush (*A. tridentata*) and sand sagebrush (*A. filifolia*) are abundant, and to the Pacific coast, the range of *A. californica*. Additional local sources are present especially about the upper Great Lakes and in Tennessee and bordering states. However, the overall importance of artemisias as allergen sources east of the Great Plains seems minor. Although pollens of sages and ragweeds appear to share certain allergens, this similarity apparently is not based on antigen E.

In many areas, small amounts of pollen derived from insect-pollinated composites become airborne. Suspected sources of these particles include asters, sneezeweeds (*Helenium*) and goldenrods (*Solidago* species) as well as dandelions and their allies. While the impact of their pollens usually is negligible, close respiratory contact with native composites or with cultivated types, including sunflowers, chrysanthemums, dahlias, and marigolds can precipitate symptoms in certain ragweed-sensitive persons. This potential is rarely evident, but probably has contributed to the enduring myth that links late summer hay fever and goldenrods. Antigen E seems absent from cantaloupe, banana, and watermelon, although these foods clearly provoke pharyngeal pruritus or rhinitis or both in certain ragweed-sensitive subjects.

Chenopodiales. The goosefoot and amaranth families (Chenopodiaceae and Amaranthaceae, respectively,) represent the order Chenopodiales and include many anemophilous types that are thought to share (certain)

pollen allergens (Weber and Nelson, 1985). Differences in pollen productivity are marked within both families. Russian thistle (*Salsola kali* var. *pestifer*) and burning bush (*Kochia scoparia*) shed copiously over much of central and western North America, while western water hemp (*Acnida tamariscina*) and Palmer's amaranth are prominent in the south central states. In the far west, several "scales" (*Atriplex* species), greasewoods, and carelessweeds contribute pollen of this type, and sugar beet (*Beta vulgaris*) may serve as an allergen source—especially where it is grown for seed. However, pollen shedding by many widely evident species including lamb's quarters (*Chenopodium album*) and redroot pigweed (*Amaranthus retroflexus*) appears limited.

Goosefoot and amaranth pollens feature spherical grains with pitted surfaces and many precisely spaced circular pores (Fig. 11–11). Although grain sizes, pore numbers, and interpore distances can distinguish some types, most observers are content to record a "chenopod-amaranth" category, relying upon field observations to implicate specific source species.

Plantains. Of the several plantains (*Plantago* species) established in North America, only one—narrow-leafed or buckhorn plantain (*P. lanceolata*)—commonly known as "English plantain" sheds sufficient pollen to warrant serious clinical attention. The species is a familiar, perennial, rosetting weed of lawns with elongate leaves and conical flower clusters on long central stalks. Plantain grains superficially resemble those of the chenopod-amaranth group but have substantially fewer (usually five to eight) scattered pores—each with an opercu-

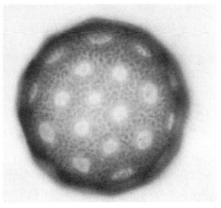

FIGURE 11–11. Pollen grain of lamb's quarters. The "golf-ball" appearance, due to numerous regularly spaced pores, is typical of the goosefoot and amaranth families (Chenopodiaceae and Amaranthaceae, respectively).

lum. Pollen shedding by plantains often extends over several months without a well-defined peak. Rates of skin reactivity to plantain pollen are high in many temperate regions, and frank pollinosis has been ascribed to this factor in the Pacific Northwest. However, the relatively low levels prevailing elsewhere suggest that the overall clinical importance of the plantains probably is low.

Sorrels and Docks. Pollens of these wind-pollinated members of the knotweed family (Polygonaceae) are allergenically distinct and appear during late spring in temperate regions. In North America, red or sheep sorrel (*Rumex acetosella*) is the principal source, and pollen shedding accompanies or precedes anthesis of the early grasses. Although other *Rumex* species are robust and familiar weeds, their pollen output is relatively low. Pollen grains typical of the genus show three or four slit-like furrows, each with a central pore, and a protoplast packed with starch granules.

Nettles. Increasing use of high efficiency impactors and spore traps has demonstrated abundant airborne nettle (*Urtica* species) pollen at sites in North America and Great Britain. Typical grains are subspheroidal with three collared pores and are small enough (12 to 17 microns) to appear rarely in gravity slide collections. In North America *U. dioica* var. *procera* appears to be the main source species. However, the classification of the nettles is controversial. Nettle pollen is shed in mid- and late summer, with peak levels just preceding the ragweed pollinosis season.

Trees

Single species of anemophilous trees commonly shed pollen briefly in a given locality. However, the "seasons" of anthesis for several types often are concurrent or overlap broadly, imposing intense exposures that involve numerous unrelated pollen allergens. This complexity often obscures specific sensitivities and can present a serious barrier to the success of immunotherapy. In temperate regions, wind-pollinated trees are the rule, and source types represent the conifers (Class Gymnospermae) as well as numerous families of more conventional flowering plants (i.e., Class Angiospermae). (The class is a taxonomic level that includes one or more orders and, in turn, is one component of a division. In this case, the divi-

sion of flower plants, Spermatophyta, comprises the classes Gymnospermae and Angiospermae.)

Conifers (Class Gymnospermae). Conifers and their allies dominate the extensive boreal forests of Canada and the contiguous states as well as the southern "pinelands," Appalachian summits and slopes of the Cascades and Rockies. Much of the huge pollen output by this group affects remote areas only.

Pollens of the pines (*Pinus*), spruces (*Picea*), and firs (*Abies*) as well as the true cedars (*Cedrus*) planted in southern states, the mountain hemlock (*Tsuga mertensiana*) and golden larch (*Pseudolarix amabilis*) of western mountains are large grains bearing two air bladders. The clinical importance of these abundant pollens generally is unproved. However, instances of pollinosis and strong skin sensitivity to them clearly do exist.

A second type of conifer grain — spherical, lacking bladders, and showing both a thick intine and a thin exine (which may be shed at anthesis) — is often encountered. Pollens of the cypress-juniper family (Cupressaceae), the yew family (Taxaceae), and sequoia–bald cypress family (Taxodiaceae) share this form, and similar grains of larger size are shed by larches (*Larix*) and Douglas fir (*Pseudotsuga menziesii*). This group includes acknowledged sensitizers, with the mountain cedars, especially *Juniperus ashei* (previously designated *Juniperus sabinoides*) serving as major factors in pollinosis. These compact evergreen trees are found from the hills of west Texas and lower elevations of central Mexico northward; they shed pollen copiously from late December to February.

Pollens of additional junipers (and of related *Cupressus* species) also deserve clinical attention. Suggested allergenic similarities among species of both genera, including the eastern red cedar (*Juniperus virginiana*), extend also to the incense cedar (*Calocedrus decurrens*) and Port Orford cedar also known as western red cedar (*Chamaecyparis lawsoniana*) of the Pacific Northwest; pollens of cultivated yews (*Taxus media* varieties) may share this activity.

Pollen of the bald cypress has uncertain allergenic activity, and much of it is shed in sparsely settled wetlands. However, a related member of the Taxodiaceae, the sugi cedar (*Cryptomeria japonica*), is an important cause of pollinosis in Japan.

Palm Family (Arecaceae). Members of this large group, including economically important species, generally are restricted to frost-free regions. Many species are anemophilous, and pollen shedding by sabal (*Sabal spp.**), date (*Phoenix dactylifera*), coconut (*Cocos nucifera*), and queen (*C. plumosa*) palms can produce moderate atmospheric contamination. The date palm has been a suspected minor and highly local source of pollinosis in southern California and Hawaii, but other palms have not been definitely implicated.

Australian Pine or Beefwood Family (Casuarinaceae). Clinical interest in this group of Australasian trees has followed introduction of a single species, *Casuarina equisetifolia* in highly populated subtropical areas. The plant is tolerant of dry, sandy soils and highly wind-resistant, whether as a tall triangular tree or sheared as a hedge. A "pine-like" aspect is imparted by reduction of leaves to minute scales that are clustered along innumerable short, slender branchlets. Flowering by this species is uniquely prolonged and sporadic, extending over several months in Florida. The 30- to 35-micron pollen grains have three-collared pores and recall those of the bayberry and the birch family. Pollen emission may be copious, and pollinosis seems definitely to result.

Willow-Poplar Family (Salicaceae). The numerous North American members of this family represent only two genera, as follows: (1) the willows (*Salix spp.*) and (2) poplars and aspens (*Populus spp.*). Many of the willows rely on insect pollination as well as wind pollination, and in a given area, sequential shedding by several species creates prolonged "seasons" of low intensity. The prevalence (if any) of willow pollinosis is problematic, although skin sensitivity is easily demonstrated.

Separate male and female trees are characteristic of both *Salix* spp. and *Populus* spp.; however, the poplars and aspens are exclusively anemophilous. In northern states, the quaking (*P. tremuloides*) and big-toothed (*P. grandidentata*) aspens are among the earliest trees to flower; although their pollen output is moderate, most is shed in rural areas. In the eastern states and Great Plains, most poplar pollen probably is derived from eastern cottonwood (*P. deltoides*). Additional regional sources include the California cottonwood (*P. fremontii*), the black cottonwood (*P. trichocarpa*) of the Northwest, and the swamp cottonwood of southern river bottoms. Female cottonwoods (and some willows) release wind-borne seeds

bearing tufted hairs in early summer. At times, this "cotton" has been indicted falsely as the cause of coexisting hay fever (generally grass pollinosis).

Pollen grains of the willows are relatively small with reticulate surfaces and prominent furrows, whereas those of the poplars are larger, lack apertures, and show a distinctive fragmentation of the thin exine. Despite their family ties, pollen allergens of the willows and poplars also appear to differ.

Walnut-Hickory Family (Juglandaceae). Pollens of the hickories (*Carya spp.*) and walnuts (*Juglans spp.*) are relatively potent sensitizers, exhibiting allergenic differences between and within genera. *Carya* species are large trees of eastern and southern states and include the pecans (*C. texana* and *C. illinoensis*), which are cultivated both for the edible nuts and as street trees in warmer regions. Pollen shedding by pecans occurs in March and April. Late spring pollination is typical of the cold-tolerant hickories (e.g., *C. laciniosa*, *C. ovalis*, and *C. glabra*). Walnuts, including the black walnut (*J. nigra*), butternut (*J. cinerea*), and California walnut (*J. californica*), also are typically late flowering spring trees. The 40- to 50-micron, three-pored hickory grains are among the largest wind-borne pollen types; those of walnuts are smaller, flattened spheres with numerous pores restricted to half of each grain's surface.

Birch Family (Betulaceae). In North America, this family includes major pollen producers such as hazelnuts (*Corylus spp.*), birches (*Betula spp.*), and alders (*Alnus spp.*) as well as hornbeams or ironwoods (*Carpinus caroliniana* and *Ostrya virginiana*), with lesser outputs. Hazelnuts and filberts, including cultivated forms, flower from January to April depending on latitude. The alders, including the naturalized European, (*A. glutinosa*), follow and, although widely established in moist locations, are associated with pollinosis mainly in the Pacific Northwest. Several native birches, including the paper birch (*B. papyrifera*) and cherry birch (*B. lenta*) are prominent in eastern states, and paper birch grows widely in western mountains as well. In many areas, varieties of the European white birch (*B. pendula*), used extensively in ornamental plantings, may serve as factors in pollinosis.

Except for the characteristic four- or five-pored grains of alders, pollens of the Betulaceae typically show three, collared pores. *B. pendula* is considered the principal source of hay fever in Scandinavia, and a heat-stable major aller-

---

* *Spp.* = species.

gen (ca 20,000 daltons mol wt) has been isolated from its pollen. A related pollen allergen reported for *Alnus glutinosa,* may indicate similarities within the Betulaceae; however, intergeneric relationships remain speculative.

Oak Family (Fagaceae). Although this family also includes the beeches *(Fagus spp.)* and remaining chestnuts *(Castanea spp.),* their pollen output is, at best, modest, leaving the true oaks *(Quercus spp.)* as the proper focus of clinical attention. Red oak *(Q. rubra)* and eastern white oak *(Q. alba)* are especially prominent in the northeast, while *Q. gambelii* is a scrubby dominant in the southwest, and *Q. garryana* is a notable oak pollen source of the Pacific Northwest. Oaks are widely planted, with pin oak *(Q. palustris)* favored in northern states; to the south the evergreen live oak *(Q. virginiana)* and partially evergreen laurel oak *(Q. laurifolia)* are favored by urban landscapers. Oaks often begin to shed pollen in the Gulf States by February, but pollination is not complete in some northern areas before early June. Rough-surfaced grains with three torn furrows are common to all of the oaks, and attempts to determine their species or groups of origin by light microscopy are not recommended. The degree of cross antigenicity among oak pollens has not been determined.

Elm Family (Ulmaceae). Although the American elm *(Ulmus americana)* has been decimated by fungus infections, trees surviving in urban "islands" still produce pollinosis. In addition, more blight-resistant species—including the slippery elm *(U. fulva),* the red *(U. serotina)* and scrub *(U. crassifolia)* elms of south central states, as well as the Chinese elm *(U. parvifolia)*—are regionally significant pollen sources. Grains of all elms have a finely undulating surface (much like a peanut) and five pores in one (equatorial) plane, imparting a somewhat pentagonal outline. In northern and eastern states, elms typically reach anthesis in early spring. However, the red (or "September") and scrub (or "cedar") elms flower in late summer, when *some* Chinese elms also shed pollen.

The hackberries *(Celtis spp.)* are unique within the Ulmaceae, shedding delicate-appearing, three-pored grains. In North America, *C. occidentalis* is common locally in the east and *C. laevigata* abundant in southern and south-central states. Pollen shedding by the last-mentioned species occurs in February and March and is an acknowledged cause of pollinosis.

Pollen of a related species, *C. tala,* has been implicated as a clinical allergen in Argentina.

Ash-Olive Family (Oleaceae). In North America, clinical interest in this large family is focused largely on the ashes *(Fraxinus spp.).* Among these, the white or American ash *(F. americana),* Oregon ash *(F. oregona),* and Arizona ash *(F. velutina)* are regionally important in pollinosis. Additional species and cultivated varieties contribute to local pollen loads; all produce four-furrowed reticulate grains of angular outline.

The olive *(Olea europaea)* often dominates ornamental and sidewalk plantings in warmer western states. Despite substantial insect pollination, wind-borne olive pollen may be abundant locally; clinical allergy results, especially in Arizona and southern California. The olive also is regarded as a major allergenic factor in the Mediterranean basin.

Sycamore or Plane Tree Family (Platanaceae). Although the native sycamore *(Platanus occidentalis)* is locally prominent in eastern river bottom floras, most exposure to sycamore pollen is related to urban plantings of the English plane tree *(P. acerifolia)* and its hybrids. This imported sycamore has been a replacement for the vanishing elms in cities such as Philadelphia, New York, and Washington. In addition, the related *P. orientalis* is a modest pollen source at points of introduction in California. All species shed small reticulate grains with flecks of exine substance on the three, wide furrow membranes. In eastern states, sycamore pollen is airborne in April and May (concurrently with many additional types), making assessment of its clinical impact difficult; skin sensitivity is easily demonstrated, however.

Maple Family (Aceraceae). Maples *(Acer spp.)* are widely prominent in North America and vary from almost exclusive insect pollination, as in the widely planted Norway maple *(A. platanoides)* to the total wind pollination of box elder *(A. negundo).* Between these extremes are familiar species, such as red maple *(A. rubrum)* and sugar maple *(A. saccharum)* of northern and eastern regions and broad-leafed maple *(A. macrophyllum)* of the Pacific coast, with uncertain clinical significance. In many areas, the flowering of staminate box elders defines the local period of maple pollen prevalence. This species is abundant in the Midwest, where it is an aggressive urban weed; in the West, it is often planted for shade or as a windbreak. Pollen grains of maples have three furrows and, at high magnification, display delicate surface striations. Although most are easily identified (to genus), those of box elders are relatively small (ca 25 to 32 microns) and short-furrowed, strongly resembling the pollens of oaks. Box elder anthesis occurs in April and causes substantial pollinosis. Additional species flower sequentially from March to mid-May; allergenic relationships remain to be studied.

Mulberry Family. This family, the Moraceae, includes several genera of variably important anemophilous trees, as follows: the mulberries *(Morus spp.)*, the paper mulberry *(Broussonetia papyrifera)*, and Osage orange *(Maclura pomerifera)*. Pollens of the true and paper mulberries are highly sensitizing and copiously produced. Furthermore, these two- and three-pored grains are quite small (generally 14 to 20 microns) and have been substantially underestimated in gravity slide samples. *M. rubra* is native to eastern North America, whereas white *(M. alba)* and paper mulberries are naturalized in warmer regions. *Morus alba* currently enjoys special favor as a residential and street tree in the arid Southwest.

Osage orange is a spiny small tree of the South-central states, attaining special abundance in Oklahoma where it is also cultivated as a hedge. The small, three-pored grains may be a source of brief symptoms in skin-reactive persons.

Two herbaceous species, hemp *(Cannabis sativa)* and cultivated hops *(Humulus japonica)*, also are generally treated with the Moraceae. Their delicate, three-pored pollens are essentially indistinguishable and both species shed in midsummer. However, hops cultivation is restricted largely to the Pacific Northwest, whereas the natural range of *Cannabis* is western Iowa and adjacent states. Separate male and female plants are a feature of the last-mentioned species, which is now sparsely established in many areas. The celebrated psychotropic components of *Cannabis* are obtained from the female flower clusters and appear to be unassociated with its pollen.

Myrtle Family (Myrtaceae). This largely tropical group includes many insect-pollinated trees, which also "spill" pollen into the atmosphere. In California, large plantings of gum trees *(Eucalyptus spp.)* can create notable levels locally with uncertain effects. The bottle-brush or "punk" tree *(Melaleuca spp.)* has been planted widely in Florida; however, little airborne pollen has resulted.

POLLEN DISTRIBUTION IN NORTH AMERICA

Table 11–2 summarizes the distribution and seasonal prevalence of wind-borne pollens in portions of North America with distinctive climate and flora. Ten regions, defined for this purpose, are shown in Fig. 11–12. Although sharp boundaries have been drawn, in most cases these "life zones" intermingle over broad transition areas, so that border sites share characteristics of the adjacent ecologic areas. Furthermore, individual regions are not uniform in pollen prevalence; however, they provide workable alternatives to more minute, or more inclusive, divisions.

A summary of pollen surveys organized by states has been presented by Chang (1980). An earlier review by Samter and Durham (1955), which includes Mexico and parts of the Caribbean, also may be helpful. The annual Statistical Report of the American Academy of Allergy's Committee on Pollen and Mold may be consulted for additional, regionally based, aeroallergen prevalence data.*

Table 11–2 necessarily is incomplete, since substantial gaps remain in our knowledge of pollen sources and distribution, and many established data must be updated. In most areas, questions of current allergen prevalence can be answered precisely only by a program of local atmospheric sampling. For brevity, many pollens are listed as "types" without indicating their (frequently multiple) source species.

INTERNATIONAL POLLEN EXPOSURE RISKS

Many North Americans experience decreased symptoms of respiratory allergy during travel abroad. This improvement commonly reflects the absence of ragweed pollen and the lower levels of dark-spored imperfect fungi in other regions; for certain individuals, differences in dust and animal allergen exposures also contribute. However, aerometric data from many areas are too scanty to allow more than suggestions of allergen exposure patterns globally.

Grasses are the most generally distributed

---

* Current copies may be obtained from the Executive Office, 411 Wells Street, Milwaukee, Wisconsin 53202.

TABLE 11–2. Pollen Distribution in the United States

Trees		Grasses	Weeds	
		NORTHERN FOREST		
A brief hectic growing season is typical, with copious shedding of pine, spruce, fir, hemlock, and arbor vitae *(Thuja occidentalis)* pollens from May to early July. In the same period, pollens of alders, birches, hazelnuts, poplars, and aspens may contribute to pollinosis where the forest climax has been disturbed.		Summer levels of grass pollen are relatively low and often insignificant.	With few late summer pollen sources, these areas have been traditional refuges for ragweed-sensitive persons.	
		EASTERN AGRICULTURAL		
Red cedar	Feb.–April	Sharply defined mid-May to mid-July grass pollen season in north; to the south, a longer season with earlier onset typical.	Sheep (red) sorrel	May–June
Hazelnut	Feb.–April		Plantain	May–Oct.
Elm	March–April		Nettles	July–Sept.
Alder	March–May	Importance of various species is difficult to determine; however, acknowledged sources include the following:	Hemp	July–Sept. (NW)
Maples	March–May		Western water hemp	July–Sept. (W)
Poplar, aspen	March–May		Russian thistle	July–Sept. (W)
Birch	March–May	Blue grasses *(Poa spp.)*	Kochia	July–Sept.
Ash	March–May	Orchard grass *(Dactylis glomerata)*	Pigweeds, amaranths	July–Sept.
Paper mulberry	March–May (S)*	Timothy *(Phleum pratense)*	Sages, mugworts	July–Oct. (L)
Willow	March–July	Red top *(Agrostis alba)*	Short ragweed	Aug.–Oct.
Box elder	April–May (W)	In eastern region, increase in Perennial rye	Giant ragweed	Aug.–Oct.
Beech		*(Lolium perenne)* and Sweet vernal grass *(Anthoxanthum odoratum)*	Southern ragweed	Aug.–Oct. (SW)
(Fagus grandifolia)	April–May (N)		Perennial ragweed	Aug.–Oct. (W)
Sycamore	April–May	In southern region, allergenically distinctive	Burweed marsh elder	Aug.–Oct. (S)
Hackberry	April–May	Bermuda grass *(Cynodon dactylon)* is dominant.	Rough marsh elder	Aug.–Oct. (S,W)
Oak	April–June			
Mulberry	April–June			
Walnut	April–June			
Hickory	April–June			

Pollens of dogwoods *(Cornus)*, sweet gum *(Liquidambar styraciflua)*, and black cherry *(Prunus serotina)* prominent locally but significance uncertain.

Shrubby species including bayberry *(Myrica carolinensis)* and sweet fern *(M. asplenifolia)* are sources in certain sandy eastern areas but not evaluated clinically.

Trees		Grasses	Weeds	
		SOUTHEASTERN COASTAL PLAIN		
Pecan, hickory	March–May (S)	Except for northeastern extremity, zone is dominated by Bermuda grass, which sheds most abundantly from March to September; lesser contributions come from species prominent in the Eastern Agricultural zone.	Sheep (red) sorrel	April–June
Sweet gum	March–May		Plantain	May–Oct.
Maples	March–May		Nettle	July–Sept.
Sycamore	March–June		Sagewort, mugwort	July–Sept. (L)
Mulberry	March–June		Western water hemp	July–Sept. (W)
Oak	March–May	More typically southern grasses, including Johnson grass *(Holcus halepensis)* and Sudan grass *(Holcus sudanensis)*, add small amounts of wind-borne pollen.	Russian thistle	July–Sept. (NW)
Walnut	April–May		Pigweeds, amaranths	July–Sept.
Red cedar	Jan.–April		Kochia	July–Oct.
Hackberry	Jan.–May		Short ragweed	Aug.–Oct.
Elm	Feb.–April		Giant ragweed	Aug.–Oct.
Willow	Feb.–May		Southern ragweed	Aug.–Oct. (W)
Poplar	March–April		Rough marsh elder	Aug.–Oct. (W)
Ash	March–May		Burweed marsh elder	Aug.–Oct. (W)
Birch	March–May			

Other, locally abundant tree pollens include those of beech, paper mulberry, alders, bald cypress *(Taxodium distichum)*, hornbeams *(Carpinus caroliniana* and *Ostrya virginiana)*, and in northern Florida types characteristic of the Florida Subtropical zone.

Pollen shedding by pines also is prominent in spring throughout much of region.

* Where a pollen type is confined largely to one portion of a region, this is indicated by the following notations: N = north; S = south; E = east; W = west; or L = local.

TABLE 11–2. Pollen Distribution in the United States (Continued)

Trees		Grasses	Weeds

FLORIDA SUBTROPICAL

Bald cypress	Jan.–March	Grass pollen is airborne throughout the year in subtropical Florida, derived largely from Bermuda grass. Other suspected sources include Johnson grass and Bahia grass (*Paspalum notatum*).	Locally variable levels of short ragweed pollen occur from July–Sept., and Baccharis (*Baccharis spp.*) contribute an apparently related type in coastal areas.
Oak	Jan.–April		
Palm	Jan.–Dec.		Pollens of chenopods and diverse amaranths are present almost perennially, peaking in late summer.
Australian pine	Oct.–April		

Additional tree pollens of variable and local occurrence include those of red maple (*Acer rubrum*), citrus (*Citrus sinensis*), pepper tree (*Schinus molle*), punk tree (*Melaleuca spp.*), and *Eucalyptus spp.*

A massive background of pine pollen (especially Jan.–April) cannot be completely ignored.

CENTRAL PLAINS

Mountain cedar	Dec.–March (SW)	Although originally this area was the province of long and short grass prairies, contemporary grass pollen levels are no greater than those of other areas.	Sheep (red) sorrel	May–July
Elm	Jan.–April		*Atriplex spp.*	June–Aug. (W)
	Aug.–Sept. (S)		Hemp	July–Sept. (NE)
Ash	Jan.–May	To the north, the June–July peak and the source species are those of the Eastern Agricultural zone; to the south, a prolonged season is dominated by Bermuda grass.	Russian thistle	July–Sept.
Oak	Jan.–May		Kochia	July–Sept.
Poplar	Feb.–April		Greasewood	July–Sept. (W)
Box elder	Feb.–April		Smotherweed (*Bassia*)	July–Sept. (NW)
Willow	Feb.–May	Additional sources of lesser importance include smooth brome (*Bromus inermis*), fescue (*Festuca elatior*), *Koeleria eristata*, and Johnson grass.	Burweed marsh elder	July–Sept.
Hackberry	Feb.–May (S)		Rough marsh elder	July–Oct. (S)
Sycamore	March–May		Sagebrush, sages	July–Oct.
Walnut	March–May		Western water hemp	July–Oct.
Hickory, pecan	March–May		Short ragweed	Aug.–Oct.
Mulberry	March–May		Giant ragweed	Aug.–Oct.
Osage orange	April–May (SE)		Western ragweed	Aug.–Oct.
			Bur ragweeds	Aug.–Oct.

Especially in western extremity of zone, a variety of additional chenopods and amaranths add small quantities of windborne pollens.

ROCKY MOUNTAIN

Mountain cedar, junipers	Jan.–March (SE)	Grass pollen levels generally decrease with elevation and are present from May to July.	Pollens of ragweeds and related herbs, chenopods, and amaranths diminish sharply above 5000-ft altitude.
Elm	Feb.–April		
Alder	March–April	Major source species are those of adjacent Central Plains region; *Poa sandbergii* also has been implicated.	At lower elevations, sources are similar to those of adjacent Central Plains, Great Basin, or Arid Southwestern zones.
Ash	March–May		
Willow	March–June		
Poplar, aspen	April–May		
Birch	April–June		
Oak	May–June (S)		

Although clinical significance unproved, bulk of tree pollen is produced by vast forests of conifers, including pines, spruces, mountain hemlock, Douglas fir, and sequoias.

ARID SOUTHWESTERN

Mountain cedar	Dec.–March (E)	Grass pollen is airborne in all warm months and is derived predominantly from Bermuda grass; some contributions from other species of southern Central Plains regions.	Burroweed (*Ambrosia dumosa*)	Feb.–June
Elm	Feb.–March		Sagebrush, sages	Feb.–May
	Aug.–Oct.		Rabbit bush (*Ambrosia deltoides*)	March–May
Arizona cypress	Feb.–March (W)			
Ash	Feb.–April	Salt grass (*Distichlis spicata*) and Canary grass (*Phalaris minor*) may shed sufficiently to warrant some attention.	Shadscale	May–Aug.
Poplar	Feb.–April		Greasewood	May–Sept.
Mulberry	Feb.–April		Burweed marsh elder	July–Sept.
Mesquite	Feb.–June		Kochia	July–Oct.
Olive	March–May		Sugar beet	July–Oct. (L)
			Short ragweed	July–Oct.
			Slender ragweed	July–Oct.

In irrigated areas, moderate numbers of sycamores, oaks, eucalyptus, pecans, and acacias may be locally important sources.

Table continued on following page

TABLE 11-2. Pollen Distribution in the United States *(Continued)*

Trees		Grasses	Weeds	

Arid Southwestern *(Continued)*

Trees		Grasses	Weeds	
Additional shrubby types include Creosote bush Palo verde *(Cercidium spp.)* Castor bean *(Ricinus communis)* Tamarisk *(Tamarix spp.)*			Several additional ragweeds as well as representatives of composite genera including *Dicorea, Hymenoclea,* and *Chrysothamnus* shed "ragweed-like" pollen in spring and fall. Pollens of chenopods and amaranths are airborne in most months; derived from drought- and alkali-resistant types (many known locally as "scales" and "creosote bushes"), including species of *Atriplex* (especially *A. canescens* and *A. polycarpas, Eurotina Snoeda,* and *Amaranthus,* as well as iodine bush *(Allenrolfia occidentalis).*	

Great Basin

Trees		Grasses	Weeds	
Juniper	Feb.–May	Although the overall levels of grass pollen appear relatively low, its sources are varied. To the north, the grasses are largely those of the Central Plains; in the southern section, species of the Arid Southwestern zone predominate.	Sagebrush, sages	June–Nov.
Elm	March–April		Russian thistle	July–Sept.
Poplar	March–April		Kochia	July–Oct.
Willow	March–May		Greasewood	July–Oct.
Sycamore	April–May		Short ragweed	Aug.–Oct.
Box elder	April–May		Bur ragweeds	Aug.–Oct.
			Poverty weed	Aug.–Nov.
At modest elevations, birches, alders, aspens, and oaks contribute additional tree pollens.			*(Iva axillaris)*	
			Many anemophilous chenopods and amaranths, native to the Arid Southwestern region, are also prominent in Great Basin, although source strengths are conjectural.	

California Lowlands

Trees		Grasses	Weeds	
Mulberry	Jan.–April	In much of region, airborne grass pollen, largely from Bermuda grass, is present from early March to November; in extreme north of zone, season is shorter, beginning in April or May.	Nettle	May–Aug. (N,W)
Alder	Jan.–April		Bur ragweeds	June–Sept. (S,W)
Ash	Jan.–April		Western ragweed	July–Oct.
Willow	Jan.–May		Sagebrush, sages	July–Oct.
Walnut	Jan.–May			
Poplar	Feb.–April	Many other species are implicated including rye grasses *(Lolium ssp.),* the brome grasses *(Bromus spp.),* wild oats *(Avena fatua),* and types present in zones to the east.	Wind-borne pollens of chenopods and amaranths are moderately abundant in summer and fall; major sources include Russian thistle, *Atriplex spp., Bassia hyssopifolia;* also *Amaranthus retroflexus* and *A. palmeri.*	
Elm	Feb.–April			
	Aug.–Oct.			
Oak	Feb.–May			
Sycamore	Feb.–April			
Birch	Feb.–May			
Olive	March–May (S)			
Many additional tree species contribute limited quantities of wind-borne pollen, including acacias, coast maple *(Acer macrophyllum),* box elder *(Acer negundo), Eucalyptus spp.,* and pecan.				

Northwest Coastal

Trees		Grasses	Weeds	
Hazelnut	Jan.–March	Ample grass pollens are present from May to August. Major source species appear to be similar to Eastern Agricultural zone; also being investigated are sweet vernal grass *(Anthoxanthum odoratum)* and velvet grass *(Holcus lanatus).*	Plantain	May–Sept.
Alders	Feb.–April		Sheep (red) sorrel	June–Aug.
Willow	Feb.–April		Poverty weed	June–Aug. (L)
Ash	Feb.–April		Nettle	July–Aug.
Box elder	March–April		Russian thistle	July–Sept.
Birch	March–May		Sagebrush, sages	July–Sept. (L)
Poplar, Aspen	March–June		Short ragweed	Aug.–Sept. (L)
Elm	March–June	Species including the rye grasses and tall oatgrass *(Arrhenatherum elatius)* may shed clinically significant pollen.		
Coast maple	April–June		Although all these contribute allergenic pollen, resulting concentrations are relatively low; more significantly, much of region remains essentially ragweed-free.	
Oak	April–June			
Walnut	April–June (L)			
Tree pollen levels vary widely according to local topography and, especially, altitude. In forested portions, conifer pollens of several types are abundant.			Levels of plantain and sorrel pollens may be higher than in northeastern states, but conclusive comparative data have not been gathered.	

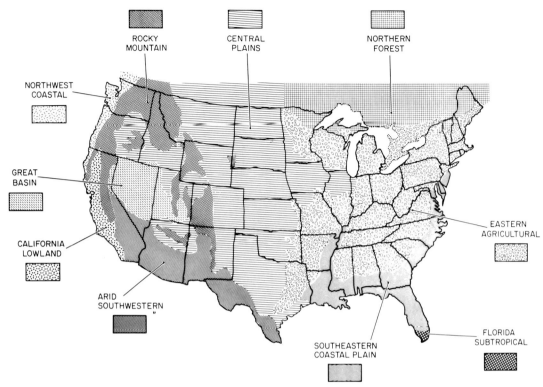

FIGURE 11–12. Floristic zones of North America. (Reproduced by permission from Solomon, W. R., Aerobiology and inhalant allergens. I. Pollens and fungi. In Middleton E., Jr., Reed, C. E., and Ellis, E. F. (eds). Allergy: Principles and Practice, 2nd ed. St. Louis, C. V. Mosby Co., 1983.)

sources of pollinosis, although groups of temperate and tropical species appear to differ allergenically. However, cosmopolitan types, such as Bermuda grass, are encountered widely in both hemispheres, and many taxa (e.g., *Phleum pratense* and *Dactylis glomerata*) are common to Europe and much of eastern North America.

Significant tree pollinosis may be reawakened in some travelers to Scandinavia by the abundant birch pollen present in spring, or, further south, by the pollen of native ashes, oaks, mulberries, walnuts, and elms. Olive pollen is a significant factor in the Mediterranean basin as well as in our own Southwest.

Insect pollination is present almost exclusively among tropical trees, although some (e.g., certain palms and mesquite) may produce endemic pollinosis. Whether recognized similarities between the temperate floras of eastern Asia and eastern North America also are relevant clinically is uncertain. However, local representatives of genera such as *Fraxinus* and *Celtis* are recognized sources of tree pollinosis in Mexico and South America. In addition, the sugi cedar of Japan is a locally well-recognized

sensitizer, and other coniferous species may be shown to have at least regional importance, in this regard.

Ragweed pollinosis is a familiar clinical problem as far south as central Mexico. However, ragweeds of several species also are variably distributed throughout lowland areas of Central and South America as well as many Caribbean islands, where their clinical impact seems small. In addition, short ragweed (*Ambrosia artemisiifolia*) has become established at several Old World sites (Charpin et al., 1975). The most notable of these stations is in the upper Rhône valley of France near the city of Lyon, where typical, late summer pollinosis now is well-recognized. Significant ragweed growth and clinical pollinosis have been evident also in the Krasnodar region of the USSR and, recently, at points in several Balkan nations. With these exceptions, the risk of ragweed pollen exposure at locations away from North America remains negligible.

Even ragweed-free regions often harbor other herbaceous sources that shed clinically relevant, wind-borne pollens. *Rumex* species (including *R. acetosella*) are widespread in Eur-asia and elsewhere, while *Urtica* species shed abundantly in Great Britain and continental Europe. Pellitory *(Parietaria officinalis* and *P. judaica)* are Mediterranean basin hay fever sources closely allied to the nettles, although apparently differing from them in pollen allergens. Many chenopods, such as Russian thistle *(Salsola)*, are widely distributed in warmer portions of the Old World, especially arid Near Eastern regions; and the numerous tropical amaranths have not been evaluated as potential pollen sources. In addition, certain nonambrosioid composites (e.g., *Parthenium spp.*) shed moderately in warmer regions and may pose minor problems for travelers with ragweed pollinosis.

REDUCING POLLEN EXPOSURE

Outdoors. Major allergenic pollens (and spores) are so well mixed throughout the lower atmosphere that avoidance measures can only hope to curtail *excessive* exposure. However, this goal seems justifiable and may be reached by attention to "common sense" considerations. Sensitive subjects should recall that just after a prolonged rain, relatively low pollen levels prevail, while extended fair weather promotes allergen dispersion. Lengthy automobile trips *with open windows* seem to augment allergen exposure and resulting symptoms and should be limited.

The tendency of ragweeds to colonize cultivated fields and flood plains defines a predictable hazard, especially during morning hours of peak pollen emission. Repeatedly disturbed vacant lots and unpaved parking areas and construction sites pose similar problems for urban children. Grass-sensitive subjects are well advised to avoid hiking through old fields during symptomatic periods and to recall that pollens of corn and various grains can provoke "grass pollinosis" on intimate exposure.

Although ambitious programs of urban ragweed eradication have not proved successful (Walzer and Siegel, 1956), sources of ragweed around the homes of sensitive persons should be manually removed or treated annually with herbicides.

Multiple, intense tree pollen sensitivities might appropriately lead the prospective home owner to choose a deforested lot over a thickly wooded one. Pollen production by single trees often is great enough to influence symptoms,

and plantings about homes should be chosen accordingly. Many splendid shade trees (e.g., locusts, lindens, mountain ashes, ginkgo, Norway maple) are insect pollinated or shed minimally, making them especially useful for multiply sensitive persons. In addition, trees such as mulberries, ashes, and poplars have separately sexed individuals, making selection of female nonpollinators practical.

Indoors. Enclosed spaces offer refuges from aeroallergens, although patients' activity patterns limit this potential. Indoor pollen prevalence may be reduced effectively by closing windows. In warm areas, however, artificial air cooling is the price of closed windows. Central air conditioning will promote reductions in indoor particle levels. Particle exclusion by window units is variable, although patients often report benefit from their use. In general, a sealed bedroom, fitted with an air conditioner that is operated only at night, should give optimal protection when a central air conditioning system is infeasible.

Devices that provide a laminar output of essentially particle-free air can be directed at the head of a sleeping individual, creating an allergenically clean microenvironment. Similar high efficiency particulate air (HEPA) filters with high capacity air movers also have been adapted for central installation recently. However, older fiber filters mounted in window openings have been poorly accepted by patients.

Centrally installed electrostatic precipitators are often viewed as panaceas by patients or by the patient's well-motivated parents, if a child. In fact, air entering these devices is effectively cleaned of pollen and even smaller particles, although overloading (e.g., due to smoke of one cigar) readily occurs. However, particles derived from factors, including open windows, at *room level* obviously can elicit symptoms uninfluenced by electrostatic cleaners, and measures to nullify pollen, dust, and animal *sources* should not be relaxed. Also, precipitators lose efficiency as particles accumulate on the collection plates, which must be removed and washed periodically—a requirement that is often overlooked. At best, however, these devices merely complement other effective particle avoidance procedures, adding relatively little to the protection from pollen afforded by central air conditioning. Considering their modest benefits as compared with their high cost and tendency to produce ozone, precipitators probably should be recommended only for carefully chosen clinical problems. A host of free-standing precipitators, air filters, and ion generators also have been marketed as aids for allergic patients. In general, except as noted for some laminar flow devices, these units have seemed ineffectual, and many impose significant electric shock or ozone hazards.

The Pollen Refuge Option. To escape one's allergies through a bold geographic move is a popular fantasy among affected persons and their families. Such relocations can be effective, if the offenders are regionally limited and newly encountered allergens are unimportant. Escape often is difficult, however, because of multiple pollen and spore sensitivities, the importance of animal or dust allergens that travel with the patient, or the vasomotor, infective, and psychological factors unimproved by relocation. In addition, the social disruption, loss of job seniority, and financial hardships involved emphasize the need for *caution in advising or condoning a major family move.* Where this option is contemplated seriously, trial periods of at least four weeks in the new area (preferably, in more than one season) should be employed before a final decision is implemented. The physician's responsibility to provide regular medication, environmental instruction, and professional liaison for these periods of adjustment is obvious.

Despite the foregoing caveats, temporary travel may be used effectively for pollen avoidance. Ragweed-sensitive subjects have long used trips abroad, ocean cruises, or sojourns on the West Coast or in northern Canada to secure late summer relief. Early in this century, extensive gravity slide data were collected to map North American ragweed-free "refuges" close to mid-continent population centers, and the resulting patterns are still cited. Unfortunately, changing land use practices have made many of these data obsolete, and their *comparative* validity was always questionable. Physicians and their patients should be wary, therefore, of communities claiming to be "pollen-free," although many portions of northern New England and Michigan as well as the southern tip of Florida afford relative relief for the allergy harassed East Coast resident. Highly ragweed-sensitive young persons contemplating several comparable job offers are justified in giving precedence to coastal Pacific Northwest and West Coast opportunities, secondarily considering those in the Southwest and judging Mid-

western and East Coast options least desirable. However, the wide distribution of grass and deciduous tree pollens in North America leaves little hope for avoiding these factors in settled areas.

REFERENCES

Arx, J.A. von: *The Genera of Fungi Sporulating in Pure Culture,* 3rd ed. Forestburg, N.Y., Lubrecht & Cramer, 1981.

Barnett, H.L., Hunter, B.B.: *Illustrated Genera of Imperfect Fungi,* 4th ed. Minneapolis, Burgess Intl Co., Inc., 1987.

Barron, G.L.: *The Genera of Hyphomycetes from Soil.* Kreger, 1977.

Bianchi, D.E., Schwemmin, D.J., Wagner, W.H.Jr.: Pollen release in common ragweed (*Ambrosia artemisiiffolia*). Bot. Gaz. 4:253, 1959.

Bruce, R.A.: Bronchial and skin sensitivity in asthma. Int. Arch. Allergy Appl. Immunol. 22:294, 1963.

Burge, H.A.: Fungus allergens. Clin. Rev. Allergy 3:319, 1985.

Chang, W.W.Y.: Pollen survey of the United States. *In* Patterson, R. (ed.): *Allergic Diseases—Diagnosis and Management,* 2nd ed. Philadelphia, J.B. Lippincott Co., 1980.

Charpin, J., Surinyach, R., Frankland, A.W.: *Atlas of European Allergenic Pollens.* Sandoz Editions, 1975.

Connell, J.T.: Quantitative intranasal pollen challenges. III. The priming effect in allergic rhinitis. J. Allergy 43:33, 1969.

Dennis, R.W.G.: *British Ascomycetes,* 3rd ed. Forestburgh, N.Y., Lubrecht & Cramer, 1978.

Durham, O.C.: The volumetric incidence of airborne allergens. IV. A proposed standard method of gravity sampling, counting and volumetric interpolation of results, J. Allergy 17:79, 1946.

Ellis, M.B.: *Dematiaceous Hyphomycetes.* Kew, Surrey, Commonwealth Mycol. Instit., 1971.

Ellis, M.B., Ellis, J.P.: *Microfungi on Land Plants. An Identification Handbook.* New York, Macmillan Publishing Co., 1985.

Gold, B.L., Burge, H.A., Muilenberg, M.L., Solomon, W.R.: Epidermal reactivity to basidiospore extracts. J. Allergy Clin. Immunol. 73:113, 1984.

Gregory, P.H.: *Microbiology of the Atmosphere,* 2nd ed. New York, John Wiley & Sons., 1973.

Hyde, H.A., Adams, K.F.: *An Atlas of Airborne Pollen Grains,* New York, St. Martin's Press, 1958.

Kapp, R.O.: *How to Know Pollen and Spores.* Dubuque, Iowa, Wm. C. Brown Co., 1969.

Ogden, E.C., Raynor, G.S., Hayes, J.V., Lewis, D.M., Haines, J.H.: *Manual for Sampling Airborne Pollen.* New York, Hafner Press, 1974.

Onions, A.S. et al: Smith's Introduction to Industrial Mycology, 7th ed., Halstead Press, 1982.

Roth, A. (ed.): *Allergy in the World,* Honolulu, The Univ. Press of Hawaii, 1978.

Santilli, J. J., Marsh, D. G., Collins, R. P., Alexander, J. F, Jr., Norman, P. S.: Basidiospore sensitivity and asthma. J. Allergy Clin. Immunol. 68:98, 1982.

Solomon, W.R.: Fungus aerosols arising from cold-mist vaporizers. J. Allergy Clin. Immunol. 54:222, 1974.

Solomon, W.R.: Assessing fungus prevalence in domestic interiors. J. Allergy Clin. Immunol. 56:235, 1975.

Solomon, W.R.: Sampling airborne allergens. Ann. Allergy 52:140, 1984.

Solomon, W.R., Mathews, K.P.: Aerobiology and inhalant allergens. *In* Middleton, E., Jr., Reed, C. E., Ellis, E. F. (eds.): *Allergy: Principles and Practice,* 2nd ed. St. Louis, C.V. Mosby Co., 1983.

Walzer, M., Siegel, B.B.: The effectiveness of the ragweed eradication campaigns in New York City. A 9-year study (1946–1954). J. Allergy 27:113, 1956.

Weber, R.W., Nelson, H.S.: Pollen allergens and their interrelationships. Clin. Rev. Allergy 3:291, 1985.

Yunginger, J.W., Gleich, G.J.: Measurement of ragweed antigen E by double antibody radioimmunoassay. J. Allergy Clin. Immunol. 50:326, 1972.

12

Other Inhalant Allergens

KENNETH P. MATHEWS, M.D.

The relative importance of the numerous inhalant allergens differs from time to time and place to place. This chapter focuses on those inhalants considered to be of prime importance, especially in the United States and Canada.

HOUSE DUST

Various types of dust frequently precipitate or aggravate respiratory symptoms. Inorganic dusts, such as road dust, often irritate the mucous membranes. Organic dusts may act as irritants or may evoke immunologically mediated responses. Hypersensitivity pneumonitis from organic dusts is considered in Chapter 47. The discussion here is limited to IgE-mediated reactions from dust of household origin.

"House dust" seems so heterogeneous that one may wonder how it could be a distinct allergen. In many instances, in fact, its allergenic properties may be due to its content of animal allergens, algae, fungi, or insect debris (see subsequent discussion). House dust also usually contains bacteria, human epidermis, fibrous materials of plant and animal origin, food remnants, and inorganic substances. Yet by the early 1920's house dust allergy was considered a distinct entity caused by a unique (but undefined) allergen. The striking immediate skin test reactions to crude extracts in some allergic patients supported this concept. Some individuals reacted to no other known allergens, while in others with multiple sensitivities, there was no relationship between the skin test reactions to house dust and to the other allergens.

Positive immmediate skin test reactions to house dust do not prove clinical sensitivity. Up to 50 percent of nonallergic subjects also react positively to intracutaneous injections of house dust, depending upon the concentration of extract used for testing (Lindblad and Farr, 1961).

However, prick skin tests or intracutaneous tests with relatively weak dilutions of house dust extract discriminate better between control subjects and atopic patients. Furthermore, inhalation of house dust extracts induces bronchospasms and nasal reactions in sensitive individuals. Bronchial responses to house dust are reported to show diurnal variation, with peak reactivity at 11 p.m. (Gerrais et al., 1977). Many asthmatic subjects have late phase reactions, as well as immediate responses, to inhalation of house dust extract (Booij-Nord et al., 1972). In sensitive subjects, house dust allergen induces positive conjunctival test results, leukocyte histamine release (May et al., 1970; Bullock and Frick, 1972; Kawai et al., 1972), skin window eosinophilia (Bullock and Frick, 1972), and positive radioallergosorbent test (RAST) results (Holford-Strevens et al., 1970). Precipitins and lymphocyte transformation with house dust extracts have been observed both in some patients and in normal controls (Romagnani et al., 1973). Worldwide observations leave little doubt that allergy to some substance or substances in house dust is common, particularly in those with perennial respiratory allergy. For example, more than 80 percent of 133 asthmatic children in Britain gave positive prick test reactions to house dust extracts (Sarsfield, 1974), and half the pollenosis patients in Holland also reacted to house dust (Voorhorst, 1972). Such observations underscore the enormous importance of identifying the allergens in house dust.

Mites in House Dust

More than 50 years ago mites in infested grains were identified as a cause of asthma. In 1928 Dekker reported that mites in bedding were a major cause of asthma in Germany. Voorhorst et al. (1967, 1969, and 1972) in Leiden undertook a comprehensive study of house dust mites. They as well as Japanese investigators developed semiquantitative techniques for recovering mites from house dust specimens. Since there are more than 50,000 species of mites, the mites in house dust had to be identified and cultured in order to carry out clinical studies.

In Holland, mites were found invariably in house dust specimens; the dominant one was

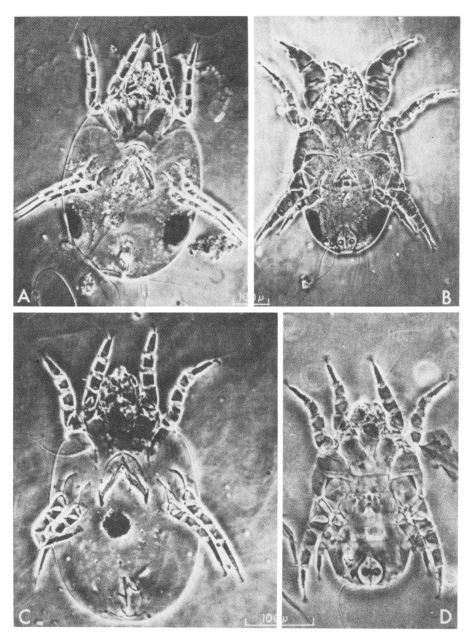

FIGURE 12–1. *Dermatophagoides farinae,* (A) female, (B) male. *D. pteronyssinus,* (C) female, (D) male. (From van Bronswijk, J.E.M.H., and Sinha, R.N.: Pyroglyphid mites (Acari) and house dust allergy. A review. J. Allergy 47:31, 1971).

Dermatophagoides pteronyssinus (Fig. 12–1). Similar observations soon were reported from Japan, the United Kingdom, Scandinavia, India, South Africa, and many other places. In several areas of North America, however, mites were not identified as frequently, and *D. farinae* (*D. culinae*) proved to be the dominant species of *Dermatophagoides* (van Bronswijk and Sinha, 1971). There was a correlation between the number of *Dermatophagoides* in many house dust specimens and the skin test activity of their extracts in house dust–sensitive subjects. Perfect correlations would not be expected, however, since mite feces have been shown to be the major source of the main allergen in house dust (Torey et al., 1981). Inoculating and incubating sterilized dust samples with living *D. pteronyssinus* produced a marked increase in their skin test reactivity, which paralleled the number of mites in the preparation (Voorhorst et al., 1967). Nevertheless, mites are not the source of allergens in a significant number of patients with positive skin test reactions to crude house dust extracts (Pauli et al., 1979).

Further studies of the house dust mites indicated that warmth and humidity enhance mite growth. Also, there may be a seasonal variation in prevalence of mites in homes in certain locations. In Leiden the peak counts of *D. pteronyssinus* occurred from August to October — a time when the largest number of house dust–sensitive patients first presented themselves for treatment. A rather similar pattern of increased mite prevalence during humid summer months also has been noted in Vancouver (Murray and Zuk, 1979) and Ohio (Arlian et al., 1979); pronounced seasonal fluctuations have been less apparent in Britain.

The mite content of house dust specimens varies greatly depending on the source of material. Mites predominate in damp houses and mattresses, perhaps in part because human epidermal scales are a preferred substrate for *Dermatophagoides.* They are rare in hospital dust, baby carriages and cribs, and on the surfaces of mattresses encased in plastic covers. Uncovered foam rubber and innerspring mattresses often harbor many mites. Sarsfield (1974) has noted that children tend to develop positive skin test reactions to house dust soon after they are transferred to ordinary beds. Somewhat in contrast to overseas experience, Arlain et al. (1982), in Ohio, found a higher house dust mite density on carpeted floors and upholstered furniture than on mattresses. Korsgaard (1983) reported that dust from the homes of 25 newly diagnosed house dust mite sensitive asthmatics had a much higher mite content than dust from the homes of 75 matched control subjects. Domestic activity greatly increases the amount of mite allergen in the air of homes (Tovey et al., 1981); this observation probably derives from the fact that the relatively large allergen-carrying mite fecal pellets (10 to 30 μm in diameter) settle quite rapidly out of still air. These observations all suggest that therapeutic benefit might accrue from programs to reduce the exposure of sensitive persons to house dust (as described in Chapter 18). Clinical improvement has been reported by some investigators (Burr et al., 1980a; Murray and Ferguson, 1983), whereas ordinary antidust procedures were ineffective in other studies (Burr et al., 1980b; Korsgaard, 1982). More complete avoidance of domestic

allergens in a hospital setting substantially benefited a group of asthmatic patients allergic to dust mites (Platts-Mills et al., 1982). A sojourn in the Alps also has been found to be beneficial for such patients. The recent report indicating the value of the acaricide, pirimiphos-methyl, in suppressing house mite allergen levels in homes may lead to enhanced clinical benefits (Mitchell et al., 1985).

Much of the evidence relating *Dermatophagoides* mites to house dust allergy is based on observations that skin test reactivity of house dust and of *D. pteronyssinus* extracts were highly correlated (Voorhorst et al., 1969). Moreover, *Dermatophagoides* extracts often produced equivalent skin test reactions at concentrations 10 to 1000 times less than house dust extracts. Extracts of *D. farinae* induced skin test reactions that correlated well with those of both house dust and *D. pteronyssinus.* Employing Prausnitz-Küstner tests, Miyamoto et al. (1968) showed that house dust and *D. farinae* extracts produced almost complete cross-neutralization of each other *in vivo* and *in vitro.* However, crossed radioimmunoelectrophoresis (CRIE) reveals that the two mite species exhibit both shared and specific allergenic determinants (LeMao et al., 1983).

Mite extracts also have been studied by several other techniques. *Bronchial inhalation challenge tests* with *D. pteronyssinus* or *D. farinae* extracts induced bronchospasm in the large majority of house dust–sensitive asthmatics in much lower concentration than house dust extracts (McAllen et al. (1970). *Nasal challenge tests* with mite extracts induce nasal symptoms in house dust–sensitive subjects. Conjunctival reactions also can be elicited.

Many laboratories have obtained positive RAST results with *D. pteronyssinus* and *D. farinae* antigens in sera of house dust–sensitive patients. RAST titers with house dust and mite extracts correlated significantly, and each allergen was active in inhibiting the other in RAST inhibition tests (Morita et al., 1975). Enzyme linked immunosorbent assays (ELISA) and reverse enzyme immunoassays also have been employed (Moneo et al. 1983). Human lung fragments, passively sensitized with such sera, released histamine *in vitro* with mite extracts (McAllen et al., 1970). Extracts of *D. pteronyssinus* or *D. farinae* also induced leukocyte histamine release *in vitro* from the cells of most house dust–sensitive donors both in the United States and Britain (McAllen et al., 1970; Bullock and Frick, 1972; Kawai et al., 1972). However, on a weight basis, substantially more dialyzed mite extract than dialyzed house dust extract was required to produce 50 percent histamine release from the leukocytes of dust-sensitive donors living in the Baltimore area.

Bullock and Frick (1972) found that *D. pteronyssinus* extract produced a significant accumulation of eosinophils at *skin windows* in 23 of 24 house dust–sensitive subjects. Some investigators have identified *precipitins* to mite extracts, but they did not correlate well with the patient's disease (Holford-Strevens et al., 1970). Late skin test reactions generally are absent. *D. pteronyssinus* extracts may induce lymphocyte transformation in both atopic and normal subjects (Romagnani et al., 1973), but more pronounced responses have been noted in patients with mite-sensitive asthma (Hiratani et al., 1981) and in patients with atopic dermatitis (Elliston et al., 1982). In the latter group, however, this response was unrelated to IgE-mediated hypersensitivity to *D. farinae*.

More recent research has emphasized the identification and purification of the allergens in mite extracts. A number of investigators have shown by radioimmunoelectrophoresis that these extracts contain numerous antigens (at least 51), and CRIE indicated that a number of these, perhaps up to 11 or more, are allergens for some patients (Krilis et al., 1984; Lind et al., 1984). Sequential fractionation of *D. pteronyssinus* extracts by gel filtration, block electrophoresis, and isoelectric focusing has yielded a 24,000 Mr fraction, P_1, which is the major allergen for many patients (Chapman and Platts-Mills, 1980). With the aid of monoclonal antibodies, it has recently been shown that this allergen has two distinct epitopes (Chapman et al., 1984). However, there also are other allergens in these extracts, such as AgX and Ag23, and an international committee has adopted an international reference preparation (NIBSC 82/518) that includes the most potent allergens (Ford et al., 1985). Meanwhile, studies of *D. farinae* extracts have shown two to four major allergens, at least one of which shares antigenic determinants with *D. pteronyssinus* (Le Mao et al., 1983; Haida et al., 1985; Chapman et al., 1985). Monoclonal antibodies to these allergens are not only valuable reagents for further immunochemical studies, but they also provide a relatively rapid means of quantitating mite allergens in the environment by radioimmunoassay. Several investigators have found purified mite allergens to be active in skin tests, RAST, RAST inhibition, and basophil histamine release. Peripheral blood mononuclear cell cultures with antigen P_1 produce stimulation predominantly of helper T cells (Rawle et al., 1984).

Besides *Dermatophagoides* species, *Euroglyphus maynei*, a closely related mite, also has been associated with house dust allergy. In addition, there is increasing evidence for the allergenicity of storage mites, including *Tyrophagus putrescentiae*, *Glycyphagus domesticus*, *Lepidoglyphus destructor*, *Tyrophagus longior*, and *Acarus siro*. Clinical difficulty related to these mites has been reported both from Southeast Asia, New Guinea, rural areas of Switzerland, Finland, and the Orkney Islands where enormous numbers of mites have been recovered from stored hay (Ingram et al., 1979).

House dust often contains substantial amounts of *human epidermis*, which is a substrate for mite proliferation. Although it has been claimed that the epidermis itself is an allergen for humans (Voorhorst, 1977), it appears unlikely that this is a frequent occurrence (Mansfield and Nelson, 1982). On the other hand, as discussed subsequently it has become clear that *cockroach allergens* are important components of house dust, particularly in the inner city. *Degeneration products* of vegetable materials, particularly *cotton linters*, also have been thought to be house dust allergens. Cohen et al. (1935) stored fresh cotton linters under various conditions for a period of about 8 months. There was a marked increase in the capacity of extracts made from these linters to elicit skin test reactions in house dust–sensitive patients. Although the increased allergenicity was attributed to breakdown products from cotton linters, in retrospect it could also have been due to mite growth under some of the conditions of storage employed in this work. A more recent study by Berrens et al. (1975) suggested the possibility that mites and microorganisms may act upon suitable substrates in such a way as to generate house dust allergens. Endotoxins, blood group active substances, and human serum proteins also can be detected in house dust (Berrens, 1970). Different commercial house dust extracts vary enormously in their endotoxin content as well as their allergenic activity (Siraganian et al., 1979). In addition, mite extracts, similar to pollen extracts, have been found to contain very low molecular weight constituents, which have hemolytic activity and produce inflammation in human skin (Freed et al., 1983).

In summary, much data suggest that *Derma-*

tophagoides mites are a major source of house dust allergen in many areas of the world, but they are not the entire source, particularly in geographic areas with low relative humidity. Immunochemical data indicate that mite extracts contain more than one allergen.

ALLERGY TO ANIMAL PRODUCTS

Type I hypersensitivity to animals, such as cats, dogs and horses, is common and well known. Frequently, the allergy becomes obvious to the patient or the patient's parent (though some resist recognizing the possibility of an adverse effect from a favorite pet). Patients with severe animal allergies, particularly to cats, may experience symptoms in households with pets even without direct contact. Contamination of the home is due not only to epidermal scales, but mammalian allergens also may be found in saliva, serum, urine, tears, semen, and amniotic fluid (Ohman, 1978).

Cat. In various studies, 9 to 36 percent of allergic patients have shown positive immediate skin test reactions to cat epidermis (Fontana et al. 1963; Ohman et al. 1977). Of course, not all skin test positive subjects have clinical intolerance to cats (Aas, 1970). The same findings apply to RAST results with cat allergens. Immunochemical studies indicate that the major allergen in cat pelts, cat allergen 1, differs from cat serum proteins, but cat albumin also may serve as a minor allergen (Ohman et al., 1974). Several other proteins also may play a minor role (Anderson and Baer, 1981). Since cat pelt and saliva extracts give identical patterns on crossed immunoelectrophoresis, it is suspected that the pelt allergen is derived largely from saliva, as a result of habitual grooming. Accordingly, very good allergen extracts can be obtained from washes of living cats (Ohman et al., 1983). There are cross-reacting allergens present in cat and dog sera (Ohman et al., 1976) and epithelia (Brandt and Yman, 1980; Viander et al., 1983). Cat urine also contains allergens but not cat allergen 1. Airborne particles bearing cat allergens are of variable size but include particles of sufficiently low aerodynamic diameter to penetrate into the peripheral lung (Findlay et al., 1983).

Dog. Five to 30 percent of allergic patients give skin test reactions to dog extracts. In assessing its possible clinical significance, historical information about lack of symptoms on exposure to domestic animals can be inaccurate when patients rarely are separated from pets or are emotionally attached to pets. Thus, a trial period of removal of the pet from the household (followed by thorough cleaning) or provocation tests may be necessary before clinical sensitivity can be properly assessed. Allergens are present in dog urine, but dog dander and saliva appear to be more abundant sources (Viander et al., 1983). Although dog serum albumin has been recognized as one of the allergens in dog dander, more recent data have indicated that other allergens commonly are important (McLean et al., 1980; Vanto et al., 1982). These are in accord with the earlier immunochemical findings of Blands et al. (1977) that dog dander contains at least five antigens not present in dog serum. Variation in allergic reactivity to different breeds of dogs was shown many years ago by skin tests and passive transfer neutralization test data (Hooker, 1944). More recently these observations have been confirmed using the RAST and RAST inhibition techniques with epidermal extracts from various breeds of dogs (Fagerberg and Wide, 1970; Moore and Hyde, 1980) and by skin testing (Lutsky et al., 1980). Such data imply the desirability of using extracts from several breeds of dogs for diagnostic testing purposes. Considering that the epidermal scales and saliva are of major importance, it is not surprising that both long-haired and short-haired breeds of dog cause allergy.

Horse. Allergy to horses obviously is less of a problem now than previously not only because there are fewer of these animals in our cities but also because of the less extensive use of horse hair–containing items, such as furniture, mattresses, mattings, padding, and felts. Nevertheless, significant exposures continue in rural areas, in persons who ride as a hobby and in persons who must work in areas contaminated with horse manure. Approximately 10 to 20 percent of allergic patients react to horse allergens on intracutaneous testing, although significant clinical sensitivity appears to be less frequent. In some studies RAST results with horse dandruff have correlated well with prick test results in children (Leegaard and Roth, 1977). Horse-sensitive patients are said also to react frequently to mule, donkey, and zebra extracts. Of particular practical importance is the relationship between allergy to horse dander and allergy to horse serum. Confirming several earlier immunochemical studies of this problem, RAST and leukocyte histamine release data, employing purified fractions of horse dandruff, have shown the presence of both horse serum albumin and unique allergens in horse dandruff (Ponterius et al., 1973; Wahn et al., 1982). By employing CRIE, sera from different patients may be found to contain IgE antibodies to dandruff proteins or serum proteins or both. This is in accord with earlier clinical observations that patients sensitive to horse dander may or may not develop allergic reactions when given equine antisera.

Other Mammalian Allergens. Antigens from virtually any mammal, including exotic species, may produce allergic symptoms. *Household pets* are an obvious source of sensitization, with hamsters and gerbils to be added to the list of more traditional dander sources in the home. Cow epidermal allergens also may be present in matting under rugs and carpets, though these have been largely supplanted by synthetic materials in newer homes. The *school environment* also may provide exposure to animals, as it is not uncommon for rabbits, mice, guinea pigs, or hamsters to be kept in classrooms. Occupational exposures also may induce symptoms. Farm family members may become sensitized to common domestic animals, such as cattle, hogs, horses, sheep, and goats. Laboratory exposures result in sensitivity to rabbits, rats, mice, guinea pigs, dogs, monkeys, or cats. Urine is a major source of rat and mouse allergens, although CRIE indicates minor allergens unique to skin and saliva (Walls and Longbottom, 1983; Lutsky et al., 1985). The value of proper animal room urine collection and disposal is implied (Taylor et al., 1977). Many garments are derived from animal epidermal sources, including various furs, cashmere, mohair, alpaca, vicuna, and camel's hair, but these processed materials are probably infrequent causes of type I hypersensitivity reactions.

Sheep's wool merits special comment, since patients not infrequently report that the fuzz from wool aggravates their allergic respiratory symptoms or contact with wool flares their eczema. However, reactivity to wool may be due to irritation rather than to true allergy because of the physical properties of wool. Indeed, in recent years there have been no serious attempts to demonstrate the existence of specific allergens in processed wool. Many sources of used wool are likely to be contaminated with human dander allergen or house dust allergen or both. It has been observed that rabbit antisera to a purified house dust allergen may cross-react with wool extract.

Feathers. Many allergic patients, particularly those afflicted with perennial respiratory symptoms, exhibit positive skin test reactions to feather extract. However, extracts of freshly plucked feathers often are inactive in patients who react strongly to extracts of aged feathers, suggesting the presence of house dust allergens in the latter. Indeed, based on skin testing with serial dilutions of house dust and feather extracts, Voorhorst and coworkers (1969) found their activities to be indistinguishable. The presence of mites in both substances could explain such results.

Regardless of the nature of the active material, aged chicken, goose, and duck feathers do in fact precipitate symptoms in some atopic individuals. The usual sources of exposure are pillows, comforters, quilts, jackets, sleeping bags, and beds. Rarely, feathers of canaries, parakeets, parrots, pigeons, turkeys, and sparrows have been reported to produce type I hypersensitivity reactions (also see Chapter 47 regarding avian hypersensitivity pneumonitis). "Feather"-sensitive patients can eat meat of the same fowl with impunity and do not experience allergic reactions from egg-containing vaccines unless they have concomitant allergies to egg proteins. It is unfortunate that package directions with egg-containing vaccines sometimes call for inquiry about "feather" allergy, as this creates unnecessary confusion and apprehension in allergic individuals who know they have positive skin test reactions to "feathers" but are not sensitive to egg proteins.

INSECT-DERIVED INHALANT ALLERGENS

In comparison with pollen and fungus allergies, the number of cases of well-documented inhalant respiratory allergies due to insect-derived material is relatively small, though this number may well expand as further knowledge is accrued. The subject is complicated by the vast numbers of insect species. Table 12–1, modified from Perlman (1958), indicates types of arthropods that have been implicated as possible causes of type I hypersensitivity.

Arthropods as Local or Indoor Allergen Sources. Some of the most convincing cases of inhalant insect allergy have involved occupational exposures; for example, entomologists and laboratory workers have become sensitized to beetles, cockroaches, grasshoppers, locusts, crickets, screwworm flies, houseflies, boll weevils, butterflies, and moths. A survey of 98 Agri-

TABLE 12-1. Arthropods Implicated as Possible Inhalant Allergens*

Class	Order	Member
Arachnida		Spiders
		Mites, ticks
Crustacea		Sowbugs
		Daphnia (water flea)
		Shrimp (plankton)
Insecta	Orthoptera	Locusts
		Grasshoppers
		Cockroaches
		Crickets
	Isoptera	Termites
	Dermaptera	Earwigs
	Ephemeroptera	Mayflies
	Hemiptera	Bedbugs
		Box elder bug
	Homoptera	Aphids
	Coleoptera	Beetles
		Bean weevil
	Neuroptera	Lancewing flies
	Trichoptera	Caddis flies
	Lepidoptera	Moths, butterflies
	Diptera	Houseflies
		Mushroom flies
		Sewer flies
		Midges
		Deer flies
		Screwworm Flies
		Black flies
	Siphonaptera	Rat fleas
	Hymenoptera	Honey bees

* Modified from Perlman, F.: Insects as inhalant allergens. J. Allergy 29:302, 1958.

cultural Research Service facilities (NIOSH, 1983) revealed that 33 percent of 507 employees who work directly with insects reported possible occupationally related allergic symptoms. Agricultural workers have experienced allergic respiratory symptoms from locally abundant concentrations of Mexican bean beetles, grain mites, and honeybees. The last inhalant sensitivity is to be distinguished from allergic reactions to Hymenoptera stings (see Chapter 52). Swarms of mushroom flies and box elder beetles (Murray et al. 1970) have penetrated homes in sufficient numbers to produce sensitization. Sewer flies have produced allergic asthma and rhinitis in sewage plant workers (Gold et al., 1985).

There are relatively rare cases of documented inhalant allergy indoors to bedbugs, houseflies, and water fleas (*Daphnia*); the last are crustaceans, which are used as fish food. *Mites* have been discussed. The *cockroach* is receiving increasing attention as an important inhalant allergen in homes. Almost half of economically disadvantaged patients in large urban areas in the United States have positive skin tests to cockroach extracts (Bernton et al., 1972), and many of these reactions can be transferred by the Prausnitz-Küstner (PK) test. Bronchial provocation tests in skin-reactive patients in many instances show immediate or dual responses, which can be inhibited by cromolyn sodium (Kang, 1976; Kang et al., 1979). Three active fractions have been purified from cockroach extracts, and antigen-induced histamine release from sensitized leukocytes has been demonstrated *in vitro* (Twarog et al., 1977). Cockroach feces and contaminated food also contain the allergen. Inhalant *silk* allergy is disappearing with the diminishing use of silk fabrics in North America and the elimination of silk filters in processing vaccines for immunization. It continues to be of potential importance in the Orient. The allergen is contained in sericin, a gelatinous substance, which binds silk fibers together.

Insect Material as Disseminated Aeroallergen. This observation was first well documented by Parlato's description (1930) of *caddis fly allergy.* The larval form of these insects develops in lakes and rivers. When mature, they rise to the surface: the adults emerge and fly to shore where mating takes place, and the females fly back over the water to deposit eggs. Although numerous varieties of caddis flies are widely distributed, these insects swarm in sufficient numbers to produce allergic symptoms primarily in the area of Buffalo, New York. The time of exposure is June to late August, with the peak in mid-August. The allergenicity of these flies is very much related to the fact that they are covered with small hairs that break off and become wind-borne. Sensitized persons have positive skin test reactions to caddis fly extracts.

At about the same time caddis fly allergy was discovered at the eastern end of Lake Erie, Figley (1929) described *mayfly* allergy at the western end of the lake. Somewhat like the caddis fly, the mayfly larvae develop in the water, and the adults emerge to swarm ashore in vast numbers in June and July. The adults live only a few hours, but during this time they shed a friable outer skin or pellicle. Debris from these pellicles and the vast numbers of dead insects accumulating near the lake shore produce sufficient airborne allergen to sensitize numbers of patients in lake shore communities near Toledo, Ohio. This disease is of diminishing importance, however, as the number of these mayflies has been decreasing, probably as a result of water pollution in western Lake Erie.

In another area, it has been recognized recently that very large numbers of persons living along the upper Nile river in the Sudan are afflicted with allergic respiratory symptoms caused by the "green nimitti" midge, *Cladotanytarsus lewisi,* which breeds in the river in vast numbers. Skin tests, RAST, and release of histamine and slow reacting substance of anaphylaxis (SRS-A) from lung fragments passively sensitized by patients' sera have documented an IgE-mediated mechanism (Gad El Rab and Kay, 1980). Larvae of closely related nonbiting midges, *Chironomus thummi thummi,* are used as food for pet fish, and investigators in Germany have documented by skin tests, RAST, and provocation tests that the respiratory symptoms occurring in some persons handling this material reflects IgE-mediated allergy (Baur et al., 1982). Furthermore, these investigators showed cross reactivity between these midge allergens and those of the green nimitti midges of the Sudan and that the source of the allergen was the hemoglobin of these chironomids! Recently another chironomid, the lake fly (*Chironomus plumosus*), has been shown to cause respiratory symptoms in atopic persons in Wisconsin (Kagen et al., 1984). In northwestern United States, the respiratory symptoms developing in persons exposed to huge numbers of Douglas fir tussock moths often represent an irritant effect, but results of prick tests and passive sensitization of monkey lung for histamine release provide evidence for true type I hypersensitivity in some cases (Perlman et al., 1976).

The possibility that many other types of insect debris might be the causes of much allergic disease has intrigued a number of investigators (Feinberg et al., 1956; Perlman, 1958). Some support for this possibility is found in the fact that skin testing of large numbers of allergic patients with a battery of insect extracts results in positive reactions in one third to one half of the subjects! Furthermore, these reactions are observed most frequently in patients with seasonal allergic symptoms and least commonly in nonallergic individuals. A more recent example is the finding that more than half of asthmatic patients in Japan have positive intracutaneous skin test reactions to moth or butterfly extracts (Kino and Oshima, 1978). In some cases RAST and bronchial provocation test results were positive. Interpretation of this kind of information, however, is more conjectural than conclusive. Correlation of hypersensitivity with the insect content of the "aerial plankton" in which we live is thwarted by the lack of technology for identifying the source of most airborne insect debris. Thus, the degree to which hypersensitivity to various inhalant insect allergens is of clinical importance remains to be clarified. Relevant entomologic information has been compiled by Frazier and Brown (1980).

MISCELLANEOUS ALLERGENS OF PLANT ORIGIN

Kapok. Imported largely from Indonesia, kapok is the seedhair from kapok trees. It has been employed as stuffing for pillows, sleeping bags, mattresses, and lifejackets and cushions for boats, the last because of its marked buoyancy. Studies many years ago suggested some relationship between kapok and cottonseed allergens, corresponding to their botanical relationship. However, the allergenicity of kapok articles is acquired largely with aging (Dhorranintra and Bunnag, 1977). Based on skin testing with serial dilutions of extracts, Voorhorst (1969) found old kapok, similar to feathers, to be indistinguishable from house dust allergen. On the other hand, there appear to be immunochemical differences (Berrens, 1966). In any case, kapok should not be employed as a substitute for feather pillows or other allergenic stuffings.

Orris Root. The powdered rhizome from certain species of iris had physical properties and a fragrance that were almost ideal for use in face powder and certain other cosmetics. Although the root was widely used for these purposes about 50 years ago, so many patients developed respiratory allergic symptoms that its use has largely been abandoned in North America.

Pyrethrum. This widely used insecticide is prepared from pyrethrum flowers. These are members of the large Compositae family and thus are botanically related to ragweed. Accordingly, skin test reactivity and clinical difficulty from pyrethrum are particularly likely to occur in ragweed-sensitive patients. Aggravation of allergic respiratory symptoms from insect sprays and powders most often is on an irritant basis, but the additional possibility of specific sensitization needs to be considered when the offending material contains pyrethrum. Some patients who travel have difficulty after the inside of an aircraft has been sprayed with pyrethrum.

Cottonseed. The water-soluble, proteinaceous material in cottonseed contains one of the most potent allergens for humans. Occasionally it contaminates inexpensive cotton stuffing in upholstery, mattresses, and cushions. More substantial exposures to the allergens arise from the use of cottonseed meal, which may be found in fertilizers and as a constituent of feed for cattle, hogs, poultry, and dogs. Symptoms usually result from inhalation, but allergic reactions also can occur from ingesting cottonseed meal used in pan-greasing compounds and in foods, such as some fried cakes, fig bars, and cookies. The processing of *cottonseed oil* generally involves washing, bleaching, and distillation at over 400°C. It is extremely unlikely that any traces of allergen would retain their activity through these procedures, and this is fortunate in view of the extremely wide usage of cottonseed oil. Patients sensitized to the water-soluble allergen tend to have explosive, intermittent symptoms depending on the source of exposure. Because of the extreme sensitivity of some individuals, casual skin testing can lead to severe or fatal reactions. Prick testing is recommended in preference to or before injection of cottonseed extracts.

Flaxseed (Linseed). This also contains potent allergens. Although varying from time to time and place to place, some of the possible inhalant sources of flaxseed exposure are cattle and poultry feed, dog food, wave-setting preparations, shampoos and hair tonics, some brands of depilatories, patent leather, insulating materials, rugs, and some cloth containing flax. Ingestant sources include Roman meal, Malt-O-Meal, flaxseed tea, milk from cows fed flaxseed meal, cough remedies, laxatives, and muffins. The numerous sources of linseed oil are not of concern for the same reasons as mentioned regarding cottonseed oil.

The precautions described in skin testing with cottonseed should be observed in testing with flaxseed.

Castor Bean. After castor oil is expressed from the beans, there remains a residual castor pomace, which contains other very potent allergens. Aside from obvious occupational exposures in handling castor beans, more occult sources of these allergens include fertilizers, used burlap sacks, felt, upholstery, and in coffee manufacturing. A colony of sensitized patients in the vicinity of a castor bean processing factory that contaminated the atmosphere with castor bean pomace has been reported. Castor beans also contain a toxin (ricin), and for skin testing it is important that detoxified material be used and that the aforementioned precautions

for dealing with potent allergens be observed. These extracts contain both high molecular weight, heat labile allergens and low molecular weight, heat stable allergens (Lehrer et al., 1981).

Other Inhalant Allergens from Bean Sources. In addition to its use in foods, *soybean* meal has many commercial uses that may permit sensitization by inhalation, as follows: fertilizer, animal food, glue and adhesives, water-based paint, paper sizing, artificial wool, fire-fighting foam, water proofing, whipping powder, soothing bath preparations, and textile dressing (Fries, 1971). Recently we observed a laboratory worker who had an acute type I hypersensitivity reaction from *Bandeiraea simplicifolia*, a bean source of anti-B lectin. Occupational allergy from *coffee bean dust* is well documented (see Chapter 46).

Vegetable Gums. Several vegetable gums have been added to a large variety of commercial products largely to improve their physical properties, but the pattern of gum usage has varied considerably at different times and in different places. For example, wave-setting lotions were the source of some of the best documented cases of vegetable gum allergy many years ago, but the lotions in common use today generally contain polyvinylpyrrolidone instead of vegetable gums. The gums most frequently reported to produce sensitization were karaya or Indian gum, tragacanth, and acacia gum or gum arabic. Other gums are derived from quince seed, locust bean (carob seed), Irish moss (carrageenin), chickle, algin, agar, bassora, gelatin, ghatti, gum guar, mesquite, and pectin. Current information about inhalant sources is difficult to obtain, but vegetable gums still may be present in some brands of denture adhesive powders, tooth powders, wave-setting preparations, face powder, rouge, adhesives, sizing materials, and other substances used in printing and paper making. The occurrence of karaya gum–induced asthma and rhinitis in an enterostomal therapist illustrates how the possibility of vegetable gum allergy should not be overlooked (Wagner, 1980). Vegetable gums also are used extensively in food products. Evaluation of possible gum allergy by skin testing requires employing several gums, since cross-reactions cannot be assumed. These allergens have not been assessed by modern immunochemical methods. The demonstration of cross-reacting IgE antibodies to gum acacia and gum tragacanth in a patient with quillaja bark (soapbark)–induced asthma raises the possibility of immunologic cross reactivity between the sapogenin quillaic acid in the bark and the structurally very similar acacic acid in the gum (Raghuprasad et al., 1980).

Miscellaneous Plant Inhalants. These include lycopodium (dusting powders), and jute (burlap, rope, carpets). Allergic reactions also have resulted from occupational exposures to chicory and tobacco leaf (Gleich et al., 1980).

OTHER INHALANT ALLERGENS

Fish odors can produce allergic respiratory symptoms in highly sensitive patients. Such persons also may be highly reactive to fish glue, such as LePage glue. Skin testing with these potent allergens can be dangerous; prick testing is recommended.

In Japan, asthma has been reported due to *buckwheat* attached to buckwheat chaff in pillows. Allergy to *papain* can develop through inhalation of meat tenderizers, laboratory reagents, and pharmaceuticals. Sensitized persons are at risk of developing anaphylaxis if treated by chymopapain chemonucleolysis. *Garlic dust* may sensitize, and inhaled *medications* also can sensitize. Indeed, this occurred so frequently with penicillin that its administration by inhalation has been largely abandoned. Intranasal insufflation of posterior pituitary preparations (Pituitrin) also caused considerable hypersensitivity. Inhalant allergy to pancreatic extract has been reported in parents of cystic fibrosis patients, caused by the parents' sprinkling the enzyme preparation on their children's food (Dolan and Meyers, 1974). Psyllium and ispaghula laxative powders also have evoked allergic respiratory symptoms. The numerous other inhalant allergens, which are related to occupational exposures, are reviewed in Chapter 46.

In summary, among the inhalant allergens other than pollens and fungi, "house dust" is of major importance, but identification of the allergenic substances in this heterogeneous material is difficult; mites appear to be important in many cases. Allergens from various mammalian species are common offenders, which usually are easily recognized. Insects can produce allergic symptoms in localized areas, but their importance as widely disseminated aeroallergens remains to be defined. There are many other substances that occasionally act as inhalant allergens, and it is incumbent upon

physicians caring for allergic patients to be familiar with these.

REFERENCES

Aas, K.: Bronchial provocation tests in asthma. Arch. Dis. Child 45:221, 1970.

Anderson, M.C., Baer, H.: Allergenically active components of cat allergen extracts. J. Immunol. 127:972, 1981.

Arlian, L.G., Bernstein, I.L., Gallagher, J.S.: The prevalence of house dust mites, *Dermatophagoides* spp., and associated environmental conditions in homes in Ohio. J. Allergy Clin. Immunol. 69:527, 1982.

Baur X., Dewair, M., Fruhmann, G., et al.: Hypersensitivity to chironomids (non-biting midges): Localization of the antigenic determinants within certain polypeptide sequences of hemoglobins (erythrocruorins) of *Chironomus thummi thummi* (Diptera). J. Allergy Clin. Immunol. 69:66, 1982.

Bernton, H.S., McMahon, T.F., Brown, H.: Cockroach asthma. Br. J. Dis. Chest 66:61, 1972.

Berrens, L.: Kapok allergens. Int. Arch. Allergy 29:575, 1966.

Berrens, L.: The allergens in house dust. Prog. Allergy 14:259, 1970.

Berrens, L., van Bronswijk, J.E.M.H., Young, E., van Dijk, A.G.: A controlled study of allergen production in cultures of *Dermatophagoides pteronyssinus.* Acta Allergo. 30:390, 1975.

Blands, J., Lowensten, H., Weeke, B.: Characterization of extract of dog hair and dandruff from six different dog breeds by quantitative immunoelectrophoresis. Identification of allergens by crossed radioimmunoelectrophoresis (CRIE). Acta Allergo. 32:147, 1977.

Booij-Nord, H., DeVries, H.J., Sluiter, H.J., Orie, N.G.M.: Late bronchial obstructive reaction to experimental inhalation of house dust extract. Clin. Allergy 2:43, 1972.

Brandt, R., Yman, L.: Dog dander allergens. Specificity studies based on radioallergosorbent technique. Int. Arch. Allergy Appl. Immunol. 61:361, 1980.

Bullock, J.D., Frick, O.L.: Mite sensitivity in house dust–allergic children. Am. J. Dis. Child. 123:222, 1972.

Burr, M.L., Neale, E., Dean, B.V., Verrier-Jones, E. R.: Effect of a change to mite-free bedding on children with mite-sensitive asthma: A controlled trial. Thorax 35:513, 1980a.

Burr, M.L., Dean, B.V., Merrett, T.G., Neale, E., et al.: Effects of anti-mite measures on children with mite sensitive asthma: A controlled study. Thorax 35:506, 1980b.

Chapman, M.D., Sutherland, W.M., Platts-Mills, T.A.E.: Recognition of two *Dermatophagoides pteronyssinus*–specific epitopes on antigen P_1 by using monoclonal antibodies: Binding to each epitope can be inhibited by serum from dust mite–allergic patients. J. Immunol. 133:2488, 1984.

Chapman, M.D., Sutherland, W.M., Platts-Mills, T.A.E.: Recognition of species-specific and cross-reacting antigenic determinants on house dust mite (*Dermatophagoides*) allergens using monoclonal antibodies. Int. Arch. Allergy Appl. Immunol. 77:166, 1985.

Chapman, M.D., Platts-Mills, T.A.E.: Purification and characterization of the major allergen from *Dermatophagoides pteronyssinus*–antigen P_1. J. Immunol. 125:587, 1980.

Cohen, M.B., Nelson, T., Reinarz, B.H.: Observations on the nature of the house dust allergy. J. Allergy 6:517, 1935.

Dekker, H.: Asthma and Milben. Munch Med Wochenschr 75:515, 1928 (translated in J. Allergy Clin. Immunol. 48:251, 1971).

Dhorranintra, B., Bunnag, C.: Cross reactions in skin tests between kapok and house dust allergenic extracts. Ann. Allergy 39:201, 1977.

Dolan, T.F., Meyers, A.: Bronchial asthma and allergic rhinitis associated with the inhalation of pancreatic extracts. Am. Rev. Respir. Dis. 110:812, 1974.

Dolovich, J., Shaikh, W., Tarlo, S., Bell, B., Hargreave, F.E.: Human exposure and sensitization to airborne papain. Ann. Allergy 38:382, 1977.

Elliston, W.L., Heise, E.A., Huntley, C.C.: Cell-mediated hypersensitivity to mite antigens in atopic dermatitis. Arch. Derm. 118:26, 1982.

Fagerberg, E., Wide, L.: Diagnosis of hypersensitivity to dog epithelium in patients with asthma bronchiale. Int. Arch. Allergy 39:301, 1970.

Feinberg, A.R., Feinberg, S.M., Beniam-Pinto, C.: Asthma and rhinitis from insect allergens. I. Clinical importance. J. Allergy 27:437, 1956.

Figley, K.D.: Asthma due to mayfly. Am. J. Med. Sci. 178:338, 1929.

Findlay, S.R., Stotsky, E., Leitermann, K., Hemady, Z., Ohman, J.L.: Allergens detected in association with airborne particles capable of penetrating into the peripheral lung. Am. Rev. Respir. Dis. 128:1008, 1983.

Fontana, V.J., Wittig, H., Holt, L.E., Jr.; Observations on the specificity of the skin test. The incidence of positive skin tests in allergic and nonallergic children. J. Allergy 34:348, 1963.

Ford, A., et al.: A collaborative study on the first international standard of Dermatophagoides pteronyssinus (house dust mite) extract. J. Allergy Clin. Immunol. 75:676, 1984.

Ford, A.W., Rawle, F.C., Lind, P., Spieksma, F.T.M., Lowenstein, H., Platts-Mills, T.A.E.: Standardization of Dermatophagoides pteronyssinus: Assessment of potency and allergen content in ten coded extracts. Int. Arch. Allergy Appl. Immunol. 76:58, 1985.

Frazier, C.A., Brown, F.K.: Insects and Allergy and What to do about Them. Norman, University of Oklahoma Press, 1980.

Freed, D.L., Buckley, C.H., Tsivion, Y., Sharon, N., Katz, D.H.: Non-allergenic haemolysins in grass pollens and house dust mites. Allergy 38:477, 1983.

Fries, J.H.: Studies on the allergenicity of soy bean. Ann. Allergy 29:1, 1971.

Gad El Rab, M.O., Kay A.B.: Widespread immunoglobulin E−mediated hypersensitivity in the Sudan to the "green nimitti" midge, Cladotanytarsus lewisi (Diptera: Chironomidae). J. Allergy Clin. Immunol. 66:190, 1980.

Gerrais, P., Reinberg, A., Gerrais, C., Smolensky, M., DeFrance, O.: Twenty-four hour rhythm in the bronchial hypersensitivity to house dust in asthmatics. J. Allergy Clin. Immunol. 59:207, 1977.

Gleich, G.S., Welsh, P.W., Yunginger, J.W., et al.: Allergy to tobacco: An occupational hazard. N. Engl. J. Med. 302:617, 1980.

Gold, B.L., Mathews, K.P., Burge, H.A.: Occupational asthma caused by sewer flies. Am. Rev. Resp. Dis. 131:949, 1985.

Haida, M., et al.: Allergens of the house dust mite Dermatophagoides farinae—immunochemical studies of four allergenic fractions. J. Allergy Clin. Immunol. 75:686, 1985.

Hiratani, M., Muto, K., Oshida, Y., et al.: Lymphocyte responsiveness to Dermatophagoides farinae extract in mite-sensitive patients: Effect of immunoglobulin E antibody (RAST score). J. Allergy Clin. Immunol. 68:205, 1981.

Holford-Strevens, V., Wide, L., Milne, J.F., Pepys, J.: Allergens and antigens of Dermatophagoides farinae. Clin. Exper. Immunol. 6:49, 1970.

Hooker, S.B.: Qualitative differences among canine danders. Ann. Allergy 2:281, 1944.

Ingram, C.G., Jeffrey, I.G., Symington, I.S., Cuthbert, D.D.: Bronchial provocation studies in farmers allergic to storage mites. Lancet 2:1330, 1979.

Kagen, S.L., Yunginger, J.W., Johnson, R.: Lake fly allergy: Incidence of chironomid sensitivity in an atopic population. J. Allergy Clin. Immunol. 73:187, 1984.

Kang, B.: Study on cockroach antigen as a possible causative agent in bronchial asthma. J. Allergy Clin. Immunol. 58:357, 1976.

Kang, B., Vellody, D., Homburger, H., Yunginger, J.W.: Cockroach cause of allergic asthma. Its specificity and immunologic profile. J. Allergy Clin. Immunol. 63:80, 1979.

Kawai, T., Marsh, D.G., Lichtenstein, L.M., Norman, P.S.: The allergens responsible for house dust allergy. I. Comparison of Dermatophagoides pteronyssinus and houe dust extracts by assay of histamine release from allergic human leukocytes. J. Allergy Clin. Immunol. 50:117, 1972.

Kino, T., Oshima, S.: Allergy to insects in Japan. I. The reaginic sensitivity to moth and butterfly in patients with bronchial asthma. J. Allergy Clin. Immunol. 61:10, 1978.

Korsgaard, J.: Preventive measures in housedust allergy. Am. Rev. Resp. Dis. 125:80, 1982.

Korsgaard, J.: Mite asthma and residency. A case-control study on the impact of exposure to house-dust mites in dwellings. Am. Rev. Resp. Dis. 128:231, 1983.

Krilis, S., Baldo, B.A., Sutton, R., Basten, A.: Antigens and allergens from the common house dust mite Dermatophagoides pteronyssinus. II. Identification of the major IgE-binding antigens by crossed radioimmunoelectrophoresis. J. Allergy Clin. Immunol. 74:142, 1984.

Leegaard, J., Roth, A.: RAST in the diagnosis of hypersensitivity to horse allergens. A comparison with clinical history and in vivo tests. Clin. Allergy 7:455, 1977.

Lehrer, S.B., Taylor, J., Salvaggio, J.E.: Castor bean allergens: Evidence for distinct heat-labile and stable entities. Int. Arch. Allergy Appl. Immunol. 65:69, 1981.

LeMao, J., Dandeu, J.P., Rabillon, J., et al.: Comparison of antigenic and allergic composition of two partially purified extracts from Dermatophagoides farinae and Dermatophagoides pteronyssinus mite cultures. J. Allergy Clin. Immunol. 71:588, 1983.

Lind, P., Weeke, B., Lowenstein, H.: A referance allergen preparation of the house dust mite D. pteronyssinus produced from whole mite culture—a part of the DAS 76 study. Comparison with allergen preparations from other raw materials. Allergy 39:259, 1984.

Lindblad, J.H., Farr, R.S.: The incidence of positive intradermal reactions and demonstration of skin sensitizing antibody to extracts of ragweed and dust in humans without history of rhinitis or asthma. J. Allergy 32:393, 1961.

Lutsky, I., Fink, J.N., Arkins, J.A., et al.: Skin test reactivity to dog-derived antigens. Clin. Allergy 10:331, 1980.

Lutsky, I., Fink, J.N., Kidd, J., Dahlberg, M.J., Yunginger, J.W.: Allergenic properties of rat urine and pelt extracts. J. Allergy Clin. Immunol. 75:279, 1985.

Mansfield, L.E., Nelson, H.S.: Allergens in commercial house dust. Ann. Allergy 48:205, 1982.

May, C.D., Lyman, M., Alberto, R., Cheng, J.: Immuno-chemical evaluation of antigenicity of house dust extract. Specificity of dermal wheal reactions and responses to injections for immunotherapy. J. Allergy 46:73, 1970.

McAllen, M.K., Assem, E.S.K., Mannsell, K.: House dust mite asthma. Results of challenge tests on five criteria with *Dermatophagoides pteronyssinus*. Br. Med. J. 2:501, 1970.

McLean, A.C., Glovsky, M.M., Hoffman, D.R., Ghekiere, L.M.: Identification of allergens in dog dander extract. I. Clinical and immunological aspects of allergenicity activity. Ann. Allergy 45:199, 1980.

Mitchell, E.B., Wilkins, S., Deighton, J.M., Platts-Mills, T.A.E.: Reduction of house mite allergen levels in the home; use of the acaricide, pirimiphos methyl. Clin. Allergy 15:235, 1985.

Miyamoto, T., Oshima, S., Ishizaki, T.: Antigenic relation between house dust and dust mite (*Dermatophagoides farinae* Hughes, 1961) by a fractionation method. J. Allergy 44:282, 1969.

Miyamoto, T., Oshima, S., Ishizaki, T., Sato, S.: Allergenic identity between the common floor mite (*Dermatophagoides farinae* Hughes, 1961) and house dust as a causative antigen in bronchial asthma. J. Allergy 42:14, 1968.

Moneo, I., Cuevas, M., Urena, V., et al: Reverse enzyme immunoassay for the determination of *Dermatophagoides pteronyssinus* IgE antibodies. Int. Arch. Allergy Appl. Immunol. 71:285, 1983.

Moore, B.S., Hyde, J.S.: Breed-specific dog hypersensitivity in humans. J. Allergy Clin. Immunol. 66:198, 1980.

Morita, Y., Miyamoto, T., Horiuchi, Y., Oshima, S., Katsuhata, A., Kamal, J.: Further studies in allergic identity between house dust and the house dust mite, *Dermatophagoides farinae* Hughes, 1961. Ann. Allergy 35:361, 1975.

Murray, A.B., Ferguson, A.C.: Dust-free bedrooms in the treatment of asthmatic children with house dust or house dust mite allergy: A controlled trial. Pediatrics 71:418, 1983.

Murray, A.B., Zuk, P.: The seasonal variation in a population of house dust mites in a North American city. J. Allergy Clin. Immunol. 64:266, 1979.

Murray, F.J., Brown, H., Bernton, H.S.: A case of asthma caused by box elder beetle. J. Allergy 45:103, 1970.

NIOSH: Health hazard evaluation report LHETA 81-121. Morgantown, W.Va., National Institute for Occupational Safety and Health, 1983.

Ohman, J.L.: Allergy in man caused by exposure to mammals. J. Am. Vet. Med. Assn. 172:1403, 1978.

Ohman, J.L., Baer, H., Anderson, M.C., et al.: Surface washes of living cats: An improved method of obtaining clinically relevant allergen. J. Allergy Clin. Immunol. 72:288, 1983.

Ohman, J.L., Bloch, K.S., Kendall, S., Lowell, F.C.: Allergens of mammalian origin. IV. Evidence for common allergens in cat and dog serum. J. Allergy Clin. Immunol. 57:560, 1976.

Ohman, J.L., Jr., Lowell, F.C., Bloch, K.J.: Allergens of mammalian origin. III. Properties of a major feline allergen. J. Immunol. 113:1668, 1974.

Parlato, S.J.: The sand fly (caddis fly) as an exciting cause of

allergic coryza and asthma. II. Its relative frequency. J. Allergy 1:307, 1930.

Pauli, G., Bessot, J.C., Hirth, C., Thierry, R.: Dissociation of house dust allergies. J. Allergy Clin. Immunol. 63:245, 1979.

Perlman, F.: Insects as inhalant allergens. Consideration of aerobiology, biochemistry, preparation of material, and clinical observations. J. Allergy 29:302, 1958.

Perlman, F., Press, E., Googins, J.A., Malley, A., Poarea, H.: Tussockosis: reactions to Douglas fir tussock moth. Ann. Allergy 36:302, 1976.

Platts-Mills, T.A.E., Tovey, E.R., Mitchell, E.B., et. al.: Reduction of bronchial hyperreactivity during prolonged allergen avoidance. Lancet 2:675, 1982.

Ponterius, G., Brandt, R., Hulten, E., Yman, L.: Comparative studies on the allergens of horse dandruff and horse serum. Int. Arch. Allergy 44:679, 1973.

Raghuprasad, P.K., Brooks, S.M., Litwin, A., et al.: Quaillaja bark (soapbark)–induced asthma. J. Allergy Clin. Immunol. 65:285, 1980.

Rawle, F.C., Mitchell, E.B., Platts-Mills, T.A.E.: T cell responses to the major allergen from the house dust mite *Dermatophagoides pteronyssinus*, antigen P_1; comparison of patients with asthma, atopic dermatitis, and perennial rhinitis. J. Immunol. 133:195, 1984.

Romagnani, S., Biliotti, G., Passaleva, A., Ricci, M.: Mites and house dust allergy. III. *In vitro* lymphocyte transformation and precipitating antibody to house dust and mite (*Dermatophagoides pteronyssinus*) extract in atopic and nonatopic individuals. Clin. Allergy 3:51, 1973.

Sarsfield, J.K.: Role of house-dust mites in childhood asthma. Arch. Dis. Child. 49:711, 1974.

Siraganian, R.P., Baer, H., Hochstein, H.D., May, J.C.: Allergenic biologic activity of commercial preparations of house dust extract. J. Allergy Clin. Immunol. 64:526, 1979.

Taylor, A.N., Longbottom, J.L., Pepys, J.: Respiratory allergy to urine proteins of rats and mice. Lancet 2:847, 1977.

Tovey, E.R., Chapman, M.D., Platts-Mills, T.A.E.: Mite feces are a major source of house dust allergens. Nature 289:592, 1981.

Tovey, E.R., Chapman, M.D., Wells, C.W., Platts-Mills, T.E.A.: The distribution of dust mite allergen in the houses of patients with asthma. Am. Rev. Resp. Dis. 124:630, 1981.

Twarog, F.J., Picone, F.J., Strunk, R.S., So, J., Colten, H.R.: Immediate hypersensitivity to cockroach. Isolation and purification of the major antigens. J. Allergy Clin. Immunol. 59:154, 1977.

van Bronswijk, J.E.M.H., Sinha, R.N.: Pyroglyphid mites (Acari) and house dust allergy. J. Allergy 47:31, 1971.

Vanto, T., Viander, M., Schwartz, B.: Dog serum albumin as an allergen. IgE, IgG and lymphocyte responses in dog dander–sensitive asthmatic children. Int. Arch. Allergy Appl. Immunol. 69:311, 1982.

Viander, M., Valovirta, E., Vanto, I., Koivikko, A.: Cross-reactivity iof cat and dog allergen extracts. Int. Arch. Allergy Appl. Immunol. 71:252, 1983.

Voorhorst R: To what extent are house-dust mites (*Dermatophagoides*) responsible for complaints in asthma patients? Allerg. Immunol. 18:9, 1972.

Voorhorst, R.: The human dander atopy. II. Human dander, a complicating factor in the study of the relationship between house dust and *Dermatophagoides* allergens. Ann. Allergy 39:339, 1977.

Voorhorst, R. Spieksma, F. Th. M., Varekamp, H.: *House-*

dust Atopy and the House-dust Mite. Leiden, Staflen's Scientific Publishing Co., 1969.

Voorhorst, R., Spieksma, F. Th. M., Varekamp, H., Lenpen, M.J., Lyklema, A.W.: The house-dust mite (*Dermatophagoides pteronyssinus*) and the allergens it produces. Identity with the house-dust allergen. J. Allergy 39:325, 1967.

Wagner, W.: Karaya gum hypersensitivity in an enterostomal therapist. J.A.M.A. 243:432, 1980.

Wahn, U., Herold, U., Danielsen, K., Lowenstein, H.: Allergoprints in horse allergic children. Allergy 37:335, 1982.

Walls, A.F., Longbottom, J.L.: Quantitative immunoelectrophoretic analysis of rat allergen extracts. II. Fur, urine, and saliva studied by cross radioimmunoelectrophoresis. Allergy 38:501, 1983.

13

Other Environmental Factors

WILLIAM E. PIERSON, M.D.
JANE Q. KOENIG, Ph.D.

Allergic individuals have an increased risk for reacting to the many environmental by-products of our complex society. Routes of contact and types of reactivity to these various agents are numerous, but this chapter focuses on the agents and factors that affect primarily the respiratory system. Major indoor air pollutants include sidestream cigarette smoke (i.e., smoke released from a burning cigarette), formaldehyde, and wood and gas stove emissions. Common outdoor pollutants include sulfur dioxide (SO_2), sulfuric acid (H_2SO_4), ozone (O_3), and nitrogen dioxide (NO_2). Humidity and temperature influence the health effects of these pollutants, and weather conditions are of importance in assessing the health effects of air pollutants in general. The presence of various ions in the atmosphere also may have important influences on the intensity by which certain environmental agents can affect humans. The health effects of exposures to various occupational agents are considered in Chapter 46.

INDOOR AIR POLLUTION

For the past decade, in addition to outdoor air pollution, the existence and effects of indoor air pollution have been recognized; both have significant impact on human health. The major sources of indoor air pollution include residential heating and cooling devices, materials used in residential construction and furnishings, radon, molds spores, and cigarette smoking. Some indoor air pollutants listed by source location are shown in Table 13–1. Symptoms associated with these pollutants include headaches, drowsiness, nausea, eye and upper respiratory tract irritation, dizziness, skin itching and eruption, difficulty in breathing, and sinus congestion.

Tobacco Smoke Inhalation

There is mounting evidence that nonsmokers suffer negative health effects by inhaling the sidestream and exhaled smoke created by smokers (mainstream smoke). The concentration of gaseous and particulate constituents of tobacco smoke often are higher in sidestream than in mainstream smoke (Table 13–2). The health effects of involuntary smoke exposure have been reviewed recently by Weiss et al. (1983). This review led to several conclusions as follows: (1) eye irritation is the most common complaint relating to *acute* effects of contact with tobacco smoke; (2) approximately one third of subjects also report headache, nasal irritation, and cough; and, (3) in general, allergic subjects report no greater irritation than do nonallergic subjects. Also, studies to date have revealed no consistent change in pulmonary function in either normal or asthmatic subjects (Dahms et al., 1981; Shephard et al., 1979). *Chronic effects* of involuntary smoking, as reviewed in Weiss et al. (1983), include bronchitis, pneumonia, and other lower respiratory illnesses that are significantly more common in the first year of life in children who live with parents who smoke. Prenatal exposure may cause the conditions that are measured postnatally, such as low birth weight. The effects of involuntary smoking on pulmonary function are shown in Table 13–3.

Ekwo and coworkers (1983) demonstrated a relationship between parental smoking and hospitalization for respiratory illness in children before the age of two years. In a survey of 1355 children 6 to 12 years of age, the risk of hospitalization for respiratory illness before age 2 years was increased when one parent smoked ($p < 0.02$) or when gas was used for home cooking ($p < 0.001$). Kraemer and associates (1983) showed that children with household cigarette smoke exposure had an increased risk of developing persistent middle ear effusions. The risk of persistent middle ear effusions was further increased in allergic children living in smoker's households. This finding has been reinforced by an epidemiologic study, which

178

TABLE 13–1. A Summary of Air Pollution Sources*

Pollutants	Sources
GROUP I — SOURCES PREDOMINANTLY OUTDOOR	
Sulfur oxides (gases, particles)	Fuel combustion, nonferrous smelters
Ozone	Photochemical reactions
Pollens	Trees, grass, weeds, plants
Lead, manganese	Automobiles
Calcium, chlorine, silicon, cadmium	Suspension of soils or industrial emissions
Organic substances	Petrochemical solvents, natural sources, vaporization of unburned fuels
GROUP II — SOURCES BOTH INDOOR AND OUTDOOR	
Nitric oxide, nitrogen dioxide	Fuel burning
Carbon monoxide	Fuel burning
Carbon dioxide	Metabolic activity, combustion
Particles	Resuspension, condensation of vapors and combustion products
Water vapor	Biologic activity, combustion, evaporation
Organic substances	Volatilization, combustion, paint, metabolic action, pesticides, insecticides, fungicides
Spores	Fungi, molds
GROUP III — SOURCES PREDOMINANTLY INDOOR	
Radon	Building construction materials (concrete, stone), water, soil
Formaldehyde	Particleboard, insulation, furnishings, tobacco smoke, gas stoves
Asbestos, mineral and synthetic fibers	Fire-retardant, acoustic, thermal or electric insulation
Organic substances	Adhesives, solvents, cooking, cosmetics
Ammonia	Metabolic activity, cleaning products
Polycyclic hydrocarbons, arsenic, nicotine, acrolein, etc.	Tobacco smoke
Mercury	Fungicides in paints, spills in dental care facilities or laboratories, thermometer breakage
Aerosols	Consumer products
Viable organisms	Infections
Allergens	House dust, animal dander

* From Yocum, J.E.: Indoor-outdoor air quality relationships. A critical review. J. Air Poll. Control Assoc. 32:500–520, 1982.

included 337 children over a 3-month period and measured indoor environmental factors and incidence of middle ear effusions (Iversen et al., 1985). The only environmental factor positively correlated with increased frequency of middle ear effusion was parental smoking.

Tager and associates (1983) measured FEV_1 for 6 consecutive years in 1156 children from 404 families. They found after one, two, and five years a 10.7, 9.5, and 7.0 percent reduction in FEV_1 in children from homes of smoking mothers compared with homes of nonsmoking mothers. The investigators concluded that passive exposure to maternal cigarette smoke may have important effects on the development of pulmonary function in children. Collishaw and associates (1984) recently reviewed the effects of exposure to tobacco smoke in the workplace and concluded that there may not be a "safe" level of exposure. Pedreira and coworkers (1985) carried out a prospective study of 1144 infants. Smoking and family histories were evaluated for incidence of lower respiratory disease during the first year of life. Tracheitis and bronchitis occurred more frequently in infants exposed to cigarette smoke in the home, especially if there was a family history of respiratory illness. These workers concluded that passive smoking is dangerous to the health of infants and that infants born to families with histories of respiratory illness (e.g., chronic cough and bronchitis) are at increased risk of developing bronchitis or other lower respiratory tract disease.

A longitudinal study of respiratory health effects of indoor and outdoor air pollutants by Ware and associates (1984a) reported pulmonary function, respiratory illness history, and symptom history of 10,106 children. They found that maternal smoking was associated with increases of 20 to 35 percent in the rates of respiratory illnesses and respiratory symptoms.

TABLE 13–2. Constituents of Cigarette Smoke.[1] Ratio of
Sidestream Smoke (SS) to Mainstream Smoke (MS)*

Gas Phase	MS	SS/MS		MS	SS/MS
Carbon dioxide	20–60 mg	8.1	Nitrogen oxides (NO_x)		
Carbon monoxide	10–20 mg	2.5	Ammonia	80 μg	73
Methane	1.3 mg	3.1	Hydrogen cyanide	430 μg	0.25
Acetylene	27 μg	0.8	Acetonitrile	120 μg	3.9
Propane propene	0.5 mg	4.1	Pyridine	32 μg	10
Methylchloride	0.65 mg	2.1	3-Picoline	24 μg	13
Methylfuran	20 μg	3.4	3-Vinylpyridine	23 μg	28
Propionaldehyde	40 μg	2.4	Dimethylnitrosamine	10–65 μg	52
2-Butanone	80–250 μg	2.9	Nitrospyrrolidine	10–35 μg	27
Acetone	100–600 μg				

B Particulate Phase	MS	SS/MS		MS	SS/MS
"Tar"	1–40 mg	1.7	Quinoline	1.7 μg	11
Water	1–4 mg	2.4	Methylquinolines	0.7 μg	11
Toluene	108 μg	5.6	Aniline	360 ng	30
Stigmasterol	53 μg	0.8	2-Naphthylamine	2 ng	39
Total phytosterols	130 μg	0.8	4-Aminobiphenyl	5 ng	31
Phenol	20–150 μg	2.6	Hydrazine	32 ng	3
Catechol	130–280 μg	0.7	N'-Nitrosonornicotine	100–500 ng	5
Naphthalene	2.8 μg	16	NNK[2]	80–220 ng	10
Methylnaphthalene	2.2 μg	28	Nicotine	1–2.5 mg	2.7
Pyrene	50–200 μg	3.6			
Benzo(a)pyrene	20–40 μg	3.4			

[1] Nonfilter cigarette.

[2] NNK = 4-(N-methyl-N-nitrosamino)-1-(3-pyridyl)-1-butanone (tobacco specific carcinogenic nitrosamine).

* From Smoking and health, a report of the Surgeon General. DHEW Publication no. (PHS) 79–50066, 1979.

FEV_1 values were significantly lower for children whose parents smoked. These results provide strong support for a causal effect of sidestream cigarette smoke for increased respiratory illness and reduced FEV_1 values in preadolescent children.

Formaldehyde

In the early 1980's, the Chemical Industry Institute of Toxicology sponsored a long-term inhalation toxicology and carcinogenicity study of formaldehyde vapor in rats and mice (Kerns et al., 1983). Approximately one half of the rats exposed to 15 ppm of formaldehyde developed squamous cell carcinomas of the nasal cavity. Since formaldehyde is a ubiquitous chemical found in many consumer goods, the results of this study raised concern for human health. At the same time, there appeared to be increasing numbers of complaints about various "illnesses" believed to be caused by indoor air pollution. Many complaints were from people who lived in mobile homes where formaldehyde levels have been measured in the range of 50 to 500 ppb. The increase in complaints occurred because energy conservation has led to better insulated homes. Three reported respiratory responses to formaldehyde are throat irritation, airway obstruction, and cancer (Gamble, 1983) (Table 13–4).

Bernstein and coworkers (1984) reviewed the toxicology, epidemiology, monitoring, and control of formaldehyde inhalation exposure. They concluded that 30 percent of the general population experience characteristic irritant symptoms from exposures to 0.5 to 1.5 ppm of formaldehyde. Guidelines for monitoring and control of formaldehyde also are included in their report.

Robertson and associates (1985) surveyed two buildings with similar populations of workers who complained of "building sickness." One building was fully air conditioned with humidification, and the other was ventilated naturally. The occupants of the air conditioned building complained of rhinitis more frequently (28 percent) than occupants of the naturally ventilated building (5 percent). Other complaints were of nasal blockage and dry throats (35 percent versus 9 percent), lethargy

TABLE 13–3. Pulmonary Function in Children and Adults Exposed to Involuntary Smoking*

Population and Age Range (Source)	Pulmonary Function Measure	Outcome	Comments
816 children 7 to 17 yr of age in CT and SC† (Schilling)	FEV_1 as percent predicted	No effect of parental smoking	No control for sibship size or correlation of siblings' pulmonary function. Child's function first adjusted for parent's function; this adjustment may have marked any effect of parental smoking
444 children 5 to 19 yr of age in East Boston, MA† (Tager)	Maximal midexpiratory flow (MMEF) in standard deviation units	Significant effect of parental smoking	Analysis controlled for sibship size and correlation of siblings' pulmonary function
650 children 5 to 9 yr of age in East Boston, MA† (Weiss)	MMEF in standard deviation units	Significant effect of parental smoking	Analysis controlled for sibship size and correlation of siblings' pulmonary function
4000 children 6 to 13 years of age (Vedal)	FEV_{75}, FVC, $Vmax_{50}$, $Vmax_{75}$, $Vmax_{90}$	FVC positively associated flows, negatively associated	Flows dose response with amount smoked by mother
271 households with complete smoking histories of both parents and pulmonary function of children 6+, Tucson, AZ† (Lebowitz)	FEV_1, FVC, $Vmax_{50}$, $Vmax_{75}$ derived from Mef_1V curves, expressed as standard deviation units	No effect of parental smoking	Suggestion that real differences in indoor levels of exposure compared to more northern climates may be occurring
558 children 8 to 10 yr of age in AZ† (Dodge)	FEV_1 by age change FEV_1/H^3 per year	No effect of parental smoking	Potential bias in participation rates. Cross-sectional data not controlled for children's height. Annual change in FEV_1/H^3 at ages 8, 9, 11 consistently greater in nonsmoking households than 2-parent smoking households; however, statistical test not significant.
16,689 children 5 to 17 yr of age, 7 geographic regions in US (Hasselbladt)	FEV_{75} as percent predicted	Significant effect of mother's smoking but not father's smoking	Large number of children excluded because of invalid pulmonary function data or missing parental smoking data
8120 children 6 to 10 years in 6 US cities (Speizer)	FVC and FEV_1 as percent predicted	No effect for FEV_1 or FVC	A recent analysis of this cohort demonstrated an effect for FVC and FEV_1
10,000 children 6 to 11 yr of age in 6 US cities (Ware)	FEV_1 and FVC	FVC positively associated with smoking, FEV_1 negatively associated	FEV_1 dose response with amount smoked by mother
2100 adults in San Diego, CA† (White)	FVC, FEV_1 and MMF as percent predicted	Significant effect of office exposure to involuntary smoke	Potential bias in selection. Only assessed current cigarette smoke exposure
1724 adults in Washington County, MD† (Comstock)	FEV_1 as percent predicted	No effect of wives' smoking on husbands' pulmonary function	Includes adults 20+
7818 adults in 7 cities in France, selected subgroups (Kauffman)	FEV_1, FVC, and MMEF	Significant effect in wives of smoking husbands in all measures. Only for MMEF in husbands of smoking wives	Not adjusted for height. Dose response to amount of husbands' smoking for MMEF in wives. No effect below age 40.

* From Weiss, S.T. et al.: The health effects of involuntary smoking: State of the art. Am. Rev. Resp. Dis. 128:933–942, 1983.
† CT = Connecticut; SC = South Carolina; MA = Massachusetts; AZ = Arizona; CA = California; MD = Maryland.

TABLE 13-4. Summary of Epidemiologic Studies of Irritation from Formaldehyde (HCHO)*

Estimated exposure (PPM)	Type of exposure	Symptoms	Comment
0.1–0.5	Customers in dress shops	Burning and stinging of eyes and nose and throat irritation, headache	
0.9–2.7	Workers in garment factory (urea-formal-dehyde resin)	Lacrimation, nose and throat irritation	Dose-related adaptation in 15 to 20 min
0.1–5.3	7 embalmers in 6 funeral homes	Eye and nose burns, sneezing, coughing, headache	Dose-related; no control group
	57 of 80 embalmers	Eye irritation (81%), nose and throat irritation (75 percent), cough (37%), skin irritation (37%), chest tightness (23%), shortness of breath (10 percent), wheezing (12%)	Self-administered questionnaire; no control group; no environmental measures
>1 No phenol detected	4 embalmer instructors	Burning of eyes and nose, dryness of mouth and throat, cough, headache, lacrimation	NIOSH Health Hazard Evaluation, no symptoms when <1 ppm; early disability retirement with asthmatic bronchitis of instructor with 5 years' exposure
0.03–1.41	83 employees of particleboard and plywood manufacturing plant	Bodily fatigue (52%), headache, sore throat, cough, stuffy or runny nose (41 percent), eye discomfort (62 percent), respiratory or eye discomfort attributed to unsatisfactory air (38%), eye fatigue (21%), odor (41%)	Not dose-related
0.1–3 (most <1)	168 mobile home residents complaining of formaldehyde (102 > 18 years old)	Eye, nose, throat irritation (78 percent), cough and wheeze (38%), respiratory problems (30%), diarrhea (28%), headache (52%), nausea and vomiting (20%)	Mean HCHO concentration highest in homes of those with eye, nose, throat irritation; concentration related to age of mobile home; no control group; investigated complaints only
None detected–2.5 (91% <1)	Residents of 68 mobile homes with complaints (n = 239)	Eye irritation (34%), nose irritation (5%), respiratory tract (24%), headache (21%), nausea (5%), drowsiness (11%)	Not dose-related; no control group; investigated complaints only
	395 urea-formaldehyde-foam insulated homes; 400 control homes	*Prevalence* (exposed versus control): Asthma (1.1% versus 0.9%), wheezing (2.0% versus 0.9%) $p = 0.02$, burning skin (0.8% versus 0.2%), headache (1.9% versus 3.2%) $p = 0.04$, burning eyes (2.1% versus 2.6%), cough (2.7% versus 3%), symptomatic persons (15% versus 17%), symptomatic households (33% versus 35%)	No obvious differences between exposed and controls; prevalence much lower than previous studies.
		Incidence (exposed versus control): Wheezing (0.6% versus 0.1%) $p = 0.01$, burning skin (0.7% versus 0.1%) $p = 0.04$, symptomatic persons (9.9% versus 9.9%), symptomatic households (23% versus 24%)	No obvious differences between exposed and controls; incidence of symptoms twice as high in exposed households reporting *any* odor compared to exposed households reporting *no* odor
		Incidence (preinsulation versus postinsulation) (#/1000): asthma (1.2 versus 0.9), wheezing (1.2 versus 2.3), burning eyes (2.4 versus 5.5), runny nose (3.1 versus 3.2), cough (1.2 versus 12.4), headache (3.1 versus 3.7), symptomatic persons (15.3 versus 45.5), symptomatic households (21 versus 70)	Tendency for incidence of symptoms in preinsulation group to be higher than controls; dose-response in that postinsulation incidence higher than preinsulation

* Gamble, J.: Effects of formaldehyde on the respiratory system. *In* Gibson, J.E. (ed.), Formaldehyde Toxicity. New York, Hemisphere Publishing Corp., 1983.

(36 percent versus 13 percent), and headaches (31 percent versus 15 percent). An environmental assessment of the offices was performed to identify factors responsible for the differences in prevalance of these symptoms. Temperature, relative humidity, air velocity, positive and negative ions, CO, O_3, and formaldehyde concentrations were measured. None of these factors differed between the buildings, suggesting that building sickness was caused by other unknown factors.

Other studies have speculated that formaldehyde exposure might be related to increased respiratory illnesses in children (Tuthill, 1984) or to a wide range of illness symptoms (Harris et al., 1981). However, formaldehyde levels were not measured in either study.

Studies evaluating sensitivity to formaldehyde in allergic subjects have been carried out by exposing them directly to the vapor. Frigas and coworkers (1984) exposed 13 patients with asthmatic symptoms who thought they were clinically sensitive to formaldehyde; exposure to concentrations of 0.1, 1, and 3 ppm of the gas was compared with exposure to clean air. No significant decrease in FEV_1 following formaldehyde exposure compared with clean air exposure could be found. Sheppard and associates (1984) also exposed asthmatic subjects to 3 ppm of formaldehyde and found no increased pulmonary resistance. In studies with nonasthmatic subjects, Nordman and associates (1985) found that 12 of 230 persons who had occupational exposure to formaldehyde showed increased bronchial sensitivity to formaldehyde challenge tests. Seventy one of the 218 workers who did not respond to formaldehyde had positive responses to histamine or methacholine bronchial challenge tests. These investigators concluded that, although formaldehyde asthma is a rare disease, it probably is under-reported. Day and associates (1984) studied 18 subjects, nine of whom had previously complained of adverse affects from urea formaldehyde foam insulation (UFFI) in their homes. These subjects were exposed both to 1 ppm formaldehyde and to 1.2 ppm formaldehyde emitted directly from the foam insulation. No clinical responses or statistically significant changes in pulmonary function were found at 1 hour or 8 hours postexposure.

Burge and associates (1985) studied 15 workers exposed to formaldehyde in their occupation. Three workers had late asthmatic responses, which may have been due to hypersensitivity. Six workers developed immediate asthmatic reactions, which were likely due to direct irritant responses. The concentration of formaldehyde ($4.8\,mg/m^3$ or 3.9 ppm) required to elicit these responses was higher than that typically encountered in buildings. Main and Hogan (1983) studied 21 subjects who had been exposed to 0.12 to 1.6 ppm formaldehyde in mobile homes along with 18 unexposed subjects using questionnaires and pulmonary function tests. Although symptoms were more common in the exposed group, spirometry revealed no decrease in pulmonary function among the mobile home dwellers.

One occupation known for substantial exposure to formaldehyde is embalming. Levine and coworkers (1984) administered questionnaires and pulmonary function tests to 105 embalmers. Their results indicate that relatively high concentrations of the gas were not associated with signs of respiratory illness. On the other hand, Alexandersson and coworkers (1982) studied 47 workers exposed to formaldehyde in a carpentry shop and compared them with 20 unexposed workers. Pulmonary functions in the exposed workers were normal on Monday morning. After an 8-hour workday, FEV_1 decreased an average of 0.2 L in the formaldehyde exposed workers, in contrast to those not exposed ($p < 0.002$), suggesting bronchoconstriction secondary to prolonged exposure to formaldehyde.

There have been several reports of contact dermatitis caused by formaldehyde. Kofoed (1984) reported the case of a woman who developed subacute eczema confined to the neck, axillae, elbow flexures, and the breast area corresponding to that covered by the brassiere. The eruption was traced to the fabric softener used, which the manufacturer stated contained 0.4 to 0.7 percent formaldehyde as a preservative. Bruze and coworkers (1985) evaluated contact sensitivity to phenol-formaldehyde resins. Of 1220 patients given patch tests to the resin, 26 had positive results. Adverse reactions included depigmentation, irritant dermatitis, chemical burns, and allergic contact dermatitis. The investigators suggest adding a battery of phenol-formaldehyde resins to the standard patch-testing screening process.

Contact dermatitis to other agents is prevalent. Weston and Weston (1984) estimate that allergic contact dermatitis accounts for up to 20 percent of all dermatitis in childhood. They list the major sources of contact allergy in children as metals, shoes, preservatives, and plants (see also Chapter 30.)

Gas and Wood Stoves

As part of a long-range prospective study of the health effects of air pollution, approximately 8000 children, 6 to 10 years of age from six communities, were given questionnaires and pulmonary function tests (Speizer et al., 1980). Comparisons were made between children living in homes with gas or electric stoves. Children from households with gas stoves had greater histories of respiratory illnesses before age two and reduced pulmonary function tests. Parental smoking did not explain the difference. NO_2 concentrations were found to be 4 to 7 times higher in the homes with gas stoves. However, this group found subsequently, looking at a larger sample, that none of the respiratory illnesses and symptoms in the 10,106 children studied was significantly associated with exposure to gas cooking (Ware et al., 1984a). Exposure to gas stoves was associated with reductions of 0.7 percent in mean FEV_1 at the first examination ($p < 0.01$) and 0.3 percent at the second examination (nonsignificant). These results suggest that exposure to gas stoves may be associated with a transitory reduced pulmonary function but that such exposure does not seem to increase respiratory illness among children.

Melia and associates (1982) also examined the possible association between respiratory illness and use of gas for cooking in 179 schoolchildren, 5 and 6 years old. NO_2 was measured for 1 week in the child's bedroom and the living room. NO_2 concentrations ranged from 4.7 to 160.8 ppb in the bedrooms and 9.0 to 292 ppb in the living rooms. No statistically significant relationship was found between respiratory illnesses and NO_2 levels, although there was a tendency for more respiratory illnesses in children from the homes with the higher NO_2 levels. A significantly positive association was found, however, between the prevalence of respiratory complaints and relative humidity. The workers concluded that there may be a weak association between NO_2 levels and respiratory illnesses. The relationship between respiratory illness and the use of gas stoves also was examined from data on 1565 infants in Dundee, Scotland, in 1980 (Ogston et al., 1985). Both hospital admissions and illness episodes were more common in infants from houses using gas for cooking, but differences were not statistically significant. This study also is consistent with the idea that there is a weak relationship between respiratory illness and gas stove emissions.

Hoek and coworkers (1984) attempted to examine the relationship between respiratory symptoms of Rotterdam, the Netherlands, schoolchildren and NO_2 levels. All six-year-old schoolchildren were examined, and those with respiratory symptoms were selected for study along with case controls. NO_2 concentrations were measured in all the children's homes, but varied so widely that comparisons between the groups based on possible differences in NO_2 concentrations could not be made. Fischer and associates (1985) found no association between NO_2 level in the house and pulmonary function decline in 97 nonsmoking adult women in the Netherlands.

Wood smoke, as well as NO_2, has been a subject of concern and study with respect to childhood respiratory health. The incidence of symptoms of respiratory illness among preschool children living in homes heated with wood-burning stoves was examined (Honicky et al., 1985). Sixty-two children were in the study group with a case-matched control group. During the winter of 1982, moderate to severe respiratory symptoms were significantly greater in the study group compared with the control group. Thus, indoor heating with wood-burning stoves may be a significant etiologic factor in the occurrence of symptoms of respiratory illness in young children.

OUTDOOR POLLUTION

Controlled, Human Studies

The six ambient air pollutants regulated by the United States Environmental Protection Agency (EPA) are sulfur dioxide (SO_2), nitrogen dioxide (NO_2), ozone (O_3), suspended particulate matter (PM), carbon monoxide (CO), and airborne lead. There is compelling evidence that asthmatic subjects are much more sensitive to effects of inhaled SO_2 than are healthy, nonasthmatic subjects. Jaeger and coworkers (1979) exposed normal and asthmatic subjects to 0.5 ppm SO_2 or ambient air for 3 hours: mid-maximal expiratory flow rates decreased only in the asthmatic subjects and lasted for the duration of the SO_2 exposures. Koenig and coworkers (1981, 1982a, and 1983a) showed that asthmatic adolescent subjects who inhaled 0.5 or 1.0 ppm SO_2 during moderate exercise demonstrated large reductions in pulmonary function, approximately 20 times greater than those seen in healthy adolescent subjects under similar conditions. Similarly increased sensitivity to SO_2 has been shown in adult asthmatic subjects (Sheppard et al., 1981; Linn et al., 1983). Koenig and coworkers (1982b) showed that allergic adolescents who never had been diagnosed as having asthma and whose only sign of airways hypersensitivity was exercise-induced bronchospasm also were hypersensitive to the effects of inhaled SO_2.

Asthmatic adolescents also show increased sensitivity to 100 $\mu g/m^3$ of sulfuric acid (H_2SO_4), a common atmospheric transformation product of SO_2 and form of suspended particulate matter (Koenig et al., 1983b). This is not so clearly the case in adult asthmatic subjects. Avol and coworkers (1979) found no difference between normal and asthmatic subjects in the pulmonary response to inhalation of 100 $\mu g/m^3$ of H_2SO_4 exposure. Utell and associates (1983) found increased airways resistance following inhalation of 1000 $\mu g/m^3$ of H_2SO_4 in adult asthmatics but saw no changes following inhalation of 100 $\mu g/m^3$. It appears, therefore, that adolescent asthmatic subjects may be more sensitive to inhaled H_2SO_4 than adult asthmatic subjects.

Cold, dry air is known to act as an irritant in asthma. Two groups have studied the effects of a combination of SO_2 and cold, dry air on adults with asthma. Linn and coworkers (1984) found that moderate cold stress (5°C) exaggerated the SO_2 effect only slightly and inconsistently. Sheppard and coworkers (1984b) challenged asthmatic subjects with colder air ($-20°C$) and found that the concentration of SO_2, which caused a 100 pecent increase in airways resistance, was significantly lower (as low as 0.1 ppm SO_2) when it was inhaled in the colder, dry air.

Increased sensitivity has not been shown for the other five criteria air pollutants (CO, NO_x, O_3, total suspended particulate (TSP) matter, lead) in asthmatics. There is one report of an exaggerated response in adult asthmatic patients to a carbachol challenge following inhalation of 0.1 ppm NO_2 (Orehek et al., 1976). Kleinman and coworkers (1983) found a variable change in bronchial reactivity following exposure to 0.2 ppm NO_2 in adult asthmatics. Other investigators (Hazucha, et al., 1983) were not able to demonstrate increased bronchial sensitivity after NO_2 exposure. Koenig and coworkers (1985) found no difference in the pulmonary response to 0.12 ppm NO_2 or 0.12 ppm O_3 between healthy and asthmatic adolescent subjects. Using a higher concentration of NO_2 (approximately 0.5 ppm), Bylin and associates (1985) did demonstrate increased bronchial sensitivity in asthmatic subjects. However, both asthmatic and healthy subjects showed changes in pulmonary function following this concentration of NO_2.

Although ozone (O_3) is toxic for the human respiratory tract (EPA, 1978, see Air quality criteria for ozone and other photochemical oxidants), adult asthmatic subjects appear to be no more sensitive than healthy subjects to inhaled O_3. Holtzman and associates (1979) found no difference in the inducibility or time course of bronchial hyperactivity between nonatopic and atopic adult subjects, following a 2-hour exposure to 0.6 ppm O_3. Linn and coworkers (1980) compared the pulmonary responses of normal and asthmatic adult subjects following exposure to approximately 0.2 ppm O_3. Slight effects were seen but there was no difference between the two groups. Silverman (1979) has shown that asthmatic subjects are quite sensitive to 0.25 ppm O_3 exposures at rest; one third of these subjects showed greater changes in maximal expiratory flow rates following the O_3 exposures, as compared with the clean air exposures.

Respiratory responses to CO or airborne lead have not been studied, since the lung is not a target organ for either pollutant.

Epidemiologic Studies

Severe air pollution, including the "killer smog" episodes of Donora, Pennsylvania and London, England, has been associated with striking increases in morbidity and mortality in individuals with respiratory tract disease. Other than such apparent associations, attempts to obtain more precise delineation of the effects of air pollution on human health have been largely inconclusive. Epidemiologic studies on this relationship are difficult to design for the following reasons: (1) aerometric monitoring data often are inadequate either because the data are not precise or because the monitoring stations are widely placed, and the results are difficult to relate to individual residences or locations; (2) health endpoint (effects) data often are inadequate because they are based on individual symptom reporting or parental recall of childhood illness; and (3) variables such as cigarette smoking history, time spent outdoors, occupational exposure, coexisting pollutants, health and nutritional status, and respiratory infections confound the issue. Nevertheless, epidemiologic studies are the only method for determining chronic effects of air pollution on human health.

Most of the historical killer smog episodes involved SO_2 and total suspended particulate (TSP) matter. The health effects of these pollutants were reviewed by the EPA (see Air quality criteria for particulate matter and sulfur oxides), the agency authorized to set ambient air quality standards that protect public health (1982) and by Ware and associates (1984b). Although there is agreement that the historically severe air pollution episodes caused numbers of deaths over predicted numbers and increased incidence of respiratory illness, the effect of current ordinary ranges of air pollutant concentrations is not so clear.

The American Thoracic Society newsletter (1978) reported increased mortality, chronic respiratory illness, episodes of asthma, lower respiratory tract infections in adults and children, upper respiratory infections in children, symptoms of coronary artery disease, and sensory irritation associated with air pollution.

Detels and his associates conducted population studies of chronic obstructive pulmonary disease in the Los Angeles area. In one phase of their studies, they found a higher prevalence of decreased FEV_1 and closing volume values in participants residing in areas of higher concentrations of air pollutants (Detels et al., 1981). The pollutants involved were photochemical oxidants, NO_2, and sulfates. Lutz (1983) examined diagnoses made in a family practice center during an episode of high air pollution in Salt Lake City. Pollutants measured were CO, O_3, and TSP matter. In this study, pollution related disease (upper and lower respiratory irritation or infection, asthma, pneumonia, and ischemic heart disease) was significantly higher with TSP matter level (r = 0.79) and percentage of smoke and fog (r = 0.79) but was not related to ozone level (r = −0.67). These results relate to the acute rather than the chronic effects of air pollution.

Ware and coworkers (1984b) concluded that the effects of acute exposure to SO_2 and TSP matter were frequently associated with excess mortality and morbidity, but that there was relatively little evidence documenting such effects at concentrations of SO_2 below 1000 $\mu g/m^3$ (1000 $\mu g/m^3$ SO_2 is equal to 0.35 ppm SO_2). This concentration was used because ambient air in the United States has not exceeded these concentrations since the early 1970's, as a result of enforcement of the Clean Air Act. Evidence for mortality caused by chronic exposure to SO_2 or particulate matter was inconclusive, although evidence for increased morbidity demonstrated by a higher prevalence of respiratory illness was more impressive. Lipfert (1985) subsequently reached the same conclusion.

Frezieres and coworkers (1982) examined severity of daytime and nighttime symptoms and medication usage in 34 asthmatic subjects and correlated these with pollutant-pollen levels and meteorologic observations over an 8-month period. Three of the 34 subjects (9 percent) appeared to report symptoms that correlated highly with suspended sulfate levels. Perry and coworkers (1983) also studied symptoms, medication usage, and peak expiratory flow rate in asthmatics during a three-month period in which Denver air pollution levels were generally high although variable. CO, SO_2, O_3, TSP matter, temperature, and barometric pressure were measured. Of the environmental variants studied, only fine nitrates were associated with increased symptom reports and aerosolized bronchodilator usage. Mazumdar and Sussman (1983) examined mortality and morbidity in Allegheny County, Pennsylvania in relation to levels of SO_2 and particulate matter (PM) obtained from three monitoring stations. Analysis indicated a possible association between heart disease mortality/morbidity and PM levels but no association between SO_2 levels and total disease mortality/morbidity was found.

The prevalence of respiratory symptoms, ascertained by questionnaire, was evaluated in 6666 nonsmokers who lived for at least 11 years in either a high photochemical pollution area (4379 individuals) or a low photochemical pollution area (2287 individuals) (Hodgkin et al., 1984). The risk estimate for chronic obstructive pulmonary disease (COPD), as defined in this study (cough or sputum production or both on most days for the previous 2 years) was 15 percent higher in the high pollution area.

Linn and associates (1983b) employed a movable environmental chamber to expose asthmatic subjects for 2 hours during intermittent exercise either to the ambient air (Los Angeles area) or to purified clean air. Subjects were studied in the summer of 1981 when the ambient O_3 was 0.156 ± 0.055 ppm. They found only a 2 percent (insignificant) drop in FEV_1 following the O_3 exposure. Lippmann and coworkers (1983) studied children attending two weeks of summer camp. Daily O_3 concentrations, spirometric values, and peak flows were measured. O_3 levels of 0.10 ppm or more appeared to be associated with diminished FEV_1 values; this reduction in FEV_1 was not seen when the O_3 concentration was below 0.08 ppm.

Meteorologic Conditions

Weather changes commonly appear to be associated with worsening of asthma. A small number of studies have attempted to correlate asthmatic attacks with various weather-related phenomena, including the concentrations of positive and negative ions. Ions always are present in the atmosphere as a result of cosmic radiation and the natural radioactivity of the earth's surface. Ion concentrations can vary significantly with marked weather changes and in some indoor environments.

Two studies have investigated the relationship between negative ions and asthmatic symptoms in the laboratory. Ben-Dov and associates (1983) studied 11 asthmatic children during exercise and histamine challenge. Children also breathed negatively ionized air or nonionized air in a double blind fashion. Exercise-induced asthma was attenuated significantly by exposure to negative ions. The response to histamine following ion exposure was variable. Nogrady and Furnass (1983) found no benefit from inhaling negative ions in a long-term study. Twenty asthmatic subjects were studied over six months. Negative or placebo ionizers were placed in the subjects' bedrooms for 8-week periods. There were no significant differences among peak flow values, symptom ratings, and medication usage associated with negative ion generation.

Klabuschnigg and associates (1981) examined the relationship between local and central European weather, pollen and spore counts, asthmatic complaints, and drug requirements in 40 asthmatic children during a 6-week summer camp. The influence of local weather patterns on asthmatic symptoms appeared to be negligible in this study. Wagner and coworkers (1983) studied the hypothesis that small changes in the concentration of positive ions that occur in association with weather fronts are responsible for aggravation of asthmatic symptoms. Pulmonary function was measured in 12 patients, four times daily, during two episodes of inclement weather. There was no significant association between mean peak flow rates and ion levels or other meteorologic factors. Chipps

and coworkers (1984) studied 54 children attending a summer camp for asthmatics. Pulmonary function was measured regularly over an 8-week period. No additive effects of changes in weather conditions on pulmonary function could be found in these children.

Packe and Ayres (1985) examined an outbreak of asthma that occurred during a thunderstorm. Acute asthmatic symptoms began at a time of sudden changes in the weather. Air pollution was low during this period. The large and sudden increase in numbers of airborne fungal spores, especially *Didymella exitialis* and *Sporobolomyces*, around the time of the outbreak suggested that these spores may have been etiologic factors. A subsequent report suggested the presence of calcium sulfate crystals may have been responsible for this outbreak of acute asthma (Morrow-Brown and Jackson, 1985).

OCCUPATIONAL EXPOSURES

In the last decade, occupational etiologies for allergic disease have been recognized (Table 13-5). Occupational asthma is discussed in Chapter 46. A summary of causes of occupational asthma also is given in Table 13–5. A recent review by Becklake (1985) discusses the relationship between occupational exposures and chronic airflow limitations. This review suggests that individual susceptibility underlies the development of chronic respiratory disease from exposure to occupational agents.

About 5 percent of workers exposed to volatile isocyanates, 10 to 45 percent of workers exposed to proteolytic enzymes, and 2 to 40 percent of workers exposed to grain dust develop asthma (Brooks, 1983). Varying degrees of self-selection may account for some of the variations in these data. For example, Broder and associates (1979) found that positive skin reactions to pollens and molds and a family history of asthma were less frequent among grain elevator workers than among control groups. In contrast to other substances encountered in the workplace, western red cedar and toluene diisocyanate cause asthma in nonatopic individuals.

Thiel and Ulmer (1980) studied a group of bakers, including healthy apprentice bakers, healthy male bakers with a mean occupational history of 32 years, and bakers with "bakers' asthma." Total IgE levels and numbers of blood eosinophilic leukocytes were significantly ele-

TABLE 13–5. Some Causes of Occupational Asthma*

Occupation	Industrial Exposures
Animal handlers	Hair, epidermal squamae, mites, small insects, danders, urine protein
Apiarist, entomologist	Bee toxin, squamae from bees, hairs, chitin
Antibiotic workers	Penicillin, ampicillin
Baker, miller, grain worker	Flour, grain dust, grain weevil
Brewer or farmer	Hops
Celery picker	Pink-rot fungus
Cheese workers	*Penicillium casei*
Coffee worker	Green coffee dust
Cotton, flax, hemp workers, weavers, textile workers	Cotton, flax, hemp
Culture oyster workers	Marine organisms
Detergent industry or laundry workers	*Bacillus subtilis*
Feather workers	Uncleaned feathers, mites, moths
Food technologist	Papain
Hairdressers	Human hair
Morticians	Formaldehyde
Outdoor workers	River flies, screwworm flies, locust, Mexican bean beetle, sewage flies
Paprika splitter	Molds
Silkworm cutters	Silk hair, butterfly squamae, silk glue (sericin)
Soybean workers	Soybean flour and dust
Spice workers	Garlic powder
Tea makers	Tea fluff
Tea workers	Green leaf tea
Tobacco workers	Green leaf tobacco
Wood workers	Wood dusts of various types

* Brooks, S.M.: Bronchial asthma of occupational origin. *In* Rom, W.N., Environmental and Occupational Medicine. Boston, Little, Brown and Co., 1983.

vated in the bakers with asthma. Asthmatic symptoms were more prevalent among apparently healthy bakers than among apprentices (50 percent versus 25 percent). Bronchial sensitivity, as measured by the methacholine challenge test, was higher in apprentices than in a control group of students. The range of susceptibility to grain dusts is broad, and the role of genetic susceptibility has not been investigated.

Nordman (1984) recently considered the relationship between atopy and occupational settings. He noted that work-related hypersensitivity symptoms cannot be eradicated by eliminating atopic individuals from the workplace. The intensity of exposure to causative agents often is extremely high in occupational settings that can trigger the production of specific IgE antibodies even in nonatopic workers.

REFERENCES

Air quality criteria for ozone and other photochemical oxidants. USEPA EPA 600/8–78–004, 1978.
Air quality criteria for particulate matter and sulfur oxides. USEPA EPA 600/8–82–029c, 1982.

Alexandersson, R., Hedenstierna, G., Kolmodin-Hedman, B.: Exposure to formaldehyde: Effects on pulmonary function. Arch. Environ. Health 37:279–284, 1982.
American Thoracic Society. Health effects of air pollution. New York, 1978.
Avol, E.L., Jones, M.P., Bailey, R.M., Chang, N-M.N., Kleinman, M.T., Linn, W.S., Bell, K.A., Hackney, J.D.: Controlled exposures of human volunteers to sulfate aerosols: Health effects and aerosol characterization. Am. Rev. Resp. Dis. 120: 319–328, 1979.
Becklake, M.R.: Chronic airflow limitation: Its relationship to work in dusty occupations. Chest 88:608–617, 1985.
Ben-Dov, I., Amirav, I., Shochina, M., Amitai, I., Bar-Yishoy, E., Godfrey, S.: Effect of negative ionization of inspired air on the response of asthmatic children to exercise and inhaled histamine. Thorax 38:584–588, 1983.
Bernstein, R., Stayner, L.T., Elliott, L.J., Kimbrough, R., Falk, H., Blade, L.: Inhalation exposure to formaldehyde: An overview of its toxicology, epidemiology, monitoring and control. Am. Ind. Hyg. Assoc. J. 45:778–785, 1984.
Broder, I., Mintz, S., Hutcheon, M., Corey, P., Silverman, F., Davies, G., Leznoff, A., Peress, L., Thomas, P.: Comparison of respiratory variables in grain elevator workers and civic outside workers in Thunder Bay, Canada. Am. Rev. Resp. Dis. 119:193–203, 1979.
Brooks, S.M.: Bronchial asthma of occupational origin. *In* Rom, W.N. (ed.), Environmental and Occupational Medicine. Boston, Little, Brown and Co., 1983.

Burge, P.S., Harries, M.G., Lam, W.K., O'Brien, I.M., Patchell, P.A.: Occupational asthma due to formaldehyde. Thorax 40:255–260, 1985.

Bruze, M., Fregert, S., Zimerson, E.: Contact allergy to phenol-formaldehyde resins. Contact Dermatitis 12:81–86, 1985.

Bylin, G., Lindvall, T., Rehn, T., Sundin, B.: Effects of short-term exposure to ambient nitrogen dioxide concentrations on human bronchial reactivity and lung function. Eur. J. Resp. Dis. 66:205–217, 1985.

Chipps, B.E., Mak, H., Menkes, H.A., Schuberth, K.C., Talamo, J.H., Talamo, R.C., Permutt, S., Scherr, M.S., Mellits, E.D.: Do weather conditions change pulmonary function of asthmatics at summer camp? J. Asthma 21:15–20, 1984.

Collishaw, N.E., Kirkbride, J., Wigle, D.T.: Tobacco smoke in the workplace: An occupational health hazard. Can. Med. Assoc. J. 131:1199–1204, 1984.

Dahms, T.E., Bolin, J.E., Slavin, R.G.: Passive smoking: Effects on bronchial asthma. Chest 80:530–534, 1981.

Day, J.H., Lees, R.E.M., Clark, R.H., Patlee, P.L.: Respiratory response to formaldehyde and off-gas urea formaldehyde foam insulation. Can. Med. Assoc. J. 131:1061–1063, 1984.

Detels, R., Sayre, J.W., Coulson, A.H., Rokaw, S.N., Massey, F.J., Tashkin, D.P., Wu, M-M.: The UCLA population studies of chronic obstructive pulmonary disease. IV. Respiratory effect of long-term exposure to photochemical oxidants, nitrogen dioxide and sulfates on current and never smokers. Am. Rev. Resp. Dis. 124:673–680, 1981.

Ekwo, E., Weinberger, M.M., Lachenbruch, P.A., Huntley, W.H.: Relationship of parental smoking and gas cooking to respiratory disease in children. Chest 84:662–668, 1983.

Fischer, P., Remjin, B., Brunekreef, B., van der Lende, R., Schouten, J., Quanjer, P.: Indoor air pollution and its effects on pulmonary function of adult non-smoking women. II. Associations between nitrogen dioxide and pulmonary function. Int. J. Epidemiol. 14:221–226, 1985.

Frezieres, R.G., Coulson, A.H., Katz, R.M., Detels, R., Siegel, S.C., Rachelefsky, G.S.: Response of individuals with reactive airway disease to sulfates and other atmospheric pollutants. Ann. Allergy 48:156–165, 1982.

Frigas, E., Filley, W.V., Reed, C.E.: Bronchial challenge with formaldehyde gas: Lack of bronchoconstriction in 13 patients suspected of having formaldehyde-induced asthma. Mayo Clin. Proc. 59:295–299, 1984.

Gamble, J.: Effects of formaldehyde on the respiratory system. *In* Gibson, J.E. (ed.), Formaldehyde Toxicity. New York, Hemisphere Publishing Corp., 1983.

Harris, J.G., Rumack, B.H., Aldrich, F.D.: Toxicology of urea formaldehyde and polyureathane foam insulation. J. Am. Med. Assoc. 245:243–246, 1981.

Hazucha, M.J., Ginsberg, J.F., McDonnell, W.F., Haak, E.D. Jr., Pimmel, R.L., Salaam, S.A., House, D.E., Bromberg, P.A.: Effects of 0.1 ppm nitrogen dioxide on airways of normal and asthmatic subjects. J. Appl. Physiol. 54:730–739, 1983.

Hodgkin, J.E., Abbey, D.E., Euler, G.L., Magie, A.R.: COPD prevalence in nonsmokers in high and low photochemical air pollution areas. Chest 86:830–838, 1984.

Hoek, G., Brunekreef, B., Meijer, R., Scholten, A., Boleij, J.: Indoor nitrogen dioxide pollution and respiratory symptoms in school children. Int. Arch. Occup. Environ. Health. 55:79–86, 1984.

Holtzman, M.J., Cunningham, J.H., Sheller, J.R., Irsigler, G.B., Nadel, J.A., Boushey, H.A.: Effect of ozone on bronchial reactivity in atopic and nonatopic subjects. Am. Rev. Resp. Dis. 120:1059–1067, 1979.

Honicky, R.E., Osborne, J.S., Akpom, C.A.: Symptoms of respiratory illness in young children and the use of wood-burning stoves for indoor heating. Pediatrics 75:587–593, 1985.

Iversen, M., Birch, L., Lundqvist, G.R., Elbrond, O.: Middle ear effusion in children and the indoor environment: An epidemiologic study. Arch. Environ. Health 40:74–79, 1985.

Jaeger, M.J., Tribble, D., Wittig, H.J.: Effect of 0.5 ppm sulfur dioxide on the respiratory function of normal and asthmatic subjects. Lung 156:119–127, 1979.

Kerns, W.D., Parkov, K.L., Donofrio, D.J., Gralla, E.J., Swenberg, J.A.: Carcinogenicity of formaldehyde in rats and mice after long-term inhalation exposure. Cancer Res. 43:4382–4392, 1983.

Klabuschnigg, A., Gotz, M., Horak, F., Jager, S., Machalek, A., Popow, C., Haschke, F., Skoda-Turk, R.: Influence of aerobiology and weather on symptoms in children with asthma. Respiration 42:52–60, 1981.

Kleinman, M.T., Bailey, R.M., Linn, W.S., Anderson, K.R., Whynot, J.D., Shamoo, D.A., Hackney, J.D.: Effects of 0.2 ppm nitrogen dioxide on pulmonary function and response to bronchoprovocation in asthmatics. J. Toxicol. Environ. Health 12:815–826, 1983.

Koenig, J.Q., Pierson, W.E., Horike, M., Frank, R.: Effects of SO_2 plus NaCl aerosol combined with moderate exercise on pulmonary function in asthmatic adolescents. Environ. Res. 25:340–348, 1981.

Koenig, J.Q., Pierson, W.E., Horike, M., Frank, R.: Effects of inhaled SO_2 on pulmonary function in healthy adolescents exposed during rest and exercise. Arch. Environ. Health 37:5–9, 1982a.

Koenig, J.Q., Pierson, W.E., Horike, M., Frank, R.: Bronchoconstrictor responses to sulfur dioxide or sulfur dioxide plus sodium chloride droplets in allergic nonasthmatic adolescents. J. Allergy Clin. Immunol. 69:399–344, 1982b.

Koenig, J.Q., Pierson, W.E., Horike, M., Frank, R.: A comparison of the pulmonary effects of 0.5 ppm versus 1.0 ppm sulfur dioxide plus sodium chloride droplets in asthmatic adolescents. J. Toxicol. Environ. Health 11:129–139, 1983a.

Koenig, J.Q., Covert, D.S., Morgan, M.S., Horike, M., Horike, N., Marshall, S.G., Pierson, W.E.: Acute effect of 0.12 ppm ozone or 0.12 ppm nitrogen dioxide on pulmonary function in healthy and asthmatic adolescents. Am. Rev. Resp. Dis. 132:648–651, 1985.

Koenig, J.Q., Pierson, W.E., Horike, M.: The effects of inhaled sulfuric acid on pulmonary function in adolescent asthmatics. Am. Rev. Resp. Dis. 128:221–225, 1983b.

Kofoed, M.L.: Contact dermatitis to formaldehyde in fabric softeners. Contact Dermatitis 11:254, 1984.

Kraemer, M.J., Richardon, M.A., Weiss, N.S., Furukawa, C.T., Shapiro, G.G., Pierson, W.E., Bierman, C.W.: Risk factors for persistent middle-ear effusions. J.A.M.A. 249:1022–1025, 1983.

Levine, R.J., DalCorso, R.D., Blunden, P.B., Battigelli, M.C.: The effects of occupational exposure on the respiratory health of West Virginia morticians. J. Occup. Med. 26:91–97, 1984.

Linn, W.S., Jones, M.P., Bachmayer, E.A., Spier, C.E., Mazur, S.F., Avol, E.L., Hackney, J.D.: Short-term respiratory effects of polluted ambient air: A laboratory study of volunteers in a high-oxidant community. Am. Rev. Resp. Dis. 121:243–252, 1980.

Linn, W.S., Venet, T.G., Shamoo, D.A., Valencia, L.M., Anzar, U.T., Spier, C.E., Hackney, J.D.: Respiratory effects of sulfur dioxide in heavily exercising asthmatics. Am. Rev. Resp. Dis. 127:278–283, 1983.

Linn, W.S., Shamoo, D.A., Venet, T.G., Bailey, R.M., Wightman, L.H., Hackney, J.D.: Comparative effects of sulfur dioxide exposures at 5°C and 22°C in exercising asthmatics. Am. Rev. Resp. Dis. 129:234–239, 1984.

Linn, W.S., Avol, E.L., Hackney, J.D.: Effects of ambient oxidant pollutants on humans: A movable environmental chamber study. In Lee, S.D., Mustafa, M.G., Mehlman, M.A. (eds.), International Symposium on the Biomedical Effects of Ozone and Related Photochemical Oxidants. Advances in Modern Environmental Toxicology, vol. 5, 1983.

Lipfert, F.W.: Mortality and air pollution: Is there a meaningful connection? Env. Sci. Technol. 19:764–770, 1985.

Lippmann, M., Lioy, P.J., Leikauf, G., Green, K.B., Baxter, D., Morandi, M., Pasternack, B.S., Fife, D., Speizer, F.E.: Effects of ozone on the pulmonary function of children. In Lee, S.D., Mustafa, M.G., Mehlman, M.A. (eds.), International Symposium on the Biomedical Effects of Ozone and Related Photochemical Oxidants. Advances in Modern Environmental Toxicology, vol. 5, 1983.

Lutz, L.J.: Health effects of air pollution measured by outpatient visits. J. Fam. Pract. 16:307–313, 1983.

Main, D.M., Hogan, T.J.: Health effects of low-level exposure to formaldehyde. J. Occup. Med. 25:896–900, 1983.

Mazumdar, S., Sussman, N.: Relationship of air pollution to health: Results from the Pittsburgh Study. Arch. Environ. Health 38:17–24, 1983.

Melia, R.J.W., Florey C. du V., Morris, R.W., Goldstein, B.D., John, H.H., Clark, D., Craighead, I.B., MacKinlay, J.C.: Childhood respiratory illness and home environment. II. Association between respiratory illness and nitrogen dioxide, temperatue and relative humidity. Int. J. Epidemiol. 11:164–169, 1982.

Morrow-Brown, H., Jackson, F.A.: Asthma outbreak during a thunderstorm. Lancet 2:562, 1985.

Nogrady, S.G., Furnass, S.B.: Ionisers in the management of bronchial asthma. Thorax 38:919–922, 1983.

Nordman, H.: Atopy and work. Scand. J. Work. Environ. Health 10:481–485, 1984.

Nordman, H., Keskinen, H., Tuppurainen, M.: Formaldehyde asthma — rare or overlooked. J. Allergy Clin. Immunol. 75:91–99, 1985.

Ogston, S.A., Florey, C du V., Walker, C.H.M. The Tayside infant morbidity and mortality study: Effect on health of using gas for cooking. Brit. Med. J. 290:957–959, 1985.

Orehek, J., Massari, J.P., Gayrard, P., Grimaud, C., Charpin, J.: Effect of short-term, low-level nitrogen dioxide exposure on bronchial sensitivity of asthmatic patients. J. Clin. Invest. 57:301–307, 1976.

Packe, G.E., Ayres, J.G.: Asthma outbreak during a thunderstorm. Lancet 2:199–204, 1985.

Pedreira, F.A., Guandolo, V.L., Feroli, E.J., Mella, G.W., Weiss, I.P.: Involuntary smoking and incidence of respiratory illness during the first year of life. Pediatrics 75:594–597, 1985.

Perry, G.B., Chai, H., Dickey, D.W., Jones, R.H., Kinsman, R.A., Morrill, C.G., Spector, S.L., Weiser, P.C.: Effects of particulate air pollution on asthmatics. Am. J. Public Health 73:50–56, 1983.

Robertson, A.S., Burge, P.S., Hedge, A., Sims, J., Gill, F.S., Finnegan, M., Pickering, C.A.C., Dalton, G.: Comparison of health problems related to work and environmental measurements in two office buildings with different ventilation systems. Brit. Med. J. 291:373–376, 1985.

Shephard, R.J., Collins, R., Silverman, F.: Passive exposure of asthmatic subjects to cigarette smoke. Environ. Res. 20:392–402, 1979.

Sheppard, D., Eschenbacher, W.L., Boushey, H.A., Bethel, R.A.: Magnitude of interaction between the bronchomotor effects of sulfur dioxide and those of cold (dry) air. Am. Rev. Resp. Dis. 130:52–55, 1984.

Sheppard, D., Saisho, A., Nadel, J.A., Boushey, H.A.: Exercise increases sulfur dioxide–induced bronchoconstriction in asthmatic subjects. Am. Rev. Resp. Dis. 123:486–491, 1981.

Sheppard, D., Eschenbacher, W.L., Epstein, J.: Lack of bronchomotor response to up to 3 ppm formaldehyde in subjects with asthma. Environ. Res. 35:133–139, 1984.

Silverman, F.: Asthma and respiratory irritants (ozone). Environ. Health Perspect. 29:131–136, 1979.

Smoking and health. A report of the Surgeon General. DHEW Publication no. (PHS) 79–50066, 1979.

Speizer, E.E., Ferris, B., Bishop, Y.M.M., Spengler, J.: Respiratory disease rates and pulmonary function in children associated with NO$_2$ exposure. Am. Rev. Resp. Dis. 121:3–10, 1980.

Tager, I.B., Weiss, S.T., Munoz, A., Rosner, B., Speizer, F.E.: Longitudinal study of the effects of maternal smoking on pulmonary function in children. N. Engl. J. Med. 309:699–703, 1983.

Thiel, H., Ulmer, W.T.: Bakers' asthma: Development and possibility for treatment. Chest 78:400–405, 1980.

Tuthill, R.W.: Woodstoves, formaldehyde and respiratory disease. Am. J. Epidemiol. 120:952–955, 1984.

Utell, M.J., Morrow, P.E., Speers, D.M., Darling, J., Hyde, R.W.: Airway responsiveness to sulfate and sulfuric acid aerosols in asthmatics. Am. Rev. Resp. Dis. 128:444–450, 1983.

Wagner, C.J., Danziger, R.E., Nelson, HS.: Relation between positive small air ions, weather fronts and pulmonary function in patients with bronchial asthma. Ann. Allergy 51:430–435, 1983.

Ware, J.H., Dockery, D.W., Spiro, A., Speizer, F.E., Ferris, B.G.: Passive smoking, gas cooking, and respiratory health of children living in six cities. Am. Rev. Resp. Dis. 129:366–374, 1984a.

Ware, J.H., Thibodeau, L.A., Speizer, F.E., Colome, S., Ferris, B.G.: Assessment of the health effects of atmospheric sulfur oxides and particulate matter: Evidence from observational studies. Environ. Health Perspect. 41:255–276, 1984b.

Weiss, S.T., Tager, I.B., Schenker, M., Speizer, F.E.: The health effects of involuntary smoking: State of the art. Am. Rev. Resp. Dis. 128:933–942, 1983.

Weston, W.L., Weston, J.A.: Allergic contact dermatitis in children. Am. J. Dis. Child. 138:932–936, 1984.

Yocum, J.E.: Indoor-outdoor air quality relationships: A critical review. J. Air Poll. Control Assoc. 32:500–520, 1982.

14

Infection and Atopic Diseases

OSCAR L. FRICK, M.D., PH.D.

An association between respiratory infections and the subsequent development of asthma has been known since ancient days and was noted by Hippocrates. Rackemann (1918) observed that "150 cases of asthma can nearly all be divided, according to the etiology of their attacks, into 'extrinsic asthma' due to inhaled antigens or 'intrinsic asthma' in which infectious agents sensitized the bronchial mucosa."

Viral respiratory infections were proved by viral isolates in 357 hospitalized children of whom 27 percent wheezed during the infections (Freeman and Todd, 1962). Wheezing occurred in infections with respiratory syncytial virus (RSV) (52 percent), parainfluenza virus (21 percent), and adenoviruses (13 percent) in children under age 2. In a 20-month mean follow-up; 50 percent of the children who wheezed with the infection, especially those with parainfluenza virus, subsequently developed asthma or other allergies, whereas this occurred in only 17 percent of the children who did not wheeze with the virus infection. When asthmatic bronchitis occurred under age 1, later allergy occurred only rarely; if asthmatic bronchitis occurred between ages 1 and 3 years and over 3 years, asthma occurred later in 25 percent and 50 percent, respectively (Boesen, 1953). Wheezing was associated with serologic evidence of infection in 27 of 84 asthmatic children studied; one third had influenza type A2 or parainfluenza virus, and one fourth had *Mycoplasma pneumoniae* (Berkovich et al., 1970). It appeared that early virus-induced asthmatic bronchitis was associated with later development of asthma and other allergies.

The association between viral infections and wheezing attacks in asthma was firmly established by the landmark studies of McIntosh et al. (1973) and Minor et al. (1974 and 1976). In 32 chronically hospitalized children under 5 years of age, each upper respiratory infection (URI) was evaluated with bacterial and viral cultures and serologic studies (McIntosh et al., 1973). In 2 years, 58 acute wheezing attacks were associated with 102 proven viral infections. At times when particular respiratory viruses were prevalent, the proportion of wheezing attacks due to infection was much higher, e.g., 85 percent during one winter with RSV parainfluenza virus, and coronavirus. Wheezing was most commonly associated with infections with RSV (24 of 25); parainfluenza types 2 and 3 viruses (12 of 32); coronavirus OC38–43 (7 of 10); and adenovirus (4 of 13). In these young children, *no* wheezing occurred with 11 influenza type A2 (Hong Kong) infections which was in contrast to other studies in older children and adults; also, there was no wheezing with infections associated with common gram-positive or gram-negative bacterial pathogens. Thus, 42 percent of episodes of wheezing in young children could be associated with identifiable virus infections, predominantly RSV, parainfluenza type 2 virus, and coronavirus.

The association between wheezing and virus infection was studied in three different patient groups by the University of Wisconsin team. In a group of 16 nonallergic, "intrinsic" asthmatic children 3 to 11 years of age, two thirds (42 of 61) of asthma attacks were coincident with severe respiratory infections (SRIs) (Minor et al. 1974a). Most common (58 percent) were rhinovirus infections that produced both asthma and severe infection (fever with rhinorrhea and/or cough). Influenza A2 (Hong Kong) caused asthma and SRI in six children. In this school-age group, no other viruses or bacteria precipitated asthma attacks. Thus, the virus spectrum associated with asthma attacks in these school-age nonatopic children differed from that found by McIntosh et al. (1973) in preschool atopic children. In fact, McIntosh et al. (1973) found parainfluenza virus type 2 but no influenza virus type A2HK associated with asthma attacks, whereas Minor et al. (1974a) found the converse. The latter suggested that the severe infections caused the respiratory inflammations required to exacerbate asthma.

Minor et al. (1974b) found a significantly greater frequency of known viral respiratory infections in the 16 asthmatic children studied, when compared with their 15 nonasthmatic siblings. Similarly, respiratory infections of

191

both proven viral etiology and unknown etiology (but most probably viral) were significantly more frequent in asthmatics than in nonasthmatics, with an incidence of 5.1 per year for the asthmatic and 3.8 per year for the nonasthmatic. Asthmatics had more symptomatic rhinovirus infections. Concurrent respiratory infections occurred in 24 instances in asthmatics and their siblings in whom the average duration of infection was 6.1 and 4.4 days, respectively. Minor et al. (1974b) suggested that the difference in infection rate in asthmatics was due to their necessarily increased indoor life in a cold climate, resulting in longer exposures to respiratory viruses shed by other family members. This increased exposure would be expected, especially to rhinoviruses, which are likely to precipitate asthma attacks. These workers also raised the possibility that slow resolution of mucus plugging of the small airways after an asthmatic attack might leave the asthmatic child more vulnerable to a new infection.

Subsequently, Minor et al. (1976) confirmed that both rhinovirus and influenza A virus infections were asthmogenic. Nasal effluent cultures were made in 41 children, aged 3 to 17 years, and 8 adults, aged 22 to 60 years, with four or more infection-induced asthmatic attacks per year. Asthma occurred in 55 percent of symptomatic respiratory infections. Pathogens were identified in 42 of 128 infections, 19 of which were associated with wheezing. Rhinoviruses of 14 different serologic types were associated with wheezing, as were five influenza type A virus and 2 RSV infections. Although type-specific rhinovirus immunity appears to be long lasting, the 113 known rhinovirus types could cause recurrent wheezing attacks in asthmatics. Certain rhinovirus types may be more asthmogenic, such as type 49 in 1972, which was associated with asthma in five of six infected individuals. Although virus identification in older children and adult asthmatics was more difficult, viruses appeared to precipitate wheezing in a wide age spectrum of asthmatics.

In summary, studies of McIntosh et al., (1973) and Minor et al. (1974 and 1976) implicate symptomatic respiratory virus infections in triggering attacks of wheezing in asthmatic individuals. RSV and parainfluenza virus are asthmogenic in preschool children, whereas rhinoviruses and influenza virus assume this role in older children and adults, although other viruses, such as coronaviruses and adenoviruses, also may be involved. Bacterial infections generally do not provoke wheezing.

Asthma may be provoked by viral infection through a number of possible individual or combined mechanisms. These include (1) denudation of bronchial epithelium by influenza, which increases absorption of allergens and exposes rapidly alternating airway epithelial receptors (irritant or cough receptors), leading to firing of these receptors with minimal stimuli; (2) impairment of β-adrenergic receptor function, resulting in an autonomic nervous imbalance, which causes hyperreactivity of bronchial smooth muscles as a result of unopposed cholinergic stimulation; (3) enhancement of allergic mediator release through stimulation of interferon production; (4) hypersensitivity of IgE antibodies to the virus itself, which acts as an allergen; and (5) viral induction of perturbations of the immunoregulatory controls on IgE antibody formation.

The first and simplest explanation of virus action in an allergic reaction may be sloughing of the respiratory epithelial cells caused by influenza viruses (Cate, 1976). These infected cells release virus particles, undergo necrosis, and slough, leaving behind only a basal layer of epithelial cells. The virus spreads from the initial infection site by cell-to-cell contact. The removal of this protective epithelial cell barrier exposes the basal cell layer to direct, facile penetration by allergens to the subepithelial mast cells. The rapidly adapting irritant receptors are directly exposed or even sloughed, leaving exposed nerves that can also fire to cause bronchospasm with minimal stimulation.

Changes in airway resistance to inhaled histamine during virus infections were found by Empey et al. (1976). In 16 normal subjects with viral upper respiratory infections, airway resistance following inhaled histamine increased by 218 ± 55 percent compared with 31 ± 6 percent in 11 healthy control subjects. It took up to 7 weeks for this increased bronchoconstrictive responsiveness in subjects with colds to return to normal. A similar result occurred with a cough response to inhaled citric acid in subjects with colds. Both responses to inhaled histamine and to citric acid in these subjects could be prevented or reversed with inhaled isoproterenol or atropine. Laitinen et al. (1977) confirmed that respiratory virus infection increased bronchoreactivity in 12 normal subjects in whom half received live attenuated influenza A and B viruses and half received placebo intranasally. Increases in airway resistance of 70 percent occurred in 4 of 6 virus-infected subjects on day 2 after histamine inhalation challenge and gradually decreased. This effect of virus infection was reversed or prevented by isoproterenol or atropine aerosols. These studies suggest an increased responsiveness of "irritant cholinergic receptors" to inhaled irritants during respiratory virus infections.

Second, reduced bronchial β-adrenergic responsiveness occurs during viral infections. Szentivanyi (1968) hypothesized that asthmatic individuals have an autonomic nervous system imbalance in airways due to an inherent β-adrenergic blockade. Asthmatics had decreased systemic metabolic responsiveness to epinephrine and β-adrenergic agonists and increased cholinergic responses of the bronchi. Lymphocytes from asthmatics also had less cyclic 3',5'-adenosine monophosphate (cAMP) and smaller increases in cAMP after catecholamine stimulation than lymphocytes from normal subjects (Parker and Smith, 1973). Also, lymphocytes from asthmatic individuals responded poorly to β-agonists during respiratory infections; the response of asthmatics' lymphocytes to prostaglandin E_1 (PGE_1), however, was normal. This response indicates β-adrenergic receptor impairment rather than adenylate cyclase involvement. Thus, asthmatic individuals appear to have an impaired target cell response to β-adrenergic agonists.

Lysosomal enzyme release from neutrophils has served as a model to study cellular β-adrenergic responsiveness (Busse, 1977). Upon ingestion of complement-activated zymosan particles, neutrophils release lysosomal enzymes, such as β-glucuronidase. Isoproterenol and PGE_1 inhibit such lysosomal enzyme release in a dose-response manner. *The isolated neutrophils* from asthmatic patients during upper respiratory infections that provoked asthmatic attacks, were tested for inhibition of lysosomal enzyme release with isoproterenol. This inhibition was decreased, leading to increased enzyme release that, in turn, correlated with increased airway irritability. The neutrophils of a group of normal volunteers infected with rhinovirus 16 also had decreases in β-adrenergic and H-2 histamine inhibitory responses; several subjects also had concomitant increases in airway reactivity to inhaled methacholine (Bush et al., 1978).

In vitro experiments confirmed that viruses cause β-adrenergic inhibition of neutrophil lysosomal enzyme release (Busse et al., 1980). Isolated human granulocytes that were incubated with either rhinovirus 16 or influenza A virus had decreased lysosomal enzyme (β-glucuronidase) inhibitory responsiveness to isoproterenol, histamine, and PGE_2. Such granu-locytes incubated directly with interferon also had increased enzyme release. Busse (1980) suggested that respiratory viruses alter the inhibitory response to a β-agonist that ablates the normal catecholamine suppression of mediator secretion. When applied to the airways with viral infections that induce inflammatory cell infiltrations, the virus-induced β-adrenergic blockade results in greater granulocyte lysosomal product release. This contributes to further local inflammation, especially in late phase responses, which in turn causes increased nonspecific bronchial hyperirritability.

A third postulated effect of viruses is upon the effector target cells — basophils and mast cells. Virus-induced β-adrenergic block negates the catecholamine inhibitory controls on mediator release from these cells. Ida et al. (1977) demonstrated that influenza A virus, herpesvirus (HSV-1), and adeno-1 viruses, whether live or killed, greatly enhanced *in vitro* histamine release from leukocytes (basophils) of ragweed atopic patients with ragweed antigen E or anti-IgE serum. Similar enhancements of specific histamine release by such sensitized basophils occurred with interferon inducers (poly I-C) and with purified human interferons (IFN-α and IFN-β). In addition, basophil chemotaxis toward C5a or a lymphocyte-derived chemotactic factor or both was reported by Lett-Brown et al. (1981) in leukocytes incubated with a parainfluenza virus or interferon. Therefore, during a viral infection of the airway, the virus or interferon or both could both recruit more basophils, and possibly mast cells, into the airway and enhance specific mediator release from such sensitized target cells. Interferons may act directly to enhance basophil and mast cell histamine release, or interferons may work by interfering with the cells' responsiveness to catecholamines. Although the mechanism is not yet clear, virus infections that induce interferon may markedly enhance specific IgE-mediated atopic reactions.

A fourth mechanism of virus involvement in asthma came from the demonstration of Welliver et al. (1980) of specific IgE antibodies to RSV and parainfluenza virus in infected children, which might cause classic allergic reactions to such viruses. They found specific IgE antibodies to RSV attached to exfoliated nasopharyngeal epithelial cells in 70 percent of all patients during the first 10 days of an RSV infection. All patients with bronchiolitis and asthma had cell-bound IgE in nasal secretions, whereas 30 percent with pneumonia or URI had such cell-bound IgE. Welliver et al. (1981)

subsequently studied 79 infants ($<$12 months of age) with proven RSV infections. Histamine and IgE antibodies to RSV in nasal secretions were measured sequentially. IgE antibodies to RSV rose significantly from 2 weeks to 3 months after RSV infections. Most striking, however, was that IgE anti-RSV antibodies were higher in infants with pneumonia and wheezing or wheezing alone and lower in infants with URI or pneumonia alone. There was a highly significant inverse correlation between peak of IgE anti-RSV and severity of illness, measured by degree of hypoxia (low arterial pO_2); a similar good inverse correlation between high nasal histamine content and low arterial pO_2 also was observed. The height of the IgE anti-RSV titer during an acute infection also appears to be predictive for the recurrence of subequent wheezing episodes; the higher the titer the more likely the recurrences (Welliver et al., 1986). This suggests a true allergic response in infants with IgE antibodies to RSV, with release of histamine from the nasal mast cells into the nasal secretions. When a similar reaction was observed in the bronchi, low arterial pO_2 was observed. Welliver et al. (1982) reported similar findings of IgE anti–parainfluenza 3 antibodies in children with severe croup and asthma.

A genetic component in allergy was known in ancient days to Maimonides who observed that several members of the Egyptian royal family had asthma. In a review of family histories of 1000 allergic patients, Cooke and VanderVeer (1916) observed that if both parents were allergic, 75 percent of the children developed allergies; if one parent was allergic, about 50 percent of the children developed allergies; and 38 percent of the children developed allergies if neither parent was allergic. This distribution of familial allergies suggested a single gene mendelian dominant or recessive inheritance. Today, we know that the genetics of atopy is polygenic. From twin studies, total serum IgE level is concordant in monozygotic, but discordant in dizygotic twins, and is controlled by a gene independent of HLA type (Bazaral et al., 1974). Similarly, bronchial hyperreactivity to methacholine inhalation in asthmatic monozygotic twins is concordant, less so in dizygotic twins; in nonasthmatic family members, there is somewhat increased sensitivity to inhaled methacholine (Konig and Godfrey, 1973).

Histocompatibility loci (HLA) on human chromosome 6 appear to control immune responsiveness (Ir genes) or immune supression

(Is genes) to certain purified allergens. Levine et al. (1972) described the "hayfever haplotype" in seven families, the first disease-oriented Ir genes described in humans. In a particular family, all the ragweed sensitive individuals had a common haplotype; no ragweed sensitive individuals in that family were missing that haplotype. However, the ragweed haplotype was different in each of the seven families. In large population studies, Freidhoff et al. (1981) found certain HLA associations with purified minor fractions of allergens, especially in individuals with low total IgE levels, in whom a major portion of their IgE was committed to that allergenic fraction. Hozouri et al. (1982) found that monozygotic twins had a high concordance of positive or negative skin test and RAST results, whether they were raised together or apart in different environments; this concordance suggested a strong genetic influence in responsiveness to certain allergens.

Responsiveness to certain viruses also appears to be HLA-related. Certain Dutch Army recruits failed to get a "take" upon repeated vaccinia vaccinations. Such individuals all had HLA-C3, and their lymphocytes failed to proliferate in culture with vaccinia. This suggested either an Is gene or a lack of a receptor for vaccinia virus (deVries et al., 1977). Individuals with HLA-Dw2 are poor T cell responders to measles virus; this observation suggests an Is gene that might make such individuals susceptible to multiple sclerosis (Visccher et al., 1981). Thus, it may be possible that certain viruses stimulate an HLA-associated Ir or Is gene for certain allergens to initiate allergic sensitization in genetically susceptible individuals.

In relation to the fifth mechanism, virally induced IgE-immunoregulation perturbations, a prospective study of 24 infants born into families with two allergic parents was started in 1975 to investigate whether other factors, more than genetic factors, influenced the onset of allergy (Frick et al., 1979). At 3-month intervals from birth, these infants were examined for clinical signs of allergy. Several immunologic tests were done for serum immunoglobulins IgE, IgM, IgG, and IgA and for IgE antibodies by RAST, leukocyte histamine release, and lymphoproliferation with a panel of six common allergens. Results were compared with those in a group of 28 well babies from nonatopic families in whom allergy had been ruled out by history. In the allergy-prone children, after 2 years, a score of 88 symptoms and signs of allergy from a possible score of 120 (five symptoms times 24 subjects), or 73 percent positive, was observed. This was significantly greater than the 21 of 140 signs and symptoms found in the 28 control children (15 percent positive).

Immunologic test results also showed a significantly greater percentage of positive results for allergy with all three tests (61 percent) compared with nonallergic controls (10 percent). In positive, control children with hayfever tested to grass pollen, 80 percent had reactions. Most striking was the timing of the onset of positive clinical and immunologic test findings, namely immediately after respiratory tract infections, such as in patient 1 (Fig. 14–1). This infant had a documented URI at 5 months, which was culture positive for pneumococcus. At 6 months, patient 1 had a positive RSV antibody titer, but negative parainfluenza virus antibody titer. However, at 6 months he had considerable persistent nasal congestion and a positive histamine release test with cat and a positive RAST with cow's milk; he had just been switched completely to cow's milk feeding. By 9 months, parainfluenza virus 3 antibody titer rose 8-fold, and cat histamine release increased; by 12 months, he was wheezing. At 23 months, the

patient was hospitalized with severe viral diarrhea, fever, and dehydration, following which in 1 month, he had a marked rise in lymphoproliferation tests with house dust mite. Such rising patterns of RAST, leukocyte histamine release, and lymphoproliferation with allergens occurred in 21 of 24 children. In 15 of 24, rising antibody titers to RSV and parainfluenza virus occurred in the 3 months spanning the start of allergic symptoms and immunologic test changes; six already had high titers, whereas, in three, there were few symptoms or changes in viral antibody titers. These results suggested a temporal association between viral respiratory and possibly intestinal tract infections and the onset of allergy, although there was no actual proof for a cause and effect relationship. Bahna et al. (1978) had observed sharp rises in total IgE levels during infectious mononucleosis, and postinfection suppression of IgE. Perelmutter et al. (1978) also found high IgE levels in patients with acute viral infections, and lower IgE levels during convalescence. Shalit et al. (1984) found that IgE levels increased > 20 percent in 56 percent of patients during the acute phase of measles which fell during recovery, while IgG

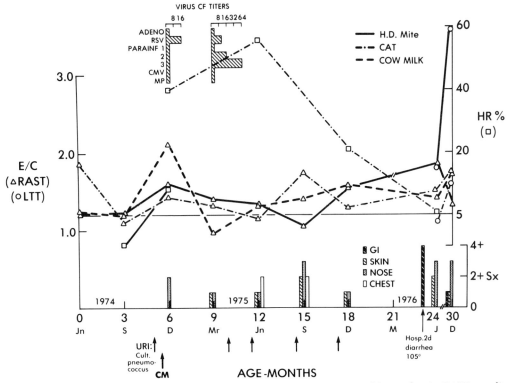

FIGURE 14–1. Clinical and immunologic course of patient 1. E/C = experimental/control ratio; RAST = radioallergosorbent test; LTT = lymphoproliferation; HR = leukocyte histamine release; URI = upper respiratory infection; CM = cow's milk; and CF = complement fixation.

and IgA levels remained unchanged. These findings all suggested an IgE immunoregulatory role for certain viral infections, especially in atopy-prone children.

An animal model was sought to test whether live viral infections could trigger the onset of allergy. Black (1977) had observed increased allergic reactions and rises in reaginic antibodies in cattle, following administration of foot and mouth disease vaccine. Dogs also develop allergic sensitivity to pollens. After screening 220 hunting dogs to mixed grass and weed pollen extracts, seven dogs were selected for breeding (Frick and Brooks, 1983). Pups from these dogs were immunized with live attenuated distemper-hepatitis virus vaccine at 4, 8, and 12 weeks of age followed each time in 2 and 9 days by subcutaneous injections of grass and ragweed pollen extract in alum. Littermate controls received only the pollen extracts and no viral vaccines until 2 weeks after the pollen injections. Consistently, the vaccinated pups made more IgE antibodies to both pollens than did their littermate controls. These IgE antibodies have persisted into adulthood in the dogs who received viral vaccines before pollen injections. There were precipitous rises in IgE antibodies to the pollens after each annual distemper-hepatitis booster inoculation. About 10 percent of the pups developed facial eczema during grass pollen season; eczema is the main manifestion of atopy in dogs.

In order to simulate natural events more closely, pups at 3, 7, and 11 weeks were given 10-fold concentrated attenuated canine parainfluenza virus vaccine intranasally, followed by four 1-hour inhalation exposures in a chamber to 2 percent aerosolized pollen extracts; littermates received only the pollen extract inhalations. The vaccinated pups made more IgE antibodies to both pollens than did their littermate controls. When the dogs reached adolescence,

those with high anti-pollen IgE antibodies developed markedly increased airway resistance to inhalation challenges with nebulized pollen extracts (Chung et al., 1985). Two thirds of these dogs experienced increased bronchial hyperreactivity to inhaled acetylcholine at 6 and 24 hours after the pollen extract inhalation. This was accompanied by increased numbers of neutrophils and eosinophils in the bronchial lavage fluids taken at these times, presumably cellular manifestations of late phase asthmatic responses. The duration of this increased bronchial hyperreactivity varied, but in some dogs, it persisted for many weeks and up to 4 months after a single pollen extract inhalation exposure.

Results of studies in atopy-prone children and inbred dogs indicate that myxovirus infections have an immunoregulatory effect on IgE antibody formation. Regulation of IgE antibodies is extremely T cell dependent and probably independent of regulation of IgM, IgG, and IgA antibodies (Ishizaka, 1984). Katz (1978) suggested an "allergic breakthrough" mechanism (Fig. 14–2) in which T-suppressor lymphocytes normally exert a "damping effect" upon IgE antibody production. The IgE system is an extremely potent homeostatic inflammatory defense system that ordinarily must be rigidly held in check. Chiorazzi et al. (1977) had shown that IgE "nonresponder" SJL mice became good IgE "responders" if pretreated 10 days before immunization, using treatments that destroy selectively T-suppressor lymphocytes, such as cyclophosphamide and low dose irradiation. This presumably permits T-helper cells to escape and to signal B cells to make IgE antibodies to antigens in the environment. IgE "nonresponsiveness" in SJL mice could be restored promptly by injecting them with syngeneic spleen cells containing IgE T-suppressor cells. The disturbance in the damping mechanism that prompted IgE antibody production was

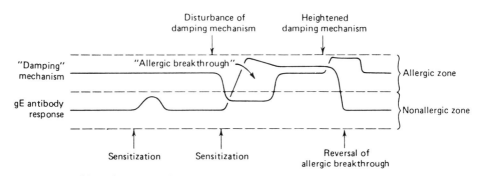

FIGURE 14–2. Possible pathogenesis of "allergic breakthrough." (From Katz, D.H., J. Immunol. 1:2191, 1979.)

termed "allergic breakthrough" by Katz. It is proposed that certain viruses, especially myxoviruses that are good interferon inducers, induce an "allergic breakthrough" either by depressing T-suppressor cells for IgE or by stimulating T-helper cells, perhaps through certain lymphokines.

PREVENTION OF VIRAL INFECTIONS

Immunizations. Current American Academy of Pediatrics Redbook recommendations for influenza vaccination (Peter, 1986) targets "high-risk" children. "The Committee recommends that the following groups of children, 6 months old or older, be considered particularly in need of yearly immunization: Children with chronic pulmonary diseases, including those with moderate to severe asthma and those with bronchopulmonary dysplasia. Children with hemodynamically significant cardiac disease. Children receiving immunosuppressive therapy. Children with sickle cell and other hemoglobinopathies."

Immunization with inactivated mixed influenza virus vaccine is routinely recommended to be given to all elderly adults and those of any age with chronic respiratory diseases, such as asthma, to prevent complications of influenza. However, the effects of influenza immunizations may vary, especially with time. Ouelette and Reed (1965) found that killed influenza A vaccination in asthmatics caused a transient, increased reactivity to inhaled methacholine, with a decrease in FEV_1 that peaked in 1 day and subsided in 5 days; such transient bronchial hyperirritability did not occur in normal individuals. Later, Kava and Laitinen (1985) found that killed influenza vaccine did not increase specific airway conductance in Finnish asthmatics. Bell et al. (1978) also found a transient fall in peak expiratory flow and an increased need for bronchodilators for 2 days after killed influenza vaccination in young asthmatics. However, such immunized asthmatics also had fewer flu-like illnesses and hospitalizations for influenza. The investigators concluded that the risk of brief transient increase in bronchial hyperreactivity after influenza vaccination was justified by decreased morbidity from influenza in a high risk group of asthmatics.

Intranasal vaccination with live attenuated influenza vaccine gives higher persistent immunity to reinfection with the same strain of influenza. Busse et al. (1986) found that asthmatics given such intranasal immunizations had a four-fold rise in antibody titer and no change in pulmonary function, so that this approach appeared to be safe in asthmatics. Johnson et al. (1986) compared protective efficacy in four groups of young children based upon prior exposure to influenza A (H3N2) as follows: (1) natural infection, (2) live attenuated cold-adapted influenza vaccine given intranasally, (3) inactivated influenza A vaccine given intramuscularly, and (4) no previous exposure (negative H3N2 antibodies). One year later, they challenged these children with homologous live attenuated vaccine. Significantly less viral shedding occurred in those with prior natural infection and those given live attenuated vaccine, in comparison to the other groups. Protection in natural and live attenuated vaccine groups was associated exclusively with the pre-challenge presence of nasal IgA antibodies to virus. Inactivated vaccine did prime patients for an enhanced secondary local antibody response to challenge with live attenuated vaccine.

Amantadine. Amantadine (Symmetrel) protects against all strains of influenza A viruses probably by interfering with viral uncoating (Fig. 14–3). Amantadine 200 mg/day orally can prevent influenza A in 70 to 90 percent of healthy adults. Dosages should be decreased for children, patients with renal dysfunction, and those with seizure disorders. Therefore, it has a potential usefulness in preventing such infections in at-risk asthmatic and other allergic patients. In addition, the use of amantadine within 48 hours of onset of infection may ameliorate symptoms. Little et al. (1976) found that amantadine used in acute influenza resulted in faster improvement of symptom scores and faster resolution of small airway obstruction. Although significant, differences were small in the 15 patients studied. These workers suggested that amantadine delayed the progressive cell-to-cell spread of the virus, thus, restricting the total amount of lung parenchyma involved and minimizing the changes in lung mechanics.

Van Voris et al. (1981) evaluated both amantadine and rimantadine in 45 college students with proven influenza A/USSR/77 H1N1 infection. By 48 hours, less fever and fewer symptoms were reported in the drug-treated groups; those treated returned to classes earlier and shed smaller amounts of virus than did placebo recipients. In a similar study, 47 subjects with influenza A/Brazil/78 H1N1 infection (Younkin et al., 1983) were treated with

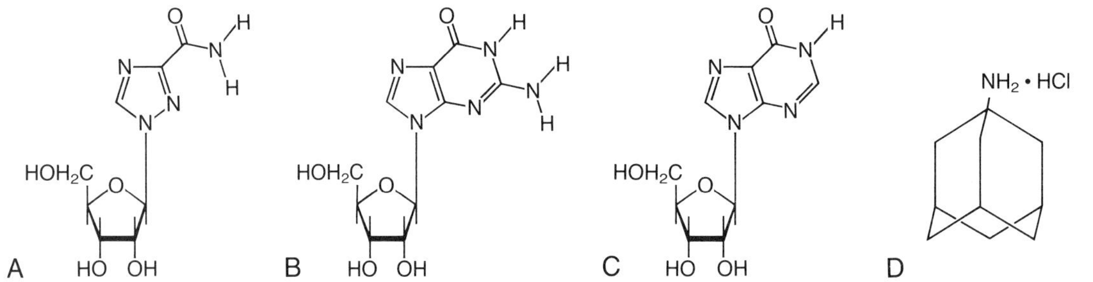

FIGURE 14–3. Structure of virucidals. A = Ribavirin (mol wt 244.21); B = guanosine; C = inosine; D = amantadine (mol wt 187.72).

200 or 100 mg amantadine or with 3.25 g aspirin per day. Both amantadine groups experienced greater symptomatic improvement, with decreased viral shedding in the 200 mg amantadine group. Side effects were insomnia, light headedness, and difficulty in concentration, which may be more troublesome in the elderly. In summary, amantadine may have a place in prophylaxis and early treatment of asthmatics for influenza A infection.

Ribavirin (Virazole). Ribavirin is a synthetic nucleoside analogue of guanosine and inosine that appears to inhibit viral nucleic acid synthesis and in so doing is virucidal (Fig. 14–3A to C) (Sidwell et al., 1979). The phosphate metabolites of ribavirin are incorporated into viral mRNA, which prevent cap formation of viral mRNA but are not incorporated into host cell RNA or DNA. Furthermore, these phosphate derivatives specifically inhibit viral, but not cellular, enzymes, the nucleic acid polymerases. Therefore, ribavirin has anti-viral activity against a broad spectrum of DNA viruses (poxvirus, herpesvirus, and adenovirus) and RNA viruses (respiratory myxoviruses — influenzavirus, parainfluenzavirus RSV, measlesvirus, arenavirus, and bunyavirus) but is less effective against enteroviruses.

Because of ribavirin's effectiveness against myxoviruses, it might be especially useful in preventing early infantile RSV and parainfluenza virus infections and, therefore, perhaps the development of asthma. Ribavirin (20 mg/ml) is administered by continuous aerosol in an oxygen hood, mask or tent using a Collison generator of particles of 1.4 μm diameter or 0.8 mg/kg/hr for about 16 to 20 hr/day for 3 to 5 days. This produces a tracheal concentration of 1000 μg/ml; 4 to 16 μg/ml concentration inhibits RSV replication. To date, no viral resistance to ribavirin has developed.

Ribavirin aerosol was devised by Knight et al.

(1981) who found a highly significant reduction in height and duration of fever, a reduction in symptoms and their duration, and early disappearance of influenza viruses from respiratory secretions during an influenza A (England/333/80 H1N1) epidemic in college students. A similar rapid clinical improvement took place with ribavirin aerosol in an influenza B (Singapore/222/79) epidemic among college students (McClung et al., 1983).

Ribavirin was tested in 16 adult volunteers who received intranasal inocula of RSV followed 2 days later by aerosol inhalations of ribavirin or placebo (Hall et al., 1983a). Fever, other symptoms, and viral shedding all were significantly less in the ribavirin-treated group. There was neither toxicity nor pulmonary function changes. Continuous ribavirin aerosol was studied by double-blind protocol in 33 infants with RSV (Hall et al., 1983b). Ribavirin-treated infants had significantly less severe illness, with greater improvement in lower respiratory tract signs, in arterial oxygen saturation, and in virus shedding. Similar degrees of improvement have been found with ribavirin aerosol therapy in RSV-infected infants who had bronchopulmonary dysplasia, congenital heart disease (Hall et al., 1985), or compromised immune function (McIntosh et al., 1984). However, in children receiving oral corticosteroids or chemotherapy, viral shedding was significantly greater and prolonged. Problems and adverse effects from ribavirin use have included ribavirin precipitation and clogging of vital ventilation equipment and some rashes, conjunctivitis, and reticulocytosis after aerosol therapy. In animals, ribavirin has been mutagenic, teratogenic, and embryotoxic.

The cost of ribavirin and of hospitalization for the constant 3 to 5 day aerosol treatment may limit its usefulness as experience develops. The potential of ribavirin therapy for RSV and infantile respiratory viral infections in the prevention of the development of subsequent asthma has yet to be studied.

Recombinant Interferons. The existence of 113 distinct strains of rhinoviruses and many strains of coronaviruses makes immunoprophylaxis of the common cold unlikely. Isaacs et al. (1981) described four children with recurrent respiratory infections with wheezing whose lymphocytes had deficient primary interferon-a (IFN-a) formation. Such a defect was demonstrated in lymphocytes cultured with viruses *in vitro* and from nasal lymphocytes in response to *in vivo* rhinovirus infections.

The increasing availability for clinical trials of recombinant interferons has shown promising results in common colds. Intranasal rIFN-a2b (1.5×10^6 IU bid for 4 weeks) and placebo were compared in 400 college students (Manto et al., 1986). Rhinovirus infections were prevented with 76 percent protective efficiency, but parainfluenza virus infections were not prevented, although symptoms were less severe than in the untreated group. At the dose of rIFN-a2b used, there were considerable nasal irritation, bleeding points, and mucosal erosions, which required reduction in dosage. Coronaviruses cause about 10 percent of common colds (Turner et al., 1986). Healthy adult volunteers were given either intranasally rIFN-a2b (2×10^6 IU/day) or placebo for 15 days, and on the eighth day, all received an intranasal inoculum of 100 $TCID_{50}$ (i.e., half the tissue culture infective dose) coronavirus 229E. Cold symptoms developed in 73 percent of the placebo group and in 41 percent of the interferon-treated group. However, mean and total symptom scores were significantly higher in the placebo group, and duration of high symptoms scores was significantly shortened in the interferon-treated group, so that interferon pretreatment shortened duration and reduced severity of common cold symptoms.

Recombinant IFN-b has similar anti-viral effects as rIFN-a but is bound to tissues more and inhibits viruses better; it also causes less skin and nasal irritation than rIFN-a. Therefore, rIFN-b$_{ser}$ (10^6 IU) or placebo was given daily intranasally for 6 days to adult volunteers, and on the third day, an intranasal inoculum of rhinovirus 9 and R 14 were given (Higgins et al., 1986). Significantly less clinical cold symptoms, viral shedding, and nasal secretion occurred in the interferon-treated group than in the control group. It was concluded that rIFN-b is nonirri-

tating and is effective as prophylaxis against experimental rhinovirus infections. Evaluation studies of the efficacy of recombinant interferons in preventing respiratory infections in susceptible children will be forthcoming.

"Killer Kleenex" for Prevention of Spread of Viral Infection. Fomites appear to be primary vehicles for spread of colds. Unenveloped rhinoviruses are acid labile. Consequently, citric acid (91 percent) and malic acid (4.5 percent) at a low pH of 2.2 were incorporated into disposable Kleenex tissues along with sodium lauryl sulfate (1.8 percent) which kills enveloped paramyxoviruses (Dick et al., 1986). These (i.e., CMS tissues) are capable of inactivating 100,000 $TCID_{50}$ of rhinovirus 16 in 1 minute. Prolonged intimate or close social contact was simulated by a series of four 12-hour poker games among 20 volunteers each including eight who had newly acquired colds from intranasal inoculations of rhinovirus 16, 2 days before. In two control groups, usual social interchange and use of cloth handkerchiefs prevailed. In two test groups, CMS tissues were used liberally to catch nasal effluents and wipe up nasal discharges. Among the controls, 14 of 24 recipients developed fresh rhinovirus 16 colds, whereas in the CMS tissue group, none of 24 developed colds. The four-table poker game format was similar to the crowding in a restaurant. Therefore, "Killer Kleenex," such as CMS tissues, may be able to control spread of colds in social gatherings and potentially prevent more serious effects of URIs in allergic and asthmatic patients.

In summary, viral infections affect allergic individuals by at least six different potential mechanisms as follows: (1) denudation of the respiratory mucosa which facilitates entry of allergens to the submucosal mast cells, firing allergic reactions, and to submucosal IgE-producing lymphoblasts, which form new IgE antibodies; (2) denudation of respiratory mucosa exposes rapidly alternating irritant cough receptors to smaller stimuli, which may lead to bronchial hyperreactivity; (3) decrease of B-adrenergic inhibitory effect on secretion of lysosomal enzymes from granulocytes that may be involved in late phase reactions; (4) increase of release of basophil and mast cell mediators; (5) true IgE-mediated allergy to viruses, such as RSV and parainfluenza virus; and (6) disturbance of IgE immunoregulation by an "allergic breakthrough" mechanism.

There are several promising means of preventing viral respiratory infections as follows: immunizations, especially via intranasal route; amantadine for influenza A; ribavirin for influenza viruses, RSV, and rhinoviruses; recombinant interferons for influenza viruses and rhinoviruses; and new virucidal tissues to prevent the spread of viruses. A combination of such measures may become keys to the prevention of virally induced asthmatic attacks, and possibly, the prevention of allergic sensitization.

REFERENCES

Bahna, S.I., Horwitz, C., Fiala, M., Heiner, D.C.: IgE response in heterophilpositive infectious mononucleosis. J. Allergy Clin. Immunol. 62:167, 1978.

Bazaral, M., Orgel, H.A., Hamburger, R.N.: Genetics of IgE and allergy: Serum IgE levels in twins. J. Allergy Clin. Immunol. 54:288, 1974.

Bell, T.D., Chai, H., Berlow, B., Daniels, G.: Immunization with killed influenza virus in children with chronic asthma. Chest 73:140, 1978.

Berkovich, S., Millian, S.J., Synder, R.D.: The association of viral and mycoplasma infections with recurrence of wheezing in the asthmatic child. Ann. Allergy 28:43, 1970.

Black, L.: Allergy in cattle after foot-and-mouth disease vaccination. Vet. Res. 100:195, 1977.

Boesen, I.: Asthmatic bronchitis in children. Acta Pediatr. 42:87, 1953.

Bush, R.K., Busse, W.W., Flaherty, D., Warshauer, D., Dick, E.C., Reed, C.E.: Effects of experimental rhinovirus 16 infection on airways and leukocyte function in normal subjects. J. Allergy Clin. Immunol. 61:80, 1978.

Busse, W.W.: Decreased granulocyte response to isoproterenol in asthma during upper respiratory infections. Am. Rev. Respir. Dis. 115:783, 1977.

Busse, W.W.: Prevention of virus-induced asthma. Proc. XII Inter. Congr. Allergy Clin. Immunol. C.E. Reed (ed.) St. Louis, C.V. Mosby Co., 1986.

Busse, W. W., Anderson, C.L., Dick, E.C.: Reduced granulocyte response to isoproterenol, histamine and prostaglandin E after in vitro incubation with rhinovirus 16. Am. Rev. Respir. Dis. 122:641, 1980.

Cate, T.R.: Influenza Viruses. In Joklik, W.K., Willett, H.P. (eds.): Zinsser Microbiology, 16th ed. New York, Appleton-Century-Crofts, 1976.

Chiorazzi, N., Fox, D.A., Katz, D.H.: Hapten-specific IgE antibody responses in mice. VII. Conversion of IgE "non-responders" by elimination of suppressor T-cell reactivity. J. Immunol. 118:48, 1977.

Chung, K.F., Becker, A.B., Lazarus, S.C., Frick, O.L., Nadel, J.A., Gold, W.M.: Antigen-induced airway hyperresponsiveness and pulmonary infiltration in allergic dogs. J. Appl. Physiol. 58:1347, 1985.

Cooke, R.A., VanderVeer, A. Jr.: Human sensitization. J. Immunol. 1:201, 1916.

deVries, R.P., Kreeftenberg, H.G., Loggen, H.G., van Rood, J.J.: In vitro immune responsiveness to vaccinia and HL-A. N. Engl. J. Med. 297:692, 1977.

Dick, E.C., Hossain, S.U., Mink, K.A., Meschievitz, C.K., Schultz, S.B., Raynor, W.J., Inhorn, S.L.L.: Interruption of transmission of rhinovirus colds among human vol-

unteers using virucidal paper handkerchiefs. J. Infect. Dis. 153:352, 1986.

Empey, D.W., Laitinen, L.A., Jacobs, L., Gold, W.M., Nadel, J.A.: Mechanisms of bronchial hyperreactivity in normal subjects after upper respiratory tract infection. Am. Rev. Respir. Dis. 113:131, 1976.

Freeman, G.L., Todd, R.H.: The role of allergy in viral respiratory tract infections. Am. J. Dis. Child. 104:330, 1962.

Freidhoff, L.R., Meyers, D.A., Bias, W.B., Chase, G.H., Hussain, R., Marsh, D.G.: A genetic-epidemiologic study of human immune responsiveness to allergens in an industrial population. I. Epidemiology of reported allergy and skin test positivity. Am. J. Med. Genet. 9:323, 1981.

Frick, O.L., Brooks, D.L.: Immunoglobulin E antibodies to pollens augmented in dogs by virus vaccines. Am. J. Vet. Res. 44:440, 1983.

Frick, O.L., German, D.F., Mills, J.: Development of allergy in children. I. Association with virus infection. J. Allergy Clin. Immunol. 64:228, 1979.

Hall, C.B., McBride, J.T., Gala, C.L., Hildreth, S.W., Schnabel, K.C.: Ribavirin treatment of respiratory syncytial virus infection in infants with underlying cardiopulmonary disease. J.A.M.A. 254:3047, 1985.

Hall, C.B., McBride, J.T., Walsh, E.E., Bill, D.M., Gala, C.L., Hildreth, S., Teneyck, L.G., Hall, W.J.: Aerosolized ribavirin treatment of infants with respiratory syncytial viral infection. N. Engl. J. Med. 308:1443, 1983b.

Hall, C.B., Walsh, E.E., Hruska, J.F., Betts, R.F., Hall, W.J.: Ribavirin treatment of experimental respiratory syncytial viral infection: A controlled double-blind study in young adults. J.A.M.A. 249:2666, 1983a.

Higgins, P.G., Al-Nakib, W., Willman, J., Tyrrell, D.A.J.: Interferon-b$_{ser}$ as prophylaxis against experimental rhinovirus infection in volunteers. J. Interferon Res. 6:153, 1986.

Hozouri, K., Hanson, B., Roitman-Johnson, B., Walsh, G., Blumenthal, M.N.: Genetics of atopic diseases in twins raised together and apart. J. Allergy Clin. Immunol. 69:121, 1982.

Ida, S., Hooks, J.J., Siraganian, R.P., Notkins, A.L.: Enhancement of IgE-mediated histamine release from human basophils by viruses: Role of interferon. J. Exp. Med. 145:892, 1977.

Isaacs, D., Clarke, J.R., Tyrrell, D.A.J., Webster, A.D.B., Valman, H.B.: Deficient production of leukocyte interferon (Interferon a) in vitro and in vivo in children with recurrent respiratory tract infections. Lancet 2:950, 1981.

Ishizaka, K.: Regulation of IgE Synthesis. Ann. Rev. Immunol. 2:159, 1984.

Johnson, P.R., Feldman, S., Thompson, J.M., Mahoney, J.D., Wright, P.F.: Immunity to influenza A virus infection in young children: A comparison of natural infection, live cold-adapted vaccine and inactivated vaccine. J. Infect. Dis. 154:121, 1986.

Katz, D.: The allergic phenotype: Manifestation of "allergic breakthrough" and imbalance in normal "damping" of IgE antibody production. Immunol. Rev. 41:77, 1978.

Kava, T., Laitinen, L.A.: Effects of killed and live attenuated influenza vaccine on symptoms and specific airway conductance in asthmatics and healthy subjects. Allergy 40:42, 1985.

Knight, V., McClung, H.W., Wilson, S.Z., Waters, B.K., Quarles, J.M., Cameron, R.W., Groggs, S.E., Zerwas,

J.M., Couch, R.B.: Ribavirin small-particle aerosol treatment of influenza. Lancet 2:945, 1981.

Konig, P., Godfrey, S.: Prevalence of exercise-induced bronchial lability in families of children with asthma. Arch. Dis. Child. 48:513, 1973.

Laitinen, L.A., Elkin, R.B., Empey, D.W., Jacobs, L., Mills, J., Gold, W.M., Nadel, J.A.: Changes in bronchial reactivity after administration of live attenuated influenza virus. Am. Rev. Respir. Dis. 113:194, 1977.

Lett-Brown, M.A., Aelvoet, M. Hooks, J.J., Georgiades, J.A., Thueson, D.O., Grant, J.A.: Enhancement of basophil chemotaxis *in vitro* by virus induced interferon. J. Clin. Invest. 67:547, 1981.

Levine, B.B., Stember, R.H., Foting, M.: Ragweed hayfever: Genetic control and linkage to HL-A haplotype. Science 178:1201, 1972.

Little, J.W., Hall, W.J., Douglas, R.G. Jr., Hyde, D.W. Speers, D.M.: Amantadine effect on peripheral airway abnormalities in influenza. Ann. Intern. Med. 86:177, 1976.

McClung, H.W., Knight, V., Gilbert, B.E., Wilson, S.Z., Quarles, J.M., Divine, G.W.: Ribavirin aerosol treatment of influenza B virus infection. J.A.M.A. 249:2671, 1983.

McIntosh, K., Ellis, E.F., Hoffman, L.S., Lybass, T.G., Eller, J.J., Fulginiti, V.A.: The association of viral and bacterial respiratory infections with exacerbations of wheezing in young asthmatic children. J. Pediatr. 82:578, 1973.

McIntosh, K., Kurachek, S.C., Cairns, L.M., Burns, J.C., Goodspeed, B.: Treatment of respiratory syncytial viral infection in immunodeficient infant with ribavirin aerosol. Am. J. Dis Child. 138:305, 1984.

Manto, A.S., Shope, T.C., Schwartz, S.A., Albrecht, J.K.: Intranasal Interferon-a2b for seasonal prophylaxis of respiratory infection. J. Infect. Dis. 154:128, 1986.

Minor, T.E., Baker, J.W., Dick, E.C., DeMeo, A.N., Ouellette, J.J., Cohen, M., Reed, C.E.: Greater frequency of viral respiratory infections in asthmatic children as compared with their non-asthmatic siblings. J. Pediatr. 85:472, 1974b.

Minor, T.E., Dick, E.C., Baker, J.W., Ouellette, J.J., Cohen, M., Reed, C.E.: Rhinovirus and influenza type A infections as precipitants of asthma. Am. Rev. Respir. Dis. 113:149, 1976.

Minor, T.E., Dick, E.C., DeMeo, A.N., Ouellette, J.J., Cohen, M., Reed, C.E.: Viruses as precipitants of asthmatic attacks in children. J. Am. Med. Assoc. 227:292, 1974a.

Ouellette, J.J., Reed, C.E.: Increased responses of asthmatic subjects to methacholine after influenza vaccine. J. Allergy 36:558, 1965.

Parker, C.W., Smith, J.W.: Alterations in cyclic adenosine monophosphate metabolism in human bronchial asthma. I. Leukocyte responsiveness to beta-adrenergic agents. J. Clin. Invest. 52:48, 1973.

Perelmutter, L., Phipps, P., Potvin, L.: Viral infections and IgE levels. Ann. Allergy 41:158, 1978.

Peter, G.: Report of the Committee on Infectious Diseases, ed 20. Elk Grove, Illinois, Academy of Pediatrics, 1986.

Rackemann, F.M.: A clinical study of one hundred and fifty cases of bronchial asthma. Arch. Intern. Med. 22:252, 1918.

Shalit, M., Ackerman, Z., Wollner, S., Morag, A., Levo, Y.: Immunoglobulin E response during measles. Int. Arch. Allergy Appl. Immunol. 75:84, 1984.

Sidwell, R.W., Robins, R.K., Hillyard, I.W.: Ribavirin: An anti-viral agent. Pharmacol. Ther. 6:123, 1979.

Szentivanyi, A.: The beta-adrenergic theory of the atopic abnormality in asthma. J. Allergy 42:203, 1968.

Turner, R.B., Felton, A., Kosak, D., Kelsey, D.K., Meschievitz, C.K.: Prevention of experimental coronavirus colds with intranasal a-2b Interferon. J. Infect. Dis. 154:443, 1986.

VanVoris, L.P., Betts, R.F., Hayden, F.G., Christmas, W.A., Douglas, R.G. Jr.: Successful treatment of naturally occurring influenza A/USSR/77/H1N1. J.A.M.A. 245:1128, 1981.

Visscher, B.R., Sullivan, C.B., Detels, R., Madden, D.L., Sever, J.R., Terasaki, P.I., Park, M.S., Dudley, J.P.: Measles antibody titers in multiple sclerosis patients and HLA-matched and unmatched siblings. Neurology (NY) 31:1142, 1981.

Welliver, R.C., Kaul, T.N., Ogra, P.L.: The appearance of cell bound IgE in respiratory tract epithelium after respiratory syncytial virus infection. N. Engl. J. Med. 303:1198, 1980.

Welliver, R.C., Sun, M., Rinaldo, D., Ogra, P.L.: Predictive value of RSV specific IgE response for recurrent wheezing after bronchiolitis. J. Pediatr. 109:776, 1986.

Welliver, R.C., Wong, R.T., Middleton, E. Jr., Sun, M., McCarthy, N., Ogra, P.L.: Role of parainfluenza virus–specific IgE in pathogenesis of croup and wheezing subsequent to infection. J. Pediatr. 101:1889, 1982.

Welliver, R.C., Wong, R.T., Sun, M., Middleton, E. Jr., Vaughan, R.S., Ogra, P.L.: The development of respiratory syncytial virus–specific IgE and the release of histamine in nasopharyngeal secretions after infection. N. Engl. J. Med. 305:841, 1981.

Younkin, S.W., Betts, R.F., Roth, F.K., Douglas, R.G., Jr.: Reduction in fever and symptoms in young adults with influenza A/Brazil/78 H1N1 infection after treatment with aspirin or amantadine. Antimicrob. Agents Chemother. 23:577, 1983.

15

Endocrine Aspects of Allergic Diseases *

HAROLD S. NELSON, M.D.
RICHARD W. WEBER, M.D.

The function of the endocrine system influences the manifestations of allergic diseases in a variety of ways. Cyclic and maturational fluctuations in hormonal levels may enhance or suppress the expression of allergic reactions through effects on effector cells of the immune system or on target tissues. On the other hand, medications used in the treatment of allergic diseases may affect the function of effector or regulatory hormones. It is not the intent of this chapter to review the complex actions and interactions of the endocrine system; rather the focus is on only those areas that are of concern in clinical allergy.

INTERACTION OF ENDOCRINE AND IMMUNE SYSTEMS

Maturational and Cyclic Fluctuations in Hormones. Diurnal fluctuations occur in several hormones. Plasma cortisol level peaks about 8 a.m. (normal values, 6 to 16 μg/dl) and falls to a nadir between 6 p.m. and midnight. This fall in plasma corticosteroid level induces the hypothalamus to secrete corticotropin-releasing factor, stimulating in turn the pituitary secretion of ACTH, and ultimately, the adrenal cortex secretion of cortisol. Endogenous catecholamines have a similar diurnal pattern with levels that peak, however, about 4 p.m.; the trough is between 2 and 4 a.m. (Barnes et al., 1980).

* The opinions or assertions contained herein are the private views of the authors and are not to be construed as official or as reflecting the views of the Department of the Army or the Department of Defense. The protocol under which this study was conducted was approved by the Clinical Research and Human Use Committee of Fitzsimons Army Medical Center and the Office of the Surgeon General, United States Army.

Maturation of the hypothalamic-pituitary-gonadal axis is attended by changes in the sensitivity of the negative-feedback loop and by the attainment of periodicity in the release of gonadotropins and secretion of sex steroids. Estrogens and testosterone are present in low amounts in the prepubertal child, but even these amounts are sufficient to prevent the exceedingly sensitive hypothalamus from producing gonadotropin releasing hormone or luteinizing hormone–releasing hormone (LHRH). Luteinizing hormone (LH) and follicle stimulating hormone (FSH) are produced, however, in very small amounts. In some fashion, puberty is triggered by the achievement of a critical body mass and is heralded by the onset of high pulsatile releases of LHRH during the sleeping hours. There follows a return of feedback sensitivities to adult levels. LH and FSH are required for normal ovarian follicular development in the female and spermatozoa formation in the male. Gonadotropin release in the female assumes a much more cyclic nature than in the male. During menses, levels of estradiol and progesterone are low. Estradiol begins to climb approximately 1 week before the LH/FSH peak; it peaks and begins to fall shortly before midcycle at which time there is a dramatic rise in LH and FSH, resulting in the rupture of the primary follicle and release of the ovum. Shortly before the LH peak, progesterone production begins but is not obvious until after ovulation, peaking about 1 week thereafter. Concomitantly, there is a second rise in estradiol, both hormones falling as menses approaches. Menopause is attended by the progressive inability of the ovary to produce estrogens and progesterone. The adrenal gland becomes, postmenopausally, the primary source of estrogens through the production of androstenedione. Although there may be a diminution in androgen production with age in the male, reproductive capability continues potentially throughout life.

Hormonal and Immune Interactions. Regulatory effects of the sex steroids on immune function have been documented, but animal studies and clinical observations are often confusing or conflicting. A recent review by Grossman (1984) has consolidated this diverse information. Estrogen receptors have been demonstrated on thymic epithelial cells and possibly on T cells as well. Estrogens are inhibitory and depress T cell subsets. Androgens alter the development of certain T cell and B cell populations; T cells have been shown to possess androgen receptors. Testosterone treatment decreases antibody levels and perhaps modulates thymic hormones. Progesterone increases suppressor cell activity and inhibits phytohemagglutinin (PHA) lymphocyte transformation. Thymic epithelial cell receptors have been demonstrated for estrogens, progesterone, and androgens. The thymus also possesses enzymes that metabolize testosterone and progesterone. Experimental work supports a stimulatory effect of thymosins on the hypothalamus, suggesting a hypothalamic-pituitary-gonadal-thymic feedback circuit.

The anti-inflammatory and immunosuppressive effects of corticosteroids are well appreciated and will be dealt with only briefly. Glucocorticoids do not require a membrane receptor for entry into the cell and pass freely through cell membranes where they bind to a cytosol receptor. The steroid-receptor complex then migrates into the nucleus and binds to DNA, causing de-repression and synthesis of mRNA, which ultimately is followed by production of a new protein within the cell. Such proteins may have either an excitatory or inhibitory effect.

Corticosteroids affect the immune system through two general mechanisms; cell traffic and mobilization and cell function. Bolus infusion of moderate doses of corticosteroids results in the following effects on blood leukocytes: neutrophilia, lymphopenia, monocytopenia, eosinopenia, and basopenia. The total white blood cell count rises 40 to 80 percent, almost entirely accounted for by increases in polymorphonuclear leukocytes (PMNs) and immature band forms. Steroids cause a premature release of PMNs from the bone marrow. Additionally, there is a decrease in the marginated pool, that is, PMNs that adhere to the vessel wall. This decrease in margination results in fewer cells leaving the vascular compartment for sites of inflammation, a larger percentage remaining in the circulation, and hence a higher neutrophil count. Lymphocyte counts, on the other hand, fall rapidly with corticosteroid administration, reaching a trough by 4 hours post dose but recovering by 24 hours. This drop in lymphocyte counts in humans is not due to lympholysis, as occurs in certain animal species, but rather to migration of the lymphocytes out of the circulation into the bone marrow, spleen, and other

tissues. Monocyte counts mirror those of the lymphocytes, resulting from decreased bone marrow delivery and tissue redistribution. Eosinopenia occurs because of a decrease in bone marrow delivery and an increase in margination. The cause for the drop in basophil counts is unknown but may be an important factor in the protection afforded by corticosteroids against recurrent anaphylactoid reactions to radiocontrast media.

Other anti-inflammatory effects of corticosteroids are mediated primarily through effects on cell functions. They are potent vasoconstrictors, possibly through potentiation of the alpha-adrenergic activity of the cathecholamines. Suppression of fever is secondary to inhibition of production or of release of interleukin-1 (endogenous pyrogen). Corticosteroids diminish mitogenic activity, in association with decreasing interleukin-2 production, and inhibit the production of a number of macrophage enzymes, such as elastase, collagenase, and plasminogen activator. Perhaps of central importance in atopic diseases is the decrease in the products of both the cyclooxygenase and lipoxygenase pathways of arachidonic acid metabolism owing to production of lipocortin, which blocks the conversion of membrane phospholipids to arachidonate by phospholipase A. Additionally, corticosteroids cause a modest fall in antibody levels due to decreased production and increased catabolism; this effect is of questionable significance since specific antibody responses to immunization remain normal despite steroid therapy (Claman, 1984).

The role of endogenous catecholamines in the course of atopic disease, while speculative, is central to the theory of beta-adrenergic dysfunction as the etiology of atopy (Szentivanyi, 1968). Evidence for and against the beta-adrenergic blockade theory will not be presented here; however, there are observations that circulating catechols do modulate beta-adrenergic responsiveness by affecting receptor function. A decrease in high affinity beta receptors after simple ambulation has been reported, presumably due to uncoupling of the beta-receptor–adenylate cyclase complex by increased circulating catecholamines. The findings were duplicated by the infusion of norepinephrine. There is a direct correlation between the nocturnal fall in pulmonary function in asthmatics and the diurnal fall in circulating epinephrine. Plasma cAMP mirrors this pattern, whereas plasma cortisol levels have their trough hours earlier and are rising when pulmonary function is still falling. A rise in plasma histamine level was observed in asthmatics but not in normal controls: this level peaked at the same time that levels of epinephrine and pulmonary function were at their nadir.

HORMONAL FLUCTUATIONS OR ABNORMALITIES AND ALLERGIC DISEASE

Premenstrual Exacerbation of Allergic Disease. Premenstrual worsening of symptoms of both asthma and chronic urticaria and angioedema has been reported. In two recent studies of female asthmatics, about 40 percent felt their asthma varied with menses, and 80 percent of these asthmatics reported worsening 1 to 5 days prior to menses (Hanley, 1981; Gibbs et al., 1984). Peak expiratory flow rates documented significantly lower morning and evening function premenstrually compared with midcycle. No changes were documented in women without complaints of premenstrual worsening. There were no correlations with premenstrual increases in asthma and premenstrual tension, aspirin consumption, use of birth control pills, cycle length, or asthma during pregnancy. The cause of the fluctuation has not been elucidated, although a hormonal factor is likely—perhaps the fall in plasma progesterone level, a hormone that may have bronchodilating properties.

Thyroid Abnormalities and Allergic Disease. Asthma has been noted to become more severe in patients with hyperthyroidism and to respond to treatment of the endocrine problem. There may be numerous mechanisms involved in this relationship. A shift in nonspecific bronchial hyperactivity measured by histamine inhalation has been demonstrated. The effects of hyperthyroidism may be mediated through alterations of metabolism at the target cell site and through differing levels of various circulating hormones due to altered clearance. Many of the signs and symptoms of the hyperthyroid state appear to be due to potentiation of adrenergic responses and are successfully treated by beta-adrenergic blockade. There are no changes in circulating levels or in urinary excretion of catecholamines, but increased levels of intracellular cAMP have been found, suggesting perhaps increased coupling of the beta receptor and adenylate cyclase. However, such changes would be expected to improve the status of asthma in hyperthyroidism rather than worsen

it, as is the case. Triiodothyronine has been used to improve asthma, but studies reported were poorly controlled. Gordon and Southren (1977) summarized the effects of thyroid hormone on steroid-hormone metabolism. Metabolic clearance rates and secretory rates of C-21 steroids (cortisol and aldosterone) are increased in hyperthyroidism and decreased in myxedema; changes in the secretory rate are most likely compensatory and keep plasma levels within the normal range. Hyperthyroidism causes a shift toward larger amounts of 11-keto metabolites. Thyroid status also affects the metabolism of C-19 and C-18 steroids (sex hormones) but in the opposite direction from that of the C-21 steroids; levels decrease with hyperthyroidism and increase with hypothyroidism, owing in part to alterations in plasma protein binding of the steroids.

An interesting association of thyroid autoimmunity with chronic urticaria and angioedema has been reported (Lentzoff et al., 1983). Seventeen of 140 (12.1 percent) consecutive patients with chronic urticaria had elevated titers (1:1600) of antithyroid microsomal antibodies. In a control population of 477 patients, 5.6 percent had similar titers. Eight of 17 had either goiter or thyroid dysfunction, three were hyperthyroid, three hypothyroid, and three had biopsy proven Hashimoto thyroiditis. All 17 patients had angioedema. The following eight patients were treated with levothyroxine (0.2 mg/day): three showed complete remission of chronic urticaria, three improved, and two were unchanged. How thyroid autoimmunity is related to the manifestations of chronic urticaria is unclear.

INTERACTIONS OF HORMONES AND DRUGS USED TO TREAT ALLERGIC DISEASE

Theophylline. Metabolism of theophylline occurs in the liver over several pathways involving both first-order and capacity-limited kinetics, with the primary route involving cytochrome P-450. This system may be saturated or enhanced by a large variety of drugs.

The cellular actions of many hormones appear to be mediated through activation of receptor-linked adenylate cyclase, with a subsequent rise in cAMP. In any particular cell type, this may have either an excitory or inhibitory effect. Theophylline inhibits phosphodiesterase, thereby retarding degradation of cAMP and increasing intracellular levels of cAMP. This action, however, has been demonstrated at concentrations ten-fold greater than those achieved therapeutically: theophylline administration in normal subjects fails to produce a rise in plasma cAMP level. Warren and associates (1983) proposed that theophylline potentiates the action of catecholamines and that the potency of the theophylline effect depends on the level of sympathetic activity. They observed that intravenous theophylline administered with the patient supine had no effect, but when administered with the patient upright, it caused significant elevations of heart rate, plasma cAMP, and glucose, and was associated with a small but significant rise in plasma epinephrine and norepinephrine levels. These investigators thought that this was consistent with theophylline acting as a phosphodiesterase inhibitor, with amplification apparent only in the face of significant beta receptor stimulation.

In several animal models, theophylline augments the action of parathyroid hormone (PTH). Whether theophylline enhances PTH action in the human is not well established, but theophylline does possess PTH-like effects in the human kidney in that it stimulates nephrogenous cAMP, which is associated with increased phosphate and calcium excretion. PTH differs in increasing cAMP (through activation of adenylate cyclase) and promoting phosphaturia but decreasing urinary calcium excretion. Theophylline appears to have no effect on the metabolic clearance rate or half-life of glucocorticoids. Theophylline causes decreased cerebral blood flow and decreased oxygen tension in the brain. Whether the lowered seizure threshold seen in some patients treated with theophylline is due to hypoxemia or an effect on neurotransmitter functioning is not clear. According to Schraa and Dirks (1982), theophylline interferes with the ability to concentrate.

Adrenergic Agonists. Several studies have demonstrated diminution of peak effect and duration of action of exogenous adrenergic agents after chronic usage (Jenne, 1982). The mechanism appears to be a decrease in the number of membrane, high affinity beta receptors and an uncoupling of the beta receptor–adenylate cyclase complex. This subsensitivity secondary to adrenergic agonist therapy can be expected to blunt the response to endogenous catechols as well. Ephedrine administration increases the metabolic clearance rate and decreases the half-life of dexamethasone;

whether it similarly affects the metabolism of endogenous steroid hormones is unknown.

Corticosteroids. Therapy with glucocorticoids has far-reaching impact on many tissues in the body (Claman, 1984). Adverse effects from long-term usage are numerous and are only summarized here (Table 15–1), with emphasis on certain hormonal interactions.

In normal tissues, hydrocortisone increases cAMP level as well as the cAMP response to isoproterenol. Increased numbers of beta receptors have been noted after oral cortisone or prednisone administration (Davies and Lefkowitz, 1984). In tissues desensitized by chronic administration of adrenergic agonists, glucocorticoids attenuate the reduced stability of the high affinity state of the agonist-receptor, receptor-adenylate cyclase complex. There are some experimental data suggesting mineralocorticoids increase beta receptor density as well.

The major effect of exogenous corticosteroids is suppression of the hypothalamus with de-

TABLE 15–1. Complications of Corticosteroid Therapy

Endocrine

Diabetes mellitus
Delayed sexual maturation
Secondary amenorrhea
Adrenal insufficiency

Metabolic

Hyperlipidemia
Hypokalemia
Sodium retention
Centripetal obesity
Negative nitrogen balance

Musculoskeletal

Growth retardation (decreased somatomedin)
Osteoporosis
Myopathy
Aseptic necrosis of bone

Immunologic

Leukocyte redistribution
Impaired macrophage function
Impaired inflammatory response
Increased susceptibility to infection

Other

Peptic ulcer
Pancreatitis
Glaucoma
Posterior subcapsular cataracts
Psychosis
Pseudotumor cerebri
Hypertension
Subcutaneous tissue atrophy
Impaired wound healing

creased release of ACTH from the pituitary and subsequent suppression of adrenal function. When utilizing glucocorticoids in therapy, therefore, an attempt should be made to minimize hypothalamic suppression by mimicking the normal diurnal pattern, utilizing a short-acting corticosteroid such as prednisone (half-life of 60 minutes) given near the normal 8 a.m. plasma cortisol peak. Prednisolone and methylprednisolone, with half-lives of 180 to 200 minutes, may be used at slightly greater risk, but long-acting preparations, such as dexamethasone and triamcinolone, with half-lives of 300 minutes should be avoided. Alternate day dosing allows further time for hypothalamic recuperation and decreases incidence of adverse side effects. The use of inhaled topical steroid preparations in place of oral preparations further minimizes systemic side effects. Basal cortisol levels and ACTH response test results improve when inhaled steroids are substituted for oral steroids, although hypophysial-adrenal recovery may be gradual. In children, doses of 300 to 400 μg/day of inhaled beclomethasone dipropionate can cause a decrease in basal cortisol levels, although the ACTH response is normal. In some adults, doses of greater than 800 μg/day of the same drug have been reported to cause adrenal suppression.

Suppression of the hypothalamic-pituitary-adrenal axis is most easily assessed by monitoring the a.m. plasma cortisol; values consistently below 10 μg/dl are indicative of at least partial adrenal suppression. In patients on alternate day corticosteroid regimens, the cortisol level should be obtained immediately before the normally scheduled dose. The response to ACTH can be used to assess suppression, but this test evaluates only the ability of the adrenals to respond and does not assess hypothalamic or pituitary function. For this reason, a stress test such as insulin-hypoglycemia may be superior: however, some steroid-treated patients may have a suboptimal response to insulin yet respond satisfactorily to a major stress, such as surgery.

Suppression of ACTH secretion by exogenous corticosteroids appears to interfere with cerebral function, adversely affecting memory attention (Schraa and Dirks, 1982). Treatment of steroid-dependent asthmatics with ACTH fragments reveals sex-related differences; men improve in visual-spatial performance, whereas women improve in verbal memory. Animal studies suggest that corticosteroids block activation of the brain stem and reticulo-limbic system by ACTH.

A major adverse consequence of corticosteroid therapy is osteoporosis. Corticosteroids can cause growth retardation in children and aseptic necrosis of the femoral head, perhaps related to the vasoconstrictive properties of steroids. Clinical manifestations of corticosteroid-induced bone loss otherwise are similar to those of aging. Trabecular bone is the most affected. Histology reveals decreased trabecular volume, increased osteoclastic resorption surface, and decreased osteoblastic apposition rate (decreased calcification rate with normal osteoid volume) (Burkhardt, 1984). Age-related bone loss in women is associated with a rise in bone resorption and no change in bone forming surfaces, presumably due to estrogen deficiency. Simple osteoporosis in men shows a decline in bone formation with no rise in resorption, probably secondary to androgen deficiency. In both sexes, accelerated osteoporosis is seen with malabsorption of calcium (Nordin et al., 1981). Estrogen or testosterone therapy improves calcium balance by lowering bone resorption. Corticosteroids stimulate osteoclasts and inhibit osteoblasts and intestinal calcium absorption by a mechanism unrelated to vitamin D. Corticosteroids appear to stimulate parathyroid hormone secretion directly. ACTH suppression caused by corticosteroid administration results in diminished adrenal synthesis of estrogen precursors, such as androstenedione, which is especially important in postmenopausal women. Alternate day therapy, while allowing greater bone growth in children, still causes osteoporosis in adults. Two studies of daily or alternate day steroids in asthmatics have shown significant trabecular bone loss, with increased incidence of fractures (Adinoff and Hollister, 1983; Ruegsegger et al., 1983). One study suggested that young adults may be at greater risk of bone loss. Recommended therapy is replacement calcium, vitamin D, and sodium fluoride, although the benefit from such therapy has been challenged. It has been suggested that hydrochlorothiazide antagonizes renal hypercalciuria.

Growth retardation will be seen in a third of asthmatic children treated with corticosteroids. This effect is due to decreased release of somatomedin. Glucocorticoids delay epiphysial closure, while increased levels of sex steroids hasten closure.

Steroid myopathy most commonly affects the pelvic girdle and proximal muscles of the lower extremities, although the upper extremities and muscles of the diaphragm and rib cage also may be involved. The latter involvement can complicate the management of the steroid-dependent asthmatic patient. Steroid myopathy involving the muscles of respiration can be assessed by the measurement of maximum inspiratory pressures. The dysphonia that may accompany use of inhaled steroids may be due to myopathy of the vocal cords. Animal studies suggest that heart muscle usually is spared and that fluorinated steroids cause a greater degree of myopathy than nonfluorinated steroids.

H₂ Receptor Antagonists. Cimetidine prolongs the serum half-life of theophylline. It also may have a profound effect on gonadotropins and sex steroids. In two studies of men using cimetidine, luteinizing hormone (LH) response to luteinizing hormone releasing factor (LHRF) was diminished while follicle stimulating hormone (FSH) and testosterone responses to LHRF were normal. Serum LH was normal and FSH, prolactin (PRL), and testosterone levels all increased. Sperm counts were appreciably diminished, but morphology and motility were unaffected. Gonadotropin secretion to clomiphene was suppressed. Cimetidine did not affect the response of thyroid stimulating hormone (TSH), PRL, growth hormone (GH), or thyroxine to thyrotropin releasing factor (Van Thiel et al., 1979; Wang et al., 1982). In contrast, another H₂ antagonist, ranitidine, does not raise testosterone levels, presumably because ranitidine does not bind to androgen receptors. It also does not increase PRL, and gynecomastia is less frequently seen. Cimetidine has modulating effects on cellular immunity, especially on suppressor cell activity, and has caused pancytopenia. Immune effects have not been reported with ranitidine. Cimetidine, but apparently not ranitidine, reacts with receptors on lymphocytes.

Macrolide Antibiotics. Troleandomycin (TAO) has a "steroid-sparing" effect in asthmatics requiring corticosteroids. This effect frequently is observed with methylprednisolone, occasionally with prednisolone, but not with prednisone. The exact nature of its action is not understood, although two mechanisms have been described. One is the interference with theophylline metabolism: a reduction of a third to half the dose of theophylline usually is necessary to avoid theophylline toxicity. Troleandomycin therefore may be useful in asthmatics with chaotic theophylline levels due to inordinately rapid metabolism. The other and probably primary mechanism of troleandomycin effect is prolongation of the serum half-life of methylprednisolone. This effect can be induced rapidly with multiple daily dosing, but is maintained ultimately with single alternate day doses of 250 mg. Whether TAO acts solely by converting methylprednisolone to a longer-acting compound is unclear and requires further study. TAO does not appear to work in all asthmatics requiring corticosteroids. In some patients, erythromycin exhibits a similar action of decreasing steroid requirements. In many patients, it will delay theophylline clearance and, in so doing, can cause toxicity when used to treat a flare in asthma symptoms, if theophylline dosage is not adjusted appropriately.

PREGNANCY AND ASTHMA

Hormonal Levels. The predominant hormone of early pregnancy is human chorionic gonadotropin, produced by the syncytiotrophoblastic layer of the placenta. The hormone rises to a peak at 60 to 90 days of gestation, then declines to a plateau, which is maintained throughout the remainder of pregnancy. This hormone plays a luteotropic role, maintaining the corpus luteum and its steroidogenesis until the placenta becomes self-sufficient. The same placental layer that produces human chorionic gonadotropin produces chorionic somatomammotropin, which peaks in the last trimester of pregnancy.

Progesterone and estrogen levels rise throughout pregnancy to plasma concentrations that are 50 and 100 times, respectively, the peak levels in the nonpregnant woman during the menstrual cycle. The exact function of these hormones in pregnancy is unknown. It has been suggested that progesterone relaxes smooth muscles, although a motor effect on bronchial smooth muscle is thought unlikely. Estrogens may function to maintain the increased uteroplacental blood flow. Increased levels of progesterone are associated with the increased sensitivity of the respiratory center to carbon dioxide; this effect is credited as the cause of hyperventilation so characteristic of pregnancy.

Total plasma cortisol level is markedly increased as is the level of cortisol-binding protein, transcortin. Throughout pregnancy, the levels of free cortisol are two to three times those in nonpregnant women due to increased production, diminished plasma clearance rates, and displacement of cortisol from transcortin by progesterone. Despite the rise in free cortisol, evidence of increased glucocorticoid effects are equivocal, and there is no indication for any modification in the dose of corticosteroids employed in the treatment of asthma or other conditions during pregnancy.

Fetal tissue contains histamine in high concentrations. Perhaps in response, large amounts of histaminase are produced by the placenta and enter the maternal circulation where levels are several hundred times those in nonpregnant women. Despite such high levels, there is no known effect on the symptoms of allergic diseases in pregnant women.

Excretion of metabolites of prostaglandin $F_{2\alpha}$ (PGF_{2a}) is elevated to two to three times normal throughout pregnancy, rising to ten to thirty times normal during labor. PGE_2 levels, on the other hand, are increased only during the last trimester. Despite the known but opposing actions of these two mediators on bronchial smooth muscle, there is no known clinical result of their increased concentrations during gestation.

Energy Metabolism. The net effect of increased levels of estrogens, progesterone, free cortisol, and human chorionic gonadotropin, particularly, is to produce an anti-insulin effect, which leads to impaired maternal glucose utilization, impaired protein synthesis, and increased lipolysis. All have the effect of making glucose, amino acids, and free fatty acids available to the fetus. In this setting, fasting may produce maternal hypoglycemia; because glucose also can pass from the fetus to the mother, prolonged maternal fasting can deplete fetal glycogen and promote fetal gluconeogenesis at the expense of its supply of amino acids. If the pregnant woman has an inadequate caloric intake during severe asthma, it is advisable to administer parenteral glucose to protect the fetus from the deleterious effects of maternal hypoglycemia.

Circulation and Fluid Balance. During pregnancy, sodium and water are retained. Most women gain over 11 kg, largely fluid. Total body water increases 6 to 8 L, two thirds are extracellular. Blood volume increases an average of 40 to 50 percent, and red blood cell mass, 20 to 40 percent. A 20 to 50 percent increase in cardiac output occurs due to increased stroke volume despite little change in heart rate. The increased cardiac output is required to supply the uteroplacental circulation, which increases from 50 ml/min in the nonpregnant state to over 500 ml/min at term. The increased extracellular fluid has been viewed as a reser-

voir to protect the increased blood volume against temporary fluid deficits. Severe attacks of asthma frequently lead to dehydration and reduced plasma volume. Fluid replacement during these acute attacks is critical to ensure adequate cardiac output.

Pulmonary Physiology and Respiration. Despite the marked elevation towards term of the resting diaphragm caused by the upward pressure of the gravid uterus, pulmonary physiology and function is altered relatively little by normal pregnancy (Weinberg et al., 1980). A decrease in functional residual capacity and residual volume begins in the fifth to sixth month and may reach 25 percent by term, but vital capacity and total lung capacity are preserved since the movement of the diaphragm is not impaired. Furthermore, there is no significant change in airflow; FEV_1, $FEV_1$1/FVC ratio and dynamic compliance all are unaltered.

Changes in respiration begin in the first trimester and progress to term. The principal alteration is an increase in minute volume, which results from an increase in tidal volume while respiratory rate is unchanged. This increase in minute ventilation, which may reach 50 percent by the end of pregnancy, exceeds the increased requirement for oxygen and appears to result from the effect of progesterone on the respiratory center, leading to a shift to the left in the ventilatory response to CO_2. As a result of hyperventilation and compensatory responses by the kidney, the maternal blood is diagnostic of compensated alkalosis with a pH of 7.4 to 7.47, $PaCO_2$ of 25 to 32 mm Hg (normal 38 to 45 mm Hg), and bicarbonate value of 18 to 21 meq/L (normal 20 to 30 meq/L).

With the decrease in residual volume and expiratory reserve capacity, the closing volume can approach or exceed the functional residual capacity. This could result in collapse of the small airways in the dependent areas of the lung during normal respiration, leading to decreased ventilation/perfusion ratios and hypoxemia. Since the PaO_2 is preserved in normal pregnancy, these effects do not appear to be important factors. However, there probably is some early closure even in uncomplicated pregnancies; the alveolar-arterial oxygen gradient when sitting is increased to a mean of 14 mm Hg near term, increasing further to 20 mm Hg when supine. This change reflects early collapse of the dependent areas of the lungs, which could be a detrimental factor in patients with asthma who already are experiencing ventilation/perfusion mismatches.

Fetal Oxygenation. Generous uteroplacental blood flow and strong affinity of fetal hemoglobin for oxygen allow the fetus to thrive in a state of relative hypoxemia. Normally, with the mother breathing room air at sea level, the maternal PaO_2 is about 91 mm Hg, and the fetal PaO_2 is about 32 mm Hg. When pregnant women were given 15 percent oxygen, the fetal oxygen level fell to 26 mm Hg; however, a further decrease in inspired oxygen to 10 percent, while reducing the maternal oxygen levels to 47 mm Hg, had no further depressing effect on fetal oxygen levels. Hyperventilation, on the other hand, has a more profound influence on blood oxygen levels. When, as a result of hyperventilation, the maternal PaO_2 increased from 91 to 100 mm Hg and the $PaCO_2$ decreased from 22 to 14 mm Hg, the fetal oxygen content decreased from 25 to 19 mm Hg (Greenberger, 1985). The deleterious effect of hyperventilation may result either from constriction of the uterine blood vessels by hypocarbia or from a shift of the maternal oxygen dissociation curve to the left by a rise in pH. In either case, in the asthmatic mother, hyperventilation and hypoxemia typical of acute asthma could substantially increase fetal hypoxemia.

Immunity of Pregnancy. The fetus and placenta contain a number of histocompatability antigens encoded by paternal genes; thus, they represent a paternal allograft to the mother. There is no simple explanation why this foreign tissue is not rejected. Explanations that the uterus represents an organ incapable of allograft rejection or that the placenta represents an impermeable barrier have been disproved. Transplacental exchange of immunogenic cells and macromolecules occurs in both directions. However, the main area of contact between mother and fetus, the syncytiotrophoblastic layer, does act at least as a partial barrier to the exchange of immunogenic material. In addition, although it does express unique antigens of paternal origin, it lacks HLA, ABO, and Rh blood group antigens. This partial barrier is supplemented by a variety of modifications in immune responses in both mother and fetus which apparently allow the pregnancy to persist.

Maternal humoral immunity appears to function normally during gestation. There are no changes in B lymphocyte numbers or in levels of IgG, IgM, or IgA. There is, in fact, evidence of specific antibody production directed towards a variety of fetal antigens of paternal origin. These include IgG antibodies directed towards paternal Class I and Class II HLA antigens, which can block the maternal lymphocytes cytotoxic for these same antigens and are therefore functionally protective of the fetal "graft." Also there are antibodies directed toward non-HLA antigens of the syncytiotrophoblast layer of the placenta, which combine with these antigens to form immune complexes in the maternal circulation. There is clearly some depression of maternal cell-mediated immunity during normal pregnancy, but it is not of a profound degree. Variable results have been reported when pregnant and nonpregnant women have been compared for the incidence of delayed hypersensitivity skin test reactions, skin graft rejections, and *in vitro* stimulation of lymphocytes with plant mitogens, recall antigens, or allogeneic lymphocytes.

Perhaps more convincing than immunologic studies is clinical evidence suggesting a "pregnancy associated immune deficiency syndrome" (Weinberg, 1984). There is epidemiologic evidence that susceptibility in the pregnant woman to clinical infection with poliomyelitis, hepatitis A, variola, and *Plasmodium falciparum* is two to seven times that in the nonpregnant woman, and deaths from hepatitis A, influenza A, variola, and *Entamoeba histolytica* are similarly increased. Carcinoma of the breast occurs almost twice as often in pregnant women and carcinoma of the cervix almost fourteen times as often as in nonpregnant women of the same age. Furthermore, patients with tumors that are discovered during pregnancy, particularly in the third trimester, have poorer prognoses, and the five-year survival in patients with malignant melanomas is reduced by each succeeding pregnancy.

This reduction in cell-mediated responses and increased susceptibility to tumors and to infections against which cell-mediated immunity normally plays a role in host defense appears to be the result of multiple factors. At a cellular level, there is ample evidence for both an increase in suppressor T lymphocytes and a decrease in helper T lymphocytes resulting in a decreased helper/suppressor ratio that is somewhat reduced in the first two trimesters but falls even further in the last trimester (0.93/1) (Sridama et al., 1982). Studies of the sera from 287 pregnant women clearly demonstrated a serum factor, appearing about the thirteenth week, which was capable of suppressing lymphocyte blastogenic responses. Although changes in T cell populations did not correlate with levels of various serum factors studied, several other substances are known to be present in increased levels during pregnancy, which are known to be capable of suppressing lymphocyte function (Weinberg, 1984). The steroid hormones cortisol, progesterone, and estradiol all can suppress some aspect of cell-mediated immunity; the last two, which are found in considerably higher concentrations in the placental circulation than in the maternal blood, could easily play a local role in reducing an immune reaction between maternal lymphocytes and fetal cells. Also, alpha-fetoprotein occurs in high concentrations in the fetal circulation in the first trimester then declines, while alpha-2-glycoprotein, produced by maternal peripheral leukocytes, rises progressively throughout pregnancy. Both are capable of blocking the lymphocyte response to allogeneic cells in concentrations encountered in normal pregnancy.

Suppression of cell-mediated responses during pregnancy is only partial. The mother does develop cytotoxic lymphocytes directed toward antigens of paternal origin on fetal cells and placental trophoblastic cells. These cytotoxic lymphocytes first appear about the fifteenth week of gestation and by the second trimester are present in 88 percent of pregnancies. There is evidence that natural killer cell activity also is reduced in the pregnant woman. Inflammatory cells function is impaired, with decreased chemotaxis and phagocytosis by PMNs and decreased phagocytosis by macrophages. These factors may account for the increased susceptibility of pregnant women to certain bacterial infections, such as *Streptococcus pneumoniae* meningitis and *Neisseria gonorrhoeae* septicemia.

The fetus is exposed to maternal antigens and is immunologically competent by the second trimester. Thus, the fetus could as well reject the mother as the reverse. There is evidence of cells in the fetal cord blood of the suppressor phenotype, which are capable of suppressing the proliferative response of both maternal and unrelated lymphocytes.

In summary, fetal survival appears to be the result of the interaction of several factors. These include the following: (1) the interface of the syncytiotrophoblast layer, lacking in HLA antigens, which reduces the crossover of immunogenic antigens between mother and fetus; (2) specific antibody that blocks potentially destructive cell-mediated responses to paternal HLA antigens and antigens on the syncytiotrophoblast; (3) nonspecific serum factors that reduce cell-mediated immunity either generally or locally in the placenta; and (4) suppressor T lymphocytes of both maternal and fetal origin, which depress immune responsiveness.

Effect of Pregnancy on the Course of Bronchial Asthma. Review of retrospective studies of the course of asthma in 1087 pregnancies revealed that 36 percent of patients were improved, 41 percent were unchanged, and 23 percent became worse. Prospective studies suggest an even greater number become worse. The change in asthma, if it occurs, appears to be more than random since it is sometimes dramatic and tends to be consistent in subsequent pregnancies (Williams, 1967). In a prospective study, those whose asthma worsened during pregnancy did so during the twenty-ninth and thirty-sixth weeks (Forsythe et al., 1985). All asthmatics tended to improve during the last few weeks of pregnancy and had few asthma-related problems during labor and delivery (Schatz et al., 1983).

The reason for the improvement or worsening of asthma in pregnancy was analyzed in a prospective study; women whose asthma improved also had rhinitis improved. However, a higher incidence of pregnancy-associated hypertension, a longer gestation, and a greater need in multiparous women for augmentation of uterine contraction were observed (Schatz et al., 1985). Schatz therefore hypothesized that those improving had the greatest gestational induced corticosteroid effects, perhaps due to induced beta-adrenergic enhancement and decreased production of prostaglandins.

Effect on Asthma of Drugs Used to Terminate Pregnancy. Since prostaglandins are used to terminate pregnancy, one must be aware of their action on patients with bronchial asthma. $PGF_{2\alpha}$ is a potent bronchoconstrictor, and asthmatics are many times more sensitive to this effect than are normal individuals. Though PGE_2 is normally a bronchodilator, both PGF_{2a} and PGE_2, when given intravenously in doses employed for inducing abortion, cause increased airway resistance, even in normal women. They should be used with special caution in women with asthma.

THE EFFECT OF PREGNANCY ON OTHER ALLERGIC DISEASES

Allergic Rhinitis. Nasal congestion is a common complaint in pregnancy, occurring in about one third of all pregnant women. Many have similar symptoms before pregnancy but experience a further increase in symptoms during pregnancy. Congestion of the nasal mucosa develops by the end of the first trimester and progresses throughout pregnancy. Mucosal edema is particularly prominent in the last two months before delivery. These changes parallel the increased levels of estrogen and progesterone, which are their probable cause. Paradoxically, some women may experience improvement in chronic rhinitis during pregnancy.

Urticaria, Angioedema, and Eczema. Occasionally women experience urticaria limited to pregnancy, with recurrences in subsequent pregnancies. This pattern was observed in three of 554 consecutive patients with urticaria evaluated by Champion et al. (1969). In addition to urticaria, an autoimmune progesterone dermatitis was described in one patient who experienced an acneform eruption, arthritis, peripheral and tissue eosinophilia, spontaneous abortion, and a delayed hypersensitivity skin test reaction to progesterone during two consecutive pregnancies (Bierman, 1973). Other patients have been described with apparent immediate or delayed sensitivity to progesterone who experienced premenstrual urticaria and bullous, eczematoid, maculopapular, or urticarial lesions (Hart, 1977).

The course of hereditary angioneurotic edema is affected favorably by pregnancy. Of 25 patients, 23 improved during their last trimester, and none had any angioedema during the course of labor and delivery (Frank, 1976).

The course of atopic dermatitis appears to be little affected by pregnancy. In a large series from the Mayo Clinic, 3 percent stated that their eczema improved during pregnancy, while only 1 percent reported exacerbation.

Effect of Bronchial Asthma on the Course of Pregnancy. Three studies which examined the outcome of pregnancy retrospectively in asthmatic women found suggestive evidence that asthma could have a deleterious effect on the fetus. An increased risk of premature birth (7.4 versus 3.7 percent) and a neonatal mortality (18.5 in 1000 versus 8 in 1000) were reported in Norwegian women with asthma (Bahna and Bjerkedal, 1972). Pregnant patients with bronchial asthma treated in a New York hospital also experienced an increased incidence of premature birth (8.9 versus 6.2 percent) (Schaefer and Silverman, 1961). In another study of 277 asthmatic women, there was no increase in the incidence of premature labor or low birthweight infants for the group as a whole, but 16 women with severe asthma had a 35 percent incidence of low birth weight infants and a 28 percent perinatal mortality (Gordon et al., 1970). Details regarding the status of the asthma in these studies is lacking, however. It is possible that the control of asthma was less

than optimal and that the trend toward prematurity and low birth weight reflects the effect of recurrent episodes of bronchoconstriction and resulting fetal hypoxia. In an ongoing prospective study in which care has been taken to avoid uncontrolled asthma, there has been no increased incidence of obstetric complications, no increase in preterm or low birth weight infants, and no increase in perinatal complications (Schatz et al., 1983b).

Effects of Drugs Used to Treat Asthma on the Development of the Fetus and the Course of Pregnancy. A primary concern regarding drugs administered during pregnancy is their possible effect on the development and survival of the fetus. Between fertilization and implantation, the embryo is resistant to all environmental agents. By the fifth week of gestation, however, placental transportation of maternal substances to the fetus is established. From that time on, substances of molecular weight less than 600 daltons readily cross the placenta by diffusion. This placental transmission is modified somewhat by the extent of protein binding and ionization of the drug, both of which impede movement across the membrane. However, since most therapeutic agents are in the range of 250 to 400 daltons, it can be assumed that they enter the fetal circulation even if at a lower concentration than in the maternal.

The most critical period for the fetus is during organogenesis, which largely is completed by the eighth to tenth week of gestation. Thereafter, drugs cannot cause gross abnormalities but can affect the fetal growth and function of organs and tissues. Examples of these late occurring drug effects include dental enamel dysplasia from tetracycline, nephrotoxicity and ototoxicity from aminoglycosides, goiter from iodides, and an increased incidence of adenocarcinoma of the vagina in females and reproductive tract abnormalities in males whose mothers received diethylstilbesterol during pregnancy. Unfortunately, animal studies of drug teratogenicity have not proved helpful to elucidating risks in humans, since there is little similarity in the effects of drugs even from one strain to another, let alone from one species to another.

Effects of Specific Drugs on Fetal Development. Documentation of teratogenic effects of drugs currently employed in the United States and Canada is sparse. The incidence of teratogenesis due to drugs is thought to be very low. However, there is suggestive evidence that women who bear children with congenital abnormalities take more drugs during the first trimester of pregnancy than do those who bear normal children. Although this could reflect the effect of the illness for which the drugs were taken rather than the effect of the drugs themselves, it seems prudent to avoid any unnecessary drugs during the critical first trimester of pregnancy.

Certain drugs are contraindicated during pregnancy. Tetracycline is capable of retarding fetal skeletal growth and causing dental enamel dysplasia and discoloration. Iodides can block fetal organic binding of elemental iodine, leading to decreased thyroid hormone systhesis, increased TSH, and goiter. Goiters have caused respiratory obstruction and death in newborns. Live viral vaccines should be avoided during pregnancy; not only is there a potential of harm to the fetus, there also is a possibility of severe infection in the mother because of her compromised ability to resist many viral infections. A number of antibiotics in addition to tetracycline should be avoided during certain periods of gestation. Aminoglycosides can cause neural arch and renal abnormalities early in pregnancy and nephrotoxicity and ototoxicity late in pregnancy. Sulfonamides given late in pregnancy compete with bilirubin for albumin binding and lead to increased diffusion of bilirubin into tissues. Trimethoprim also may cause hyperbilirubinemia when given late in pregnancy (Holt and Mabry, 1983).

The principal information on the safety of drugs used in the treatment of asthma during pregnancy is derived from the Collaborative Perinatal Project Study, which was conducted at twelve medical centers during the years 1959 to 1965 (Heinonen et al., 1977). A total of 50,282 maternal-fetal pairs were studied, in which there were 3248 congenital malforma-

tions. On the basis of these data, standardized risks were calculated on an expected frequency of 1.00. The results for a number of drugs relevant to the treatment of asthma and rhinitis are given in Table 15-2.

Several points are clear as follows from perusal of this table: first is the small number of mothers exposed to several of these drugs and second is the absence of many of the drugs most commonly employed today, such as selective beta-2 adrenergic agonists, cromolyn, and inhaled corticosteroids. In addition, considering the number of drugs examined, it would be anticipated that several would be implicated by chance alone. Therefore, these retrospective associations can be, at best, only the basis for further studies. Unfortunately, no similar extensive studies have been conducted since.

What about drugs used in the treatment of asthma and rhinitis which were not in use at the time of the Collaborative Perinatal Project Study (CPPS)? Data have been presented on the use of cromolyn in nearly 300 pregnant women; there is no evidence of an increased incidence of birth defects (Greenberger et al., 1985). Information also was reported on 42 women who used inhaled beclomethasone dipropionate during the first trimester; the only malformed infant was in a mother who was also diabetic and schizophrenic (Greenberger et al., 1983). There is no information to date concerning the outcome of use of beta-2 adrenergic bronchodilators during early pregnancy even though many exposures must have occurred, considering the popularity of these drugs.

Effects on Uterine Function. In addition to possible effects on fetal development, as discussed, drugs can influence the fetus indirectly through alterations in uterine blood flow or

Table 15-2. Safety of Allergy Medications in Pregnancy

Drug	Number Exposed	Standardized Risk	Significance
Epinephrine	189	1.71	<.05
Theophylline	117	1.38	
Ephedrine	373	1.07	
Atropine	401	1.04	
Isoproterenol	31	0.94	
Corticosteroids	145	0.67	
Brompheniramine	65	2.34	<.05
Hydroxyzine	50	1.44	
Diphenhydramine	595	1.25	
Chlorpheniramine	1070	1.20	
Tripelennamine	100	0.81	
Phenylpropanolamine	726	1.40	<.01
Phenylephrine	1249	1.31	<.05

uterine contractility and the progress of labor.

A possible deleterious effect of sympathomimetic amines could be constriction of blood vessels supplying the uterus, particularly if combined with dilatation of the vascular beds supplying the skeletal muscles. Although this is only a theoretic consideration, it should be noted that the three sympathomimetic amines with alpha-adrenergic agonist properties listed in Table 15–2 (epinephrine, phenylpropanolamine, and phenylephrine) all were found to be associated with significantly increased incidences of malformations.

A second property of the beta-2 adrenergic agonists, and to a lesser extent theophylline, that might prove deleterious to the fetus is relaxation of the uterine smooth muscle. Beta-adrenergic agonists have been employed frequently in doses exceeding those employed for the treatment of asthma to control premature labor. No deleterious effects on the fetus have been reported, including one long-term follow-up. Recent data from the Kaiser-Permanente study of pregnancy and asthma have shown a prolongation of labor in multiparous women receiving theophylline (Schatz et al., 1983b). Although no complications resulted, this information suggests that bronchodilator drugs, administered orally or parenterally, may have some retarding effect on the progress of labor.

Treatment of Bronchial Asthma and Rhinitis in Pregnancy. The objective in treating bronchial asthma during pregnancy should be to control asthma and to avoid severe attacks that might result in significant fetal hypoxemia. In general, the approach to therapy is the same as that in the nonpregnant asthmatic, with a few exceptions. First, certain drugs, such as tetracycline and iodides, must be avoided. These drugs actually are peripheral to and unnecessary for the treatment of asthma. Second, to the extent consistent with adequate control of asthma, those drugs that have not been demonstrated to be safe in pregnancy should be avoided. Unfortunately, these include selective beta-2 adrenergic bronchodilators, which are extremely important in the treatment of asthma.

The mainstay of asthma therapy in pregnancy is theophylline. This may be supplemented, if needed, with intermittent use of beta-adrenergic bronchodilators by inhalation. Drugs that appear to have an adequate safety record, which may be added progressively if needed for asthma control, are cromolyn, inhaled beclomethasone diproprionate, inhaled atropine, and prednisone or methylprednisolone. Safety data, particularly in regard to teratogenesis, are lacking for the selective beta-2 agonists. The unknown potential for risk must be balanced against the known risk of fetal hypoxemia. If regular beta-adrenergic therapy appears necessary, the inhaled route is not only more effective but will expose the fetus to much lower blood levels.

If severe asthma does develop during the course of pregnancy, injected terbutaline is preferred to injected epinephrine, since the latter was associated with an increased incidence of fetal malformations (see Table 15–2). Because of the special conditions of fluid and energy balance and the tenuous state of fetal oxygenation, particular attention should be given to the use of oxygen and to adequate fluid and glucose administration during any severe episodes of asthma.

The patient should be brought to an optimal state of asthma control in preparation for delivery. The preferred anesthetic is local or spinal anesthesia for caesarean sections. If general anesthesia is required, nitrous oxide and halothane are preferred. When the patient has received systemic corticosteroids during pregnancy, supplemental steroids should be administered at the time of delivery to protect the mother against stress should the adrenal-pituitary axis be suppressed. An acceptable schedule is cortisone acetate 100 mg, intramuscularly, every 8 hours throughout labor and delivery. The infant should be observed for adrenal insufficiency, but this is encountered very rarely, and routine administration of steroids to the infant is not indicated. Theophylline passes freely across the placenta, and cord blood and neonatal serum levels are fully as high as maternal. Because of the immaturity of the hepatic cytochrome P-450 system, theophylline levels fall slowly in the newborn, with serum half-life frequently longer than 10 hours. Nevertheless, therapeutic maternal theophylline blood levels at delivery (10 to 20 μg/ml) uncommonly have been associated with symptoms in the newborn, usually transient jitteriness and mild tachycardia (Schatz et al., 1983a).

Rhinitis frequently is a troublesome if not dangerous problem during pregnancy. Information on the safety of antihistamines comes largely from the Collaborative Perinatal Project Study (CPPS) (Heinonen et al., 1977), which found an overall increase of malformations in offspring of mothers who had taken brompheniramine and of selected malformations in those of mothers who had taken chlorpheniramine, although the overall incidence with the latter drug was not significantly increased. Tripelennamine was the antihistamine with the lowest incidence of malformations, but also had very limited use. A subsequent study of drug intake by mothers of 458 children with congenital anomalies, and two matched groups, revealed that the mothers of the children with malformations had actually taken significantly fewer antihistamines than did the controls (Nelson and Forfar, 1971), emphasizing that if enough statistical comparisons are performed some probably meaningless "significant" associations will be found. In another study of 6837 women, 80 infants were born with fetal abnormalities (1.2 percent). Among the several hundred women who employed either pseudoephedrine or brompheniramine, there was a slightly less then expected incidence of malformations (Jick et al., 1981.) Thus, it is not clear that any of the commonly employed antihistamines should be regarded with great suspicion, although it seems wise to minimize their use in the first trimester of pregnancy. Decongestants, on the other hand, were more strongly implicated in the CPPS. However, the low incidence of abnormalities with pseudoephedrine makes it the preferred decongestant if one must be used. Finally, it has been reported that nasal beclomethasone provides excellent relief to the majority of women with rhinitis in pregnancy and perhaps should be the preferred choice in the first trimester (Parkin, 1983).

Immunotherapy. Severe systemic reactions to injections of allergy extract can be accompanied by lower abdominal cramping and uterine bleeding. Although abortion has been reported in a very few such instances, the administration of allergy immunotherapy throughout pregnancy increases neither the risk of fetal loss, even in the face of systemic reactions, nor the risk of congenital malformation (Metzger et al., 1978). Nevertheless, to maximize safety, allergy immunotherapy should be administered with caution during pregnancy. Doses should be increased slowly while building to maintenance. During the patient's pollen season when the possibility of inducing a constitutional reaction is increased, dosage probably should be reduced. There rarely is an indication to initiate immunotherapy during pregnancy. Generally, institution of this procedure can be delayed until after delivery.

There would appear to be no danger associated with immunotherapy during nursing of those of mothers who had taken chlorphenirasensitization of the infant or of allergic reactions in the infant. Allergic sensitivity that occurs early in infancy usually is directed towards food allergens either from maternal ingestion of foods which can be secreted in breast milk or from supplemental feeding in the nursery or later.

BREAST-FEEDING

Immunology of Breast Milk. Colostrum and breast milk provide important immune defenses for the infant's gastrointestinal tract, particularly during the early neonatal period. Breast-feeding during this period should be viewed as a further contribution of the mother to the infant's ability to survive in an extrauterine environment and not merely as a source of nutrition. The incidence of enteric and respiratory infections, meningitis, and gram-negative sepsis is decreased in breast-fed infants. This is true not only in underdeveloped countries but has been found in the United States where hospitalization for bacterial infections in the first few months of life has been shown to be markedly reduced by exclusive breast-feeding (Fallot et al., 1980).

Human breast milk contains a number of substances that may account for this beneficial effect, as follows: (1) nonspecific anti-infective components, such as lysozyme, lactoferrin, and nonspecific antiviral activity; (2) secretory IgA specific for enteric bacteria, viruses, and food antigens; (3) a growth stimulating factor contributing to differentiation of the gastrointestinal mucosa; (4) viable macrophages, and B and T lymphocytes; and (5) chemical factors that produce and maintain a low pH, which favors colonization of the gut with *Lactobacillus bifidus* to the exclusion of gram-negative organisms. The last property is lost with the addition of either supplementary formula or solid food.

Drug Excretion in Breast Milk. Most drugs are secreted in the mother's milk, often in concentrations that approach those of maternal serum. Despite this secretion, medications used for the treatment of asthma and rhinitis rarely present a problem for the infant. Less than 1 percent of the dose of theophylline administered to the mother appears in breast milk. It has been estimated that the infant would receive between 0.7 and 2.8 mg/kg/24 hours with the mother who has therapeutic theophylline serum levels. This dose is well under that prescribed for infants for treatment of apnea.

There is one reported case of irritability in an infant whose mother was receiving a rapidly absorbed theophylline preparation. Prednisone also passes into the milk in low concentrations; it has been estimated that following a 50 mg oral dose of prednisone to the mother, an infant would receive less than 20 percent of its daily physiologic corticosteroid requirement. Beta-adrenergic agonists and antihistamines are excreted in the milk in small amounts, but there are no reports of significant side effects in nursing infants. There is a single report of crying and poor sleeping pattern in an infant whose mother ingested an oral decongestant, isoephedrine.

Food proteins also can be excreted in human milk. A number of instances have been documented in which gastrointestinal, respiratory, or cutaneous symptoms in nursing infants responded to the removal of a particular food from the diet of the mothers (Kilshaw and Cant, 1984). This was specifically examined by feeding nursing mothers one egg or ½ pint of cow's milk. Analysis of the mother's milk revealed detectable ovalbumin in 13 of 22 specimens, and beta-lactoglobulin in 10 of 19 specimens. Thus the avoidance of intake of highly allergenic food proteins may be a more important consideration than the avoidance of drugs in infants with a strong family history of atopy.

MISCELLANEOUS ASPECTS OF REPRODUCTION WITH IMMUNE FEATURES

Spontaneous Abortion. Fifteen percent of diagnosed pregnancies end in spontaneous abortion, which are caused by infection and genetic, anatomic, and hormonal abnormalities. However, some workers believe that the most frequent cause of recurrent spontaneous abortion is immune (Mowbray and Underwood, 1985). Couples who have had recurrent spontaneous abortions share more HLA and DR antigens than do control couples, and lymphocytes of the woman have a decreased proliferative response to lymphocytes of the man but not to those of other men. It has been suggested that in these couples there also is greater sharing of antigens between the fetal trophoblast layer and the mother, resulting in a failure on the part of the mother to mount a vigorous humoral response to these paternally derived antigens. The failure to make this response, which is considered to be protective ("blocking antibod-

ies"), then allows the rejection of the fetal allograft. This concept is supported by the success of immunization with either their husbands' lymphocytes (Mowbray et al., 1985) or multiple third party donor lymphocytes (Taylor et al., 1985). Those women who develop cytotoxic antibodies as a result of this treatment have a high incidence of subsequent successful pregnancies.

Infertility. Several abnormal immune responses have been reported in infertile couples. These include an increased incidence in women of cell-mediated immunity toward sperm antigen, increased titers of antisperm antibodies, and presence of sperm-immobilizing antibodies. The significance of these responses to sperm antigens is unknown.

Preeclampsia. Preeclamptic women have been reported to possess circulating immune complexes in the third trimester of pregnancy more frequently than do other women. In one study, 80 percent of preeclamptic women had circulating immune complexes compared with only 11.7 percent of normal pregnant women at the same stage of gestation.

Immediate Hypersensitivity to Semen. Asthma, urticaria, and angioedema occurring in women following sexual intercourse have been shown to be due to immediate hypersensitivity to proteins in their partners' seminal secretions. The diagnosis, suspected on epidemiologic grounds, is readily confirmed by immediate skin test reactivity to the partner's semen. In several instances, this condition has responded to immunotherapy that employed standard allergen immunotherapy protocols (Friedman et al., 1984).

Immune Consequences of Vasectomy. Following vasectomy, a number of men develop spermatozoa-agglutinating antibodies, which may persist for as long as 20 years. In prospective studies, circulating immune complexes have been detected several months following vasectomy but then disappear; studies several years after surgery show no increased incidence of complexes. Review of all available information by Kevacs and Francis in 1983 led to the conclusion that there is no evidence that vasectomy has deleterious health effects in humans.

REFERENCES

Adinoff, A.D., Hollister, J.R.: Steroid-induced fractures and bone loss in patients with asthma. N. Engl. J. Med. 309:265, 1983.

Bahna, S.L., Bjerkedal, T.: The course and outcome of pregnancy in women with bronchial asthma. Acta Allergol. 27:397, 1972.

Barnes, P.J., Fitzgerald, G., Brown, M., et al.: Nocturnal asthma and changes in circulating epinephrine, histamine and cortisol. N. Engl. J. Med. 303:263, 1980.

Bierman, S.M.: Autoimmune progesterone dermatitis of pregnancy. Arch. Dermatol. 107:896, 1973.

Burkhardt, P.: Corticosteroids and bone: A review. Hormone Res. 20:59, 1984.

Champion, R.H., Roberts, S.B., Carpenter, R.G., Roger, J.H.: Urticaria and angioedema. Br. J. Dermatol. 81:588, 1969.

Claman, H.N.: Anti-inflammatory effects of corticosteroids. Clin. Immunol. Allergy 4:317, 1984.

Davies, A.O., Lefkowitz, R.J.: Regulation of beta-adrenergic receptors by steroid hormones. Ann. Rev. Physiol. 46:119, 1984.

Fallor, M.E., Boyd III, J.L., Oski, F.A.: Breast-feeding reduces incidence of hospital admissions for infections in infants. Pediatrics 65:1121, 1980.

Forsythe, A., Schatz, M., Harden, K., et al.: Effect of stage of pregnancy on asthma course (abstract). J. Allergy Clin. Immunol. 75:133, 1985.

Frank, M.M.: Hereditary angioedema: The clinical syndrome and its management. Ann. Intern. Med. 84:580, 1976.

Friedman, S.A., Bernstein, I.L., Enrione, M., Marcus, Z.H.: Successful long-term immunotherapy for human seminal plasma anaphylaxis. J.A.M.A. 251:2684, 1984.

Gibbs, C.J., Coutts, I.I., Lock, R., Finnegan, O.C., White, R.J.: Premenstrual exacerbation of asthma. Thorax 39:833, 1984.

Gordon, G.G., Southren, A.L.: Thyroid-hormone effects on steroid-hormone metabolism. Bull. N.Y. Acad. Med. 53:241, 1977.

Gordon, M., Niswander, K.R., Brendes, H., Kantor, A.G.: Fetal morbidity following potentially anoxigenic obstetric conditions. VII. Bronchial asthma. Am. J. Obstet. Gynecol. 106:421, 1970.

Greenberger, P.A., Patterson, R.: Beclomethasone dipropionate for severe asthma during pregnancy. Ann. Intern. Med. 98:478, 1983.

Greenberger, P.A.: Pregnancy and asthma. Chest 87:85s, 1985.

Grossman, C.J.: Regulation of the immune system by sex steroids. Endo. Rev. 5:435, 1984.

Hanley, S.P.: Asthma variation with menstruation. Br. J. Dis. Chest 75:306, 1981.

Hart, R.: Autoimmune progesterone dermatitis. Arch. Dermatol. 113:426,1977.

Heinonen, O.P., Slone, D., Shapiro, S.: Birth defects and drugs in pregnancy. Littleton, Massachusetts, P.S.G. Publishing Co., 1977.

Holt, G.R., Mabry, R.L.: ENT medications in pregnancy. Ototolaryngol. Head Neck Surg. 91:338, 1983.

Jenne, J.H.: Whither beta-adrenergic tachyphylaxis? J. Allergy Clin. Immunol. 70:413, 1982.

Jick, H., Holmes, L.B., Hunter, J.R., et al.: First-trimester drug use and congenital disorders. J.A.M.A. 246:343, 1981.

Kilshaw, P.J., Cant, A.J.: The passage of maternal dietary proteins into human breast milk. Int. Arch. Allergy Appl. Immunol. 75:8, 1984.

Kovacs, G.T., Francis, M.: Vasectomy: What are the long term risks? Med. J. Austral. 2:564, 1983.

Lentzoff, A., Josse, R.G., Denburg, J., Dolovich, J.: Association of chronic urticaria and angioedema with thyroid autoimmunity. Arch. Dermatol. 119:636, 1983.

Metzger, W.J., Turner, E., Patterson, R.: The safety of immunotherapy during pregnancy. J. Allergy Clin. Immunol. 61:268, 1978.

Mowbray, J.F., Gibbings, C., Liddell, H., et al.: Controlled trial of treatment of recurrent spontaneous abortion by immunisation with paternal cells. Lancet 1:941, 1985.

Mowbray, J.F., Underwood, J.L.: Immunology of abortion. Clin. Exp. Immunol. 60:1, 1985.

Nelson, M.M., Forfar, J.O.: Associations between drugs administered during pregnancy and congenital abnormalities of the fetus. Br. Med. J. 1:523, 1971.

Nordin, B.E.C., Marshall, D.H., Francis, R.M., Crilly, R.G.: The effects of sex steroid and corticosteroid hormones on bone. J. Steroid Biochem. 15:171, 1981.

Parkin, J.L.: Topical steroids in nasal disease. Otolaryngol. Head Neck Surg. 91:713, 1983.

Ruegsegger, P., Medici, T.C., Anliker, M.: Corticosteroid-induced bone loss. A longitudinal study of alternate day therapy in patients with bronchial asthma using quantitative computed tomography. Eur. J. Clin. Pharmacol. 25:615, 1983.

Schaefer, G., Silverman, F.: Pregnancy complicated by asthma. Am. J. Obstet. Gynecol. 82:182, 1961.

Schatz, M., Wasserman, S., O'Conner, R.D., et al.: Distinguishing clinical and biochemical characteristics associated with improvement or deterioration of asthma during pregnancy (abstract). J. Allergy Clin. Immunol. 75:133, 1985.

Schatz, M., Harden, K., Saunder, B., Porreco, R., Hoffman, C., O'Patry, D., Sperling, W., Mellon, M., Zieger, R.S.: The placental transfer of theophylline at term and its effect on the infant (abstract). J. Allergy Clin. Immunol. 71:130, 1983a.

Schatz, M., Zeiger, R.S., Mellon, M., Porreco, R.P.: Asthma and allergic diseases during pregnancy: Management of the mother and prevention in the child. In Middleton E., Jr., Reed, E.D., Ellis, E.F. (eds.): Allergy: Principles and Practice. St. Louis, CV Mosby Co., 1983b.

Schraa, J.C., Dirks, J.F.: The influence of corticosteroids and theophylline on cerebral function. Chest 82:181, 1982.

Sridama, V., Pacini, F., Yang, S-L., et al.: Decreased levels of helper T cells: A possible cause of immunodeficiency in pregnancy. N. Engl. J. Med. 307:352, 1982.

Szentivanyi, A.: The beta-adrenergic theory of the atopic abnormality in bronchial asthma. J. Allergy 42:203, 1968.

Taylor, C.G., Faulk, W.P., McIntyre, J.A.: Prevention of recurrent spontaneous abortions by leukocyte transfusions. J. Roy. Soc. Med. 78:623, 1985.

Van Thiel, D.H., Gavaler, J.S., Smith, W.I. Jr., Paul, G.: Hypothalamic-pituitary-gonadal dysfunction in men using cimetidine. N. Engl. J. Med. 300:1012, 1979.

Wang, C., Lai, C.L., Lam, K.C., Yeung, K.K.: Effect of cimetidine on gonadal function in man. Br. J. Clin. Pharm. 13:791, 1982.

Warren, W.J., Turner, C., Dalton, N., Thomson, A., Cochrane, G.M.: The effect of posture on the sympathoadrenal response to theophylline infusion. Br. J. Clin. Pharm. 16:405, 1983.

Weinberg, E.D.: Pregnancy associated depression of cell-mediated immunity. Rev. Infect. Dis. 6:814, 1984.

Weinberg, S.E., Weiss, S.T., Cohen, W.R.: Pregnancy and the lung: State of the art. Am. Rev. Respir. Dis. 121:559, 1980.

Williams, D.A.: Asthma and pregnancy. Acta Allergol. 22:311, 1967.

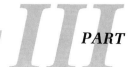
PRINCIPLES OF DIAGNOSIS AND TREATMENT OF ALLERGIC DISEASES

16

Medical Evaluation of Allergic Diseases

R. MICHAEL SLY, M.D.

The purposes of the medical evaluation are to establish the diagnosis, to estimate the severity of the illness, to determine responses to previous treatment, to identify possible complications, and thus to guide appropriate further management. A thorough medical history is the most helpful tool in achieving these objectives in the field of allergy.

ALLERGY HISTORY

The chief complaint directs questioning concerning the history of the present illness. Occasionally, the patient's chief complaint even may differ from the reason for referral. Often there is more than one illness present. Both should be explored in detail. For example, the patient with asthma may also have symptoms of allergic rhinitis and allergic conjunctivitis.

To facilitate exchange of information, permit the patient or parent to describe the history of the present illness in the sequence he or she deems appropriate. Later direct questioning can establish the chronologic sequence of events. When was there first any problem of any kind? What was that problem? How severe was it? How long did it last? How often did it recur initially? Has there been a change in the frequency of recurrences or in the severity? How was it treated? What was the response to treatment? Were there any side effects of treatment? What was the next problem and when did it occur? Such details not only guide initial ther-

apy but also provide a basis for evaluation of subsequent improvement or worsening and response to future treatment.

Additional specific questions depend on the nature of the complaints. Are respiratory symptoms perennial or seasonal? Are symptoms worse at night or during the day? Are they worse indoors or outdoors? Are they related to exposure to potential allergens? Did they begin shortly after a change in residence? Does improvement occur during overnight trips away from home? Do symptoms occur only on weekends when the patient is home or only during the week at work or at school?

As the interview proceeds, one can explore the various possibilities in the differential diagnosis. When the complaint is coughing it is helpful to know whether the cough has been loose (productive of sputum) or dry. The cough of asthma is usually dry or, occasionally, productive of clear mucus. A cough productive of copious secretions may suggest chronic bronchitis. A chronic cough productive of purulent sputum in a child may be that of bronchiectasis or cystic fibrosis. Viscid sputum that a parent must remove from an infant's pharynx because of choking suggests cystic fibrosis. A sudden onset of coughing with choking may be due to aspiration of a foreign body. Association of coughing with swallowing may indicate tracheoesophageal fistula, achalasia, or poor coordination of swallowing and breathing with secondary aspiration. Coughing with aphonia or dysphonia suggests a hypopharyngeal or laryngeal foreign body or laryngeal papilloma. A harsh, barking cough evokes glottic or subglottic obstruction. Recurrent coughing with wheezing is a sign of obstruction of the lower airway due to asthma, a bronchial foreign body, or a neoplasm. A paroxysmal cough raises the possibility of pertussis or a foreign body. A paroxysmal, staccato cough without fever during the first three months of life is consistent with chlamydial pneumonia.

217

When a complaint of wheezing raises the possibility of asthma, ask whether symptoms have been associated with the following factors that commonly trigger episodes of asthma: changes in weather, fumes or odors, smoke, exercise, tension or frustration, laughing or crying, or infection. The nasal congestion, nasal discharge, and sneezing of allergic rhinitis are often mistaken for symptoms of an upper respiratory infection, and physicians may ascribe the coughing and wheezing of asthma to bronchitis. Segmental or subsegmental atelectasis due to asthma may simulate pulmonary infiltrates due to pneumonia. Eliciting the history of recurrent sneezing and nasal itching suggestive of allergic rhinitis and persistent nocturnal coughing and coughing or wheezing after exercise typical of asthma permits correct interpretation of the history of recurrent colds, sinusitis, bronchitis, and pneumonia. Association of symptoms with respiratory symptoms in other family members and fever implicates infection, but viral respiratory infection can trigger episodes of asthma. Infection can also occur as a complication of asthma or allergic rhinitis.

A chronic or recurrent, clear nasal discharge is most suggestive of allergic rhinitis, whereas a purulent discharge is suggestive of infection. An abundance of eosinophils also can cause discoloration of the discharge in a patient with allergic rhinitis, however. A history of itching of the palate or throat suggests allergic rhinitis. Frequent clearing of the throat, nocturnal coughing, or hoarseness may be caused by the postnasal drip of allergic rhinitis or sinusitis.

Allergic conjunctivitis is often associated with allergic rhinitis. It is appropriate to inquire about conjunctival itching and injection, excessive tearing, and periorbital edema. There may be a history of chemosis. Extremely intense conjunctival itching associated with photophobia and a viscid, white conjunctival discharge may be indicative of vernal conjunctivitis.

Environmental History

The purpose of the environmental history is to establish exposure to potential allergens and irritants, to identify relationships between symptoms and exposure, and to determine the feasibility of modifications to minimize allergenic exposure. It also directs the attention of patients and parents to sources of allergens that they may not have considered important previously (Table 16–1).

TABLE 16–1. Environmental History

Home

Location: urban, suburban, rural
Length of time at present location
Previous locations
Trees, grass, weeds
Basement or crawl space
Heating and cooling systems
    Type of filters and frequency of changes
    Humidification
Exhaust fans: kitchen, bathroom
Carpeting and rugs: material, length of pile
    Pads: material
    Type of vacuum cleaner: central, portable

Patient's Bedroom

Location: basement or which floor
Other occupants
Floor covering
Beds
    Mattress: type of stuffing, encasing
    Box springs
    Pillows: type of stuffing, encasing
    Quilts or quilted mattress pad: type of stuffing
Stuffed toys and whether kept in bed
Other furniture: upholstered furniture, bookcases
Curtains: whether washable and frequency of washing
Venetian blinds or shutters
Closet: contents, door open or closed

Pets

Past, present, future
How long in household
Indoors or outdoors

Indoor plants

Type and location

Smoking

Patient or relative
Locations allowed

Hobbies

Patient or relative

Other Environments

Workplace
    Occupation
School
Daycare facility or home of babysitter
Vacation home
Home of other parent or relatives

It may be possible to correlate changes in symptoms with changes in the location of the patient's home. One may then be able to identify major differences in allergenic exposure between different homes. A damp basement or crawl space suggests exposure to fungi. Wood-burning stoves, fireplaces, and kerosene heaters are frequent sources of irritants that can cause respiratory symptoms in patients with asthma or allergic rhinitis as well as in otherwise healthy subjects. Both active and passive smoking can cause respiratory symptoms.

The patient's bedroom is an appropriate focus of attention because of daily exposure to its contents for 8 to 10 consecutive hours while sleeping. Allergic respiratory symptoms during the night or upon arising in the morning are consistent with the prolonged exposure to house dust mite allergens. It is helpful to know whether dogs or cats characterized as living outdoors are ever permitted indoors. Occasional trips by pets into the house may deposit allergens to which anyone indoors subsequently has continual exposure. Occasional patients know whether previous occupants of their homes had pets that may be responsible for allergens that remain after their departure. Most indoor plants do not produce airborne pollens, such as those commonly responsible for allergic respiratory symptoms, but fungi may grow on the plants or in the soil around the plants. When plants have been placed near open windows or air vents, drafts can carry such fungi to the patient. The patient's employment may be a vital clue to a cause of occupational asthma or hypersensitivity pneumonitis. Also ask what materials they are exposed to in the course of their work. Allergens or irritants carried home on clothing by others in the household may be relevant when the patient is not employed in such an environment. Furthermore, a spouse or child may occasionally visit a household member at the workplace.

Past History

The past history includes the patient's immunization status and any adverse reactions to immunizations, drugs, or insect stings or bites. The review of systems may disclose additional complaints that may or may not be related to the presenting allergic complaint. There may be a potential for interactions of drugs prescribed for other complaints with those prescribed for the present complaint.

The developmental history of a child may indicate an effect of chronic illness, such as delayed speech due to impairment of auditory acuity. This type of history may also indicate a delay that may affect ability to cooperate with diagnostic or therapeutic procedures, such as pulmonary function testing or inhalation of medication from a metered-dose inhaler. Information about the child's placement in school is helpful.

Inquiry about a child's relationships with siblings, other children, parents, and teachers may elicit disclosure of possible problems with psychologic adjustment. Asking the parent to characterize the child's psychologic profile by choosing between paired adjectives presented sequentially not only provides further information about psychologic adjustment but also gives the parent further opportunity to express concerns about behavior (Table 16–2).

Family History

It is the immediate family history that is of greatest relevance for atopic allergy. Ask not only about allergic rhinitis, hay fever, asthma, eczema, and hives but also about sinusitis and a constant stuffy nose. The immediate family history of each parent is also of interest not only because of possible hereditary transmission of an allergic disorder that has not yet been expressed but also because of the insight it may provide into the degree of sophistication or anxiety of the parent. A parent whose own siblings and parents have had asthma is likely to be able to recognize wheezing in his or her child. A parent whose father or mother has died during an acute asthmatic attack is likely to view asthma differently from one who has had no previous experience with an asthmatic patient.

The ages at death and causes of death of siblings, parents, aunts, uncles, and grandparents also may help suggest other hereditary conditions of significance, including some that may require consideration in the differential diagnosis, such as cystic fibrosis. Absence of a family history of cystic fibrosis does not exclude the possibility of cystic fibrosis or other autosomal recessive disorders, of course.

The ages of living siblings, parents, and grandparents may provide insight into possible family interactions relevant to a chronic illness, such as asthma.

TABLE 16–2. Psychologic Profile*

Is he (she) generally more timid or aggressive?
shy or forward?
introverted or extroverted?
hostile or passive?
happy or depressed?
dependent or independent?
anxious or calm?
tense or relaxed?
quiet or bustling?
maladjusted or well adjusted?

* Permit intermediate responses and ask for further details when indicated by responses.

PHYSICAL EXAMINATION

A complete physical examination is necessary to identify all abnormalities whether related to the chief complaint or not.

Height and Weight

Height and weight should be compared with normal values for age. Severe asthma can suppress both height and weight in children, and treatment with adrenal corticosteroids can suppress linear growth. Weight loss occurs in adults with emphysema. Weight gain is poor in most children with cystic fibrosis.

Vital Signs

Accurate determination of respiratory rate, pulse rate, and blood pressure, which is a part of every complete physical examination, requires the patient be in a stable, resting state. Normal values vary with age. Comparison of respiratory rates, with normal values for age is especially helpful in patients with pulmonary disease because of the association of tachypnea with restrictive pulmonary diseases, such as pneumonia, pleural effusion, and pneumothorax as well as atelectasis (Fig. 16–1). Other possible causes of tachypnea include anxiety, exercise, fever, anemia, metabolic acidosis, and respiratory alkalosis.

Pulsus Paradoxus

Pulsus paradoxus, the difference in systemic arterial blood pressure during inspiration and expiration, is exaggerated in heart failure, cardiac tamponade, and pulmonary diseases associated with excessive decreases in intrathoracic pressure during inspiration, such as asthma and cystic fibrosis. When blood pressure is measured with a sphygmomanometer and stethoscope, the pulsus paradoxus is readily determined as the difference in systolic blood pressure between the pressure at which pulse sounds are initially heard, intermittently, and that at which every pulse sound is heard. The pulsus paradoxus is normally less than 5 mm Hg, but is often greater than 10 mm Hg during acute asthma. A value greater than 20 mm Hg indicates moderate or severe airway obstruction when due to asthma.

General Appearance

Inspection may disclose cyanosis if arterial oxygen saturation is less than 80 to 85 percent. Anemia may permit detection of cyanosis only at lower levels of arterial oxygen saturation. Cyanosis of the lips, mouth, face, and trunk usually indicates cardiorespiratory disease except in chilled newborn infants. Possible causes of cyanosis include alveolar hypoventilation due to airway obstruction, depression of the

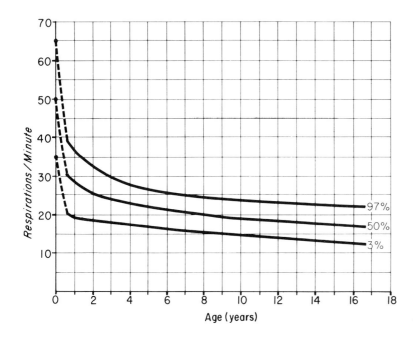

FIGURE 16–1. Normal resting respiratory rates in infants and children. (From Sly, R.M.: *Textbook of Pediatric Allergy*, New Hyde Park, N.Y., Medical Examination Publishing Co., 1985; used with permission of Elsevier Science Publishing Co., Inc.)

respiratory center, or respiratory muscle weakness; inequities of ventilation and perfusion, such as may occur with pneumonia; anatomic right to left shunts, such as those that cause cyanotic congenital heart disease; and rare disturbances of alveolocapillary diffusion, as in interstital pneumonia or pulmonary fibrosis. Failure of cyanosis to improve with administration of supplemental oxygen suggests an anatomic right to left shunt.

Flaring of the alae nasi indicates recruitment of accessory muscles of respiration. A requirement for excessive decreases in intrapleural pressure to initiate inspiration through obstructed airways may cause supraclavicular and intercostal retractions. Abnormal increases in intrapleural pressure during expiration may cause bulging of intercostal spaces. Head bobbing with each inspiration in an infant lying with the head unsupported except for the suboccipital area is a sign of dyspnea.

Mouth breathing, a blue or black discoloration in the orbitopalpebral grooves beneath the lower eyelids (allergic shiners), nose wrinkling, and the allergic salute may suggest allergic rhinitis. A transverse nasal crease at the junction of the bulbous tip of the nose and the more rigid bridge also suggests allergic rhinitis, but a familial transverse nasal groove unrelated to rhinitis can also occur, inherited as a mendelian dominant. Dennie's line, a wrinkle just below the lower eyelids, is associated with allergic rhinitis, asthma, and atopic dermatitis (see Chapter 29).

Digital clubbing is recognized most readily by comparison of the depth of the index finger at the base of the nail with that at the distal interphalangeal joint (Fig. 16–2). The depth at the base of the nail is normally less; when it is equal or greater, digital clubbing is present. Digital clubbing is rare in uncomplicated asthma, so its detection should suggest another diagnosis (Table 16–3). Hereditary digital clubbing often has its onset at or after puberty but occurs much less frequently than acquired clubbing.

Skin

Examination of the skin may disclose the erythematous maculopapular eruption, the fine scaling, or the weeping and oozing eruption of atopic dermatitis. Scratching is usually obvious and incessant, and excoriations may be evident. Crusting may be present with superimposed infection. The distribution often varies with

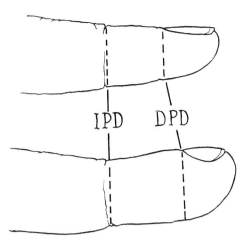

FIGURE 16–2. Measurement of distal phalangeal depth (DPD) and distal interphalangeal depth (IPD) on index fingers for detection of digital clubbing. Normal DPD/IPD = 0.895 (S.D. 0.041). A ratio of 1 is 2.5 S.D. above normal, indicative of slight digital clubbing. The upper finger is normal. Digital clubbing is evident in the lower finger. (From Sly, R.M.: *Textbook of Pediatric Allergy,* New Hyde Park, N.Y., Medical Examination Publishing Co., 1985; used with permission of Elsevier Science Publishing Co., Inc.)

age, with involvement of the cheeks and extensor aspects of the extremities in infants and predilection for antecubital spaces, popliteal spaces, and the neck in older children and adults. Lichenification and hyperpigmentation or hypopigmentation may be evident in older children and adults. Contact dermatitis appears as an erythematous or papulovesicular eruption at the area of exposure to the contactant. Urticarial lesions can vary from the multiple, 1 to 3 mm wheals with flares of cholinergic urticaria to the giant wheals of angioedema.

TABLE 16–3. Diseases Associated with Acquired Digital Clubbing

Pulmonary	Cardiac
Abscess	Cyanotic congenital heart
Bronchiectasis	disease
Chronic pneumonia	Subacute bacterial
Empyema	endocarditis
Malignant neoplasms	**Gastrointestinal**
Tuberculosis	Chronic dysentery
Pleural	Chronic ulcerative colitis
Mesothelioma	Multiple polyposis
Hepatic	Regional enteritis
Biliary cirrhosis	**Other**
	Thyrotoxicosis

Eyes

Conjunctival injection, excessive tearing, and periorbital edema of allergic conjunctivitis may be evident. A tenacious, ropy, white conjunctival discharge and pseudoptosis with photophobia suggest vernal conjunctivitis.

Nose

Examination of the nose may disclose the enlarged, edematous nasal turbinates of allergic rhinitis with pale or blue, moist nasal mucosa. Nasal polyps are a rare complication of allergic rhinitis but occur in more than 6 percent of children with cystic fibrosis and may occur in more than 50 percent of patients with aspirin sensitivity.

Ears

Chronic middle ear effusion can be secondary to allergic rhinitis with eustachian tube dysfunction (see Chapters 33 and 36). The tympanic membrane is usually retracted but may appear normal or bulging. It is often dull and may appear thickened or wrinkled. It may be gray, pink, amber, slightly yellow, or deep blue. A fluid level or bubbles are evident occasionally. The handle of the malleus may appear chalky white, or bony landmarks may be completely obliterated. Pneumatic otoscopy usually discloses limitation of mobility.

Tonsils

Tonsillar and adenoidal hypertrophy is a common complication of allergic rhinitis in young children. Rarely, extreme upper airway obstruction may cause alveolar hypoventilation and cor pulmonale, one of the few indications for tonsillectomy. With maturity and adequate allergy management, tonsils usually regress.

Chest

Examination of the chest may disclose the increase in the anteroposterior diameter associated with chronic obstructive lung disease. Measurement of the depth and width of the chest with chest or obstetric calipers permits objective evaluation of the chest configuration.

The chest of a newborn infant is almost circular in cross section, but as the infant grows the depth (anteroposterior diameter) increases less than the width (transverse diameter). By the time the child has attained a height of 95 cm at approximately 3 years of age the ratio of depth to width has decreased to 0.75 in normal children and remains between 0.70 and 0.75 thereafter. Plotting depth and width on published graphs (Sly et al., 1981) permits immediate comparison with normal populations of girls and boys. Administration of a bronchodilator to an asthmatic patient with an abnormal increase in the ratio of depth to width usually causes a return of the ratio toward normal. Persistent, progressive increases in depth to width may occur in frequently recurrent or continual asthma but are more typical of conditions that cause more persistent airway obstruction, such as cystic fibrosis and emphysema.

Auscultation of the lungs may reveal the expiratory wheezing or sibilant rales and prolongation of the expiratory phase typical of asthma

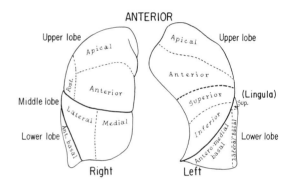

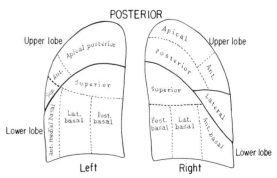

FIGURE 16–3. Normal distribution of bronchopulmonary segments available for auscultation. The medial basal segment of the right lower lobe does not abut against the chest wall. (From Sly, R.M.: *Textbook of Pediatric Allergy*, New Hyde Park, N.Y., Medical Examination Publishing Co., 1985; used with permission of Elsevier Science Publishing Co., Inc.)

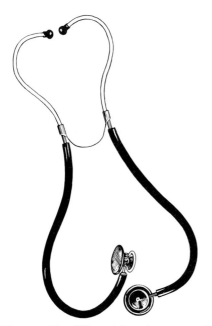

FIGURE 16–4. The differential stethoscope or double stethoscope. (From Sly, R.M.: *Textbook of Pediatric Allergy*, New Hyde Park, N.Y., Medical Examination Publishing Co., 1985; used with permission of Elsevier Science Publishing Co., Inc.)

or the fine crepitant rales (crackles) of hypersensitivity pneumonitis. The wheezing of uncomplicated asthma is usually generalized, although there may be minor differences in intensity from one segment to another. Many pulmonary diseases tend to be segmental, however, and examination of the lungs is not complete until one has auscultated each of the 18 bronchopulmonary segments that abut against the chest wall (Fig. 16–3). Use of a differential stethoscope facilitates examination of the lungs, permitting detection of differences in ventilation of corresponding segments of the two lungs with simultaneous auscultation (Fig. 16–4). This may be especially helpful in the diagnosis of a bronchial foreign body, a congenital lobar emphysema, an airway obstruction due to a neoplasm, a segmental atelectasis, or a lobar consolidation.

LABORATORY FINDINGS

Certain laboratory procedures are often helpful even after the most thorough medical history and the most thoughtful physical examination. Results of the history and physical examination determine which laboratory procedures are appropriate. These may include hemoglobin concentration; hematocrit value; leukocyte count with differential; platelet count; examination of the blood smear for platelet morphology; nasal or sputum smears for cytologic examination; audiometry; tympanometry; evaluation of eustachian tube function; pulmonary function testing (with or without challenge with exercise or inhalation of methacholine or histamine and before and after administration of a bronchodilator); radiographs of the chest or paranasal sinuses; barium swallow examination; sweat test; determination of serum immunoglobulin concentrations (IgG, IgA, IgM, IgE); determination of serum diphtheria and tetanus antibody titers after immunization; determination of serum isohemagglutinin titers; determination of serum complement; skin testing for delayed hypersensitivity to *Candida albicans,* tetanus toxoid, purified protein derivative (PPD), histoplasmin, and coccidioidin; patch testing, allergy prick and intradermal skin testing; and, occasionally, *in vitro* tests for specific IgE. Details concerning procedures and indications are described in other chapters of this text.

REFERENCES

Sly, R.M.: *Textbook of Pediatric Allergy,* New Hyde Park, N.Y., Medical Examination Publishing Co., 1985.

Sly, R.M., Farhadian, H., Waring, W.W., McConnell, M.C.: Objective assessment of chest configuration in children with asthma or cystic fibrosis. Ann. Allergy 47:278–287, 1981.

Waring, W.W.: The History and Physical Examination. *In* Kendig, E.L., Jr., Chernick, V. (eds.): *Disorders of the Respiratory Tract in Children,* 4th ed., Philadelphia, W.B. Saunders Co., 1983.

17

Diagnostic Methods for Assessing the Patient With Possible Allergic Disease

GAIL G. SHAPIRO, M.D.

The history and physical examination are the most important elements of the evaluation for possible allergic disease. If after completing such an interview and examination, the physician suspects strongly that the patient's complaints are due to allergy to environmental factors, further investigation is not always necessary; general environmental control measures with or without medications, such as antihistamines, may control symptoms sufficiently to avoid further diagnostic tests.

Often such an approach is not sufficient either because the patient is not convinced that an allergy is really the cause or because a direct causal relationship is not clear. Specialized diagnostic procedures then may be valuable adjuncts to the history and physical examination. The physician must formulate a differential diagnosis that will serve as a guide for selection of appropriate tests. For example, nasal cytology can be a helpful clue to the likelihood of nasal allergy in patients with seasonal or perennial rhinitis. A predominance of eosinophils in the secretions supports this diagnosis, whereas a predominance of polymorphonuclear cells and bacteria is more consistent with infectious rhinitis and sinusitis and may suggest the need to obtain sinus radiographs. It is not unusual for children with chronic rhinitis to have middle ear dysfunction, so that audiometry and tympanometry may be indicated. Pulmonary function test results may provide the differential diagnosis between bronchitis and asthma in the patient with chronic coughing. Pulmonary function test results serve also as baselines for future care in the patient with asthma. If pulmonary function is normal, bronchoprovocation testing with methacholine, for example, can help establish whether or not the patient does indeed have asthma. In cases of nasal and pulmonary disease in which the patient is reacting to environmental allergens, testing for specific IgE antibody can help identify the allergens. The physician needs to select the appropriate test or tests which differ in sensitivity, specificity, and expense.

DIAGNOSTIC TESTS AND METHODS

Nasal Cytology. The cellular composition of nasal secretions is an easily assessable clue to what pathophysiologic phenomena are occurring in the nose and paranasal structure. Normal nasal secretions typically contain epithelial cells, some mononuclear cells, some polymorphonuclear cells, and very few eosinophils. The presence of greater than 5 to 10 percent eosinophils suggests allergic disease. Less commonly, however, eosinophils can occur in the absence of allergy, presumably caused by nonallergic release of mast cell eosinophil chemotactic factors.

Patients with acute viral upper respiratory infections will sometimes show karyolysis, a fragmenting of the ciliated epithelial cells, with round bases being sheared from the elongated stem of the cell. Often some polymorphonuclear cells will be present. Patients with bacterial sinusitis are likely to have nasal secretions that appear purulent. They contain, microscopically, sheets of polymorphonuclear cells and bacteria, often present intracellularly.

A single specimen reflects the pathophysiologic process occurring in the nose at one point in time and must be viewed in that context. Diagnostically, it can be helpful or misleading when, for example, the subject who has allergic rhinitis has an upper respiratory infection at that moment in time, since eosinophils may appear only after recovery.

Nasal Cytologic Technique. For this procedure, the patient should blow his or her nose into plastic wrap. In cases of young children who cannot perform this maneuver voluntarily and in situations of patients who cannot provide nasal secretions, a cotton swab applicator can be placed in the nasal vault for a brief interval. Secretions can be rubbed from the plastic wrap or applicator onto a glass slide. After briefly heat-fixing the material, Hansel stain (an eosin-methylene blue stain) is used according to the protocol in Table 17–1. An alternative technique involves the use of a plastic curette, which is gently scraped in the midanterior portion of the middle turbinate. The epithelial scraping that is obtained can be stained with Hansel stain and may show mast cells in addition to the other above mentioned cell types.

Nasal Resistance Measurements. One can elucidate pathophysiologic mechanisms with nasal provocation challenge or study the effects of pharmacologic intervention by performing resistance studies before and after therapy by measuring nasal resistance to air flow. Nasal resistance is defined as the ratio of the pressure change between the nose and nasopharynx (ΔP) and the airflow through the nose ($R = \Delta P/V$). Two methods of measurement are anterior and posterior rhinomanometry. With anterior rhinomanometry, flow is measured with a pneumotagraph placed in one nostril. Pressure differential is determined from pressure transducers located at the occluded and patent nares. Thus, all measures are obtained from the anterior airway. Although there may be some artifact introduced by altering the nares, this technique is easier to perform than posterior rhinomanometry. For performing posterior rhinomanometry, the patient wears a diving mask, which contains a flowmeter and pressure transducer. Another pressure transducer is attached to a mouthpiece. The patient must breathe without obstructing the mouthpiece and must be cooperative with the cumbersome diving mask in place. While the patient breathes, pressure change and flow are measured. Detailed explanations of these techniques can be found in Georgitis (1985). In general, allergic individuals have higher nasal resistance than do nonallergic subjects, but there is some overlap between the two popula-

tions. There also is some variability in measurements from the same individual at different times. Variation in the same individual generally will be less than 20 percent. Nevertheless, since there is considerable variability from hour to hour or day to day, conclusions about the effectiveness of a particular mode of therapy probably should be drawn only with a 50 percent or greater change in resistance measurements.

Ear Function. Many adults and up to 50 percent of children with respiratory allergy have middle ear dysfunction or otitis media with effusion (see Chapter 36) (Friedman et al., 1983; Kraemer et al., 1983; Walker, 1985). When individuals have had chronic upper respiratory complaints that suggest allergy, this link between the nose and ear should be explored with the history and then possibly with diagnostic tests. There are three principal tools for examining middle ear function; pneumatic otoscopy, pure-tone audiometry, and tympanometry.

Pneumatic Otoscopy. During the physical examination a fiberoptic otoscope should be used to observe the tympanic membranes. The head of the scope must have an airtight seal and an attachment for rubber tubing, through which air may be blown into the ear canal to exert pressure on the tympanic membrane. In the absence of middle ear fluid, a normal membrane will move in response to positive and negative pressure. The presence of effusion will diminish this response. Pneumatic otoscopy allows visual assessment of the tympanic membrane and some information concerning middle ear status.

Pure-Tone Audiometry. Screening audiometry is a useful means to estimate hearing acuity. Ordinarily, the patient is tested at 15 or 20, 40, and 60 decibels of volume and at frequencies that incorporate pitches from 400 to 4000 hertz. Conductive hearing loss due to middle ear effusion will produce a low frequency hearing deficit. A sensorineural loss typically affects the higher frequencies.

Tympanometry. In patients with histories of recurrent ear effusions or intermittent hearing losses, tympanometry can add information in regard to middle ear function. A tympanometer utilizes a probe that is inserted into the ear canal. The probe possesses three parts; (1) an air pressure control to alter the pressure in the external ear canal from negative to positive, (2) a device to transmit a low frequency tone to the tympanic membrane, and (3) a microphone to receive the signal when it is reflected from the

TABLE 17–1. Technique of Staining Nasal Secretions

---

1. Transfer the specimen to a glass slide, dry, and fix with heat.
2. Stain for 30 seconds with Hansel stain (1:500 eosin and 1:200 methylene blue in alcohol).
3. Add distilled water to take up the stain for 30 seconds.
4. Wash with water.
5. Decolorize with methanol or 95 percent ethyl alcohol (do not overdecolorize).
6. Dry and examine under oil immersion.

membrane. Tympanometry utilizes the fact that compliance of the tympanic membrane is maximal when pressure in the external canal and middle ear are equal. By varying external canal pressure and recording compliance, the point of maximal compliance can be determined, which defines the air pressure within the middle ear. If maximum compliance is at a pressure more negative than 150 mm H_2O, there is an abnormally negative middle ear pressure, usually indicating eustachian tube dysfunction. If maximum compliance occurs in the positive range, it suggests acute otitis media. A flat tracing with no peak in compliance indicates the presence of fluid in the middle ear (Fig. 17–1).

Nine-step tympanometry (involving *five* actual tympanograms) is a method for evaluating eustachian tube function by determining the tube's ability to equalize positive and negative pressures (Bluestone, 1981). After a baseline tympanogram is obtained (no. 1), a positive pressure of 200 mm H_2O is applied to the middle ear. The patient swallows three times to equilibriate pressure and another tympanogram is obtained (no. 2). Middle ear pressure normally will be slightly negative at this time. The patient then takes several swallows of water and a tympanogram is obtained (no. 3) again to see if the negative pressure is equilibrated by the eustachian tube. Next, a negative pressure of 200 mm H_2O is applied. The patient swallows three times and again a tympanogram is obtained (no. 4); this time it should be slightly positive. The patient again swallows several times and the tracing is repeated to see if positive pressure is equilibriated (no. 5). These functional test results are often abnormal in individuals with normal baseline tympanometry who complain of the sensation of plugged or

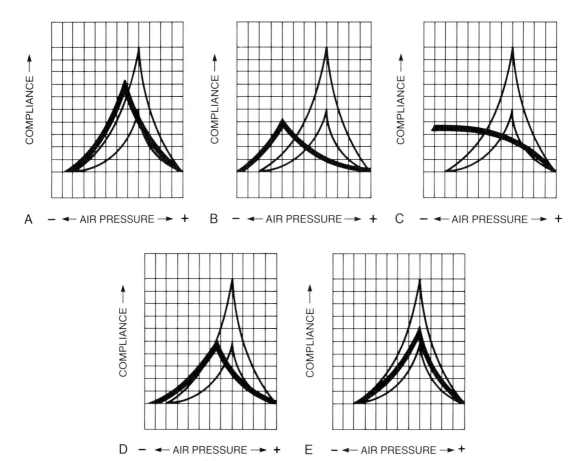

FIGURE 17–1. Tympanometry is a useful technique for following the pathophysiology of middle ear effusion. A near normal tympanogram is represented in A; negative middle ear pressure and reduced compliance often accompany an upper respiratory problem B; middle ear effusion is present in C; and return of the middle ear to its proper condition is shown in D and E.

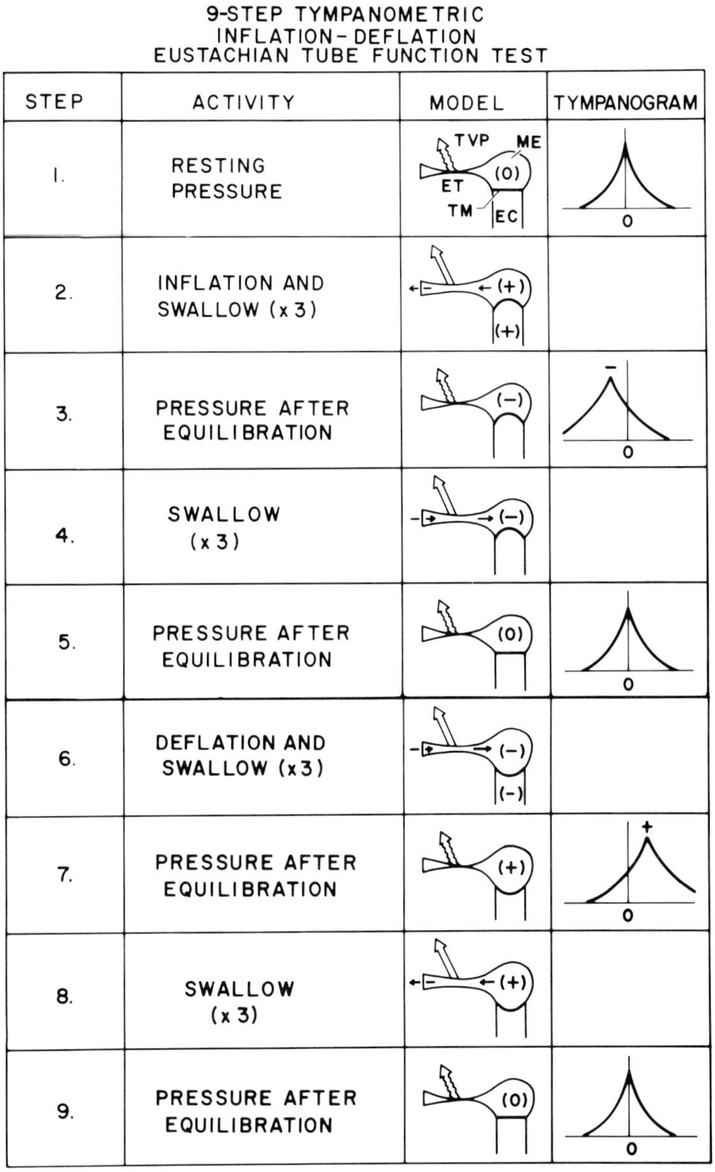

9-STEP TYMPANOMETRIC INFLATION–DEFLATION EUSTACHIAN TUBE FUNCTION TEST

STEP	ACTIVITY	MODEL	TYMPANOGRAM
1.	RESTING PRESSURE	TVP ME (0) ET TM EC	
2.	INFLATION AND SWALLOW (x 3)	(+) (+)	
3.	PRESSURE AFTER EQUILIBRATION	(−)	
4.	SWALLOW (x 3)	(−)	
5.	PRESSURE AFTER EQUILIBRATION	(0)	
6.	DEFLATION AND SWALLOW (x3)	(−) (−)	
7.	PRESSURE AFTER EQUILIBRATION	(+)	
8.	SWALLOW (x 3)	(+)	
9.	PRESSURE AFTER EQUILIBRATION	(0)	

FIGURE 17–2. The nine step tympanometry technique is more sensitive than ordinary tympanometry for detecting eustachian tube dysfunction.

popping ears. It has provided the sensitivity needed to study the effects of inhaled allergens and irritants on eustachian tube physiology (Fig. 17–2).

Pulmonary Function Testing. When wheezing, shortness of breath, or cough is the patient's main complaint, it is important to have a functional assessment of pulmonary physiology. The initial measures of pulmonary function aid the physician's assessment of whether the patient has obstructive or restrictive lung disease. This baseline becomes a point from which future progress can be measured. Subsequent follow-up studies will reveal whether ab-

normalities are static or reversible and whether they respond to therapy.

It is common to see mild or moderate pulmonary airflow obstruction on a spirometric tracing in a patient who denies symptoms and is unaware of pulmonary dysfunction. As an example, Figure 17–3A is spirometry of a 10-year-old girl who claimed that she felt well and that she was asthma free. The child's mother asked to speak to the physician prior to her daughter's visit to express her concern regarding the child's denial of asthma and overuse of beta-adrenergic inhaler therapy. The spirometric curve shows marked obstruction. Had spir-

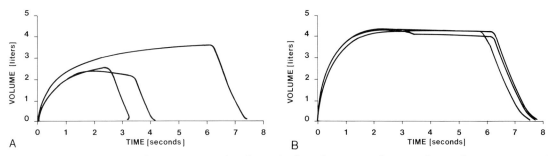

FIGURE 17-3. *A*, Spirometry from a patient with asthma who denied symptoms; however, her mother was concerned about her overuse of a beta agonist metered dose inhaler. *B*, Pulmonary function from the same patient after her therapeutic regimen was revamped.

ometry not been obtained, the physician might have undervalued the mother's concern. One week later, after appropriate changes in therapy, the patient's spirometric function has improved (Fig. 17-3B).

History and physical examination cannot replace pulmonary function testing (and vice versa). Since patients vary greatly in the way they perceive and describe their diseases, pulmonary function tests provide objective measurements, which aid the physician in deciding how aggressive to be in managing asthma (see Chapters 38 and 41).

Peak Expiratory Flow Rates. Children as young as 3 years of age can perform peak expiratory flow rate (PEFR) maneuvers (Fig. 17-4), although some children and adults at any age may have difficulty coordinating their breath-

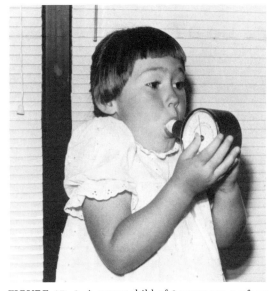

FIGURE 17-4. A young child of 3 years can perform peak flow maneuvers.

ing to perform the maneuver appropriately. The PEFR is an assessment of air flow through all airways. While the most durable and best known measuring devices cost hundreds of dollars, small plastic units helpful in monitoring peak flow rates are available for a fraction of that price. These inexpensive peak flow meters are useful for home monitoring of lung function, especially in patients with poor perception of obstruction. Keeping a home peak flow diary with PEFR determinations, two or three times a day, gives the family, patient, and physician an understanding of the patient's airway lability pattern and provides an early warning of severe obstruction. Such home monitoring allows for early intervention to avert a crisis.

Spirometry. Usually by 5 years of age, a child can be instructed and encouraged to perform spirometry with a forced expiratory maneuver that will yield adequate and reproducible tracings (Fig. 17-5). Such measurements yield information on flow and obstruction in large and small airways and on possible pulmonary restrictive disease (see Chapter 38). As the patient performs a forced expiration into the spirometer, a stylus is deflected at a rate and to an extent that are proportional to the expiratory volume over time. One usually has the patient perform this maneuver two or three times to be certain that he or she has used maximal effort and that the best effort has been selected for analysis. Expiratory volume is plotted against time in seconds. The highest volume expired is the forced vital capacity. In general, a normal individual will expire 79 percent or more of vital capacity within 1 second (FEV_1). The FEV_1 is the most commonly followed spirometric value. It will be low when there is obstruction to air flow; it represents flow mainly in the larger airways. By determining the slope of the points drawn at 25 percent and 75 percent of vital capacity, the forced expiratory flow at 25 to 75 percent of

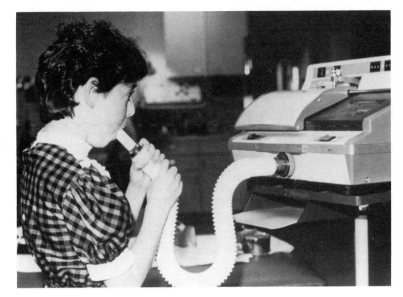

FIGURE 17-5. Children aged 5 years and older can perform spirometry.

vital capacity (FEF$_{25-75\%}$) can be determined, a measure that appears to represent air flow through the smaller airways (Fig. 17-6).

In order to interpret pulmonary function data, results are compared with normal standards for race, sex, and height. Predicted normal values are different for children and adults, and one cannot simply extrapolate downward from adult values to arrive at correct pediatric values (Polgar, 1971). Once normal values for the patient are established, comparisons can be

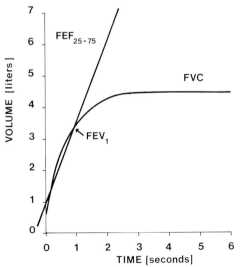

FIGURE 17-6. Commonly obtained information from the spirogram includes forced vital capacity (FVC), forced expiratory volume in 1 second (FEV$_1$), and forced expiratory flow at 25 to 75 percent of vital capacity (FEF$_{25-75\%}$).

made between the actual values for patients and standard predictions for normal individuals. Absolute values of flow rates must be kept in mind when interpreting the FEV$_1$: FVC ratio. For example, a normal adult with a vital capacity of 3.0 L might have an FEV$_1$ of 2.4 L as follows: $2.4/3.0 \times 100\% = 80\%$. A patient with acute asthma may have severe obstructive changes with superimposed restrictive changes and be unable to exhale to reasonable normal vital capacity as follows: FVC of 1 L (only 33 percent of the normal value) and FEV$_1$ of 0.8 may be recorded as $0.8/1.0 \times 100\% = 80\%$. Thus, the ratio of FEV$_1$: FVC is deceptively normal, whereas airway obstruction is severe.

Spirometry that is performed in the physician's office is a relatively inexpensive commitment. Reliable wedge spirometers cost about $1000, although more sophisticated computerized machines can cost more than $10,000. The less expensive devices are extremely cost effective for following patients with asthma. (Pulmonary function measurements are considered in detail in Chapter 38.)

Bronchoprovocation Tests. There are certain instances when specialized bronchial challenge tests are necessary additions to the patient's evaluation. Although some of these tests require sophisticated equipment that limits their availability to a few medical centers, most can be adapted for general use.

Bronchodilator Evaluation. If a patient's spirometric data show obstructive and restrictive changes, another spirometric effort after bronchodilator inhalation will measure the degree of reversibility of the abnormality. A variety of bronchodilators may be used; two inhalations of albuterol or its equivalent from a metered dose inhaler will provide efficient bronchodilation within minutes. If the patient's pulmonary dysfunction is longstanding, beta agonist inhalation may provide little or no change in pulmonary function. A short course of relatively high dose corticosteroid therapy, e.g., prednisone 1 to 2 mg/kg daily for 1 week, may be necessary to accomplish reversibility.

Exercise tolerance testing (ETT) to evaluate the presence of exercise induced bronchospasm (EIB) should be considered in the evaluation of patients with rhinitis as well as asthma. Up to 90 percent of asthmatics have bronchoconstriction after strenuous exercise, as do about 40 percent of children with allergic rhinitis. Thus, EIB is a common problem in children (Kawabori et al., 1976).

If unrecognized, EIB can lead to a child's failure to participate in school and leisure time sports, frustration about suboptimal physical performance, and poor self image. When EIB is suggested by history, an ETT should be performed. However, the history often is deficient in documenting this problem (especially when it occurs in children at school or elsewhere out of parents' sight), and an ETT should be considered when a history is at all suspicious. In addition, since EIB is extremely common in patients with chronic asthma, an ETT should be performed when a patient with chronic asthmatic symptoms denies the need for bronchodilator therapy prior to or after exercise. This type of patient may be coping unnecessarily with impairment, does not exercise, or is unaware of his or her exercise-related problems or wishes for one reason or another to deny it.

The ETT involves running for approximately 5 or 6 minutes at a speed that raises the heart rate to 80 to 90 percent of maximal oxygen consumption (Eggleston and Guerrant, 1976). Typically, bronchoconstriction follows a brief period of bronchodilation postexercise and is most severe 5 to 15 minutes postexercise. For clinical diagnosis, free running exercise around buildings or through corridors also is useful and is somewhat more sensitive than other modes of exercise for evoking EIB (Shapiro et al., 1979). Exercise-induced asthma is discussed in detail in Chapter 44.

Bronchial challenge with specific antigen can be performed to identify environmental factors that produce bronchospasm. Although a standardized protocol has been available for some time (Chai et al., 1975), antigen challenge is performed infrequently for a variety of the following reasons: (1) it is cumbersome to prepare material for challenge that is similar to the environmental antigen that is suspect; (2) there can be a "nonspecific" bronchial response to antigen in individuals who appear to have only upper respiratory symptoms on natural exposure (Bruce et al., 1975); and (3) approximately half of patients who react immediately to antigen challenges may have more severe late phase reactions, which occur 4 to 12 hours after the challenge and after recovery from the early challenge. Therefore, prolonged observation after challenge is necessary.

Bronchial challenge with histamine or methacholine is employed to determine whether there is "abnormal" bronchial hyperreactivity of the airways. Bronchoprovocation of this type can reveal underlying asthma when the history, physical examination, and resting pulmonary function tests are inconclusive. For example, this test can be helpful particularly in patients with persistent cough who do not have sufficient upper airway disease to explain their symptoms and who have no evidence for lower airway obstruction on physical examination and resting pulmonary function testing. A variety of provocative agents are useful for eliciting bronchial reactivity. Hyperventilation of cold air has been used in adults and children. Inhalation of hypertonic and hypotonic saline or distilled water is similarly informative. These agents rely on the observation that a range of alterations in airway heat and water loss and molarity can induce bronchospasm in asthmatic subjects but not in normal ones. Methacholine or histamine chemical bronchoprovocation has been performed extensively for both diagnostic and research purposes. Standardized protocols are in use (Tables 17–2 and 17–3), which allow for delivery of the provocative chemical by a tidal volume breathing or intermittent inhalation technique (Hargreave et al., 1983; Shapiro et al., 1983).

With the tidal volume method, the agent is nebulized continually and the subject breathes sequential concentrations, for 2 minutes each concentration, with tidal volume breathing. Pulmonary function tests are performed after each 2 minute challenge, until the appropriate range of concentrations has been completed, or the FEV_1 drops 20 percent or more. With the intermittent method, the patient inhales while actuating a solenoid valve dosimeter, which allows the agent to be nebulized for a specific

TABLE 17-2. Breath Units* for Methacholine on a mg/ml Basis†

Methacholine Concentrations (mg/ml)	Cumulative no. Breaths	Units Breath	Units/5 Breaths	Cumulative Units/5 Breaths‡
0.075	5	0.075	0.375	0.375
0.15	10	0.15	0.750	1.125
0.31	15	0.31	1.55	2.68
0.62	20	0.62	3.10	5.78
1.25	25	1.25	6.25	12.0
2.50	30	2.50	12.50	24.5
5.00	35	5.00	25.00	49.5
10.00	40	10.00	50.00	99.5
25.00	45	25.00	125.00	225.00

* One breath unit = 1 inhalation of 1 mg/ml.

† Chai, H. et al.: Standardization of bronchial inhalation challenge procedures. J. Allergy Clin. Immunol. 56:323–327, 1975.

‡ If final FEV$_1$ test is performed at other than a 5-breath interval (i.e., 23 breaths), the cumulative units are calculated by adding 3 × 0.62 = 1.86 to 5.78 = 7.64.

period of time. The patient takes five breaths of one concentration, performs pulmonary function tests, and then proceeds to the next concentration if the FEV$_1$ has not declined at least 20 percent. These two techniques are fairly comparable, and the dose or concentration of agent that induces a reduction in FEV$_1$ of 20 percent is called the PD$_{20}$ or PC$_{20}$.

Bronchoprovocation challenge should not be done soon after respiratory viral infections, since they can induce transient bronchial hyperreactivity for up to 8 weeks even in nonasthmatic individuals. When children are tested, they must be encouraged to put out maximal effort. The technician who works with them must be inventive to prevent their boredom and restlessness. Younger children may find the tidal volume method easier to perform, since this does not require synchronization of inhalation with the dosimeter actuation. Children who are too young for pulmonary function testing, obviously, cannot have proper chemical inhalation challenges. Preliminary work suggests, however, that following the very young patient's auscultatory findings or peak expiratory flow rates may give valuable information (Adinoff and Strunk, 1984).

Radiography. When an adult or a child wheezes for the first time, it is wise to obtain anteroposterior and lateral chest films. These allow identification of inflammatory processes, which may or may not be infectious. Structural abnormalities also may be detected. Individuals with repeated episodes of pneumonia require follow-up films to document resolution of episodes and whether recurrences affect the same or different parts of the lung. Whereas repeated transient upper or middle lobe atelectasis is not

TABLE 17-3. Breath Units* for Histamine on a mg/ml Basis†

Histamine Concentrations (mg/ml)	Cumulative no. Breaths	Units Breath	Units/5 Breaths	Cumulative Units/5 Breaths‡
0.03	5	0.03	0.15	0.15
0.06	10	0.06	0.30	0.45
0.12	15	0.12	0.60	1.05
0.25	20	0.25	1.25	2.30
0.50	25	0.50	2.50	4.80
1.00	30	1.00	5.00	9.80
2.50	35	2.50	12.50	22.30
5.00	40	5.00	25.00	47.30
10.00	45	10.00	50.00	97.30

* One breath unit = 1 inhalation of 1 mg/ml.

† Chai, H. et al.: Standardization of bronchial inhalation challenge procedures. J. Allergy Clin. Immunol. 56:323–327, 1975.

‡ If final FEV$_1$ test is performed at other than a 5-breath interval (i.e., 23 breaths), the cumulative units are calculated by adding 3 × 0.25 = 0.75 to 2.30 = 3.05.

uncommon in individuals who have severe asthma exacerbations, structural abnormalities may predispose them to this problem. Recurrent or persistent localized pneumonia is particularly worrisome. Tomography, radiocontrast studies, or bronchoscopy may be indicated.

Sinus disease is a common finding among allergic individuals. Although there are no controlled evaluations that document the incidence of sinusitis in a nonallergic person compared with an allergic person, up to 70 percent of youngsters presenting to an allergist's office for chronic rhinitis may have abnormal sinus radiographs (Rachelefsky et al., 1978). The majority respond specifically to antimicrobial therapy, possibly indicating bacterial disease.

Even in infancy, ethmoid and maxillary sinuses are pneumatized. In asymptomatic children under 1 year of age, maxillary antra may be cloudy on radiographs, minimizing their value. In children over age 1 year, however, abnormal findings are likely to correlate with disease. *Crying will not cause clouding of the sinuses* (Kovatch, 1984).

A sinus radiograph should be considered when an older patient complains of chronic purulent rhinorrhea or localized facial pain and tenderness or when a child has symptoms of chronic rhinorrhea and cough, particularly if nasal cytology shows a predominance of polymorphonuclear cells and bacteria.

For optimal visualization of the sinuses, the three following views should be performed: (1) the anteroposterior (Caldwell), (2) occipitomental (Waters), and (3) lateral. The ethmoid and frontal sinuses are best visualized with the Caldwell, the maxillary antra with the Waters, and the sphenoid sinuses with the lateral, which also is useful for visualizing the frontal sinuses. Actually, one can often obtain adequate information from one or two views. For example, young children do not yet have sphenoid and frontal sinuses; a Waters view often adequately demonstrates ethmoid sinuses and provides the best view of the maxillary antra. The clinician should give careful consideration to the history and physical examination in order to determine the views that will be most helpful.

Lateral head films are useful for a gross estimate of adenoid size (Fig. 17–7). A variety of methods for measuring the adenoid shadow have been used, e.g., distance from the anterior adenoid shadow to the posterior turbinate and distance from the anterior adenoid to the maxillary antrum. Commonly, adenoid size is interpreted from the degree that they impinge upon the nasopharyngeal airway. Although the lateral head film provides only a two dimensional estimate of adenoid size, it may provide important information when the nasal airway is patent but the voice is markedly hyponasal.

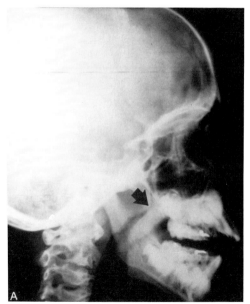
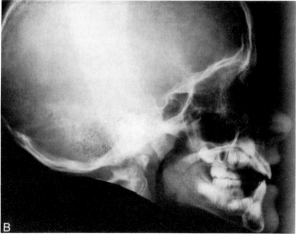

FIGURE 17–7. *A,* The airway is markedly narrowed by the large adenoid mass, which almost abuts on the palate. Nasal breathing is compromised by this degree of adenoidal enlargement. *B,* There is an ample nasal airway in this patient, in whom the adenoid shadow is quite small.

Gastroesophageal Reflux (GER). The patient with possible asthma may present with unusual symptoms that should alert the physician to the possibility of GER (Shapiro and Christie, 1983). The young child who has chronic vomiting, recurrent pneumonia, nocturnal spasmodic cough and wheeze, and failure to thrive represents the archetype of this problem. Results of a barium swallow are obtained to evaluate swallowing function, presence of structural abnormalities, and gross reflux. Radionuclide gastroesophagoscopy may be used to evaluate gastric emptying and aspiration of radiolabeled material into the pulmonary tree. Manometry may be performed to evaluate lower esophageal sphincter pressure, which tends to be less in patients with reflux than in normal individuals.

Intraluminal pH monitoring provides the most sensitive means of diagnosing GER and provides the opportunity for correlating symptomatic episodes with presence of reflux. A pH probe is placed in the lower esophagus, and pH is monitored for a controlled period of time. Acid is introduced into the stomach by way of a nasogastric tube. Monitoring of pH may be done for 1 hour or continued for up to 24 hours. During a 1 hour evaluation, two episodes of a decrease in esophageal pH to less than 4.0 indicate the presence of significant reflux in children. For adults, a drop in pH to less than 4.0 that lasts for 5 seconds or longer is diagnostic. The 24-hour tracing can be evaluated for the number of reflux episodes, the acid clearance time, and the relationship of coughing or cyanotic spells to changes in esophageal pH.

IMMUNODEFICIENCY

One group of patients that presents for allergy evaluation is characterized by a history of repeated or chronic infections. The chronic infections of the upper airways and related areas (sinusitis, otitis, pharyngitis) and of the lower airways (pneumonia, bronchitis) may have been due in part to the patient's allergic status. Simple viral syndromes in patients with excessive secretions, mucosal edema, and airways reactivity may evolve into more complicated disease states. Alternatively, other sorts of immune dysfunction may have predisposed the individual to these complications.

If the history and physical examination suggest an immune evaluation, the physician can screen the patient's immune status with several tests for humoral and cellular immunity, phagocyte function, and complement function (Bahna, 1985). (These are discussed in Chapters 3 and 4.) Briefly, a complete blood count will provide information concerning anemia, lymphopenia, neutropenia, and thrombocytopenia. An erythrocyte sedimentation rate is a useful indication of active infection or inflammation or both. Screening for humoral immunity should begin with quantitative measurement of IgG, IgA, and IgM. IgG subclass deficiency should be considered. IgE measurement will be important if recurrent skin infections and eczema suggest a hyper-IgE syndrome.

Specific humoral responses to antigen stimulation can be assessed by obtaining sera before and several weeks after routine immunization, for example, with diphtheria, tetanus, polio, mumps, rubeola, or rubella. Delayed hypersensitivity skin testing provides a screening assessment of T cell function. Antigens most commonly used are shown in Table 17–4. When 0.1 ml of the standardized concentration of antigen is injected intradermally, a positive response is at least 5 mm diameter of induration and 10 mm erythema after 24 to 72 hours. About 90 percent of normal adults will show a positive response to at least one of several antigens tested. Young children may have insufficient sensitization, and the elderly may be anergic.

Phagocytic function can be screened, assessing neutrophil morphology and number, with nitroblue tetrazolium test or chemiluminescence tests of cellular oxidative metabolism. Overall complement activity is measured by total serum complement activity (CH_{50}), which will be depressed if there is appreciable reduction of any of the complement components (see Chapter 4).

A child or young adult with recurrent sinopulmonary disease should have a sweat chloride test to rule out cystic fibrosis, especially if there are recurrent gastrointestinal complaints. A ciliary biopsy should also be considered in children with recurrent severe sinusitis and pneumonia, to screen for immotile ciliary syndrome.

If the aforementioned screening evaluation leaves doubt as to the patient's immune integrity, a more thorough immunologic evaluation is indicated (see Chapter 3.)

Total Serum IgE. In certain situations it is valuable to measure a patient's total serum IgE concentration. Approximately 45 percent of the

TABLE 17-4. Antigens Commonly Used for Delayed Hypersensitivity Skin Testing*

| Antigen | Trade Name | Strength | |
		FIRST	SECOND
Candida	Dermatophytin "0"	1:100	1:10
Trichophyton	Dermatophytin	1:30	—
Tetanus	Tetanus Toxoid Fluid (8 Lf/ml)	2 Lf/ml	8 Lf/ml
	Tetanus Toxoid Fluid (15 Lf/ml)		
Mumps	Mumps Skin Test Antigen	As is	—
Staphylococcus	Staphage Lysate	1:5	—
Phytohemagglutinin	Phytohemagglutinin	20 μg/ml	100 μg/ml
Tuberculin	Alpisol (Tuberculin PPD)	5 TU	250 TU
	Tubersol (Tuberculin PPD)	5 TU	250 TU
Histoplasma	Histoplasmin	1:100	1:10
Coccidioides	Coccidioidin	1:100	1:10

* Adapted from Bahna, S.L.: Office diagnosis of immunodeficiency diseases. Immunol. Allergy Pract. 7:252–258, 1985.

patients with allergic rhinitis will have a total serum IgE level that is greater than one standard deviation from the nonatopic population's mean. Approximately 75 percent of the patients with allergic asthma also will have had an elevated level of IgE. Therefore, an elevated total IgE level is helpful confirmatory evidence, but does not exclude allergy if normal. Considering this limitation, obtaining IgE levels on all patients is unnecessary.

In certain patients with eczema-like dermatitis and frequent staphylococcal skin infections, unusually high total serum IgE levels are found. Documenting such a situation clarifies the type of patient one is managing. In the patient whose history and physical examination suggest allergy but whose skin test reactions to common antigens are negative, a high serum IgE concentration may direct one toward more historical probings and skin testing; a low IgE concentration may help one to diagnose that disease as intrinsic rather than extrinsic. In allergic bronchopulmonary aspergillosis, the serum IgE concentration provides an important indicator of the course of the disease; the concentration should decline as remission occurs. There is a strong correlation between elevated serum IgE levels and the occurrence of wheezing in children with viral upper respiratory infections (Stempel et al., 1980). Thus, a serum IgE level may provide a better understanding of disease in certain patients with asthma or rhinitis.

In Vivo **Tests for IgE (Allergy Skin Testing).** The history provides the information on possible environmental or dietary factors that may be inciting or aggravating the patient's difficul-

ties. In order to identify which factors may be causative, one may need to determine the allergens to which the patient has specific IgE antibodies.

Allergy skin testing is an extraordinarily sensitive bioassay for specific allergic homocytotropic antibody. This so-called skin sensitizing or reaginic antibody usually belongs to the IgE class. There usually is a good correlation between antibody found in the skin and in the respiratory tract and blood. The interaction of antigen introduced into the skin with antibody fixed to dermal mast cells results in local release of mediators, such as histamine, which induce local vasodilation with wheal and flare formation peaking after 10 to 15 minutes. Although this "immediate" reaction fades after 20 minutes, patients occasionally will experience "late" cutaneous reactivity hours after initial antigen application. This late reactivity may be similar to the clinical late phase reaction, which can occur with allergic asthma and rhinitis.

A positive skin test reaction usually indicates that the subject has IgE directed toward the antigen that has been tested. This does not prove, however, that this sensitization causes clinically significant disease. The likelihood that the IgE antibody present has clinical importance correlates with the amount of antibody present and, therefore, roughly with the intensity of the skin test reaction. In other words, the weaker the antigen necessary to provoke a positive skin test reaction, the greater the likelihood that it is clinically relevant.

Determinants of Reactivity. The degree of skin test reactivity that an individual shows after antigen injection depends on the (1) non-

TABLE 17–5. Commonly Used Pharmacologic Agents and Their Effects on Skin Test Reactivity

No Effect	Partial Suppression	Marked Suppression
Corticosteroids	Oral sympathomimetics*	Epinephrine (marked alpha adrenergic
Cromolyn	(mild alpha adrenergic ac-	activity)
Theophylline	tivity)	Antihistamines
Beta-2 agonists	Ephedrine	Astemizole
Albuterol	Phenylephrine	Hydroxyzine
Metaproterenol	Phenylpropanolamine	Terfenadine
Isoproterenol	Most antihistamines	Anti-anxiety drugs (antihistamine char-
Terbutaline		acteristics)
		Doxepin
		Trimeprazine tartrate

* Infrequently significant at usual dosages.

specific reaction to the trauma of the test; (2) degree of antibody sensitization of dermal mast cells towards the specific antigen; (3) quantity and specificity of antigen injected; (4) medications recently taken, especially antihistamines; and (5) age, with infants and the elderly being less reactive than other age groups.

Reliable skin test results depend on careful attention to a variety of aspects of the procedure. Skin test antigens must be purchased from laboratories with commitment to quality control. Since extract composition is not yet standardized for most antigens, purity and potency of allergenic material may vary from lot to lot. Antigen must be preserved properly to minimize deterioration and must be replaced when shelf life has expired. Diluting antigen speeds its loss of potency. The addition of glycerin at 10 percent or 50 percent concentration or of 0.03 percent human serum albumin increases stability of most antigens significantly (Nelson, 1981).

Grading systems for skin test reactions depend on specific quantities of material being injected intradermally or applied epicutaneously. Injection of too much or too little antigen or injection too deeply can cloud results. Grading depends upon comparison with positive and negative controls, usually histamine (1 mg/ml for prick tests, 0.01 mg/ml for intradermal tests) and saline, respectively. Placing the tests too close together may cause overlapping wheals and resultant misinterpretation.

Drug effects may alter skin reactivity (Table 17–5). Antihistaminic medication can suppress skin wheals and erythema. Although these effects are greatest with hydroxyzine and astemizole (Gendreau-Reid, 1986; Ting et al., 1985), it is best to withhold all antihistamines for at least 48 hours prior to testing. (Hydroxyzine should

be withheld 96 hours and astemizole for 4 weeks!) One should be aware of all medication that the patient is taking, since some sedative or antianxiety drugs, such as trimeprazine tartrate (Temaril) and doxepin (Sinequan), may bind to the skin's histamine receptors. If one is uncertain whether a patient's medication may alter test results, a histamine control should be performed before skin testing. Selective beta-2 agonists and corticosteroids do not appear to alter skin test reactivity. Adrenergic agents with alpha activity will partially suppress wheal formation for a short period of time, and an injection of epinephrine may completely block a skin test response.

Infants and young children can be skin tested reliably if one appreciates that wheal size will be smaller in response to both histamine and antigen (Van Asperen et al., 1984; Menardo et al., 1985; Zeiger, 1985). The elderly will also manifest decreased reactivity that can be put in perspective with use of saline and histamine controls.

GENERAL GUIDELINES FOR TESTING

There are several general guidelines regarding the physician's approach to the patient who is to be tested. First, tests should be based on information gleaned from the history, as a positive reaction is only corroborative evidence and cannot stand alone as proof of clinical disease. Second, testing should be limited to pertinent allergens that interact with specific IgE antibodies and not to substances such as formaldehyde and newsprint ink, which are irritating to the skin but not specific antigens. Similarly, food testing for nonimmune substances, such as monosaccharide and disaccharide sugars, is spurious. Third, only a limited number of skin tests should be performed at one time, particularly in the very sensitive patient, to minimize the possibility of a systemic reaction. Fourth, patients with histories of anaphylaxis from known substances should only be tested for those substances when there are benefits to be gained for the patients as follows: Hymenoptera testing when immunotherapy may be lifesaving; penicillin testing when the history is equivocal, and it is essential to use penicillin; and food testing when dietary restriction is difficult, and enough time has elapsed that sensitivity may well have decreased. In these situations and whenever skin testing is performed, there is a risk of anaphylaxis for which the physician must be prepared. Epinephrine, oxygen, and antihistamine must be immediately available. Further emergency therapy including an oral airway, intravenous fluids, pressors, and corticosteroids should be accessible (see Chapter 51.)

Techniques of Testing. Testing is done using an epicutaneous or intradermal method. Epicutaneous refers to the direct application of antigen extract to the epidermis. An intradermal test involves injection of a small quantity of antigen into the superficial dermis. In either case, the skin to be tested is wiped clean with alcohol. A felt-tip or ball-point pen is used to indicate where tests will be placed.

For the epicutaneous method known as prick testing, the back or volar surface of the forearm is used. A drop of antigen in fairly high concentration, usually $1/10$ to $1/50$ dilution, is placed on the skin. A sterile needle is then passed through the extract at an angle of approximately 60 degrees with the skin, and the skin is slightly raised. This allows antigen to make contact with superficial mast cells but does not draw blood. The procedure is repeated for each antigen. A new needle may be used each time, or an alcohol pad can be used to clean the needle between each test. The puncture test is similar to the prick test except for the use of a two-pronged needle for lightly puncturing the skin. Scratch testing, which involves scratching the skin and applying antigen on top of the abrasion, is similar but less sensitive. Scarifiers and needles of many types have been used successfully in epicutaneous testing.

Skin tests are evaluated 15 to 20 minutes after antigen is applied. To grade reactivity, a normal saline test ("negative control") and histamine test ("positive control") using a concentration of 1 mg/ml are used and applied in the same way as the antigen. Most test results are considered positive if the wheal diameter exceeds that of the saline control by at least 3 mm. If epicutaneous test results are positive, further testing need not be done. If they are negative in the face of a suggestive history, intradermal tests may be helpful (Fig. 17–8).

When intradermal tests are performed as a second step after epicutaneous testing, a small amount (0.02 ml) of dilute antigen (1:1000) is injected into the dermis. Though the antigen is 100-fold weaker than that used for prick testing, the direct injection into the proximity of

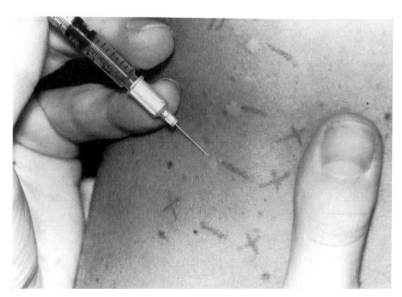

FIGURE 17–8. A 27-gauge needle is used for the intradermal injection of a small amount (0.2 ml) of allergen extract.

dermal mast cells makes the intradermal test more sensitive than the epicutaneous and also more likely to induce a systemic reaction. Intradermal testing at 1:1000 dilution is unsafe unless prior epicutaneous test reactions have been negative (or only questionably positive).

For grading intradermal test reactions, a saline control and histamine control (0.01 mg/ml) are necessary. One commonly used grading system defines wheals that are 5 mm greater in diameter than those of the saline control as 3+ and larger wheals with pseudopods as 4+. Wheals smaller than 5 mm in diameter are graded subjectively as 1+ or 2+.

The grading system used is less important than a knowledge of the limitations of one's techniques. Epicutaneous tests are highly specific for detecting mast cell–bound IgE and possibly IgG4. Positive prick test results for inhalant factors correlate well with results of nasal provocation (Brown et al., 1977; Cavanaugh et al., 1977). Positive prick test results for a number of food antigens show reasonable correlation with ingestion challenge (Sampson and Albergo, 1984). With the increased sensitivity of intradermal testing at 1:1000 weight/volume concentration of antigen, in the face of a negative epicutaneous test result, the correlation between positive intradermal testing results and clinically relevant symptoms after antigen exposure is not as high as that of epicutaneous testing (Cavanaugh et al., 1977; Reddy et al., 1978). This factor must be considered when counseling patients about environmental control and immunotherapy.

Intradermal testing with a dilution weaker than 1:1000 does not have this limited specificity. An alternative approach to epicutaneous testing is to begin with intradermal injection at 1:100,000 and to proceed at 15 minute intervals with tests at ten-fold higher concentrations, until there is a significant wheal response or until the 1:1000 dose (the most concentrated dilution tested) is interpreted. This titration approach gives valuable quantitative information regarding the patient's degree of sensitization.

Strict attention should be paid to sterile techniques in order to minimize the transmission of blood-borne infectious agents from patient to patient. The sterile epicutaneous needle should be discarded after use on a single patient. A separate sterile needle and syringe should be used for each antigen on each patient and discarded after use to avoid transfer of microorganisms from patient to patient (Lutz et al., 1984).

In Vitro **Testing for IgE.** As an alternative to assessing mast cell–fixed IgE with skin testing, specific serum IgE antibody can be measured by means of the radioallergosorbent test or RAST. Antigen is coupled covalently to an inert carrier, such as latex particles, a cellulose disk, or polystyrene microtiter tubes. These are incubated with the patient's serum. If there is serum IgE directed against the antigen, antigen-antibody complexes will be formed which can be isolated. A radiolabeled or monoclonal antibody to IgE is then added to interact with the antigen-antibody complexes. The resulting combination of antigen IgE and anti-IgE can now be assessed with a gamma scintillation counter.

Modifications of the RAST are numerous (e.g., MAST and FAST). These are variations on the same procedure that utilize different carriers for antigen, such as radiolabeled or enzyme labeled anti-IgE (enzyme-linked assays or ELISAs), which are detected with a fluorometer (Tsay and Halpern, 1984). There are few clinical situations in which serologic tests are preferable to skin tests, since skin tests generally are more sensitive, less expensive, and potentially offer more comprehensive information. When a patient has extensive skin disease, extreme dermatographism, or a history of anaphylactic sensitivity, a serologic test may be the diagnostic method of choice (Position Statement, 1983). The lesser sensitivity of a serologic test, however, also raises the possibility that it may miss the presence of antibody in a patient at risk of a severe allergic reaction to a substance.

Serologic tests do have several advantages over skin tests as follows: (1) the patient time and discomfort are minimized; (2) the subjective aspect of skin test reading is decreased (but the physician must still interpret the results which are expressed in counts per minute); (3) the antigen is stable in solid state unlike skin test solutions; (4) the patient with a skin disorder, such as widespread eczema, can be assessed; and (5) the use of antihistaminic drugs will not alter results. The disadvantages of serologic tests, however, include the following: (1) not all laboratories performing RAST or other serologic tests are reliable, and quality control standards are not required; (2) expense is significantly greater than for skin tests; (3) sensitivity is significantly less than for skin tests; (4) attempts to modify RAST by increasing the scale to enhance sensitivity have resulted in significant loss of specificity; (5) results are not immediately available to the patient; and (6) not all antigens are readily coupled to insoluble materials.

REFERENCES

Adinoff, A., Strunk, R.: Methacholine inhalation challenge (MC) in young children: Results of testing and follow-up. J. Allergy Clin. Immunol. (Abstract) 73:124, 1984.

Bahna, S.L.: Office diagnosis of immunodeficiency diseases. Immunol. Allergy Pract. 7:252–258, 1985.

Bluestone, R.D., Cantekin, E.I.: Panel of experience with testing eustachian tube function. Ann. Otol. Rhinol. Laryngol. 90:552–562, 1981.

Brown, W.G., Halonen, M.J., Kaltenborn, W.T., Barbee, R.A.: The relationship of respiratory allergy, skin test reactivity and serum IgE in a community population sample. J. Allergy Clin. Immunol. 63:328–335, 1977.

Bruce, C.A., Rosenthal, R.R., Lichtenstein, L.M., Norman, P.S.: Quantitative inhalation bronchial challenge in ragweed hay fever patients: A comparison with ragweed allergic asthmatics. J. Allergy Clin. Immunol. 56:331–337, 1975.

Cavanaugh, M.J., Bronsky, E.A., Buckley, J.M.: Clinical value of bronchial provocation testing in childhood asthma. J. Allergy Clin. Immunol. 59:41–47, 1977.

Chai, H., Farr, R.S., Froehlich, L.A., Mathison, D.A., McLean, J.A., Rosenthal, R.R., Sheffer III, A.L., Spector, S.L., Townley, R.G.: Standardization of bronchial inhalation challenge procedures. J. Allergy Clin. Immunol. 56:323–327, 1975.

Eggleston, P.A., Guerrant, J.L.: A standardized method of evaluating exercise-induced asthma. J. Allergy Clin. Immunol. 58:414, 1976.

Friedman, R.A., Doyle, W.J., Casselbrant, M.L., Bluestone, C., Fireman, P.: Immunologic-mediated eustachian tube obstruction: A double-blind crossover study. J. Allergy Clin. Immunol. 71:442–447, 1983.

Gendreau-Reid, L., Simons, K.J., Simons, F.E.R.: Comparison of the suppressive effect of astemizole, terfenadine, and hydroxyzine on histamine-induced wheals and flares in humans. J. Allergy Clin. Immunol. 77:335–340, 1986.

Georgitis, J.W.: The applicability of rhinomanometry in nonatopic children: Comparison of three techniques. J. Allergy Clin. Immunol. 75:614–620, 1985.

Hargreave, F.E., Dolovich, J., Boulet, L.P.: Inhalation provocation tests. Semin. Resp. Med. IV: 224–236, 1983.

Kawabori, I., Pierson, W.E., Conquest, L.L., Bierman, C.W.: Incidence of exercise-induced asthma in children. J. Allergy Clin. Immunol. 58:447–455, 1976.

Kovatch, A.L.: Maxillary sinus radiography in children with nonrespiratory complaints. Pediatrics 73:306–308, 1984.

Kraemer, M.J., Richardson, M.A., Weiss, N.S., Furukawa, C.T., Shapiro, G.G., Pierson, W.E., Bierman, C.W.: Risk factors for persistent middle ear effusions. J.A.M.A. 249:1022–1025, 1983.

Lutz, C.T., Bell Jr., C.E., Wedner, H.J., Krogstad, D.J.: Allergy testing of patients should no longer be performed with a common syringe. N. Engl. J. Med. 310:1335–1337, 1984.

Menardo, J.L., Bousquet, J., Rodiere, M., Astruc, J., Michel, F-B.: Skin test reactivity in infancy. J. Allergy Clin. Immunol. 75:646–651, 1985.

Nelson, H.S.: Effect of preservatives and conditions of storage on potency of allergy extracts. J. Allergy Clin. Immunol. 67:64–69, 1981.

Polgar, G., Promadhat, V. (eds.): *Pulmonary Function Testing in Children,* Philadelphia, W.B.Saunders Co., 1971.

Position Statement: Skin testing and radioallergosorbent testing (RAST) for diagnosis of specific allergens responsible for IgE medical diseases. J. Allergy Clin. Immunol. 72:515–517, 1983.

Rachelefsky, G., Goldberg, M., Katz, R.M., Borris, G., Gyepes, M.T., Shapiro, M.J., Mickey, M.R., Finegold, S.M., Siegel, S.C.: Sinus disease in children with respiratory allergy. J. Allergy Clin. Immunol. 61:310–314, 1978.

Reddy, P.M., Nagaya, H., Pascual, H.C., Lee, S.K., Gupta, S., Lauridsen, J.I., Jerome, D.C.: Reappraisal of intracutaneous tests in the diagnosis of reaginic allergy. J. Allergy Clin. Immunol. 61:36–41, 1978.

Sampson, H.A., Albergo, R.: Comparison of results of skin tests, RAST, and double-blind, placebo-controlled food challenges in children with atopic dermatitis. J. Allergy Clin. Immunol. 74:26–33, 1984.

Shapiro, G.G., Bierman, C.W., Furukawa, C.T., Pierson, W.E.: Allergy skin testing: Science or quackery? Pediatrics 59:495–498, 1977.

Shapiro, G.G., Christie, D.L.: Gastroesophageal reflux and asthma. Clin. Rev. Allergy 1:39–56, 1983.

Shapiro, G.G., Furukawa, C.T., Pierson, W.E., Bierman, C.W.: Methacholine bronchial challenge in children. J. Allergy Clin. Immunol. 69:365–369, 1982.

Shapiro, G.G., Pierson, W.E., Furukawa, C.T., Bierman, C.W.: Comparison of the effectiveness of free running treadmill exercise for assessing exercise-induced bronchospasm in a clinical practice. J. Allergy Clin. Immunol. 64:609–611, 1979.

Stempel, D.A., Clyde Jr., W.A., Henderson, F.W., Collier, A.M.: Serum IgE levels and the clinical exposure of respiratory illness. J. Pediatr. 97:185–190, 1980.

Ting, S., Rauls, D.O., Reiman, B.E.F.: Inhibitory effect of hydroxyzine on antigen-induced histamine release in vivo. J. Allergy Clin. Immunol. 75:63–66, 1985.

Tsay, Y.G., Halpern, G.: IgE fluoroallergosorbent test: Concept and clinical applications. Immunol. Allergy Pract. 6:27–32, 1984.

Van Asperen, P.P., Kemp, A.S., Mellis, C.M.: Skin test reactivity and clinical allergen sensitivity in infancy. J. Allergy Clin. Immunol. 73:381–386, 1984.

Walker, S.B., Shapiro, G.G., Bierman, C.W., Morgan, M.S., Marshall, S.G., Furukawa, C.T.: Induction of eustachian tube dysfunction with histamine nasal provocation. J. Allergy Clin. Immunol. 76:158–162, 1985.

Zeiger, R.S.: Atopy in infancy and early childhood: Natural history and role of skin testing. J. Allergy Clin. Immunol. 75:633–639, 1985.

18

Controlling the Environment for Allergic Diseases

JEROME M. BUCKLEY, M.D.
DAVID S. PEARLMAN, M.D.

The word environment is derived from Old French, environer, which means "to surround or encompass." Maimonides (1135–1204) recorded the following observation in his *Treatise on Asthma* (Muntner, 1963): "Your Highness (the King of Egypt) has already confided in me that the air in Alexandria is harmful to you and whenever you fear an attack of asthma, you prefer to move to Cairo where the air is much drier and calmer, making the attack more tolerable for you." Maimonides later lists as one of his Six Obligatory Regulations For His Highness' Illness, "keeping clean the air which you breathe." Thus, as early as the twelfth century, a "governmental body" was aware of the relationship between the environment and human respiratory disease.

BACKGROUND

Many airborne substances in the environment can induce allergic reactions. In addition, numerous environmental pollutants can precipitate or aggravate "allergic" symptoms by nonimmune mechanisms. For example, sneezing and burning or itching of the nose and eyes, which can be induced by allergic reactions to pollens and animal danders, can be induced by airborne irritants, such as cigarette smoke and petrochemical or formaldehyde fumes. These airborne irritants also can aggravate preexistent allergic reactions of the eyes or the respiratory tract.

Irritants as well as allergens in the indoor environment are now recognized as causes of disease. As the cost of energy for home heating has risen, the increased use of kerosene heaters and wood stoves coupled with increased insulation and decreased indoor air exchange have produced a general elevation in indoor air pollution. At the same time other new devices, such as the functional central high efficiency particulate air (HEPA) filters (see subsequent discussion), have helped to offset such adverse pollution.

The purpose of environmental control measures is to minimize contact with allergens or irritants that precipitate or aggravate that patient's disease. Decreased exposure may reduce bronchial hyperreactivity in the patient with asthma (Cockroft et al., 1977) or reduce nasal obstruction in the patient with rhinitis. Appropriate environmental control depends first upon identifying the offending factors. Often the patient or parents are unaware of many allergic and irritant factors. Although an environmental history is the first step in their identification, addressing where symptoms occur (home, school, workplace, vacation cabin, friends' homes) and when (time of day, week, month, or year) provides a beginning to the understanding of environmental relationships. (Chapter 16 discusses environmental history and Chapter 17 discusses allergy tests.) Allergy tests, and when appropriate, elimination and reexposure, can help determine the importance of putative factors. Since environmental irritants also may exacerbate allergic symptoms, it is important to remember that "allergy tests" may not identify all relevant factors.

A visit to the home, school, or workplace can reveal unusual or unexpected environmental factors (Weiseman and Weiseman, 1964). The surrounding neighborhood, nearby industrial plants, as well as factors related to the home, such as quality of housekeeping, presence of animals or animal danders, filled ashtrays, musty odors, or cluttered bedroom, can provide the physician with additional information on which to base specific advice on environmental control. Also such a visit may have a positive effect on compliance of the patient and family with environmental control measures.

APPROACH TO ENVIRONMENTAL CONTROL

General Considerations. Environmental control must be rational, based on a knowledge

239

of the patient's sensitivities, and individualized, according to the physical, psychologic, and financial resources of the patient and his or her family. Environmental restrictions must not be so rigid that other family members are neglected over concern for the patient but should protect the patient from allergens to which he or she is very allergic. Often, reduced exposure rather than total elimination may control symptoms adequately. When environmental control involves extensive household alterations, purchase of expensive equipment, or total changes in life style, the physician must be confident that these changes will be beneficial and must convince the patient and family that these changes should be carried out. The wise physician will take a middle road, recommending first those changes that are easily accomplished and accepted by the family. If the initial changes are not sufficiently effective, more extensive environmental manipulation may then be encouraged. This approach will tend to make difficult environmental changes more acceptable.

The physician in his or her recommendations for environmental control must consider the effect that these alterations may have both on the patient and on the family. For example, compromises can be effected in which the patient who is only mildly allergic to animals may be allowed outdoor contact with an animal, which is kept but excluded from the house. Every effort must be made to avoid family resentment toward the patient because of allergies while promoting normal psychosocial development. Similarly, it is essential to avoid undue limitation of physical activity. The ultimate goal should be full participation in sports and recreational activities.

In approaching the home environment, the physician must consider the basic home construction; heating and cooling systems; potential problems of moisture or mildew in the basement, bathrooms, or attic; cleaning methods; and presence of pets or smokers. Particular emphasis should be placed on that part of the environment in which the patient spends the greatest amount of time. Attention should be focused especially on the bedroom in which young children may spend half of their time, and older children and adults may spend over a third.

Generally, next in importance is the family or "TV room," with less intense attention to other rooms of the house. However, for patients with severe allergic disease, attention may have to be extended to relatives' homes, babysitters' homes, schoolrooms, workplaces, and any other places the patients frequent.

"House dust" is a composite of various potentially allergenic materials of which the Pyroglyphid dust mites (present globally in moist climates) and animal allergens in homes with domestic animals are the most significant. However, house dust may contain other insect emanations (e.g., cockroach) and rodent, bird, and mold allergens (see Chapter 12). House dust also is a universal irritant, and minimizing dust exposure is desirable for all patients with allergic disorders. Since house dust control and control of various indoor allergens is related to heating and cooling systems and particularly to methods of cleaning, these are discussed in the following sections. Systems that regulate other qualities of the indoor environment, such as humidity which also can influence allergic symptoms, are addressed in addition. Since the prevalence of many of the allergens and irritants found indoors are related to methods of controlling indoor environments, an understanding of these systems is essential.

CONTROL OF TEMPERATURE AND HUMIDITY

Heating Systems. There are four basic types of central controlled heating systems as follows: (1) forced air, in which air is heated and then forced (blown) throughout the house via a duct system; (2) electric heat, with separate electric heating units in each room, in which heating occurs by radiation and convection from heated metal; (3) hot water or steam heat, in which water is heated and distributed to pipes in individual rooms, and heating occurs by radiation and convection; and (4) heat pump, in which the effect is a variation of the forced air system. There also are radiant heating systems similar to hot water systems except that metal conductors transfer heat from the energy source (hot water pipe or electrically heated metal) to the environment. Other heating systems include space heaters or floor furnaces, with or without fans, which usually are placed in a central location in the house. Various energy sources—natural gas, oil, kerosene, coal, and electricity—can be used for each of these. In some, air is moved passively by heating it; in others, air is moved by blade-type fans or by quieter "squirrel cage"–type fans. Some systems employ filters.

Generally, all can be improved without a great deal of cost.

Hot water, electric, and other radiant heating systems are the most desirable home heating methods for individuals with allergic disorders since they do not require the movement of large volumes of air. Forced air systems, especially those without filters, are less desirable because moving air carries with it house dust and other allergens or irritants and has a drying effect on respiratory mucosa. However, air that does not circulate cannot be filtered, cooled, humidified, or dehumidified effectively without the use of numerous room units. Thus, the least expensive all-purpose system, which allows heating, humidification if appropriate, cooling, and most importantly filtration, is a properly designed and maintained forced air system. Mechanical filters on the cold air return of such systems must be changed at least monthly during the heating season. Methods of air filtration are discussed subsequently. Periodic (yearly) cleaning of the duct system may be important, as is thorough cleaning of the duct system in a new house prior to use, when the duct system frequently serves as a garbage and waste disposal system during construction. Vents in the patient's bedroom should be closed at night to minimize air turbulence if adequate heating can still be maintained; keeping the bedroom door open may help as may covering the vent opening with a portion of a standard furnace filter. Special attention should be given to proper insulation—walls, doors, windows, and attic —not only to conserve energy but also to minimize air turbulence and "nonfiltered" leaks.

A heat pump can be an appropriate option for purposes of energy conservation. A heat pump works on the principle of heat exchange, utilizing refrigerant contained within the unit to remove or to add heat to a source; compression of the refrigerant increases its temperature, providing a source of heat; and expansion of the refrigerant absorbs heat and allows it to extract heat from a source. There are two types of heat pumps as follows: an air-source type that uses outside air for its operation and a water-source type that uses water-filled pipe coils as its source for heat exchange. Heat is added to the house in the winter from compression of expanded refrigerant. Heat is removed from the inside air in the summer by letting the compressed refrigerant expand. A heat pump in effect is a form of forced air system. Fans and ductwork are the same as in other forced air systems and require the same yearly cleaning and maintenance. *There is no environmental advantage of heat pumps* except for possible energy efficiency.

Other Heating Systems. Kerosene heaters pose a fire hazard in general and produce indoor pollutants in high concentrations (Consumer Reports, 1982). Cooper and Alberti (1984) studied 14 homes with asthmatic patients in which kerosene heaters with "water clear" kerosene were used. In six homes, maximal 8-hour concentrations of SO_2 far exceeded the 0.1 to 0.2 ppm concentrations of SO_2 shown to cause bronchospasm in asthmatics.

Wood and coal burning stoves also have created problems (Honicky, 1985). Burning of wood or coal produces significantly more pollutants per unit of heat than does oil or gas and also forms large amounts of carbon monoxide, hydrocarbons, and solid and liquid particulates (Consumer Reports, 1985). Wood stoves have been implicated specifically in increasing respiratory illness in children (Honicky, 1985). In order to minimize indoor pollution, the wood stove must be installed properly (professionally), operated correctly, and maintained properly. It is important that the damper be opened fully before adding wood since most of the indoor pollution occurs during this time period. The chimney should be cleaned yearly to prevent accumulation of combustible material, which can lead to fire. The cost involved in proper installation and maintenance of these units may offset any anticipated reduction in fuel costs.

Cooling Systems. Cooling systems include everything from simple fans to sophisticated air conditioning systems. Cooling systems also include attic exhaust fan systems of two types as follows: one that cools by pulling air into all rooms via open windows through the entire house and out the attic and another that simply cools only the attic air by replacing hot inside air with cooler outside air. In the first type, the system pulls more outside particulate matter, including pollens, molds, and "dirt," through the house. Such cooling systems are not advisable for most patients. However, since pollens and most molds are sufficiently large that they can be trapped and removed by simply using regular furnace filters (Figure 18–1), we have advised the use of furnace filters in the bedroom windows of the allergic patient. Since submicroscopic allergens from pollens may pass through ordinary filters, it is better to wait until dusk to open windows when pollen concentrations decrease and to turn fans off in the

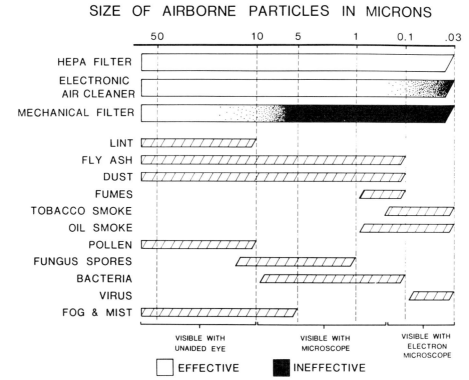

FIGURE 18–1. Effectiveness of various filtering systems in eliminating airborne particles that may precipitate or aggravate allergic diseases.

morning when pollen concentrations increase. The second system, which cools only the attic, decreases the heating of the bedroom by the sun and decreases the need to open the windows overnight for cooling.

Evaporative coolers are used in some parts of the country where humidity is low as alternatives to refrigeration systems. Because they utilize water evaporation, they are frequent sources of mold spores and may increase mite growth. When ambient temperatures are extremely high, they also can cause hypersensitivity lung disease due to growth of thermophilic actinomycetes. They should not be used by individuals with actual or potential mold sensitivities. Mold growth tends not to be a problem when a cold water cooling device is used in which a fan is employed to blow air over coils cooled by cold water, completely enclosed in the coils.

The most common type of air conditioning in use is the refrigeration type, available as window or central units. Window air conditioners cool only a room or several rooms of the home and can be especially effective for a bedroom if the door is kept closed (Seebohm, 1973). Using the fan without refrigeration can bring in fresh filtered air during the cooler time of the night. Filters must be changed regularly.

A central air conditioner can be an efficient filter, trapping larger allergens and irritant particles if it is used continuously. However, the system frequently is used only intermittently by patients, i.e., only in the hottest weather or during the day because of the cost of operation, thus losing its effective filtering potential. Pollen-sensitive and mold-sensitive individuals should keep the bedroom windows closed during "problem seasons" to minimize any allergen and irritant exposure (Seebohm, 1973). A heat pump can also be used for cooling.

The least expensive method that combines adequate temperature control with allergen reduction is the most desirable. For example, the patient whose bedroom is comfortable at night with windows closed for most of the year but who, nevertheless, needs air conditioning some of the time, may do well with a refrigerated window air conditioning unit for the occasional hot nights during the pollen season.

Humidification Systems. In some areas, humidification of air in the home is desirable, whereas in others, dehumidification may be needed. Warm air is capable of holding more moisture than is cold air. When a furnace heats a home it also reduces the relative moisture content of air, called "relative humidity," which is expressed as the amount of moisture in the air as a percent of the moisture-holding capacity, unless water is added to the air. An illustration of the potential drying effects of this process follows: heating outdoor air that has a temperature of 20°F (−6.7°C) and 80 percent relative humidity to 70°F (21.1°C), without adding water to the air, reduces its relative humidity to 12 percent. Although the actual amount of moisture in the air did not change, the capacity of the warmer air to hold moisture increased. Consequently, the air became "drier" with an increased propensity to remove moisture from household items and the mucous membranes and skin of the occupants of the house. A humidity level of 25 to 40 percent is recommended as optimal.

There are three types of humidifiers; reservoir, evaporator, and jet spray. The reservoir type is the most common. A wheel rotates in a reservoir of water, and air is blown over the wheel, which picks up moisture as it passes by. In *any* humidifier, excess moisture can encourage mold growth, although there is less risk of mold growth at the site of humidification in a nonreservoir type, e.g., jet spray. In areas of hard water, precipitation of minerals and malfunction of humidifiers can be minimized by using water from the hot water heater for humidification. This increases the cost of humidification (which then uses heated water) and may shorten the life of the hot water heater. On the other hand, using this "softened" hot water can markedly extend the life of the central humidifier. In order to determine the most appropriate system for a particular house, it is necessary to know the size, design, and heating system of the house, as well as the meteorologic conditions in the area (Consumer Reports, August, 1984).

Portable humidifiers can be selected for either hot or cold humidification. True humidifiers have a humidistat control that shuts them off when the relative humidity attains a certain level. A vaporizer, on the other hand, adds hot or cold moisture to the atmosphere without respect to the level of humidity. Without control of humidification, excessive moisture will facilitate mold growth. If rugs, beddings, windows, or walls become damp, humidity is excessive; if there is static electricity, humidity is inadequate.

Humidifiers and vaporizers must be cleaned regularly to control mold growth. If not, the humidifier itself can become a major source of airborne mold spores and bacteria, which can worsen asthma and allergic rhinitis and even induce hypersensitivity pneumonitis (Sweet et al., 1971; Tourville et al., 1972).Vaporizers are difficult to clean adequately and to keep mold free. Ultrasonic vaporizers and humidifiers appear to be more desirable since they are more easily disassembled and cleaned. They also are relatively inexpensive, quiet, and possibly more effective in adding moisture to the air.

For individuals who are mold sensitive, any humidification system may pose a potential problem, especially in moister areas of the country because of mold growth within the system. Molds grow best in a moist environment, especially in humidity greater than 50 percent and temperatures above 37°C. Certain molds, however, survive in less favorable conditions. Cold walls in winter time in poorly insulated houses or single-pane windows encourage condensation and increased mold growth. Double-pane or triple-pane insulated glass and well-insulated walls can be helpful in controlling potential indoor mold growth.

Dehumidification. Dehumidification may be necessary when a patient's symptoms are aggravated by excessive humidity itself or by mold or mite growth that the humidity facilitates (Villaveces, 1971). This is an important factor not only in homes in humid climates, but also in homes with damp crawl spaces, leaks, poor insulation, and condensation of moisture on inside walls in the winter, and humidifiers. Most dehumidifiers are portable and use calcium chloride or cold refrigeration coils to remove moisture from air that is passed through them.

Additives that come with humidifiers or dehumidifiers contain sodium nitrite, a toxic chemical, or a bleach. It is advisable rather to use water without additives in operating the units and to clean the units periodically with chlorine bleach, rinsing thereafter to remove any irritating materials otherwise contained in these units.

Improving ventilation may eliminate the need for a dehumidifier, especially in kitchens, showers, laundry rooms, and basements. Wrapping cold water pipes can prevent condensation and dripping. In crawl spaces, covering the earth with plastic sheeting or insulating the spaces with a vapor barrier can eliminate these areas as significant sources of mold. Dehumidifiers the size of stereo speakers can extract as little as 12 or as much as 41 pints of water per day from the air. The Association of

Home Appliance Manufacturers claims that a model with a capacity of 25 pints per day can handle most problems of excessive moisture. It is important, however, to obtain a unit with adequate capacity. Larger units that do not need to work to capacity are more efficient than smaller units that must work to maximum capacity. It is also important to recognize that in very cold climates, coil-type dehumidifiers can freeze. An excellent review can be found in *Consumer Reports,* August, 1984, which contains information on heating, cooking, humidification, and dehumidification load estimates and includes a map of the United States with climate correction factors. Consumers Union of the United States, a nonprofit organization that publishes an annual *Buying Guide* and the monthly *Consumer Reports* magazine, also is an excellent source of information regarding specific equipment.

CONTROL OF INDOOR ALLERGENS AND IRRITANTS THROUGH FILTRATION

Home Air Filtration Units. The air contains two physically different groups of substances that may be harmful, particulate matter and gases. Removal of *particulate matter* can be achieved by several methods; the efficiency of each depends upon the size of the particles it must filter. Straining or sieving is based on filtration through a device woven with sufficient density that air passages are smaller than the particulate matter to be removed. (An analogy is a fly and a screen.) Impingement or impaction uses filtering elements (fibers or vanes) positioned so that the air must change direction as follows: larger (> 5 microns) particles travel in a straight path because of inertia and impinge on the fibers or vanes, which usually are coated with mineral oil or an adhesive to cause them to stick. (An analogy is a fly and flypaper). Filtration by these simple types of systems employs straightforward mechanical principles. Mechanical filters are the kind used in most standard furnaces. Particles as small as 10 microns (see Fig. 18–1) can be removed by the closely knit fibers. Mechanical filters are suitable, therefore, for filtration of most soil mold spores (these usually exceed 10 microns) and most pollens (these usually exceed 30 microns). However, smaller pollen fragments and mold-derived allergens are not removed by these filters. House dust allergens (mites and animal dander) tend to be too small (< 10 microns) to be filtered adequately by mechanical filters; this inadequacy applies also to cigarette smoke, various aerosols, and other environmental allergens and irritants. Mechanical filters should be changed frequently for proper operation, generally once a month. More frequent changes may be necessary in areas with high pollen and mold counts or with heavy dust problems.

Electrostatic Filtration

Electrostatic filtration is capable of removing particles to 1 micron in size. There are three types of electronic air filters as follows: (1) polystyrene charged–media type; (2) self-charging, single-stage type; and (3) two-stage type. Polystyrene-type devices employ a thermoplastic film in which the plastic film media is charged "permanently" with a positive charge on one side and a negative charge on the other. It is nonconducting but retains its charge which is dielectric, thus attracting both positively and negatively charged particles. These filters in effect are the electric counterparts of magnets. Particles filtered by these devices are those already naturally charged, since there is no power source involved for ion generation or charging particles. Polystyrene filters resemble mechanical filters in appearance. They are more efficient than the standard furnace filters, since they are capable of collecting smaller particles than are simple mechanical filters. Unlike the two-stage type of electrostatic filters, arcing does not occur, and ozone is not generated. Unfortunately, these filters are useful only when humidity is very low and are inefficient in moist climates.

A recently developed filtering system of some promise is the Electret or the 3M Filtrete filtering system. In this system the air is first "cleaned" by means of a dielectric filter, which attracts oppositely charged contaminants passing through the system. When fibers are covered by particulates and gradually lose their charge, the filter in effect becomes a "tight" mechanical filter incorporating straining or sieving, impingement, and diffusion. In this system, it would still be advisable to utilize a standard mechanical filter to precede the Electret or Filtrete in order to remove the large particles from the air so as to extend the life of the electrostatic component of the system. A newer portable unit, Bionaire, also adds negative ions to the air by charging neutral particulate matter, which enhance its filtering capabilities.

Another type of electrostatic filter uses highly static prone monofilament plastics that generate an internal charge when exposed to moving air and, in so doing, attract particulate matter. This single-stage type of filter is marketed by Hi-Tech of North Quincy, Massachusetts, and by Newton or Sanditron of Houston, Texas.

The two-stage electrostatic filter requires a power source and works by charging particles in an electric field (the first stage), then by trapping them on an oppositely charged filter plate (the second stage). Such electrostatic filters may arc and generate ozone, a respiratory irritant; room electrostatic units of this type have been criticized because they may generate sufficient ozone, and even with charcoal air filters they can intensify asthma. Because of this concern and the fact that there are better filtering units available (e.g., HEPA units, see subsequent discussion), they are not generally recommended now. Central furnace units in which two-stage electrostatic filters located in the cold air return farther away from the patient do not appear to generate much ozone in the house and would not seem to be as much of a problem in this regard. Self-cleaning and manually cleaned two-stage electrostatic filtration units are available. Self-cleaning is not generally satisfactory, however, and the units with filtration cells that can be removed for manual cleaning are recommended, especially if the cells can be cleaned in a dishwasher. All electrostatic filters require mechanical prefilters.

Ionization filtration is based upon delivering large numbers of ions to the air stream, causing particles with which they associate to precipitate from the air onto naturally and oppositely charged surfaces. Generation of negative ions tends to be more advantageous than generation of positive ions because of the higher mobility of negative ions. For whatever reason, some patients also claim to "feel better" in a highly concentrated negative ion environment, although no medical benefits have been demonstrated objectively. A drawback of this particular type of system, however, is the resulting highly apparent dust on walls, particularly in areas surrounding the ionizers. The Bionaire is an example of a portable unit that adds negative ions to the air.

High Efficiency Particulate Air (HEPA) Filters. Filtration of very small (<1 micron) particles, which move by random diffusion (brownian movement), requires a different approach to remove such particles from air. In many respects, however, HEPA filtration is similar to simple mechanical (sieve) filtration. HEPA filters are some of the most effective filters available for removing particulate matter. The HEPA filter is an extremely fine sieve of densely packed small fibers. This construction results in high resistance to air flow, with large air flow and pressure drops, and requires a great deal of force to propel air through this type of filter. Because of the force necessary to propel air through such filters, satisfactory central HEPA filtration units have become available only recently; HEPA filtration units also are more expensive than electrostatic filters. Since HEPA filters are not electrostatic, ozone generation is not a problem

Portable HEPA units have been available for years. Extremely effective air filtration is possible for a few feet directly in front of the portable HEPA unit (Zwemer and Karibo, 1973). Generally, the flow of air is minimal, creating little feeling of blowing air and relatively little noise. A "squirrel cage"–blower rather than a blade-type fan is used. This makes the use of portable units practical in offices, near desks, for filtration of dust and smoke.

A newly marketed central unit, the CRSI-600H Air Purification System, available from Control Resource Systems, Inc., Michigan City, Indiana, has an accessory blower and attaches to the return duct of the furnace. It takes only part of the air per pass and filters it through the HEPA filter. After several passes, the air eventually is filtered completely. Although efficient in removing particulate matter from the air, its clinical effectiveness remains to be determined (Swanson and Reed, 1985).

Negative Ion Machines. Positive ions appear to inhibit bronchociliary clearance, thus potentially increasing respiratory tract problems; a greater number of negative ions may have a beneficial effect by increasing bronchociliary clearance. Generators produce electronegatively charged ions that collide with pollutant particles in the air, conveying to them a negative charge. The particles are then drawn to surfaces with lower electric potential and "precipitate" out on these surfaces, for example, walls and floors. Krueger (1982) suggests that there is a promising role for negative ion generators. However, there is no evidence that such generators are effective clinically (Jones, 1976). Until evidence for substantial clinical benefit is produced, there is little justification for recommending their use.

Gases. Removal of gases is more difficult than removal of particulate matter from the air. Filtration devices including activated carbon filters and air scrubbers, are too inefficient or expensive or both for practical consideration at this time. Identification of the sources of contaminants and their removal are the primary effective methods for reducing exposure to problematic gases. Increasing ventilation so as to dilute the concentration of gases indoors is a less desirable alternative (see Chapter 13).

Filtration Masks. Effective filtration masks that diminish industrial exposures to small molecular weight allergens and irritants or toxic particles or gases are available, and special masks for specific toxic materials can be obtained. In North America, the North Safety Equipment Company, Cranston, Rhode Island, and Rexdale, Ontario, is an excellent source of information and equipment. For a given mask, the optimal protection factor for most allergens or irritants is in excess of 1000 fold (i.e., if the usual work exposure to a substance is increased 1000 times, the mask would be totally protective). The fit of the mask is critical to its performance and should be selected specifically for the individual.

CLINICAL EFFECTIVENESS OF ENVIRONMENTAL CONTROL

Short-term analyses of the effect of environmental control (with or without air filtration devices) on asthma and allergic rhinitis have led to somewhat differing conclusions. Improvement in asthma symptoms has been reported in children in a "dust-free" environment (Murray and Ferguson, 1983), including those of mite-induced asthma (Burr et al., 1980) and mold-induced asthma (Villaveces et al., 1971). Using conventional methods without adding air filtration, Kooistra et al. (1978) concluded that HEPA filtration in an air conditioned environment produced minimal additional benefit over the air conditioning alone for patients with hay fever. Zwemer and Karibo (1973) reached similar conclusions in a study of children with asthma, but the effect of air conditioning alone was not assessed. The concentration of indoor allergens clearly can be decreased by air filtration devices, including air conditioning (Chafee, 1985). This fact, in itself, neither establishes that significant clinical benefit is the result of the use of such devices nor that substances effectively filtered are problematic in the first

place (Patterson et al., 1985). In the absence of more conclusive information, it is difficult to be enthusiastic about prescribing expensive air filtration equipment for allergic patients. On the other hand, for individuals with marked sensitivity to airborne inhalants, aggressive environmental control, which may include air filtration, is warranted.

Environmental Control of Specific Allergens and Irritants

Fungi and Molds. Fungi are ubiquitous. The major fungal allergens of classic importance are the airborne spores from these organisms (see Chapter 11). Molds, yeasts, rusts, and smuts are found on decaying vegetation, in soil, and on various plants (Wyse and Malloch, 1970). Allergic symptoms associated with lawn mowing can be due to sensitivity to molds that "contaminate" the lawn, rather than sensitivity to grass pollen. Sudden increases in certain mold spores during thunderstorms have been implicated as causes of acute asthmatic attacks (Packe, 1985).

As previously noted, fungal growth flourishes in damp areas of the home, such as in basements or crawl spaces, in areas where there have been leaks in the house, in rubber carpet underpads soiled by leaks in plumbing or by urine from animals, in bathrooms (especially shower stalls), on window sills in moist climates, in utility rooms (especially those with washing machines), and in humidifiers and vaporizers.

Window frames, baths, showers, and other areas in which fungi grow should be treated periodically with a chlorine bleach solution (available commercially as X-14 or Tilex). The frequency is determined by the climate and household conditions, but such cleaning should be done at least monthly. These areas also may be rinsed with zephiran chloride, using a 17 percent solution which can be purchased without prescription.

Particular attention should be directed to crawl spaces in moist areas of the country. The ground should be covered by black polyethylene sheets as a vapor barrier to decrease fungal spores in the house. Standing water in the crawl space can be eliminated by installation of effective drains. To decrease fungi in basements and crawl spaces, the use of trioxymethylene (crystalline paraformaldehyde) can be effective. Crystals are placed in open petri dishes in various areas of the house, but the area must be closed as tightly as possible for 24 hours, making certain that the family (including domestic animals) are out of the house during the procedure. The number of petri dishes depends on several factors, such as air circulation, humidity, and amount of mold. Details and recommendations must be followed carefully. The rooms should be well ventilated afterwards, since formaldehyde is toxic and even small amounts of the vapor can be extremely irritating to respiratory membranes. Food should not be left exposed during the formaldehyde treatment. The frequency of this procedure also depends on climatic and household conditions and can be determined by repeated mold cultures. Moisture reduction is the most effective means of eliminating mold. Increased ventilation, repair of cracks in the foundation, use of dehumidifiers, and avoidance of vaporizers and humidifiers will aid in reduction of mold growth. The same treatment is suitable for summer or winter homes that are closed for a portion of the year. (See Chapter 11 for other discussion on mold control.)

Animals. For the most part, it is the dandruff, serum, saliva, and urinary proteins from animals that are responsible for allergy rather than the hair. Individuals allergic to one species of animals tend to be allergic to all members of that species, although the degree of cross sensitivity may vary. Some animals tend to be more sensitizing than others. Although very large animals may produce more dander and other potentially allergic material, the degree of allergenicity and the amount of potential allergen produced are not necessarily related to size. Smaller, younger animals may be more problematic before they are housebroken. It is a common belief that certain dogs (poodles, for instance) are "nonallergenic" or "hypoallergenic" and rarely cause sensitization. Unfortunately, this belief is incorrect, and severe sensitivity can occur to virtually all animals, including poodles and Chihuahuas (the animals associated with the myth of "taking one's asthma away").

As with allergy in general, the degree of animal sensitivity varies from patient to patient. Consequently, for one patient total elimination of the animal from the environment may be necessary whereas, for another reduced contact, such as keeping the animal out of the allergic patient's bedroom at all times or keeping the animal strictly outdoors, may suffice. If animals are allowed even limited indoor contact, for in-

stance confinement to the utility room or basement, allergen dissemination throughout the house still can occur, especially if there is a forced air heating-cooling system. In cases of severe animal sensitivity or of severe asthma with even mild animal sensitivity, there is a strong argument for eliminating animals from the environment altogether, since the animal may both provoke allergic inflammation and increase mite allergens in the environment. In addition, since bronchial reactivity can be heightened by exposure to allergens (Cockroft et al., 1977), reduced exposure to animals that can serve as major sources of allergens may substantially reduce hyperreactivity.

The animals should not be groomed in the house, nor by the person allergic to the animal. Simply wearing a mask is not adequate protection, since the patient's entire body can be covered with the allergen during grooming. Other animal contacts, at a babysitter's home or at school for instance, may present a major problem. Elimination of the animal from the classroom or changing to another babysitter may be necessary. A babysitter who has animals at home and comes to the child's home should be encouraged to wear clothes with which the animals have had little or no contact. Family members in contact with animals to which the patient is highly allergic should change clothes before or upon entering the house or avoid visiting the home of friends who have those animals.

Occasional contacts with animals for the patient who is not highly allergic to them are permissible. For instance, an individual who is only mildly sensitive to horse dander can ride a horse occasionally if the respiratory symptoms are controlled with simple medication. The patient should not groom the horse, however, and should not enter the barn. In order that a patient who is allergic to animals may visit a home with animals, especially to stay overnight, the animals should be removed temporarily, the rooms to be occupied should be cleaned thoroughly before the visit, and the bedding should be changed. Frequently, these measures together with pretreatment of the patient with antihistamine, bronchodilators, or cromolyn will permit limited exposure to offending allergens, while allowing the patient to participate in normal activity. Similar principles apply to camping. If animals are a normal part of the camping experience, they should not sleep in the same cabin or tent with allergic individuals nor travel in the same vehicle with the campers. Vehicles used for the campers' transport should be cleaned thoroughly before use.

A strong effort should be made to keep animals known to cause allergic problems out of the classroom. *There is no justification for classroom animals if they make any child ill.* When a patient who is allergic to animals moves to a home that previously had animals, it is essential that the home be cleaned thoroughly before moving in. The furnace ducts should be vacuumed commercially, the carpeting should be steam cleaned, and the drapes should be dry cleaned. If the odor of animals persists, it may be necessary to replace the carpeting.

Pollens. Pollen and mold spores float for considerable distances, hence foliage in the general area is of greater significance than the particular grass, trees, or shrubs in the patient's yard. Pollen concentrations in the air reach peaks early in the morning and at dusk. It is wise to keep windows closed at these times though they may be opened after darkness falls if necessary for ventilation and cooling. A tree or shrub just outside an open window also can serve as a source of intense allergen exposure, and removal of such foliage, particularly near a bedroom window, may be warranted.

The location of the bedroom in which the patient sleeps can be important. Selecting a room on the opposite side of the prevailing wind direction or the "cooler" side of the house in summer to maximize the feasibility of keeping windows closed can be helpful. Patients highly sensitive to weed and other plant pollens should be discouraged from working or playing in the midst of fields in which these plants grow, keeping in perspective the importance of allowing and encouraging normal activity in children. Open fields near the house invite the growth of weeds that cause allergic symptoms; if possible, weeds should be cut short before and during the weed pollen season to minimize pollination. Patients with severe pollen or mold sensitivities should be discouraged from mowing lawns and similar activities. Pollen masks are useful while engaging in these activities for patients with moderate sensitivity, especially if combined with the use of prophylactic medication.

Although there is no data concerning its effectiveness, we encourage patients to bathe and change clothes after playing or working outside in grass or weeds. We also suggest that clothes worn by the patient while outside in that environment should be kept outside the bedroom until laundered. A family member in daily contact with allergens to which a patient is highly allergic should be encouraged to change clothes and bathe upon entering the house to the extent feasible.

Flowers are insect pollinated and generally are not significant problems for allergic patients because of the heaviness and poor dissemination of the pollen. However, since pollen from flowers can be sensitizing and, with sufficiently close contact, can be a source of significant respiratory tract symptoms, large quantities of flowers in the house are discouraged. Sensitivity to pollen from flowers sometimes constitutes a major problem for florists, especially if greenhouses are involved. Some flowers can be more of a problem than others. It is wise to remember that ragweed is related to chrysanthemums, zinnias, marigolds, and dahlias, which all are part of the sunflower (Composite) family. (See the previous discussion of air filtration and cooling systems and Chapter 11 for additional details regarding pollen control.)

House Dust. Although it is impossible to provide a completely dust-free environment, the aim is to minimize house dust exposure, particularly in the patient's bedroom since bedding is a major source of mites. The *bedroom* should be cleaned thoroughly at least weekly and lightly wet-dusted daily. Furnishings not essential to the bedroom that "catch" dust, such as toys, models, and books, should be minimized. A few books can be allowed in the bedroom (bookcases should have closed doors), and the bedroom closet should be used to store only the patient's present seasonal clothes.

Particular attention should be directed to the bedding. *Pillows* should be made of synthetic fibers which are washable, and *mattresses and box springs* should be encased in zippered impermeable plastic or vinyl covers. A waterbed can be an excellent substitute for a box spring and mattress (Sarsfield, 1974). A polyester mattress pad or several sheets doubled over should be used over a plastic cover, especially for patients who have atopic dermatitis with itching exacerbated by sweating. If possible, bunk beds should be separated since the individual in the lower bunk receives increased dust exposure from the upper bunk. *Bedding* should be of washable synthetic or synthetic blend material. Blankets, bedspreads, and pillows should be washed in hot water at least monthly. In dry climates, where mites seldom grow in abundance, furniture brought from mite-infested areas can be a continuing source of even live mites at least 2 years later and therefore can pose a clinical problem in a mite sensitive patient (Moyer et al., 1985).

Curtains should be of smooth material that can be washed or tumbled in the clothes dryer via the "air-only" cycle to remove dirt and dust. Window shades are preferable to other types of blinds. If metal blinds are used, they can be cleaned conveniently by immersing them in a bathtub full of soapy water. *Short-pile carpeting* is easier to clean and traps fewer particles. Shag carpets appear to be an especially important source of mites (Arlian, 1982). The physician should encourage the family to try other control measures, including frequent vacuuming, before urging the replacement of bedroom carpeting. Linoleum, vinyl, or wood floors are easier to clean than carpeted floors. Area rugs may be desirable, particularly in winter. Easily washed synthetic area rugs are advised.

The patient particularly sensitive to "house dust" should be encouraged to keep his or her room neat but, if possible, should not do the actual dusting and vacuuming of the room (Clark, 1976). Alternatively, an appropriate mask can be worn, which may be sufficiently effective to allow dusting activities (Tovey, 1981). The bedroom should be closed off to the extent compatible with keeping the room at a comfortable temperature. *Windows* should be closed, and electric fans should be avoided. A *humidity* of less than 40 percent is one of the most effective ways of controlling mite growth (Korsgaard, 1983).

Cleaning Procedures

Methods of cleaning and the actual equipment used are of great importance. Sweeping with a broom or dusting with a dry cloth increase airborne dust. Treated dust cloths or damp cloths should be used exclusively to avoid increasing airborne dust. Damp mopping is an efficient means of cleaning impermeable floors without adding to airborne dust. Vacuum cleaners should have adequate air filters to minimize the recirculation of dust. Filter paper collecting bags are essential, and units with only cloth bags should be avoided. The choice of an upright versus a canister vacuum depends on the house and its furnishings.

Bags from the vacuum cleaner should be emptied outside the house. A central vacuuming system which exhausts outside is the ideal, as no air circulation nor dust discharge from the vacuum bag occurs in the house. These systems are easily and economically installed during home construction. Alternatives include water-filtered vacuum cleaners, such as those made by Rainbow. However, they are nearly as costly as central units and are not as effective nor as powerful. The allergic individual should avoid vacuuming procedures, if possible, and allergic children should not be in the room when it is being cleaned.

Other Household Allergens

Animal Products

Fur coats, pillows, sleeping bags, and down-filled jackets should not be kept in the patient's closet or near the bedroom. However, it usually is permissible to wear a down-filled jacket outdoors. Rug pads, mattresses, and furniture stuffing made of various kinds of animal hair, including horse, cow, and hog, were common years ago and are still found in some homes. The extent to which hair in these products constitutes a significant allergenic source is unclear, however, since the hair shaft generally is not the allergen. However, such organic material is a haven for mold and mite growth.

Plant Products

Pyrethrum. For individuals sensitive to ragweed, contact with pyrethrum, an insecticide derived from plants related to the ragweed family, should be avoided.

Kapok. Kapok is a plant fiber used in inexpensive pillows and mattresses and in some stuffed toys. It also is found in some old sleeping bags, in flotation vests, and in antique furniture stuffing. Sensitivity to kapok can be severe, and the material should be eliminated from the immediate environment.

Cottonseed. Cottonseed is part of unrefined cotton and can be the source of extreme hypersensitivity. Refined cotton, as in cotton sheets, does not present a problem, but cottonseed associated with cotton linters used in innerspring mattresses and upholstered furniture can be a source of inhalant allergens. Cottonseed also is used in fertilizers and certain animal foods and baked goods. Because it is so highly refined, cottonseed oil rarely is a problem. However, cottonseed flour, the use of which is increasing as a protein supplement in foods, can induce life-threatening allergic reactions in sensitive individuals.

Orrisroot. Orrisroot was once a frequent component of cosmetics and still is found in some inexpensive cosmetics, some tooth powders, and bathing salts. Sensitivity can be severe.

Flaxseed. Sensitivity to flaxseed is uncommon but can be severe. Flaxseed is found in chicken feeds, in feeds for other animals including dogs, in hair setting lotions, shampoos, some insulating materials, rugs, and some food items, such as Roman Meal Bread.

Vegetable Gums. Karaya, tragacanth, carob seed, acacia, chicle, and quince seed gums are found in wave setting lotions (these flake off the hair when dry and can be irritative as well as allergenic), in medications as fillers, in sizing, in print drying powders, and in hand lotions, chewing gums, chocolate substitutes, gelatin preparations, soft center candies, pie fillings, ice cream, gravies, cake icing, salad dressings, laxatives, toothpastes and powders, and mouthwashes. These products may be allergenic for some.

Cigarette Smoke and Other Irritants

Although there are claims of allergic sensitivity to cigarette smoke, the significance of smoke as an allergen is unclear. On the other hand, smoke is a universal irritant and can exacerbate upper and lower respiratory tract problems (Lim, 1973) and predispose some individuals to middle ear effusions (Pedreira, 1985). Contact with smoke should be minimized in all individuals with allergic diseases (Nadel and Comroe, 1961). Smoking should not be permitted by family members or visitors. Passive smoke inhalation can increase the number, severity, and duration of respiratory illnesses in nonallergic nonasthmatic children (National Research Council, 1984; Pedreira, 1985). These effects are magnified in children with allergic rhinitis or asthma and are associated in adult asthmatics with a more rapid loss of airflow than that of nonasthmatics (see Chapter 41). It is hoped that a greater awareness of the increased health care costs associated with exposure to smoke will aid in efforts to remove this ubiquitous irritant from all environments.

Perfumes, cosmetics, various other odors, and hair sprays can exacerbate allergic respiratory disease either as allergens or irritants (Rosen, 1978; Engebretson, 1971). Fish odors are especially dangerous (Horesch, 1966). Direct and indirect contact with these materials should be minimized particularly in the home. Exposure to irritating or sensitizing chemicals constitutes a growing problem in our society. One practical approach to the evaluation of suspected environmental exposures, especially to chemicals, has been proposed by Selner (1985). (Consideration of occupational allergens, other environmental factors, and irritants can be found in Chapter 46.)

OTHER ENVIRONMENTAL PROBLEMS

Travel. Travel poses a potential problem for allergic individuals. Patients should take along a polyester pillow to avoid feathers, mold, and mite exposure when travelling. The animal allergic patient should select a motel or hotel that does not permit animals. The importance of taking along appropriate medication, if necessary, and of continuing the regular medication schedule should be emphasized. A clinical summary and medication schedule from the patient's physician can be especially helpful in case medical care is needed while away from home. Highly allergic patients would be wise to select a time of year for travel when airborne allergens in the area to be visited are at a minimum (Samter and Durham, 1955).

Change of Location. Only rarely should patients be advised to move to another geographic area, though an actual change of housing may be essential for control of factors such as mold or mite exposure (Burr et al., 1980; Korsgaard, 1983). Only in severe disease, in which inclement weather, cold damp climates, or long intense pollen seasons clearly are responsible for intractable symptoms, should a change in geographic location be considered. Such a move should be encouraged only if compatible with the psychosocial and financial well-being of the family. There is evidence that such a move may be helpful (Skoogh et al., 1976), but long-term studies are necessary for a better perspective on the value of changing location because of allergic disease. An allergic disorder commonly will remit or significantly improve for an interval after a move until additional allergic sensitization develops to factors in the new environment. On the other hand, moves from highly allergenic environments, such as ranches or farms, can be very important in highly allergic patients. Job-related exposure may require a transfer to an area free of the allergens or irritant factors either within the building or to another geographic area.

REFERENCES

Al-Doory, Y.: The indoor airborne fungi. N.E.R. Allergy Proceedings 6:140–150, 1985.

Arlian, L.G., Bernstein, I.L., Gallagher, J.S.: The prevalence of house dust mites *Dermatophagoides* and associated environmental conditions in homes in Ohio. J. Allergy Clin. Immunol. 69:527–532, 1982.

Burr, M.I., Dean, B.V., Merrett, T.G., Neale, E., St. Leger, A.S., Verrier-Jones, E.R.: Effects of anti-mite measures on children with mite-sensitive asthma: A controlled trial. Thorax 35:506–512, 1980.

Chafee, F.H.: Pollen studies in a hospital air-conditioned room. N.E.R. Allergy Proceedings 6:150–152, 1985.

Chipps, B.E., Mak, H., Menkes, H.A., Schuberth, K.C., Talamo, J.H., Talamo, R.C., Permutt, S., Scherr, M., Mellits, E.D.: Do weather conditions change pulmonary function of asthmatic at summer camp? J. Asthma 21:15–20, 1984.

Clark, R.P., Preston, T.D., Gordon-Nesbitt, D.C., Malka, S., Sinclair, L.: The size of airborne dust particles precipitating bronchospasm in house dust sensitive children. J. Hygiene 77:321–325, 1976.

Cockroft, D.W., Ruffin, R.E., Dolovich, J., et al.: Allergen-induced increase in non-allergic bronchial reactivity. Clin. Allergy 7:503–513, 1977.

Consumer Report: Consumers Union of the U.S., Inc., 256 Washington St., Mt. Vernon, New York 10550.

Cooper, K.R., Alberti, R.R.: Effect of kerosene heater emissions on indoor air quality and pulmonary function. Am. Rev. Respir. Dis. 129:629–631, 1984.

Dowse, G.K., Turner, K.J., Stewart, G.S., Alpers, M.P., Woolcock, A.J.: The association between *Dermatophagoides* mites and the increasing prevalence of asthma in village communities within the Papua New Guinea highlands. J. Allergy Clin. Immunol. 75:75–83, 1985.

Engebretson, G.R.: Allergies and odors arising from indoor environments. Am. J. Public Health 61:366–375, 1971.

Feinberg, S.M.: Environmental factors and host responses in asthma. Acta Allergol. 29:7–14, 1974.

Honicky, R.E.S., Osborne, J.S., Akron, C.A.: Symptoms of respiratory illness in young children and the use of woodburning stoves for indoor heating. Pediatrics 75:587–593, 1985.

Horesch, A.J.: The role of odors and vapors in allergic disease. J. Asthma Res. 4:125–136, 1966.

Jones, D.P., O'Connor, S.A., Collins, J.W., Watson, B.W.: Effect of long-term ionized air treatment on patients with bronchial asthma. Thorax 31:428–432, 1976.

Klabuschnigg, A., Gotz, M., Horak, F., Jager, S., Machaclek, A., Popow, C., Haschke, F., Skoda-Turk, R.: Influence of aerobiology and weather on symptoms in children with asthma. Respiration 42:52–60, 1981.

Kooistra, J.B., Pasch, R., Reed, C.E.: The effects of air cleaners on hay fever symptoms in air-conditioned homes. J. Allergy Clin. Immunol. 61:315–319, 1978.

Korsgaard, J.: House-dust mites and absolute indoor humidity. Allergy 38:84–92, 1983.

Korsgaard, J.: Preventive measures in mite asthma. Allergy 38:93–102, 1983.

Krueger, A.P.: Air ions as biological agents: Fact or fancy. Immunol. Allergy Pract. 4:129–140 and 173–183, 1982.

Lim, T.P.K.: Airway obstruction among high school students. Am. Rev. Respir. Dis. 108:985–988, 1973.

Moyer, D.B., Nelson, H.S., Arlian, L.G.: Housedust mites in Colorado. Ann. Allergy 55:680–682, 1985.

Munter, S. (ed.): Treatise on Asthma. (Maimonides, M.) Medical Writings, vol. 1. Philadelphia, J.B. Lippincott, Co., 1963.

Murray, A.M., Ferguson, A.B.: Dust free bedrooms in the treatment of asthmatic children with house dust or house dust mite allergy: A controlled study. Pediatrics 71:418–422, 1983.

Nadel, J.A., Comroe, J.H., Jr.: Acute effects of inhalation of cigarette smoke on airway conductants. J. Appl. Physiol. 16:713–716, 1961.

National Research Council, Committee on Indoor Pollutants. Washington, D.C., National Academy Press, 1984.

Nogrady, S.C., Furnass, S.B.: Ionizers in the management of bronchial asthma. Thorax 38:919–922, 1985.

Packe, G.E., Ayres, J.G.: Asthma outbreak during a thunderstorm. Lancet 2:199–204, 1985.

Patterson, R., Beltrane, V.S., Singal, M., Gorman, R., Zeiss, C.R., Harris, K.E.: Creating an indoor environmental problem from a non-problem: A need for cautious evaluation of antibodies against Hapten-protein complexes. N.E.R. Allergy Proceedings 6:135–139, 1985.

Pauli, G., Bessot, J.C., Thierry, R.: Dissociation of house dust allergies. J. Allergy Clin. Immunol. 63:245–252, 1979.

Pedreira, F.A., Gaundold, V.L., Feroli, E.J., Mella, G.W., Weiss, I.P.: Involuntary smoking and incidence of respiratory difficulty during the first year of life. Pediatrics 75:594–597, 1985.

Platt-Mills, T.A.E.: House dust mites. N.E.R. Allergy Proceedings 6:158–159, 1985.

Rosen, H.: Hydrocarbons and other Gases as Related to the Field of Allergy. Clinical Allergy Based on Provocative Testing. Hicksville, New York, Exposition Press, 1978.

Samter, M., Durham, O.C.: Regional Allergy of the United States, Canada, Mexico, and Cuba. Springfield, Illinois, Charles C Thomas, 1955.

Sarsfield, J.K., Gowland, G., Toy, R., Norman, A.: Mite-sensitive asthma of childhood: Trial of avoidance measures. Arch. Dis. Child. 49:716–721, 1974.

Seebohm, P.M.: Management of respiratory problems by nonallergists. 1. Allergic rhinitis. 2. Asthma. Postgrad. Med. 53:52–63, 1973.

Selner, J.C., Staudenmayer, H.: Practical approach to the evaluation of suspected environmental exposures: Clinical statement. Ann Allergy 55:665–673, 1985.

Skoogh, B.E., Simonsson, B.G., Beiggren, A.G., Bergstrom, M.J.: Climate and environment change in patients with chronic airway obstruction. Arch. Environ. Health 31:15–20, 1976.

Soyka, F., Edmonds, A.: The Ion Effect. New York, E.P. Dutton & Co., Inc., 1977.

Swanson, M.C., Reed, C.E.: Effect of HEPA filtration installed in a hot air furnace on the concentration of cat allergens in the air of a home. Presented at The 1985 Aspen Allergy Conference, Aspen, Colorado.

Sweet, L.C., Anderson, J.A., Callies, Q.C., Coates, E.O., Jr.: Hypersensitivity pneumonitis related to a home furnished humidifier. J. Allergy Clin. Immunol. 48:171–178, 1971.

Tovey, E.R., Chapman, M.D., Wells, C.W., Platt-Mills, T.A.E.: The distribution of dust mite allergen in the houses of patients with asthma. Am. Rev. Respir. Dis. 124:630–635, 1981.

Tovey, E.R., Chapman, M.D., Wells, C.W., Platt-Mills, T.A.E.: Mite faeces are a major source of house dust allergens. Nature 289:592–593, 1981.

Tourville, D.R., Weiss, W.I., Wertlake, P.T., Lendemann,

G.M.: Hypersensitivity pneumonitis due to contamination of home humidifier. J. Allergy Clin. Immunol. 49:245–251, 1972.

Villaveces, J.W.: The dehumidifier: Its indoor use in controlling molds and mold asthma — a personal case history. Ann. Allergy 29:93–98, 1971.

Wagner, C.J., Danziger, R.E., Nelson, H.S.: Relation between positive small air ions, weather fronts and pulmonary function in patients with bronchial asthma. Ann. Allergy 51:430–435, 1983.

Weiseman, R.D., Weiseman, J.R.: Value of home visits in the treatment of the allergic patient. N.Y. State J. Med. 64:1948, 1964.

Wharton, G.W.: House dust mites. J. Med. Entomol. 12:577–581, 1976.

Wyse, D.M., Malloch, D.: Christmas tree allergy: Mold and pollen studies. Can. Med. Assoc. J. 103:1272–1276, 1970.

Zweiman, B., Slavin, R.G., Feinberg, A.J., Falliers, C.J., Aaron, T.H.: Effect of air pollution on asthma: A review. J. Allergy Clin. Immunol. 50:305–314, 1972.

Zwemer, R.J., Karibo, J.: Use of laminar flow device as an adjunct to standard environmental control measures in symptomatic asthmatic children. Ann. Allergy 31:284–290, 1973.

19

Pharmacologic Management of Allergic Diseases
MILES WEINBERGER, M.D.
LESLIE HENDELES, PHARM.D.

PRINCIPLES OF MANAGEMENT

Asthma

A rational approach to the management of asthma requires a conceptual understanding of the disease and a definition of its particular clinical pattern in the patient to be treated. Because of variability in both clinical pattern and severity, the treatment of asthma must be individualized according to frequency, severity, and chronicity of symptoms.

Management of acute asthma that occurs infrequently and intermittently requires only measures that relieve respiratory distress rapidly and effectively. Rapidity of drug action, potency, and safety over a short time are the major considerations, without concern for long-term toxicity. Thus, an inhaled beta-adrenergic agonist is the preferred bronchodilator, and one need not be concerned about duration of action or potential for tolerance. In contrast, an orally administered drug, such as theophylline, which requires time to be absorbed and is slower in onset of action, is used as a secondary bronchodilator. The same reasoning, i.e., maximal efficacy without concern for long-term toxicity, justifies the short-term use of high-dose systemic corticosteroids when acute symptoms are not relieved by maximal use of bronchodilators.

On the other hand, continuous administration of theophylline or cromolyn has been shown to be highly effective in managing chronic asthma. Although cromolyn is generally less effective than theophylline in severe asthma, it often is adequate in milder asthma and has the advantage of standardized dosage and virtual absence of toxicity. Oral or inhaled sympathomimetic bronchodilators also are used to treat chronic asthma. Data supporting control of symptoms with continuous use of these agents are limited, however, and their relatively rapid decrease in effect over time gives reason for concern during extended use. Corticosteroids also may be needed when continuous or frequently recurring symptoms of chronic asthma are unresponsive to bronchodilators. Because of the potential long-term adverse effects of daily corticosteroid therapy, alternative strategies for increased safety have been developed; these include the short-acting oral steroids on alternate mornings and the newer generation of inhaled corticosteroids.

As might be expected, more medications may be required for adequate control of more severe disease. Management of intermittent asthma may require only inhaled sympathomimetic bronchodilators, but those asthmatics whose symptoms progress rapidly to require care or hospitalization may need early corticosteroid administration to prevent severe acute airway obstruction. Most patients with chronic asthma require a single medication, such as regular use of an inhaled sympathomimetic, cromolyn, or oral slow-release theophylline. Patients with histories of more severe disease, however, are likely to require additional medication for control of chronic asthma (Fig. 19–1).

Rhinitis

Although removal of the allergen is the most effective method of avoiding symptoms of allergic rhinitis and injection therapy with allergenic extracts may decrease sensitivity to inhalant allergens, pharmacologic management often is necessary to relieve symptoms, particularly in patients with chronic rhinitis.

For almost four decades, antihistamines have been the drugs used most commonly to treat allergic rhinitis. They can relieve symptoms of sneezing, nasal itching, rhinorrhea, and associated conjunctivitis. However, their use may be associated with annoying side effects, including sedation and dry mouth. Regular administration, however, generally leads to tolerance of side effects while providing considerable clinical efficacy, and some newer agents have no central nervous system (CNS) effects.

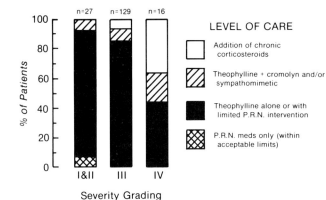

FIGURE 19-1. Relationship between severity of chronic asthma and maintenance medication required for disease control in 172 patients. Severity of disease increases from grades I through IV. Not shown are treatment requirements of patients with intermittent symptoms who need only intervention measures without maintenance medication. (Adapted from Ekwo and Weinberger: Evaluation of a program for the pharmacologic management of children with asthma. J. Allergy Clin. Immunol. 61:240, 1978.)

Whereas H_1 antihistamines relieve sneezing, itching, and runny nose, they fail to relieve congestion. Orally active sympathomimetic agents, such as ephedrine, pseudoephedrine, and phenylpropanolamine may decrease nasal congestion.

Sodium cromolyn, an anti-asthmatic drug that prevents mast cell degranulation and subsequent histamine release, also can reduce symptoms of allergic rhinitis and conjunctivitis when applied topically, particularly in patients with high serum levels of IgE. However, frequent administration of the drug is required for maximal effectiveness. Intranasal insufflation of the new generation of potent topical corticosteroids is highly effective in controlling symptoms, particularly nasal congestion. In selected patients whose predominant symptom is rhinorrhea, the use of an anticholinergic drug may offer symptomatic relief.

Anaphylaxis

The most appropriate initial therapy for anaphylaxis is prompt administration of a rapid acting physiologic antagonist of the effects of histamine; the classic and most potent drug for this purpose is parenteral epinephrine. Antihistamines may be useful following parenteral epinephrine, since antigenic exposure may be continuing (as with an ingested food that is not yet completely absorbed). However, they are inappropriate drugs to treat the acute manifestations of anaphylactic reactions, since they cannot reverse the rapid action of histamine already released. Antihistamines may partially prevent anaphylactic reactions, if administered prior to allergen exposure and release of histamine. Corticosteroids are of unproven value in treating the initial reactions of acute anaphylaxis but are effective in decreasing the late reactions.

Chronic Urticaria

Urticaria responds promptly but briefly to injected epinephrine, and oral epinephrine-like agents, including ephedrine and pseudoephedrine which have been used for chronic urticaria, may have some effectiveness. The H_1 antihistamines have been major pharmacologic agents to treat chronic urticaria.

THERAPEUTIC AGENTS

Sympathomimetic Bronchodilators

Since 1906, when epinephrine was found to be a potent bronchodilator, adrenergic drugs have been studied extensively and a relationship identified between structure and function of sympathomimetic amines (Fig. 19-2). Epinephrine has multiple actions on both the bronchial smooth muscle and the cardiovascular system. The vasoconstrictor action of epinephrine is retained in agents such as phenylephrine and longer-acting nasal decongestants, but the therapeutic goal for newer drugs has been greater selectivity for beta-2 adrenergic receptors (bronchial smooth muscle) for improved specificity of bronchodilator effect (Table 19-1). Additionally, newer agents can be used orally because of the resistance to degradation by intestinal and hepatic enzymes. In contrast to the general adrenergic effects of epinephrine, isoproterenol has relatively specific activity for beta adrenergic receptors. Isoetharine and metaproterenol, which was developed later, pos-

PHENYLETHYLAMINE

CATECHOLAMINE

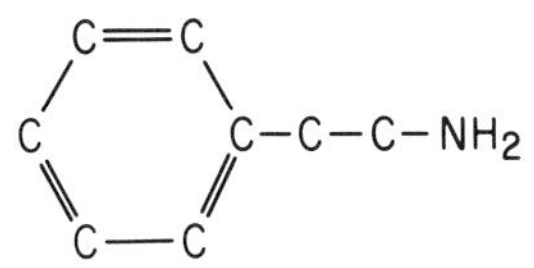

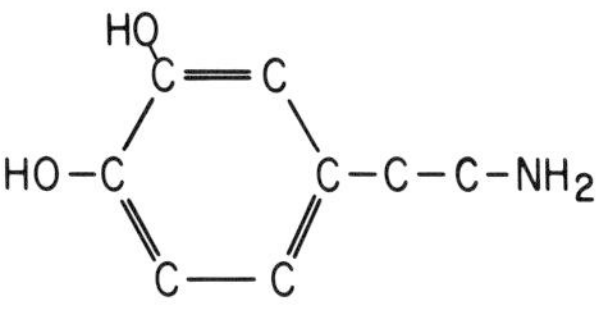

Drug Name	Structure	Major Receptor Activity	Oral Bioavailability In Conventional Doses	Approximate Duration Of Apparent Effect
NOREPINEPHRINE	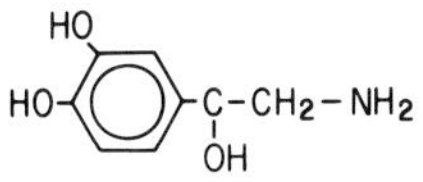	α	NO	<1 HOUR
PHENYLEPHRINE	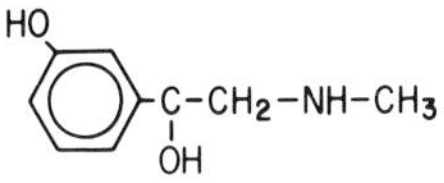	α	NO	<1 HOUR
EPINEPHRINE	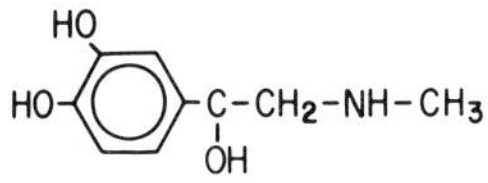	α, β_1, β_2	NO	<1 HOUR
EPHEDRINE	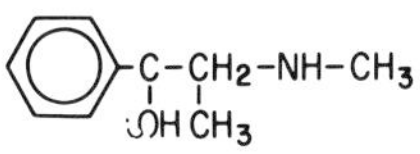	α, β_1, β_2 CNS	YES	2-4 HOURS
ISOPROTERENOL	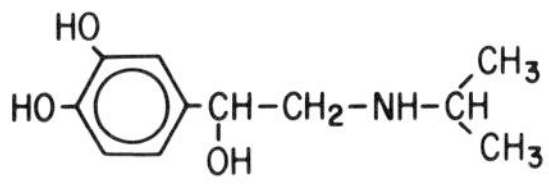	β_1, β_2	NO	<1 HOUR
ISOETHARINE	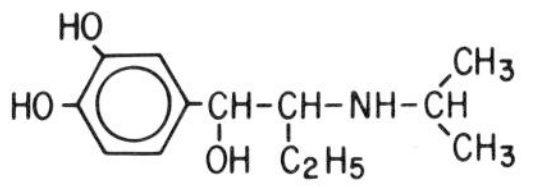	β_2	SOME	1 HOUR
METAPROTERENOL	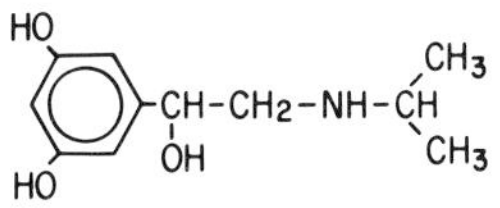	β_2	YES	2-4 HOURS
TERBUTALINE	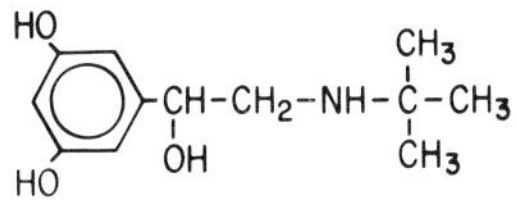	β_2	YES	4-6 HOURS
ALBUTEROL	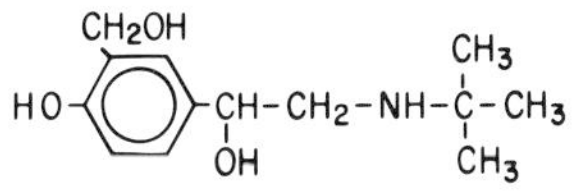	β_2	YES	4-6 HOURS
FENOTEROL	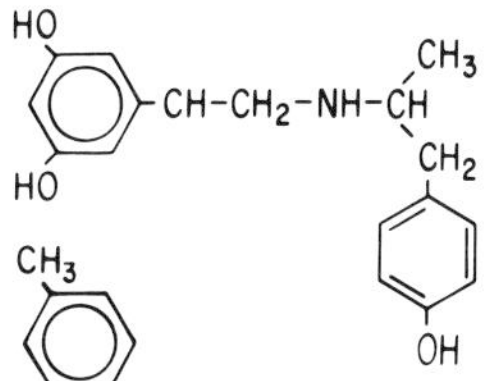	β_2	YES	4-6 HOURS
BITOLTEROL	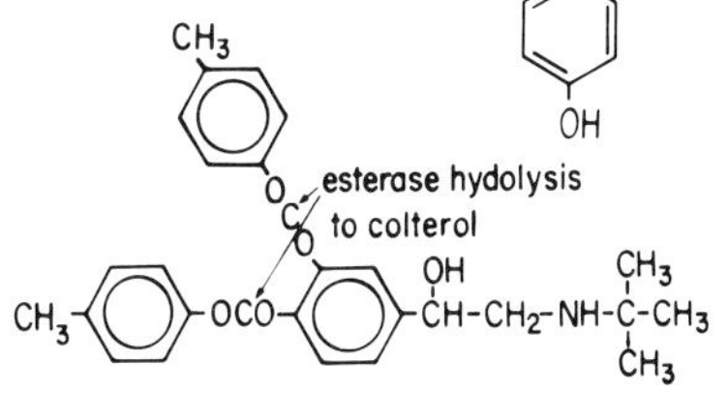	β_2	YES	4-6 HOURS

FIGURE 19-2. Structure and function of sympathomimetic amines. Adrenergic receptor activity is indicated by the conventional α, β_1, and β_2. Pharmacologic effects associated with the stimulation of these receptors are indicated in Table 19-1. Note that oral bioavailability is relative; many of the oral formulations are only 10 to 20 percent bioavailable because of first pass hepatic degradation. Estimates of duration of effect relate to usual doses. (See text for discussion of this complex issue.)

255

TABLE 19–1. Selected Pharmacologic Effects of Sympathomimetics

Clinical Effect	Receptor
Bronchodilation	Beta-2
Tremors	Beta-2
Tachycardia and arrhythmias	Beta-1
Hypertension	Alpha
Pallor	Alpha
Urinary retention	Alpha
CNS stimulation	Not defined (dependent upon crossing blood-brain barrier).

sessed a greater degree of beta-2 receptor specificity. The newest agents, including albuterol, terbutaline, fenoterol, and bitolterol, appear to have even greater degrees of beta-2 receptor specificity. It is these agents with their greater degree of specificity for bronchial smooth muscle action and potentially longer duration of action that are of the greatest clinical interest today for treatment of asthma.

TOPICAL AEROSOLIZED SYMPATHOMIMETIC BRONCHODILATORS

Sympathomimetic drugs delivered by inhalation can provide the most rapid and effective means of relief from acute asthmatic symptoms. Many are at least as effective as parenterally administered medications, have fewer side effects, and are more suitable for self-administration. Exceptions appear to be commercially available formulations of epinephrine metered dose inhalers (e.g., Primatene and Medihaler-Epi), which have only a very modest degree of transient bronchodilator effect compared with other agents (Chatterjee and Perry, 1971); the weak potency of these preparations is further evidenced by the absence of cardiovascular effects (Riding et al., 1970).

In order for inhaled beta-2 agonists to exert their anti-asthmatic effects, they must reach appropriate receptors, which appear to be located in the lower airways (Ruffin et al., 1978). Inhaled beta-2 agonists exert their effect topically rather than by way of the systemic circulation after absorption from the oral mucosa or gastrointestinal tract (Newman et al., 1981; Davies, 1984). The major effect is probably mediated by direct action on the receptors on the surface of smooth muscle cells throughout the conducting airways, but effects on neural structures (Rich-

ardson, 1977), mast cells (Lichtenstein and Margolis, 1968; Howarth et al., 1985), or other structures also may play a clinical role.

The degree and duration of therapeutic effect of the inhaled bronchodilators depends upon the intrinsic potency of the pharmacologic agent, the dose administered, the dose actually delivered to receptors, and the subsequent rate of removal or degradation of the drug (or both) in the airways. Since these are not readily measurable, it is the measure of the effects, i.e., the pharmacodynamics, that is used to assess the pharmacokinetics, i.e., the time course of the drug in the body

The catecholamine bronchodilators isoproterenol and isoetharine exert their maximal effect within 5 minutes after aerosol administration (Ahrens and Smith, 1984; Svedmyr, 1985). The peak effects of newer noncatecholamine bronchodilators occur somewhat later; nonetheless, they produce about 80 percent of their maximal effect within the first 5 minutes. Thus, although the newer agents have a "later" peak effect, the difference in rate of onset of bronchodilator effect is generally of trivial clinical importance.

The duration of effect of an inhaled beta agonist is a function of the rate of disappearance and the degradation of the drug at airways receptors, the dose of the drug given, as well as the relative potency of the drug; the higher the dose of a drug given, the greater the effect at any given point in time. It should then be apparent that effect may still be measured following a higher dose when effect following a lower dose is no longer detectable. Similarly, the more potent of two drugs given at equal doses may appear to have a longer duration of effect (and actually have a longer clinical effect) even though the rate of disappearance of effect may not be different.

Measurements of duration of bronchodilatation effect based on only examination of the intensity and duration of bronchodilatation, however, may be deceptive. Examination of the effect of a drug on airway responsiveness (i.e., the ability of a drug to protect against bronchoconstriction) permits an ability to detect the rapid decline of the effect of the drug at the receptor, thereby giving a potentially more accurate picture of the pharmacokinetics of drug effect at the receptor level than does measurement of duration of bronchodilatation alone. This methodology has been used to examine various of the currently marketed aerosol bronchodilator medications. Differences in apparent duration of action of bronchodilatation compared with protection against bronchoconstriction have been found in some cases to be differences in intensity of effect (i.e., failure to use equipotent doses) and, in other cases, to be differences in rates of disappearance from the receptor site (Harris et al., 1986a; Harris et al., 1986b; Ahrens et al., 1985).

Various strategies for delivery of inhaled sympathomimetic bronchodilators have been used. The pressurized, metered dose inhaler is the most convenient means of administration; however, the desired response may be difficult to obtain in a severely dyspneic patient or a young child who is unable to coordinate inhalation with aerosolized release of the drug. Various strategies therefore have been developed. These range from the careful instruction in technique for timing inhalation from end tidal volume to maximal inspiration with the burst of spray that is ejected by actuation of the metered dose inhaler to the use of spacers and aerosol receiving chambers of various designs. Valved devices can minimize the problems of coordination. Spacers and aerosol-receiving chambers may minimize the amount of high velocity particles impacting on the posterior pharnyx and thereby improve delivery to the airways. The use of solutions of these drugs in compressed air–driven nebulizers can permit administration even to totally uncooperative patients such as infants and toddlers. However, *delivery by intermittent positive pressure equipment gives no additional benefit* (Moore et al., 1972), *and it may increase the risk of pneumothorax when used for acute exacerbations of asthma* (Karetzky, 1975).

Concern has been expressed regarding the potential development of tolerance or "subsensitivity" with repeated use of sympathomimetic bronchodilators (Jenne et al., 1977; Nelson et al., 1977; Plummer, 1978). This phenomenon involves decreases in apparent duration and intensity of effect with repeated use. Alarming observations of actual paradoxical bronchospasm were described from extensive overuse of isoproterenol and even from one case of intravenous albuterol (Paterson et al., 1971). Routine use (four times daily) of the newer inhaled sympathomimetic bronchodilators, although not showing progressive loss of effect, does demonstrate some decrease in effect from initiation of therapy over the first month of treatment but apparently not beyond that (Weber et al., 1982).

When used in recommended dosage and under appropriate medical supervision, inhaled sympathomimetic bronchodilators have a very high margin of safety. However, epidemics of fatalities were reported during the mid-1960's in both England and Australia in association with apparent laxity in medical supervision and nonprescription availability of these agents (Campbell, 1976; Inman et al., 1969). Upon reviewing the experience of these epidemics, Inman (1974) commented, "It seems possible that we are dealing with an entirely new type of hazard caused, paradoxically, by the provision of a highly effective rather than an intrinsically dangerous form of self-treatment." *A major concern of potential overuse of this form of medication is an over-reliance on this medication alone and serious delay in obtaining other treatment necessary for reversing progressive bronchial obstruction.* It thus is important that these medications not be dispensed casually, without adequate instruction for proper use and contingency measures when response is inadequate, and with sufficient appropriate maintenance measures as needed to prevent chronic or frequently recurring symptoms.

TOPICAL DECONGESTANTS

Sympathomimetics with predominant vasoconstrictor activity are used as nasal decongestants. Phenylephrine (Neo-Synephrine) is most commonly used, but others such as oxymetazoline (Afrin) have longer duration of action. Topical decongestants should be used for only *short* periods of time (less than 5 days) to prevent development of *rhinitis medicamentosa*, i.e., severe chronic nasal congestion. They should *not* be used for rapidly recurring rebound congestion in chronic rhinitis.

PARENTERAL SYMPATHOMIMETIC DRUGS

In acute asthma, epinephrine and terbutaline can be administered by subcutaneous injection as an alternative to inhaled sympathomimetic drugs. This is the route of choice in an asthmatic who is so dyspneic that aerosolized administration is ineffective. Terbutaline has a higher therapeutic index because of its beta-2 specificity and permits safe, progressive dosing to well above that conventionally used, with less risk of toxicity. Additionally, terbutaline has an inherently longer duration of action than epinephrine. *Injected epinephrine, however, is the drug of choice for anaphylaxis because of its alpha-adrenergic activity, which acts as a physiologic antagonist against anaphylactic-induced vascular col-*

lapse. Parenteral terbutaline (or other newer beta-2 agonists when available as parenteral solutions) is probably the drug of choice when an injected sympathomimetic is needed for bronchospasm. Although isoproterenol has been administered intravenously with considerable success as an alternative to mechanical ventilation in children with respiratory failure (Perry et al., 1976), it requires special precautions to avoid serious complications, especially in older children and adults in whom cardiac complications are particularly greater potential hazards. Intravenous terbutaline (or albuterol when available) is probably generally as effective with less associated cardiac risk (Johnson et al., 1978).

ORAL SYMPATHOMIMETIC BRONCHODILATORS

The first oral sympathomimetic bronchodilator developed was ephedrine; it has a relatively weak bronchodilator effect and historically was used extensively in combination with theophylline. In fixed dose combinations of ephedrine and theophylline, ephedrine added only a small degree of bronchodilator effect but was associated with synergism for toxicity (Weinberger and Bronsky, 1974 and 1975). Newer agents appear to exceed the bronchodilator effects of ephedrine and avoid the central nervous system effects because of their decreased transport across the blood-brain barrier. However, they share with ephedrine only modest and transient clinical action and still possess the annoying systemic effect of tremor (due mainly to an effect on skeletal muscle). Because of the frequency of annoying adverse effects and the considerably lesser potency, as compared with the same agent given by inhalation, the best of the oral sympathomimetics still have limited clinical applicability. Moreover, they are not free of at least a degree of tolerance, i.e., decreasing effect with continuous therapy (Nelson et al., 1977; Plummer, 1978).

Oral sympathomimetics with alpha-adrenergic activity have some nasal decongestant activity and also may be of benefit in treating urticaria. Single doses of pseudoephedrine (Cantekin et al., 1977) or phenylpropanolamine (Dressler et al., 1977) decrease nasal airway resistance. The efficacy of these drugs in chronic therapy has not been well studied, however. Conventionally, ephedrine is used in doses up to 50 mg (depending on the size of the patient and clinical response); pseudoephedrine is used

in doses of 30 to 120 mg, and phenylpropanolamine in doses of 12.5 to 50 mg for nasal decongestion, administered at intervals of 4 to 8 hours. Phenylephrine, also used orally as a nasal decongestant for some time, is not orally bioactive at recommended doses (Elis et al., 1967).

Theophylline

Theophylline is one of various xanthine bronchodilators (Fig. 19–3), and the only one so far with important clinical use for asthma. Enprophylline, a 3-propyl xanthine derivative, is of potential interest because of apparent greater specificity of action. Although five times more potent than theophylline, it does not share theophylline's adenosine receptor inhibition and has less potential for CNS toxicity, diuresis, and cardiac sphincter relaxation. Nausea and headache, however, appear to be common side effects, and a 2-hour half-life of elimination may complicate clinical use.

PHARMACODYNAMICS

Theophylline has been used in the past mainly for its acute bronchodilatory effect. Since the early 1970's, definition of its pharmacokinetics and pharmacodynamics has provided greater safety and efficacy. Most importantly, studies of theophylline have demonstrated its efficacy as maintenance therapy in the prevention of asthmatic symptoms (Fig. 19–4). Although newer drug regimens for maintenance therapy have been demonstrated to be effective, comparative studies continue to demonstrate the high degree of efficacy of theophylline for this purpose. In a multi-center, comparative study with cromolyn, theophylline was associated with a greater frequency of asymptomatic days among children chosen for the study because of their relatively severe chronic asthma (Hambleton et al., 1977). However, subsequent studies of children with milder disease have shown little difference between these two regimens (Shapiro and Konig, 1985; Weinberger, 1985). Comparison with an oral beta-2 agonist similarly has shown therapeutic advantage for theophylline. When compared with the more potent route of sympathomimetic administration, inhaled delivery, theophylline has still demonstrated therapeutic advantage. The explanation for the difference in clinical effect was not an advantage of inten-

GENERIC NAME	STRUCTURE	Oral Bioavailability (%)	Mean Adult Elimination Half-Life (hrs.)	Estimated Potency
Theophylline	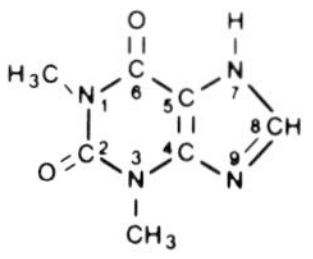 1,3 dimethylyanthine	100	7.7	1
Caffeine	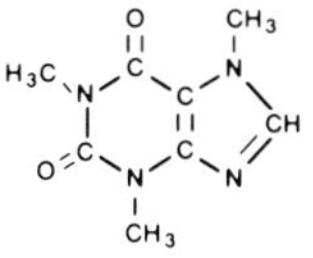 1,3,7 trimethylxanthine	100	6	0.2
Dyphylline	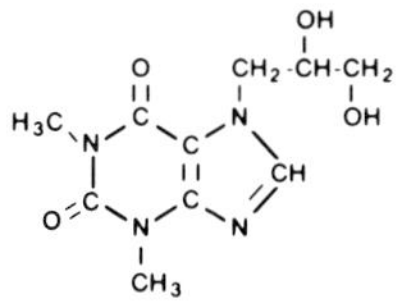 dihydroxypropyl theophylline	88	2.1	0.1
Etophylline	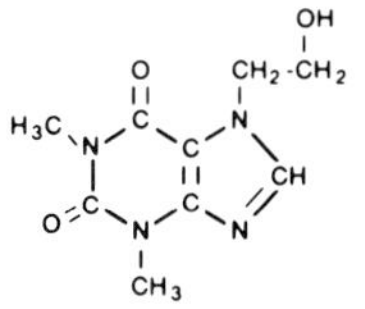 β-hydroxyethyl theophylline	80	4.1	0.14
Proxyphylline	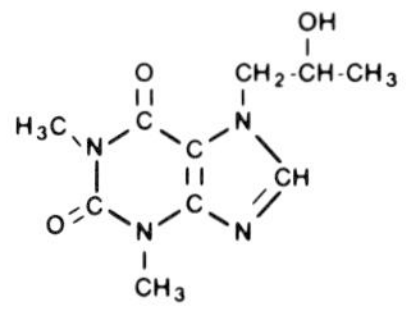 β-hydroxypropyl theophylline	100	6.8	15
Acephylline Piperazine	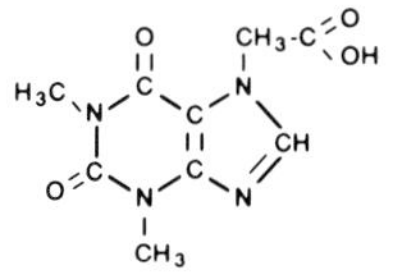 theopylline-7-ylacetic acid	2.5	0.8	0
Bamifylline	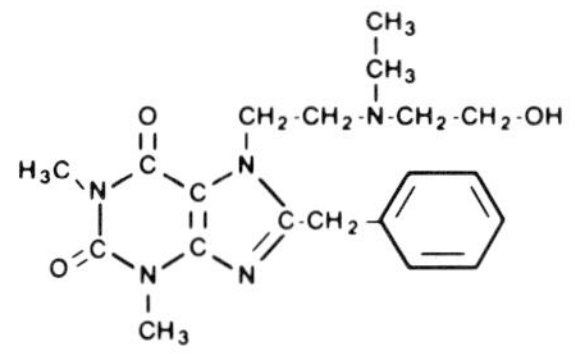 8-Benzyl-7- [2-(N-ethyl-N-2-hydroxyethyamino)ethyl] theophylline	21	20.5	3
Enprofylline	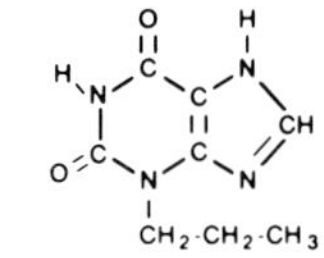 3-propylxanthine	100	2	5

FIGURE 19–3. Comparison of methylxanthines. The various stable derivatives of theophylline are formed by substitution of larger functional groups on the 7-nitrogen of the 1,3 dimethylxanthine structure except for enprofylline, which is 3-propylxanthine. Oral bioavailability and half-life data were obtained from various sources that used an intravenous reference product. *In vitro* potency was determined from the reported ability of these compounds to relax stimulated tracheal strips. (Acephylline piperazine is also called acepiphylline, i.e., the British approved name.) (From Weinberger: The pharmacology and therapeutic use of theophylline. J. Allergy Clin. Immunol. *73*:525, 1984.)

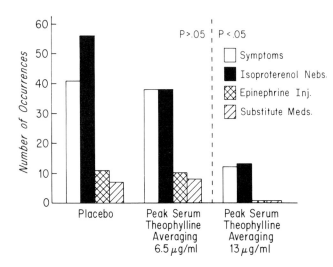

FIGURE 19–4. Frequency of symptoms (measured as the number of asthma attacks) and need for intervention among 12 children with chronic asthma treated (double-blind) with placebo, an ephedrine-theophylline combination in doses once considered conventional and individually titrated doses of theophylline that averaged twice the formerly conventional recommendations. (From Weinberger: Theophylline for treatment of asthma. J. Pediatr. 92:1, 1978.)

sity of effect, in which the inhaled beta-2 agonist is far superior, but in sustained duration of effect from maintained blood levels (Joad et al., 1987). The rapid fall-off of effect on the airways was associated with the progressive increase in symptoms at periods beyond 4 hours after the inhalation of albuterol in this study. The clinical importance of this observation was apparent from the greater than two-fold frequency of nocturnal symptoms in association with maintenance therapy during the inhaled albuterol as compared with the slow-release theophylline regimen (Joad et al., 1987).

The degree of clinical effect from theophylline described in the aforementioned studies is most readily seen when serum concentrations are maintained between 10 and 20 μg/ml. Response in the airways can be demonstrated to parallel changes in the serum concentrations (Fig. 19–5). In a similar fashion, inhibition of exercise-induced asthma is related closely to serum concentration (Pollack et al., 1977). This relationship between bronchodilatation and airway responsiveness to serum concentration is reflected in the relationship between serum concentration and symptoms. A more recent study has confirmed the relationship between control of symptoms and serum concentrations (Fig. 19–6).

On the other hand, theophylline clearly has the greatest potential for serious toxicity of any medication used for asthma. An extensive review of the world's English language medical literature of reported cases of theophylline toxicity is recorded elsewhere (Hendeles and Weinberger, 1983a). Toxicity is related to serum concentration and increases in likelihood and

degree as serum concentrations exceed 20 μg/ml (Fig. 19–7). Obvious or subtle CNS side effects (e.g., behavioral change and interference with learning) and other types of side effects can occur at significantly lower levels.

FORMULATION

Selection of formulation for treatment with theophylline is an important issue. Although theophylline still is used occasionally for acute therapy when the rapid onset of action of the intravenous route may be indicated, oral treatment is used predominantly for maintenance prophylactic therapy, with sustained action of slow-release theophylline preparations. During the 50 years that theophylline has been used, many formulations have been marketed as drug companies vie for perceived commercial advantage, and many available preparations have been chosen because of marketing perception rather than scientific justification. Some formulation selections may also have been a result of misguided notions of the chemistry of theophylline. Certainly, the use of the many so-called "salts" of theophylline has little rationale. Theophylline is largely unionized at physiologic pH, so its ability to form salts with ethylenediamine, choline, or other compounds at divergent pH is of little clinical interest. Even the traditional parenteral use of "aminophylline," the so-called ethylenediamine salt of theophylline, is no longer justified. The ethylenediamine simply raises the pH of the solution which increases the solubility of theophylline. A theophylline solution, marketed by Travenol Labs Inc., is becoming increasingly popular be-

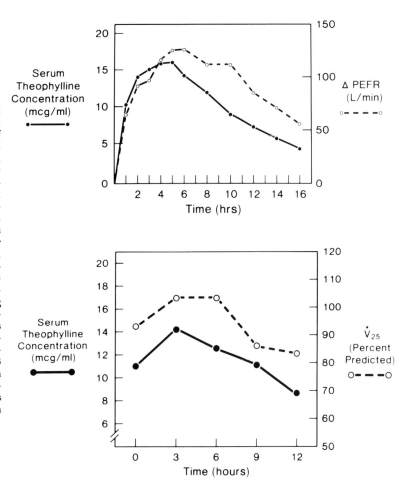

FIGURE 19-5. Relationship between serum theophylline concentration and pulmonary function. In a study by Richer and coworkers (1982), 31 adults received a single 7.5 mg/kg dose of a rapid release, plain tablet. Pulmonary function, as measured by the change in peak expiratory flow rate (ΔPEFR) closely paralleled the rise and fall in serum concentration. In the data illustrated in the lower part of the figure, Simons and coworkers (1982) demonstrated a similar parallel relationship between serum concentration and pulmonary function ($\dot{V}_{25}$, flow rate at 25 percent at a maximal forced expiration) among 10 children receiving a slow release theophylline preparation every 12 hours. Symptoms of asthma requiring inhaled albuterol occurred in 7 of the 10 children exclusively during the last 3 hours of the dosing interval when serum concentrations were generally falling below 10 mcg/ml; this intervention blunted further fall in pulmonary function.

cause it does not contain ethylenediamine, which has been associated with occasional allergic reactions (Petrozzi and Shore, 1976; Folli and Cupit, 1978; Elias and Levinson, 1981; Provost and Jillson 1967).

Slow-release formulations are the most clinically relevant formulations for maintenance therapy today. Because of their widespread clinical use, many unique formulations have been developed and marketed under an even wider variety of brand names. Despite commercial claims for formulation-specific dosing intervals, *it is the characteristic rate of absorption of the product combined with the rate of elimination of the individual patient at a selected dosing interval that results in the consequent fluctuations in serum concentration.* The methodology for evaluating products is reviewed elsewhere (Hendeles et al., 1984). Theophylline formulations reliably and completely absorbed at the rate described for Theo-Dur tablets and Slo-Bid capsules permit 12-hour dosing for most patients with fluctuations that generally can maintain

serum concentrations between 10 and 20 μg/ml. Patients with more rapid theophylline elimination (identifiable by above average dose requirements), however, may benefit from the decreased fluctuations expected during an 8 hour dosing schedule (Hendeles et al., 1984; Weinberger and Hendeles, 1983). Most other reliably absorbed formulations are absorbed more rapidly than these two formulations, whereas more slowly absorbed formulations have thus far been erratic or incomplete or both in their absorption characteristics (Hendeles and Weinberger, 1986). Slow release formulations available as bead-filled capsules have been extensively used in young children, who are unable to swallow the capsules or tablets intact, by opening the capsules and sprinkling the contents on spoonfuls of soft food.

Although previously described methodology permits reasonably accurate prediction of fluctuations in serum concentration during multiple dosing at defined rates of theophylline elimination based on single dose absorption studies

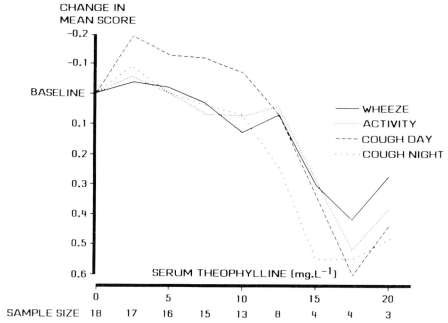

FIGURE 19–6. Relationship between 4-hour postdose peak serum theophylline concentrations during slow release theophylline administration and change in mean symptom scores among children treated with 3 different levels of maintenance theophylline for 2 weeks each in a crossover manner (From Neijens et al.: Clinical and bronchodilating efficacy of controlled release theophylline as a function of its serum concentrations in preschool children. J. Pediatr. 107:811, 1985.)

(Hendeles et al., 1984), confounding factors complicate clinical decision making. Specifically, absorption from some formulations may not be the same for doses given at different times of the day. For example, absorption of Slophyllin was found to be significantly greater when given at midnight than in the morning or afternoon, and to be somewhat greater when given at 8 a.m. than at 4 p.m. Moreover, food has specific effects on some formulations that may result in adverse consequences but no effects on others (Table 19–2).

One of the more recent developments in slow release theophylline marketing has been the

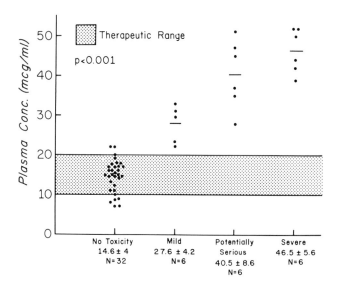

FIGURE 19–7. Relationship between serum theophylline concentration and adverse effects. Mild toxic symptoms = nausea or headache; potentially serious symptoms = vomiting, tachycardia, or both; severe symptoms = arrhythmias, seizures, or both. Seizures occurred in two patients with severe symptoms, and one died. (From Hendeles et al.: Frequent toxicity from intravenous aminophylline infusions in critically ill patients. Drug Intell. Clin. Pharm. 11:12, 1977.)

TABLE 19-2. Summary of the Effects of Food on Theophylline Absorption from Various Formulations*

Formulation	Extent of Absorption	Rate of Absorption	Reference
Plain tablets and liquids	None	Slightly slower	Welling et al., 1975
Slo-bid	None	Somewhat slower	Weinberger and Milavetz, 1986
Somophyllin-CRT Somophyllin-12	None	Slightly slower	Pedersen et al., 1985
Theobid Duracap	None	Slightly slower	Osman et al., 1983
Theo-Dur tablets Pulmi-dur Sustaire Theolin Retard	None	Slightly slower	Sips et al., 1984; Leeds et al., 1982; Osman et al., 1983; Karim, 1985
Theo-Dur Sprinkle Caps	Reduced from 91 percent fasting to 40 percent after food	Much slower	Pedersen and Moller-Petersen, 1984; Karim et al., 1985
Theo-grad	Increased from 64 percent fasting to 90 percent after food	Slightly slower	Lagas and Jonkman, 1983
Theolair SR Neulin Depot Neulin Retard Respid	None	Much slower	Pedersen and Moller-Petersen, 1982
Theo-24	Increased from 71 percent fasting to 100 percent after food	Precipitously increased (dose dumping)	Hendeles et al., 1985; Karim et al., 1985
Uniphyl	Increased from 61 percent fasting to 83 percent after food	Slightly slower	Karim et al., 1985; Milavetz et al., 1986a

* Formulations with variability in extent of absorption or where rate is affected to a major degree should not be used because of increased risk of toxicity or excessive variations in efficacy.

commercial obfuscation associated with claims for 24-hour dosing. This subject has been reviewed extensively elsewhere (Weinberger, 1984b and 1986). Regardless of marketing claims, however, the principles of product selection remain the same. The rate and extent of absorption need to be identified, and then fluctuations in serum concentrations for patients with defined rates of elimination can be predicted, as previously described (Hendeles et al., 1984). This information provides at least a minimal estimate of expected fluctuations in serum concentration at the dosing interval to be selected. A more precise estimate could be made by the same methodology if the rate of absorption following an evening dose of the formulation were incorporated into the equation; unfortunately, these data are not available for most products. Formulations with major effects in rate or extent of absorption resulting from food are best avoided.

DOSAGE

In the selection of dosage for theophylline, one must consider the rate of theophylline elim-

ination which varies, on average, with age and is mirrored by the consequent wide range of dosage (Fig. 19-8). An additional confounding factor that influences dosing schedule is the observation that the frequency of minor adverse effects is greatly diminished when initial dosage is low and the final therapeutic dosage is approached slowly by clinical titration over a 1 to 2 week period (Fig. 19-9). When this is done, the frequency of even minor adverse effects detectable by history is only about 2 percent, as long as serum concentrations are under 20 μg/ml (Milavetz et al., 1986b).

Once dosage is established by measurement of serum concentration, dosage requirements generally remain stable for extended periods. However, sustained fever, some viral infections, macrolide antibiotics (erythromycin, troleandomycin), cimetidine, oral contraceptive, heart failure, and liver disease slow theophylline elimination and thus increase steady state serum concentration (Hendeles and Weinberger, 1983b). On the other hand, phenytoin, phenobarbital, and cigarette (or marijuana) smoking will increase the rate of theophylline elimination thereby decreasing steady state

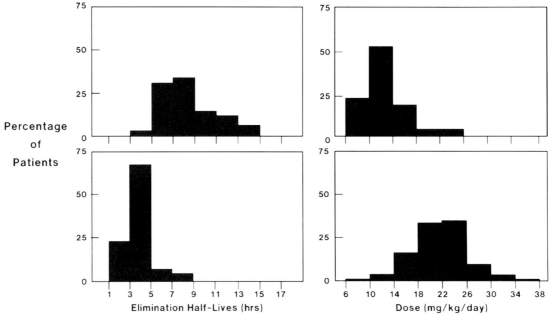

FIGURE 19-8. Frequency distribution for elimination half-life (left) and dose requirements (right) for adults (upper) and children (lower). In the absence of identifiable exogenous factors (see text), elimination rate and dose requirements generally remain stable for extended periods. (Reproduced in part from Milavetz et al.: Evaluation of a scheme for establishing and maintaining dosage of theophylline in ambulatory patients with chronic asthma. J. Pediatr. 109:351, 1987.)

serum concentrations. (It is important to consider that patients whose therapy was initially titrated to appropriate dosage based on serum concentration while they were smoking or receiving phenytoin or phenobarbital will develop slower theophylline elimination and increased serum concentration should these exogenous factors be discontinued.)

The long-term effects of maintenance therapy with a systemic medication such as theophylline, particularly in growing children, has been of concern. In fact, both neuropsychologic and metabolic effects of theophylline can be detected during maintenance therapy (Joad et al., 1986). The effects appear to be similar to those associated with caffeine and include improved performance on a task requiring mental alertness, such as remembering a number sequence; decreased motor steadiness; and an increased frequency of various affective and somatic responses on a questionnaire designed to detect mood and behavior changes (Hopkins Symptom Checklist). Interestingly, however, none of these were detectable from daily symptom diaries (Joad et al., 1986; Furakawa et al., 1984b; Weinberger and Hendeles, 1985), even over extended periods, suggesting that these findings are generally of limited clinical impor-

tance for most patients. Joad et al. (1986) also reported detectable metabolic effects, including slight but statistically significant decreases in serum bicarbonate level, with even smaller but statistically significant increases in serum creatinine, serum calcium, urine calcium, and uric acid levels. These findings suggest that there may be occasional patients who have clinically important effects and support the need for further investigation. Certainly, selected patients are seen in whom the neuropsychologic effects of theophylline are sufficiently troublesome that alternative therapy is indicated.

MANAGEMENT OF THEOPHYLLINE POISONING

Despite more than a decade of clinical experience with theophylline, iatrogenic overdosage continues to occur (Mountain and Neff, 1984; Woodcock et al., 1983). Ingestion of an excessive dose of theophylline obviously requires discontinuation of the drug followed by activated charcoal (Sintek, 1979). If less than 30 minutes have elapsed after ingestion, syrup of ipecac should be given first to evacuate the stomach; charcoal should then be given after vomiting occurs. If more than 30 minutes has

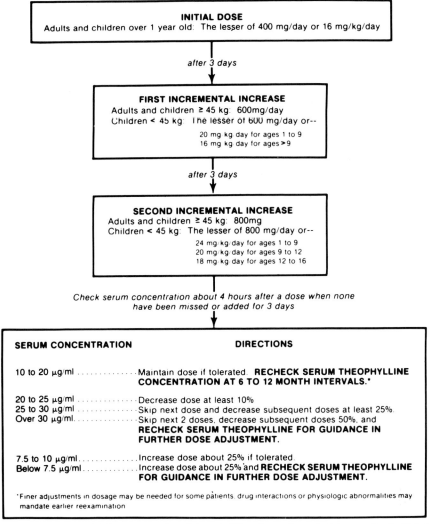

INITIAL DOSE
Adults and children over 1 year old: The lesser of 400 mg/day or 16 mg/kg/day

after 3 days

FIRST INCREMENTAL INCREASE
Adults and children ≥ 45 kg: 600mg/day
Children < 45 kg: The lesser of 600 mg/day or--

20 mg/kg/day for ages 1 to 9
16 mg/kg/day for ages >9

after 3 days

SECOND INCREMENTAL INCREASE
Adults and children ≥ 45 kg: 800mg
Children < 45 kg: The lesser of 800 mg/day or--

24 mg/kg/day for ages 1 to 9
20 mg/kg/day for ages 9 to 12
18 mg/kg/day for ages 12 to 16

*Check serum concentration about 4 hours after a dose when none
have been missed or added for 3 days*

SERUM CONCENTRATION	DIRECTIONS
10 to 20 µg/ml	Maintain dose if tolerated. **RECHECK SERUM THEOPHYLLINE CONCENTRATION AT 6 TO 12 MONTH INTERVALS.**
20 to 25 µg/ml	Decrease dose at least 10%
25 to 30 µg/ml	Skip next dose and decrease subsequent doses at least 25%.
Over 30 µg/ml	Skip next 2 doses, decrease subsequent doses 50%, and **RECHECK SERUM THEOPHYLLINE FOR GUIDANCE IN FURTHER DOSE ADJUSTMENT.**
7.5 to 10 µg/ml	Increase dose about 25% if tolerated.
Below 7.5 µg/ml	Increase dose about 25% and **RECHECK SERUM THEOPHYLLINE FOR GUIDANCE IN FURTHER DOSE ADJUSTMENT.**

*Finer adjustments in dosage may be needed for some patients, drug interactions or physiologic abnormalities may
mandate earlier reexamination

FIGURE 19-9. Scheme for establishing optimal oral theophylline dosage in ambulatory patients. This is a conservative application of recommendations incorporated into the FDA-approved package inserts. Ideal body weight should be used for obese patients. Initial dosage (mg/kg/day) for infants from 6 weeks to 1 year is 0.2 × age in weeks + 5; average dose to attain serum concentrations of 10 to 20 µg/ml will be 0.3 × age in weeks + 8. (From Weinberger and Hendeles: Slow release theophylline—rationale and basis for product selection. N. Engl. J. Med. *308*:760, 1983.)

elapsed, ipecac should not be given, and charcoal should be given immediately. Charcoal both stops further absorption of theophylline in the gut and also serves as a gastrointestinal hemoperfusion system by absorbing theophylline from the intestinal capillary bed. This action appears to double the rate of theophylline elimination (Berlinger et al., 1983). The addition of a cathartic will shorten the mouth to anus transit time of the charcoal but does not reduce the amount of theophylline absorbed from a slow release product (Massanari, 1985). Since the addition of sorbitol to activated charcoal does not enhance the removal of theophylline and, in fact, appears to cause gastrointestinal distress and vomiting, large surface area charcoal dissolved in water (SuperChar Liquid) should be used in preference to commercial formulations containing sorbitol. Doses are 1 gm/kg up to 30 gm for children and 50 gm for adults. Serum concentrations should be measured frequently, and all patients with levels greater than 30 µg/ml should be monitored in an intensive care unit. Treatment with charcoal should be repeated every 2 to 4 hours until serum concentrations fall to 20 µg/ml.

Many patients survive very high serum theophylline concentrations unscathed. However, when seizures occur, death and permanent brain damage are common sequelae (Zwillich et al., 1975; Helliwell and Berry, 1979; Culberson et al., 1979). Charcoal hemoperfusion can more rapidly remove theophylline (Weinberger and Hendeles, 1980; Park et al., 1983) and may be clinically indicated when the serum concentration is very high, even in the absence of obvious signs of toxicity. Seizures may thereby be prevented by promptly reducing the serum concentration to safe levels. If risks of the procedure such as hypotension and thrombocytopenia are not judged to be excessive and the patient is large enough to gain vascular access, treatment should be instituted promptly prior to obvious clinical toxicity. This step probably is not warranted when the serum concentration is less than 40 $\mu g/ml$, since the risk of the procedure probably outweighs the potential benefit. In the range of 40 to 60 $\mu g/ml$, the decision must be individualized, depending upon the availability of clinicians experienced with charcoal hemoperfusion and the presence of severe clinical symptoms, such as resistant cardiac arrhythmias. In patients intoxicated with multiple doses over time, seizures have occurred at concentrations greater than 40 $\mu g/ml$ (Zwillich et al., 1975; Hendeles et al., 1977; Culberson et al., 1979), whereas they are rare at concentrations less than 100 $\mu g/ml$ in patients with single overdoses in suicide attempts (Helliwell and Berry, 1979; Gaudreault et al., 1983; Olson et al., 1983). Thus, the duration of the intoxication must be taken into consideration and may alter the decision to perform hemoperfusion.

Phenobarbital has been shown to protect laboratory animals from theophylline-induced seizures (Gardner et al., 1950), but this effect has not been evaluated clinically. Nonetheless, a 10 mg/kg intravenous loading dose administered slowly over 30 minutes can be considered for patients of all ages with serum theophylline levels greater than 40 $\mu g/ml$, even if asymptomatic. This procedure would result in phenobarbital blood levels approaching the low end of the therapeutic range. A second identical loading dose 1 hour later would provide greater assurance that a serum concentration within the therapeutic range of 15 to 30 $\mu g/ml$ has been attained. Phenytoin does not protect laboratory rats against theophylline-induced seizures and should not be considered as an alternative to phenobarbital until there is clinical data to the contrary. When seizures occur, they should be terminated rapidly with intravenous diazepam, paraldehyde, thiopental, or a general anesthetic, if necessary, while oxygenation and respiratory support are maintained. Halothane should be avoided because of sensitization of the myocardium to endogenous catecholamines.

Cromolyn Sodium

Cromolyn sodium was introduced into the United States market in 1973, 5 years after its introduction in the United Kingdom. This drug was promoted initially for patients with severe steroid-dependent asthma, with less than impressive results. Subsequent studies and greater clinical experience have permitted cromolyn to be placed into appropriate clinical perspective as an extremely safe form of treatment for many patients. This drug can largely normalize life styles of responsive patients who have had daily symptoms of asthma with virtually no risk of serious toxicity. For reasons not entirely clear, some patients seem to derive great therapeutic benefit from cromolyn whereas others do not (vide infra). Its relative absence of toxicity has also made it attractive therapy for topical use in the nose and eyes as treatment for allergic rhinitis and conjunctivitis.

Cromolyn is unique among the classes of anti-asthmatic drugs in that it has no bronchodilator, anti-inflammatory, or antihistaminic effect. As a result, cromolyn sodium has no effect on acute symptoms. Cromolyn's major and best understood mode of action appears to be its protective effect on mast cell degranulation, with prevention of the release of chemical mediators that result in bronchospasm and mucous membrane inflammatory changes. Whether or not this potential actually is an explanation for the clinical effectiveness, however, is far from clear. The drug is administered topically as a dry powder via a Spinhaler device, as an aerosol solution via a nebulizer, or as a fine mist via a metered dose inhaler. Topically applied cromolyn has been demonstrated to prevent antigen-induced bronchospasm in addition to bronchospasm induced by other bronchial challenges thought to be mediated by nonantigen-induced mediator release. Specifically, exercise-induced bronchospasm, cold air–induced bronchospasm, and sulfur dioxide–induced bronchospasm have been inhibited partially by cromolyn. There is controversy about whether cromolyn will inhibit nonspecific airway reactivity induced by methacholine or histamine (Shapiro and Konig, 1985). There are reports that cromolyn can decrease nonspecific bronchial hyperresponsiveness after weeks or months of usage, but this result appears to be neither consistent nor profound.

Multiple controlled studies have demonstrated that cromolyn decreases the frequency and severity of daily wheezing, cough, and shortness of breath when used at a dose of 20 mg, 4 times daily, by the Spinhaler device through which cromolyn is administered with lactose-filler as a dry powder or at a dose of 2 mg (two inhalations) by the pressurized metered dose inhaler. Open, uncontrolled studies have suggested that less frequent administration may maintain efficacy in many patients (Furukawa, 1984a), and there is limited data to suggest that higher doses may provide greater degrees of efficacy for some patients. Cromolyn appears to be similar to theophylline in degree of efficacy for patients with milder asthma (Newth et al., 1982; Edmonds et al., 1980; Furukawa et al., 1984a). Newth and coworkers (1982) even suggested an unsustained trend toward somewhat greater efficacy of nebulized cromolyn over theophylline in young children. On the other hand, a study of patients with severe asthma demonstrated greater frequency of asymptomatic days in association with theophylline (Hambleton et al., 1977). Theophylline also has been associated with clinically important additive effects in those who could not be adequately controlled without the use of maintenance corticosteroids (21 receiving beclomethasone dipropionate and 10 receiving alternate day prednisone) (Nassif et al., 1981). Cromolyn appeared to add no therapeutic benefit to patients receiving maintenance therapy with inhaled corticosteroids (Hiller and Milner, 1975; Dawood et al., 1977; Toogood et al., 1981). In contrast to these placebo-controlled studies, some open trials have suggested a steroid-sparing effect for patients receiving oral steroids.

Many clinicians and investigators experienced in the use of cromolyn have been impressed that, to a large extent, cromolyn tends to be an "all or nothing" drug in that efficacy either is impressively present or, for a substantial number of patients, is strikingly absent. This observation is in contrast to the bronchodilator and anti-inflammatory medications, with which degrees of efficacy are more readily apparent. This has resulted, therefore, in considerable efforts to identify "responders." In spite of the well-defined mechanism of action by preventing antigen-induced mast cell release of chemical mediators, cromolyn has not been consistently more effective in preventing symptoms in patients with "extrinsic asthma," as compared with those with "intrinsic asthma." In fact, at least one controlled study demonstrated statistically significant clinical benefit in a group of 30 patients identified as having "instrinsic perennial asthma" but not in a group of 29 patients with well-defined and characterized seasonal allergic asthma (Blumenthal et al., 1973). The influence of age of patients on responsiveness to cromolyn also is not completely clear. The clinical impression of many has been that efficacy is greater in children and young patients than in older patients, but controlled studies have shown that older patients may also benefit (Toogood et al., 1978).

Side effects from cromolyn appear to be relatively infrequent and minor (Settipane et al., 1979), with at least some rarely reported side effects' being immunologically mediated (Sheffer et al., 1975). Symptoms that include transient airway irritation, skin eruptions, myositis, and pulmonary infiltrates have been very rare.

Cromolyn thus appears to be a clinically useful first line drug for patients with chronic disease, i.e., daily symptoms of asthma, particularly if the disease is relatively mild or no more than moderate in severity. It should be initiated for asthma as four times daily therapy in one of its three currently available forms. Acute symptoms of asthma need to be cleared initially with other measures, such as inhaled sympathomimetic bronchodilators or corticosteroids or both, if the patient is unresponsive to bronchodilators. In at least one study there was no decrease in the frequency or severity of viral-induced acute exacerbations of asthma in preschool children whose daily symptoms were controlled with nebulized cromolyn. Thus, it is important that acute exacerbations of asthma be promptly and appropriately treated in the child whose asthma is controlled by cromolyn.

It would appear reasonable to abandon therapy if clearly evident clinical effect is not apparent within 1 month of initiation of cromolyn therapy. Moreover, the need to add additional maintenance measures can be interpreted as evidence of cromolyn "failure," although there is little data to indicate whether cromolyn has a bronchodilator or steroid sparing effect or not. Although many clinicians have observed that the frequency of cromolyn use can be decreased to as little as twice daily once a good response has been observed, others suggest that absence of asthmatic symptoms on reduced dosage actually indicates remission of disease and the lack of need for any cromolyn.

Cromolyn also appears to be effective for a substantial number of patients with allergic rhinitis and conjunctivitis when topically applied. Frequent administration is needed, and response appears to be neither as consistent nor as impressive as that seen with topically applied corticosteroids. However, the apparent absence of potential for adverse effects makes this medication an attractive option.

Since the development and introduction of cromolyn sodium, other drugs with cromolyn-like activity have been sought, and several have reached varying stages of clinical investigation. Ketotifen is an orally administered drug with both antihistaminic and cromolyn-like activity. The data supporting the efficacy of this agent has thus far been equivocal with the antihistaminic effects along with accompanying drowsiness being more prominent than antiasthmatic effects. To the extent that anti-asthmatic effects are qualitatively present, they appear to be generally small in magnitude, almost certainly less than that of cromolyn (Shapiro and Konig, 1985; Loftus and Price, 1987). Other cromolyn-like drugs are under investigation but generally seem less effective than cromolyn.

Corticosteroids

Corticosteroids are the only drugs currently used for asthma that can reverse airway obstruction unresponsive to bronchodilators. In fact, return of bronchodilator responsiveness as early as 1 hour after a dose of parenteral prednisolone has been described in stable adult asthmatics unresponsive to inhaled bronchodilators (Fig. 19–10), whereas change in pulmonary function usually begins slowly and progresses to peak effect over 9 to 12 hours (Ellul-Micallef et al., 1974). Corticosteroids are more frequently used, however, during acute exacerbations of disease when response is typically slower (Harris et al., 1987). However, not all studies have consistently shown clinical effects from corticosteroids during acute exacerbations of disease, and some have shown only equivocal results. The apparent explanation for the conflict over the clinical efficacy of corticosteroids for acute asthma (Fiel, 1985; Mok et al., 1985) probably relates to either brief periods of observations or observations in patients in whom short self-limited episodes were suffi-

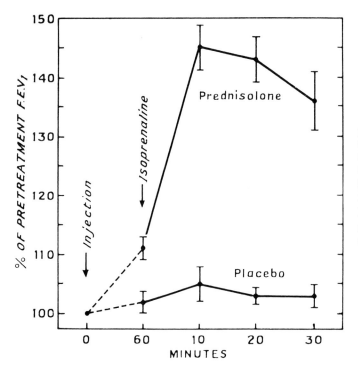

FIGURE 19–10. Effect of inhaled isoproterenol (isoprenaline) 1 hour after intravenous injection of placebo or 40 mg prednisolone to 8 patients with chronic bronchial asthma no longer responding to brochodilator therapy, but not acutely ill. (From Ellul-Micallef and Fenech: Effect of intravenous prednisolone in asthmatics with diminished adrenergic responsiveness. Lancet 2:1260, 1975.)

ciently common that the rate of spontaneous improvement frequently rivaled corticosteroid effect.

The well-recognized potential for adverse effects has served to make corticosteroid therapy often controversial. An examination of available data, however, enables benefits and risks to be put into proper perspective. Although corticosteroid usage can be associated with potentially serious adverse consequences, including suppression of endogenous adrenal function, cushingoid changes in appearance, growth suppression, posterior subcapsular cataracts, osteoporosis, aseptic necrosis of the femoral head, and others, all appear to be predominantly related to extended daily therapy. Short courses, i.e., up to 10 to 14 days, appear to be associated with little more than some occasional mood changes along with some facial edema and erythema that may develop by the end of a course of this duration. However, the use of a short course of high dose steroids for acute exacerbations of asthma may avoid the necessity of emergency care or hospitalization or both (Fiel et al., 1983; Littenberg and Gluck, 1986; Harris et al., 1987).

Whereas toxicity is minimal when short-term courses of corticosteroids are used to treat infrequent acute exacerbations of asthma, toxicity becomes of major importance when steroids are used for long-term courses. Indications for maintenance steroids must be carefully considered; dosage and formulation strategies have been developed to increase the safety of long-term use (Table 19–3). One of the earlier strategies developed was based on the observation that suppression of corticosteroid responsive diseases could be obtained by intermittent therapy. Single doses of a short-acting steroid, such as prednisone, prednisolone, or methylprednisolone, on alternate mornings appear not to cause persistent adrenal suppression. This therapy is relatively free of the more serious adverse effects associated with long-term therapy. Studies as early as the late 1960's showed little in the way of cushingoid changes or adrenal suppression, and growth in children appeared to be normal at doses averaging 40 mg every other morning (Ackerman and Nolan, 1968; Sadeghi-Nejad and Senior, 1969).

More recently, a new generation of inhaled corticosteroids with potent topical effect at usual therapeutic doses that have little systemic effect has become available for clinical use. Although not totally free of measurable systemic effects, these drugs nonetheless have a high

TABLE 19–3. Indications and Therapeutic Strategies for Maintenance Corticosteroids

Indications

Repeated relapse of bronchodilator-unresponsive symptoms after short course of high-dose oral steroids.

Therapeutic alternatives

Oral prednisone (or prednisolone or methylprednisolone) on alternate mornings.
Inhaled topically active steroids
  Beclomethasone dipropionate
  Budesonide
  Flunisolide
  Triamcinolone acetonide

Dosages

Start high
Lower slowly to establish maintenance dose
Mean (usual range) dosage*
  Alternate day prednisone—30 (20–40) mg QOD[†]
  Inhaled beclomethasone—550 (200–900) μg/day

---

* At University of Iowa.
[†] QOD—every other morning.

margin of safety in clinical use. We compared alternate morning prednisone with inhaled beclomethasone, the first of the new generation of inhaled corticosteroids. In our hands, doses required for control of disease have ranged most commonly from 20 to 40 mg (mean 30 mg) of alternate morning prednisone and from 400 to 800 μg/day (mean 550 μg/day) of inhaled beclomethasone dipropionate. At these doses, little difference in adrenal suppression or growth has been observed (Wyatt et al., 1978; Nassif et al., 1980). There also appears to be similar minor effects on cortisol secretion. Specifically, early morning serum cortisol levels, although transiently depressed 24 hours after a dose of prednisone in children on alternate day prednisone, were essentially identical before the next dose of prednisone to those of children receiving inhaled corticosteroids. In addition, free cortisols excreted into the urine were suppressed equally in children receiving alternate day prednisone and in those inhaling beclomethasone dipropionate.

Relative efficacy of two regimens often is similar, although some patients inadequately controlled on acceptable doses of alternate day prednisone may be better controlled with inhaled agents (Wyatt et al., 1978). Our experience also supports studies by others that have demonstrated that high doses of inhaled corticosteroids can be given with substantial benefit and little risk despite the measurable adrenal suppression that almost certainly will occur

(Toogood, 1977; Smith and Hodson, 1983; Editorial, 1984).

The same inhaled steroids used for asthma also have been used for rhinitis by topical spray. Unlike the older dexamethasone preparation (Turbinaire Decadron), which readily causes measurable adrenal suppression at usual therapeutic doses (Norman et al., 1967), the greater degree of topical effect from the newer preparations, at doses sufficiently low to minimize systemic effect, provides an apparent wide margin of safety for use in rhinitis. Topical steroids are of particular value for relief of nasal blockage from inflamed nasal mucosa since antihistamines have little effect on nasal obstruction, and the oral sympathomimetic decongestants are only weakly potent.

Antihistamines (H₁ Receptor Antagonists)

Classic antihistamines (H_1 blockers) competitively inhibit the physiologic effects of histamine that cause vascular smooth muscle relaxation with resulting vasodilatation, possible increases in microvascular permeability, and contraction of smooth muscle in the gastrointestinal and respiratory tracts (Levi et al., 1982). The more recently introduced blockers of the H_2 histamine receptors, cimetidine and ranitidine, competitively block histamine-induced stimulation of gastric acid secretion primarily (Fig. 19–11). H_1 antihistamines often possess additional phamacologic activities, including antiemetic, anticholinergic, and sedative, or occa-sionally CNS stimulating properties. It has been apparent that these last mentioned effects differ greatly among various antihistamines. Two antihistamines, terfenadine and astemizole, recently were introduced with claims for the absence of all CNS effects because of their inability to cross the blood-brain barrier (Howarth and Holgate, 1984; Nicholson and Stone, 1982).

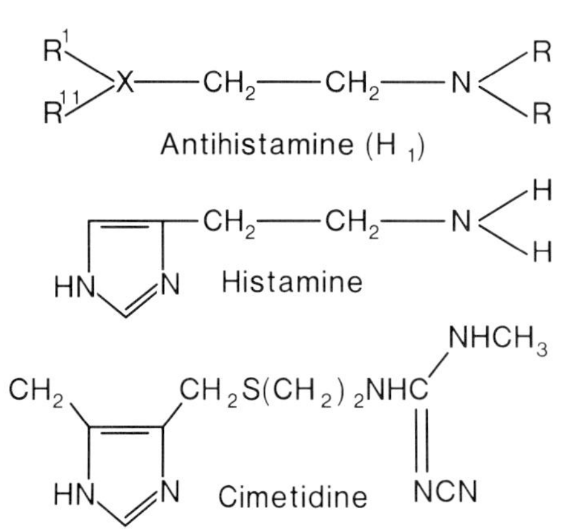

Previous attempts have been made at categorizing antihistamines according to chemical structure, but data do not support that differences in effect among the antihistamines relate to structure. Thus, these traditional categories have limited functional importance since they predict neither relative efficacy nor side effects of individual drugs. Half-lives and consequent durations of effect also differ greatly among antihistamines within the same chemical class.

Despite the plethora of antihistamines commercially available as single entities or in combination with other agents, few have been subjected to scientific study using double-blind placebo controlled techniques. Cook et al. (1973) did present evidence that hydroxyzine is more effective than diphenhydramine and other antihistamines in suppressing histamine-induced wheal size, both in extent and duration of action. Hydroxyzine also was shown to be more effective than diphenhydramine and cyproheptadine in inhibiting histamine-induced pruritus (Rhoades et al., 1975). When administered on a constant daily basis, hydroxyzine is highly effective in preventing symptoms of allergic rhinitis and conjunctivitis (Schaaf et al., 1979). In this same study, mild side effects of drowsiness and xerostomia occurred initially but were transient. Beyond the initial period of observation, hydroxyzine generally was unassociated with detectable side effects in doses as high as 150 mg daily. The strategy of beginning with low doses in the evening and increasing doses slowly appears to minimize sedative and anticholinergic side effects that may be observed initially.

Terfenadine was the first antihistamine without apparent potential for even initial sedative effect introduced on the United States market. In one study, this drug was considered to be "slightly less effective than or as effective as chlorpheniramine" (Connell, 1985). In another study that compared the same dosage of terfenadine, 60 mg twice daily, with astemizole at a maintenance dosage of 10 mg once daily preceded by a larger loading dose, and hydroxyzine 50 mg once daily, terfenadine was the

FIGURE 19–11. Structure-function comparison of histamine with the general structure of the H_1 antihistamines and the first of the marketed H_2 antihistamines (cimetidine).

least effective, whereas astemizole and hydroxyzine had similar degrees of both efficacy and relative absence of adverse effects (Gendreau-Reid et al., 1986). Thus, terfenadine, despite its lack of apparent CNS effect, may be limited in clinical efficacy compared with the newer nonsedating agent astemizole or even the older antihistamine, hydroxyzine.

Hydroxyzine had long been used for its clinical action on urticaria and pruritus. In fact, studies had shown it to be more effective than other classic H₁ antagonists in suppressing pruritus, wheal, and flare from intracutaneously injected antigen or histamine (Cook et al., 1973; Rhoades et al., 1975). Controlled studies also showed a high degree of clinical effect in suppressing the symptoms of seasonal allergic rhinitis (Schaaf et al., 1979; Wong et al., 1981). When doses titrated up to 150 mg were compared with 24 mg/day of chlorpheniramine or placebo, both antihistamines were more effective than placebo in suppressing symptoms of allergic rhinitis, but the data also demonstrated a degree of greater effectiveness for hydroxyzine over chlorpheniramine. Moreover, both antihistamine regimens were not associated with detectable adverse findings when compared with placebo during the sustained maintenance therapy of the trial. This study suggested that the relative results of antihistamines in suppressing histamine or antigen-induced skin reactions might reflect clinical efficacy. Hydroxyzine also appears to be the most effective antihistamine for controlling exercise-induced anaphylaxis and cholinergic urticaria (Kaplan, 1984).

The pharmacokinetics of antihistamines have had only limited and often not very systematic study despite the fact that pharmacokinetics may have important therapeutic implications (Paton and Webster, 1985). Dosage and dosing intervals for antihistamines traditionally have been empirical. Four times daily dosing has been common, and slow release preparations of some antihistamines have been marketed with the purpose of permitting longer dosing intervals. However, many antihistamines have very long durations of effect. For example, the commonly used chlorpheniramine and brompheniramine antihistamines have reported half-lives ranging from one-half to one and one-half days, suggesting that doses not more than twice daily might be sufficient for clinical use. This argues against any rationale for slow release preparations (which are marketed for both). In comparison, diphenhydramine, clemastine, and triprolidine appear to be eliminated rapidly (Simons et al., 1986). Of interest and relevance for dosing is the 7 to 20 day half-life of the new nonsedating antihistamine, astemizole. Without an initial loading dose, the very slow accumulation of this antihistamine (50 percent of steady state levels attained after one half-life; 75 percent after two half-lives, 85 percent after three, and so forth) will be associated with a long delay in optimal effect (Gendreau-Reid et al., 1986). Moreover, cessation will be associated with long duration of continued effect.

Tolerance to side effects, common with initial therapy of the older antihistamines, unquestionably occurs. In our hands, tolerance to suppression of wheal and flare from intracutaneous antigen and clinical symptoms appears not to occur (Fig. 19–12), although others have reported the development of partial tolerance with repeated antihistamine use (Taylor et al., 1985).

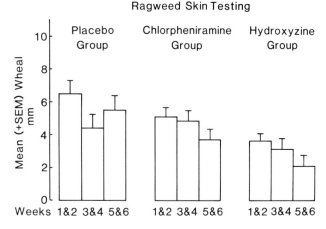

FIGURE 19–12. Mean (±SEM) wheal diameter from serial ragweed skin testing among 3 groups of subjects (approximately 30 in each group) receiving placebo, 24 mg/day of chlorpheniramine, 150 mg/day of hydroxyine. No evidence of tolerance to the antihistamines is apparent; to the contrary, a suggestion of progressive decrease in mean wheal size from the ragweed skin testing was apparent in the 2 groups receiving antihistamines, whereas this was not apparent in the placebo group.

The use of antihistamines as combination products with oral sympathomimetic decongestants has long been popular. Observations that antihistamines significantly decrease symptoms of sneezing, itchy nose, rhinorrhea, and conjunctivitis without affecting nasal obstruction that can be decreased with the oral sympathomimetic agents support the rationale for the combination *when nasal obstruction is a prominent part of the symptomatology* (Hendeles et al., 1980). Combination products containing pseudoephedrine or phenylpropanolamine are rational convenient preparations, although using these agents separately may allow better individualization of dosage. Moreover, preferred antihistamine agents are inherently long-acting and probably do not need sustained action preparations, whereas the sympathomimetic preparations are relatively short-acting and could potentially benefit from slow release formulations. It is important to note that phenylephrine, a sympathomimetic agent in a number of combination products, is not orally bioactive and has no measurable clinical efficacy in the doses used.

Based on available data, it appears that chlorpheniramine or brompheniramine is a good choice for routine antihistamine therapy because of low cost; relatively long half-life to permit once or twice daily dosing; long experience with clinical use in patients of all ages, including pregnant women; and general absence of side effects during chronic therapy. Aside from the generally greater cost and need for a prescription, hydroxyzine appears to be a more efficacious choice with no greater frequency of side effects. Its prolonged duration of effect, its greater degree of efficacy than chlorpheniramine, and its relative freedom from adverse effects during chronic therapy should be weighed against its generally higher cost and absence of a product containing an oral sympathomimetic decongestant.

The nonsedating antihistamine, terfenadine, might have advantages over older antihistamines for "prn" therapy when the duration of usage is insufficient to permit slow titration of evening doses to minimize the initial drowsiness until tolerance develops. High cost (at least when first marketed) and limited efficacy compared with hydroxyzine or astemizole are negative factors in the selection of this medication.

Astemizole is also nonsedating and is more efficacious than terfenadine. Although it compares favorably with hydroxyzine in a dose of 50 mg daily in suppressing a histamine-induced wheal, dose response data that would permit comparison with higher doses of hydroxyzine, shown to be tolerated and effective in suppressing symptoms of seasonal allergic rhinitis, are not available. An interesting feature of astemizole is its extraordinarily slow rate of elimination; this feature has prompted different dosing strategies than for other antihistamines. Slow rate of elimination dictates a long period of drug accumulation. Astemizole and its metabolites, with their 7 to 20 day half-life of elimination, therefore can result in accumulation during constant maintenance dosing until a steady state is attained at approximately four to five half-lives. More prompt optimal effect is attained by using higher initial doses to "load" patients (Gendreau-Reid et al., 1986). The slow elimination may cause some complications for physicians wishing to do skin testing since periods of a month or longer without medication may be required to eliminate the drug sufficiently to allow valid testing.

Anticholinergic Agents

The use of anticholinergic, antimuscarinic compounds as bronchodilators for asthma is a relatively new approach for modern pharmacotherapy of asthma but one that has its roots in 19th century medicine. The leaves of *Datura stramonium* were smoked until the middle of this century for its anticholinergic bronchodilating effects. Although subsequently replaced by more potent adrenergic bronchodilators, there has been renewed interest in the topical use of atropine and its derivatives. This has been reinforced by animal and human studies demonstrating a role for vagally mediated reflex bronchospasm in asthma. Greatest interest has been focused on the quaternary ammonium congeners, atropine methylnitrate and ipratropium bromide, since these are poorly absorbed by inhalation and have little ability to cross the blood-brain barrier. Consequently, they are relatively free of systemic side effects that can occur from inhaled atropine sulfate.

Studies of both agents are in the medical literature (Gross and Skorodin, 1984) particularly ipratropium (Pakes et al., 1980). Ipratropium bromide has been marketed extensively throughout the world. Despite the extensive medical literature documenting the bronchodilator effect of these medications, many questions remain regarding their clinical use. Most investigators have considered the effects to be predominantly in the large central airways both in normal and in asthmatic subjects. These findings are in contrast to inhaled beta-2 agonists, which have major effects in the more peripheral airways. While the bronchodilator effects of anticholinergic agents have been clearly and consistently documented, their ability to stabilize hyperresponsive airways to various stimuli is less clear. Full protection is offered against cholinergic stimulation of the airways, since these drugs are specific pharmacologic antagonists of acetylcholine. Protection against bronchospasm induced by histamine and various other clinical precipitants of asthma (inhaled irritants, antigens, exertion, hyperventilation, cold air), however, is partial at best. The only activity of potential clinical importance for which the inhaled cholinergic bronchodilators appear to have greater effect than beta-2 agonists is protection against bronchospasm induced by beta blocking agents. In fact, most of the apparent effect of the anticholinergic bronchodilators in partially blocking airway hyperresponsiveness appears to reflect only its antagonism by the normal bronchomotor tone of acetylcholine without actually affecting post-challenge bronchoconstriction, in contrast to the effects of inhaled beta-2 agonists. Various studies have demonstrated additive effects from these two classes of drugs.

Unfortunately, studies of the pharmacodynamics and pharmacokinetics of these drugs are limited. What studies exist suggest that these drugs have longer durations of action than inhaled beta-2 agonists and enhance both the intensity and duration of effect of inhaled beta-2 agonists. Questions regarding the potential for tolerance, i.e., decreasing effect with continuous usage, need to be adequately resolved before recommending these drugs for maintenance therapy. Moreover, in spite of the extensive evaluations of the bronchodilator effect of these drugs, little data have demonstrated actual decreases in symptoms and control of disease (although some degree of clinical benefit could be inferred and would be expected from continuously maintained bronchodilatation).

Since anticholinergic drugs are less potent than inhaled beta-2 agonists and newer inhaled beta-2 agonists are being developed with longer durations of activity, a major issue involving a place for anticholinergic bronchodilators in asthma therapy relates to the issue of whether certain patients might uniquely benefit from anticholinergic bronchodilators. Patients with

"chronic bronchitis" are reported to respond better to these agents than do patients with asthma. However, the failure to define clearly chronic bronchitis with bronchospasm, as a unique and distinct entity from asthma, limits both the interpretability and the usefulness of data obtained in these studies. Until subsets of patients can be identified with more specific criteria, only selected clinical trials with careful observation will determine if there is any therapeutic benefit to be obtained from these medications over other classes of drugs. On the other hand, the new agents in this class appear to be remarkably nontoxic and free of adverse effects, and their ability to enhance the duration of inhaled beta-2 agonists warrants further investigation of this combination as maintenance therapy for chronic disease. Further studies examining the issue of tolerance and actual control of symptoms are needed to provide further therapeutic guidance.

Interest in the use of anticholinergic drugs for rhinorrhea has been supported by the demonstration of decreased rhinorrhea from the use of ipratropium (Borum et al., 1981). The onset of action is rapid, and side effects appear to be limited to minor irritation and dryness of the nose. Sustained usage probably should await more extensive data.

Calcium Channel Blockers

During the past few years, numerous investigations have examined the effects of verapamil, diltiazem, and nifedipine on experimentally induced asthma (Barnes, 1985). None of these agents affects resting bronchomotor tone, and their effectiveness in preventing bronchospasm is a function of the agent, dose, route of administration, and method of provocation. Diltiazem appears to be the least effective, even by the inhaled route (Harman et al., 1985; Moore et al., 1985), whereas nifedipine is potentially the most active (Cerrina et al., 1981). By the sublingual route, nifedipine blocks bronchospasm induced by exercise (Cerrina et al., 1981), cold air (Henderson et al., 1983), deep inspiration (Rolla et al., 1982), leukotrienes C_4 and D_4, prostaglandin F_2 (Kohrogi et al., 1985), histamine (Cuss and Barnes, 1985), methacholine (Gonzalez et al., 1983), and inhaled antigen (Russi et al., 1985). With the exception of verapamil, which causes bronchoconstriction when inhaled at higher concentrations (Hill et al., 1985), the inhaled route allows administration of larger doses that provide greater efficacy without clinically important systemic effects (Ahmed et al., 1985).

In the only clinical study published thus far on the ability of a calcium antagonist in controlling asthmatic symptoms, nifedipine 60 mg/day sublingually was significantly more able than placebo in reducing the severity of symptoms and the number of puffs of inhaled beta-agonists when added to other anti-asthmatic medication, but did not decrease the frequency of "attacks" (Ozenne et al., 1985). This result may have been due in part to the prolongation of the duration of bronchodilatation from inhaled albuterol (Lever et al., 1984).

At the present time, there is insufficient data upon which to base any recommendations about the use of these agents in the management of patients with chronic asthma. Rather, additional studies are needed to determine if the observed effects on experimentally induced bronchoconstriction can be extrapolated to the control of symptoms of chronic asthma. At the least, however, it would seem prudent to use a calcium antagonist such as nifedipine for the treatment of hypertension or angina in a patient with airway obstruction in whom beta-receptor antagonists may be contraindicated. The effectiveness of currently available calcium channel blockers in the therapy of asthma seems relatively unimpressive. Even if the present generation of calcium antagonists prove ineffective as prophylactic agents, future members of this class of drugs might have greater specificity for the lungs and thus offer potential benefit under yet undefined circumstances.

REFERENCES

Ackerman, G.L., Nolan, C.M.: Adrenocortical responsiveness after alternate-day corticosteroid therapy. N. Engl. J. Med. 278:405–409, 1968.

Ahmed, T., Russi, E., Kim, C.S., Danta, I.: Comparative effects of oral and inhaled verapamil on antigen-induced bronchoconstriction. Chest 88:176–180, 1985.

Ahrens, R.C., Bonham, A.C., Maxwell, G.A., et al.: A method for comparing the peak intensity and duration of action of aerosolized bronchodilators using bronchoprovocation with methacholine. Am. Rev. Respir. Dis. 129:903–906, 1984.

Ahrens, R.C., Harris, J.B., Annis, L.: Effect of metaproterenol and albuterol administered by metered dose inhaler on non-specific airway responsiveness. J. Allergy Clin. Immunol. 75:161, 1985.

Ahrens, R.C., Smith, G.D.: Albuterol: An adrenergic agent for use in the treatment of asthma; pharmacology, pharmacokinetics and clinical use. Pharmacotherapy 4:105–121, 1984.

American Conference of Governmental Industrial Hygienists: Air Sampling Instruments. Cincinnati, Ohio, Edition 5:F9–F10, 1978.

Anderson, S.D., Seale, J.P., Rozea, P., Bandler, L., Theobald, G., Lindsay, D.A.: Inhaled and oral salbutamol in exercise-induced asthma. Am. Rev. Resp. Dis. 114:493–500, 1976.

Barnes, P.J.: Clinical studies with calcium antagonists in asthma. Br. J. Clin. Pharmacol. 20:289S–298S, 1985.

Berlinger, W.G., Spector, R., Goldberg, M.J., et al.: Enhancement of theophylline clearance by oral activated charcoal. Clin. Pharmacol. Ther. 33:351–354, 1983.

Blumenthal, M.N., Schoenwetter, W.F., MacDonald, F.M., McHugh, R.B.: Cromolyn in extrinsic and intrinsic asthma. J. Allergy Clin. Immunol. 52:105–113, 1973.

Borum, P., Olsen, L., Winther, B., Mygind, N.: Ipratropium nasal spray: A new treatment for rhinorrhea in the common cold. Am. Rev. Respir. Dis. 123:418–420, 1981.

Campbell, A.H.: Mortality from asthma and bronchodilator aerosols. Med. J. Aust. 1:386–391, 1976.

Cantekin, E.I., Bluestone, C.D., Welch, R.M., et al.: Nasal decongestant activity of pseudoephedrine. Ann. Otol. Rhinol. Laryngol. 86:235, 1977.

Cerrina, J., Denjean, A., Alexandre, G., Lockhart, A., Duroux, P.: Inhibition of exercise-induced asthma by a calcium antagonist, nifedipine. Am. Rev. Respir. Dis. 123:156–160, 1981.

Chatterjee, S.S., Perry A.E.: Salbutamol: Clinical application as pressure-packed aerosol. Postgrad. Med. J. 47:53–55, 1971.

Chipman, P., Glover, W.E.: Histamine H_2-receptors in the human peripheral circulation. Br. J. Pharmacol. 56:494, 1976.

Cogswell, J.J., Simpkiss, M.J.: Nebulised sodium cromoglycate in recurrently wheezy preschool children. Arch. Dis. Child. 60:736–738, 1985.

Connell, J.T.: Pharmacology and clinical efficacy of terfenadine, a new H_1-receptor antagonist. Pharmacotherapy 5:201–208, 1985.

Cook, T.J., MacQueen, D.M., Witting, H.J., et al.: Degree and duration of skin test suppression and side effects with antihistamines. J. Allergy Clin. Immunol. 51:71, 1973.

Culberson, C.G., Langston, J.W., Herrick, M.: Aminophylline encephalopathy: Clinical, electroencephalographic and neuropathological analysis. Trans. Am. Neurol. Assoc. 104:224–226, 1979.

Cuss, F.M., Barnes, P.J.: The effect of inhaled nifedipine on bronchial reactivity to histamine in man. J. Allergy Clin. Immunol. 76:718–723, 1985.

Dawood, A.G., Hendry, A.T., Walker, S.R.: The combined use of beta-methasone valerate and sodium cromoglycate in the treatment of asthma. Clin. Allergy 7:161–165, 1977.

Davies, D.S.: The fate of inhaled terbutaline. Eur. J. Resp. Dis. 65:141–147, 1984.

Dressler, W.E., Meyers, T., London, S.J., et al.: A system of rhinomanometry in the clinical evaluation of nasal decongestants. Ann. Otol. Rhinol. Laryngol. 86:310, 1977.

Dusdieker, L., Green, M., Smith, G.D., Ekwo, E.E., Weinberger M.: Comparison of orally administered metaproterenol and theophylline in the control of chronic asthma. J. Pediatr. 101:281–287, 1982.

Editorial: High-dose corticosteroid inhalers for asthma. Lancet 2:23–24, 1984.

Edmunds, A.T., Carswell, F., Robinson, P., Hughes, A.O.: Controlled trial of cromoglycate and slow-release aminophyllin in perennial childhood asthma. Br. Med. J. 281:842, 1980.

Ekwo, E., Weinberger, M.: Evaluation of a program for the pharmacologic management of children with asthma. J. Allergy Clin. Immunol. 61:240, 1978.

Elias, J.A., Levinson, A.I.: Hypersensitivity reactions to ethylenediamine in aminophylline. Am. Rev. Respir. Dis. 123:550–552, 1981.

Elis, J., Laurence, D.R., Mattie, H., et al.: Modification by monoamine oxidase inhibitors of the effect of some sympathomimetics on blood pressure. Br. Med. J. 2:75, 1967.

Ellul-Micallef, R., Borthwick, R.C., McHardy, G.J.R.: The time-course of response to prednisolone in chronic bronchial asthma. Clin. Sci. Mol. Med. 47:105–117, 1974.

Ellul-Micallef, R., Fenech, F.F.: Effect of intravenous prednisolone in asthmatics with diminished adrenergic responsiveness. Lancet 2:1269–1270, 1975.

Fiel, S.B.: Should corticosteroids be used in the treatment of acute, severe, asthma? I. A case for the use of corticosteroids in acute, severe asthma. Pharmacotherapy 5:327–335, 1985.

Fiel, S.B., Swartz, M.A., Glanz, K., Francis, M.E.: Efficacy of short-term corticosteroid therapy in outpatient treatment of acute bronchial asthma. Am. J. Med. 75:259–262, 1983.

Folli, H.L., Cupit, G.C.: Ethylenediamine hypersensitivity. Drug Intell. Clin. Pharm. 12:482–483, 1978.

Furukawa C.T., DuHamel T., Weimer L., Shapiro G.G., Pierson W.E., Bierman C.W.: Cognitive and behavioral findings in children taking theophylline versus cromolyn. J. Allergy Clin. Immunol. 77:186, 1986.

Furukawa, C.T., Shapiro, G.G., Kraemer, M.J., Pierson, W.E., Bierman, C.W.: A double-blind study comparing the effectiveness of cromolyn sodium and sustained-release theophylline in childhood asthma. Pediatrics 74:453–459, 1984a.

Furukawa, C.T., Shapiro, G.G., DuHamel, T., et al.: Learning and behaviour problems associated with theophylline therapy. Lancet 1:621, 1984b.

Gardner, R.A., Hansen, H., Ewing, P.L., et al.: Unexpected fatality in a child from accidental consumption of antiasthmatic preparation containing ephedrine, theophylline and phenobarbital. Tex. Med. 45:516–520, 1950.

Gaudreault, P., Wason, S., Lovejoy, F.H.: Acute pediatric theophylline overdose: A summary of 28 cases. J. Pediatr. 102:474–476, 1983.

Gendreau-Reid, L., Simons, K.J., Simons, F.E.R.: Comparison of the suppressive effect of astemizole, terfenadine, and hydroxyzine on histamine-induced wheals and flares in humans. J. Allergy Clin. Immunol. 77:335–340, 1986.

Gonzalez, J.M., Morice, R.C., Bloom, K., et al.: Inhibition of airway reactivity by nifedipine in patients with coronary artery disease. Am. Rev. Respir. Dis. 127:155–157, 1983.

Gross, N.J., Skorodin, M.S.: Anticholinergic, antimuscarinic bronchodilators. Am. Rev. Respir. Dis. 129:856–870, 1984.

Haltom, J.R., Szefler, S.J.: Theophylline absorption in young asthmatic children receiving sustained-release formulations. J. Pediatr. 107:805–810, 1985.

Hambleton, G., Weinberger, M., Taylor, J., et al.: Comparison of cromoglycate (cromolyn) and theophylline in controlling symptoms of chronic asthma. Lancet 1:381, 1977.

Harman, E., Peeler, D., Hill, M., Hendeles, L.: The effect of single dose oral diltiazem on methacholine responsiveness in adult asthmatics. Am. Rev. Respir. Dis. 131:50, 1985.

Harris, J.B., Ahrens, R.C. Milavetz, G. et al.: Relative potencies and rates of decline in effect of inhaled albuterol (A) and terbutaline (T). J. Allergy Clin. Immunol. (Abstract). 77:148, 1986a.

Harris, J.B., Ahrens, R.C., Milavetz, G.M., et al.: Relative potencies and rates of decline in effect of albuterol and bitolterol using bronchial provocation with histamine. Ann. Allergy (Abstract.) 56:520, 1986b.

Harris, J.B., Weinberger, M., Nassif, E., et al.: Early intervention with short courses of prednisone to prevent progression of asthma in ambulatory patients incompletely responsive to bronchodilators. J. Pediatr. 110:627–644, 1987.

Helliwell, M., Berry, D.: Theophylline poisoning in adults. Br. Med. J. 2:1114, 1979.

Hendeles, L., Bighley, L., Richardson, R.H., et al.: Frequent toxicity from IV aminophylline infusions in critically ill patients. Drug Intell. Clin. Pharm. 11:12–18, 1977.

Hendeles, L., Iafrate, R.P., Weinberger, M.: A clinical and pharmacokinetic basis for the selection and use of slow-release theophylline products. Clin. Pharmacokinet. 9:95–135, 1984.

Hendeles, L., Weinberger, M.: Theophylline. *In* Middleton, E., Reed, C., Ellis, E. (eds.), Allergy: Principles and Practice, 2nd ed. St. Louis, C.V. Mosby, 1983a.

Hendeles, L., Weinberger, M.: Theophylline: A state-of-the-art review. Pharmacotherapy 3:2–44, 1983b.

Hendeles, L., Weinberger, M.: Nonprescription sale of inhaled metaproterenol—deja vu. N. Engl. J. Med. 310:207–208, 1984.

Hendeles, L., Weinberger, M.: Selection of a slow-release theophylline product. J. Allergy Clin. Immunol. 78:743, 1986.

Hendeles, L., Weinberger, M., Milavetz, G., Hill, M., Vaughan, L.: Food-induced dose dumping from a "once-a-day" theophylline product as a cause of theophylline toxicity. Chest 87:758–765, 1985.

Hendeles, L., Weinberger, M., Wong, L.: Medical management of noninfectious rhinitis. Am. J. Hosp. Pharm. 37:1496–1504, 1980.

Henderson, A.F., Heaton, R.W., Costello, J.F.: The effect of nifedipine on bronchoconstriction induced by inhalation of cold air. Thorax 38:512–515, 1983.

Hill, M., Hendeles, L., Moore, P., Harman, E., Pieper, J.A., Peeler, D.: The effect of increasing doses of inhaled verapamil on airway reactivity to methacholine in mild asthmatics: a paradoxical response. Drug Intell. Clin. Pharm. 19:464, 1985.

Hiller, E.J., Milner, A.D.: Betamethasone 17 valerate aerosol and disodium cromoglycate in severe childhood asthma. Br. J. Dis. Chest 69:103–106, 1975.

Howarth, P.H., Durham, S.R., Lee, T.H., et al.: Influence of albuterol, cromolyn sodium and ipratorium bromide on the airway and circulating mediator responses to allergen bronchial provocation in asthma. Am. Rev. Respir. Dis. 132:986–992, 1985.

Howarth, P.H., Holgate, S.T.: Comparative trial of two non-sedative H₁ antihistamines, terfenadine and astemizole, for hay fever. Thorax 39:668–672, 1984.

Inman, W.H.W.: Recognition of unwanted drug effects with special reference to pressurized bronchodilator aerosols. *In* Burley, D.M., Clarke, S.W., Cuthbert, M.F., Paterson, J.W., Shelley, J.H. (eds.), Evaluation of bronchodilator drugs. An asthma research council symposium, October 1973, London: The Trust for Education and Research in Therapeutics, 191–201, 1974.

Inman, W.H.W., Adelstein, A.M.: Rise and fall of asthma mortality in England and Wales in relation to use of pressurized aerosols. Lancet 2:279–284, 1969.

Jenne, J.W., Ahrens, R.C.: Pharmacokinetics of inhaled beta$_2$ adrenergic compounds. In Jenne, J.W., Murphy, S., (eds.). Drug Therapy for Asthma: Research and Clinical Practice. New York, Marcel Dekker, 1987.

Jenne, J., Chick, T., Strickland, R., et al.: Subsensitivity of beta responses during therapy with a long acting beta-2 preparation. J. Allergy Clin. Immunol. 59:383–390, 1977.

Joad, J., Ahrens, R.C., Lindgren, S.D., Weinberger, M.M.: Relative efficacy of maintenance therapy with theophylline, inhaled albuterol, and the combination for chronic asthma. J. Allergy Clin. Immunol. 79:78–85, 1987.

Joad J., Ahrens, R., Lindgren, S., Weinberger, M.: Extrapulmonary effects of maintenance therapy with theophylline and inhaled albuterol in patients with chronic asthma. J. Allergy Clin. Immunol. 78:1147–1153, 1986.

Johnson, A.J., Spiro, S.G., Pidgeon, J., et al.: Intravenous infusion of salbutamol in severe acute asthma. Br. Med. J. 1:1013, 1978.

Kaplan, A.P.: Exercise-induced hives. J. Allergy Clin. Immunol. 73:704–707, 1984.

Karetzky, M.S.: Asthma mortality associated with pneumothorax and intermittent positive-pressure breathing. Lancet 1:828, 1975.

Karim, A., Burns, T., Wearley, L., Streicher, J., Palmer, M.: Food-induced changes in theophylline absorption from controlled-release formulations. Part I. Substantial increased and decreased absorption with Uniphyl tablets and Theo-Dur Sprinkle. Clin. Pharmacol. Ther. 38:77, 1985.

Kohrogi, H., Horio, S., Ando, M., Sugimoto, M., Honda, I., Araki, S.: Nifedipine inhibits human bronchial smooth muscle contractions induced by leukotrienes C$_4$ and D$_4$, prostaglandin F$_2$, and potassium. Am. Rev. Respir. Dis. 127:155–157, 1983.

Lagas, M., Jonkman, J.H.G.: Greatly enhanced bioavailability of theophylline on postprandial administration of a sustained release tablet. Eur. J. Clin. Pharmacol. 24:761, 1983.

Leeds, N.H., Gal, P., Purohit, A.A., Walter, J.B.: Effect of food on the bioavailability and pattern of release of a sustained-release theophylline tablet. J. Clin. Pharmacol. 22:196, 1982.

Lever, A.M.L., Corris, P.A., Gibson, G.J.: Nifedipine enhances the bronchodilator effect of salbutamol. Thorax 39:576–578, 1984.

Levi, R., Owen, D.A.A., Trzeciakowski, J.: Actions of Histamine on the Heart and Vasculature. In Ganellin, C.R., Parsons, M.E. (eds.), Pharmacology of Histamine Receptors. Littleton, Massachusetts, John Wright P.S.G., Inc., 1982.

Lichtenstein, L.M., Margolis, S.: Histamine release in vitro: Inhibition by catecholamines and methylxanthines. Science 161:902–903, 1968.

Littenberg, B., Gluck, E.H.: A controlled trial of methylprednisolone in the emergency treatment of acute asthma. N. Engl. J. Med. 314:150–152, 1986.

Loftus, B.G., Price, J.F.: Longterm placebo-controlled trial of ketotifin in the management of preschool asthma. J. Allergy Clin. Immunol. 79:350–355, 1987.

Massanari, M., Hendeles, L., Neims, A., et al.: The effect of cathartics on drug absorption from a slow-release formulation. Drug Intell. Clin. Pharm. 19:462, 1985.

Milavetz, G., Vaughan, L., Weinberger, M., Harris, J., Mullenix, T.: Bioavailability of oral theophylline: Single and multiple dose studies of Uniphyl. J. Allergy Clin. Immunol. (Abstract). 77:146, 1986a.

Milavetz, G., Vaughan, L., Weinberger, M., Hendeles, L.: Evaluation of a scheme for establishing and maintaining dosage of theophylline in ambulatory patients with chronic asthma. J. Pediatr., 109:359–364, 1986b.

Mok, J., Kattan, M., Levison, H.: Should corticosteroids be used in the treatment of acute, severe asthma? II. A case against the use of corticosteroids in acute, severe, asthma. Pharmacotherapy 5:327, 1985.

Moore, P., Hill, M., Harman, E., Peeler, D., Hendeles, L.: The effect of inhaled diltiazem on exercise-induced bronchoconstriction. Chest 88:32, 1985.

Moore, R.M., Cotton, E.K., Pinney, M.A.: The effect of intermittent positive-pressure breathing on airway resistance in normal and asthmatic children. J. Allergy Clin. Immunol. 49:137, 1972.

Morse, J.L., Jones, N.L., Anderson, G.D.: The effect of terbutaline in exercise-induced asthma. Am. Rev. Resp. Dis. 113:89–92, 1976.

Mountain, R.D., Neff, T.A.: Oral theophylline intoxication. A serious error of patient and physician understanding. Arch. Intern. Med. 144:724–727, 1984.

Nassif, E., Weinberger, M., Thompson, R., Huntley, W.: The value of maintenance theophylline for steroid dependent asthma. N. Engl. J. Med. 304:71–75, 1981.

Nassif, E., Weinberger, M., Thompson, R., Sherman, B.: Effects of continuous corticosteroid therapy on children with chronic asthma. J. Allergy Clin. Immunol. 65:219, 1980.

Neijens, H.J., Duiverman, E.J., Braatsma, B.H., Kerrebijn, K.F.: Clinical and bronchodilating efficacy of controlled-release theophylline as a function of its serum concentrations in preschool children. J. Pediatr. 107:811–815, 1985.

Nelson, H.S., Raine, D., Jr., Doner, H.C., Posey, W.C.: Subsensitivity to bronchodilator action of albuterol produced by chronic administration. Am. Rev. Respir. Dis. 116:871, 1977.

Newman, S.P., Pavia, D., Clarke, S.W.: How should pressurized aerosols be inhaled? Eur. J. Resp. Dis. 62:3–21, 1981.

Newth, C.J.L., Newth, C.V., Turner, J.A.P.: Comparison of nebulised sodium cromoglycate and oral theophylline in controlling symptoms of chronic asthma in preschool children; a double-blind study. Aust. N.Z. J. Med. 12:232–238, 1982.

Nicholson, A.N., Stone, B.M.: Performance studies with the H$_1$-histamine receptor antagonists, astemizole and terfenadine. Br. J. Clin. Pharmacol. 13:199–202, 1982.

Norman, P.S., Winkenwerder, W.L., Agbayani, B.F., Migeon, C.J.: Adrenal function during the use of dexamethasone aerosols in the treatment of ragweed hay fever. J. Allergy 40:57, 1967.

Norman, P.S.: Review of nasal therapy: Update. J. Allergy Clin. Immunol. 72:421–432, 1983.

Olson, K.R., Benowitz, N., Woo, O., et al.: Clinical features of acute and chronic theophylline intoxication. (Abstract). Vet. Hum. Toxicol. 25:269, 1983.

Osman, M.A., Patel, R.B., Irwin, D.S., Welling, P.G.: Absorption of theophylline from enteric coated and sustained release formulations in fasted and non-fasted subjects. Biopharm. Drug Dispos. 4:63, 1983.

Ozenne, G., Moore, N.D., Leprevost, A., et al.: Nifedipine in chronic bronchial asthma: a randomized double-blind crossover trial against placebo. Eur. J. Respir. Dis. 67:238–243, 1985.

Pakes, G.E., Brogden, R.N., Heel, R.C., Speight, T.M., Avery, G.S.: Ipratropium bromide: A review of its pharmacological properties and therapeutic efficacy in asthma and chronic bronchitis. Drugs 20:237–266, 1980.

Park, G.D., Spector, R., Roberts, R.J., et al.: Use of hemoperfusion for treatment of theophylline intoxication. Am. J. Med. 74:961–966, 1983.

Paterson, J.W., Evans, R.J.C., Prime, F.J.: Selectivity of bronchodilator action of salbutamol in asthmatic patients. Br. J. Dis. Chest 65:21–38, 1971.

Paton, D.M., and Webster D.R.: Clinical pharmacokinetics of H_1-receptor antagonists (the antihistamines). Clin. Pharmacokinet. 10:477–97, 1985.

Pedersen, S., Moller-Petersen, J.: Influence of food on the absorption rate and bioavailability of a sustained release theophylline preparation. Allergy 37:531, 1982.

Pedersen, S., Moller-Petersen, J.: Erratic absorption of a slow-release theophylline sprinkle product caused by food. Pediatrics 74:534, 1984.

Pedersen, S., Moller-Petersen, J.: Influence of food on the absorption of theophylline from a sustained release formulation (Somophyllin). Clin. Allergy 15:253, 1985.

Perry, W.H., Martorano, F., Cotton, E.K.: Management of life-threatening asthma with intravenous isoproterenol infusions. Am. J. Dis. Child 130:39, 1976.

Petrozzi, J.W., Shore, R.N.: Generalized exfoliative dermatitis from ethylenediamine. Arch. Dermatol. 112:525–526, 1976.

Plummer, A.L.: The development of drug tolerance to beta₂ adrenergic agents. Chest 73:949s, 1978.

Pollock, J., Kiechel, F., Cooper, D., et al.: Relationship of serum theophylline concentration to inhibition of exercise-induced bronchospasm and comparison with cromolyn. Pediatrics 60:840, 1977.

Provost, T.T., Jillson, O.F.: Ethylenediamine contact dermatitis. Arch. Dermatol. 96:231–234, 1967.

Rhoades, R.B., Leifer, K.N., Cohan, R., et al.: Suppression of histamine induced pruritus by three antihistaminic drugs. J. Allergy Clin. Immunol. 55:180, 1975.

Richardson, J.B.: The Neural Control of Human Bracheobronchial Smooth Muscle. *In* Lichtenstein, L.M., Austen, K.F. (eds.), Asthma: Physiology, Immunopharmacology, and Treatment. New York, Academic Press, 1977.

Richer, C., Mathier, M., Bah, H., et al.: Theophylline kinetics and ventilatory flow in bronchial asthma and chronic airflow obstruction: Influence of erythromycin. Clin. Pharm. Ther. 31:579, 1982.

Riding, W.D., Dinda, P., Chatterjee, S.S.: The bronchodilator and cardiac effects of five pressure-packed aerosols in asthma. Br. J. Dis. Chest 64:37–45, 1970.

Rolla, G., Bucca, C., Polizzi, S., Maina, A., Giachino, O., Salvini, P.: Nifedipine inhibits deep inspiration–induced bronchoconstriction in asthmatics. Lancet 1:1305–1306, 1982.

Ruffin, R.E., Montgomery J.M., Newhouse, M.: Site of beta-adrenergic receptors in the respiratory tract. Chest 74:256–260, 1978.

Russi, E., Danta, I., Ahmed, T.: Modification of antigen induced bronchoconstriction by the calcium antagonists nifedipine and verapamil. Chest 88:74–78, 1985.

Sadeghi-Nejad, A., Senior, B.: Adrenal function, growth, and insulin in patients treated with corticoids on alternate days. Pediatrics 43:277–283, 1969.

Schaaf, L., Hendeles, L., Weinberger, M.: Hydroxyzine suppression of symptoms of seasonal allergic rhinitis. J. Allergy Clin. Immunol. 13:129–133, 1979.

Settipane, G.A., Klein, D.E., Boyd, G.K., Sturam, J.H., Freye, H.B., Weltman, J.K.: Adverse reactions to cromolyn. J.A.M.A. 241:811–813, 1979.

Shapiro, G.G., and Konig, P.: Cromolyn sodium: A review. Pharmacotherapy 5:156–170, 1985.

Sheffer, A.L., Rocklin, R.E., Goetzi, E.J.: Immunologic components of hypersensitivity reactions to cromolyn sodium. N. Engl. J. Med. 293:1220–1224, 1975.

Simons, F.E.F., Luciuk, G.H., Simons, K.J.: Sustained-release theophylline for treatment of asthma in preschool children. Am. J. Dis. Child. 136:790, 1982.

Simons, K.J., Singh, M., Gillespie, C.A., Simons, F.E.R.: An investigation of the H_1-receptor antagonist tripolidine: Pharmacokinetics and antihistaminic effects. J. Allergy Clin. Immunol. 77:326–330, 1986.

Sintek, C., Hendeles, L., Weinberger, M.: Inhibition of theophylline absorption by activated charcoal. J. Pediatr. 94:314–316, 1979.

Sips, A.P., Adelbroek, P.M., Kulstad, S., et al.: Food does not affect bioavailability of theophylline from Theolin Regard. Eur. J. Clin. Pharmacol. 26:405, 1984.

Smith, M.J., Hodson, M.E.: High-dose beclomethasone inhaler in the treatment of asthma. Lancet 1:265–269, 1983.

Svedmyr, N.: Fenoterol: A beta₂-adrenergic agonist for use in asthma. Pharmacology, pharmacokinetics, clinical efficacy, and adverse effects. Pharmacotherapy 5:109–125, 1985.

Taylor, R.J., Long, W.F., Nelson, H.S.: The development of subsensitivity to chlorpheniramine. J. Allergy Clin. Immunol. 76:103–107, 1985.

Toogood, J.H., Jennings, B., Lefcoe, N.M.: A clinical trial of combined cromolyn/beclomethasone treatment for chronic asthma. J. Allergy Clin. Immunol. 67:317–324, 1981.

Toogood, J.H., Lefcoe, N.M., Haines, D.S.M.: A graded dose assessment of the efficacy of beclomethasone dipropionate aerosol for severe chronic asthma. J. Allergy Clin. Immunol. 59:298–308, 1977.

Toogood, J.H., Lefcoe, N.M., Wonnacott, T.M., McCourtie, D.R., Mullin, J.K.: Cromolyn sodium therapy: Predictors of response. Adv. Asthma Allergy Pulm. Dis. 5:2–15, 1978.

Trzeiakowski, J.P., Levi, R.: Antihistamines. *In* Middleton, E., Reed, C., Ellis, E. (eds.), Allergy: Principles and Practice, 2nd ed. St. Louis, C.V. Mosby Co., 1983.

Weber, R.W., Smith, J.A., Nelson, H.S.: Aerosolized terbutaline in asthmatics: development of subsensitivity with long-term administration. J. Allergy Clin. Immunol. 70:417, 1982.

Weinberger, M.: Theophylline for treatment of asthma. J. Pediatr. 92:1–7, 1978.

Weinberger, M.: The pharmacology and therapeutic use of theophylline. J. Allergy Clin. Immunol. 73:525–766, 1984a.

Weinberger, M.: Theophylline QID, TID, BID, and now QD? A report on 24-hour dosing with slow-release theophylline formulations with emphasis on analysis of data used to obtain Food and Drug Administration approval for Theo-24. Pharmacotherapy 4:181–198, 1984b.

Weinberger, M.: Commentary. Pharmacotherapy 5:169–170, 1985.

Weinberger, M.: Clinical and pharmacokinetic concerns of 24-hour dosing with theophylline. Ann. Allergy 56:2–8, 1986.

Weinberger, M., Bronsky, E.A.: Evaluation of oral bronchodilator therapy. J. Pediatr. 84:421–427, 1974.

Weinberger, M., Bronsky, E.A.: Interaction of ephedrine and theophylline. Clin. Pharmacol. Ther. 17:585–592, 1975.

Weinberger, M., Hendeles, L.: Management of asthma. Post. Med. 61:85, 1977.

Weinberger, M., Hendeles, L.: Role of dialysis in the management and prevention of theophylline toxicity. Dev. Pharmacol. Ther. 1:26–30, 1980.

Weinberger, M., Hendeles, L.: Slow-release theophylline—Rationale and basis for product selection. N. Engl. J. Med. 308:760–764, 1983.

Weinberger, M., Hendeles, L.: Theophylline usage: An overview. J. Allergy Clin. Immunol. 76:277–284, 1985.

Weinberger, M., Hendeles, L., Wong, L., Vaughan L.: Relationship of formulation and dosing interval to fluctuation of serum theophylline concentration in children with chronic asthma. J. Pediatr. 99:145–152, 1981.

Weinberger, M., Milavetz, G.: Influence of formulation on oral drug delivery: Considerations for generic substitution and selection of slow-release products. Iowa Med. 76:24–28, 1986.

Weinberger, M., Milavetz, G., Vaughan, L.: Rate and extent of absorption of Slo-Bid fasting and following a large breakfast (unpublished data on file at Rorer Pharmaceuticals), 1984.

Welling, P.G., Lyons, L.L., Craig, W.A., Trochta, G.A.: Influence of diet and fluid on bioavailability of theophylline. Clin. Pharmacol. Ther. 17:475, 1975.

Wong, L., Hendeles, L., Weinberger, M.: Pharmacologic prophylaxis of allergic rhinitis: Relative efficacy of hydroxyzine and chlorpheniramine. J. Allergy Clin. Immunol. 67:223–228, 1981.

Woodcock, A.A., Johnson, M.A., Geddes, D.M.: Theophylline prescribing, serum concentrations, and toxicity. Lancet 2:610–613, 1983.

Wyatt, R., Weinberger, M., Hendeles, L.: Oral theophylline dosage for the management of chronic asthma. J. Pediatr 92:125–130, 1978.

Zwillich, C.W., Sutton, F.D., Neff, T.A., et al.: Theophylline-induced seizures in adults: correlation with serum concentrations. Ann. Intern. Med. 82:784–787, 1975.

20

Injection Therapy for Allergic Diseases

C. WARREN BIERMAN, M.D.
DAVID S. PEARLMAN, M.D.
BERNARD A. BERMAN, M.D.

DESENSITIZATION, HYPOSENSITIZATION, AND IMMUNOTHERAPY

In 1903, Dunbar introduced the concept of injection treatment of allergic disease. He attempted to develop a passive "antitoxin," *pollantin,* which could be administered topically, by injecting "pollen toxin" into geese and horses; therapeutic results from this procedure were inconsistent. Subsequently, Freeman and Noon (1911) attempted to develop active "immunity" in patients with hay fever by injecting extracts of boiled grass pollen. These investigators reported beneficial results in the 20 grass pollen hay fever patients so treated, and this therapy soon was tried in America. In 1915, Cooke reported the first study in the United States on the successful treatment of hay fever by active immunization. Cooke believed, as had Noon and Freeman, that hay fever was caused by a toxin to which pollen injections induced an antitoxin that "desensitized" the patient to the pollen. By 1922, however, Cooke noted that in spite of clinical improvement, patients still had skin reactions to pollen injections. This reactivity he believed to be due to "unneutralized antibody," and he suggested the term "hyposensitization" in place of "desensitization."

By 1935, Cooke had discovered a substance in the blood of treated patients that could inhibit the Prausnitz-Küstner (PK) test. He called this factor "blocking antibody" and demonstrated that patients with ragweed hay fever would improve clinically if they were transfused with serum from treated patients. Loveless (1940) further characterized blocking antibody as a substance different from reaginic ("allergic") antibody, in its heat stability at 56°C and its failure to bind to human skin. These observations led to a widespread belief that pollen injections ameliorated symptoms of hay fever by producing "nonallergic" antibody that neutralized pollen antigen.

The induction of circulating blocking antibody by allergy injection therapy has been documented extensively, but recent studies suggest that clinical improvement following injection therapy is not due simply to production of blocking antibody. Although the exact mechanism or mechanisms by which injection therapy works are not known, beneficial effects from therapy appear to be antigen-specific. In 1968, Norman et al. suggested "immunotherapy" as a more appropriate term for the treatment of allergic disease by antigen injections. Immunotherapy has become the preferred term for the procedure, though it is used interchangeably with the older term, "hyposensitization," and with "allergy injection therapy."

ANTIGENS USED FOR IMMUNOTHERAPY

A wide variety of antigens have been employed for immunotherapy, ranging from housedust to foods. Many, but not all, have been subjected to controlled clinical trials, primarily in the past two decades. These studies have helped to define the effectiveness of therapy with certain specific antigens and to provide insights into the possible mechanism or mechanisms by which such therapy acts.

Housedust and Housedust Mites. Several controlled studies carried out both in the United States and in Europe have evaluated the efficacy of housedust immunotherapy with positive results generally reported for children and adults who received injections of housedust extracts (Bruun, 1949; Aas, 1971). More recently, it has become apparent that the major allergenic ingredients are housedust mites, allergens from domestic animals, or both (see Chapter 12), although current contention by many clinicians is that there are other allergenic ingredients of importance for selected patients. The fact that definable allergenicity of housedust can be attributed to mites in particular in areas in which their infestation occurs, and otherwise to animal allergens for the most part, has led to the

279

planned withdrawal of approval by the United States Food and Drug Administration (USFDA) for marketing "housedust" per se for injection therapy.

Immunotherapy to housedust mites has been examined extensively in the treatment of allergic rhinitis and asthma and found efficacious in children and adults in some studies but not in all (Bousquet et al., 1985). Of particular interest is a study by Warner et al. (1978) who found that housedust mite–sensitive asthmatic children, injected with extracts of *Dermatophagoides pteronyssinus*, not only improved symptomatically compared with placebo-treated children but tended to lose late bronchial reactions to allergen challenge more than immediate reactivity. Whether this finding has implications regarding reduction in nonspecific bronchial hyperreactivity, with which late responses appear to have some relationship, is unclear. It is of interest, however, that Bousquet et al. (1985), using the same mite allergen but employing a method of "rush" desensitization (see subsequent section), did show reduction in specific bronchial reactivity to the allergen.

Pollens. Ragweed has been the primary pollen studied in the United States. Johnstone (1957), in a placebo-controlled evaluation of immunotherapy for ragweed hay fever showed that patients who received the highest tolerated dose of antigen had significantly greater improvement in symptoms than patients who received low-dose therapy or placebo injections, indicating both efficacy of treatment and antigen dose–dependency for effectiveness of therapy.

In another study, 18 children were given immunotherapy for ragweed hay fever and 17 served as controls (Sadan et al., 1969). Symptom and medication scores were supplemented with measurements of antigen-induced histamine release *in vitro*. IgE levels, antigen-induced histamine release *in vitro*, and blocking antibody also were measured before and after treatment. Thirteen of the 18 treated children had fewer symptoms than any of the control children, and two became completely asymptomatic. The treated group showed a decrease of *in vitro* histamine release in most patients and an increase of blocking antibody, whereas there was little change in these measurements in most of the untreated patients. There were no group differences in changes in IgE levels. In a second study of 24 of these children, all were treated. Those patients who had received placebo during the first year of therapy had significant de-

creases in symptoms, whereas those previously treated maintained their protection (Levy et al., 1971).

A study carried out in both ragweed- and grass-allergic adults evaluated the specificity of pollen immunotherapy by treating with only ragweed antigen and showed that hyposensitization was specific for the antigen used (Norman et al., 1978). Other more recent studies have corroborated and extended previous findings (Norman et al., 1982).

Animal Allergens. In general, there is little indication for immunotherapy with animal allergens. *Animals to which patients are allergic should be removed from their immediate environment.* Evidence for the efficacy of currently available animal extracts is meager. However, Taylor et al. (1978) and Ohman et al. (1984) did demonstrate a reduction in symptoms and specific bronchial reactivity as well as skin test reactivity to cat extract in asthmatic subjects treated by conventional immunotherapy. Ocular but not nasal symptoms also were reduced or delayed in these patients. Other investigators also have found efficacy of treatment to a variable degree utilizing cat and dog allergens with conventional and "rush" immunotherapy techniques (Sundin, 1986). A commercial animal allergen extract may not have sufficiently high concentration of the specific animal allergen to which the patient is most sensitive to be maximally effective, however (Ohman et al., 1984). Immunotherapy to allergens from rodents and other laboratory animals also has been employed in treatment of laboratory workers sensitized to these animals, with some success. Contamination with animal viruses is a potential hazard of immunotherapy to animal allergens, and some cat dander extracts have been found to contain feline leukemia virus, which poses an unknown risk to the recipient.

Mold. Mold antigens are commonly used in the treatment of patients with rhinitis or asthma, when history and allergy test results suggest that these agents play an etiologic role in the illness. Mold antigens appear to be effective in selected cases, but few well-controlled studies on these antigens have been published to date, although a recent one does indicate efficacy (Dreborg et al., 1986).

Foods. Elimination of offending foods from the diet is the primary therapy of food allergy. Not only is there a lack of evidence for benefit from food immunotherapy, but also the possibility of causing or exacerbating food allergy must be kept in mind. For example, in the past, egg-based vaccines that contained significant amounts of egg albumin have been implicated in inducing allergic reactions in egg-sensitive recipients, although most newer egg-based vaccines tend to be sufficiently free of egg allergen that this is a potential problem only in the most highly egg-sensitive recipients. Egg allergy patients should be skin tested to the specific vaccines before administration (Miller et al., 1983). Similarly, patients who have been treated with milk injections to induce fever ("fever therapy") frequently have become allergic to milk and beef products. Oral desensitization of food allergens in general has not been efficacious and is attendant with the risk of provoking anaphylactic reactions in highly sensitive patients.

Insects. Immunotherapy for hypersensitivity to stinging insects of the Hymenoptera group (bees, wasps, hornets, fire ants) is considered in Chapter 52. Although the whole body extract antigens used in years past were of dubious value, specific venom antigens are highly effective in protecting against anaphylaxis (Hunt et al., 1978). The effects of immunotherapy for large reactions to mosquito bites studied many years ago were unimpressive, and such immunotherapy is utilized rarely for mosquito hypersensitivity. Immunotherapy for inhaled insect antigens, such as mayfly and caddis fly, has not been evaluated.

Drugs. Immunotherapy or desensitization may be useful in drug reactions that involve IgE antibody. Patients with penicillin allergy who require penicillin for effective therapy may be given the drug by "rush desensitization" techniques. Similarly, patients with insulin allergy may be "desensitized" to insulin. This topic is discussed more fully in Chapter 53. These techniques tend to produce short-term tolerance to the drug rather than long-term hyposensitization, which can be produced by conventional immunotherapy to inhaled allergens.

Bacterial Vaccines. The use of bacterial vaccines to control "infectious" asthma has been the subject of controversy for years. Numerous clinical studies in children have shown that asthma results from viral rather than bacterial infections (McIntosh et al., 1973). A double-blind study carried out in children showed no benefit for bacterial vaccine treatment (Fontana et al., 1965), as have numerous other studies. One pediatric study (Mueller et al., 1969) suggested that selected children might benefit from the procedure, although there was no overall difference between the treated and placebo

groups. Bacterial vaccines have been withdrawn by the USFDA. Autogenous vaccines, that is, vaccines made from the patient's own flora (e.g., throat culture), have not been subject to scientific scrutiny; there is no credible evidence for their effectiveness. In addition, there is a theoretic risk of inducing arthritis from the injection of killed bacterial antigens.

CONDITIONS THAT MAY RESPOND TO IMMUNOTHERAPY

Immunotherapy can be beneficial in the treatment of certain IgE-mediated disorders as follows: *seasonal allergic rhinitis* (hay fever) (Frankland and Augustin, 1954; Johnstone, 1957; Sadan et al., 1969; Levy et al., 1971), *perennial allergic rhinitis* (Bruun, 1949), and the *allergic component of asthma* (Johnstone, 1968; Aas, 1970 and 1971; Warner et al., 1978; Taylor et al., 1978; Fink, 1985). Less clear is its usefulness in managing the complications of rhinitis, such as *otitis media with effusion, middle ear dysfunction,* and *sinusitis.* These complications occur in part because of nasal obstruction and obstruction of the eustachian tubes or sinus ostia by edematous nasal mucosa, and it is reasonable to expect that any therapy that decreases rhinitis may lead to improved middle ear and paranasal sinus functions (see Chapters 34 to 36).

The effectiveness of immunotherapy in asthma is more controversial. Recent findings suggest that reactions to allergens are responsible for aspects of bronchial hyperreactivity that characterize asthma (Lichtenstein et al., 1984). Larsen and colleagues (1985) have developed an animal model of both early and late reactions in asthma. IgG antibody from active or passive immunizations ablates the late response but has relatively less and possibly no significant effect on the early response to antigen challenge. Studies in humans are consistent with this finding using *Alternaria* (Metzer et al., 1983), *D. pteronyssinus* (Warner et al., 1978), and grass pollen (Reid et al., 1986; Adler et al., 1985); these studies have shown a decrease in the late phase response, associated with inflammation and bronchial hyperreactivity, which is believed to play a major role in the pathogenesis of asthma.

There is little evidence that immunotherapy will benefit atopic dermatitis although there are anecdotal reports of benefit. If used for coexisting respiratory allergy, immunotherapy should be administered cautiously, since it is commonly accepted that dermatitis may be exacerbated if antigen concentration is increased too rapidly, especially during pollen season. Immunotherapy has been administered for many other conditions, including food allergy, migraine headache, vasomotor rhinitis, intrinsic (nonallergic) asthma, and chronic urticaria. There is no evidence that it is beneficial in any of these conditions.

Immunotherapy decreases but, rarely, totally eliminates symptoms; its beneficial effects vary widely from patient to patient. Some may show dramatic improvement, whereas others may show negligible or no improvement. It is most likely to be successful if the number of problematic allergens can be limited, the therapeutic dosages to offending allergens can be maximized, and the concomitant exposures to allergens and irritants can be minimized.

MECHANISMS OF ACTION

Immunotherapy induces a number of immune changes in the host. The induction of "blocking antibody," described by Cooke (1935) and Loveless (1940), presumably results in interception of antigen before it has an opportunity to interact with cell bound–specific IgE, thereby diminishing the opportunity for antigen-induced IgE-mediated histamine release. The correlation between blocking antibody titers and symptom improvement is relatively poor, however, and recent investigations suggest that the effects of immunotherapy involve considerably more than the production of IgG antibodies.

Immunologically, a variety of changes have been demonstrated that may in part be responsible for the relief of allergic symptoms. Among these changes are (1) a rise in serum IgG "blocking" antibodies; (2) a suppression in the usual seasonal rise in IgE antibodies, which follows environmental exposure, and a slow decline during several years in the level of specific IgE antibodies (although complete disappearance is rare); (3) an increase in blocking IgA and IgG antibodies in secretions; (4) a reduction in basophil reactivity and sensitivity to allergens (as determined by *in vitro* leukocyte histamine release studies); and (5) a reduction of *in vitro* lymphocyte responsiveness to allergens (Norman, 1985).

Patients receiving immunotherapy for hay fever show an initial rise in specific IgE antibody levels for pollen antigen. As treatment progresses, specific IgE antibody levels gradually decline. Treated patients no longer demonstrate the seasonal increases in specific IgE antibody seen in untreated populations (Berg and Johannson, 1971; Yunginger and Gleich, 1973). Long-term treatment also produces a decrease in the sensitivity of mediator cells in many patients, with a resulting decrease in antigen-induced basophil histamine release; a stimulation of IgA and IgG blocking antibody in nasal secretions (Norman, 1978); a decrease in the proliferative response of T cells to antigen; and other changes, such as decreased numbers of T lymphocytes with IgM antibody markers on their surfaces in some patients (Neiburger 1978; Rocklin, 1980); and generation of antigen-specific T suppressor cells.

Of these changes, suppression of specific IgE antibody synthesis and development of secretory "blocking" antibodies would appear to be of particular importance in reducing mucosal reactivity to aerosolized antigen. These blocking antibodies are capable of binding to specific antibody and presumably thereby of inhibiting IgE antibody–induced histamine release. Immunotherapy produced a four-fold increase in blocking antibody titers of both IgG and IgA class antibodies but did not alter the ratio of IgG to IgA blocking antibodies or to IgE antibodies in one study (Platts-Mills et al., 1976). Serum blocking antibody titers, in other words, do not accurately reflect local blocking antibody production. Most important to this discussion, several studies in humans, previously cited, indicate that immunotherapy changes the late-phase reaction to bronchial challenge more than it changes the immediate reaction. Since the late-phase reaction may be partially inflammatory, it may be particularly important in the development of nonspecific reactivity, and immunotherapy could favorably influence it. *Thus, recent evidence makes a somewhat different case for immunotherapy from the traditional one and indicates that bronchial hyperreactivity is susceptible to improvement by proper management of allergic reactions* (Norman, 1985).

STANDARDIZATION OF ANTIGENS USED FOR IMMUNOTHERAPY

The lack of highly specific potent antigens has been a limiting factor to effective immunotherapy. All commercially produced pollen extracts, for example, contain a number of protein antigens, but only a few are associated with the specific biologic activity of the extract. Some of the clinically unimportant material may produce adverse immune reactions that limit the amount of extract the patient can tolerate. The standardization of allergenic extracts has been a major problem since Noon first initiated pollen injections. Specific methods of standardization have varied from laboratory to laboratory, and the reactivity of a group of extracts may appear to differ by ten- to 100-fold in one test, but only two- or three-fold in another test (Baer, 1978).

Initially, antigens were standardized on the basis of the amount of soluble protein that could be extracted from a given quantity of pollen. Noon defined his pollen unit as one one-millionth of the quantity of protein that could be extracted from 1 gm of pollen. This unit was superseded by a weight to volume system in which a given weight of dried extracted protein was diluted in a volume of solution. A further refinement converted the weight to volume system to a protein-nitrogen unit system in which the protein content of the solutions was determined and expressed in terms of protein nitrogen units (1 PNU = 0.00001 mg of protein-nitrogen). Though all three systems are still in use, none determines the *specific allergen content*, so that different lots of antigen, even from the same firm, may vary widely in allergen potency. Accordingly, new methods of standardization are being developed, and in the United States federal standards are being set and gradually being made more stringent as techniques improve.

Identification of several of the allergenic components of ragweed pollen and the development of specific antisera have allowed the FDA to initiate a program for standardization of short ragweed, which has greatly improved the uniformity of commercial products. This approach has yet to be applied to the many other extracts of airborne allergens being marketed in the United States. The Protein Laboratory in Denmark has successfully applied crossed immunoelectrophoresis and crossed radioimmunoelectrophoresis with allergic human serums to the problem of characterization of a variety of extracts. These methods, coupled with isoelectric focusing and radioallergosorbent test (RAST) inhibition, are being employed to develop well-characterized standards for a number of common allergens by a committee of the International Union of Immunologic Societies. At the same time, techniques for testing production batches for their ability to match the standard are being normalized. Thus, the technology is at hand to standardize the complex reagents required for definitive clinical studies and to make available to clinicians those materials that prove to be efficacious (Lichtenstein et al., 1984).

PRINCIPLES OF IMMUNOTHERAPY

Immunotherapy is an adjunct to allergic management, not a substitute for it. The overall goal of allergic management is to minimize symptoms and reduce the need for drugs. The first priority is to identify major offending allergens and irritants and to eliminate them from home, school, or work environment. *Immunotherapy should be reserved for those allergic factors that cannot be eliminated and that appear to play a major role in the patient's allergic disease.* The patient or parent should be presented with the facts of what immunotherapy can and cannot do. They should understand that *immunotherapy can help control but not cure symptoms.* Furthermore, they should be offered a choice as to whether or not the benefits are worth the time, effort, inconvenience, and expense. Immunotherapy may be of greatest benefit to patients with the most severe symptoms and in whom skin and nasal sensitivity is the most pronounced (D'Souza et al., 1973).

Patient Selection. Severity and duration of the disease will have a strong bearing on recommending immunotherapy (Rocklin, 1983). Patients who have moderate or even severe respiratory symptoms during short, well-defined pollen seasons of 1 to 3 weeks may well elect medications, such as antihistamines, topical intranasal cromolyn or corticosteroid sprays, or even *short courses* of parenteral steroids, rather than immunotherapy.

Patients with multiple seasonal allergic symptoms may be candidates for immunotherapy, especially if the symptoms induce physical or emotional hardships that interfere with normal daily activities or reduce substantially the quality of life. For example, the patient may be unable to sleep or may cough so much at night that no one else in the house can sleep. Immunotherapy may relieve the symptoms sufficiently to allow the patient to function effectively at school or at work. It also may lessen some of the complications of chronic allergic rhinitis, such as sinusitis, recurrent upper respiratory infections, and recurrent otitis media or effusion. Johnstone and Dutton (1968) suggested that immunotherapy may lessen the development of allergic asthma, though no comparable study can confirm or refute this suggestion.

Selection of Antigens. Any physician involved in the formulation of programs for immunotherapy should be familiar with the principal allergen sources in the geographic area (see Chapters 11 and 12). Extracts of local varieties of grass and weeds should be included in the injections if the clinical and laboratory results indicate sensitivities to these substances. Allergen sources with minor roles in the patient's clinical symptoms, such as trees that pollinate only 2 or 3 weeks each year, may be omitted in favor of symptomatic treatment during these critical periods. In cases in which different members of the same plant family are known to strongly cross-react, the physician can select the most prevalent members of the group for inclusion in the treatment program and exclude the others, keeping in mind, however, that cross-reactivity of clinically important allergens may not be complete. Whereas several antigens may be combined safely in the same mixture, the use of an excessive number of antigens should be avoided, especially those of minor importance. Attempts to include extracts of every possible allergen may diminish the overall effectiveness of immunotherapy. Patients may receive suboptimal doses of the clinically significant allergens and get little benefit from the others. In treating young children, a special effort should be made to combine extracts into one vial to minimize the number of injections per visit.

To be condemned is the practice by some firms and by some physicians who market allergens by making up treatment mixtures arbitrarily on the basis of a skin test or RAST sheet submitted by a physician, without regard to the patient's history, symptoms, or clinical course.

PRINCIPLES OF TECHNIQUE

Preparation of Solutions. Treatment antigens should be prescribed individually for each patient by the physician supervising therapy, and a copy of the prescription retained by the consultant physician, preferably on the patient's chart. The antigen set and its container should be labeled clearly with the patient's name, specific contents, antigen concentrations, and expiration date. Color coding labels according to concentration further safeguard against a mistake in dosage. Clearly written instructions for administration should accompany the antigen set (Table 20–1) and should include a general description of antigen content (e.g., tree, grass, and weed pollen), a schedule that lists the dose and frequency of injections during the period of increasing antigen concentration, the projected maintenance dosage, the frequency of maintenance injections, and the specific emergency procedures to be followed in case of adverse reactions (Table 20–2). If more than one antigen mixture is used, a separate sheet should be used for each.

Perennial and Preseasonal Immunotherapy. The selection of an appropriate treatment schedule involves a choice between two forms of therapy, *perennial* and *preseasonal.* Both approaches involve weekly or biweekly injections of allergen in increasing doses until a maximum tolerated dose is reached.

In preseasonal therapy, injections are begun 3 to 4 months before the anticipated onset of the pollen season. The goal is to reach the maximum tolerated dosage by the beginning of the season, at which point the treatment is discontinued until the following year. (Coseasonal therapy in which an attempt is made to decrease allergen sensitivity by a form of immunotherapy strictly within the problem season has been abandoned for the most part, because of poor therapeutic results.)

With perennial immunotherapy, the patient is placed on a year-round maintenance schedule with the highest tolerated dose. Clinical and immunologic evidence suggest that perennial treatment allows the patient to tolerate a higher cumulative dose of antigen, which results in better clinical protection than preseasonal treatment. Once maintenance dosage has been reached, the frequency of maintenance injections depends on the patient's symptoms. An advantage of preseasonal therapy is in maximizing the motivation of the patient to follow through with an immunotherapy schedule since it is instituted in a relatively short time before and in anticipation of the problematic allergen season. On the other hand, the total number of injections required during the course of 3 to 5 years of therapy tend eventually to be substantially less in perennial therapy. In addition, the goal in perennial immunotherapy is to reach a monthly maintenance schedule, though some allergists prefer to increase the injections to every 1 to 2 weeks immediately before the pollen season.

Though perennial treatment for pollen aller-

TABLE 20–1. Antigen Dosage Sheet*

Name _____ Date _____ Doctor _____
Direction for Administration of _____ antigen

Read Carefully: Roll bottle and shake. Measure accurately with a tuberculin syringe. Give subcutaneously in the triceps area (outer arm). *In the event of a systemic reaction call this office for further instruction. The patient should remain under observation 20 minutes after injection.*

If a Systemic Reaction Occurs: (diffuse redness, itching, hoarseness, dyspnea, or wheezing):
(1.) Apply a tourniquet above the site of the injection. (2.) Give 0.2 ml 1 : 1000 aqueous epinephrine into the injection site. (3.) Give 0.2 ml epinephrine into opposite arm. (4.) Have oxygen readily available.

In Case of Question Regarding Antigen Administration: Please call (prescribing physician's telephone number). You should attempt to follow the schedule outline below, vials No. 1, No. 2, No. 3, and No. 4 should be given weekly until maintenance dose is reached. In case of a significant local reaction (greater than ¾ in) resulting from the injection, the dosage must be dropped back two doses. This is repeated once, then again attempt to follow the schedule as outlined.†

Warning: Do not increase dosage during pollen season if patient has severe hay fever or asthma.	These injections should be administered under a physician's supervision. All other arrangements are at patient's own risk.

VIAL NO. 0		VIAL NO. 1‡		VIAL NO. 2		VIAL NO. 3		VIAL NO. 4	
1 : 1,000,000		1 : 100,000		1 : 10,000		1 : 1,000		1 : 100	
DOSE NO.	ML	DOSE NO.	ML	DOSE NO.	ML	DOSE NO.	ML	DOSE NO.	ML
1	0.05	1	0.05	8	0.05	16	0.05	24	0.03
2	0.10	2	0.10	9	0.07	17	0.07	25	0.05
3	0.20	3	0.15	10	0.10	18	0.10	26	0.07
4	0.30	4	0.20	11	0.15	19	0.15	27	0.10
5	0.40	5	0.30	12	0.20	20	0.20	28	0.15
6	0.50	6	0.40	13	0.30	21	0.30	29	0.20
		7	0.50	14	0.40	22	0.40	30	0.25
				15	0.50	23	0.50	31	0.30

Maintenance Dosage: _____ ml, 1 : 100 every _____ weeks. Replace this vaccine by _____

DATE	DILUTION	DOSAGE	NOTES	DATE	DILUTION	DOSAGE	NOTES

* Immunotherapy for moderately sensitive patients.
† Number of intervals can be decreased for less sensitive patients or increased for very sensitive ones.
‡ The bars under the vial numbers should be color coded to match the labels on the corresponding vials.

TABLE 20-2. General Information and Precautions for Injections of Allergen Solutions

1. Treatments should be administered under the direct supervision of a licensed physician.
2. Keep all solutions in the dark, in the refrigerator.
3. Never give an injection unless you have on hand a syringe and epinephrine hydrochloride (Adrenalin) 1:1000 for use in case of a reaction.
4. Cleanse the skin with 70 percent alcohol before injection. Use a 0.5 or 1.0 cc tuberculin syringe and administer in the arm subcutaneously. *Always pull back the piston of the syringe before an injection of allergen solution.* If blood appears in the syringe, always change the position of the needle point to make sure that the solution is not injected into a blood vessel.
5. Always keep the patient under observation for at least 20 minutes after an injection.
6. Reduce the dosage 50 percent during the pollen season if the patient is having moderate to severe symptoms.
7. If a systemic reaction occurs (usual manifestations of hives, acute hay fever, paroxysmal coughing, asthma, cyanosis, flushing, perspiration, nausea, vomiting, dizziness, fainting, or collapse), place a tourniquet around the patient's arm above the site of the injection and inject 0.25 cc of epinephrine into the site of the allergy injection and 0.25 cc in the opposite arm. Repeat the epinephrine at 15-minute intervals for three doses as necessary, and release the tourniquet occasionally so that you do not embarrass the circulation. Administer oxygen by mask. Give 200 mg of hydrocortisone or equivalent by iv injection. An antihistamine (e.g., chlorpheniramine 10 mg) should be injected intramuscularly or slowly and intravenously.
7a. If the patient continues to have respiratory distress or hypotension, begin an intravenous infusion with 5 percent glucose in normal saline, insert oral airway, if necessary, and transfer to nearest hospital for further treatment.
7b. *Subsequent doses of allergen must be reduced.*
8. If the patient experiences trouble because of injections, such as sore arms or more general forms of reactions, it may not be possible to proceed as rapidly as indicated in the schedule. Under such circumstances, it is better practice to go back to a well-tolerated dose and to increase, if possible, by smaller increments than those originally suggested. Conversely, some patients may be able to tolerate more rapid increases than those indicated on the schedule. This depends upon the judgment of the attending physician.
9. In our experience, the perennial method of treatment is the most effective regimen for the patient. With this technique, injections are continued all year. The frequency is determined by the patient's clinical response. Usually, if the patient is doing well after the initial program of immunization is completed, the frequency can be reduced to every 2 weeks, then every 3 weeks, and finally to once a month.
10. *In the event that treatments are inadvertently missed and the patient's injections are spaced more than 4 weeks apart, the dose should be reduced to avoid the possibility of a systemic reaction.* For each week beyond 4 weeks, we recommend the dose be decreased by 50 percent. For example, if the patient had last received 0.50 cc and the interval between injections was 8 weeks, then the patient's dosage should be reduced one full bottle (to 0.50 ml of a tenfold lower concentration).
11. The presence of mild upper respiratory allergic symptoms is not a contraindication for administering the injection. Active wheezing demands other treatment.

gies may be started during the pollen season, if the initial dose is small, it probably is wiser to wait until the end of the season, especially if the patient has extreme sensitivity or if the symptoms are severe. Pollen-sensitive patients who have reached a maintenance level before the season begins should receive a slightly reduced dose during the season. This procedure minimizes the chance of a sudden systemic reaction due to the combination of injected and inhaled pollens.

A third treatment technique, "rush desensitization," developed originally in the 1930's, may be used for certain specific substances, such as penicillin and insulin, or for anaphylactic sensitivity to stinging insects. This procedure usually requires that the patient be hospitalized, with an intravenous infusion running and appropriate emergency equipment immediately at hand. Injections of allergen extract are

administered every 15 to 30 minutes for up to 2 days. The rationale behind this approach for desensitization to drugs is to gradually bind circulating IgE antibodies and to achieve a state of "antigen excess." Patients subjected to rush desensitization must be monitored very carefully for the appearance of severe local and systemic reactions. In general, only life-threatening clinical conditions justify the risk associated with this procedure.

Initial Dose. The initial dose of allergen extract must be adjusted carefully to the sensitivity of the patient. The severity of clinical symptoms, the intensity of skin test reactions, the prior history of systemic reactions, and the patient's age should be considered. Young children usually tolerate a more concentrated initial dose than do adolescents or adults. For patients with moderate sensitivity, the customary starting dose is in the range of 1:10,000 to

1:100,000 weight by volume (w/v) of the anticipated final dose.* Some allergists prefer to determine the starting point by performing serial skin tests, beginning at 1:1,000,000 and increasing the concentrations ten-fold with each skin test, selecting as the beginning dose a solution that is 5 to 10 times as dilute as that producing a positive test result. If the patient tolerates the first injection of dilute extract without a significant local reaction, therapy can proceed at weekly or biweekly intervals with increments of 0.05 to 0.10 ml or with increments of approximately 50 percent greater than the preceding dose, depending on the individual treatment schedule. When the dose reaches 0.50 ml, the entire process should begin again, with 0.05 to 0.10 ml injection of an extract that is 5 to 10 times stronger than the original. Any reaction larger than a 2-cm local reaction or a systemic reaction requires an adjustment in the dosage schedule (see Reactions).

Maintenance levels usually are reached in 3 to 6 months, depending on the sensitivity of the patient. At that time, the interval between injections may be increased gradually, depending on the patient's symptoms. For many patients, the maintenance dose is 0.50 ml of a 1:50 or 1:100 w/v extract. In many cases, however, this dose or concentration cannot be reached without severe reaction, necessitating a lower dose for maintenance.

Who Should Administer Allergy Injections? Allergy injections should be administered only by trained personnel *under the direct supervision of the physician, with the physician immediately available.* Appropriate emergency equipment including a syringe and an aqueous 1:1000 epinephrine must be within reach. Once the consulting physician has established a diagnosis and a suitable treatment program, the administration of immunotherapy may be turned over to the patient's primary physician. If not unduly inconvenient for the patient, it may be wise to supervise the procedure in the consulting physician's office until maintenance dosage is reached, however, in order to facilitate a rapid but safe progression of therapy. Because of the risk of anaphylaxis, *parents or patients never should be permitted to administer injections at home.* It is important that the patient return once or twice a year to the consultant for follow-up examination to review the patient's clinical status and progress with treatment and to adjust the immunotherapy and other treatment program if necessary.

Pre-Injection Precautions. Vials containing allergenic extracts should be stored in a refrigerator but not in the freezer compartment. Color-coded labels and dosage sheets provide safeguards against mistakes. Serious reactions can occur if the wrong extract or wrong concentration of the right extract is administered; always crosscheck the vial against the treatment card and ask the patient to repeat his or her name and address and, perhaps, birth date.

Administration. The injection of antigen should be given in the upper, outer aspect of the arm, midway between the shoulder and elbow, staying away from the elbow and shoulder joints. This area permits sufficient space for a tourniquet in the event of a systemic reaction. To minimize the pain of injection, it is suggested that the extract be administered with a 26- or 27-gauge ⅝-in needle. The injection should be given deep subcutaneously, and great care should be taken *not* to inject antigen directly into the blood stream, drawing back the plunger to be certain that a blood vessel has not been entered before administering the antigen.

Long-term storage of allergenic extracts diminishes their potency; thus, special precautions are necessary when changing vials. Since the exact degree of potency loss is not predictable empirically, the dose generally is reduced to one half the maintenance dose or to as much as one full dilution (e.g., from 1:100 to 1:1000), on changing from an old to a newly prepared antigen. It is then increased weekly back to the maintenance dose. If the treatment schedule is disrupted by such events as a patient's vacation or illness, the dose should be adjusted based on the time elapsed. We suggest that if 2 to 4 weeks have passed, the previous dose should be repeated; beyond 4 weeks, the dose should be dropped 50 percent for every week missed.

Reactions. Following the injection, the patient should be instructed to wait 20 to 30 minutes before leaving the physician's office. Severe reactions can occur after this time period, but the vast majority of life-threatening reactions will occur within this time period (Lockey et al., 1987). The patient should be examined by the physician or by the medical assistant before being permitted to leave.

---

* Since most allergen solutions are mixtures of various allergens in unequal amounts, any terminology including weight by volume is misleading. It is employed, however, to represent a general order of magnitude of allergen concentration.

If the patient does experience a systemic reaction — rhinorrhea, nasal itching, hoarseness, tight chest, generalized hives, or extreme weakness — 0.1 to 0.25 ml of 1:1000 aqueous epinephrine should be administered subcutaneously into the injection site and an equal amount into the opposite arm. A tourniquet should be applied proximal to the site to slow the absorption of the antigen. If necessary, additional epinephrine and injectable antihistamines may be used (see Chapter 51). Emergency equipment should be readily available, and the physician and trained personnel immediately accessible to treat any patient with a reaction.

Many patients develop small wheals at the injection sites, resembling mosquito bites. These do not require any attention in the treatment schedule. However, it is recommended that the dose be repeated rather than increased (if not on maintenance dosage) if swelling 2 cm or greater in diameter occurs or if swelling persists for 24 hours. If swelling is larger than 2 cm, the next injection should be reduced by 0.10 to 0.30 ml. Continued local reaction should be discussed with the allergist. If reactions occur after 3 or 4 months of therapy, the patient may have reached the maximal tolerated dose.

Large local reactions indicate that the patient has a significant potential for developing a systemic reaction, and the dose must be reduced accordingly. *Systemic reactions can occur even in the absence of prior local reactions, however.*

Delayed reactions generally appear between 12 and 24 hours after the injection and may be either local or systemic. Delayed local reactions resemble large soft bruises and can be treated with oral antihistamine, aspirin (in patients in whom aspirin use is permitted), or local application of an ice pack. If a delayed local reaction occurs, the dosage should be adjusted by the consultant.

Delayed systemic reactions are the most difficult to recognize. They usually appear as a slight or moderate flare-up of the patient's symptoms, with increased rhinorrhea or sneezing, for example. This type of reaction is not serious, but it indicates that the patient has received too large a dose of antigen and that the dose should be reduced to a level that does not induce symptoms.

Duration of Therapy. The first year of immunotherapy generally is considered a trial period. If the patient responds favorably, the maintenance injections are continued until the patient has been relatively free of symptoms for a year or more. The entire treatment program may last from 2 to 5 years, with an average duration of 3 years. Some patients relapse when injections are stopped and must resume therapy for continued relief.

Not all patients benefit from immunotherapy, and some patients may not improve until the second year of treatment. Treatment failures may be due to inadequate dosage, inactive extracts, incorrect diagnosis, or continued exposure to allergens, such as domestic animals that contribute substantially to symptomatology. Patients who improve initially and then experience an increase in symptoms in a later season may have acquired additional allergies, may have developed another condition, or may have experienced significant environmental change, introducing increased exposure to similar or other allergens.

It cannot be emphasized enough that treatment failures often are due to neglect of environmental controls. The patient or parent may believe that immunotherapy negates the need to eliminate allergenic factors from the environment or permits unlimited exposure to the allergens to which the patient is being treated. If this is the case, the physician must educate the patient or parent again about the goals of allergic management and the limitations of immunotherapy.

TYPES OF ANTIGEN PREPARATIONS AVAILABLE

Aqueous Extracts. The original antigen administered by Noon and Freeman was protein, extracted from grass pollen by boiling. Because boiling inactivated some proteins, extraction at room temperature was substituted using buffered saline solution. Such buffered aqueous antigens have had the most widespread use, and their clinical and immune effects have been studied in greatest depth.

There have been no well-documented adverse effects other than the occurrence of local or systemic reactions to injections (Rocklin, 1983 and Negrini et al., 1985). Although these cannot be avoided entirely when high dose therapy is used, these reactions can be handled easily if appropriate emergency equipment is immediately available. Aqueous immunotherapy has been studied in pregnancy, and no adverse maternal or fetal effects have appeared (Metzger et al., 1978). (Nevertheless, it is wise to be conservative with regard to *instituting* immunotherapy during pregnancy). Aqueous extracts have a major disadvantage in that therapeutic effectiveness requires multiple injections over a prolonged period of time. Local and systemic reactions also limit the total amount of antigen that can be administered. With ragweed, for example, 50 to 100 μg antigen E is the maximal amount that can be administered in a year of therapy (Norman and Lichtenstein, 1978).

Alum-Precipitated, Pyridine-Extracted Antigens. In an effort to increase the antigenic stimulus while decreasing the number of local and systemic reactions, a pyridine-extracted, alum-precipitated antigen was introduced (Allpyral). This antigen became the center of great controversy in the late 1960's when a study of ragweed immunotherapy showed it to be without potency for ragweed antigen (Lichtenstein et al., 1968). At the same time, other investigators showed inhibition of histamine release and development of blocking antibody to grass pollen antigens (Weinstock and Starr, 1970). The differences in immunogenicity appeared to be related to a step in the extraction process that denatured the ragweed antigen but not grass antigen. A subsequent study of alum-precipitated, pyridine-extracted grass antigen confirmed that it was equivalent clinically and immunologically to aqueous grass antigen (Bierman et al., 1972). Studies of other alum-pyridine antigens have not been performed.

Alum-Precipitated, Aqueous-Extracted Antigens. Though alum-precipitated pollen antigens were first introduced more than four decades ago (Stull et al., 1940), in-depth studies were not carried out until the 1970's. Therapy with alum-precipitated ragweed antigens showed them to be effective in stimulating blocking antibodies. Amelioration of symptoms was similar to that attained with aqueous extracts, with fewer injections and fewer local and systemic reactions (Norman and Lichtenstein, 1978). Similar results were obtained using alum-precipitated grass antigens (Bierman et al., 1972). The effectiveness of other alum-precipitated antigens has yet to be determined.

SAFETY AND COMPLICATIONS OF IMMUNOTHERAPY

Short-term Effects

Both the physician and patient must realize that immunotherapy is a potentially dangerous treatment, since the margin between optimal dosages and those that induce adverse reactions is narrow. Some local swelling, itching, and redness at the injection site is inevitable. In a large study, systemic reactions, such as increased rhinitis, worsening of asthma, generalized urticaria, and anaphylaxis, were observed in 0.1 percent of subjects (Vervloet et al., 1980). In this series only two of more than 150,000 injections resulted in anaphylaxis, which required (and responded to) epinephrine injection. Other workers, however, have reported that the risk of anaphylaxis may range from 8 to 30 percent per patient course (Levy, 1980).

Umetsu et al. (1985) reported one patient who had anaphylaxis from immunotherapy that progressed to serum sickness with fever, arthralgia, urticaria, and eventually hemorrhagic rash, splenomegaly, abdominal pain, proteinuria, and neurologic symptoms suggestive of cerebral vasculitis. This appears to be an extremely unusual adverse reaction to immunotherapy.

Lockey et al. (1987) conducted a retrospective study of patients who died from skin testing or immunotherapy in the last 40 years in the United States. Of the 30 subjects whose records were complete enough for analysis, 24 deaths resulted from immunotherapy injections. Eleven of the 24 were unusually sensitive to the injected allergens. Of the 30 subjects, the records of 24 permitted an estimation of the time that elapsed between the injection and the onset of the systemic reaction. Twenty had symptoms in 20 minutes or less (half in less than 10 minutes), one in approximately 30 minutes, and three in more than 30 minutes.

Long-term Effects

Murray et al. (1985) reported that long-term immunotherapy with *Dermatophagoides farinae* can lead to increased bronchial reactivity to histamine not seen in control subjects. Asthma in the treated patients in Murray's report did not improve. As reflected by twice or thrice daily peak flow measurements, they postulated that this increased bronchial reactivity was caused by iatrogenic subclinical mite-induced pulmonary inflammation. An increase in bronchial reactivity from mite immunotherapy has been reported by others (Gabriel et al., 1977; Davies et al., 1979).

Other studies of mite immunotherapy, however, have reported a decreased responsiveness to bronchial challenge by specific antigen and improvement in asthma symptoms, as judged by symptom scores and medication diaries (Warner et al., 1978; Newton et al., 1978). Formgren et al. (1985) reported that bronchial sensitivity to allergen was significantly less in mite-treated patients as compared with placebo-treated patients. Histamine sensitivity increased similarly in both groups.

In studies of cat-1 immunotherapy, 50 treated patients showed a significant decrease in histamine bronchial reactivity, as compared with placebo-treated patients whose reactivity did not change (Sundin, 1986).

Safety during Pregnancy

Studies carried out on 90 atopic mothers who received immunotherapy through 121 pregnancies revealed no adverse effects on the offspring (Metzger et al., 1978; Greenberger et al., 1978). Specifically, the incidence of prematurity, abortion, neonatal death, and congenital malformation in this group did not differ from that of the general population. Nevertheless, it would be prudent to withhold immunotherapy from untreated patients who are pregnant until after delivery, to minimize the risk of potential systemic reactions on the fetus.

Studies of children at 10 years of age or older born to women receiving immunotherapy during pregnancy showed no adverse effects of treatment. Immunotherapy did not prevent the development of atopic disease, such as rhinitis or asthma, in the offspring (Settipane et al., 1987).

CONTROVERSIAL ANTIGENS AND TECHNIQUES

In allergy treatment, a number of techniques evolved, enjoyed a period of popularity, and were discarded ultimately, when they were proved to be ineffective, naively conceived in the light of new knowledge, or potentially harmful.

Histamine "Desensitization." With the identification of histamine as a mediator of the allergic reaction, histamine injections were introduced to treat a variety of "allergic" disorders between 1930 and 1950. Histamine was administered either intravenously or by serial injections for such disorders as vascular headache, known as "histamine cephalgia" (Hanes,

1969; Horton, 1941). This form of therapy is no longer employed.

Antigen Emulsification in Oil. Antigens were emulsified in mineral oil to slow absorption and permit the administration of a large total dose in a single injection. This procedure was popularized as a "one-shot" treatment for hay fever. In addition to significant systemic reactions, local reactions consisting of sterile abscesses or mineral oil tumors are associated with such therapy. Evidence that mineral oil injections can induce myelomas in mice led to abandonment of this procedure (Potter, 1962).

Oral Desensitization to Foods. Another technique popularized for treatment of food allergy was oral desensitization, that is, the administration of progressively increasing amounts of the food to which the child is allergic. Though this is still practiced by some physicians, there is no immunologic evidence of effectiveness.

Other Controversial Techniques. Techniques such as antigen titration ("Rinkel method") (Van Metre et al., 1980) and sublingual drops have never been of proven benefit. These are discussed in Chapter 57.

PROSPECTS FOR THE FUTURE

Current research on therapeutic antigens involves their chemical modification by such substances as formalin (allergoids), ultraviolet light, urea, and polymerization; isolation of purified specific antigens; and therapeutic techniques, such as topical (intranasal) immunotherapy. These are reviewed by Grammer et al. (1985).

Allergoids. Allergoids are pollen antigens that have been modified by formalin. They are able to stimulate blocking antibodies while they induce fewer allergic reactions because they react poorly with IgE. Clinical studies of both ragweed and grass antigens showed that patients developed higher titers of IgG antibodies the first 2 years of treatment with allergoids as compared with conventional antigen preparations and also had fewer symptoms during the pollen season (Marsh et al., 1972). Recent studies of therapy with ragweed allergoids (Meriney et al., 1986) and high molecular weight grass pollen allergoids show effective suppression of symptoms when compared with placebo injections (Bousquet et al., 1987).

Urea Denatured Antigens. Urea treatment dissociates the two noncovalently bound chains of ragweed antigen E to reduce its allergenicity 10,000 fold. In mice, dissociated chains suppress IgE antibody responses possibly by stimulating suppressor T cells. In humans, limited clinical trials have shown only minimal efficacy (Norman et al., 1980).

Polymerized Antigens. Polymerized antigens were developed on the hypothesis that equal weights of polymerized allergens and monomeric allergens would be similarly immunogenic but that polymerized allergens would be less allergenic. This difference would enable the safe administration of large doses of allergens in a few injections. Studies of polymerized whole ragweed and of polymerized ragweed antigen E showed that such antigens can induce clinical and immune protection equivalent to that obtained with aqueous antigen, with fewer local or systemic reactions (Metzger et al., 1976; Patterson et al., 1978; Bacal et al., 1978). Subsequent double-blind multicenter studies of polymerized ragweed antigen have indicated efficacy in ragweed pollenosis (Hendrix et al., 1980; Grammer et al., 1982). Polymerized grass pollen antigens have been studied in double-blind fashion and appear to be safe and effective in grass-sensitive patients (Grammer et al., 1983 and 1986).

Ultraviolet Irradiated Antigens. These have been studied primarily in Europe (Henocq et al., 1973). Housedust antigens irradiated with ultraviolet light lose their ability to induce positive skin test results or induce bronchial reactions. When used for immunotherapy they appeared to protect as well as standard antigens. No studies in the United States have been carried out.

Isolation of Purified Specific Antigens. This technique has already improved the effectiveness of immunotherapy for Hymenoptera anaphylaxis (Hunt et al., 1978); the identification of the specific allergen of ragweed pollen has improved the quality of ragweed antigens. The progress in identification and purification of other specific antigens should advance the specificity and effectiveness of immunotherapy in general.

Topical (Intranasal) Immunotherapy. Intranasal immunotherapy is one example in the search for new therapeutic techniques. The success of intranasal immunization for certain viral diseases (e.g., influenza) stimulated trials of this technique for hay fever. Though initial studies showed some induction of local blocking antibodies, results in general have been inconsistent (McLean et al., 1979; Nickelson et al., 1979).

However, more recent studies with aqueous grass antigens suggest that they can significantly reduce symptoms of allergic rhinitis (Georgitis et al., 1984). Further studies will make use of more potent topical antigens.

REFERENCES

Aas, K.: Bronchial provocation tests in asthma. Arch. Dis. Child. 45:221, 1970.

Aas, K.: Hyposensitization in house dust asthma. Acta Paediat. Scandinav. 60:264, 1971.

Adler, T.R., Beall, G.N., Heiner, D.C., Sabharwal, U.K., Swanson, K.: Immunologic and clinical correlates of bronchial challenge responses to Bermuda grass pollen extracts. J. Allergy Clin. Immunol. 75:31–36, 1985.

Bacal, E., Zeiss, C.R., Suszko, I., et al.: Polymerized whole ragweed: An improved method of immunotherapy. J. Allergy. Clin. Immunol. 62:289, 1978.

Baer, H.: Standardization of antigens. J. Allergy Clin. Immunol. 6:206, 1978.

Berg, T., Johansson, S.G.O.: *In vitro* diagnosis of atopic allergy. IV. Seasonal variations of IgE antibodies in children allergic to pollens. Int. Arch. Allergy 41:452, 1971.

Bierman, C.W., Pierson, W.E., Van Arsdel, P.P., Jr.: The effect of long-term pollen immunotherapy in children on leukocyte histamine release. J. Allergy Clin. Immunol. 59:111, 1972.

Bousquet, J., Calvayrac, P., Guerin, B., Hejjaoui, A., Dhivert, H., Hewitt, B., Michel, F.B.: Immunotherapy with a standardized *Dermatophagoides pteronyssinus* extract. J. Allergy Clin. Immunol. 76:734–744, 1985.

Bousquet, J., Frank, E., Soussana, M., Wahl, R., Maasch, H., Michel, F.B.: Comparison of parameters assessing the efficacy of immunotherapy with allergoid in grass pollenosis. (Abstract.) J. Allergy Clin. Immunol. 79:134, 1987.

Bruun, E.: Control examination of the specificity of specific desensitization in asthma. Acta Allergy 2:122, 1949.

Chakrabarty, S., Ekramoddoullah, A.K.M., Kisil, F.T., Sehon, A.H.: Isolation of a highly purified allergen from Kentucky blue grass pollen. J. Allergy Clin. Immunol. 63:192, 1979.

Cooke, R.A.: The treatment of hay fever by active immunization. Laryngoscope 25:108, 1915.

Cooke, R.A.: Studies in specific hypersensitiveness. IX. On the phenomenon of hyposensitization. J. Immunol. 7:219, 1922.

Cooke, R.A., Barnard, J.H., Hebard, S., et al.: Serologic evidence of immunity with co-existing sensitization in a type of human allergy (hay fever). J. Exper. Med. 62:733, 1935.

Davies, D., Berry, G., Hills, E., McAllen, M., Morrison-Smith, J., Pepus, J.: A trial of house dust mite extract in bronchial asthma. Br. J. Dis. Chest 260–270, 1979.

DeMeo, A.N., Ouellette, J.J., Cohen, M., Reed, C.E., Minor, T.E., Baler, J., Dick, E.: Greater frequency of viral respiratory infections in asthmatic children as compared with their nonasthmatic siblings. J. Pediat. 85:472–477, 1974.

Dreborg, S., Agrell, B., Foucard, T., Kjellman, N.I.M., Koivikko, A., and Nilsson, S.: A double-blind, multicenter immunotherapy trial in children using a purified and standardized *Cladosporium herbarum* preparation. Allergy 41:131–140, 1986.

D'Souza, M.F., Pepys, J., Wells, I.D., et al.: Hyposensitization with *Dermatophagoides pheronopsinus* in house dust allergy: A controlled study of clinical and immunological effects. Clin. Allergy 3:177, 1973.

Dunbar, W.P.: Zur Urache und Specifischen Heilung des Heufiebers. Munich, Roldenbourg, 1903.

Fink, J.N.: Immunotherapy of asthma. J. Allergy Clin. Immunol. 76:402–404, 1985.

Fontana, V.J., Salanitro, A., Wolfe, H., Moreno, F.: Bacterial vaccine and infectious asthma. J.A.M.A. 193:895–900, 1965.

Formgren, H., Lanner, Å., Lindholm, N., Löwhagen, O., Dreborg, S.: Effects of immunotherapy on specific and non-specific sensitivity of the airways. J. Allergy Clin. Immunol. 73:140, 1984.

Frankland, A.W., Augustin, R.: Prophylaxis of summer hay fever and asthma. Lancet 1:1055, 1954.

Freeman, J., Noon, L.: Further observations on treatment of hay fever by hypodermic innoculation of pollen vaccine. Lancet 2:814, 1911.

Gabriel, M., Ng, H.K., Allan, W.G.L., et al.: Study of prolonged hyposensitization with *D. pteronyssinus* extract in allergic rhinitis. Clin. Allergy 7:325–336, 1977.

Georgitis, J.W., Clayton, W.F., Wypych, J.I., Barde, S.H., Reisman, R.E.: Further evaluation of local intranasal immunotherapy with aqueous and allergoid grass extracts. J. Allergy Clin. Immunol. 74:694–700, 1984.

Grammer, L.C., Shaughnessy, M.A., Finkle, S.M., Shaughnessy, J.J., Patterson, R.: A double-blind placebo-controlled trial of polymerized whole grass administered in an accelerated dosage schedule for immunotherapy of grass pollinosis. J. Allergy Clin. Immunol. 78:1180–1184, 1986.

Grammer, L.C., Shaughnessy, M.A., Patterson, R.: Modified forms of allergen immunotherapy. J. Allerg. Clin. Immunol. 76:397–401, 1985.

Grammer, L.C., Shaughnessy, M.A., Suszko, I.M., Patterson, R.: A double-blind histamine placebo controlled trial of polymerized grass for immunotherapy of grass allergy. J. Allergy Clin. Immunol. 72:448–453, 1983.

Grammer, L.C., Shaughnessy, M.A., Suszko, I.M., Shaughnessy, J.J., Patterson, R.: Persistence of efficacy after a brief course of polymerized ragweed allergen: A controlled study. J. Allergy Clin. Immunol. 73:484–489, 1984.

Grammer, L.C., Zeiss, C.R., Suszko, I.M., Shaughnessy, M.A., Patterson, R.: A double-blind, placebo controlled trial of polymerized whole ragweed for immunotherapy of ragweed allergy. J. Allergy Clin. Immunol. 69:494–499, 1982.

Greenberger, P., Patterson, R.: Safety of therapy for allergic symptoms during pregnancy. Ann. Intern. Med. 89:234–237, 1978.

Hanes, W.J.: Histamine cephalgia resembling tic douloureux. Headache 8:162, 1969.

Hendrix, S., Zeiss, C.R., Suszko, I.M., et al.: Polymerized ragweed allergens: multi-institutional study of the safety and efficacy of an improved form of immunotherapy (Abstract). J. Allergy Clin. Immunol. 65:164, 1980.

Henocq, E., Garcelon, M., Berrens, L.: Photo-inactivated allergens. Clin. Allergy 3:461, 1973.

Horton, B.: The use of histamine in the treatment of specific types of headaches. J.A.M.A. 116:377, 1941.

Hunt, K.J., Vallentine, M.D., Sobotka, A.K., Benton, A.W., Amodio, E.J., Lichtenstein, L.M.: A controlled trial of immune therapy in insect hypersensitivity. New Engl. J. Med. 299:157–161, 1978.

Johnstone, D.E.: Study of the role of antigen dosage in the treatment of pollenosis and pollen asthma. Am. J. Dis. Child. 94:1, 1957.

Johnstone, D.E., Dutton, A.: The value of hyposensitization therapy for bronchial asthma in children—a 14-year study. Pediatrics 42:793, 1968.

Larsen, G.L.: Late phase reactions: Observations of pathogenesis and prevention. J. Allergy Clin. Immunol 76:665–669, 1985.

Levy, D.A.: Hazards and adverse reactions associated with administration of allergenic extracts. *In* Brede, H.D., Going, H., (eds.), Regulatory control and standardization of allergenic extracts. New York, Gustav Fischer Verlag, 1980.

Levy, D.A., Lichtenstein, L., Goldstein, E.O., Ishizaka, K.: Immunologic and cellular changes accompanying the therapy of pollen allergy. J. Clin. Invest. 50:360–369, 1971.

Lichtenstein, L.M., Norman, P.S., Winkenwerder, W.L.: Antibody response following immunotherapy in ragweed hay fever. Allpyral vs. whole ragweed extract. J. Allergy 41:49–57, 1968.

Lichtenstein, L.M., Valentine, M.D., Norman, P.S.: A reevaluation of immunotherapy for asthma. Am. Rev. Respir. Dis. 129:657–659, 1984.

Lockey, R.F., Benedict, L.M., Turkeltaub, P.C., Burkantz, S.C.: Fatalities from immunotherapy (IT) and skin testing (ST). J. Allergy Clin. Immunol. 79:660–677, 1987.

Loveless, M.H.: Immunologic studies in pollenosis. The presence of two antibodies related to the same pollen antigen in the serum of treated hay fever patients. J. Immunol. 38:25, 1940.

Marsh, D.G., Lichtenstein, L.M., Norman, P.S., et al.: Induction of IgE-mediated immediate hypersensitivity to group I rye grass pollen allergen and allergoids in nonallergic man. Immunology 22:1013, 1972.

McIntosh, K., Ellis, E.F., Hoffman, L.S., Lybass, T.G., Eller, J.J., Fulginiti, U.A.: The association of viral and bacterial respiratory infections with exacerbations of wheezing in young asthmatic children. J. Pediatr. 82:578, 1973.

McLean, J.A., Mathews, K.P., Bayne, N.K., Brayton, P.R., Solomon, W.R.: A controlled study of intranasal immunotherapy with short ragweed extract. J. Allergy Clin. Immunol. (Abstract). 63:166, 1979.

Meriney, D.K., Kothar, I.H., Chinoy, P., Grieco, M.H.: The clinical and immunologic efficacy of immunotherapy with modified ragweed extract (allergoid) for ragweed hay fever. Ann. Allergy 56:34–38, 1986.

Metzger, W.J., Donnelly, B.A., Richardson, H.B.: Modification of late asthmatic responses (LAR) during immunotherapy for Alternaria-induced asthma (Abstract). J. Allergy Clin. Immunol. 71:119, 1983.

Metzger, W.T., Patterson, R., Zeiss, C.R., Irons, J.S., Pruzansky, S.S., Suszko, I.M., Levitz, D.: Comparison of polymerized and unpolymerized antigen E in immunotherapy of ragweed allergy. New Engl. J. Med. 295:1160, 1976.

Metzger, W.J., Turner, E., Patterson, R.: The safety of immunotherapy during pregnancy. J. Allergy Clin. Immunol. 61:268–272, 1978.

Miller, J.R., Orgel, H.A., Meltzer, E.O.: The safety of egg-containing vaccines for egg-allergic patients. J. Allergy Clin. Immunol. 71:568–573, 1983.

Mueller, H.L., Lang, M.: Hyposensitization with bacterial vaccine in infectious asthma. J.A.M.A. 208:1379, 1969.

Murray, A.B., Ferguson, A.C., Morrison, B.J.: Non-allergic bronchial hyperreactivity in asthmatic children decreases with age and increases with mite immunotherapy. Ann. Allergy 54:541–544, 1985.

Negrini, A.C., Troise, C., Voltini, S., Siccardi, M., Grassia, L.: Long-term hyposensitization and adverse immunologic responses. Ann. Allergy 54:534–537, 1985.

Neiburger, R.G., Neiburger, J.B., Dockhorn, R.J.: Distribution of peripheral blood T and B lymphocyte markers in atopic children and changes during immunotherapy. J. Allergy Clin. Immunol. 61:88–92, 1978.

Newton, D.A.G., Maberley, D.J., Wilson, R.: House dust mite hyposensitization. Br. J. Dis. Chest 72:21–28, 1978.

Nickelson, J.A., Wypuch, J.I., Arbesman, C.E.: Clinical and immunological response to local nasal immunotherapy (Abstract). J. Allergy Clin. Immunol. 63:166, 1979.

Noon, L.: Prophylactic inoculation against hay fever. Lancet 1:1952, 1911.

Norman, P., Winkenwerder, W., Lichtenstein, L.: Immunotherapy of hay fever with ragweed antigen E. J. Allergy 42:93–108, 1968.

Norman, P.S.: Bronchial reactivity and immunotherapy. J. Allergy Clin. Immunol. 61:281–282, 1978.

Norman, P.S.: Role of immunotherapy in asthma. Chest 87:625–645, 1985.

Norman, P.S., Ishizaka, K., Lichtenstein, L.M., Adkinson, N.F.: Treatment of hay fever with urea-denatured antigen E. J. Allergy Clin. Immunol. 66:336–341, 1980.

Norman, P.S., Lichtenstein, L.M.: Comparison of alum-precipitated and unprecipitated aqueous ragweed pollen extracts in the treatment of hay fever. J. Allergy Clin. Immunol. 61:384–389, 1978.

Norman, P.S., Lichtenstein, L.M., Kagey-Sobotka, A., Marsh, D.G.: Controlled evaluation of allergoid in the immunotherapy of ragweed hay fever. J. Allergy Clin. Immunol. 70:248–260, 1982.

Norman, P.S., Lichtenstein, L.M., Tignall, J.: The clinical and immunologic specificity of immunotherapy. J. Allergy Clin. Immunol. 61:370–377, 1978.

Ohman, J.L., Jr., Findlay, S.R., Leitermann, K.M.: Immunotherapy in cat-induced asthma. Double-blind trial with evaluation of in vivo and in vitro responses. J.A.C.I. 74:230–239, 1984.

Patterson, R., Suszko, I.M., Zeiss, C.R., Pruzansky, J.J., Bacal, E.: Comparison of immune reactivity to polyvalent monomeric and polymeric ragweed antigens. J. Allergy Clin. Immunol. 61:28–35, 1978.

Platts-Mills, T.A.E., Norman, P.S., Lichtenstein, L.M., von Maur, R.G., Ishizaka, K.: IgA and IgC antiragweed antibodies in nasal secretions. J. Clin. Invest. 57:1041–1050, 1976.

Potter, M., Boyce, C.R.: Induction of plasma cell neoplasm in strain BALB/C mice with mineral oil and mineral oil adjuvants. Nature 193:1086, 1962.

Reid, M.J., Moss, R.B., Hsu, Y-P., Kwanicki, J.M., Commerford, T.M., Nelson, B.L.: Seasonal asthma in Northern California: Allergic causes and efficacy of immunotherapy. J. Allergy Clin. Immunol. 78:590–600, 1986.

Rocklin, R.E.: Clinical and immunologic aspects of allergen-specific immunotherapy in patients with seasonal allergic rhinitis and/or allergic asthma. J. Allergy Clin. Immunol. 72:323–334, 1983.

Rocklin, R.E., Sheffer, A.L., Greineder, D.K., Melmon, K.L.: Generation of antigen-specific suppressor cells during allergy desensitization. N. Engl. J. Med. 302:1213–1219, 1980.

Sadan, N., Rhyne, M.B., Mellits, E.D., Goldstein, E.O., Levy, D.A., Lichtenstein, L.M.: Immunotherapy of pollenosis in children: New Engl. J. Med. 280:623–627, 1969.

Settipane, R.A., Chafee, F.H., Settipane, G.A: Allergy immunotherapy in pregnancy: Long-term effect on offspring (Abstract). J. Allergy Clin. Immunol. 79:134, 1987.

Stull, A., Cooke, R.A., Sherman, W.B., Hebald, S.: Experimental and clinical study of fresh and modified pollen extracts. J. Allergy 11:439–465, 1940.

Sundin, B.: Immunotherapy with animal dander extracts in a double-blind cross-over study. Clinical and immunological results after 3 years treatment (Abstract). J. Allergy Clin. Immunol. 77:212, 1986.

Taylor, W.V., Ohman, J.L., Lowell, F.C.: Immunotherapy in cat-induced asthma. J. Allergy Clin. Immunol. 61:283–287, 1978.

Umetsu, D.T., Hahn, J.S., Perez-Atayde, A.R., Geha, R.S.: Serum sickness triggered by anaphylaxis: A complication of immunotherapy. J. Allergy Clin. Immunol. 76:713–718, 1985.

Vervloet, D., Khairallah, E., Arnaud, A., Charpin, J.: A prospective national study of the safety of immunotherapy. Clin. Allergy 10:59–64, 1980.

Van Metre, T.E., Adkinson, N.F., Lichtenstein, L.M., Mardiner, M.R., Jr., Norman, P.S., Jr., Rosenberg, G.L., Sobotka, A.K., Valentine, M.D.: A controlled study of the effectiveness of the Rinkel method of immunotherapy for ragweed pollen hay fever. J. Allergy Clin. Immunol. 65:288–297, 1980.

Warner, J.O., Price, J.F., Soothill, J.F., Hey, E.N.: Controlled trial of hyposensitization to Dermatophagoides pteronyssinus in the children with asthma. Lancet 2:912–915, 1978.

Weinstock, M., Starr, M.S.: Studies in pollen allergy. II. Comparison of leucocyte sensitivity and levels of blocking antibody in hay fever subjects administered Allpyral or Pollaccine. Int. Arch. Allergy 37:385, 1970.

Yunginger, J.W., Gleich, G.J.: Seasonal changes in serum and nasal IgE concentrations. J. Allergy 51:174–186, 1973.

21

Prevention of Allergic Diseases

DOUGLAS E. JOHNSTONE, M.D.

Because there appears to be an important genetic component to atopic disease, there is potential for preventing such disease by "genetic engineering." As a practical matter, however, capabilities of influencing the development of atopic disease appear to be restricted to manipulating the effect of the environment, largely by reducing the allergenic load or contact with other factors, which are associated with the development of atopic disease.

FACTORS THAT PREDISPOSE TO ATOPIC DISEASE

Heredity. The risk of developing atopic disease in infants is about 70 percent if there is a bilateral family history of atopy; it is 54 percent if there is a unilateral history. Parental allergic disease affects the incidence, age of onset, and type of atopic disease in offspring (Kjellman and Johansson, 1976). In addition, IgE hyperresponsiveness to specific antigens has been associated with specific HLA haplotypes; associations have been documented for responsiveness to the ragweed antigen Ra5 and the haplotype Dw2, and for rye I, B8, and Dw3 (Marsh et al., 1980). Associations between specific tissue types and various atopic syndromes were reported by Soothill et al. (1976) who found that HLA types A1 and B8 were more frequent in patients with eczema, and A3 and B7 were more frequent in those with hay fever. On the other hand, concordance of atopic disease in identical twins is far less than 100 percent. Bronchial reactivity in monozygotic twins seems to be acquired rather than strictly inherited (Falliers et al., 1971). This observation suggests that environmental factors play as important a role as inheritance in the development of atopy.

Intrauterine and Prenatal Factors

Drugs. Progesterone administered during pregnancy increases the risk of atopy in offspring. Of newborns born of mothers given this drug, 53 percent had detectable IgE in their cord blood compared with only 24 percent of newborns born of mothers not given progesterone (Michel et al., 1980). The effects of drugs to be avoided during pregnancy that may otherwise harm the infant have been reviewed by Schatz et al. (1983).

Smoking. Parental smoking increases the risk of respiratory tract symptoms in infants and children and increases the risk of and rate of decline in bronchiolar airflow in children and nonsmoking adults with hyperreactive airways. These decreases in airflow are greater in asthmatic than in nonasthmatic individuals. Pregnant women should be made aware of the adverse effects of smoking on the baby as well as the mother (Magnusson, 1986). This information may permit the physician to convince a woman to stop smoking during pregnancy.

Level of Maternal IgE. The concentration of IgE in a mother's serum has been shown to be a factor correlating with the future development of atopy (Michel et al., 1980). In this study, if a mother had a serum IgE level of more than 100 IU/ml, the serum IgE level of her newborn's cord blood was significantly higher than that of a newborn whose mother's serum IgE level was lower. In the same study, IgE levels of the infants' fathers did not seem to influence cord blood IgE levels.

A History of Maternal Asthma, Symptomatic during Pregnancy. This history is associated with an increased incidence of respiratory disease or jaundice or both in newborns (Light and Wortley, 1980).

Food Sensitization *In Utero*. This possibility has been suspected on the basis of animal experimentation (Ratner et al., 1927). Supporting evidence in humans was reported by Michel et al. (1980), who found three newborns with specific IgE antibodies against cow's milk in their cord blood. Mothers of these infants did not have the same anti-milk antibodies in their sera. Maternal avoidance of certain foods (generally the more sensitizing) has been suggested to reduce fetal contact and may prevent sensitization (Kuroume et al., 1976).

294

Perinatal Factors

Season of Birth. This seems to have a bearing on atopic sensitization. Infants in Scandinavia born between February and April were reported to be at greater risk of developing birch pollen allergy than those born at other times of the year (Björksten et al., 1980). In England, bronchial asthma was found more frequently in children born in late autumn (Soothill et al., 1976). In the United States, adolescents born in the months of May through September have shown the greatest susceptibility to ragweed pollenosis (Settipane and Hagy, 1979).

Place of Birth. This factor also may influence the development of atopy. In a study of immigrants to Great Britain, a lower incidence of bronchial asthma than the overall population was found in children of African origin who were born outside Great Britain; offspring of parents of African origin who were born in Great Britain had at least as high a prevalence of atopic disease as non-African children (Morrison-Smith, 1973). This finding again suggests an environmental rather than a purely genetic influence on the prevalence of asthma.

The usefulness of elevated *cord blood IgE* level in predicting the development of atopic disease was demonstrated by the finding that from 52 to 82 percent of infants with elevated cord blood IgE levels developed allergic disease during childhood compared with 5 to 30 percent of those with normal cord blood IgE levels (Michel et al., 1980; Croner et al., 1982; Businco et al., 1983; Kjellman and Croner, 1984).

Perinatal Complications in Mother or Child. These complications in mother and child may affect significantly the chances of developing bronchial asthma. Salk et al. (1974) examined the birth records of three groups of children born on the same day in the same obstetric unit, as follows: one group of 5-year-old children with asthma and two groups without asthma. These investigators found a significantly greater frequency of neonatal complications of mothers or children among the asthmatic children. Only half as many children in each of the control groups had perinatal complications.

Factors that may be Operative once a Child is Born

Dietary Factors. In my opinion, an important place where the physician can influence the development of atopy is through intervention in the amount and type of allergenic load in the infant through dietary manipulation. For centuries, this was a less complicated matter when all newborns were breast-fed. Kaufman (1972) reported an early onset of atopic dermatitis associated with early cessation of breast-feeding in a prospective study of infants of atopic parents. In this study, more than 70 percent of mothers either did not breast-feed or did so for less than 6 weeks. Atopic eczema was reported seven times more frequently in cow's milk–fed infants than in breast-fed infants (Grulee and Sanford, 1936). Other studies reported that breast-feeding significantly protects children from developing atopic disease (Chandra, 1979; Saarinen et al., 1979). This effect is maximized if the breast-feeding continues for at least the first 6 months of life. In a prospective controlled study of antigen avoidance, Matthew et al. (1977) showed that exclusively breast-fed infants developed less eczema; also, at 6 months of age, serum IgE levels were significantly lower. It should be noted, however, that not all investigators have found that dietary manipulation influences the development of allergic diseases (Halpren, 1973).

Since human milk may contain foreign food antigens (Kaplan and Solli, 1979), allergen avoidance by lactating mothers also may be an important consideration in allergy prevention. Specific IgE anti-cow's milk antibodies have been demonstrated both by positive prick skin test and by radioallerosorbent test (RAST) results on the sera of infants exclusively breast-fed. Several anaphylactic reactions to foods have been reported after the very first feeding of a food, suggesting either antenatal sensitization or sensitization via breast-feeding (Schwartz et al., 1985). Clearing of atopic dermatitis was reported in some infants when their mothers stopped eating eggs; the dermatitis recurred when their mothers began eating eggs again (Warner, 1980). Similarly, other investigators reported that "colic" disappeared in 13 of 19 breast-fed "colicky" infants when the mothers of these infants were put on a diet free of cow's milk (Jacobsson and Lindberg, 1978). In 12 of these 13, the colic reappeared when the mothers resumed drinking cow's milk. These findings suggest that perhaps mothers of potentially allergic infants should be on a diet free of cow's milk while they breast-feed their offspring. Other studies of *dietary prophylaxis* based on withholding cow's milk, wheat, and egg from newborns of allergic families have suggested that such regimens will lessen the incidence of atopic disease in offspring. Glaser (1953) and Hill (1929) independently first popularized the recommendation of deliberately withholding specific foods from the diets of potentially atopic infants from the time of birth until 6 to 9 months of age. The earlier of such studies (Glaser and Johnstone, 1953; Johnstone and Dutton, 1966) found that fewer children from atopic families who had been placed on a diet free of cow's milk, eggs, and wheat developed bronchial asthma and perennial allergic rhinitis than did siblings or other children of atopic families permitted to eat these foods in the first few months of life. Kajosaari and Saarinen (1983) have emphasized the importance of delaying the introduction of foods for the prevention of food allergy. However, this cannot be expected to prevent the development of allergies in those infants already sensitized antenatally or through breast milk.

Since dietary prophylaxis of atopic disease was first proposed, no satisfactory explanation for the mechanism of its effects has been presented to support the assumptions of its authors or their clinical findings. Information accumulated in recent years may be relevant, however. Taylor et al. (1973) have suggested that a transient IgA deficiency might be an important factor in the development of atopy. They studied a group of infants of atopic families to test their thesis and found that infants of atopic families who had low serum IgA levels at 3 months of age were more likely to have positive prick test results and to develop atopic disease than infants of atopic families who had normal serum IgA levels at that age. The investigators interpreted their findings to support the argument of withholding commonly allergenic foods from the diets of these children until the intestinal tract was capable of producing food-specific IgA immunoglobulin, which in turn might exclude antigen from contact with IgE-antibody producing tissues. In other words, they theorized that withholding certain foods until this happens might lessen the likelihood of "turning on" the IgE system, which sets the stage for clinical atopic disease.

Juto (1980) presented an alternative theory to explain the clinical findings in children of allergic families fed cow's milk compared with similar children not fed cow's milk. He studied serum IgE levels at various ages during the first year of life and found that these levels appeared to be related to the number of T cells assessed at 1 month of age and the type of feeding the infant had received. Babies fed cow's milk who had low T cell counts at 1 month of age had higher serum IgE levels at 3 and 6 months of age than breast-fed babies who had normal T cell counts. Initiation of cow's milk feeding before 3 months of age in babies with low T cell counts was associated with continuously elevated serum IgE levels during the first year of life compared with the levels in babies with normal T cell counts. Juto concluded that in T cell–deficient infants there might exist a crucial time period during which the onset of cow's milk feeding can be associated with a subsequent increase in IgE synthesis and, presumably, the subsequent development of atopic disease.

The importance of elevation of serum IgE level in the first 6 months of life was demonstrated clearly by the studies of Kjellman (1976) who examined a group of 207 healthy children without known family histories of atopy in order to determine whether a relationship exists between serum IgE levels and atopic disease. Seventy-five percent of the children studied who had an initial serum IgE level greater than 1 standard deviation (SD) above the mean developed atopic disease in the first year of life. By contrast, allergic disease developed in only 6.4 percent of those from the same age group with a serum IgE level lower than 1 SD above the mean. Even among children in the 2- to 14-year old age group, it was noted that a high serum IgE level was predictive of subsequent atopic disease (Hamburger et al., 1974).

Early Surgery or Hospitalization or Both. In early infancy, factors other than diet seem to "turn on" the allergic diathesis. The pioneer pediatric allergist, Oscar Schloss, suspected that infants who had pyloric stenosis were at increased risk of developing asthma or hay fever (personal communication). A three-part study was carried out in Rochester, New York, to test the thesis that surgery in infancy predisposes to atopic disease (Johnstone et al., 1975). In the first part of the study, 115 children who had been operated on for pyloric stenosis were traced and found to have had an above-average prevalence of atopic disease as follows: 20 percent had developed bronchial asthma in the first 5 years of life; 21 percent had developed hay fever, that is, a total of 36 percent of the children who had surgery developed one or both of these conditions. These cumulative prevalences are much higher than those found in household interviews in the Rochester Child

Health Study investigation of a random sample of children from birth to 17 years of age in Monroe County, New York (Haggerty et al., 1975). That study showed a cumulative prevalence of 3 to 4 percent for bronchial asthma, 8.5 percent for hay fever, and 10.6 percent for one or both of these conditions. In the second part of the study of Johnstone and coworkers, 47 boys who had hernia repair were followed. Of those who had undergone herniorrhaphy in the first year of life, 35 percent developed asthma, 21 percent developed hay fever, and a total of 55 percent developed one or the other condition or both. In the third part of the study, 202 children from the Rochester Child Health Study reported by their parents to have had asthma or hay fever were surveyed for evidence of early hospitalization or surgery. Significantly more early operations involving general anesthesia as well as more early hospitalizations for medical reasons were found for the "allergic" group compared with nonasthmatic children of the same age from the same random population group.

Home Environmental Factors. It is apparent that exposure to household allergens and irritants is important in investigating systems of allergic disease as well as in propagating them. Of particular importance are the following household factors shown to be problematic in atopic disease and to which exposure can be avoided or at least can be reduced: house dust, house dust mites, indoor mold, animal allergens, and cigarette smoke. Detailed consideration of environmental manipulation to control these factors can be found in Chapter 18.

Role of Infection. Respiratory viral infections are among the most common triggers provoking episodes of asthma. In infants the most important infectious agents are respiratory syncytial virus (RSV) and parainfluenza virus (McIntosh et al., 1973). In older children and adults, rhinoviruses and influenza viruses predominate. Not only do viral infections provoke episodes of asthma, they often seem to usher in the asthmatic state itself. Welliver et al. (1981) studied the development of respiratory syncytial virus–specific IgE antibody and the release of histamine in the nasopharyngeal secretions of 79 infants with illness due to RSV. Children with wheezing or bronchiolitis associated with this infection were more likely to have more histamine in their secretions and to produce significant amounts of virus-specific IgE antibodies. These children were thought to be most at

risk to develop asthma. It is possible that vaccination against major respiratory viruses associated with the onset of asthmatic symptoms will prove to be beneficial in preventing the development of asthma. However, Ouelette et al. (1965) found that an injection of killed influenza virus vaccine in fact increased nonspecific bronchial hyperreactivity in nine of the ten asthmatics inoculated. Nonatopic patients had no such response. Thus, it is not clear whether the beneficial effects of immunization against respiratory tract viruses can be separated from the asthmogenic effects associated with human responsiveness to such viruses in those predisposed to asthma (see Chapter 14).

OTHER IMPORTANT FACTORS IN ATOPIC DISEASE

Choice of Career. Atopic individuals with propensities to develop IgE antibodies to common inhalant antigens are prone to develop respiratory disease when working in highly sensitizing industrial environments. Exclusion of such individuals from certain types of employment has led to the successful reduction in the incidence of disease among workers in the enzyme detergent and platinum industries (Juniper et al., 1977). Just as children who are highly sensitive to animal danders should be discouraged from veterinary medicine or other careers or associations with animals, to the extent feasible, individuals with allergic disorders are wise to avoid careers, vocations, or hobbies that will result in exposure to extremes of temperature, pollens, dampness, molds, enzymes, strong chemicals, or odors.

Early Immunotherapy for Pollen Rhinitis in Children. The immunotherapy may prevent the development of allergic asthma. Seasonal allergic rhinitis due to pollen allergy is one of the most common and undertreated types of allergy in American children (Appel et al., 1961). A study I undertook, on the value of immunotherapy for pollenosis in children, revealed that approximately half of the children with hay fever treated with placebo developed pollen asthma during the 5-year period of the study; although not all the antigen-treated children lost their hay fever symptoms, *none* developed asthma during this period (Johnstone, 1957). In addition, Pedvis et al. (1962) reported that the longer one delayed in giving immunotherapy to children with ragweed hay fever, the greater the risk of their developing asthma. Although the ability to prevent (pollen) asthma by immunotherapy in children with pollen-induced upper respiratory symptoms has not been universally accepted, in my opinion, it seems desirable to begin specific immunotherapy as soon as the diagnosis of pollen "hay fever" is made in children, regardless of the severity or mildness of their symptoms. Reduction of risk for developing asthma by immunotherapy for pollen hay fever does not appear to apply to adults.

Early Immunotherapy for Inhalant Sensitive Bronchial Asthma in Children. This type of immunotherapy increases the likelihood that a child will "outgrow" asthma. In each of three long-term studies on the follow-up of untreated asthmatic children, approximately 75 percent of the children experienced persistent asthmatic symptoms until late adolescence (Flensborg, 1945; Ryssing, 1959; Johnstone, 1968). By contrast, in a 20-year follow-up study of 688 asthmatic children, all of whom had received specific immunotherapy, Rackemann and Edwards (1952) reported findings nearly the opposite of those in the three previous studies of untreated children. These findings suggested that immunotherapy might significantly influence the natural history of asthma in children.

To test the thesis that immunotherapy significantly affects the end result of childhood asthma, Johnstone and Dutton (1968) carried out a 14-year prospective controlled study. A total of 220 asthmatic children were studied who were given either specific immunotherapy or placebo injections. In the treated group, the proportion of children free from asthma for at least 1 year by 16 years of age was close to that found in Rackemann and Edwards's study of treated children. In the placebo group, the proportion of children free from asthma resembled that found in the three long-term follow-up studies of untreated children. In addition, in those treated with antigen, the persistence of asthmatic symptoms seemed inversely related to the antigen dose given in hyposensitization injection therapy. That is, the higher the antigen dose administered, the greater the chance a child would become symptom free. The likelihood that a child in this study would "outgrow" asthma did not seem to be significantly increased by sex, age at the onset of asthma, or severity of asthma when first identified. However, a previous history of seasonal hay fever was associated with the significantly increased

likelihood of persistence of asthma into adulthood (Johnstone, 1968).

REFERENCES

Appel, S., Szanton, V., Rapaport, H.: Survey of allergy in a pediatric population. Penn. Med. 64:621, 1961.

Björksten, F., Saarinen, U.: IgE antibodies to cow's milk in infants fed breast milk and milk formulae. Lancet 2:624, 1978.

Björksten, F., Suoniemi, I., Koski, V.: Neonatal birch pollen contact and subsequent allergy to birch pollen. Clin. Allergy 10:585, 1980.

Buckley, R., Dees, S.: Correlation of milk precipitins with IgA deficiency. N. Engl. J. Med. 281:456, 1969.

Buffum, W., Settipane, G.: Prognosis in asthma in children. Am. J. Dis. Child. 112:214, 1968.

Businco, L., Marchetti, F., Pelligrini, B., Berlini, R.: Predictive value of cord blood IgE levels in "at risk" newborn babies and influence of type of feeding. Clin. Allergy 13:503, 1983.

Chandra, R.: Prospective studies of the effect of breast feeding on incidence of infection and allergy. Acta Paediatr. Scand. 68:691, 1979.

Croner, S., Kjellman, N., Ericksson, B., Roth, A.: IgE screening in 1701 newborn infants and the development of atopic disease during infancy. Arch. Dis. Child. 57:364, 1982.

Falliers, C., Cardoso, R., Bane, N., Coffey, B., Middleton, E.: Discordant allergic manifestations in monozygotic twins: genetic identity vs. clinical physiologic and biochemical differences. J. Allergy 47:207, 1971.

Flensborg, E.: Prognosis for bronchial asthma arising in infancy after non-specific treatment hitherto applied. Acta Paediatr. 33:4, 1945.

Glaser, J., Johnstone, D.: Prophylaxis of allergic disease in children. J.A.M.A. 253:620, 1953.

Grulee, C., Sanford, H.: The influence of breast and artificial feeding on infantile eczema. J. Pediatr. 9:223, 1936.

Haggerty, R., Roghmann, K., Pless, I.: Child Health and the Community. New York, Wiley and Sons, 1975.

Halpren, S.R., Sellars, W.A., Johnson, R.B., Anderson, D.W., Saperstein, S., Reisch, J.S.: Development of childhood allergy in infants fed breast milk, soy or cow milk. J. Allergy Clin. Immunol. 51:139, 1973.

Hamburger, R., Lenoir, M., Groshong, R., Miller, J.R., Wallace, W., Orgell, H.: Development of IgE and allergy during the first year of life: Preliminary data. J. Allergy Clin. Immunol. 53:94, 1974.

Hill, L., Stuart, H.: A soy bean food preparation for feeding patients with milk idiosyncrasy. J.A.M.A. 93:986, 1929.

Jacobsson, I., Lindberg, R.: Cow's milk as a cause of infantile colic in breast fed infants. Lancet 1:437, 1978.

Johnstone, D.: Study of the role of antigen dose in the treatment of pollenosis and pollen asthma. Am. J. Dis. Child. 94:1, 1957.

Johnstone, D.: A study of the natural history of bronchial asthma in children. Am. J. Dis. Child 115:213, 1968.

Johnstone, D., Dutton, A.: Dietary prophylaxis of allergic disease in children. New Engl. J. Med. 274:715, 1966.

Johnstone, D., Dutton, A.: The value of hyposensitization therapy for bronchial asthma in children: a fourteen year study. Pediatrics 42:793, 1968.

Johnstone, D., Roghmann, K., Pless, I.: Factors associated with the development of asthma and hay fever in children: the possible risks of hospitalization, surgery, and anesthesia. Pediatrics 56:398, 1975.

Juniper, C., Howe, M., Goodwin, B., Kinshott, A.: Bacillus enzymes: A seven year clinical, epidemiological, and immunological study on an industrial allergen. J. Soc. Occup. Med. 27:3, 1977.

Juto, P.: Elevated serum immunoglobulin E in T cell–deficient infants fed cow's milk. J. Allergy Clin. Immunol. 66:402, 1980.

Kajosaari, M., Saarinen, U.: Prophylaxis of atopic disease by six months total solid food elimination. Acta Paediatr. Scand. 72:411, 1983.

Kaplan, M., Solli, N.: Immunoglobulin E in breast fed atopic children. J. Allergy Clin. Immunol. 64:122, 1979.

Kaufman, H.: Diet and heredity in infantile atopic dermatitis. Arch. Dermatol. 105:400, 1972.

Kjellman, M.: Predictive value of high IgE levels in children. Acta Paediatr. Scand. 65:465, 1976.

Kjellman, N., Croner, S.: Cord blood IgE determination for allergy prediction—a follow-up to seven years of age in 1651 children. Ann. Allergy 53:167, 1984.

Kjellman, N., Johansson, S.: IgE and atopic allergy in newborns and infants with a family history of atopic disease. Acta Paediatr. Scand. 65:495, 1976.

Korsgaard, J.: Preventative measures in house dust allergy. Am. Rev. Resp. Dis. 125:80, 1982.

Kuroume, T., Oguri, M., Matsumura, T., Iwasaki, I., Kanbe, Y., Yamada,T., Kawabe, S., Negiski, K.: Milk sensitivity and soya sensitivity in the production of eczematous manifestations in breast fed infants with practical reference to intrauterine sensitization. Ann. Allergy 37:41, 1976.

Light, W., Wortley, G.: Effect of maternal asthma on the newborn. J. Allergy Clin. Immunol. 65:204, 1980.

Magnusson, C.: Maternal smoking influences cord serum IgE and IgD levels and increases the risk for subsequent infant allergy. J. Allergy Clin. Immunol. 78:898, 1986.

Marsh, D., Hsu, S., Hussain, R., Meyers, D., Friedhogg, L., Bias, W.: Genetics of human immune response to allergens. J. Allergy Clin. Immunol. 65:322, 1980.

Matthew, D., Taylor, B., Norman, A., Turner, M., Soothill, J.: Prevention of eczema. Lancet 1:321, 1977.

McIntosh, K., Ellis, E., Hoffman, L., Lybass, T., Eller, J., Fulginiti, V.: The association of viral and bacterial respiratory infections with exacerbations of wheezing in young asthmatic children. J. Pediatr. 83:578, 1973.

Michel, F., Bousquet, J., Greillier, P., Robinet-Levy, M., Coulomb, Y.: Comparison of cord blood immunoglobulin E and maternal allergy for the prediction of atopic disease in infancy. J. Allergy Clin. Immunol. 65:422, 1980.

Minor, R., Baler, J., Dick, E., Demateo, A., Ouellette, J., Cohen, M., Reed, C.: Greater frequency of viral respiratory infections in asthmatic children as compared with nonasthmatic sibs. J. Pediatr. 85:472, 1974.

Morrison-Smith, J.: Skin tests and atopic allergy in children. Clin. Allergy 3:269, 1973.

Murray, A., Ferguson, A., Morrison, B.: Sensitization to house dust mites in different climatic areas. J. Allergy Clin. Immunol. 76:108, 1985.

O'Connell, E., Logan, G.: Parental smoking in childhood asthma. Ann. Allergy 32:142, 1971.

Ouelette, J., Reed, C.: Increased response of asthmatic subjects to methacholine after influenza vaccine. J. Allergy 36:558, 1965.

Pedvis, S., Fox, Z., Bacal, H.: Long-term follow-up of ragweed hay fever in children. Ann. Allergy 20:596, 1962.

Platts-Mills, T.: Dust mite avoidance in the treatment of asthma. Ann. Allergy 55:419, 1985.

Rackemann, R., Edwards, M.: Asthma in children: A follow-up study of 688 patients after an interval of 20 years. N. Engl. J. Med. 246:858, 1952.

Ratner, B., Jackson, C., Gruehl, H.: Transmission of protein hypersensitiveness from mother to offspring. V. Active sensitization in utero. J. Immunol. 14:303, 1927.

Ryssing, E.: Continued follow-up investigation concerning the fate of 298 asthmatic children. Acta Paediatr. 48:255, 1959.

Saarinen, U., Kajosaari, M., Backman, A., Sumes, M.: Prolonged breast feeding as a prophylaxis for allergic disease. Lancet 2:163, 1979.

Salk, L., Grelling, B., Straus, W., Dietrich, J.: Perinatal complications in the history of asthmatic children. Am. J. Dis. Child. 127:30, 1974.

Sarsfield, J., Gowland, G., Toy, R., Norman, A.: Mite sensitive asthma of childhood. Trial of avoidance measures. Arch. Dis. Child. 49:716, 1974.

Schatz, M., Zeiger, R., Mellon, M., Porreco, R.: Asthma and allergic diseases during pregnancy: Management of the mother and prevention in the child. In Middleton, E., Reed, C., Ellis, E. (eds.): Allergy Principles and Practice. St. Louis, C.V. Mosby Co., 1983.

Schwartz, R., Kubicka, M., Dreyfus, E.: Extreme sensitization to cow's milk (CM) in infants fed breast milk (BM) or soy milk (SM). J. Allergy Clin. Immunol. 75:177, 1985.

Settipane, G., Hagy, R.: Effect of atmospheric pollen on the newborn. R.I. Med. J. 62:477, 1979.

Soothill, J., Stokes, C., Turner, M., Norman, A., Taylor, B.: Predisposing factors and development of reaginic allergy in infancy. Clin. Allergy 6:305, 1976.

Taylor, B., Norman, A., Orgel, H., Stokes, C.: Transient IgA deficiency and pathogenesis of infantile atopy. Lancet 2:111, 1973.

Tosato, F., Magrath, I., Koski, I., Dooley, N., Blaese, M.: Activation of suppressor T cells during Epstein-Barr virus–induced infectious mononucleosis. N. Engl. J. Med. 301:1133, 1979.

Warner, J.: Food allergy in fully breast fed infants. Clin. Allergy 10:133, 1980.

Welliver, R., Wong, D., Sun, M., Middleton, E., Vaughan, R., Ogra, P.: The development of respiratory syncytial virus–specific IgE antibodies and the release of histamine in nasopharyngeal secretions after infection. N. Engl. J. Med. 305:841, 1981.

Wiseman, R., Wiseman, J.: Value of home visits in the treatment of the allergic patient. N.Y. State J. Med. 64:1948, 1964.

22

Psychologic Factors and Allergic Diseases

SANFORD E. AVNER, M.D.
ROBERT A. KINSMAN, Ph.D.

Just as allergic diseases vary in their pathophysiologic and clinical manifestations, patients with allergic diseases vary considerably in their psychologic dimensions. There are remarkable differences by which patients experience illness and cope with treatment. At all ages, beginning even early in life, patients possess diverse and individual ways of dealing with problems in their lives; psychologic resources to meet those problems, i.e., coping skills, can vary widely. Coping skills can affect medical management of allergic diseases in at least two ways as follows: (1) in perception of illness, and thus the historical and clinical presentation of illness can be influenced significantly by psychosocial orientation, which, in turn, can affect physicians' medical decisions and (2) in patient behaviors during treatment, particularly the requirements of self-management, which may affect control of the illness.

This chapter considers the role of psychologic factors in the management of allergic diseases. Its objective is to promote a sensitive approach towards better treatment by exploring the psychologic effects of allergic diseases upon patients and the psychologic factors that may contribute to the illness. Because of the critical role that the psychologic orientation of patients (and their families) can play in the presentation of an illness and results of treatment, much emphasis will be placed on examining those factors that either can perpetuate illness by undermining treatment plans or can promote successful medical management by improving compliance with treatment plans.

Several terms are used that refer to concepts of causal relationships between physical (somatic) and psychologic (psychic) domains. The term "somatopsychic" is applied to psychologic changes arising from an illness. "Psychosomatic," often used without any implication of

causality, is employed here to refer specifically to the indirect triggering of physical symptoms by psychologic events, such as elicitation of airways obstruction by suggestion (Luparello et al., 1968). "Illness psychomaintenance" refers to the maintenance of illness, i.e., causing the illness to persist, by the operation of specific psychologic factors that lead to nonbeneficial behaviors, such as noncompliance in medication use. A single psychologic factor can function simultaneously in each of these roles. For example, anxiety is a common reaction to respiratory difficulties in asthma (somatopsychic). For some asthmatic patients, anxiety concomitant with increased physical activity and hyperventilation may exacerbate the airways obstruction (psychosomatic) while interfering with the patient's ability to remember and execute the steps needed to resolve the attack (illness psychomaintenance).

HISTORICAL PERSPECTIVE— THEORIES AND HYPOTHESES IN PSYCHOSOMATIC MEDICINE

A variety of etiologic theories and hypotheses have been introduced in an attempt to help clarify the roles of psychologic factors of disease and disease factors on patients' psychologic state. The most appealing is the *summation hypothesis* (Alexander, 1950), which postulates an interrelationship of three factors as follows: (1) a somatic predisposition, (2) a psychologic predisposition, and (3) a precipitating event. It is of interest that a relationship among these factors has been implicated as being important in other diseases as well (Friedman et al., 1974).

Psychosomatic theories can be categorized into three *specificity hypotheses*. The first assumes that there is a distinction between "psychosomatic" and "physical" illnesses. An obvious implication is that psychologic issues are involved in some illnesses but not in others. The second holds that specific psychologic factors are unique to "psychosomatic" patients. A recent example is Nemiah's (1975) concept of alexithymia, an inability to describe feelings in words which has been suggested to be a feature common to patients with "psychosomatic" disorders (including asthma). However, a major problem arises in clearly identifying a "psychosomatic patient" and a psychosomatic illness. The third hypothesis describes a distinct psychologic factor specific to each psychosomatic illness, as portrayed, for example, by the personality profiles theory of Dunbar (1943) and the nuclear conflict theory of Alexander (1950). Dunbar (1938), Fenichel (1945), Rees (1956), and Israel (1954) describe patients with asthma as having hysteric and dependent personality traits; other investigators describe patients with asthma as overly sensitive, often depressed, and shy (Kerman, 1946; Knapp and Nemetz, 1957). Although these early reports suffered in design and interstudy definitions, they did contribute to the now generally accepted position that patients with allergic disease run the gamut of personality types found in the population at large. It is important to note, though, that certain patients may cope poorly with illness in ways which selectively bring them to the attention of psychologists or psychiatrists (Jones et al., 1979). This position will be addressed subsequently.

Both the second and third hypotheses presuppose the first hypothesis, i.e., that there is a fundamental distinction between "psychosomatic" and "physical" illnesses. By promoting such an artificial dichotomy, investigative attention was diverted from potentially important and productive lines of inquiry of psychologic and physical interrelationships, and physicians began to dismiss psychosomatic medicine altogether.

The concept of illness psychomaintenance evolved more recently from studies of patients with asthma (Jones et al., 1979; Kinsman et al., 1982). This approach does not address the etiology of illness, but rather how psychologic factors can affect the perceived severity of illness and its intractability. While accepting the possibility that psychologic factors can be involved in triggering episodes of an allergic disease once it has developed, or even have some role in the initial onset of illness, it focuses on psychologically determined factors which can be involved in the maintenance of illness. Hypotheses related to illness psychomaintenance reject all specificity hypotheses and disclaim any arbitrary distinction between "psychosomatic" and "physical" illness. In agreement with the best evidence available, these hold that allergic diseases affect individuals who are psychologically heterogeneous. Given this heterogeneity, it is assumed that psychologic differences among patients need to be examined in order to understand why some patients do well,

whereas others do poorly, given similar treatment for similar problems. Illness psychomaintenance accepts the evidence that allergic diseases can lead to emotional, intellectual, and behavioral changes. However, it also addresses how somatopsychic effects of illness differ among individual coping styles, and how these differences affect medical management.

Figure 22–1 illustrates the illness psychomaintenance model (Kinsman et al., 1982) with six levels of involvement. At Level 1, the patient's behavior is assumed to be a function both of the pre-illness personality coping style and of the onset, type, and severity of the illness. For example, a dependent person will likely be yet more dependent with a chronic illness and present as a demanding, clinging, fearful patient. At Level 2, the attitudes of such a patient toward illness and its treatment will coincide with the personality features of pessimism about his or her own ability to master the illness and will manifest an excessive reliance upon medical care to the exclusion of what the patient needs to do on his or her own. At Level 3, these attitudes in combination with a dependent personality will be linked to characteristic ways of experiencing the illness. The patient is likely to experience excessive anxiety during each exacerbation of the illness. By understanding the patient's personality, attitudes, and experiences of illness, the physician can understand and predict behavior during illness and its treatment shown at Level 4. Thus, the dependent patient with asthma may exhibit a variety of behaviors, such as erratic use or overuse of medications, exaggerated distress from symptoms, hyperventilation during exacerbations of illness, and omissions of self-management procedures.

The psychologic bases underlying these behaviors are well understood. Since such abnormal responses to illness do occur, the potential for illness psychomaintenance is greater at Level 5, which increases the intractability of the illness (Level 6). An important implication of this approach is that there are diverse psychologic routes through which the intractability of an illness may be increased, each of which may be identified by this type of analysis; in turn, each potentially is susceptible to modification. Also, any particular illness behavior, such as underuse of medication, can arise from more than one psychologic base. Treating an adverse illness behavior directly, without an appreciation of its psychologic base, makes no more sense than treating fatigue without careful

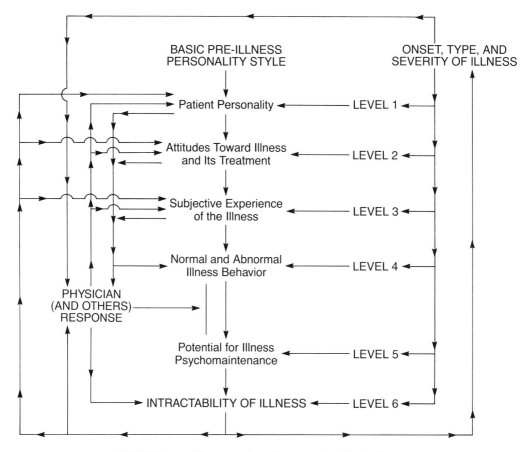

FIGURE 22–1. Illness psychomaintenance in allergic disease.

medical assessment of its pathophysiologic base. The model is applicable to any allergic disease, as well as any other illness. For example, among asthmatics in whom assessment has been refined by the Battery of Asthma Illness Behavior (Kinsman et al., 1982), repeated hospitalization for asthma has been predicted successfully in blind studies (Dirks and Kinsman, 1981; Dirks et al., 1981; Dirks, 1982).

PSYCHOLOGIC EFFECTS OF ALLERGIC DISEASE

The emotional, intellectual, and behavioral effects of an allergic disease or its treatment are a function both of the nature and severity of the illness and the preexisting psychosocial attributes and resources of a particular patient. As a consequence, symptoms and experiences differ among allergic diseases as well as among patients with the same allergic disease. It is these differences, along with the requirements of

treatment, that are central to an understanding of the psychologic factors that operate to affect medical management and how they do so. The following section examines illness psychomaintenance in asthma as an example of this process in allergic disorders, since it has been studied in greatest depth and is the disease about which the most information is available. Where possible, allergic rhinitis and atopic dermatitis will be similarly discussed in order to illustrate how specific psychologic factors may differ, yet be understood within the same general model of illness psychomaintenance.

Asthma

Subjective experiences during an asthma attack are among the most immediate somatopsychic reactions to this illness. These can be measured by the Asthma Symptom Checklist (ASC) (Kinsman et al., 1973; Kinsman et al., 1977). For children and adults, physical symptoms of airways obstruction are woven into a tapestry of other symptoms and experiences, as shown in Table 22–1.

Symptom categories shown in Table 22–1 characterize the asthma attack from the patient's point of view, as an often fatiguing, irritating, and frightening experience. For some patients, an asthma attack is accompanied by the physiologic concomitants of anxiety, including rapid breathing, heart "pounding," hyperventilation symptoms, and concerns about isolation or abandonment. Thus, the cardinal emotional feature of an asthma attack is anxiety, focused on the possibility of incapacitation and helplessness, which the patient experiences in various ways. Patients have been classified according to different patterns of perception of symptoms that occur during typical asthma attacks (Kinsman et al., 1974). These differences are independent of age of onset of asthma (Dirks and Kreischer, 1982), level of airways hyperreactivity assessed by histamine and methacholine inhalation challenge (Dirks and Brown, 1982), and daily pulmonary function measurements (Dirks, Ruback et al., 1982). Rather, with the exception of dyspnea and congestion, the target physical symptoms of asthma, the symptom reports vary according to the personality type of the patient (Kinsman et al., 1980). Such symptoms, related to patient personality, then influence physician decisions including aggressiveness of medication regimens prescribed to manage the condition, independent of any objective evidence of the illness severity (Kinsman et al., 1977).

For predisposed patients, anxiety inherent to asthma can trigger dependency conflicts, which also are unrelated to age at onset of asthma (Dirks et al., 1977). The existence of a dependency conflict and how it is resolved rest upon aspects of the patient's emotional development separate from the illness. However, the mode of resolution of the dependency conflict, either passive or active, identifies various subgroups of patients, two of which differ extremely in how patients experience and cope with asthma (Dirks et al., 1979). The passive patient yields to anxiety, tends to give up easily in the face of difficulty, withdraws, exaggerates the distress of breathing, and clings dependently to others. Children and adults who react this way conceive of themselves as having a fragile body, which contributes further to a sense of personal helplessness, dependency, and depression. Approximately 22 percent of adolescent and adult asthmatic patients hospitalized for intensive treatment display this excessively dependent style (Kinsman et al., 1982). At the other extreme, some confront this same anxiety by attempting actively to prove their competence in an excessively independent way, by minimizing symptoms stoically during acute asthma and refusing to carry out appropriate treatment, including the use of medications or the observance of important environmental restrictions. Such patients are rigidly overconfident in their own physical and personal resources and may show unusually low levels of anxiety or depression. Approximately 16 percent of adolescent and adult patients hospitalized for asthma dis-

TABLE 22–1. Symptoms and Experiences Reported to Occur During Acute Episodes of Breathing Difficulty in Asthma*

Symptom Category	Description	Scale Value Mean (SD)†
Dyspnea	Breathing difficulty	4.29 (0.69)
Fatigue	Reduced energy level	3.65 (0.88)
Congestion	Chest congestion	3.60 (0.81)
Rapid breathing	Rapid breathing, heart pounding, and panting	3.45 (0.91)
Worry	Concern about self	3.22 (0.94)
Irritability	Edginess and irritability	2.96 (0.87)
Panic-Fear	Anxiety focused on asthma	2.86 (0.87)
Anger	Anger during the attack	2.32 (0.84)
Hyperventilation-hypocapnia	Hyperventilation symptoms	2.25 (0.72)
Loneliness	Concern about being alone	2.21 (0.90)

* Based on 374 asthma patients ranging in age from 12 to 72 years who were administered the Asthma Symptom Checklist (ASC).

† Mean value of 5-point scale (1 = never; 5 = always) for each of the discrete symptom items within the symptom category.

play this excessively independent style (Kinsman et al., 1982). These extreme behavioral responses are evident in levels of personality, in attitudes towards treatment, in symptom reports, and in illness behaviors (Kinsman et al., 1982). Thus, the patient's personality, in fact, affects emotional aspects of illness and ultimately may affect the outcome of treatment, in some cases. This places the patient at much greater risk from the disease process.

Asthma or its treatment also may affect cognitive functioning. In a recent study, 65 percent of a sample of 95 adult patients, 21 to 55 years of age, with intractable asthma were found to have equivocal or definite Bender-Gestalt signs indicative of cerebral dysfunction (Shraa et al., 1981). The majority (53 percent) had clear-cut memory deficits. Dunleavy and Baade (1980), using the Halstead-Reitan Neuropsychological Battery, found seven of a group of 20 severely asthmatic children, 9 to 14 years of age, to be impaired neurologically, with deficits noted in visualizing and remembering spatial configurations and in incidental memory. Several reasons, none mutually exclusive, may account for cognitive or memory deficits as follows:

1. Four of the seven asthmatic children whom Dunleavy and Baade identified as "neuropsychologically impaired" had histories of cyanosis or loss of consciousness during asthma attacks, whereas only one of the 13 unimpaired children had similar histories. Thus, hypoxic episodes may have caused permanent brain damage in these children, although controls for medication were not included in the study.
2. Suess and Chai (1981) reported that theophylline and steroid medications used to treat asthma lead to mnemonic impairments which are largely, if not totally, reversible (Shraa and Dirks, 1982).
3. Fatigue or mood changes secondary to asthma or asthma medications, including anxiety and depression, may interfere with attention and other aspects of cognitive functioning.

Any or all of these factors can operate together to affect cognitive or memory functioning on psychologic tests. To our knowledge, there has not been research exploring the relationship of these factors and impaired academic or vocational functioning. Certainly, academic or vocational difficulties experienced by asthmatic patients can be a direct result of absenteeism from work or school due to illness. According to the National Health Survey for 1963, 64,000,000 days were lost to work and school due to asthma and hay fever. Resolution of such real life problems due to absenteeism hinges on effective, total management of these illnesses.

Severe asthma also can affect family and peer relationships. In one study, 53 percent of parents of hospitalized asthmatic children reported that they had met serious social or economic difficulties (or both) due to the child's asthma; 42 percent said they were overprotective of their child; and 39 percent admitted that they resented the child's asthma because of its affect on them and other family members (Creer et al., 1983). These families cope poorly with the child's asthma in ways that can set up a vicious cycle, which further complicates management. Specifically, noncompliance, secondary gain from asthma, and generally poor self-management are most evident for asthmatic children and adults imbedded in an unhappy family situation. Consequently, patients may benefit from family or individual psychologic treatment aimed at resolving serious impediments to medical management.

Allergic Rhinitis

Signs and symptoms of allergic rhinitis include sneezing, nasal discharge, pressure over paranasal sinus areas, mouth breathing, snorting, coughing, throat clearing, and nose wiping. If anxiety is less significant an issue than for asthma, irritability and alienation are more so. Symptoms can be nagging and distracting to the point of interfering with work or school activities. Sleeplessness and fatigue are common. Intermittent hearing loss due to ear involvement often occurs and may be interpreted as deliberate inattention by parents, teachers, or others. Together, these symptoms and experiences predictably give some patients with rhinitis an absent-minded, preoccupied, and spiritless quality that obstructs interest in activities and strains relationships. Nose wiping, open-mouthed breathing and eating, and constant sniffing can be unattractive to parents or peers, contributing to subtle and even blatant rejection. Children who are rejected by parents or peers often are unable to identify that the reasons for this rejection are related to the rhinitis and blame themselves instead. The distraction of this illness can be compounded by increased absenteeism from school or work, which impairs academic or vocational performance. Cognitive effects that occur secondary to rhinitis or its treatment are more transient and benign than the psychologic problems of severe asthmatics.

Atopic Dermatitis

Inasmuch as the principal symptom of atopic dermatitis is itching, which in turn leads to scratching that can cause bleeding, scabbing, and secondary infections of the skin, the role of scratching cannot be underestimated. Skin changes may be marked and embarrassing. The constant scratching and unappealing changes in skin may lead to rejection by parents, teachers, or peers. The likelihood of rejection is influenced by severity of dermatitis and parts of the body affected. For subgroups of patients, an important conflict centering on their need for attention, affection, and support from others may be triggered by the illness (Wittkower and Edgell, 1951). This conflict may be handled either actively or passively. The coping style adopted then will influence the patient's attitudes toward the illness and its treatment, how the illness is experienced, the significance attached to the signs and symptoms of dermatitis, and ultimately the behaviors during treatment. The passive approach is characterized by submission, docility, and helplessness. For such patients, the attitudes toward the dermatitis and its treatment may parallel this passive style; for example, a pessimism about their own ability to manage the illness or an over reliance upon physicians to the exclusion of what they themselves can do and an exaggerated belief that they are stigmatized by the illness. To the extent that they fail to assume effective self-management responsibilities and continue to yield to every itch with a scratch, the illness may be more difficult to manage. Those adopting the active style may conceal the same needs for attention, affection, and support behind a self-assertive, ambitious, or belligerent façade. The attitudes of these patients towards illness and its treatment derive from an active, confronting stance. The patients display an overconfidence in their own ability to manage the illness without medical help, a reluctance to follow medical advice, and a denial that the dermatitis causes any difficulties in their interpersonal relationships. These patients are likely to scratch in defiance of medical advice. For both of these extreme styles, various manifestations of treatment noncompliance may serve to undercut medical management.

PSYCHOLOGIC FACTORS AS TRIGGERS FOR PHYSICAL SYMPTOMS

For each of the allergic diseases discussed previously, immune abnormalities and a variety of other precipitating factors can trigger symptoms by activating biochemical mediators with close links to the autonomic nervous system that act through final common pathways (Szentivanyi and Williams, 1980). The role of psychologic factors in triggering symptoms has been noted clinically for various allergic disorders but considered most extensively for asthma. Models that have been predominant in these considerations are based on classic conditioning and suggestion. Both of these models have evolved to include a mediating role for anxiety in the triggering of asthma attacks.

Classic Conditioning Studies

Although clinical reports favor the expectation that airways obstruction can be conditioned in asthmatics, a critical appraisal of the related literature reveals that conditioned airways obstruction in humans remains to be demonstrated convincingly. The earliest account of asthma as a conditioned response was reported by MacKenzie (1886). MacKenzie's patient wheezed in the presence of real roses — but also wheezed in the presence of an artificial rose. However, MacKenzie's case report, cited in the asthma-related literature repeatedly, provides little evidence for the generality of classic conditioning in asthma symptoms. During the first half of this century, there were major developments in research and theory in classic conditioning (Pavlov, 1927 and 1941). A number of investigators came to apply the classic conditioning model to asthma using animals and human subjects.

Studies in Animals. With animals, Noelpp and Noelpp-Eschenhagen (Noelpp and Noelpp-Eschenhagen, 1952; Noelpp-Eschenhagen and Noelpp, 1954) and Ottenberg and coworkers (1958) were able to show that asthma-like breathing patterns could be elicited in sensitized guinea pigs by an initially neutral stimulus alone after pairing the neutral stimulus with histamine or antigen. In general, studies such as these failed to measure possible changes in airways caliber and thus to differentiate between "asthma" and conditioned breathing patterns, such as hyperventilation, which could result from simple exposure to any fear provoking stimulus (Stein, 1962). Presumably, repeated presentation of a neutral stimulus with an aversive event, such as anaphylaxis, could render the initially neutral cue as fear provoking, thus evoking a pattern of hyperventilation. This breathing pattern, consisting primarily of rapid or irregular breathing or both, could be regarded erroneously as conditioned asthma. Furthermore, Ottenberg and his coworkers did not specify the effective stimulus during conditioning, thereby making it difficult to assess whether true conditioning had occurred. Somewhat later, Justesen and coworkers (1970) elicited changes in airways caliber in guinea pigs by classic conditioning methods and demonstrated differential pharmacologic blocking of allergic and of "conditioned" asthma attacks: isoproterenol blocked both responses, whereas diphenhydramine blocked the allergic but not the conditioned response. In contrast, atropine was effective against only conditioned asthma attacks. As Bouhuys (1971) pointed out, Justesen and coworkers failed to differentiate between fear-provoked hyperventilation and conditioned asthma, since both responses could lead to the changes observed in measured peak pressures. Nevertheless, the differential blocking of conditioned and allergic responses supports the possibility of true conditioning, albeit conditioning that may be mediated by fear or anxiety. Such a model, in fact, was proposed by Justesen and his coworkers and independently derived later by Kinsman and his coworkers (1974) from their work with asthma symptoms in humans. Their model holds that internal body cues associated with the response of anxiety gain the ability to elicit or perpetuate airways obstruction, as an inherent byproduct of repeated asthma attacks; in effect, this contributes an "interoceptive-interoceptive" classic conditioning trial of the type described by Razran (1961). Precisely this type of conditioning happens for subgroups of asthma patients, sharing important features of the atopic (autonomic) defect depicted by Szentivanyi and Williams (1980), in later bronchoconstrictive suggestion studies.

Studies in Humans. Research addressing classic conditioning in human asthma is sparse. In addition, designs of earlier studies were poor in general, resulting in little useful data from which to draw any conclusions concerning the possible role of conditioning in the induction or propagation of asthma. Knapp (1963), in a series of studies, was unable to demonstrate classically conditioned asthma in humans. Dekker and coworkers (1957) previously had reported successful conditioning in the laboratory. However, their study represented the distillation of only two selected cases from at least 31 subjects earlier studied by Dekker and Groen (1956). Conditions were not controlled nor were subjects treated comparably at similar times without conditioning. Also, the conditioned stimulus was not specific. The conclusion from information to date would seem to be that a conditioned attack is an unusual phenomenon in asthma. It is paradoxical that numerous autonomic responses have been shown repeatedly to be readily conditioned in animals and humans (Razran, 1961; Kimble, 1961). Thus, the apparent exception of airways obstruction in human asthmatics is a bit puzzling. To our knowledge, there has not been a new study of classic conditioning in asthma using human subjects reported in the literature in the past 22 years. Studies using a highly analogous suggestion model (see subsequent discussion) picked up the thread dropped when classic conditioning in human asthma was essentially dismissed as undemonstrated, if not undemonstrable. Given the results from studies supporting the role of suggestion in some asthmatics and the dearth of information available supporting conditioning specifically, the possible role that conditioned responses may play in human asthma remains an open question.

Suggestion Studies

Luparello and coworkers (1968) first adopted the model of bronchoconstrictive suggestion to study the role of anxiety as a trigger for airways obstruction in asthmatics. Briefly, bronchoconstrictive suggestion involves a ruse, i.e., a neutral substance is presented to the asthmatic patient with instructions that it is something that will cause an asthma attack. For humans, cognition makes suggestion identical to classic conditioning, except that a person is told that the neutral agent is capable of inducing an asthma attack, rather than taught that it can do so by repeated conditioning trials. Using effort-independent pulmonary function measurements by means of whole body plethysmography, a series of studies demonstrated that broncho-constrictive suggestion can induce rapid and clinically significant changes in airways caliber in some patients. Furthermore, these changes were susceptible to differential pharmacologic blocking, lending support to the position that the changes induced were vagally mediated (McFadden et al., 1969; Luparello et al., 1970; Luparello et al., 1971). The initial work was subsequently replicated by Spector and his co-workers (1976). Increases in airways resistance of up to 90 percent relative to baseline measures were observed. Corroborative results also have been obtained by Strupp et al. (1974) and Phillip et al. (1972).

It is important to note that one third to two thirds of the asthmatic patients studied in various reports displayed meaningful decreases in airways caliber. That is, not all asthmatic patients respond to an identical stressor ("suggestion") with airways obstruction. A later study by Horton and coworkers (1978) found differences in responses to suggestions among 22 patients involved, ranging from a small increase to a marked decrease in specific airways conductance (SGaw). More importantly, the magnitude of the airways response to suggestion varied according to two classes of variables as follows: (1) airways hyperreactivity, measured by prior methacholine and histamine inhalation challenge, and (2) physiologic indices of the emotional reaction to suggestion, measured by changes in diastolic blood pressure, finger pulse amplitude, and forehead electromyelographic (EMG) activity. The relationships between the physiologic indices of the emotional reaction were not dependent upon the level of the subject's airways hyperreactivity. Thus, by taking both factors into consideration, the airways response to suggestion could be predicted with the best accuracy.

In summary, at least two factors appear to be involved in determining whether or not an asthmatic will respond to a potentially stressful situation with bronchoconstriction. The first involves the patient's appraisal of a threat and the magnitude of his or her emotional response (i.e., the situation elicits the physiologic concomitants of anxiety). If the person appraises the threat as being high and reacts strongly, the probability of airways obstruction is increased. Although not as yet confirmed, those asthmatics most likely to respond in this way would seem to be those who characterologically are anxious, that is, predisposed to react with anxiety to various situations (Dirks et al., 1978).

However, the airways response may be dependent ultimately upon a second factor, namely, the intrinsic hyperreactivity (lability) of the airways. In brief, asthmatics who have the greatest airways lability and who are most prone to react to various stressors emotionally, are those most likely to have clinically significant emotional triggers for asthma. In such patients, in particular, selection of therapeutic modalities that reduce anxiety would be especially important, as would recognition that anxiety can affect their illness in a variety of ways (Kinsman et al., 1980).

PSYCHOLOGIC FACTORS THAT MAINTAIN ILLNESS

Although anxiety is a normal central emotion resulting from acute asthma, it also can serve to induce airways obstruction in a subgroup of patients and may play an important role in increasing the intractability of asthma. In this section, we will address what is known about psychologic factors that undermine treatment in conformance to the illness psychomaintenance model presented in Figure 22–1. It is important first to distinguish between two different types of anxiety in asthma, both called Panic-Fear, at the level of patient personality (Level 1) or at the level of symptom reports (Level 3).

Panic-Fear in Asthma

The illness psychomaintenance model has been applied clinically as the Battery of Asthma Illness Behavior (BAIB) by Kinsman et al. (1982). This battery consists of the following three psychometric tests, each conforming to a level of measurement in Figure 22–1: (1) Minnesota Multiphasic Personality Inventory (MMPI; Greene, 1980) at Level 1; (2) Respiratory Illness Opinion Survey (RIOS; Kinsman et al., 1976; Staudenmayer et al., 1978) at Level 2; and (3) Asthma Symptom Checklist (ASC; Kinsman et al., 1973; Kinsman et al., 1973, 1974 and 1977) at Level 3. The BAIB simplifies the assessment of the role of psychologic factors in continuing disease by using two measures to classify asthma patients into nine psychologic subtypes based on two forms of anxiety. This is shown in Table 22–2 as follows: (1) general anxiety, indexed by the Panic-Fear Personality Scale of the MMPI (Dirks et al., 1977) and (2)

TABLE 22–2. Asthma Response Styles Based on Panic-Fear Symptoms (PF-S) and Panic-Fear Personality (PF-P) and Effect on Medical Treatment and Outcome

| | Type of Anxiety | | | Response Style | | Influence upon Medical Treatment and Its Outcome | | |
PATTERN NUMBER	ILLNESS FOCUSED ANXIETY (PF-S)	GENERAL ANXIETY (PF-P)	PATIENTS (PERCENT)*	ATTENTION TO SYMPTOMS	RESPONSE TO ATTACKS	INTENSITY OF PRESCRIBED MEDICATIONS	LENGTH OF HOSPITAL STAY	FREQUENCY OF HOSPITALIZATION
1	Low	Low	8.5	Disregard	Rigid independence	Decreased	Short	High
2	Low	Moderate	16.4	Disregard	Generally adaptive	No Effect	Moderate	Moderate to High
3	Low	High	2.0	Disregard	Anxious dependency and helplessness	ND†	ND†	High
4	Moderate	Low	6.3	Typical	Rigid independence	No Effect	Short	High
5	Moderate	Moderate	33.4	Typical	Generally adaptive	No Effect	Moderate	Moderate
6	Moderate	High	8.3	Typical	Anxious dependency and helplessness	Increased	Long	High
7	High	Low	1.3	Vigilant	Rigid independence	ND†	ND†	ND†
8	High	Moderate	12.2	Vigilant	Generally adaptive	No Effect	Moderate	Low
9	High	High	11.6	Vigilant	Anxious dependency and helplessness	Increased	Long	High

* These percentages reflect incidence for asthmatic patients treated at National Jewish Hospital and Research Center in Denver, Colorado.
† ND: Not documented: These patients were too few in number to permit documentation of the effect.

illness-focused anxiety, indexed by the Panic-Fear Symptom Scale of the ASC. Table 22-2 also depicts how each subtype may influence several aspects of medical treatment and its outcome: frequency of hospitalization, length of hospital stay, and intensity of the medical regimen prescribed to manage the asthma (Jones et al., 1979).

The Panic-Fear Symptom Scale measures the frequency of reported panic and fear symptoms during typical asthma attacks (Fig. 22-1, Level 3), a type of anxiety focused directly upon the illness. Increased levels of anxiety that are focused on the illness seem potentially helpful and may be consistent with appropriate vigilance toward breathing difficulties. In contrast, unusually low levels of illness-focused anxiety are related to disregard of symptoms and may be harmful (Dirks et al., 1979; Staudenmayer et al., 1979). The Panic-Fear Personality Scale measures stable personality characteristics of the patient (Fig. 22-1, Level 2) and reflects a predisposition to react to various situations including (but not limited to) asthma attacks with anxiety and helplessness (Dirks et al., 1977). This test predicts the kind of reaction expected when the patient develops trouble breathing. As Table 22-2 implies, the degrees of illness-focused anxiety and general anxiety relate to patient behaviors that influence not only the physicians' decisions but also long-term outcomes of medical treatment.

For example, Pattern 1 of Table 22-2 includes 8.5 percent of asthmatic patients studied who are normatively low on both types of anxiety. These patients have two problems that can defeat treatment as follows: (1) their anxiety focused on the illness is too low, leading them to disregard symptoms; (2) when symptoms finally progress beyond the point where disregard is possible, they then try to "tough out" their physical distress without medication or medical assistance. Behaviorally, they use medications such as aerosolized bronchodilators too infrequently to relieve asthma, even when significant airways obstruction is present (Dahlem et al., 1977). Because these patients minimize their symptoms, physicians typically treat them less intensively than other patients with airways obstruction, hospitalizing them for shorter periods (Dirks et al., 1977). Their long-term outlook is poor, and they are hospitalized frequently even after intensive treatment (Dirks et al., 1978 and 1980). Patient response styles are independent of actual disease severity and can obscure objective measurements of severity

to reduce the effectiveness of medical treatment or increase the intractability of the asthma. Specific psychologic mechanisms that often are associated with the response styles (listed in Table 22-2) tend to perpetuate the illness.

Mechanisms of Illness Psychomaintenance

Personality, attitudes toward treatment, and reported symptoms and experiences are useful in describing the patient and identifying response styles. Illness is maintained, however, much more directly by various mechanisms including the patient's behaviors, the ability or inclination to use symptoms as cues for action, the manner in which the patient presents, and, ultimately, the physician's decisions in view of these parameters. Table 22-3 lists a number of the mechanisms studied in asthma and shows their relationship to each of the nine response styles of Table 22-2.

Emotions as Triggers for Symptoms. This was described in detail previously as a mechanism for illness psychomaintenance. In brief, those patients who react to stress with strong emotional responses and who have the most highly reactive airways are at most risk to have emotional responses as triggers for airways obstruction. Mechanical (physical) factors related to emotional reactions, including hyperventilation and crying, may exacerbate bronchoconstriction through well-described reflexes. Patients at greatest risk to respond with strong emotional responses to real or perceived stress factors appear to be those who are anxious, dependent, and helpless (i.e., high Panic-Fear personality), as shown in Table 22-3.

Medication Noncompliance. Medication misuse remains a universal and serious problem, involving 46 to 58 percent of patients in long-term treatment (Sackett and Snow, 1979; Haynes, 1982). The related literature has focused almost exclusively on one type of misuse, i.e., underuse of medications. Dirks and Kinsman (1982) have pointed out that this focus on medication underuse has been perpetuated by methods to measure medication underuse (e.g., biochemical assay), which actually create artificial dichotomies of "compliers" and "noncompliers." By so doing, this approach ignores factors such as actual usage patterns and differences in metabolism, leading to misclassification of patients. For example, the patient's actual usage can conform to one of four pat-

TABLE 22-3. Asthma Response Styles and Known Mechanisms of Illness Psychomaintenance

	Response Style		Medication Compliance		Symptom Recognition		Clinical Presentation	
Number	Attention to Symptoms	Response to Attacks	Routinely Scheduled Medications	As-needed (PRN) Medications	Symptom Labeling	Symptom Perception	Clinical Presentation	Approach to Medical Care
1	Disregard	Rigid independence	Underuse	Underuse	Correct	Good	Minimize Severity	Avoids
2	Disregard	Generally adaptive	NP*	Underuse	Correct	Fair	Realistic Severity	Accepts
3	Disregard	Anxious dependency and helplessness	ND†	ND†	ND†	ND†	ND†	ND†
4	Typical	Rigid independence	Underuse	NP*	Correct	Good	Minimize Severity	Avoids
5	Typical	Generally adaptive	NP*	NP*	Correct	Fair	Realistic Severity	Accepts
6	Typical	Anxious dependency and helplessness	Erratic Overuse and Underuse	Arbitrary and Overuse	Errors	Poor	Maximize Severity	"Clings"
7	Vigilant	Rigid independence	ND†	ND†	ND†	ND†	ND†	ND†
8	Vigilant	Generally adaptive	Compliant	Appropriate Use	Correct	Fair	Realistic Severity	Accepts
9	Vigilant	Anxious dependency and helplessness	Erratic Overuse and Underuse	Arbitrary and Overuse	Errors	Poor	Maximize Severity	"Clings"

* NP = Not predicted: Compliance cannot be predicted solely on the basis of this style.

† ND = Not documented: These patients are too few in number to permit documentation of the mechanism and effects.

terns as follows: (1) appropriate usage, the patient takes medications according to the prescribed schedule; (2) underusage, the patient fails to take as much medication as prescribed; (3) overusage, the patient takes more medication than prescribed; and (4) erratic usage, the patient both underuses and overuses the medications at different times. Continuous monitoring of medication use is required to identify actual patterns. This monitoring is possible for aerosolized medications (Spector et al., 1983) and for pills taken orally by using medication "chronologs" to record each usage time electronically. (The latter currently is in developmental stages). Each type of medication use is likely to be associated with a specific response pattern (see Table 22–3) and to exert a unique effect upon the risk-benefit ratio, for both regularly scheduled and "as needed" (prn) medications (Dirks and Kinsman, 1982).

For regularly scheduled medications, Kleiger and Dirks (1979) found that 28 percent of a small sample (N = 54) of asthma patients reported that they underuse medications at times; 11 percent reported that they overused medications; and 15 percent reported that they underused and overused medications at different times. Excessively independent patients typically reported underuse (87.5 percent), whereas erratic usage, (e.g., overusage and underusage at different times) was more characteristic of helpless, dependent patients (50 percent).

For as needed (prn) aerosolized medications commonly prescribed for asthma, certain prn usage patterns bear no relationship to those intended. Among a group of 88 asthmatic inpatients, only 33 percent requested prn medications appropriately, judged as taking prn medications more frequently on days when airways obstruction was present and rarely when airways obstruction was not present. The remaining 67 percent took medications in clearly inappropriate ways; 20 percent overused medication by taking them frequently on days when no airways obstruction was present, 20 percent underused them by taking them rarely on days when airways obstruction was significant, and 27 percent used them in erratic, arbitrary ways with respect to airways obstruction (Kinsman et al., 1980). Such misuse of prn medications affects treatment for asthma. Overusage and underusage influence medical decisions related to amount and frequency of medications prescribed and to length of hospitalization (Dahlem et al., 1979). Additionally, for certain aerosolized bronchodilators, overusage has been

related to a paradoxical pulmonary response with potentially serious consequences to the patient (Bierman and Pierson, 1974). Although no differences were found in the actual severity of asthma among these various groups, sharp differences did exist for the personality styles measured by the Battery of Asthma Illness Behavior. The prn medication underusers presented themselves unrealistically as independent, capable, and optimistic about their ability to manage their asthma attacks (i.e., low Panic-Fear personality). In contrast, overusers were more helpless, less able to cope effectively, unusually pessimistic about their ability to master asthma successfully, and intolerant and fearful of discomfort (i.e., high Panic-Fear personality). Both of these personality styles are known to be related to poor medical outcome in asthma (see Table 22–2; Jones et al., 1979).

Symptom Disregard. As described, anxiety focused directly upon the illness is related to behaviors that reflect the patient's level of attention toward respiratory trouble (Jones et al., 1979). In this case, low levels, not high, are maladaptive.

Dahlem and coworkers (1977) found that asthmatic inpatients with exceptionally low anxiety regarding difficulties in breathing requested few prn aerosolized bronchodilators even on days when marked airways obstruction was present. In contrast, asthmatics with exceptionally high levels of anxiety focused on difficulties in breathing requested frequent prn medications even when no airways obstruction was present. Subsequent analyses indicated that such overusage was primarily due to personality features related to general anxiety. One way to view the results of Dahlem's study is that low, illness focused anxiety is related to symptom disregard. Presumably, vigilance towards symptoms is adaptive, whereas disregard towards symptoms is maladaptive. The results of Staudenmayer et al. (1979) support this interpretation. Dahlem's symptom disregarders, i.e., asthma patients with unusually low levels of illness focused anxiety, were rehospitalized within 6 months at exceptionally high rates after intensive treatment, most notably when their low, illness focused anxiety coexisted with highly reactive airways (47 percent). In contrast, those asthma patients with high levels of illness focused anxiety, i.e., Dahlem's vigilant patients, were the least likely to be rehospitalized, and none were rehospitalized when this vigilant stance coexisted with relatively low airways reactivity. Procedures to reduce anxiety never should address illness focused anxiety alone, since this type of anxiety is appropriate and adaptive in asthma. A lack of anxiety about difficulty breathing may delay effective action to resolve incipient attacks. In effect, illness focused anxiety acts as a signal, energizing the patient to react. The nature of the subsequent actions then may be of critical importance (Dirks et al., 1979), but any adjunctive interventions should leave intact the appropriate symptom vigilance associated with illness focused anxiety (Kinsman et al., 1980).

Symptom Mislabeling. Using the Asthma Symptom Checklist (ASC), Dirks, Schraa, and Robinson (1982) found that over 27 percent of a group of 587 adult asthmatics mislabeled one or more symptoms unrelated to airways obstruction as an asthma attack. Of the ten ASC symptom categories (see Table 22–1), fatigue was most frequently mislabeled as an asthma symptom, followed by worry, rapid breathing, and irritability. Symptom mislabelers were 40 percent more likely than nonmislabelers to be rehospitalized for asthma during a 6-month period after discharge from intensive treatment. The likelihood of rehospitalization grew linearly, as more symptoms were mislabeled as being those of an asthma attack. Symptom mislabeling can affect all the response styles shown in Tables 22–2 and 22–3, but it is nearly three times as likely to be characteristic of the helpless, ineffective patients with high general anxiety than the excessively independent patients with low general anxiety. Symptom mislabelers were an average of 5 years older than "nonmislabelers." Only one response style benefited from mislabeling; the relatively few excessively independent patients who were symptom mislabelers were less likely to be rehospitalized than nonmislabelers who shared this response style. Dirks regards this single exception as indicative that anything, including symptom mislabeling, that brings overly optimistic, counterdependent asthma patients to a physician for treatment is beneficial. For all other patients, symptom mislabeling serves only to confuse the clinical picture, encouraging them to act on the wrong cues, which ultimately undermine treatment.

Symptom Perception. There is marked variability among asthma patients in their ability to detect added inspiratory resistive loads to breathing; some are grossly deficient in their perception of changes in airways caliber (Rubinfeld and Pain, 1976 and 1977; Burki et al., 1978). It has been suggested that some patients

do poorly during treatment and may be at increased risk for the rare cases of death in asthma because they simply cannot detect airways obstruction early enough to relieve asthma (Nana and Pain, 1985). Poor detection of airways constriction also may contribute to symptom mislabeling.

Hudgel and coworkers (1982) found that added inspiratory resistive loads to breathing were detected most poorly by asthma patients with a response style characterized by high anxiety, helplessness, and dependency, the same patients at greatest risk for symptom mislabeling. In a second study, Hudgel and Kinsman (1983) found a strong inverse relationship between the resting inspiratory neuromuscular activity reflecting ventilatory drive and the amount of added resistance required for recognition. Higher ventilatory drives were related to lower levels of added inspiratory resistance needed for detection. Anxious, dependent asthma patients (i.e., high Panic-Fear personality) had resting ventilatory drives that were less than 50 percent of those of the excessively independent patients (i.e., low Panic-Fear personality). As a result, they required more added inspiratory resistance for recognition than other patients. Since anxious, dependent patients do not appear to breathe more forcefully when faced with added inspiratory resistance to breathing, it follows that they then may experience little dyspnea early in the progression of attacks. This characteristic may contribute to confusion about what symptoms require a response and therefore to symptom mislabeling, further compromising their already poor ability to react effectively to breathing difficulties.

Memory Deficiencies. Any chronic physical illness places demands on the patient for self-management. Depending on the nature of the allergic disease and the treatment requirements, the patient will be asked to keep appointments, to follow a specified diet, to reduce exposure to conditions that exacerbate physical symptoms, to follow orally conveyed directions and to retain them, and to take daily medications according to a prescribed schedule. Ultimately, the patient's medical status and course of illness depend on how well he or she manages to do what is required. There is strikingly little information available that bears on the relationship of memory and compliance. However, there is information that demonstrates that many patients with severe asthma have serious memory problems, as indicated by their performance on psychometric tests (Shraa et al., 1981). As many as 35 percent of hospitalized patients give accounts of their treatment programs immediately after discharge discrepant from those given by their physicians (Parkin et al., 1976). Patients may remember less than 50 percent of medical instructions given orally only 2 hours before (Ley and Spelman, 1965). Medication compliance can be abysmally poor for patients on long-term medical treatment (Dirks and Kinsman, 1982). Despite this fact, the precise role of memory deficiencies on behaviors during treatment (e.g., medication usage) is neither well studied nor well understood in any disease. The influence of memory deficiency undoubtedly is substantial. In our own experience, those asthma patients with serious deficiencies in short-term memory documented by testing were the only group to show no gain in knowledge whatsoever after an intensive, formal patient education program about their illness. In the absence of empiric information, logic dictates that memory deficiencies, often affecting older patients, compromise treatment through poor retention of medical information, as well as the daily forgetfulness of what to do next and when.

Patient-Physician Relationships. The remarkable differences among patients with an identical illness include the role of anxiety as a trigger for symptoms, the ability to recognize key physical changes giving rise to symptoms, the ability to correctly label symptoms, and the ability to attend to them appropriately. Also, there are significant differences in the ability to retain medical information and to remember what to do and when. Finally, there are variations in the nature of the reactions to acute episodes of illness. These color the clinical presentation during treatment and affect the outcome of a treatment plan, in part by the influence exerted upon the physician's perception of the problem. The way patient differences affect physician perceptions depends in turn on the frame of reference and personality profile of the physician.

For example, in an inpatient setting for asthmatics, physicians rated highest in "sensitivity to patients as whole persons" by their medical supervisors altered their prescribed steroid regimens proportionately more to the degree of their patients' anxiety, than to objective measures of severity. In contrast, physicians rated low in "sensitivity" based their judgments on objective pulmonary function measurements and not patient anxiety (Kinsman et al., 1977; Dirks et al., 1978). The amount and intensity of steroid usage for similar clinical situations actually was ultimately less in the group of patients treated by "sensitive" physicians than those treated by physicians with low "sensitivity" (Dirks et al., 1978). Thus, the "organically oriented" physician whose orientation does not allow an appreciation of the patient's psychologic needs may in fact provide more medical therapy in the long run to help relieve the problem for the patient. Distinctions also need to be made between a poor treatment response due to a particularly malignant pathophysiologic process and one due to psychologic factors that alter the patient's presentation or serve to defeat medical management.

MANAGEMENT OF PSYCHOLOGIC ISSUES

Recognition of potential problems in management due to the operation of psychologic factors is a key to their resolution. General and specific strategies follow only from the identification of these issues and their causes. Treating a behavior directly, without considering its causes, is a poor approach. For example, a patient may underuse medications simply because of poor memory. Another may do so because of a strong need to be independent and competent that leads him or her to regard medications as a crutch or a sign of weakness. Some may underuse medications because of depression so deep that they see no reason to make the effort; others may do so out of an unreasonable fear of side effects. For each of these patients, treatment is compromised in precisely the same way. However, resolution of their identical noncompliance patterns depends upon understanding and addressing the different psychologic causes.

As a general starting point in patient management, it is useful to assess the way that the patient presents with the illness. Does the presentation conform to one of the two extreme personality styles associated with a poor treatment response (see Table 22–2)? Does the patient appear to be excessively demanding, prone to exaggerate his or her needs, unreasonably pessimistic about being able to manage the illness, unusually anxious, helpless, or dependent in relation to various problems including the illness (high Panic-Fear personality)? If so, the patient's adherence to medication regimens needs to be monitored carefully, with special effort given to education in the proper use of medication. Careful comparisons should be made between the patient's self-reports of breathing difficulty and objective indices of the illness to avoid being misled by the patient's tendency to exaggerate. Diaphragmatic breathing training for asthmatic patients with this personality style is useful to overcome anxiety and combat any tendency toward hyperventilation. Relaxation techniques may help to contain anxiety, although the real benefit may be to convince the patient that he or she has some control over the disease. Continuous efforts to educate the patient about effective self-care responsibilities need to be made. Some asthmatic patients with this style respond exceptionally well simply to reassurance and guidance and can be shown to raise air flow rates significantly by firm reassurance, supportive concern, and a few minutes' instruction on how to breathe diaphragmatically (Kinsman et al., 1981).

At the other extreme, the patient may present in a stoic way, with a tendency to minimize the distress, with an unrealistic optimism about being able to manage the illness, and with an exceptionally calm and confident independence towards the illness (low Panic-Fear personality). This patient may profit by a careful exploration of actions and activities preceding recent exacerbations of the illness, emergency room visits, or hospitalizations, for the purpose of identifying how the patient's own attempts to "tough out" the illness without help actually led to increased helplessness and unwelcomed dependency. Clear information then should be shared with the patient about the personal costs of this style of coping, stressing that the effect of inappropriate short-term independence ultimately may be long-term dependence because of the disease. Because of the tendency of this type of patient to minimize illness, self-reports of symptoms should be compared carefully with objective measurements. Additionally, emphasis should be placed on the need to respond to symptoms expeditiously. Sometimes it is useful to equip asthma patients of this type with a home spirometer, e.g., minipeak flow meter (assuming it is possible to convince them to use it), instructing them to use it daily and to take prescribed actions whenever the values fall below a certain point irrespective of their subjective feelings. It may be helpful to give some patients permission to go directly to the hospital if acute symptoms do not respond to home self-management.

Specific problems around symptom identification, including disregard, mislabeling, and lack of recognition, often are related to the extreme Panic-Fear personality styles as indicated in Table 22 – 3. Problems also can occur for patients who respond more adaptively. Each form of misinterpretation or denial of symptoms interferes with the appropriate use of symptoms as signals for expeditious action. To resolve the issue of symptom mislabeling, careful inquiry as to what the patient really means when reporting a symptom is needed. Information from this inquiry can obviate the administration of unnecessary medical treatment with its attendant risks due to mislabeled and miscommunicated symptoms. This is a circumstance for home spirometer use for asthmatics, which has the added advantage of providing instruction to the patient so that he or she can recognize symptoms and treat them more appropriately as time goes on.

There are several situations that should lead one to consider problems with memory as a cause for treatment failure. These include elderly patients, patients treated with combined theophylline and corticosteroid medications, patients who have had repeated or serious hypoxic episodes or both, patients with decreased intellectual resources, and patients who frankly complain about forgetting. When possible, give written instructions to these patients. In conveying oral information to them, special efforts are needed to present the most important information first, to emphasize the most important points concerning what the patient needs to do, to use simple language, to make specific and concrete statements rather than general ones (e.g., do not say "Take the medication twice a day," rather, "Take the medication at noon and at bedtime"), and to repeat the same information over several meetings, as well as to provide clear written instructions. Additionally, for the memory-impaired patient, retest the patient's retention at later times by inquiring about the treatment regimen and information conveyed. For those with exceptionally severe impairments, the involvement of other family members may be needed. For these severely impaired patients, a simple strategy is sometimes useful as follows: instruct the patient to obtain an alarm wrist watch set to ring at regular times, cuing the patient to look in a prepared daily diary, laying open and flat on a desk, to find the correct time in the diary, and to follow what is written for that time. In such a case, another family member needs to be responsible for writing the actions to be taken next to the appropriate times in the diary.

It is important to acquire information from all patients about medication compliance. In a study by Kleiger and Dirks (1979), although 54 percent of asthmatic patients reported some form of medication misuse, only 27 percent of the physicians treating these patients said that they routinely inquired about medication misuse. When a patient acknowledges medication misuse, the report can be believed; self-reported compliance, however, always must be viewed with skepticism. *Noncompliance is the rule rather than the exception in treating chronic diseases.* Inquiry and monitoring always need to be considered when the treatment response is unexpected or unfavorable.

Gaps in information about an illness by the physician and by the patient, as well as gaps in information and application of therapy, have been suggested as some of the several contributing factors in the recent rise in number of catastrophic asthma attacks (Benatar, 1986). Numerous proposals have been offered to help narrow these gaps, not the least of which includes the formation of patient support groups so that information and particular difficulties surrounding the illness can be articulated and shared. Participants in patient support groups may include not only the patient, but also the physician, key members of his or her staff, school nurses, teachers (especially physical education teachers), close family members, and even employers. Such an activity should have a well-conceived program and proper supervision. Help with this can be obtained from regional, state, and national lung or asthma and allergy associations, as well as from psychiatrists, psychologists trained in this field, and appropriately supervised social workers. Additionally, specific information can be obtained from major centers for allergic diseases.

Finally, for some patients the psychologic issues unrelated to the illness may be so pronounced that referral to a psychologist or psychiatrist for individual or family therapy is required. In these cases, it can be assumed that the severity of the psychologic problems also affects medical management. For other patients, situational issues may confound treatment temporarily, and a referral may be helpful. The role of psychologic factors in the maintenance of illness is by no means limited to the seriously disturbed patient or to the patient in a serious situational crisis. The physician needs to consider the role psychologic factors may play in treatment outcome and effectively deal with them as a routine parameter of medical practice.

REFERENCES

Alexander, F.: Psychosomatic Medicine. New York, Norton, 1950.

Benatar, S.R.: Fatal asthma. N. Engl. J. Med. 314:423–428, 1986.

Bierman, C.W., Pierson, W.E.: Hand nebulizers and asthma therapy in children and adolescents. Pediatrics 54:668–670, 1974.

Bouhuys, A., Justesen, D.R.: Allergic and classically conditioned asthma in guinea pigs. Science 173:82, 1971.

Burki, N.K., Mitchell, K., Chaudhary, B.A., Zechman, F.W.: The ability of asthmatics to detect added resistive loads. Am. Rev. Respir. Dis. 117:71–75, 1978.

Creer, T.L., Marion, R.J., Creer, P.P.: Asthma problem behavior checklist: Parental perceptions of the behavior of asthmatic children. J. Asthma 20:97–104, 1983.

Dahlem, N.W., Kinsman, R.A., Horton, D.J.: Panic-fear in asthma: Requests for as-needed (PRN) medications in relation to pulmonary function measurements. J. Allergy Clin. Immunol. 60:295–300, 1977.

Dahlem, N.W., Kinsman, R.A., Horton, D.J.: Requests for as-needed (PRN) medications by asthmatic patients: Relationships to prescribed oral corticosteroid regimens and length of hospitalization. J. Allergy Clin. Immunol. 63:23–27, 1979.

Dekker, E., Groen, J.: Reproducible psychogenic attacks of asthma. J. Psychosom. Res. 1:58–67, 1956.

Dekker, E., Pelser, H.E., Groen, J.: Conditioning as a cause of asthmatic attacks: A laboratory study. J. Psychosom. Res. 2:97–108, 1957.

Dirks, J.F.: Bayesian prediction of psychomaintenance related to rehospitalization in asthma. J. Pers. Assess. 46:159–163, 1982.

Dirks, J.F., Brown, E.L., Robinson, S.K.: The Battery of Asthma Illness Behavior. II. Independence from airways hyperreactivity. J. Asthma 19:79–83, 1982.

Dirks, J.F., Jones, N.F., Fross, K.H.: Psychosexual aspects of panic-fear personality types in asthma. Can. J. Psych. 24:731–739, 1979.

Dirks, J.F., Jones, N.F., Kinsman, R.A.: Panic-Fear: A personality dimension related to intractability in asthma. Psychosom. Med. 39:120–126, 1977.

Dirks, J.F., Kinsman, R.A.: Clinical prediction of medical rehospitalization: Psychological assessment with the Battery of Asthma Illness Behavior. J. Pers. Assess. 45:608–613, 1981.

Dirks, J.F., Kinsman, R.A.: Nondichotomous patterns of medication usage: The yes-no fallacy in compliance measurement. Clin. Pharmacol. Therapeut. 31:413–417, 1982.

Dirks, J.F., Kinsman, R.A., Horton, D.J., Fross, K.H., Jones, N.F.: Panic-fear in asthma: Rehospitalization following intensive long-term treatment. Psychosom. Med. 40:4–13, 1978.

Dirks, J.F., Kinsman, R.A., Jones, N.F., Spector, S.L., Davidson, P.T., Evans, N.W.: Panic-fear: A personality dimension related to length of hospitalization in respiratory disease. J. Asthma Res. 14:61–71, 1977.

Dirks, J.F., Kinsman, R.A., Staudenmayer, H., Kleiger, J.H.: Panic-fear in asthma: Symptomatology as an index of signal anxiety and personality as an index of ego resources. J. Nerv. Ment. Dis. 167:615–619, 1979.

Dirks, J.F., Kreischer, H.: The Battery of Asthma Illness Behavior. I. Independence from age of asthma onset. J. Asthma 19:75–78, 1982.

Dirks, J.F., Robinson, S.K., Moore, P.N.: The prediction of

psychomaintenance in chronic asthma. Psychother. Psychosom. 36:105–115, 1981.

Dirks, J.F., Ruback, L.A., Covino, N.A., Feiguine, R.J.: The Battery of Asthma Illness Behavior. III. Independence from longitudinal pulmonary functions. J. Asthma 19:85–89, 1982.

Dirks, J.F., Schraa, J.C., Robinson, S.K.: Patient mislabeling of symptoms: Implications for patient-physician communication and medical outcome. Internat. J. Psych. Med. 12:15–27, 1982.

Dirks, J.F., Schraa, J., Brown, E.L., Kinsman, R.A.: Psychomaintenance in asthma: Hospitalization rates and financial impact. Brit. J. Med. Psychol. 53:349–354, 1980.

Dunbar, H.F.: Psychoanalytic notes relating to asthma and hayfever. Psychoanal. Q. 7:25, 1938.

Dunbar, H.F.: Psychosomatic Diagnosis. New York, Harper, 1943.

Dunleavy, R.A., Baade, L.E.: Neuropsychological correlates of severe asthma in children 9–14 years old. J. Consult. Clin. Psychol. 48:214–219, 1980.

Fenichel, O.: The Psychoanalytic Theory of Neurosis. New York, Norton, 1945.

Friedman, M., Rosenman, R.H.: Type A Behavior and Your Heart. New York, Knopf, 1974.

Greene, R.L.: The MMPI: An Interpretive Manual. New York, Grune and Stratton, 1980.

Haynes, R.B.: Improving patient compliance: An empirical view. In Stuart, R.B. (ed.), Adherence, Compliance, and Generalization in Behavioral Medicine. New York, Bruner/Mazel, 1982.

Horton, D.J., Suda, W.L., Kinsman, R.A., Southrada, J., Spector, S.L.: Bronchoconstrictive suggestion in asthma: A role for airways hyperreactivity and emotions. Am. Rev. Resp. Dis. 117:1029–1039, 1978.

Hudgel, D.W., Cooperson, D., Kinsman, R.A.: Behavioral style as a factor in recognition of external resistive loads. Am. Rev. Respir. Dis. 126:121–125, 1982.

Hudgel, D.W., Kinsman, R.A.: Interactions among behavioral style, ventilatory drive, and load recognition. Amer. Rev. Respir. Dis. 128:246–250, 1983.

Israel, M.: Rorschach responses of a group of adult asthmatics. J. Ment. Science 100:735, 1954.

Jones, N.F., Kinsman, R.A., Dirks, J.F., Dahlem, N.W.: Psychological contributions to chronicity in asthma. Med. Care 17:1103–1118, 1979.

Justesen, D.R., Braun, E.W., Garrison, R.G., Pendleton, R.B.: Pharmacological differentiation of allergic and classically conditioned asthma in guinea pig. Science 170:864–866, 1970.

Kerman, E.F.: Bronchial asthma and affective psychoses. Psychosom. Med. 8:53, 1946.

Kimble, G.: Hilgard and Marquis' Conditioning and Learning. New York, Appleton-Century-Crofts, 1961.

Kinsman, R.A., Dahlem, N.W., Spector, S.L., Staudenmayer, H.: Observations on subjective symptomatology, coping behavior, and medical decisions in asthma. Psychosom. Med. 39:102–119, 1977.

Kinsman, R.A., Dirks, J.F.: Psychomaintenance in chronic physical illness: A new direction for psychosomatic medicine. Advances in Psychol. 1:1–8, 1982.

Kinsman, R.A., Dirks, J.F., Dahlem, N.W.: Noncompliance to prescribed as-needed (PRN) medication use in asthma. J. Psychosom. Res. 24:97–107, 1980.

Kinsman, R.A., Dirks, J.F., Jones, N.F.: Levels of psychological experience in asthma: General and illness-specific concomitants of panic-fear personality. J. Clin. Psychol. 36:552–561, 1980.

Kinsman, R.A., Dirks, J.F., Jones, N.F.: Psychomaintenance of chronic physical illness: Clinical assessment of personal styles affecting medical management. In Millon, T., Green, C., Meagher, R. (eds.), Handbook of Clinical Health Psychology. New York, Plenum, 1982.

Kinsman, R.A., Dirks, J.F., Jones, N.F., Dahlem, N.W.: Anxiety reduction in asthma: Four catches to general application. Psychosom. Med. 42:397–405, 1980.

Kinsman, R.A., Dirks, J.F., Schraa, J.C.: Psychomaintenance in asthma: Personal styles affecting medical management. Resp. Therapy March/April, 1981.

Kinsman, R.A., Jones, N.F., Matus, I., Schum, R.A.: Patient variables supporting chronic illness: A scale for measuring attitudes toward respiratory illness and hospitalization. J. Nerv. Ment. Dis. 163:159–165, 1976.

Kinsman, R.A., Luparello, T.J., O'Banion, K., Spector, S.L.: Multidimensional analysis of the subjective symptomatology of asthma. Psychosom. Med. 35:250–267, 1973.

Kinsman, R.A., O'Banion, K., Resnikoff, P., Luparello, T.J., Spector, S.L.: Subjective symptoms of acute asthma within a heterogeneous sample of asthmatics. J. Allergy Clin. Immunol. 52:284–296, 1973.

Kinsman, R.A., Spector, S.L., Shucard, D.W., Luparello, T.J.: Observations on patterns of subjective symptomatology in asthma. Psychosom. Med. 36:129–143, 1974.

Kleiger, J.H., Dirks, J.F.: Medication compliance in chronic asthmatic patients. J. Asthma Res. 16:93–96, 1979.

Knapp, P.H.: Emotional expression—past and present. In Knapp, P.H. (ed.), Expressions of the Emotions in Man. New York, New York University Press, 1963.

Knapp, P.H., Nemetz, S.J.: Personality variations in bronchial asthma. Psychosom. Med. 19:443, 1957.

Ley, P., Soelman, M.S.: Communications in an out-patient setting. Br. J. Soc. Clin. Psychol. 4:114–116, 1965.

Luparello, T.J., Leist, N., Lourie, C.H., Sweet, P.: The interaction of psychologic stimuli and pharmacologic agents on airway reactivity of asthmatic subjects. Psychosom. Med. 32:509–513, 1970.

Luparello, T.J., Lyons, H.A., Bleecker, E.R., McFadden, E.R.: Influence of suggestion on airway reactivity in asthmatic subjects. Psychosom. Med. 30:819–825, 1968.

Luparello, T.J., McFadden, E.R., Lyons, H.A., Bleecker, E.R.: Psychologic factors and bronchial asthma. N.Y. State J. Med. 71:2161–2165, 1971.

MacKenzie, J.N.: The production of "rose asthma" by an artificial rose. Am. J. Med. Science 91:45–47, 1886.

McFadden, E.R., Luparello, T.J., Lyons, H.A., Bleecker, E.R.: The mechanism of the action of suggestion in the induction of acute asthma attacks. Psychosom. Med. 31:134–143, 1969.

Nana, A., Pain, M.: Clinical importance of evaluating the asthmatic patient's sense of breathlessness. Pract. Cardiol. 11:83–93, 1985.

Nemiah, J.: Denial revisited: Reflections on psychosomatic theory. Psychother. Psychosom. 26:140–147, 1975.

Noelpp, B., Noelpp-Eschenhagen, I.: Das experimentelle asthma bronchiale des meerschweinchens. III. Studien zur bedeutung bedinger reflexe, bahnungsbereitschalt und haftigkeit unter stress. International Arch. Psychiat. 3:108, 1952.

Noelpp-Eschenhagen, I., Noelpp, B.: New contributions to experimental asthma. Prog. Allergy 4:361–436, 1954.

Ottenberg, P., Stein, M., Lewis, J., Hamilton, C.: Learned asthma in the guinea pig. Psychosom. Med. 20:395–400, 1958.

Parkin, D.M., Henney, C.R., Quirk, J., Crooks, J.: Deviation from prescribed drug treatment after discharge from hospital. Br. Med. J. 2:686, 1976.

Pavlov, I.P.: Conditioned Reflexes. London, Oxford University Press, 1927.

Pavlov, I.P.: Lectures on conditioned reflexes, vol. 2: Conditioned reflexes and psychiatry. New York, International Publishers, 1941.

Phillip, R.J., Wilde, G.J.S., Day, J.H.: Suggestion and relaxation in asthmatics. J. Psychosom. Res. 16:193–204, 1972.

Razran, G.: The observable unconscious and the inferable conscious in current Soviet psychophysiology. Psychol. Rev. 68:81–147, 1961.

Rees, L.: Physical and emotional factors in bronchial asthma. J. Psychosom. Res. 1:98, 1956.

Rubinfeld, A.R., Pain, M.C.F.: Perception of asthma. Lancet 1:882–884, 1976.

Rubinfeld, A.R., Pain, M.C.F.: How mild is mild asthma? Thorax 32:177–181, 1977.

Sackett, D.L., Snow, J.C.: The magnitude of compliance and noncompliance. *In* Haynes, R.B., Taylor, D.W., Sackett, D.L. (eds.), Compliance in Health Care. Baltimore, Johns Hopkins University Press, 1979.

Schraa, J.C., Dirks, J.F.: The influence of corticosteroids and theophylline on cerebral function. Chest 82:181–185, 1982.

Schraa, J.C., Dirks, J.F., Jones, N.F., Kinsman, R.A.: Bender-Gestalt performance in an asthmatic sample. J. Asthma 18:7–9, 1981.

Spector, S.L., Katz, R., Siegel, S., Rachelefsky, G., Fitzgerald, J., Hardick, H., Kinsman, R.A., Dirks, J.F.: The use of the nebulizer chronolog as a monitoring device for compliance. Poster Session Abstract No. 32. American College of Allergists Meeting, February, 1983.

Spector, S.L., Luparello, T.J., Kopetzky, M.T., Souhrada, J., Kinsman, R.A.: Response of asthmatics to methacholine and suggestion. Am. Rev. Resp. Dis. 113:43–50, 1976.

Strupp, H.H., Levenson, R., Manuck, S.B., et al.: Effects of suggestion on total respiratory resistance in mild asthmatics. J. Psychosom. Res. 18.337–346, 1974.

Suess, W.M., Chai, H.: Neuropsychological correlates of asthma: Brain damage or drug effects? J. Consult. Clin. Psychol. 49:135–136, 1981.

Staudenmayer, H., Kinsman, R.A., Dirks, J.F., Spector, S.L., Wangaard, C.: Medical outcome in asthmatic patients: Effects of airways reactivity and symptom-focused anxiety. Psychosom. Med. 41:109–118, 1979.

Staudenmayer, H., Kinsman, R.A., Jones, N.F.: Attitudes toward respiratory illness and hospitalization in asthma: Relationships with personality, symptomatology, and treatment response. J. Ner. Ment. Dis. 166:624–634, 1978.

Stein, M.: Etiology and mechanisms in the development of asthma. *In* Nodine, J.H., Moyer, J.H. (eds.), Psychosomatic Medicine, The Hahnemann Symposium. Philadelphia, Lea and Febiger, 1962.

Szentivanyi, A., Williams, J.F.: The constitutional basis of atopic disease. *In* Bierman, C.W., Pearlman, D.S. (eds.), Allergic Diseases of Infancy, Childhood and Adolescence. Philadelphia, W.B. Saunders Co., 1980.

Wittkower, E.D., Edgell, P.G.: Eczema: A psychosomatic case study. Arch. Derm. Syph. 63:207, 1951.

23

Antimicrobial Agents in Allergic Diseases

JAMES K. TODD, M.D.

Since the introduction of penicillin in 1940, literally hundreds of antimicrobial agents have been discovered, synthesized, and evaluated for clinical usefulness and safety. Although the great majority have never proved to be commercially viable, enough have that the clinician is faced with an imposing array of possible therapeutic alternatives, only some of which represent logical and effective choices.

Although advertisements of new antibiotics almost always claim some element of theoretic superiority over the competition, we currently have an array of appropriate drugs for treatment of most bacterial infections. Consequently, it is unnecessary to assume that a new antibiotic agent being introduced, often with a higher price and with less known about its true clinical efficacy and side effects, should have an immediate favorable impact on the treatment of most infections. It also is easy to be misled by reading the package inserts, containing the usual information provided in advertisements or detail literature, of most new antibiotics. Most of these sources claim a wide range of *in vitro* organism susceptibility and a broad range of generalized clinical applications (e.g., "respiratory infections"). The implication is that if a group of patients with respiratory illness has been successfully treated with the drug in question (even if the illness was not proved to be bacterial infection), any respiratory infection caused by any organism that is susceptible to the antibiotic *in vitro* might be successfully treated with that antibiotic. This implication requires a leap of faith on the part of the clinician, something which is not ordinarily necessary if reasonable alternative drugs of proven efficacy exist. Thus, although the clinician will continue to be inundated with new antimicrobial agents appearing on the market, it generally is appropriate to be patient and await the increasing experience that only time can bring as long as

appropriate standard therapies exist for the common infections encountered.

CHARACTERISTICS OF COMMON ANTIMICROBIAL AGENTS

Table 23–1 lists many of the common antimicrobial agents currently available (excluding antiparasitic drugs). Because agents have different degrees of intestinal absorption some may be given orally (po), whereas others may only be given parenterally (iv, im). Dosages similarly will vary depending upon age-related absorption and excretion of the particular drug and the blood levels that are required to inhibit organisms. Thus, the dose, route, and frequency will vary for each antibiotic, depending upon its pharmacologic characteristics. In addition, many antimicrobial agents will require restriction or modification of use in patients with liver or renal failure, which might interfere with the normal excretion of the drug, or of use during pregnancy or in newborns for whom the pharmacology and safety of the drug may not have been established. It always is important when using an unfamiliar antimicrobial agent to thoroughly review specific, reliable drug information prior to prescribing the agent (Abramowicz, 1984; Nelson, 1983).

ANTIMICROBIAL SUSCEPTIBILITY TESTING

Broth Dilution Technique

The basic standard of antimicrobial susceptibility testing is the broth dilution minimum inhibitory concentration (MIC) (Jones et al., 1985), which is performed by inoculating a standardized volume and concentration of a pure bacterial isolate into tubes or microtiter wells containing two-fold dilutions of each antibiotic in a standardized broth growth medium. These mixtures of antibiotic, broth, and bacteria are incubated for 18 to 24 hours at 35 to 37°C (not in CO_2) and examined for cloudiness, indicating growth (the original inoculum is not sufficient to make the broth cloudy). The lowest concentration of antibiotic ($\mu g/ml$) to prevent growth is considered the MIC. If one wishes,

TABLE 23–1. Common Antimicrobial Agents:* Route, Dose, and Frequency of Administration

Antibiotic	Route	Dosage† mg/kg/day	Dosage† Maximum Daily	Interval (hr)
Acyclovir	IV (PO)‡	15–30	1500 mg/m²	q8
Amantadine	PO	5–8	200 mg	q12
Amikacin§	IM, IV	15–30	1.5 gm	q8
Amoxicillin	PO	20–40	3 gm	q8
Amoxicillin clavulanate	PO	20–40	1.5 gm	q8
Amphotericin§	IV	0.3–1	1 mg/kg	q24
Ampicillin	PO, IM, IV	50–200	12 gm	q4–6
Azlocillin	IV	300–450	24 gm	q4–6
Bacampicillin	PO	25–50	1.6 gm	q12
Carbenicillin	IV (PO)	400–600 (30–50)‡	40 gm	q4–6
Cefaclor	PO	40	2 gm	q8
Cefamandole	IM, IV	50–150	6 gm	q4–6
Cefazolin	IM, IV	50–100	6 gm	q8
Cefoperazone	IM, IV	100–150	10 gm	q8–12
Cefotaxime	IM, IV	100–200	10 gm	q6–8
Cefoxitin	IM, IV	80–160	12 gm	q4–6
Ceftriaxone	IM, IV	50–100	4 gm	q12–24
Cefuroxime	IM, IV	75–150	6 gm	q6–8
Cephalexin	PO	25–50	3 gm	q6
Cephalothin	IM, IV	75–125	10 gm	q4–6
Cephradine	PO, IM, IV	25–100	8 gm	q6
Chloramphenicol§	PO, IV	25–100	4 gm	q6
Clindamycin§	PO, IM, IV	10–40	4 gm	q6–8
Cloxacillin	PO	50–100	3 gm	q6
Dicloxacillin	PO	12–25	2 gm	q6
Doxycycline§	PO	5	200 mg	q12
Erythromycin	PO (IV)§	20–40	2 gm	q6–8
Erythromycin-sulfa	PO	50 (Eryth)	2 gm (Eryth)	q8
Flucytosine§	PO	50–150	150 mg/kg	q6
Furazolidone	PO	5	8.8 mg/kg	q6
Gentamicin§	IM, IV	3–7.5	300 mg	q8
Griseofulvin	PO	15	1 gm	q24
Kanamycin§	IM, IV	15–30	1 gm	q8
Ketoconazole	PO	5–10	1 gm	q12–24
Methicillin	IM, IV	100–200	12 gm	q6
Metronidazole	PO, IV	15–35	4 gm	q6–8
Miconazole	IV	20–40	3.6 gm	q8
Minocycline§	PO (IV)	4	200 mg	q12
Moxalactam§	IV	150–200	12 gm	q6–8
Nafcillin	IM, IV	50–100	12 gm	q6
Netilmicin§	IM, IV	3–6.5	300 mg	q8
Nitrofurantoin	PO	5–7	400 mg	q6
Nystatin	PO	2–6 [ml/dose]	24 ml	q6
Oxacillin	PO, IM, IV	50–200	10 gm	q6
Oxytetracycline§	PO	40–50	4 gm	q6
Penicillin G	IV	50,000–250,000 [units/kg]	20 × 10⁶ units	q4
Penicillin G (procaine)	IM	25,000–50,000 [units/kg]	4.8 × 10⁶ units	q12–24
Penicillin V	PO	25–50	4 gm	q6
Penicillin (benzathine)	IM	50,000 [units/kg]	2.4 × 10⁶ units	1 dose
Piperacillin	IV	200–300	24 gm	q4–6
Rifampin	PO	10–20	600 mg	q12–24
Sulfonamides	PO	See specific drug		
Tetracycline§	PO (IV)§	25–50 (30)	2–3 gm	q6–12
Ticarcillin	IV	200–300	30 gm	q4–6
Tobramycin§	IM, IV	3–5	300 mg	q8
Trimethoprim-sulfa	PO (IV)§	6–20 (TRI)	20 (TRI)	q6–12
Vancomycin§	IV	40	4 gm	q6
Vidarabine§	IV	15	15 mg/kg	q24

* Not including antiparasitic drugs, some newly released drugs, or ones not widely used. Always consult package insert for complete prescribing information.
† Dosage may differ for alternate route, newborns or patients with liver or renal failure and may not be recommended for use in pregnant women or newborns.
‡ Parentheses indicate less common route and dosage.
§ Indicates drug with special toxicity considerations.

the tubes or wells without growth can be subcultured subsequently to agar plates and reincubated to see if the original inoculum was killed and not just inhibited. The lowest concentration of antibiotic to kill 99.9 percent of the bacterial inoculum is considered the minimum bactericidal concentration (MBC). If the MIC is approximately equal to the MBC, the antibiotic-organism combination is considered to be bactericidal (i.e., the antibiotic kills the organism in concentrations that also inhibit it). If the MIC is much less than the MBC, the interaction is considered bacteriostatic (i.e., the organism is inhibited but not killed).

It is important to understand that many *in vitro* conditions can alter the broth dilution antibiotic susceptibility test result. Such considerations as organism strain, inoculum size and purity, characteristics of the growth media, conditions altering antibiotic activity or concentrations (e.g., pH, protein binding), and timing of reading and interpretation might significantly influence the result. It is especially true that the broth medium and conditions suitable for routine testing of many common organisms (e.g., *Staphylococcus aureus, Escherichia coli*) may not be adequate for more fastidious ones (e.g., *Haemophilus influenzae, Streptococcus pneumoniae*). Widely discrepant results can be obtained, therefore, if the wrong conditions are used. Consequently, all certified hospital and commercial laboratories are required to adhere to rigidly standardized procedures, with daily or weekly quality control (standard test organisms).

Disc Diffusion Technique

A carefully regulated inoculum of a single bacterial strain is streaked on a standardized (nutrients, depth, pH) agar plate, and paper discs impregnated with a defined concentration of antibiotic are subsequently placed on the plate and incubated for 18 to 24 hours at 35 to 37°C (Barry and Thornsberry, 1985). The zone of inhibition of growth around the antibiotic disc is inversely proportional to the MIC of the organism; the larger the zone of inhibition the lower is the MIC and hence more "susceptible" is the organism. Again, every condition must be carefully standardized, and all of the potential problems previously outlined apply. As in the case of the broth dilution test, the commonly used medium for disc susceptibility testing (Mueller-Hinton agar) is not adequate for growth and susceptibility testing of many fastidious organisms. Any *ad hoc* media modifications could result in serious errors in interpretation. It must also be emphasized that for some organism-antibiotic combinations a substantial zone of inhibition may exist even though the MIC correlates with a blood level that cannot ordinarily be achieved with that antibiotic in the patient. Thus, each organism-antibiotic combination requires a separate defined interpretive standard; a zone of inhibition does not necessarily imply susceptibility of the organism to the antibiotic.

Enzymatic Degradation of Antibiotic

Many (but by no means all) resistant bacterial organisms produce enzymes that in various ways alter specific antibiotics such that they lose all or part of their activity. Some of these enzymes (e.g., beta-lactamase) can be detected in the laboratory using commercial reagents. Although growth conditions may not be as critical as for the broth dilution or agar disc diffusion tests, and overnight incubation is not usually necessary, there are several important limitations to these enzymatic methods. Even if one determines enzymatic resistance of an organism to one group of antibiotics, its susceptibility to others can only be confirmed by additional testing, and other mechanisms of resistance to the same antibiotic may be missed. For instance, some strains of *H. influenzae* are resistant to ampicillin but do not produce beta-lactamase.

Interpretation

The clinical interpretation of antibiotic susceptibility tests requires a knowledge of antibiotic pharmacology correlated with laboratory estimates of *in vitro* susceptibility. The usual cut-off points used in susceptibility testing by reference laboratories assume that an organism is resistant to an antibiotic if the MIC of the organism is greater than the peak blood level of that antibiotic (usually assumed to be given parenterally). Thus, a susceptible organism is defined as one with a MIC that is less than the antibiotic concentration usually achieved in serum. The critical assumptions inferred by this interpretation are as follows: (1) the organism being tested is actually the cause of the pathologic process; (2) the *in vitro* susceptibility test accurately approximates the *in vivo* growth conditions and inoculum size; and (3) the antibiotic levels achieved at the site of infection in that particular patient using the selected route, dose, and frequency of administration of antibiotic will approximate the expected peak systemic levels.

Thus, there are a number of limitations associated with *in vitro* antimicrobial susceptibility testing which qualify the assumption that the antimicrobial susceptibility guarantees clinical efficacy. For those circumstances in which extensive clinical experience has confirmed this assumption, such antibiotics can be used with confidence. For newer antibiotics, however, or for unusual infections or sequestered foci of infection, it is critically important to continue to monitor the patient to assure clinical improvement.

PRINCIPLES OF SELECTING ANTIMICROBIAL THERAPY

The initial treatment of most infections is based on an orderly consideration of the anatomic site infected, the organisms likely to be associated with such a focus of infection, and the antimicrobial susceptibility patterns of the suspected organisms. For infected sites that have limited potential etiologies with predictable susceptibility patterns, empirical therapy can be based on clinical judgment, with cultures reserved for those patients who do not respond. Although cultures might be taken for academic interest in such patients, they are not necessary if their results are unlikely to alter therapy or affect outcome. In cases in which more than one organism or antimicrobial susceptibility pattern is likely or in which the severity of illness makes a definitive etiologic diagnosis more urgent, appropriate material should be obtained for culture before initiation of presumptive therapy. Thus, the following progression of events should occur prior to the prescription of any antimicrobial therapy (Todd, 1985).

1. Consider the clinical diagnosis (e.g., otitis, sinusitis, pneumonia, and so forth).
2. Consider the organisms likely to cause such an infection. Be certain to give special consideration to those patients who do not

have normal host defenses (e.g., immune deficiency, neoplasm, cancer chemotherapy), as the etiology of such infections may be much broader.
3. Obtain appropriate cultures for all infections that are not likely to have a predictable etiology with a predictable susceptibility pattern. It should be remembered that nonpermissive cultures (i.e., those that are obtained directly from the site of infection without contamination with the normal flora) are critical for those infections that have an unpredictable etiology or an unpredictable susceptibility pattern. Culturing of normally colonized surface sites (e.g., skin, nasopharynx, and so forth) may be misleading.
4. Prescribe presumptive antimicrobial therapy that encompasses the likely organisms and their susceptibility patterns, taking into consideration those drugs known to be of proven efficacy for similar infections in such patients.
5. Modify therapy based upon the results of appropriate cultures and the patient's clinical response. *The final test of success is not the* in vitro *susceptibility pattern but rather the patient's* in vivo *response to therapy.*

Table 23–1 lists the common antibiotics currently available and the general dosage information for the treatment of common infections. Table 23–2 lists those antibiotics that have proved useful for various microorganisms, and Table 23–3 lists the microbial etiology of common outpatient infections encountered in practice. By combining the information in these tables using the aforementioned process, one can come to a reasonable estimate of appropriate antimicrobial therapy for a particular infection, as illustrated by the examples that follow. It should be reemphasized that a clinician should gain experience with a limited number of antimicrobial agents and should substitute newer agents only when there is a clear indication that the usual antimicrobial therapy would be inappropriate, either because of a particular isolate that has been cultured with an unusual susceptibility pattern or because of failure of the patient to respond to the more conventional therapy. Thus, of the list of antibiotics in Table 23–1, it is likely that only five or ten would be commonly used.

TABLE 23–2. Susceptibility of Common Pathogenic Microorganisms to Various Antimicrobial Drugs

Organism	Potentially Useful Antibiotics*
Anaerobic bacteria†	Penicillins, chloramphenicol, clindamycin, cefoxitin, metronidazole
Bordetella pertussis	Erythromycin, tetracyclines
Branhamella catarrhalis	Newer cephalosporins,‡ tetracycline, trimethoprim-sulfa, erythromycin, ampicillin** (if beta-lactamase negative), amoxicillin clavulanate
Candida spp.§	Amphotericin B, flucytosine, ketoconazole, miconazole
Chlamydia spp.	Tetracyclines, erythromycin, chloramphenicol
Campylobacter fetus	Erythromycin, tetracyclines, furazolidone
Clostridium spp.	Penicillin, tetracyclines, clindamycin
Clostridium difficile	Vancomycin (PO), metronidazole
Corynebacterium diphtheriae	Penicillin, erythromycin
Enterobacteriaceae	Aminoglycosides, newer cephalosporins,‡ ampicillin,** trimethoprim-sulfa
Fungi, systemic§	Amphotericin B, ketoconazole, miconazole
Dermatophytes	Griseofulvin, topical antifungals
Gardnerella vaginalis	Metronidazole, ampicillin
Haemophilus influenzae	Newer cephalosporins,‡ chloramphenicol, ampicillin (if beta-lactamase negative),** trimethoprim-sulfa, amoxicillin clavulanate
Herpes simplex§	Acyclovir, vidarabine
Influenza A virus§	Amantadine
Neisseria gonorrhoeae	Penicillin, ampicillin, tetracyclines, cefoxitin, newer cephalosporins,‡ spectinomycin
Neisseria meningitidis	Penicillin, ampicillin, chloramphenicol
Pseudomonas spp.	Antipseudomonas penicillins,‖ aminoglycosides
Rickettsia	Tetracyclines, chloramphenicol
Salmonella spp.	Ampicillin, chloramphenicol, trimethoprim-sulfa
Shigella spp.	Ampicillin, chloramphenicol, trimethoprim-sulfa
Staphylococcus aureus	Beta-lactamase resistant penicillins ¶, vancomycin, cephalosporins, erythromycin, clindamycin
Staphylococci (coagulase negative)	Vancomycin, cephalosporins, rifampin
Streptococci (most species)	Penicillins, ampicillin,** erythromycin, cephalosporins
Streptococcus pneumoniae	Penicillin, ampicillin,** erythromycin, cephalosporins
Streptococcus (group D)	Ampicillin plus aminoglycoside, vancomycin
Varicella-zoster virus§	Acyclovir, vidarabine

* Selection dependent on age, diagnosis, site of infection, severity of illness, antimicrobial susceptibility of subjected organism, and drug hypersensitivity.
† Species dependent.
‡ Newer cephalosporins that are not affected by gram-negative beta-lactamase.
§ Organisms not effectively treated by common antimicrobials.
‖ Carbenicillin, ticarcillin, mezlocillin, piperacillin.
¶ Nafcillin, oxacillin, cloxacillin, methicillin.
** Also applies to amoxicillin.

ANTIMICROBIAL THERAPY OF COMMON OUTPATIENT CONDITIONS

Otitis Media

The common agents causing otitis media are listed in Table 23–3. Nasopharyngeal cultures are not recommended because of the lack of correlation with the actual cause of the otitis. For children, these causative organisms include *Streptococcus pneumoniae*, *Haemophilus influenzae*, and *Branhamella catarrhalis*. *S. pneumoniae* is the most common cause in older children and adults. Both *B. catarrhalis* and *H. influenzae* may produce a beta-lactamase, which makes them

TABLE 23–3. Microbial Etiology of Common Outpatient Infections*

Anatomic Diagnosis	Clinical Clues	Virus	Streptococcus pneumoniae	Group A Streptococcus	Staphylococcus aureus	Haemophilus influenzae	Other
				Usual Causative Organisms			
UPPER RESPIRATORY INFECTIONS							
Acute otitis media			1	+	+	2	Branhamella catarrhalis
Chronic otitis media					+		Enterobacteriaceae Pseudomonas spp. Anaerobes
Periorbital cellulitis			+	+	+	1 (type b)	
Acute sinusitis			2	+	+	1	Branhamella catarrhalis
Chronic sinusitis					+	+	Anaerobes
Febrile nasopharyngitis (children < 3 years)		1	?	+		?	
Primary purulent nasopharyngitis		1	?	?		?	
Acute rhinitis		1					
Acute tonsillopharyngitis		1		2			Corynebacterium diphtheriae
LOWER RESPIRATORY INFECTIONS							
Epiglottitis						1 (type b)	
Laryngotracheobronchitis		1			?	+ (type b)	
Bronchiolitis		1					
Pneumonia							
Age < 5 years		1	2	+	+	3 (type b)	
Age > 5 years		+	+	+	+	+	Mycoplasma pneumoniae
SKIN AND SOFT TISSUE INFECTIONS							
Impetigo contagiosa	Warm climate			1	(+)		
bullous	Diaper area, local injury				1		
Dermatitis	Diaper				(+)		Candida albicans
	Eczema			+	1		
Infected wound				1	1		Clostridium Enterobacteriaceae

Table continued on following page

TABLE 23–3. Microbial Etiology of Common Outpatient Infections* (Continued)

				Usual Causative Organisms			
ANATOMIC DIAGNOSIS	CLINICAL CLUES	VIRUS	*Streptococcus pneumoniae*	GROUP A STREPTOCOCCUS	*Staphylococcus aureus*	*Haemophilus influenzae*	OTHER
Cellulitis							
Traumatic	Local injury			1	2		*Clostridium perfringens*
	Animal bite				+		*Pasteurella spp.*
	Human bite			+	+		Mouth flora
Spontaneous	Facial, periorbital		+	+	+	1 (type b)	
					+		Mouth flora
	Nontraumatic, nonfacial			1	+	+	Herpes, varicella
Furuncle					1		
Abscess	Local injury				1		Enterobacteriaceae Anaerobes
Lymphangitis				1	+		
Lymphadenitis							
Cervical				1	1		*Mycobacterium spp.*
Other site							*Francisella tularensis* *Yersinia pestis* Cat scratch agent
OTHER							
Urinary tract							Enterobacteriaceae Streptococci *Staphylococcus* (coagulase negative)
Vagina							*Neisseria gonorrhoeae* *Candida* *Trichomonas* Gardnerella Herpes
Stool		1					*Salmonella* *Shigella* *Campylobacter* Rotavirus *Escherichia coli*

* 1, 2, and 3 = first most common organism, second, and third; + = occasional cause; ? = unknown.

relatively resistant to treatment with amoxicillin or ampicillin. Nonetheless, these drugs remain the treatment of choice for acute otitis media (McCracken, 1984) because they are still effective against most of the common organisms (cefaclor is recommended for infants less than 6 weeks of age because of the more common occurrence of staphylococci) and because the treatment of acute otitis media involves drainage, as much as it does antimicrobial therapy. Unfortunately, the use of oral antihistamines or decongestants has been shown not to be beneficial in improving drainage (Wald, 1984b). Regardless of the antibiotic selected, most patients improve in time; although, over 50 percent of patients may still show middle ear effusion after the completion of 7 to 10 days of antimicrobial therapy (Bluestone, 1984). This effusion, if cultured, often is sterile but occasionally will grow an organism that may still be susceptible to the original antibiotic selected. It therefore is common practice to consider continued antimicrobial therapy after 10 days, if a middle ear effusion persists, or to change to a different antibiotic, such as cefaclor, trimethoprim-sulfa, amoxicillin clavulanate, or erythromycin-sulfa). These last mentioned antibiotics may be more efficacious against beta-lactamase producing organisms. However, they are not recommended for routine use in the initial therapy of acute otitis media because of increased cost or side effects or both.

Although the antibiotics combined with sulfonamides (trimethoprim-sulfa, erythromycin-sulfa) have proved to be efficacious in treating otitis media, the increased risk of severe hypersensitivity reaction (i.e., Stevens-Johnson syndrome) suggests that they should be used only as secondary therapy for patients who are likely to have a resistant organism present (Gutman, 1984) or for those known to be allergic to the penicillins.

Those patients who have acute otitis media that remain febrile with significant inflammation of the middle ear after several days of antimicrobial therapy might benefit from tympanocentesis and drainage of the ear as well as culture of the middle ear fluid to determine more appropriate antimicrobial therapy (Bluestone, 1984; Wald, 1984a). Nonetheless, most patients with acute otitis media do respond over time, although it may take several months for the middle ear effusion to resolve. If a persistent middle ear effusion is resulting in a significant hearing loss, many practitioners favor the insertion of middle ear drainage tubes, although the true long-term benefit of such a procedure has not been well documented (Bluestone, 1984).

For those children who have chronic otitis media, especially with perforation and drainage in the external auditory canal, it is clear that other more resistant organisms may play an important role, including Pseudomonas, Proteus, and other Enterobacteriaceae. Cultures of the external auditory canal may be misleading. It is appropriate to consider maximizing drainage either by repeated suction or by using a cotton wick to actively remove infected fluid from the middle ear. Many otolaryngologists favor the use of topical antimicrobial eardrops as an adjunct to drainage therapy; however, controlled trials suggest that saline irrigation may be as effective.

For those children who experience frequent recurrent otitis media, prophylactic antimicrobial therapy may be considered as an alternative to insertion of middle ear drainage tubes. Those antibiotics proved to be successful include ampicillin and sulfisoxazole given twice a day. One study suggests an additive benefit of prophylactic antibiotics and pneumococcal vaccine in asthmatic children (Schuller, 1983).

It should be emphasized that the great majority of patients with acute otitis media improve on empiric therapy and that the objectives of such therapy should include the control of the infectious process (to prevent further invasion) and the promotion of drainage of the middle ear to protect hearing.

Acute Sinusitis

The causes of acute sinusitis in both adults and children are similar to the causes of acute otitis media. H. influenzae, S. pneumoniae, and B. catarrhalis are commonly found on needle punctures of the sinuses. As in otitis, nasopharyngeal cultures or even sinus ostium cultures do not correlate well with the actual organism isolated on needle puncture. Therefore, empirical therapy for acute sinusitis usually is indicated, focusing on organisms commonly isolated (Wald, 1983). The use of amoxicillin in children or tetracycline in adults appears to be a reasonable first selection, again emphasizing the promotion of drainage. Pharmacologic methods of promoting drainage are not well established. It has been shown that the use of systemic decongestants and antihistamines often is accompanied by undesirable side effects without any noticeable promotion of drainage. Whether the local application of topical decongestants or steroids effectively promotes such drainage is yet to be proved.

In chronic sinusitis additional organisms, such as *S. aureus* and anaerobes, may play a role for which longer term therapy with an alternative antibiotic may be indicated. Promotion of drainage is probably still the critical therapeutic modality. For those patients who have progression of sinus infection to cheek or periorbital cellulitis, osteomyelitis, or central nervous system infection, more invasive culture procedures are definitely indicated to identify the pathogen involved, to drain the focus, and to allow the selection of optimal antimicrobial therapy based upon culture susceptibility results.

Pharyngitis

Recurrent acute pharyngitis is a common complaint in both children and some adults. Although commonly assumed to be caused by resistant group A streptococci, such organisms are extremely uncommon; it is well documented that most acute pharyngitis episodes are caused by viruses (Wannamaker, 1972). There is some evidence that early treatment of acute severe streptococcal pharyngitis may result in more rapid resolution of symptoms. This does not appear to be true for those patients who have milder symptoms, however. Nonetheless, it is considered appropriate for any patient with pharyngitis to obtain a "strep only" culture (Todd, 1982). The use of rapid methods for detecting streptococcal antigen has recently been promoted; however, these tests are not so sensitive that they can solely take the place of culture (Radetsky et al., 1985). Any patient with a positive culture or antigen test result should be treated. Even after treatment, 5 to 15 percent of patients will continue to grow group A streptococcus from their pharynges. These patients should be considered carriers and do not require retreatment because they do not appear to be at any greater risk of developing rheumatic fever or of transmitting the organism to others. *It is not currently recommended to routinely reculture treated patients or to culture contacts of patients with streptococcal pharyngitis nor is it considered appropriate to culture asymptomatic patients to identify carriers.* For those patients who do seem to have a continued problem with streptococcal pharyngitis, treatment with an alternative drug, such as erythromycin or clinda-

mycin, may be effective in eradicating the carrier state. It is important to reemphasize, however, that the carrier state in general is not a threat to the patient or to others (Kaplan, 1980).

Because *S. pneumoniae, H. influenzae,* and *S. aureus* are common components of the normal upper respiratory flora, these organisms often are isolated from the throat of a patient who has pharyngitis. There is very little evidence that these or other bacteria (except for the very rare *Corynebacterium diphtheriae*) cause pharyngitis. Consequently, culture for these other organisms or treatment when they are present is not indicated (Hable et al., 1971).

Pneumonia

Pneumonia in very young children is usually caused by viruses, but occasionally can be caused by *S. pneumoniae, H. influenzae,* and rarely group A streptococcus or *S. aureus.* The same organisms can be seen in older children who, like adults, are more likely to have *S. pneumoniae* or *Mycoplasma pneumoniae* infections. Thus, age plays an important role in considering the etiology of pneumonia. It also should be emphasized that pneumonia, which occurs in hospitalized adults or children, can be caused by various other organisms; appropriate diagnostic cultures may be much more important to obtain in these patients. For the average patient with a mild to moderate case of pneumonia not requiring hospitalization, empirical therapy and close follow-up is indicated (Todd, 1977). Nasopharyngeal or "sputum" cultures do not always reflect the cause of pneumonia and may in fact be misleading. Thus, it is more appropriate to consider the potential etiologies, as shown in Table 23–3, and consider empirical therapy. More invasive culturing (e.g., lung aspirate, direct tracheal aspirate with quantitative culturing) should be reserved for those patients who are ill enough to require hospitalization, those who have host defense deficiencies, or those who have failed to respond to empirical outpatient therapy (Donowitz and Mandell, 1985).

Infections of Skin and Soft Tissue

Table 23–3 summarizes some of the common skin and soft tissue conditions caused by infectious agents. If there is any break in the skin associated with the infection, group A streptococcus or *S. aureus* organisms are found most commonly; for an animal or a human bite, any of a variety of organisms can be involved. Spontaneous cellulitis caused by *H. influenzae* can occur in younger children. For treatment of group A streptococcus or *S. aureus,* an oral beta-lactamase resistant penicillin, cephalosporin, or erythromycin is indicated. For minor infections, culture of the infected site is not necessarily indicated, except in patients with deficient host defense mechanisms or in other patients in whom there are reasons for suspecting organisms other than *S. aureus* or group A streptococcus; a direct needle aspirate culture prior to initiating therapy would be indicated (Todd, 1985). Patients with more severe infections should have appropriate cultures taken (remember that swab cultures of surface sites may be misleading), initiating at that time appropriate parenteral therapy for the organisms suspected.

REFERENCES

Abramowicz, M. (ed.): Handbook of Antimicrobial Therapy, New Rochelle, N.Y., The Medical Letter, 1984.

Barry, A.L., Thornsberry, C.: Susceptibility Tests: Diffusion Test Procedures. *In* Manual of Clinical Microbiology, 4th ed. Lennette, E.H., Balows, A., Hausleu, W.J., Jr., Shadomy, H.J. (eds.), Washington, D.C., American Society for Microbiology, 1985.

Bluestone, C.D.: Surgical management of otitis media. Pediatr. Infect. Dis. 3:392–396, 1984.

Donowitz, G.R., Mandell, G.L.: Acute pneumonia. *In* Principles and Practice of Infectious Diseases, 2nd ed. Mandell, G.L., Douglas, R.G., Jr., Bennett, J.E. (eds.). New York, John Wiley & Sons, 1985.

Gutman, L.T.: The use of trimethoprim-sulfamethoxazole in children: a review of adverse reactions and indications. Pediatr. Infect. Dis. 3:349–357, 1984.

Hable, K.A., Washington, J.A., II, Herrmann, E.C., Jr.: Bacterial and viral throat flora: comparison of findings in children with acute upper respiratory tract disease and in healthy controls during winter. Clin. Pediatr. 10:199–203, 1971.

Jones, R.N., Barry, A.L., Gavan, T.L., Washington, J.A., III.: Susceptibility Tests: Microdilution and Macrodilution Broth Procedures. *In* Manual of Clinical Microbiology, 4th ed. Lennette, E.H., Balows, A., Hausleu, W.J., Jr., Shadomy, H.J. (eds.), Washington, D.C., American Society for Microbiology, 1985.

Kaplan, E.L.: The group A streptococcal upper respiratory tract carrier state: an enigma. J. Pediatr. 97:337–345, 1980.

McCracken, G.H., Jr.: Antimicrobial therapy for acute otitis media. Pediatr. Infect. Dis. 3:383–386, 1984.

Nelson, J.D.: Pocket Book of Pediatric Antimicrobial Therapy. Baltimore, Williams & Wilkins, 1987.

Radetsky, M., Wheeler, R.C., Roe, M.H., Todd, J.K.: Comparative evaluation of kits for rapid diagnosis of group A streptococcal disease. Pediatr. Infect. Dis. 4:274–281, 1985.

Schuller, D.E.: Prophylaxis of otitis media in asthmatic children. Pediatr. Infect. Dis. 2:280–283, 1983.

Todd, J.K.: Office laboratory diagnosis of skin and soft tissue infections. Pediatr. Infect. Dis. 4:84–87, 1985.

Todd, J.K.: Pneumonia in children. Postgrad. Med. 61:251–258, 1977.

Todd, J.K.: Throat cultures in the office laboratory. Pediatr. Infect. Dis. 1:265–270, 1982.

Wald, E.R.: Changing trends in the microbiology of otitis media with effusion. Pediatr. Infect. Dis. 3:380–383, 1984a.

Wald, E.R.: Antihistamines and decongestants in otitis media. Pediatr. Infect. Dis. 3:386–388, 1984b.

Wald, E.R.: Acute sinusitis in children. Pediatr. Infect. Dis. 2:61–68, 1983.

Wannamaker, L.W.: Perplexity and precision in the diagnosis of streptococcal pharyngitis. Am. J. Dis. Child. 124:352–358, 1972.

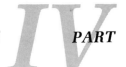

MANAGEMENT OF GASTROINTESTINAL TRACT AND FOOD-INDUCED DISEASES

24

Diagnosis and Treatment of Gastrointestinal Tract Diseases

DENNIS L. CHRISTIE, M.D.

The discussion of the gastrointestinal tract is divided into two sections since disorders of each section can result in quite different clinical syndromes due to or aggravating allergy. Disorders of the esophagus and stomach may be manifested by pulmonary symptoms, such as aspiration of gastric contents with recurrent pneumonia or asthma. Disorders of the small and large bowel are manifested by nutritional disorders, diarrhea, or both, ranging from malabsorption syndromes with failure to thrive to a number of different diarrheal diseases.

THE ESOPHAGUS AND STOMACH

Abnormalities in esophageal function have been associated with aspiration pneumonia for several decades (Urschel, 1967). However, the spectrum of pulmonary diseases caused by esophageal dysfunction has not been evaluated critically in a pediatric or an adult population. Many of the symptoms of patients with abnormal esophageal function can be confused with allergic respiratory disease and must be differentiated from other diseases associated with similar symptoms.

Physiology

The esophagus is a hollow, muscular organ that extends from the pharynx at the sixth cervical vertebra to the stomach at the gastroesophageal junction. The length of the esophagus varies from 7 to 14 cm in the infant to approximately 35 cm in the adult. It is lined by stratified squamous epithelium and has two muscle layers, an inner circular and an outer longitudinal. In the upper third of the esophagus, the muscle layers are composed of striated voluntary fibers; the remaining esophagus contains only smooth muscle.

Two sphincters are present in the esophagus. The upper esophageal sphincter consists of the muscle of the cricopharynx. This muscle arises from the cricoid cartilage of the larynx and forms a band of muscle that acts as a sphincter. This sphincter is approximately 3 cm long and has a resting pressure of up to 140 mm Hg. The upper esophageal sphincter relaxes with swallowing, which occurs in a sequence after pharyngeal contraction but before esophageal peristalsis (Fig. 24–1). The upper esophageal sphincter acts as a barrier to reflux of gastric contents into the hypopharynx.

The lower esophageal sphincter is a physiologic zone of high pressure, separating the body of the esophagus from the fundus of the stomach. No anatomic sphincter has been demonstrated at the gastroesophageal junction, but intraluminal esophageal manometrics have shown that this area has a resting pressure of approximately 15 to 30 mm Hg (Fig. 24–2). Lower esophageal sphincter pressure will drop to 0 within 2.5 seconds after swallowing is initiated. The pressure will return to its normal elevated state approximately 10 seconds after deglutition when the esophageal peristaltic wave passes the lower esophagus. The lower esophageal sphincter is believed to be the most important barrier to prevent reflux of gastroduodenal contents into the esophageal lumen.

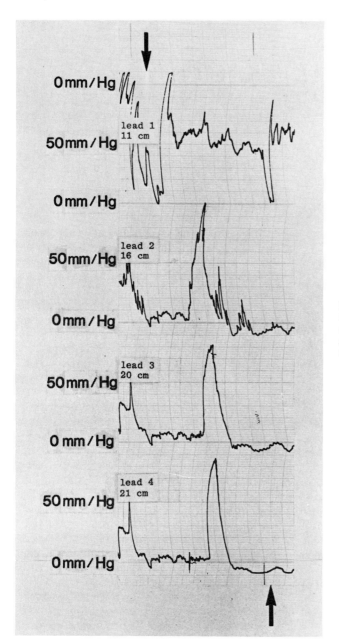

FIGURE 24–1. Esophageal manometer tracing of a normal swallow, showing relaxation of the upper esophageal sphincter in Lead 1 followed by a peristaltic wave in the body of the esophagus in Leads 2, 3, and 4.

Symptoms and Signs of Esophageal Dysfunction

Since the major function of the esophagus is the transportation of food from mouth to stomach and prevention of reflux of gastric material back into its lumen, most symptoms of esophageal disease are related to eating.

Regurgitation and vomiting are the most common symptoms of gastroesophageal disease in infants. Regurgitation refers to the ef-

fortless expulsion of gastric contents during or after eating. Regurgitation can occur whether the infant is upright, supine, or prone and can range in amount from a few milliliters to several ounces. The vomiting that occurs with esophageal dysfunction is secondary to an incompetent lower esophageal sphincter. The vomitus is forceful and projectile and usually appears during or within 1 hour after eating. No clinical distinction can be made from the vomiting secondary to gastroesophageal reflux, pyloric ste-

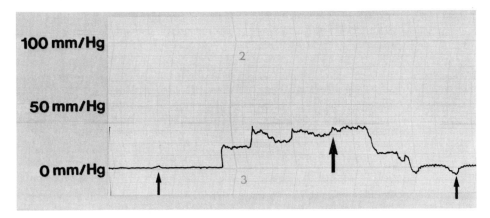

FIGURE 24–2. A high pressure zone (large arrow) of approximately 26 mm Hg separating the stomach (positive deflection on left) from the esophagus (negative deflection on right).

nosis, peptic ulcer disease, duodenal web, or food allergy.

"Colic" is a symptom so vague and difficult to characterize that many different etiologies have been incriminated, including gastroesophageal reflux, food allergy, and renal disease. Infants with significant regurgitation or vomiting may fail to thrive or may gain weight slowly in the first several months of life because they fail to retain sufficient calories.

Dysphagia is a symptom unique to the esophagus. Dysphagia is defined as a difficulty in swallowing and is seen characteristically when solid material is swallowed. Adults will describe the feeling of food "catching" in their throats, and they may be able to point to a location in the substernal area. The symptom of dysphagia can mean esophageal narrowing secondary to esophageal stricture.

Heartburn is the sensation of burning beneath the substernal area, with radiation to the neck. It occurs primarily when the patient is lying supine or when the patient increases intra-abdominal pressure by positional changes or exercise.

Aspiration of swallowed food particles and liquid secondary to reflux of gastric contents may induce respiratory symptoms. Aspiration is experienced because of abnormalities in function of the pharyngeal and laryngeal swallowing mechanisms or because of esophageal obstruction, gastroesophageal reflux, or esophageal motor disorders. Severe lung damage can develop when gastric fluid with a pH of 2.5 or less is aspirated. Aspiration pneumonia and an "asthma-like" syndrome with dyspnea, cyanosis, wheezing, rales, rhonchi, and occasional gross pulmonary edema were recognized with aspiration of gastric contents following general anesthesia (Mendelson, 1946). Aspiration of smaller quantities of gastric contents may induce significant bronchospasm (Wynne and Modell, 1977). Children with esophageal reflux and aspiration may have nocturnal episodes of coughing, shortness of breath, tachypnea, and vomiting (Carre, 1960), a symptom complex that occurs also in adults. Their recurrent attacks of wheezing and coughing may be associated with radiographic evidence of pneumonitis over a period of months to years, though they may be free of symptoms between attacks. Though many individuals with recurrent pulmonary disease due to gastroesophageal reflux have such esophageal symptoms as vomiting, regurgitation, dysphagia, or heartburn (Christie et al., 1978), some may not (Danus et al., 1976).

Patients with repeated episodes of aspiration are commonly diagnosed as having "asthmatic bronchitis," bronchitis, or asthma. A useful diagnostic sign in patients with reflux of gastric contents is the finding of an inflamed (red, irritated) epiglottis.

Differential Diagnosis

Pharyngeal and laryngeal disorders are common causes of aspiration. Anomalies, such as cleft lip and palate, choanal atresia, Pierre Robin syndrome, or laryngeal cleft, are associated with oropharyngeal dysphagia and can be associated with aspiration. Patients with neurologic abnormalities, such as cerebral palsy, familial dysautonomia, Werdnig-Hoffmann disease, and cranial nerve paralysis, which are associated with incoordinated laryngeal or pharyngeal swallowing, may aspirate during eating (Fig. 24-3).

Esophageal obstruction occurs in children or adults with achalasia, esophageal stricture, or an upper esophageal foreign body. Up to 10 percent of patients with achalasia develop aspiration pneumonia with symptoms of wheezing or chronic bronchitis with recurrent pneumonia (Anderson, 1953) (Fig. 24-4). A chest x-ray film may show aspiration pneumonitis. Complications include lung abscesses, bronchiectasis, asthma, emphysema, and pulmonary fibrosis.

Esophageal stricture, a complication of gastroesophageal reflux, can cause aspiration if the esophagus above the stricture becomes grossly dilated. Such patients may awaken at night coughing and choking because of "overflow of food" and secretions from the esophagus into the posterior oropharynx during sleep (Fig. 24-5).

Abnormal esophageal motility can result in aspiration pneumonia if food and acid are not cleared from the esophagus during deglutition. These so-affected patients are also at risk for severe esophagitis with subsequent stricture and esophageal ulcer because the esophageal mucosa is exposed to acid for prolonged periods of time. In infants and children this occurs with tracheoesophageal fistula, trisomy 21, or spastic cerebral palsy (Parker et al., 1979).

Gastroesophageal reflux can result in aspiration because an incompetent lower esophageal sphincter will not prevent reflux of gastric contents when patients are in a recumbent position. Acid gastric contents can trigger airway bronchospasm by several mechanisms, as follows: (1) through aspiration of large quantities of liquid gastric contents into the bronchopulmonary tree, (2) through aspiration of minute quantities of gastric liquid that may stimulate upper airway receptors, and (3) through stimulation of esophageal receptors by gastric acid content. In addition to the fact that gastroesophageal reflux can be a trigger mechanism for bronchospasm, bronchospasm itself also may be a trigger mechanism for significant gastroesophageal reflux (Boyle et al., 1985).

Some patients with aspiration of gastric contents present with recurrent pneumonias and have episodes of cough, fever, and tachypnea, usually worse at night. In such patients, interstitial pneumonia or lobar consolidation generally is found on chest radiographs. Aspiration tends to be episodic, and patients may be completely well between periods of aspiration.

Gastroesophageal reflux can cause acute and chronic respiratory symptoms (Nelson 1984; Mitsuhashi et al., 1985), and patients often present with recurrent episodes of bronchitis and coughing, sometimes with wheezing. Whether asthma may be worsened or precipitated by gastroesophageal reflux and aspiration remains to be determined. Before one can attribute significant asthmatic symptoms to reflux, all other causes of respiratory pulmonary disease must be excluded. Some investigators have demonstrated gastroesophageal reflux in children with severe asthma (Byrne et al., 1978; Shapiro and Christie, 1979). A significant consideration in patients with asthma is whether the effect of asthma therapy worsens reflux. Some medications used in the treatment of asthma, particularly theophylline, have been shown to decrease gastroesophageal sphincter pressure and could contribute to gastroesophageal reflux by doing so (Barish et al., 1985). However, Berquist et al. (1984) demonstrated that standard oral bronchodilator therapy in asthmatic children did not worsen gastroesophageal reflux or pulmonary function.

Tests of Esophageal Dysfunction

Cineradiography of the pharynx and esophagus is a basic screening mechanism for evaluation of the function of the posterior oropharynx and the esophagus (Donner, 1985). The barium swallow should be used to exclude abnormalities in cricopharyngeal function or abnormalities in the oropharynx that may lead to aspiration. There is a definite correlation between severity of gastroesophageal reflux by barium esophagram and protracted pulmonary disease (Darling et al., 1978).

Gastroesophageal scintiscan may be useful, if a barium esophagram does not show evidence of reflux, to demonstrate episodes of reflux into the esophagus in pediatric patients (Christie et al., 1978) (Fig. 24-6). It has not proved to be an effective test in adolescents and adults. This test consists of instilling water with a small amount of ^{99m}technetium sulfur colloid into the stomach. Reflux of material into the esophagus is measured with a gamma camera. Patients can be scanned for 60 minutes after ingestion of the ^{99m}technetium sulfur colloid to determine whether gastroesophageal reflux is present. Recent studies have demonstrated that 24 hour

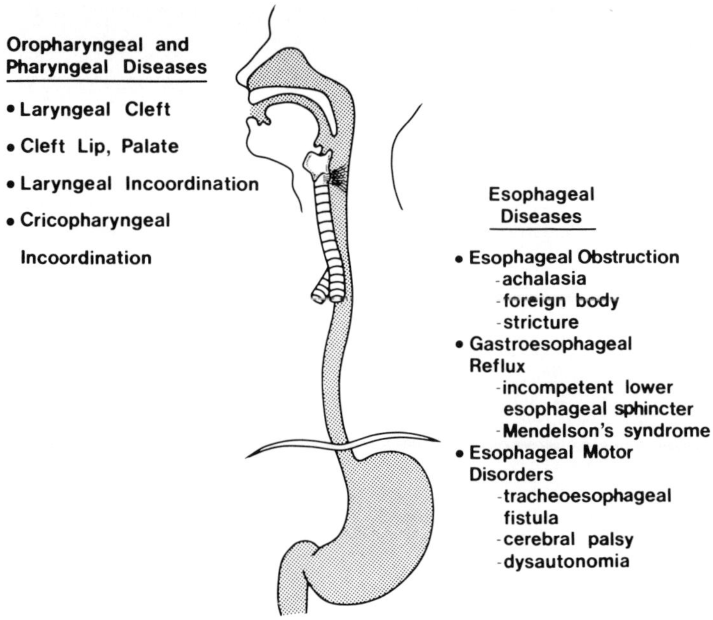

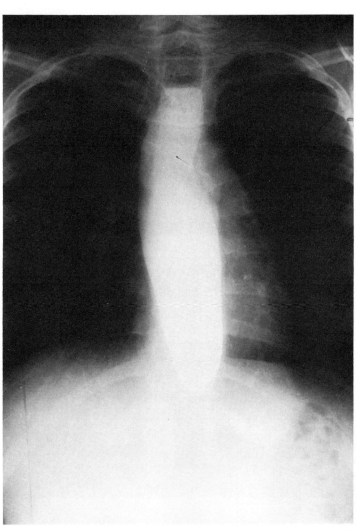

Oropharyngeal and Pharyngeal Diseases

- Laryngeal Cleft
- Cleft Lip, Palate
- Laryngeal Incoordination
- Cricopharyngeal Incoordination

Esophageal Diseases

- Esophageal Obstruction
  - achalasia
  - foreign body
  - stricture
- Gastroesophageal Reflux
  - incompetent lower esophageal sphincter
  - Mendelson's syndrome
- Esophageal Motor Disorders
  - tracheoesophageal fistula
  - cerebral palsy
  - dysautonomia

FIGURE 24–3. Causes of aspiration pneumonia.

FIGURE 24–4. Barium esophagram demonstrates dilated esophagus in a child with recurrent pneumonia from achalasia with aspiration.

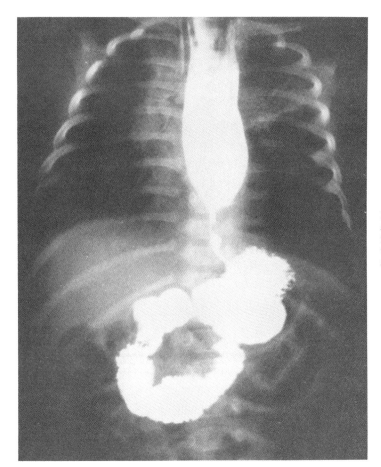

FIGURE 24-5. Narrow esophageal stricture at gastroesophageal junction is identified by barium esophagram. Fifteen-month-old child had dysphagia and recurrent pneumonia.

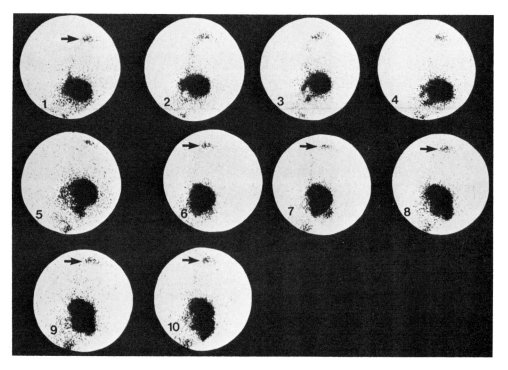

FIGURE 24-6. Gastroesophageal scintiscan demonstrates reflux into oropharynx (arrows).

pH monitoring also may be useful in some patients with recurrent aspiration secondary to esophageal disease (Joley et al., 1978) (Fig. 24–7).

The acid reflux test is the most sensitive means to diagnose gastroesophageal reflux and consists of instilling a 0.1 N HCl in the stomach and of placing a pH probe above the lower esophageal sphincter (Christie and Mack, 1978). Pressure is applied to the abdomen, or the patient performs certain maneuvers to increase abdominal pressure. A drop in pH to less than 4 in the body of the esophagus is diagnostic of gastroesophageal reflux. Esophageal manometrics with open-tipped tubes with side orifices measure esophageal peristalsis accurately. Motility data can easily be obtained of normal swallowing, relaxation of the upper and lower esophageal sphincters, and quantitation of lower esophageal sphincter pressure and peristaltic wave amplitude and duration. A variation in the acid reflux test is the instillation of acid in the esophagus to see if bronchospasm can be initiated (Wilson, 1985). Intraesophageal instillation of acid may provoke increased pulmonary flow resistance in asthmatic patients (Mansfield and Stein, 1978).

Treatment

Treatment of pulmonary disease associated with esophageal dysfunction is medical. Surgery should not be considered unless the episodes of pneumonia or bronchospasm are life-threatening or therapy has failed. Adult patients should have the head of the bed elevated on 6-in blocks, have no food after 6 p.m., and avoid offending foods that worsen reflux. H2 receptor antagonists can be added. Infants can be treated with positioning, thickened feedings, and H2 receptor medications.

THE GASTROINTESTINAL TRACT

Physiology

Normal absorption and digestion of fats, carbohydrates, and proteins from the diet depend upon three stages of digestion as follows: the intraluminal stage, the intestinal stage, and the removal stage. The intraluminal stage is characterized by secretion of pancreatic enzymes and bile salts into the lumen of the small intestine. Long chain triglycerides are hydrolyzed by pancreatic enzymes and formed into water soluble micelles. During the intestinal stage, disaccharides are digested at the surface of the small bowel mucosa. Subsequently, the by-products of carbohydrates, fat, and protein are transported across the small bowel and removed to capillaries or lymphatics.

Normally, approximately 60 to 100 gm of fat is ingested daily in the adult diet, the majority being long chain triglycerides. These long chain triglycerides are insoluble in water and must be acted upon by pancreatic lipase to form free fatty acids, 2-monoglycerides, and free glycerol. The by-products of lipase action on triglycerides are formed into water soluble micelles by the action of bile salts. Absorption of these lipo-

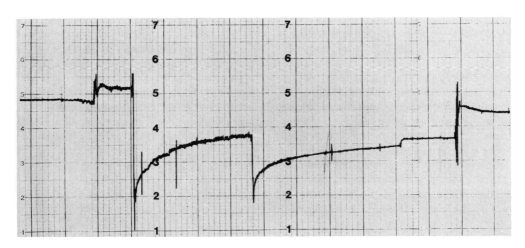

FIGURE 24–7. A section of a record of twenty-four hour pH monitoring that demonstrates reflux in an infant with a drop in pH to 3. The vertical axis indicates pH units, and the horizontal axis, time. Each large square equals two minutes.)

lytic products from the micelles takes place in the duodenum and jejunum (Gray, 1978).

The main carbohydrate constituents in the diet in the adult are starch, sucrose, and lactose. Approximately 400 mg of carbohydrate is ingested daily, usually in the form of starch and sucrose. However, in infants the majority of carbohydrate is lactose. A quart of cow's milk contains about 50 gm of lactose. Starch is composed of two polysaccharides, amylose and amylopectin. Amylase from the pancreas will break the 1,4 bonds of amylose, yielding maltose and maltotriose. Hydrolysis of amylopectin yields alpha limit dextrins, maltose, and maltotriose. The alpha limit dextrins are further hydrolyzed by the action of isomaltase, an enzyme found at the brush border of the small bowel. Sucrose is digested by the action of sucrase to glucose and fructose. Finally, lactose is digested by lactase, yielding galactose and glucose. Deficiency in isomaltase, sucrase, or lactase in young infants can result in watery, acid diarrhea with dehydration and failure to thrive (Gray, 1975).

Protein digestion starts in the stomach by the activity of pepsin upon the peptide bonds of the aromatic L-amino acids. Pancreatic proteases are secreted into the duodenum in an inactivated form. Trypsinogen is activated into trypsin by enterokinase, an enzyme found in the brush border of the duodenal mucosa. Trypsin then stimulates inactive peptidases from the pancreas. These endopeptidases are capable of breaking peptide bonds to form free amino acids and peptides. The peptides and free amino acids are then transported across the intestinal mucosa.

The majority of absorption and digestion of food occurs in the upper part of the small intestine, which is approximately 280 cm long and 5 cm in diameter in a male adult. The small intestine is composed of serosa, muscularis, submucosa, and mucosa. The mucosal surface of the small bowel is lined with columnar epithelium. The surface of the absorptive cells is covered by a microvillous membrane, which comes into contact with luminal contents. This membrane facilitates absorption of nutrients and contains disaccharidases and peptidases for digestion of disaccharides and peptides. Outpouchings of mucosal epithelium, called villi, are present to increase the absorptive and digestive surfaces that are exposed to the intraluminal nutrients.

In the premature and term infant, digestive processes can be much different than those later in life. Efficiency of fat absorption does not reach normal adult standards until after 6 months of age. Several factors seem to be involved. Lipase activity is low in the neonate, and bile acid concentrations present in the lumen of the small intestine are below the critical micellar concentration necessary for normal fat absorption. Carbohydrate digestion and absorption also may not be normal, as compared with the adult. Lactase activity does not fully develop until the end of gestation, so that lactose intolerance can occur in the first few days of life. Also, amylase activity is below normal in the full-term infant, and remains low during the first several months of life. Protein absorption also is unique, because the neonate can absorb whole protein through the small bowel mucosa. This function may be an important route of antigen absorption. The significance of macromolecular absorption in early infancy, as it relates to disease states, has yet to be determined.

Maldigestion is defined as a failure to absorb a dietary constituent because of abnormal or inadequate digestion. Malabsorption is defined as a failure to transport food by-products across the small bowel mucosa into the lymphatics or portal vein branches. Normal daily stool weight averages approximately 200 gm of which 80 percent is water. An increase in the weight of the stool can be defined as diarrhea. This increased stool weight can be secondary to increased water content as well as fat, electrolytes, or carbohydrates.

Diarrhea. There are four types of diarrhea as follows: (1) osmotic diarrhea, (2) secretory diarrhea, (3) diarrhea secondary to abnormal intestinal motility, and (4) diarrhea caused by the absence of a normal active ion absorption process. Osmotic diarrhea is due to an accumulation of poorly absorbable products in the lumen of the small intestine. Usually osmotic diarrhea is caused by failure to transport a carbohydrate, such as lactose. The osmotic pressure of the luminal contents within the small bowel results in a pressure gradient that causes water to be secreted into the lumen of the duodenum and jejunum. Osmotic diarrhea can be distinguished clinically because fasting stops the diarrhea. The osmolality of the diarrheal stool generally is greater than twice the concentration of the sodium and potassium found in the diarrheal stool (mEq Na + mEq K × 2). Reducing substances in osmotic diarrhea can be identified by placing a Clinitest tablet into an equal volume of liquid stool and water.

Secretory diarrhea usually is caused by small

bowel disease. This diarrhea results from increased hydrostatic and tissue pressure, causing passive secretion into the small intestine or active secretion by small bowel mucosal cells. Secretory diarrhea stools are extremely large and will continue even after the patient has fasted. The osmolality of the stool in secretory diarrhea generally is equal to twice the concentration of the sodium and potassium of the stool.

Diarrhea secondary to an abnormality in intestinal motility is seen predominantly in patients who have either an extremely rapid transit time or in patients who have stasis syndrome with bacterial overgrowth and secondary steatorrhea. Diarrhea may result from failure to absorb ions normally because electrolytes are not transported actively across the small bowel mucosa (Phillips, 1972; Krejs and Fordtran, 1978). (Specific diarrheal diseases and their management are discussed in Chapter 25.)

Diagnostic Tests

History and physical examination are important in the diagnosis of chronic diarrhea caused by gastrointestinal allergy, as noted in Table 24–1. Table 24–2 lists the laboratory tests useful in evaluation of allergic gastrointestinal disease.

Xylose Tolerance Tests. Several tolerance tests have been devised to assess small bowel mucosal function. The 1-hour serum D-xylose test was originally conceived to evaluate small bowel mucosal disease in infants and children with celiac sprue. Xylose is a 5-carbon monosaccharide that is absorbed across the small bowel mucosa. The xylose absorption test is used to differentiate small bowel mucosal disease from intraluminal causes of steatorrhea. Abnormal renal function and ascites invalidate the urinary test. Vomiting and delayed gastric emptying of xylose also can cause abnormally low blood and urinary concentrations. The 1-hour serum xylose test is performed by giving patients who weigh less than 30 kg, 5 gm of D-xylose after an overnight fast. For patients over 30 kg, the dosage is 14.5 gm/m^2 of body surface area to a maximum of 25 gm. The xylose levels are obtained prior to the xylose challenge and 1 hour later. Serum xylose levels of less than 20 mg/dl are abnormal. The 1-hour serum xylose level will be less than 20 mg/dl in the majority of patients with severe small bowel mucosal disease, whether it is caused by celiac sprue, cow's milk protein, or soy protein sensitivity. However, it may be normal in patients with mild to moderate villous abnormalities of the small bowel mucosa (Christie, 1978).

Lactose Tolerance Test. The lactose tolerance test is a screening test for lactase deficiency in the small intestine. The patient fasts overnight and then is given 2 gm/kg of lactose, to a maximum of 50 gm, in a 10-percent solution. Blood glucose levels are measured every 15 minutes for an hour. All stools passed within 24 hours after the lactose challenge are analyzed for the presence of reducing substances. Reducing substances are evaluated by obtaining 10 drops of liquid stool. To this is added 20 drops of water and a Clinitest tablet. Any more than a trace of reducing substance is abnormal. Blood levels should rise to greater than 20 mg/dl over fasting levels. Another way to evaluate lactose malabsorption is the breath hydrogen method. Patients with greater than 20 ppm hydrogen excretion have lactose malabsorption (Kolars et al., 1984). Patients with small bowel mucosal disease can have secondary disaccharidase deficiency and, therefore, abnormal lactose tolerance test results. The test results will also be

TABLE 24–1. Approach to Diagnosis of Gastrointestinal Disease Associated with Allergy

Step 1—Obtain Data Base

"Allergic" symptoms
Compatible gastrointestinal symptoms
Exposure to milk protein, soy, gluten
Family history of allergy
Evidence of allergic disease or IgA deficiency, e.g., nasal eosinophils, bronchospasm

Step 2—Document Abnormal Gastrointestinal Function

Serum D-xylose
Lactose tolerance
Serum carotene
Stool-reducing substances
Fecal leukocytes
72-hour stool fat
Serum albumin

Step 3—Confirm Diagnosis

Observe response to allergen-free diet
Rechallenge when gastrointestinal tests are normal and observe
Symptoms
Effects on gastrointestinal function
Changes in small bowel biopsy

Step 4—Treatment

Avoid offending antigen (soy and milk until age 2; gluten for life)
Systemic steroids for eosinophilic gastroenteritis, if necessary

TABLE 24–2. Laboratory Tests Useful in Evaluation of Allergic Gastrointestinal Disease

Test	Normal	Meaning of Test
TOLERANCE TESTS		
Serum D-xylose (5 gm orally <30 kg or 14.5 gm/m² to maximum of 25 gm)	>20 mg/dl at 1 hr	Abnormal in severe small bowel mucosal disease
Lactose tolerance test (2 gm/kg to maximum of 50 gm)	No diarrhea, abdominal distention, cramps following challenge; rise in blood glucose level of >20 mg/dl Breath hydrogen concentration <20 ppm	Abnormal response with deficiency of lactase enzyme in small bowel mucosa
Sucrose tolerance test (2 gm/kg to maximum of 50 gm)	Same as lactose tolerance test. Rise in blood of >40 mg/dl Breath hydrogen concentration <20 ppm	Abnormal response with deficiency of sucrase-isomaltase enzyme in small bowel mucosa
BLOOD TESTS		
Carotene (must be on carotene diet: green, yellow vegetables)	>100 μg/dl	Low in any disease where fat malabsorption is present, especially in small bowel mucosa
Histamine	No significant rise in plasma histamine	
Albumin	>3.2 gm	Low in diseases causing protein loss in gastrointestinal tract
Red blood cell folate	<60 ng/ml	Decrease in small bowel mucosal disease
Gliadin antibodies	Fluorescence on immunosorbent test	Diagnostic of celiac disease (Burgin-Wolff et al. 1983)
STOOL TESTS		
Fecal leukocytes	No leukocytes by methylene blue stain	Increased in inflammatory diseases of intestine, primarily colon
Reducing substances	0 to trace reducing substance in stool	Indicates malabsorption of carbohydrate
A 72-hour fecal fat	>3.5 gm fat/day (coefficient fat absorption: >95 percent over 6 months; >90 percent 0 to 6 months)	Quantitates fat malabsorption
A 24-hour stool weight	<200 gm	Formed stool >400 gm usually means steatorrhea Stool <100 gm, steatorrhea unlikely

abnormal in patients with primary lactase deficiency. It is important to make sure that a patient with suspected cow's milk protein sensitivity has a normal lactose tolerance test prior to challenge with a cow's milk protein formula that contains lactose.

Sucrose Tolerance Test. The sucrose tolerance test is performed by giving a patient 2 gm/kg of sucrose in a 10-percent solution after an overnight fast. The maximum dose for adults is 50 gm. Serum levels of glucose are obtained at 15-minute intervals for 1 hour. A rise greater than 40 mg/dl in the serum is considered normal for the sucrose tolerance test. Liquid stools are again collected for analysis of sucrose. However, if sucrase deficiency is suspected, the stool must first be hydrolyzed with dilute hydrochlo-

ric acid before the Clinitest tablet is added. Patients with the rare sucrase-isomaltase deficiency will have abnormal sucrose tolerance test results and some patients with small bowel mucosal disease from other causes may also have abnormal results. One needs also to consider fructose and sorbitol intolerance as causes of watery diarrhea. Sorbitol is commonly used as a sugar substitute in food products and can be a factor causing diarrhea, bloating, and abdominal pain (Hyams, 1983; Ravich et al., 1983; Jain et al., 1985).

A sucrose or lactose tolerance test is not considered to have an abnormal result unless the patient has clinical symptoms after the challenge. Most infants with disaccharidase enzyme deficiency will have diarrhea, cramping, abdominal pain, and abdominal distention immediately following the challenge. Some patients receiving lactose will not show normal rises in blood glucose levels after the oral dose is given (Paige et al., 1978). However, unless clinical symptoms are present, these patients should not be considered lactase deficient.

Fat Absorption Test. Only two fat absorption tests are used widely in the United States. Serum carotene is used as a screening test for fat malabsorption in patients who are eating diets containing adequate amounts of vegetables. Carotene is a precursor of vitamin A, and its absorption depends upon normal fat transport across the small bowel mucosa. Normal plasma carotene levels are greater than 100 μg/dl. Levels between 50 and 100 μg/dl are borderline; levels less than 50 μg/dl are considered to be unequivocally abnormal. Serum carotene will be low with pancreatic insufficiency, small bowel mucosal disease, and impaired intraluminal micelle formation. A 72-hour quantitative fecal fat measurement is useful to document the presence of steatorrhea. Patients must have adequate fat-containing diets before the test is contemplated. Normally, there is less than 3.5 gm of stool fat per 24 hours.

Stool Fecal Leukocyte Test. Obtaining a stool smear for fecal leukocytes is useful in patients with inflammatory bowel disease involving the colon predominantly. In an infant with a diagnosis of cow's milk or soy milk protein colitis, a methylene blue stain for fecal leukocytes should be obtained prior to proctosigmoidoscopic examination or rectal biopsy. Fecal leukocytes are not seen in patients with small bowel mucosal disease unless acute inflammation is present, as can be seen in a small percentage of infants with acute viral enteritis.

When blood and fecal leukocytes are present in the stools, proctosigmoidoscopic examination is performed to evaluate the possibility of colitis. The absence of ramifying blood vessels and the presence of friability are indications of inflammation.

Biopsy. Small bowel biopsy is performed by passing a multipurpose biopsy capsule to the ligament of Trietz. Two specimens are obtained for analysis. For proper interpretation, the biopsy must be oriented and mounted properly. Only the central core of the specimen should be evaluated (Perera et al., 1975). If done properly, a small bowel biopsy can provide a specific diagnosis, such as lymphangiectasia, eosinophilic gastroenteritis, *Giardia,* or immunodeficiency. A flat small bowel biopsy usually indicates sprue or, less commonly, severe cow's milk or soy milk protein sensitivity.

The use of small bowel biopsy is indicated in any infant with significant diarrhea and failure to thrive, even when screening tests are equivocal. This biopsy is especially needed in patients found to have isolated deficiency of a specific nutrient, such as folate, vitamin B_{12}, calcium, or iron.

Rectal biopsy should be performed to look for granulomas, crypt abscesses, and ganglion cells.

Radiographic Examination. Upper gastrointestinal and small bowel follow-through radiographs are less useful in evaluation of chronic diarrhea in young infants than in older children and adults. Small bowel mucosal detail is difficult to interpret. However, the findings of thickened folds in the duodenum, jejunum, or ileum are indications for small bowel biopsy. When the possibility of a structural abnormality such as malrotation with volvulus exists, radiographs are indicated.

A barium enema should be done only when there is no evidence of acute inflammation in the colon and at least 1 week after rectal biopsy. The barium enema is less useful in allergic gastrointestinal disease, except in the rare patient with soy or milk protein colitis or in the patient with ileocolitis with eosinophilic gastroenteritis.

Food Challenges. Food challenges are useful in identifying food to which the patient specifically is allergic (Bock, 1985; Chapters 26 and 27). However, since anaphylaxis can occur in some patients, such food challenges should not be performed unless emergency equipment is on hand (Chapter 51, anaphylaxis). Food challenge is best avoided if there is a likelihood of anaphylaxis. Recently, patients with atopic dermatitis and protein sensitivity were shown to have increased plasma histamine levels after food challenge. A significant number of these patients had diarrhea, nausea, and vomiting (Sampson et al., 1984). Biopsies of the organ suspected to be involved (stomach, small bowel, colon) should be done before and after challenge.

Other Tests of Intestinal Function. Other tests that can be useful in selected patients with allergic disease of the gastrointestinal tract are prothrombin time, serum albumin, and serum folate. Prothrombin time is prolonged in patients with vitamin K malabsorption, which can be secondary to small bowel mucosal disease or abnormal micelle formation in the small bowel mucosa. The serum folate level may be abnormal when the upper small intestine is damaged. It will be normal in pancreatic insufficiency or when micelle formation is abnormal. After performing screening tests of gastrointestinal function, challenge with the offending protein is required for definitive diagnosis.

Principles of Care

After the specific diagnosis of a gastrointestinal disease has been made, appropriate therapy should be initiated. An infant with definite cow's milk or soy milk protein sensitivity should not be fed this protein until approximately 2 years of age. All labels on any packaged foods must be read before allowing the infant to eat these foods. Any foods containing casein, lactalbumin, whey, or cow's milk protein must be avoided. Soy protein is found commonly in junior baby foods and cereals, and all labels again must be scrutinized (Tables 24–3 and 24–4; Chapter 27). The child diagnosed as having celiac sprue must be on a gluten-free diet for life (Table 24–5).

A patient found to have eosinophilic gastroenteritis can first be treated by diet elimination, if there is a reasonable history of a specific food precipitating gastrointestinal symptoms. As a general rule, elimination diets are not consistently useful in stopping symptoms in patients with eosinophilic gastroenteritis. The

TABLE 24–4. Soybean Protein–Free Diet

Allowed	Avoid
Cow's milk protein formulas	Soy milk formulas
Enfamil	Soy flour
SMA	Textured vegetable protein
Similac	Soy sauce
Low Birth Weight Similac	Coffee substitutes
Advance	Soya ice cream products
	Meat extenders
Special formulas	Worcestershire sauce
Pregestimil	Hollywood bread
Portagen	
Nutramigen	
Vivonex	
Meat base	

standard therapy for eosinophilic gastroenteritis is a trial of low-dose corticosteroids. Generally, 0.5 mg/kg/day is indicated. Patients can often be managed on less than 10 mg prednisone per day. Sometimes, patients who can be managed on alternate-day, low-dose therapy will become asymptomatic in a period of weeks to months.

Patients found to have specific nutrient deficiencies, such as folate, vitamin B_{12}, or iron, should be treated with appropriate doses of these substances. As a rule, once the nutritional deficiency has been reversed, further therapy on a long-term basis will not be indicated.

On rare occasions, an infant may be intolerant to both cow's milk and soy milk protein as well as special hydrolyzed protein formulas. In this case, long-term breast milk therapy or an elemental diet, such as Vivonex, is indicated. The elemental diet contains only free amino acids and glucose polymers, with a small amount of linoleic acid to eliminate the possibility of essential fatty acid deficiency. Elemental diets should be reserved for the patient who has definitely demonstrated intolerance to other standard and specialized formulas and for whom human breast milk cannot be supplied on a long-term basis.

Oral sodium cromolyn has been advocated as a form of therapy for patients who have adverse reactions to specific foods (Vaz et al., 1978). No data are available as to long-term use of this drug for food sensitivity. Controlled double-blind studies comparing cromolyn with placebo are necessary before routine use can be advocated.

TABLE 24–3. Cow's Milk Protein–Free Diet

Allowed	Avoid
Soy milk formulas	Cow's milk formulas
Isomil	Fresh milk
Soyalac, Soyalac-I	Cream
ProSobee	Canned milk
Neo-Mull-Soy	Cheese
	Casein
Special formulas	Lactalbumin
Pregestimil	Cured whey
Portagen	Malted milk
Nutramigen	Butter
Meat base	Margarine
Vivonex	Milk-based pudding
	Flour mixtures
	Lunch meats
	Commercial meat patties
	Hamburgers
	Sweets
	Creamed foods
	Gravies

TABLE 24–5. Gastrointestinal Diseases Associated with Allergy

Cow's Milk Protein Sensitivity

Eosinophilic gastroenteritis of infancy
Nonspecific small bowel mucosal disease
   Acute onset
   Delayed onset
Intractable diarrhea syndrome of early infancy
Nonspecific colitis
Iron deficiency anemia associated with gastrointestinal
   blood loss
Enterocolitis in low-birth-weight infants

Soy Protein Sensitivity

Nonspecific small bowel mucosal disease
Nonspecific colitis

Eosinophilic Gastroenteritis

Stomach and small bowel
   Allergic
   Nonallergic
Colon
Esophagus

Celiac Sprue

REFERENCES

Anderson, H.A., Holman, C.B., Olsen, A.M.: Pulmonary complications of cardiospasm. J.A.M.A. 151:608, 1953.

Barish, C.F., Wu, W.C., Castell, D.O.: Respiratory complications of gastroesophageal reflux. Arch. Intern. Med. 145:1882, 1985.

Berquist, W.E., Rachelefsky, G.S., Rowshan, N., et al.: Quantitative gastroesophageal reflux and pulmonary function in asthmatic children and normal adults receiving placebo, theophylline, and metaproterenol sulfate therapy. J. Allergy Clin. Immunol. 73:253, 1984.

Bock, S.A.: Natural history of severe reactions to foods in young children. J. Pediatr. 107:676, 1985.

Boyle, J.T., Tuchman, D.N., Altschuler, S.M., et al.: Mechanisms for the association of gastroesophageal reflux and bronchospasm. Am. Rev. Respir. Dis. 131:S16, 1985.

Burgin-Wolff, A., Bertele, R.M., Berger, R., et al.: A reliable screening test for childhood celiac disease: Fluorescent immunosorbent test for gliadin antibodies. J. Pediatr. 102:655, 1983.

Byrne, W.J., Euler, A.R., Strobel, C.T.: Recurrent pulmonary disease in children: A complication of gastroesophageal reflux. Gastroenterology 74:1016A, 1978.

Carre, I.J.: Pulmonary infections in children with a partial thoracic stomach ("hiatus hernia"). Arch. Dis. Child. 35:481, 1960.

Christie, D.L.: Use of the one-hour blood xylose test as an indicator of small bowel mucosal disease. J. Pediatr. 92:725, 1978.

Christie, D.L., Mack, D.V.: Evaluation of the pH probe test for gastroesophageal reflux in pediatric patients. Clin. Res. 26:173A, 1978.

Christie, D.L., Rudd, I.G.: Radionuclide test for gastroesophageal reflux (GER) in children. Pediatr. Res. 12:432, 1978.

Christie, D.L., O'Grady, L.R., Mack, D.V.: Incompetent lower esophageal sphincter and gastroesophageal reflux in recurrent acute pulmonary disease of infancy and childhood. J. Pediatr. 93:23, 1978.

Danus, O., Casar, C., Lanain, A., et al.: Esophageal reflux —an unrecognized cause of recurrent obstructive bronchitis in children. J. Pediatr. 89:220, 1976.

Darling, D.B., McCauley, R.G.K., Leonidas, J.C.: Gastroesophageal reflux in infants and children: Correlation of radiological severity and pulmonary pathology. Radiology 12:735, 1978.

Donner, M.W.: Radiologic evaluation of swallowing. Am. Rev. Respir. Dis. 131:S20, 1985.

Gray, G.M.: Mechanisms of digestion and absorption of food from gastrointestinal disease. *In* Sleisenger, M.H., Fordtran, J.S. (eds.), Gastrointestinal Disease: Pathophysiology, Diagnosis, Management. Philadelphia, W.B. Saunders Co., 1978.

Gray, G.M.: Carbohydrate digestion and absorption: Role of the small intestine. N. Engl. J. Med. 292:1225, 1975.

Hyams, J.S.: Sorbitol intolerance: An unappreciated cause of functional gastrointestinal complaints. Gastroenterology 84:30, 1983.

Jain, N.K., Rosenberg, D.B., Ulahannan, M.J., et al.: Sorbitol intolerance in adults. Am. J. Gastroenterol. 80:678, 1985.

Jolley, S.G., Johnson, D.G., Herbst, J.J., et al.: An assessment of gastroesophageal reflux in children by extended pH monitoring of the distal esophagus. Surgery 84:16, 1978.

Kolars, J.C., Levitt, M.D., Aouji, M., et al.: Yogurt—An autodigesting source of lactose. N. Engl. J. Med. 310:1, 1984.

Krejs, G.J., Fordtran, J.S.: Diarrhea. *In* Sleisenger, M.H., Fordtran, J.S. (eds.), Gastrointestinal Disease: Pathophysiology, Diagnosis, Management. Philadelphia, W.B. Saunders Co., 1978.

Liebman, W., Thaler, M.M.: Pediatric consideration of abdominal pain and the acute abdomen. *In* Sleisenger, M.H., Fordtran, J.S. (eds.), Gastrointestinal Disease: Pathophysiology, Diagnosis, Management. Philadelphia, W.B. Saunders Co., 1978.

Mansfield, L.E., Stein, M.R.: Gastroesophageal reflux and asthma: A possible reflex mechanism. Ann. Allergy 41:224, 1978.

Mendelson, C.L.: The aspiration of stomach contents into the lungs during obstetric anesthesia. Am. J. Obstet. Gynecol. 50:191, 1946.

Mitsuhashi, M., Tomomasa, T., Tokuyama, K., et al.: The evaluation of gastroesophageal reflux symptoms in patients with bronchial asthma. Ann. Allergy 54:317, 1985.

Nelson, H.S.: Gastroesophageal reflux and pulmonary disease. J. Clin. Allergy Clin. Immunol. 73:547, 1984.

Paige, D.M., Mellitis, E.D., Chiu, F.: Blood glucose rise after lactose tolerance testing in infants. Am. J. Clin. Nutr. 31:222, 1978.

Parker, F., Christie, D.L., Cahill, J.: Incidence and significance of gastroesophageal reflux in tracheoesophageal fistula. J. Pediatr. Surg. 14:5, 1979.

Perera, D.R., Weinstein, W.M., Rubin, C.E.: Small intestinal biopsy. Human Pathol. 6:157, 1975.

Phillips, S.F.: Diarrhea: A current review of the pathophysiology. Gastroenterology 63:495, 1972.

Ravich, W.J., Bayless, T.M., Thomas, M.: Fructose: Incomplete intestinal absorption in humans. Gastroenterology 84:26, 1983.

Sampson, H.A., Jolie, P.L.: Increased plasma histamine concentrations after food challenges in children with atopic dermatitis. N. Engl. J. Med. 311:372, 1984.

Shapiro, G.G., Christie, D.L.: Gastroesophageal reflux in steroid dependent asthmatic youths. Pediatrics 63:207, 1979.

Urschel, H.C., Jr., Paulson, D.L.: Gastroesophageal reflux and hiatal hernia. J. Thorac. Cardiovasc. Surg. 53:20, 1967.

Vaz, G.A., Tan, L. K-T., Gerrard, J.W.: Oral cromoglycate in treatment of adverse reactions to foods. Lancet 1:1066, 1978.

Wilson, N.M., Charette, L., Thomson, A.H., et al.: Gastrooesophageal reflux and childhood asthma: The acid test. Thorax 40:592, 1985.

Wynne, J.W., Modell, J.H.: Respiratory aspiration of stomach contents. Ann. Int. Med. 87:466, 1977.

25

Diagnosis and Treatment of Diarrheal Disorders

JANE L. TODARO, M.D.

Disorders involving the gastrointestinal tract usually are manifested clinically by vomiting and diarrhea, although pulmonary symptoms can be secondary problems. Diseases affecting primarily the esophagus, stomach, and respiratory system are discussed in detail in Chapter 24. This chapter concentrates largely on diarrhea as a symptomatic expression of a gastrointestinal disturbance.

Disorders involving the gastrointestinal tract may interface with other diseases, involving virtually all parts of the body. Allergy in particular can cause confusion for the patient and the physician. Allergic processes can be confined to the gastrointestinal tract or may involve the gastrointestinal tract as well as various other organ systems. Also, there are clearly recognized adverse reactions to foods and food additives for which no clear mechanism has been elucidated, and there are "food-associated syndromes" in which the associations claimed are controversial. Each of these topics is discussed elsewhere (see Chapters 10, 26, and 27, in particular).

The differential diagnosis of chronic diarrhea in infants, children, and adults is extensive, and some sort of reasoned approach to the evaluation of these patients is mandatory. The major categories to be considered when evaluating such patients include:

1. Infections and infestations
2. Post-infectious and antibiotic-related causes
3. Carbohydrate malabsorption (primary and secondary)
4. Pancreatic disorders
5. Celiac disease
6. Immune defects
7. Inborn errors of metabolism
8. Anatomic abnormalities
9. Inflammatory bowel disease
10. Maternal deprivation (under and over feeding of infant)
11. Food intolerance (allergic and nonallergic)
12. Irritable bowel syndrome

In order to begin a reasoned approach to the evaluation of the patient with chronic diarrhea, it is necessary to have some knowledge of the normal physiology of the gastrointestinal tract. In the adult, approximately 9 L of fluid passes through the intestine per day (Table 25–1). Note that only 2 L of this fluid is supplied by the diet, and note also that maximal absorptive efficiency occurs in the colon, less in the ileum, and even less in the jejunum. These facts become important when we think of postoperative patients or of patients with disease in specific locations of the intestinal tract. The intestine is uniquely adapted to enlarging its absorptive capacity to a maximal degree in a limited space. The addition of the folds of Kerckring, the villi, and the microvilli magnifies the absorptive capacity of the bowel 600 times, so that the absorptive field in an adult is 2 million square centimeters, about the size of a tennis court. Any injury to the bowel, either at the microvillus level or more grossly at the villus level, or even more grossly at the level of the folds (e.g., resection surgery) will alter the absorptive capacity both selectively and grossly. Most of the major components of food, vitamins, and trace elements are absorbed in the upper gastrointestinal tract, specifically in the duodenum and jejunum. The ileum serves as a reserve area for absorption should there be injury to or loss of the jejunum. In the terminal ileum, vitamin B_{12} and bile acids are actively absorbed. Bile acids are predominantly reabsorbed in the ileum by an active absorptive process and in the jejunum and colon by a passive one. The degree of absorption of bile salts is affected by the polarity and solubility of the salts, the presence of food residue, and the intestinal transit time. The enterohepatic pool circulates six times a day. If the ileum is resected or diseased, there is increased fecal sequestration of bile acid and compensatory increase of bile acid synthesis in the liver.

Figure 25–1 illustrates the mechanism of absorption of the components of food, i.e., fat,

343

TABLE 25-1. Approximate Volumes of Fluid Entering and Leaving the Human Intestinal Tract Daily

Source	Liters into Lumen	Liters Reabsorbed	Approximate "Efficiency"
Diet	2	4–5 (jejunum)	50 percent
Saliva	1		
Gastric	2	3–4 (ileum)	75 percent
Bile	1		
Pancreatic	2	1–2 (colon)	>90 percent
Small intestine	1		
Total	9	Total 8–9*	

* The stools normally contain 0.1 to 0.2 L of fluid daily. If they contain more than 0.3 L per day, diarrhea usually is present. (Adapted from Phillips, S.: Diarrhea: A broad perspective. Viewp. Digest. Dis. 7(5):1975.)

protein, and carbohydrate, and the role played by the pancreas, liver, intestinal cells, and lymphatics (Silverman and Roy, 1983). Clearly, loss or injury of any one of these will cause secondary malabsorption of specific components of food. The pancreas plays a primary role in the lipolysis of fat, reducing triglycerides to fatty acids; in the breakdown of protein, reducing whole proteins to peptides and amino acids; and in the breakdown of carbohydrates. The primary role of the liver is in the micellar solubilization of bile acids, making them water soluble. The intestinal phase of digestion is impor-

tant both at the brush border level for the transport of amino acids and the breakdown of disaccharides into monosaccharides and at the intracellular level for esterification and chylomicron formation of fat, transport of amino acids, and passive transport of monosaccharides. The intestinal cell forms a very important barrier to the absorption of unwanted antigens. Factors contributing to the pathologic absorption of antigens include a large antigen load, a decrease in intraluminal digestion, a disrupted mucosal barrier, and a decrease in IgA-producing cells in the lamina propria.

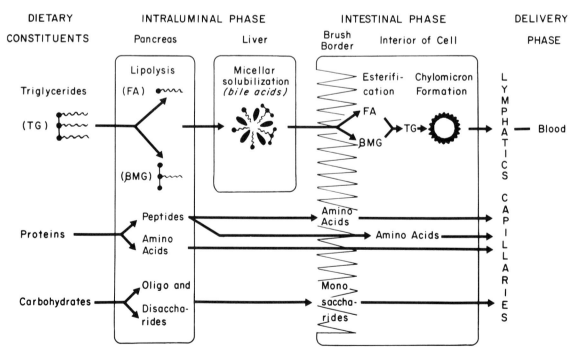

FIGURE 25-1. Digestion and absorption of triglycerides, proteins, and carbohydrates. (Reproduced by permission from Silverman, A., Roy, C.C.: Pediatric Clinical Gastroenterology, 3rd ed. St. Louis, C.V. Mosby Co., 1983.)

In beginning the evaluation of a patient with chronic diarrhea, a careful history is of the utmost importance, and this must include a dietary history. In children by far the most important piece of information that can be obtained is the pattern of growth. Figure 25–2A represents a point on a growth curve. If one were merely to observe this patient one would clearly see a well-developed and well-nourished toddler in about the middle range for his age group in height and weight. If this was the only information obtained, one would conclude that the illness had no impact on the child's growth and development but rather was an irritation to the parents and caretakers. If, however, we look at Figure 25–2B, the next growth chart on this same patient, we realize that there has been a tremendous impact on this individual and, indeed, that it has occurred at a fairly specific time. Thus, it is absolutely mandatory in the care of infants, children and adolescents that adequate and complete growth records be obtained before any evaluation is undertaken.

IRRITABLE BOWEL SYNDROME

The irritable bowel syndrome is a symptom complex characterized by altered bowel function, with or without chronic abdominal pain. Presentation can be categorized broadly into three characteristic patterns. Painless diarrhea is the most common form in the toddler age group. As patients get older, diarrhea may alternate with constipation, or patients may have abdominal pain and constipation. Older children and adults with this symptom complex often complain of associated problems, such as dyspepsia, gas, bloating, nausea, and headache. The irritable bowel syndrome represents 40 to 70 percent of gastrointestinal referrals in the adult population (Goligher et al., 1969; Drossman et al., 1977) and probably close to that percentage in the pediatric population.

The child with an "irritable bowel" often is the child who was "colicky" at birth. For example, beginning at about the age of 6 months, the infant develops unexplained diarrhea, usually no more than 4 to 6 stools a day, often firmer in the morning but becoming looser as the day progresses. The diarrhea becomes irritating, but mainly to the parents and not to the child. The buttocks rarely are burned. The child's activity, humor, and behavior remain good, and there is no impact on growth and development. Many children with these "irritable bowels" are subjected to extensive dietary manipulation to no avail. If elimination diets and food withdrawals are prolonged, the children may then suffer iatrogenic failure to thrive, thus confusing the issue considerably (Lloyd-Still, 1979). The toddler usually outgrows this so-called toddler diarrhea by 36 months of age. Therapy requires reassurance on the part of the physician and patience on the part of the parents (Davidson and Wasserman, 1966).

As children grow into their school age years, the mixed diarrhea and constipation pattern may take hold, or chronic abdominal pain may predominate. Again, there are no specific patterns to these bowel dysfunctions; pain can awaken a child at night but usually does not and usually is centered in a nonspecific pattern across the midabdomen.

Studies performed in adults suggests that emotion and stress can play significant roles in bowel motility (Almy et al., 1949). A weepy, depressed person is said to have weeping bowels, and an angry, hostile individual has "tight bowels." Thomas Almy (1951) described some remarkable experiments on the role of stress in the irritable bowel syndrome. He recorded motility changes during a stress interview by noting vascularity and contractility of the rectosigmoid during sigmoidoscopy and by balloon kymography. He described a fourth-year medical student who was a volunteer in an experiment that required sigmoidoscopy. After 10 minutes of observation and measurement, the student was told that a carcinoma of the rectum had been discovered serendipitously. At that time the rectum became suffused with blood, and heightened contractile tension was measured. Subsequently, when the student was told of the hoax, the bowel relaxed and returned to its normal color (Almy, 1951). Numerous sophisticated studies subsequently have documented alterations in motility in both the large and small bowel in patients with this disorder (Horowitz and Farrar, 1962; Snape et al., 1977; Whitehead et al., 1980).

Adult patients who manifest this clinical syndrome are usually treated with bulk-forming agents, anticholinergic agents, sedatives, antidiarrheal medications or laxatives, and most importantly reassurance and psychologic support (Sullivan et al., 1978). In infants and children, anticholinergic agents, sedatives, and symptomatic medications rarely are given;

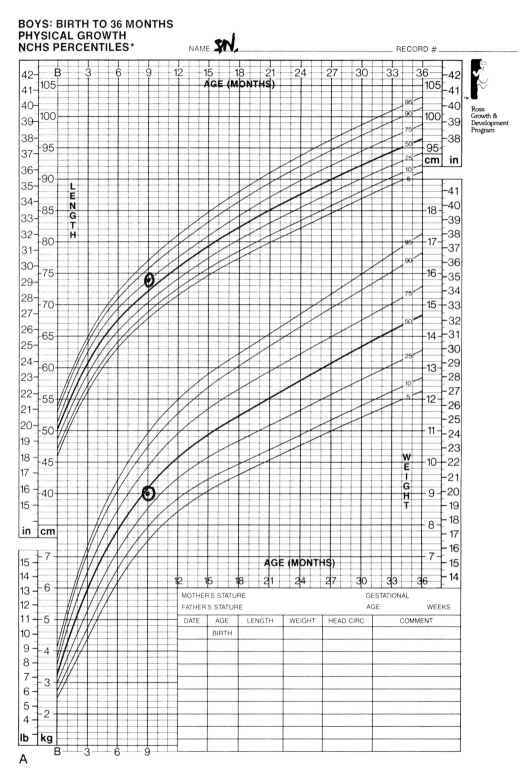

FIGURE 25-2. *A,* Patient at 9 months of age.

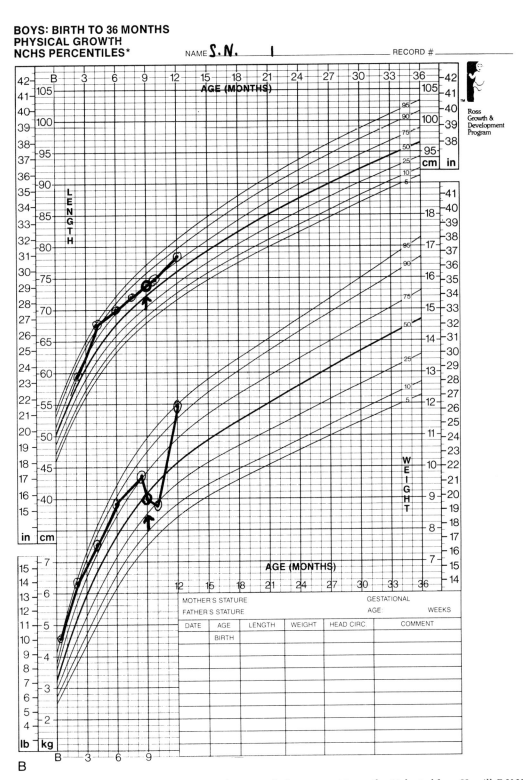

B

FIGURE 25–2 *Continued. B,* Same patient's complete growth chart at age 12 months. (Adapted from Hamill, P.V.V. et al.: Physical growth: National Center for Health Statistics percentiles. Am. J. Clin. Nutr. 32:607–629, 1979. Data from the Fels Research Institute, Wright State University School of Medicine, Yellow Springs, Ohio. © 1982 Ross Laboratories.)

bulk-forming agents and reassurance form the mainstays of therapy.

INFECTIONS AND INFESTATIONS

The more common pathogens affecting the gastrointestinal tract include viruses, parasites, and enteric bacterial pathogens. "New" pathogens are reported with surprising regularity. Not every patient with chronic diarrhea requires a stool culture, and not every patient with documented infectious disease requires antibiotic treatment. However, there are special considerations in the evaluation of patients with acute or chronic diarrhea that would lead one to look for an infectious etiology. These patients include neonates, infants in day care centers or in institutions, children or adults who have been treated recently with antibiotics or who have traveled recently, those who have compromised immune systems, and those who have been exposed to a known common diarrheal outbreak. To obtain stool cultures from every patient with loose bowel movements is not cost effective. This fact is elegantly illustrated in a study in which 2468 stool cultures were obtained, at an approximate cost of $10.00 per culture; 58 or 2.4 percent were positive, thus the cost per positive culture was $426.00 (Radetsky, 1986). This compared with the cost of $148.00 for a positive blood culture, $50.00 for a positive urine culture, and $38.00 for a positive throat culture, suggesting that we are not good at predicting those patients in whom cultures will be positive. The factors that these investigators believed best predicted the presence of an enteric pathogen included abrupt onset, frequent stools (greater than four per day), no vomiting before the onset of diarrhea, and polymorphonuclear leukocytes in a stool smear. The right question must be asked of a capable laboratory staff. If special media are required, that special media must be requested and special culture conditions required must be noted. Table 25–2 notes the common enteric pathogens (excluding viruses), the accepted treatment of these pathogens today, and the effectiveness of treatment (Pickering, 1985). A number of the enteric pathogens can cause signs and symptoms that are not localized to the gastrointestinal tract and may be confused with an allergic diathesis. When stool cultures for enteric pathogens are ordered, sensitivity testing should be requested. The secondary consequences of enteric infection, either treated or untreated, are discussed in further detail subsequently.

CELIAC DISEASE

Celiac disease is a disorder of the upper small intestine and is directly due to the toxic effect on the small intestine of the gliadin component of gluten contained in the protein of wheat, rye, barley, and probably oat. Patients with celiac disease are usually diagnosed early in infancy, but occasionally a school age child or an adolescent is diagnosed largely because of failure to grow properly. More occasionally, adult patients are diagnosed, presenting with longstanding, unexplained diarrhea or iron deficiency anemia.

The growth pattern in the infant or toddler is characteristic. Growth is normal until gluten-containing products are introduced into the diet. Some months after, there is an apparent decreasing velocity of growth in height and a leveling off or loss of weight.

Gliadin is toxic to the small intestine. The mucosa is damaged and flattened, with a loss of absorptive surface, a loss of disaccharidases that are present in the microvilli of the intestine, and an apparent inflammatory response composed largely of IgA-containing plasma cells (Rubin et al., 1960).

Because malabsorption of fat is characteristic of celiac disease, stools are overwhelmingly foul smelling and may float. Patients also may be intolerant to milk and milk products because of a secondary lactase deficiency caused by disruption of the brush border of the villous membrane. There clearly is a genetic component to celiac disease. A greater number of patients are HLA-B8 positive than the normal population, and there is an increased incidence of celiac disease in families. The exact genetic transmission has not been identified, however (Strober, 1976). Gliadin is toxic in celiac disease, and antigliadin antibody levels have been used as screening tests for celiac disease in some medical centers (Levenson et al., 1985). There probably is an allergic/immune basis for celiac disease, but the pathogenesis has not been elucidated clearly (Ferguson et al., 1984).

In addition to growth failure, patients with celiac disease present with stigmata of chronic malabsorption and malnutrition on physical examination. The young child is irritable and wasted. Abdominal distention and loss of subcutaneous tissue are most prominent on the

TABLE 25–2. Antimicrobials in Enteric Infections*

Organism	Antimicrobial Agent	Clinical Improvement	Contagious-ness	Comments
Shigellosis	Trimethoprim-sulfamethoxazole (TMP-SMX), tetracycline, or ampicillin	+	↓	TMP-SMX is drug of choice if susceptibility of organism is unknown. Not recommended for children. Effective against susceptible strains.
Salmonella gastroenteritis	None (or ampicillin, amoxicillin, or TMP-SMX)	+	0/↑	Patients with hyperpyrexia and systemic toxemia should be treated as if they have bacteremia; a 7- to 10-day course of therapy is probably sufficient.
Salmonella bacteremia or typhoid fever	Ampicillin, chloramphenicol, or TMP-SMX	+	0/↑	All three drugs are acceptable. Susceptibility testing should be performed.
Dissemination of *Salmonella* with localized suppuration (osteomyelitis)	Ampicillin, chloramphenicol, or TMP-SMX	+	−	Therapy should be provided for at least 4 to 6 weeks.
Clostridium difficile (antimicrobial associated colitis)	Vancomycin or metronidazole	+	↓	Offending antimicrobial agent must be stopped.
Campylobacter jejuni gastroenteritis	None (or erythromycin)	0	↓	Erythromycin reduces fecal excretion but does not alter clinical symptoms.
Sepsis	Gentamicin, chloramphenicol, or erythromycin	+	↓	Optimum therapy has not been established.
Yersinia enterocolitica gastroenteritis	Probably none	?	?	Infection generally self-limited: value of therapy is unknown.
Sepsis	Gentamicin, chloramphenicol, or TMP-SMX	+	↓	Optimum therapy has not been established.
Escherichia coli 0157	Probably none	+	−	Frequently associated with hemolytic-uremic syndrome.
Giardia lamblia	Furazolidone, metronidazole, or quinacrine	+	↓	Furazolidone is the only one of these drugs in liquid form.
Entamoeba histolytica	Metronidazole	+	↓	

* Adapted from Pickering, L.K.: Evaluation of patients with acute infectious diarrhea. Pediatr. Infect. Dis. S13–S19, 1985. (With permission of Williams & Wilkins.)

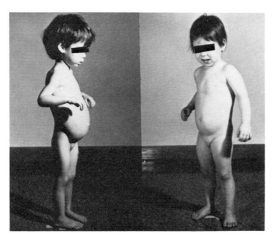

FIGURE 25–3. *A*, A 22-month-old patient with celiac disease. Note distended abdomen and emaciated extremities. *B*, Patient after introduction of a strict gluten-free diet for 3 months.

inner thighs (Fig. 25–3). Treatment is remarkably effective; it consists simply of removing wheat, rye, barley, and oat totally from the diet. This, however, requires a sophisticated approach to reading labels of food. Almost immediately upon withdrawal of gluten from the diet, the child feels better and becomes less irritable. This change in mood is followed by disappearance of the intestinal disorder and, finally, an excellent increase in growth velocity.

There is some suggestion that celiac disease may be a premalignant state, with cancers occurring both within and outside of the gastrointestinal tract (Stokes and Holmes, 1974). Most of this data is derived from symptomatic adults; it is unclear whether these adults actually have had celiac disease from birth and have been

untreated, or whether their syndrome represents a form fruste of the pediatric illness. Thus, it is not known if celiac disease that begins in infancy is premalignant nor if dietary manipulation has an effect on the subsequent development of cancer. It is clear, however, that growth is affected. Most investigators in this field agree that avoidance of gluten-containing foods should be lifelong.

CYSTIC FIBROSIS

Cystic fibrosis is one of the most common and the most severe of the chronic intestinal diseases of children and young adults (see Chapter 48). It is a disease of protean manifestations, the most imporant of which involves the pancreas and the lungs. The disease is rare in the American black population but occurs in the white population in an incidence of about 1 in 1600 live births (MacLusky et al., 1985). The risk of producing a child with cystic fibrosis is noted in Table 25–3. This extremely high incidence makes cystic fibrosis the most frequently occurring lethal genetic disease for white children. It is considered to be an autosomal recessive disorder. The primary biochemical defect in cystic fibrosis remains unknown. No unifying concept for the abnormality in exocrine secretions has been advanced. The gastrointestinal tract manifestations are secondary to the disease in the pancreas, causing pancreatic insufficiency with subsequent malabsorption of protein, fat, and carbohydrate, and subsequent development of severe diarrhea and failure to thrive.

The "typical" patient with cystic fibrosis is

TABLE 25–3. Risks of Producing a Child with Cystic Fibrosis (CF)*

One Parent	Other Parent	Risk of CF in each Pregnancy
With no CF history	With no CF history	
White		1/2300
Black		1/19,000
Oriental		1/90,000
With no CF history	With first cousin having CF	1/320
With no CF history	With aunt or uncle having CF	1/240
With no CF history	With sibling having CF	1/120
With no CF history	With CF child by previous marriage	1/80
With no CF history	With parent having CF	1/80
With no CF history	With CF history	1/40
With sibling having CF	With sibling having CF	1/9
With CF child	With CF child	1/4

* Reproduced with permission from Shwachman, H.: Current Problems in Pediatrics VIII. Cystic fibrosis. 1978.

relatively easy to identify, since the child manifests chronic, severe diarrhea and recurrent pulmonary disease. On the other hand, the presentation of the "atypical" patient may be subtle; respiratory symptoms may be confused with allergic bronchitis or asthma, whereas intestinal symptoms may mimic those of food intolerance. Gastrointestinal manifestations of cystic fibrosis, as well as their frequency of occurrence, are listed in Table 25–4 (Hubbard, 1985). Diagnosis is by a sweat test, employing pilocarpine iontophoresis. This test is reliable in general, but occasional false positive and false negative reactions can occur. Its reliability is enhanced if it is performed in a laboratory with experience performing sweat tests, and sufficient sweat is obtained. Sweat electrolytes are elevated from birth. The test is safe, simple, and painless. Rarely, a false negative test reaction is obtained, owing to inadequate sweat or hypoproteinemia. False positive results occasionally are present in malnutrition, glycogen storage disease, mucopolysaccharidoses, ectodermal dysplasia, adrenal insufficiency, and hypothyroidism. A sweat chloride value greater than 60 mEq/L is abnormal.

Children with cystic fibrosis live longer than ever before, and young adults with mild cystic fibrosis are being newly diagnosed. The mean survival age has increased to greater than 20 years, whereas in 1960 less than 50 percent of children survived 5 years after diagnosis. Prolongation of life probably is best attributed to pancreatic replacement therapy and to vigorous pulmonary toilet. Cystic fibrosis should be considered in the young adult manifesting severe pulmonary disease or unexplained chronic diarrhea and weight loss. These "late onset cases" may imply significant genetic variability in this disorder (di Sant'Agnese and Davis, 1979).

Although there is no known "allergic" basis for cystic fibrosis, the symptom complex of diarrhea and pulmonary disease often is confused with allergic disease, as noted. In addition, asthma coexists with cystic fibrosis with some frequency, and wheezing in a patient with cystic fibrosis may be a manifestation of coexistence of the two conditions. Moreover, many such patients also are allergic. Again, growth pattern and characteristics of the stool, as well as careful examination of the patient, are mandatory in making appropriate clinical distinctions.

SUGAR INTOLERANCE

The inability to digest certain sugars in foods may be the result of various intestinal disorders as follows: inborn errors of metabolism, such as glucose-galactose malabsorption; congenital enzymatic deficiencies, such as sucrase-isomaltase deficiency; and primary or acquired enzymatic deficiencies, such as lactase, the most common. Primary lactase deficiency (hypolactasia) develops at varying times throughout the lifetime of many members of the population (Table 25–5). Asian children, particularly those

TABLE 25–4. Gastrointestinal and Hepatobiliary Manifestations of Cystic Fibrosis*

Organ	Manifestation	All Ages (Percent)	More than 12 years of Age (Percent)
Pancreas	Total achylia	80–90	95
	Partial or normal function	10–20	5
	Pancreatitis	0.1–0.2	?
	Abnormal gamma glutamyl transpeptidase	40	60
	Glucosuria	?	8
	Clinical diabetes	1	1–13
Intestine	Meconium ileus		
	Newborn period	10–15	—
	Equivalent	3–7	24
	Intussusception	1	5
	Rectal prolapse	22	Rare
Gallbladder	Nonvisualizable	23	15
	Microgallbladder	16	18
	Cholelithiasis	0.4	4–12
Liver	Steatosis	15–30	15–30
	Focal biliary cirrhosis	19	25
	Multilobular biliary cirrhosis	2	2–5

* Silverman, A, Roy, C.C.: Pediatric Clinical Gastroenterology. St. Louis, C.V. Mosby Co., 1983.

TABLE 25–5. Frequency of Isolated Lactase Deficiency in Various Human Populations*

Population	Percent
North American (white)	5–20
North American (black)	70–75
North American (Indian)	66
Danish	3
African Bantu	50
Nigerian	58–99
Asians	
Filipino	95
Indian	55
Thai	97
Chinese	87
Eskimo	88
Israeli Jews	61
Israeli Arabs	81
Mexican	74

* From Gray, G.M. In Stanbury, J.B., Wyngaarden, J.B., Goldstein, J.L., Brown, M.S. (eds.) *The Metabolic Basis of Inherited Disease,* 4th ed. New York, McGraw-Hill Book Co., with permission. 1978.

living in Thailand, are intolerant to lactose by the age of four, whereas the vast majority of Danes can tolerate lactose for a lifetime. Since lactose is the primary sugar in breast milk and cow's milk, the ability to digest lactose is a key to the perpetuation of the species (Johnson et al., 1974).

Disaccharide-associated diarrheas are characterized by bloating, abdominal pain, and watery, acidic diarrhea. The sugar is retained in the intestinal lumen, since it is not broken down by the disaccharidases in the brush border of the intestine and, therefore, is not digested normally. When sugar remains in the intestine, water is drawn in and diarrhea is produced through an osmotic effect. The colonic bacteria digest the unabsorbed sugar and produce lactic acid and hydrogen, so that the resulting stool is watery, acidic, and often burns the buttocks of young infants. Because the gastrointestinal symptoms noted above clearly follow the ingestion of foods, lactose intolerance often is confused with food allergy. To further complicate the issue, several studies have documented disaccharide deficiency secondary to intestinal food allergy in blind trials. This finding probably is due to direct injury to the microvillous membrane, but the pathophysiology has not been fully elucidated (Harrison et al., 1976; Ament and Rubin, 1972). Although most infants and young children can digest lactose adequately and the relative hypolactosemia does not occur until teenage or adult years, a secondary lactose intolerance frequently is encoun-

tered. Every pediatrician knows the vicious cycle of diarrhea, followed by clear-liquid feedings, then by half-strength formula, full-strength formula, and followed in turn by recurrent diarrhea. This cycle may produce a chronic, recurrent pattern in itself and leads to an erroneous diagnosis of "chronic intractable diarrhea."

There are many agents that can injure the small bowel mucosa, and one of the most common is the rotavirus in infancy. In older children and adults, *Giardia* is a prime candidate; celiac disease is an example of an inborn error causing the same result. When the intestinal villi are damaged and flattened, the disaccharidases that exist in the microvillous tips are destroyed and the ability to digest lactose is lost. Figure 25–4 compares normal intestinal mucosa with injured intestinal mucosa, as it appears on biopsy.

The acquired form of disaccharidase deficiency usually is transient and involves a quantitative decrease in the disaccharidases. Histologic studies may or may not show gross microscopic changes, although damage to the villi usually is apparent by electron microscopy (Hyams et al., 1980). Since symptoms are secondary to the lack of absorption of sugar, a careful dietary history is imperative.

Diagnosis is made by examining the stool for pH (acid) and for reducing substances (glucose) and by breath hydrogen test, following the ingestion of a test dose of lactose or sucrose. The basis of this test is that of the pathophysiology described previously. Once the undigested sugar reaches the colon, it is fermented by the colonic bacteria. Lactic acid and hydrogen are formed, and the hydrogen is reabsorbed in the blood stream and excreted in the lungs and can be measured in the breath. This is an accurate test and reliable at all ages. In small children, a nasal prong can be used (Newcomer et al., 1975; Barr et al., 1978). Venous blood lactose and sucrose absorption tests have been abandoned for the most part. These are dependent on intestinal motility, gastric emptying, and a host of other factors, and require repeated drawing of blood.

The treatment of secondary disaccharidase deficiency is removal of the offending sugar from the diet. In theory, the bowel regenerates in 48 hours and within a few days at most should be able to accept a lactose load again. In practice, however, this often is not the case, and small infants may require a lactose-free diet for 4 to 8 weeks following an episode of acute diar-

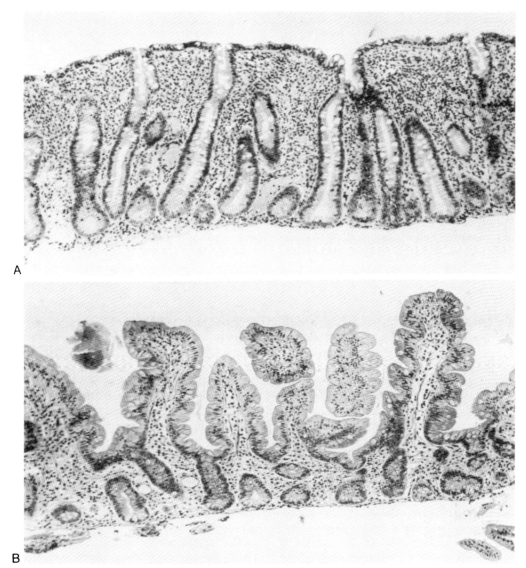

FIGURE 25–4. *A*, Initial biopsy section of a 2-year-old child showed total villous atrophy. *B*, Repeat biopsy section 6 months later shows a normal mucosa. (Reproduced by permission from Silverman, A., Roy, C.C.: Pediatric Clinical Gastroenterology, 3rd ed. St. Louis, C.V. Mosby Co., 1983.)

rhea. It is judicious to begin treatment following an acute diarrheal episode with a glucose-containing formula, such as ProSobee. If soy protein is a problem, a more elemental formula, such as Pregestimil, can be utilized.

INFLAMMATORY BOWEL DISEASE

Ulcerative colitis and Crohn disease are the two major inflammatory bowel diseases of children, adolescents, and adults (Kirsner and Shorter, 1980). Ulcerative colitis is a disease limited to the large intestine. It usually begins distally and may involve the entire large intestine or only the distal segments. The disease is confined to the mucosa and is confluent. Symptoms include tenesmus, bright red blood, and urgency. In infants, cow's milk colitis may be indistinguishable on sigmoidoscopy from ulcerative colitis (Gryboski, 1967); ulcerative colitis may be difficult to distinguish from infectious colitis at any age (Goligher et al., 1969).

Crohn disease is a chronic inflammatory bowel disease potentially affecting the entire intestine from mouth to anus. This is a transmural disease and differs from ulcerative colitis in location and depth, and in having "skip areas." Thirty percent of children with Crohn disease may present with growth failure. The extracolonic manifestations of these illnesses are protean; the arthritis and rash (most commonly erythema nodosum) have on occasion been confused with an allergic diathesis.

The chronic inflammatory bowel diseases have a symptom complex sufficiently characteristic that they rarely are confused with allergic disease, except in the instance noted. However, as many as 40 percent of patients may show decreased lactase activity during the first few months of the disease and may warrant a trial on a milk-free diet. No other dietary manipulations have been proved to be therapeutic except that adequate nutrition is imperative in these often malnourished children and adults.

SPECIFIC FOOD INTOLERANCES

Allergic reactions to food and foodstuffs are discussed in more detail elsewhere (Chapters 10, 26, and 27). Cow and soy protein sensitivity are particularly common in young infants. It is estimated that as many as 0.3 to 7.5 percent of children may be allergic to cow's milk protein (Adverse Reactions to Foods, 1984). This differs from primary or secondary sugar sensitivities as noted previously and is not a reflection of an inborn error of metabolism. The cow's milk protein as a prototype of protein sensitivity may affect the intestinal tract in one of many ways, for example, by an allergic (i.e., immune-mediated) reaction and by a direct, toxic affect on the bowel, much like that in celiac disease. The effect of cow's milk protein on the intestinal tract may result in acute gastroenteritis, eosinophilic gastroenteropathy, acute colitis, protein-losing enteropathy, or celiac disease–like syndrome.

Acute gastroenteritis caused by food intolerance may be due directly to a toxin as in food poisoning or to the toxic effect of protein on the intestine in a manner similar to that of gluten in celiac disease. Acute manifestations include vomiting and diarrhea, and in those cases in which true colitis ensues, the presentation is indistinguishable from acute infectious colitis or from acute or chronic inflammatory colitis. On sigmoidoscopy the bowel mucosa is reddened, inflamed, and friable, and there are the markers of acute inflammation. Fecal smears contain white blood cells, some eosinophils, and even colonic epithelium. Biopsy specimens

taken during the acute stage show nonspecific proctitis with edema and infiltration of round cells and polymorphonuclear leukocytes or may show changes consistent with acute ulcerative colitis, with destruction of mucosa, marked inflammatory cellular infiltration, and crypt abscesses (Gryboski, 1967).

Infants with milk-induced allergic colitis tend to present at any age between the second day and sixth month of life. The babies often are critically ill, and challenge with small amounts of milk may induce shock. This acute colitis secondary to milk protein is not usually seen in older infants, children, and adults, and protein sensitivity in older patients is an unlikely consideration in the differential diagnosis of acute colitis. Infants presenting with possible milk-induced colitis should have milk and milk products removed from their diets immediately. Unfortunately, skin testing, radioallergosorbent test (RAST), IgE titers, and hemagglutination titers are not especially valuable in diagnosis, and false negative reactions can occur. Clinical challenge with milk should not be attempted for at least 6 and probably 12 months. Since such infants are prone to anaphylaxis when challenged with milk, challenge should be performed with a small amount and in a setting in which care for acute reactions is available. An intravenous infusion should be initiated before challenge. Treatment is by a rigid milk protein–free diet. Most milk allergic infants are exquisitely sensitive to milk up to 12 months of age; some remain sensitive for 5 or 6 years, and perhaps as many as 15 percent will later develop allergic respiratory disease (Gryboski, 1967).

The acute form of cow's milk protein sensitivity (colitis/anaphylaxis) is generally limited to the young infant. However, the more common clinical manifestation of "cow's milk intolerance" is that of chronic mucoid diarrhea. Although growth usually is maintained, this is not always the case, and severe malnutrition can develop. Older infants may develop milk protein–induced enteropathy, usually secondary to an episode of acute enteritis in which there has been mucosal damage and "antigen leak." This may be confused with or, indeed, resemble celiac disease in which the patient has failure to thrive, abdominal distention, subcutaneous wasting, and clinical sensitivity either to milk protein or to wheat protein. Biopsy of the small intestine will distinguish this celiac disease–like syndrome from true celiac disease, but the issue may be complicated in milk protein sensitivity since milk protein can directly injure the small bowel mucosa (Fontaine and Navarro, 1975).

PROTEIN-LOSING ENTEROPATHY

The term protein-losing enteropathy is not a specific diagnosis but rather a condition in which protein is lost through the bowel. This condition may be a reflection of malnutrition, maldigestion, or malabsorption. In some instances, serum protein levels are reduced, owing to increased mucosal permeability or reduced lymphatic flow or both. Both gamma-globulins and albumin are lost into the bowel lumen in contradistinction to the kidney, which is selective for small molecular weight proteins. Clinically, the most obvious findings of protein-losing enteropathy are diarrhea and peripheral edema. Despite the fact that immunoglobulins are lost, systemic infection is rare because of increased immunoglobulin synthesis. Thus, hypoproteinemia may complicate a number of primary and secondary disorders of the small intestine. These disorders include anatomic lesions, inflammatory disorders, allergic disorders in which the bowel mucosa is disrupted, and increased lymphatic pressure or increased lymphatic losses. It is imperative to evaluate the protein status of a patient, since therapy and prognosis are dependent upon it.

EOSINOPHILIC GASTROENTERITIS

Eosinophilic gastroenteritis is a symptom complex that, when originally described, was thought to be due to allergy or to intolerance to specific foods (Waldmann et al., 1967). However, more recent studies indicate that less than half the patients with this disorder have specific food intolerances (Katz et al., 1984). The exact pathogenesis of eosinophilic gastroenteritis is not clearly understood. Basically, the criteria for initial diagnosis require infiltration of the gut wall with eosinophils and peripheral eosinophilia. Patients with this disorder are clustered into three major subgroups. The first is that of predominantly mucosal disease, characterized by iron deficiency anemia, increased fecal blood loss, hypoproteinemia due to protein-losing enteropathy, and malabsorption. The second is that of a disease which affects predominantly the smooth muscle layer of the bowel. There may be pyloric narrowing and obstruction, incomplete small or large bowel obstruction or both, which may mimic regional enteritis or lymphoma or both. Eosinophilic granulomas may be found in the stomach, small bowel, or colon. The third pattern is that of subserosal disease predominantly, in which the patient has eosinophilic ascites. Finally, a patient may present with all or various combinations of the aforementioned (Klein et al., 1970).

In some patients, abdominal pain and diarrhea have been convincingly and repeatedly related to the ingestion of specific foods and associated with raised serum IgE levels to these foods, indicating an immediate hypersensitivity reaction. However, as indicated previously, other patients with this syndrome do not have evident allergic manifestations, and they are not relieved by elimination diets (Katz et al., 1984).

Eosinophilic gastroenteritis is not an easy diagnosis to make. Peripheral eosinophilia is not always present. Diagnosis is made usually by intestinal biopsy. Although the lesion may be patchy, gastric antral mucosal biopsies are relatively reliable in small children. The differential diagnosis of eosinophilic gastroenteritis includes a large number of disorders of the gastrointestinal tract that may cause malabsorption. Polyarteritis nodosa, regional enteritis, and visceral lymphoma may mimic this disorder, as can the rare syndrome of hypereosinophilia. The last is characterized by persistent hypereosinophilia with widespread damage to many organs of the body (Chusid et al., 1975).

Treatment of eosinophilic gastroenteritis is simple when a specific offending food can be identified and removed from the diet. Unfortunately, elimination diets are not consistently effective in ameliorating symptoms. Steroids are widely used, beginning with an initial prednisone dosage of 20 to 30 mg/day for adults, employed for 10 days to control acute symptoms. This dosage then is reduced to 5 to 10 mg daily or 10 to 15 mg every other day, to control chronic disease, particularly in those patients with mucosal involvement. Different steroid regimens may be employed. All agree that the disease may recur when medication is discontinued, and repeated steroid trials may be necessary to control symptoms. Abnormal small bowel mucosal patterns revert to normal as early as 2 months after initiation of corticosteroid therapy in some studies (Sleisenger and Fordtran, 1983). Antihistamine, antispasmodic drugs, and antacids have not been beneficial. Cromolyn sodium may be useful in children with gastrointestinal protein allergy (Kocoshis and Gryboski, 1979), but it has not been of proven benefit in eosinophilic gastroenteritis either in children or in adults.

PSYCHOLOGIC DISTURBANCES

Psychologic disturbances may be manifested by eating disorders with secondary changes in gastrointestinal function. The most common of these are anorexia nervosa and bulimia; these occur most commonly in young women. Gastrointestinal symptoms in young infants may result from disturbed parent-child interaction, as in the "rumination" syndrome. In this syndrome, which occurs predominantly but not exclusively in infants, the child drools, vomits repeatedly at will, and characteristically "fails to thrive." A warm, loving caretaker and counselling of parents ultimately "cure" the problem. Overfeeding may induce vomiting and diarrhea as a result of inappropriately prepared formulas. Infants and children may exhibit learned food aversions. The psychologic causes of feeding disorders must be considered in the evaluation of any patient who exhibits gastrointestinal dysfunction.

APPROACH TO THE DIAGNOSIS AND MANAGEMENT OF THE PATIENT WITH CHRONIC DIARRHEA

History. A very careful and detailed history must be obtained and should include adequate and dynamic growth records in young children and good dietary records in both children and adults. Travel, medications, exposure, and family history of gastrointestinal or allergic diseases all are essential to an adequate history. A diet-symptom diary is helpful for establishing the nutritional intake as well as symptoms over several weeks.

Physical Examination. Special attention should be paid to certain manifestations of gastrointestinal disease, such as abdominal distention, subcutaneous wasting, pallor, and peripheral edema, as well as to evidence of atopic disease, such as periorbital edema, nasal mucosal edema, otitis media, pulmonary disease, and eczema.

Laboratory Evaluation. The laboratory evaluation of the patient with chronic diarrhea must begin with a careful thought process as to (1) what part of the gastrointestinal tract may be responsible for this diarrhea and (2) what, if any, foods or components of food are being inadequately absorbed? What follows is a general screening procedure we have found useful for most infants and children whose cases fit into the category of chronic, unexplained diarrhea and whose growth has been adversely affected. Useful tests are outlined, and details of their performance are given in Chapter 24.

1. *Stool.* Stool screening should include tests for ova and parasites, since *Giardia* is ubiquitous and unpredictable. Rotazyme (ELISA test for rotavirus) should be performed in an infant with acute symptoms. Stool pH and reducing substances are useful in sugar malabsorption syndromes. Sudan stain for fat in the stool is useful as a screening test when fat malabsorption is suspected, e.g., celiac disease and cystic fibrosis. A 72-hour stool fat, although difficult to obtain, when available with a concomitant diet history, is most useful. Stool trypsin is a good screening test for cystic fibrosis or pancreatic insufficiency in an infant; polymorphonuclear leukocytes in the stool are useful as markers of acute and chronic inflammation at all ages. Charcot-Leyden crystals are "footprints" of eosinophils.

2. *Blood Tests.* A complete blood count and differential should be obtained in all patients, and a reticulocyte count should be obtained as well if occult bleeding is suspected. An erythrocyte sedimentation rate is useful if chronic inflammation is suspected. Total serum protein albumin, immunoglobulins, and IgE levels are recommended in those cases with clinical suspicion of protein loss and poor nutritional status to help detect some of the basic immune gastrointestinal problems, allergic manifestations of disease, or protein-losing enteropathies. A sweat test should be performed on all infants with failure to thrive, possible malabsorption, or associated chronic pulmonary disease. Liver function tests should be ordered for all infants with failure to thrive when no etiology has been elucidated. Liver disease can be subtle and can occur without jaundice. The xylose absorption test is a useful marker of upper small bowel mucosal integrity. Sigmoidoscopy and upper and lower gastrointestinal radiologic studies are reserved for

those instances in which acute or chronic inflammation is suspected. Small bowel biopsy is indicated in specific cases when mucosal damage is suspected, such as in celiac disease.

3. *Allergy Skin Tests.* IgE antibodies to food are associated with most immediate and some delayed food reactions. Specific IgE antibody can be detected by skin prick testing or by serologic tests, such as RAST. Conventional scratch or prick tests are useful and generally correlate well with double-blind challenge (Sampson and Albergo, 1984). The best test for sensitivity to a particular food is elimination of the food followed by food challenge.

In sum, the "nonspecific" symptoms of vomiting and diarrhea in infants, children, and adults may be manifestations of a large number of illnesses in which the gastrointestinal tract may be involved as the primary or secondary target. Careful attention to history and physical examination, as well as some knowledge of the physiology of the gastrointestinal tract, is imperative in the approach to diagnosis and treatment.

REFERENCES

Adverse Reactions to Foods. American Academy of Allergy and Immunology Committee on Adverse Reactions to Foods. NIAID versus Department of Health and Human Services. Anderson, J.A., Sogn, D.D. (eds.) NIH Publication No. 84–2442, July, 1984.

Almy, T.P.: Experimental studies on the "irritable colon." Am. J. Med. 10:60, 1951.

Almy, T.P., Kern, F., Jr., Tulin, M.: Alteration in colonic function in man under stress. II. Experimental production of sigmoid spasm in healthy persons. Gastroenterology 12:425–436, 1949.

Ament, M.E., Rubin, C.E.: Soy protein—another cause of the flat intestinal lesion. Gastroenterology 2:227–234, 1972.

Barr, R.G., Perman, J.A., Schoeller, P.A., Watkins, J.R.: Breath tests in pediatric gastrointestinal disorders: new diagnostic opportunities. Pediatrics 62:393–401, 1978.

Chusid, M.J., Dale, D.C., West, B.C., Wolff, S.M.: The hypereosinophilic syndrome. Medicine 54:1–27, 1975.

Davidson, M., Wasserman, R.: The irritable colon of childhood (chronic nonspecific diarrhea syndrome). J. Pediatr. 6:1027–1038, 1966.

diSant'Agnese, P.A., Davis, P.B.: Cystic fibrosis in adults (Review). Am. J. Med. 66:121–132, 1979.

Drossman, D.A., Powell, D.W., Sessions, J.T., Jr.: The irritable bowel syndrome. Gastroenterology 73:811–822, 1977.

Ferguson, A., Ziegler, K., Strobel, S.: Gluten intolerance (celiac disease). Ann. Allergy 53:637–642, 1984.

Fontaine, J.L., Navarro, J.: Small intestinal biopsy in cows milk protein allergy in infancy. Arch. Dis. Childhood 50:357–362, 1975.

Goligher, J.C., DeDombal, F.T., Watts, J.M., Watkinson, G.: Ulcerative Colitis. Baltimore, Williams & Wilkins Co., 1969.

Gray, G.M.: In Stanbury, J.B., Wyngaarden, J.B., Fredrickson, D.S., Goldstein, J.L., Brown, M.S.: The Metabolic Basis of Inherited Disease, 4th ed. New York, McGraw-Hill Book Co., 1978.

Gryboski, J.D.: Gastrointestinal milk allergy in infants. Pediatrics 40:351–360, 1967.

Harrison, M., Kilby, A., Walker-Smith, J.A., France, N.E., Wood, C.B.S.: Cow's milk protein intolerance: a possible association with gastroenteritis, lactose intolerance, and IgA deficiency. Brit. Med. J. 1:1501–1504, 1976.

Horowitz, L., Farrar, J.T.: Intraluminal small intestinal pressure in normal patients and in patients with functional gastrointestinal disorders. Gastroenterology 42:455–464, 1962.

Hubbard, V.S.: Gastrointestinal complications in cystic fibrosis. Semin. Resp. Med. 6:299–307, 1985.

Hyams, J.S., Stafford, R.J., Grand, R.J., Walters, J.B.: Correlation of lactase breath hydrogen test, intestinal morphology and lactase activity in young children. J. Pediatr. 97:609–612, 1980.

Johnson, J.D., Kretchmer, N., Simoons, F.J.: Lactose malabsorption: Its biology and history advances. Adv. Pediatr. 21:197–237, 1974.

Katz, A.J., Twarog, F.J., Zeiger, R.S., et al.: Gastroenteropathy: Similar clinical features with contrasting mechanisms and clinical course. J. Allergy Clin. Immunol. 74:72–78, 1984.

Kirsner, J.B., Shorter, R.G.: Inflammatory Bowel Disease, 2nd ed. Philadelphia, Lea & Febiger, 1980.

Klein, N.C., Hargrove, R.L., Sleisenger, M.H., et al.: Eosinophilic gastroenteritis. Medicine (Baltimore) 49:299–319, 1970.

Kocoshis, S., Gryboski, J.D.: Use of cromolyn in combined gastrointestinal allergy. J.A.M.A. 242:1169–1173, 1979.

Krvis, W., et al.: A diagnostic score for the irritable bowel syndrome. Gastroenterology 87:1–7, 1984.

Levenson, S.D., Austin, R.K., Dietter, M.D., et al.: Specificity of antigliadin antibody in celiac disease. Gastroenterology 89:1–5, 1985.

Lloyd-Still, J.D.: Chronic diarrhea of childhood and the misuse of elimination diets. J. Pediatr. 95:10–13, 1979.

MacLusky, I., McLaughlin, F.J., Levison, H.: Cystic fibrosis. I and II. Cur. Prob. Pediatr. 15:1985.

Newcomer, A.D., McGill, D.B., Thomas, P.J., Hofmann, A.F.: Prospective comparison of indirect methods for detecting lactase deficiency. N. Engl. J. Med. 293:1232–1236, 1975.

Pickering, L.K.: Evaluation of patients with acute infectious diarrhea. Pediatr. Infect. Dis. Suppl:S13–S19, 1985.

Radetsky, M.: Laboratory evaluation of acute diarrhea. Pediatr. Infect. Dis. 5:230–238, 1986.

Rubin, C.E., Brandborg, L.L., Phelps, P.C., et al.: Studies of celiac disease. I. Gastroenterology 38:28–49, 1960.

Sampson, H.A., Albergo, R.: Comparison of results of skin tests, RAST, and double-blind, placebo-controlled food challenges in children with atopic dermatitis. J. Allergy Clin. Immunol. 74:26–33, 1984.

Schwachman, H.: Cystic fibrosis. Curr. Prob. Pediatr. 8:10, 1978.

Silverman, A., Roy, C.: Pediatric Clinical Gastroenterology. C.V. Mosby Co., 1983. p 250.

Sleisenger, M.H., Fordtran, J.S.: Gastrointestinal Disease, 3rd ed. Philadelphia, W.B. Saunders Co., 1983.

Snape, W.J., Jr., Carlson, G., Matarayze, S., Cohen, S.: Evidence that abnormal myoelectric activity produces colonic dysfunction in the irritable bowel syndrome. Gastroenterology 72:383–387, 1977.

Stokes, P.L., Holmes, G.K.T.: Malignancy. Clin. Gastroenterol. 3:159–170, 1974.

Strober, W.: Gluten-sensitive enteropathy. Clin. Gastroenterol. 5:429–452, 1976.

Sullivan, M.A., Cohen, S., Shape, W.J., Jr.: Colonic myo-electric activity in irritable bowel syndrome: effect of eating and autocholinergics. N. Engl. J. Med. 298:878–883, 1978.

Waldmann, T.A., Wochmer, R.D., Lester, L., et al.: Allergic gastroenteropathy: A cause of excessive gastrointestinal protein loss. N. Engl. J. Med. 276:762–769, 1967.

Whitehead, W.E., Eugel, B.T., Shuster, M.M.: Irritable bowel syndrome. Physiological and psychological differences between diarrhea-predominant and constipation-predominant patients. Dig. Dis. Sci. 25:404–413, 1980.

26

Evaluation of Patients with Adverse Reactions to Foods

S. ALLAN BOCK, M.D.

Many patients present with a complaint of "allergy to food." When the term "allergy" is used, the patient usually is referring to some untoward event that has been associated with food ingestion, whereas the physician usually is thinking about an immune reaction to a specific substance. Since "symptoms" and "sensitization" often are equated with "allergy," there has been much confusion about food allergy in both the medical and lay literature.

In addition to immune-mediated adverse reactions to foods, there is a substantial list of adverse reactions to foods by other mechanisms (Table 26–1) (Chapter 10). It is probable that the most common adverse reaction to food in North America, and perhaps throughout the world, is lactase deficiency leading to intolerance to lactose contained in milk products. Other less common enzyme deficiencies also may be responsible for adverse reactions to ingested foods. Since these affect the gastrointestinal tract, they can be mistaken for food sensitivity. When symptoms are limited to the gastrointestinal tract, it is important to consider the possibility that enzyme deficiency, rather than adverse reactions to proteins, may be the causative factor. Our food supply contains a long list of both natural and added substances, which may be toxic to human beings when ingested in large quantities. There is a vast literature on the subject of food toxicology. One may speculate that most transient reactions to food, affecting both children and adults, are due to unidentified inherent or generated toxins and other pharmacologically active agents present in the food in sufficient concentration to produce symptoms. Since such substances are not easily identified, the reactions cannot be readily reproduced by challenge. As we acquire more knowledge concerning mediators of inflammation and factors that induce their release, it is probable that some adverse food reactions also will be shown to be due to effects of mediators released by nonimmune mechanisms. For example, there is increasing evidence in the respiratory system that "allergic-like symptoms" result from nonimmune mechanisms.

Adverse reactions to foods induce strong emotional responses from both patients and physicians who draw conclusions based on little or no definitive data. Much of the confusion over "food allergy" or reactions to foods in general probably has to do more with patient and physician biases than with reliable scientific information. The practitioner frequently will encounter patients who want confirmation of their strongly held beliefs rather than "the truth" (which may sometimes constitute a threatening revelation concerning the origin of the patient's symptoms). Medicine also has been plagued by practitioners who attribute almost any symptom or disease to food ingestion. The vast majority of these claims, which are regarded as confusing or controversial, simply have not been confirmed by acceptable scientific methods. By rigorous application of fairly simple methodology and by proper interpretation of results, almost any reaction may be verified or refuted objectively. The diagnosis and treatment of "food allergy," in other words, need not and should not be based on preformed opinions or beliefs held by patients or physicians.

HISTORY

The objective of taking a thorough history of an adverse reaction to a food is slightly different than the usual purpose of acquiring a history. In most situations, the patient's history leads directly to the diagnosis. The purpose of a detailed history in patients who complain of food reactions is to equip the physician with sufficient facts so that a diagnostic trial may be carried out. In this way, an objective evaluation of the patient's complaints can be arranged by challenges. The specific points in such a history are noted in Table 26–2. Whenever possible, the patient should be encouraged to relate a free flowing description of the symptoms of the adverse reaction. It is most important to determine the timing between the ingestion of the food

359

TABLE 26–1. Categories of Adverse Reactions to Foods

Enzyme deficiency
Toxic reaction
Immune reaction
Psychologic reaction
Inflammatory reaction

and the appearance of symptoms. Ascertaining the quantity of food, particularly the minimum quantity, required to produce the symptoms is important. Determining the frequency with which the reaction has occurred, and particularly the occasion of the most recent reaction, also is of great importance. The practitioner will have a different opinion about an impressive set of symptoms that occurred three times over a short and recent time, than he or she will have about vague symptomatology that last occurred many years previously. Depending upon which system is involved, one may need an accurate description of nasal discharge, sputum production, and stool character. Until all of these facts have been acquired, it is impossible to proceed with attempts to determine whether a relationship between the ingestion of food and symptoms exists. Acquiring enough detail about these facts has at times been difficult because of the too often held idea that the history contains the answer. That is, when histories are impressive, there is a natural tendency to accept the patient's diagnosis and to move on to other areas, neglecting the fact that possible consequent dietary alterations actually may be deleterious and unnecessary. It is wise to bear in mind that even impressive histories may be misleading!

PHYSICAL EXAMINATION

The purpose of the physical examination is to identify signs that support the patient's description of various kinds of symptoms. The main areas of concentration include the respiratory system, skin, and gastrointestinal tract.

Height, weight, position, and change of posi-

TABLE 26–2. History Ascertained for Challenge

Description of symptoms
Timing of onset and duration
Frequency of occurrence
Quantity of food involved

tion on a growth chart for children, state of nutrition and signs of acute or chronic illness all should be noted. A thorough examination of the eyes, ears, nose, and throat may reveal specific stigmata of respiratory allergy, which potentially could be produced by food allergens. It will be important for the physician to determine not only the condition of these areas through initial examination, but through ongoing examinations as well, if a baseline is to be established and comparisons are to be made as food challenges are administered. Thorough auscultation of the lungs, particularly including forced expiration as well as pulmonary function measurements, is essential in determining the status of any airway obstruction about which the patient may complain. The abdomen should be examined thoroughly, in particular, so that important illnesses in the differential diagnosis are not overlooked in the patient's enthusiasm to blame problems on food ingestion. A detailed examination of the skin sometimes requires disrobing the patient so that areas not easily seen will not be missed. The character of any existing erythematous rashes, eczema, and urticaria is important to note at the outset so that changes over time can be ascertained.

TECHNIQUE OF CLINICAL EVALUATION

Elimination Diet

The initial step in evaluating a patient's complaint is to control or eliminate the symptoms. Often the patient will have eliminated the suspected food or foods from the diet already. However, the history frequently is so vague that the patient is uncertain which foods to eliminate. The goal of any elimination diet is to resolve symptoms and to obtain an accurate baseline. The patient may have triggers other than foods that produce symptoms, especially skin and respiratory symptoms. In this case, symptoms may not be entirely eliminated, but the maintenance of a symptom diary over a period of 7 to 14 days can demonstrate a baseline symptom level. Documentation of a baseline symptom pattern is particularly important for conditions such as atopic dermatitis and chronic rhinitis. If an accurate baseline can be obtained, food challenges have potential for demonstrating significant changes in symptoms. Without an accurate baseline, symptom exacerbations otherwise can be misinterpreted easily.

The easiest types of elimination diets to use are those that contain a few foods that reputedly are highly unlikely to produce the symptoms (Chapter 27). It should be realized, however, that even such foods as chicken and rice (which are considered benign) have been reported to be responsible for adverse reactions (Strunk et al., 1978; Bock and May, 1983). In fact, in our series of patients, we encountered more problems with chicken and rice than we did with corn and chocolate (Bock and May, 1983). The ultimate elimination diet is an elemental diet. There are several of these on the market of which a product containing crystalline amino acids, dextrose, simple fats derived from oils, and vitamins and minerals (Vivonex) may be considered to be the optimal elemental diet. For young children, the elemental formulas, Nutramigen and Pregestimil, can provide adequate nutrition while eliminating all possible problematic foods. With a strict elimination diet accompanied by the persistence of symptoms over a period of 7 to 14 days, it is unlikely that foods are responsible for the patient's symptoms. Many times, 2 to 4 days on an elimination diet will result in a dramatic change in symptoms if a dietary substance is responsible for the illness. Usually an elimination diet can be carried out at home accompanied by maintenance of a symptom diary. It rarely is necessary to have the patient record all foods eaten if a prescribed diet is being followed. Instead, the patient may be asked to list food infractions, that is, ingestion of foods that are not on the diet.

At the end of the elimination diet period, the physician may arrive at a definite opinion regarding the accuracy of the patient's history. Patients with strong needs to have symptoms attributed to reactions to food are likely to resist any device that might interfere with the conclusion they desire and, in so doing, frustrate diagnostic attempts in one way or another. It may be wise to suggest to these patients that pursuit of further evaluation is not warranted if they are comfortable with their current restrictions. Children are an exception to this. Every effort should be made to determine accurately and objectively both current symptoms that may be due to food and also the natural history of the food-related problem. Children may have strong, negative feelings about their elimination diet and, in some children, this can lead to emotional problems related to peer interaction. The use of an elimination diet, therefore, is not problem-free and should be used on a selective basis. In some cases, the need for psychologic evaluation and therapy is apparent early in the course of evaluation, and recommendation for this course of action should be considered.

SKIN TESTS FOR FOODS

Technique

Properly performed skin tests may be undertaken by the puncture (prick), scratch, or intradermal technique. At the present time, the literature pertaining to food allergy strongly supports the notion that the prick puncture test is most likely to yield useful information (Bock, 1977 and 1978; Sampson, 1982; Sampson et al., 1984; Atkins et al., 1985a and b). In most circumstances, foods tested should be those under suspicion by the patient. If there is a vague history or numerous foods are suspected, the ones tested should include a list of the most commonly identified food offenders. Wholesale food testing with hundreds of foods is inappropriate. Most of the commercially available extracts are useful if the physician is certain that each bottle of extract actually contains material likely to elicit a skin response in a sensitized person. As with any extract or reagent, it is important to ascertain that the material being used is biologically active. Attempts at standardization by extract manufacturers will be helpful in this area, but at the present time responsibility for determining that the bottle contains the material specified on the label remains with the physician.

Interpretation of Skin Tests

Research in the area of food skin testing has shown that a wheal at least 3 mm in diameter greater than the diluent control, identifies patients who have immunologically significant quantities of IgE antibody in the skin (Bock, 1977; Sampson, 1982; Sampson et al., 1984; Atkins et al., 1985a and b). Prick puncture skin tests correlate well both with the radioallergosorbent test (RAST) (Sampson, 1982; Sampson et al., 1984; Atkins et al., 1985a and b) and the leukocyte/histamine-release assays (Bock, 1977 and 1978; Bernstein et al., 1982). It has been shown that the vast majority of children, at least over 3 years of age, and adults with negative skin test reactions will not have adverse reactions to a food during a properly performed challenge. However, the converse is not necessarily true. The use of prick puncture skin testing will identify those patients in whom objective food challenges are likely to be useful. The proportion of patients with positive skin test reactions who will be challenge-positive varies from 0 to more than 50 percent in different series. Although it would be desirable to have a more sensitive and specific test, the use of a proper history, skin testing, and open challenges will limit the number of patients who require blind food challenges. Foods selected by positive prick puncture skin test results are the most likely to cause reactions to food challenge. Most investigators currently recommend that if the prick puncture skin test result in a child over 3 years of age is negative, the food can be given, since it is very unlikely that a reaction to that food will occur. Current studies suggest that intradermal skin testing is less accurate than prick puncture skin testing for identifying clinically relevant food sensitivity in children 3 years or older. Intradermal skin tests may be needed in younger children because of smaller size reactions to prick puncture skin tests. Research in the area of both *in vivo* and *in vitro* allergy testing is proceeding in a number of centers for better and more accurate methods of diagnosis.

Comparison of Skin Tests and Other Tests

Although many *in vitro* tests have been used for the diagnosis of food allergy, there are only two in widespread use shown to be efficacious, serologic tests exemplified by RAST, and histamine-release from peripheral blood leukocytes. As with skin testing, these tests measure antibodies to the food in question. In the case of the RAST, antibodies are in the circulation; in the case of the leukocyte/histamine-release, they are attached to circulating basophils. Also, as with the skin test, these tests are not diagnostic; test results must be correlated with histories or with properly performed challenge tests or both. Neither of these methods is more sensitive or more specific than skin testing for detecting clinically significant food sensitivity in patients. Moreover, they are significantly more expensive than skin testing. They are primarily excellent research tools. In today's climate of cost containment in health care, physicians should be circumspect about the widespread use of tests, the cost of which are excessive,

unless they provide information that cannot be obtained by less expensive methods. At the present time, the properly performed and properly interpreted skin test is still the best method for detecting antibodies to food allergens.

OPEN FOOD CHALLENGE

Open food challenges are easy to administer and in many instances are useful in demonstrating an absence of relationship between ingested food and purported symptoms. Open food challenges may be undertaken either at home or, in certain circumstances, under observation in the physician's office. In either case, a record of clinical manifestations should be kept either by the patient or an observer. More than half the time in young children, the combination of an elimination diet and an open challenge will be all that is necessary to dismiss an incriminated food as the cause of symptoms (Bock and May, 1983). For young children, foods often are blamed for many symptoms that subsequently are found to be due to some other cause or for which a cause of very transient symptoms is never established (Bock, 1987).

An open food challenge should begin with a quantity of food less than that reported by the patient as the smallest amount previously required to produce symptoms. If the history has been vague and the patient is uncertain about the amount of food that may cause symptoms, a small arbitrary amount may be chosen by the physician or the patient. In circumstances in which the history has been vague but the elimination of multiple foods has been associated with improvement, foods are added back to the diet at intervals of 1 to 3 days, depending on the nature of the history and the patient's and physician's suspicions (see Chapter 27 for alternative schedules). If a strict elimination diet has been employed, it can be useful to begin adding foods of low suspicion to the diet so that a more liberal, nutritious, and palatable diet may be provided quickly. This should be done by choosing representatives of major food groups, such as wheat, corn, dairy products, soy, and beef. Foods that are more highly suspected can be added later. As foods are incriminated by open challenge, they should be eliminated from the diet. Once a food has been added without apparent problems, it should be left in the diet. It should be noted that in most studies, patients who have true food allergies have been found to react to only one or two foods (Bock, 1978; Bernstein and Day, 1982; Sampson, 1982; Bock and May, 1983; Sampson and Albergo, 1984; Atkins et al., 1985a and b). The longer the patient's list becomes, the more suspicious the physician should be that the patient's symptoms may be due to factors other than foods.

At the end of the open food challenge, the patient should be able to present a list of one or more foods that have caused particular symptoms. These also should be sufficient recorded information so that the quantity of food ingested and timing of ingestion in relation to symptoms have been determined. Minimal supervision by the physician (often by telephone) can ensure that these open food challenges proceed smoothly and reasonably rapidly. It is not helpful to the patient to have the elimination and open food challenge portion of the evaluation extend for many months. In the vast majority of patients, food elimination, demonstration of improvement, and reintroduction of foods should be accomplished within a few weeks.

BLIND FOOD CHALLENGE

The technique of blind food challenge is neither complicated nor difficult. It is a procedure most likely to be undertaken by a specialist in allergy and clinical immunology. Undertaking blind food challenges in a physician's office is less time consuming and requires less office staff time than is required to provide and monitor allergy injection therapy.

Each physician planning to employ this procedure should have a supply of food challenge material on hand and should not plan to obtain the food challenge material each time a patient requires blind food challenge. I prefer the use of opaque food-containing capsules for blind food challenge. This is a desirable form of challenge for several reasons. First, dehydrated foods in capsules provide fairly large quantities of protein (the most likely offending allergenic ingredient) for each food, without requiring that the patient ingest huge quantities of the foods (Table 26–3). The larger the quantity of food required, the more difficult the blind challenge becomes. For example, a whole egg without the shell may weigh approximately 100 g. However, egg in dehydrated form may weigh 4 to 5 g and is much easier to administer to a patient in a few capsules. Second, dried food in capsules has the virtue of being easily stored in a small area. Dehydrated foods, either in capsules or in

TABLE 26–3. Quantity of Food for Blind Challenge

Food	Equivalent in Dehydrated Powder Form
1 Whole egg (100 gm)	4–5 gm
Milk (1 oz)	2.8 gm
Wheat	Flour weighed directly
Peanuts	Crushed and weighed directly
Nuts	Crushed and weighed directly

bulk, may be kept refrigerated; this usually is unnecessary if they have been properly dehydrated, however. Third, dehydrated foods are now readily available for most substances for which challenges are likely to be necessary. Cereal grains may be obtained in the dry state at local grocery or health food stores. Nuts are easy to powder and place in capsules. Although they are not completely dehydrated, they seem to have a long shelf life. Powdered milk is readily available; powdered egg also is easy to obtain.

As overnight camping becomes a more popular sport in the United States, camping stores have an ever increasing supply of dehydrated foods, which are easily powdered and placed in capsules. For example, freeze-dried beef patties have few preservatives, are readily available, and are easily encapsulated. Recently, fruits and vegetables that are lyophilized and contain few preservatives have appeared on camping store shelves. Substances that are the most difficult to obtain include fish and shellfish. It may be necessary periodically for the physician to contact a local biochemist in possession of a lyophilizer and arrange to have a fairly substantial quantity of material prepared that may then be stored for prolonged periods. Another method for producing challenge materials (particularly fish) is to put a desired quantity of the food in a microwave oven, where it is cooked until it is extremely dry. This preparation then can be placed in capsules and administered. Children can be induced to swallow capsules by making it a game. In my experience, school-age children are more likely to view the consumption of large numbers of capsules as a challenge, especially if a small reward is offered, and to object less to the process than adults who often complain about being asked to swallow a few capsules.

Other vehicles are available but are more cumbersome to use because they require more preparation at the time of challenge. Examples include milk shakes, tapioca-fruit mixtures, and iced Vivonex. The last is useful for certain food challenges in adults who require challenges with liquids that are impossible to encapsulate. For example, I have undertaken challenges with vinegar, salad oil, and white wine, by hiding those substances in iced, flavored Vivonex without the patient (or me) being able to detect their presence. In young children, many foods may be hidden in applesauce or mixed into a formula that the child already consumes. Some foods may be hidden in hamburger. There are some elaborate and dramatic reports in the literature of food challenges undertaken through nasogastric tubes; however, this is a research procedure and is not practical or recommended.

Blind challenges undertaken in the physician's office are straightforward. Depending on the timing, the patient is asked to plan to stay in the office for 4 to 8 hours and bring enough entertainment to be well occupied during that time (whether an adult or a child). If the challenge is provided by the physician, a nurse should be asked to maintain a clinical score sheet. The frequency of recording the score depends on the patient's history, and observations and questioning should be carried out at appropriate intervals. Often the history predicts that the reaction will occur within minutes or an hour or so following the challenge. The interval reported during the initial history is used to determine both the interval for symptom scoring and also for times at which challenges are repeated. It is optimal if the person providing the capsules to the patient and keeping the score is blind to the challenge along with the patient. It has been shown many times that if the observer or challenger is aware of the contents of the challenge, the results may be biased through both verbal and nonverbal communication to the patient.

The challenge is begun with an amount of food less than the smallest amount thought likely to produce the reaction. Ordinarily, it is appropriate to begin with about half the quantity of food suspected of producing a reaction. Incremental challenges should be undertaken at an interval slightly longer than that reported by the patient to produce a reaction. Incremental quantities can be doubled in the vast majority of situations. The severity and persistence of any symptoms reported by the patient will determine whether or not the challenge is continued or stopped at that point. Whenever possible, objective signs and verifiable symptoms are sought. Within limits of safety and patient comfort, the natural history of reaction to the food

may be allowed to proceed so that this information is available to the patient at the end of the challenge.

Despite extensive evaluation of patients with complaints of late or delayed onset food reactions, for the most part numerous investigators have been unsuccessful in reproducing these reactions (Bock, 1978; Bernstein et al., 1982; Bock and May, 1983; Sampson, 1982; Sampson and Albergo, 1984; Atkins et al., 1985a and b). The exception to this is protein-related enteropathy in young children. Nevertheless, many patients present to the physican with specific complaints about late or delayed onset food reactions. These reactions may be evaluated by providing the patient with several sets of capsules that are coded so the patient cannot determine their contents. The patient may be allowed to consume these capsules at home one or more times a day for several days, to see if the reaction is reproduced. In some circumstances, it may be best to have the patient report to the physician's office at the initiation of the challenge to ingest the first set of capsules. Some patients report that a quantity of food taken on one day will be responsible for symptoms 2 or 3 days later; if so, they are instructed to return to the physician's office at the appropriate time for observation. In any of these circumstances, certain considerations are important. A placebo must be used in evaluating problems outside the office; the best placebo is dextrose, which is available for human consumption and is easily placed in capsules. It may be necessary to give the patient several sets of capsules with one or more of these sets being a placebo. The patient also may need to take sets of capsules in different weeks. Whatever arrangements are required, they should attempt to reproduce the circumstances of reaction as acquired by history. Patients who are poor candidates for physician's observation include those who have obvious firmly fixed beliefs about their reactivity or who are unlikely to cooperate, for example, by attempting to determine the contents of the capsules. In most situations, both physicians and patients find the procedure both entertaining and enlightening.

At the end of the period of a blind challenge, if the symptoms have not been reproduced, it is important to *reintroduce the food openly into the diet in the usual and customary portions prepared in the usual and customary fashion and, whenever possible, under observation of the physician. The patient's ability to consume a once suspected food without any untoward reaction eliminates all questions about cooking, digestion, and any other points of preparation that may in some way alter the nature of the food.* Although the procedures outlined at first glance may appear cumbersome or overly involved, in fact these procedures for elimination, open challenge, and blind food challenge have been extremely helpful in resolving questions of food-related symptoms and in resolving the problems for which the patients presented in the overwhelming proportion of cases.

It is emphasized that none of the described challenge procedures is to be used in patients with a life-threatening history of an adverse reaction to food. These patients require special arrangements and their challenges, when undertaken, must be performed in specially equipped medical facilities. Although challenges of these patients are not recommended generally, unfortunate accidental ingestion of foods does occur followed by severe reaction to the unknown ingestion. Particularly in children, some life-threatening sensitivities to food can be diminished or can be lost in time (see subsequent discussion). In appropriate circumstances and under properly controlled conditions, therefore, challenges may be useful in determining whether or not a frightening sensitivity may have resolved (Bock, 1985).

INTERVAL CHALLENGES TO DETERMINE NATURAL HISTORY

Once an adverse reaction has been demonstrated, it is not sufficient to merely eliminate that food from the patient's diet indefinitely. Studies of the natural history of food sensitivity in children indicate that the majority of proven offending foods can be tolerated as time passes (Bock, 1983). This is particularly true for young children. The following recommendations, therefore, are offered. When a food with a brief history of causing problems has been documented by elimination and open food challenge, it should be eliminated from the diet for 1 to 3 months, depending on the severity of the initial reaction. At the end of that time, a systematic open challenge should be provided to determine whether or not the food is still a problem. If symptoms occur during this subsequent challenge, then the food should again be eliminated for 1 to 3 months. If two or three challenges at 1- to 3-month intervals produce symptoms, there is a risk that the patient will begin to acquire a strong belief about subse-

quent reactivity to that food. In these circumstances, subsequent challenges should be blind. If the food produces symptoms in a blind challenge, it is time that the mechanism of reaction be sought by appropriate laboratory means.

At this stage of our knowledge, it should be considered inappropriate for patients to be placed on prolonged elimination diets without attempts to reintroduce the food into the diets, until it is clear that the food is likely to continue producing symptoms over a long period of time. For foods such as nuts, with a propensity to produce symptoms for many years, challenges should be undertaken at yearly intervals (unless symptoms have been severe or life-threatening) until it is apparent that the food reaction is not going to be "outgrown." It is worth restating that children develop strong feelings about adherence to elimination diets. Peer interactions related to problems associated with requiring food avoidances often result in emotional difficulties, some of which may be avoided by adherence to the above recommendations, which seek to reintroduce eliminated foods as soon as it is safe to do so. Adults are more likely to adjust to dietary exclusions than are children.

REFERENCES

Atkins, F.M., Steinberg, S.S., Metcalfe, D.D.: Evaluation of immediate adverse reactions to foods in adult patients. I. Correlation of demographic, laboratory, and prick skin test data with response to controlled oral food challenge. J. Allergy Clin. Immunol. 75:348–355, 1985a.

Atkins, F.M., Steinberg, S.S., Metcalfe, D.D.: Evaluation of immediate adverse reactions to foods in adult patients. II. A detailed analysis of reaction patterns during oral food challenge. J. Allergy Clin. Immunol. 75:356–363, 1985b.

Bernstein, M., Day, J.H.: Double-blind food challenge in the diagnosis of food sensitivity in the adult. J. Allergy Clin. Immunol. 70:205–210, 1982.

Bock, S.A.: Proper use of skin tests with food extracts in diagnosis of hypersensitivity to food in children. Clin. Allergy 7:375–383, 1977.

Bock, S.A.: Appraisal of skin tests with food extracts for diagnosis of food hypersensitivity. Clin. Allergy 8:559–564, 1978.

Bock, S.A.: The natural history of food sensitivity. J. Allergy Clin. Immunol. 69:173–177, 1983.

Bock, S.A.: The natural history of severe reactions to foods in young children. J. Pediatrics 107:676–680, 1985.

Bock, S.A.: Adverse reactions to foods. 79:683–688. 1987.

Bock, S.A.: A prospective appraisal of complaints of adverse reactions to foods in children during the first 3 years of life. Pediatrics 79:683–688, 1987.

Bock, S.A., Lee, W-Y., Remigio, L.K., May, C.D.: Studies of hypersensitivity reactions to foods in infants and children. J. Allergy Clin. Immunol. 62:327–334, 1978.

Bock, S.A., May, C.D.: Adverse reactions to food due to hypersensitivity. *In* Allergy: Principles and Practice, 2nd ed., Middleton, E., Reed, C., Ellis, E. (eds.), St. Louis, C.V. Mosby Co., 1983.

Sampson, H.A.: Role of immediate food hypersensitivity in the pathogenesis of atopic dermatitis. J. Allergy Clin. Immunol. 71:473–480, 1982.

Sampson, H.A., Albergo, R.: Comparison of results of skin tests, RAST, and double-blind, placebo-controlled food challenges in children with atopic dermatitis. J. Allergy Clin. Immunol. 74:26–33, 1984.

Strunk, R.C., Pinnas, J.L., John, T.J., Hansen, R.C., Blazovich, J.L.: Rice hypersensitivity associated with serum complement depression. Clin. Allergy 8:51–58, 1978.

27

General Nutritional Considerations and Diet for Adverse Food Reactions

L. KATHLEEN MAHAN, R.D., M.S.
CLIFTON T. FURUKAWA, M.D.

Although obesity is more prevalent in the United States than is nutritional deficiency, various psychologic and medical conditions can predispose to nutritional deficiency. For instance, caloric deficiency (starvation) may occur from the prolonged use of elimination diets or from excessive concern about food sensitivity or being overweight. Thus, it is important to appreciate certain basic principles *before* recommending any kind of restrictive diet.

1. A varied diet usually is best in order to avoid nutrient deficiency.

2. Foods should be prepared in a traditional manner with as little processing as possible.

3. If whole food groups are eliminated, the diet is likely to be inadequate in certain nutrients, and nutrient replacement may be necessary.

4. Continued need for dietary restrictions should be reassessed periodically.

BASIC NUTRITIONAL REQUIREMENTS

Calories

Adequate caloric intake is easy to assess using growth and fat fold measurements. Infants up to 1 year of age require 105 to 115 kcal/kg; children 1 to 3 years of age need about 100 kcal/kg, and older children, about 85 kcal/kg. Teenagers require between 40 to 60 kcal/kg, depending on their stage of growth; adults usually require about 30 kcal/kg, but this is greatly influenced by activity level. Adequate caloric intake usually is not a problem for allergic children and adults, except when food restrictions are severe.

Proteins

Protein sources may be limited by special restrictions of meats, grains, and nuts. It can be difficult to achieve protein adequacy in a diet that restricts eggs, fish, milk, and meats. Corn is low in the amino acids tryptophan, threonine, and lysine; rice and wheat are low in threonine; and soy is low in methionine. Therefore patients who receive protein only from vegetable sources should have the protein adequacy of the diet assessed. Complementation of protein sources which do not supply all the essential amino acids is important. In addition, these diets may be low in iron, calcium, zinc, vitamin D, riboflavin, and vitamin B_{12}.

Although amino acids may be purchased as supplements from "health food" stores and "allergy" catalogs, claims that specific amino acids have unusual protective properties are without foundation, for example, that lysine will prevent viral illness; methionine and arginine will detoxify; and cysteine will combat radiation damage and heavy metals.

Vitamins

There is no evidence that more than the recommended daily allowances (RDA) for vitamins is beneficial. Deficiency of water soluble vitamins is rare in the United States, since these are added to flour, bread products, and many cereal products. The fat soluble vitamins (A, D, E, and K) are sometimes insufficient in restricted diets. However, excess of these vitamins also can be detrimental. Therefore, daily supplementation should not exceed the RDA. *Vitamins derived from special sources (e.g., ascorbic acid from rose hips) have no benefit over less expensive sources.*

Minerals

Calcium and vitamin D deficiency may result when milk and milk products are omitted from the diet; therefore, it is common practice to add calcium and vitamin D to the diet of milk-restricted children. This should be considered in adults as well. Iron deficiency is a problem in infants and rapidly growing children, so that iron fortified formulas and cereals are recommended by the American Academy of Pediatrics.

Zinc deficiency may occur in some food-restricted eczema patients. This can be assessed by a serum zinc determination possibly combined with a hair zinc analysis. Copper deficiency is relevant only in infants receiving hyperalimentation. The relevance of other minerals, particularly trace elements, is difficult to assess. Thus, a varied diet is important to allow the greatest possibility that needs for these minerals are met.

Carbohydrates

The major energy source from foods is carbohydrates. Although nutritionists recommend complex carbohydrates, preferring starches to simple sugars, the allergic patient has yet to be shown to experience harm from refined sugars (except for dental caries from excessive sucrose intake and poor oral hygiene which are unrelated to allergic status).

Fats

Excessive fat intake is discouraged because of associations with obesity, arteriosclerosis, and cancer.

MISCELLANEOUS "FOODS"

Bee pollen, queen bee jelly, kelp, selenium, special enzymes (e.g., bromelain, a protease from pineapples), caprylic acid (a coconut oil derivative touted to combat *Candida*), algae products (e.g., quercetin, a flavonoid claimed to be an antihistamine and antioxidant), and all sorts of herbal teas are examples of products sold directly to allergy patients with *claims of beneficial effects totally unsubstantiated other than by advertising.*

MODIFYING THE DIET IN ATTEMPTING TO DIAGNOSE FOOD ALLERGY

The diagnosis of food allergy can begin with the elimination of suspect foods yet still allow a liberal and effective diet. The restricted diet is followed by reintroduction of eliminated foods either singly or in groups, with documentation of resulting symptoms, if any.

In the case of suspicion of many foods, an elimination diet with severe restrictions may be tried first (Table 27–1). A diet of pears, lamb, squash, and rice that eliminates all foods and drinks except these four foods also is an option. Another example would be to choose one food in each of the four food groups (grain, fruit, vegetable, and meat) and allow only those four foods. This "oligoantigenic diet" is strict, may be nutritionally inadequate, is boring and difficult, and should be used only for a short period. When and if symptoms clear, single foods are added back to the diet one at a time every 4 to 7 days, with the continued recording of intake and symptoms. Because of the relative nutritional inadequacy of the base diet, initial challenges should include foods selected to maximize the nutritional content of the diet.

The elimination diet can be used after allergy test results indicate which foods are suspiciously problematic, selecting these foods first for elimination. With clearing of symptoms, each eliminated food is reintroduced singly, every 4 to 7 days. Another approach to food elimination and challenge in suspected food allergy, which recommends the addition of foods at shorter intervals, can be found in Chapter 26.

Modifying the diet, even severely, does not require nutritional supplementation unless the diet continues for more than a month. In that case, a daily multivitamin with iron should be recommended along with attention to calcium, iron, and zinc intake if necessary (Table 27–2).

A highly restricted type of elimination diet consists of an elemental diet of amino acids, glucose, and lipid. A common form is the liquid formula Vivonex, although others also are available (Table 27–3). This diet is utilized particularly when so many foods are suspect and symptomatology is so severe that an adequate diet cannot otherwise be provided even for a short period. Elemental diets are fortified with vitamins and minerals and are nutritionally adequate, providing that an adequate amount is consumed. For Vivonex, this amounts to 6 packages or 1800 ml full strength or 1800 kcal/day for the older child or adult. When used, an elemental diet should be initiated at one-fourth strength for 2 days, followed by one-half strength, three-fourths, and finally full strength by the sixth or seventh day.

However, in infants less than 6 months of

TABLE 27–1. Two Stages of Elimination Diets*

ELIMINATION DIET 1 (MILK-, EGG-, AND WHEAT-FREE)		
	ALLOWED FOODS	PROHIBITED FOODS‡
Animal protein sources	Lamb, chicken, turkey, beef, pork	Cow's milk, chicken eggs
Vegetable protein sources	Soy milk, soybeans, peas, other beans, lentils, peanuts	
Grains or alternate	White potato, sweet potato, yams, rice, tapioca, arrowroot, buckwheat, corn, barley, rye, millet, oats	Wheat
Vegetables	All vegetables	
Fruits	All fruits and juices	
Sweeteners	Cane or beet sugar, maple syrup, corn syrup	
Oils	Soy oil, corn oil, safflower oil, coconut oil, vegetable oil, olive oil, peanut oil, milk-free margarines	Butter and margarines that include milk
Other	Salt, all spices	

ELIMINATION DIET 2 (MINIMAL ELIMINATION DIET)		
	ALLOWED FOODS	PROHIBITED FOODS‡
Animal protein sources	Lamb	All other animal protein: meat, fish, poultry, eggs, and milk
Vegetable protein sources		Soy milk, soybeans, peas, other beans, lentils, peanuts, bean sprouts, all nuts
Grains or alternate	White potato, sweet potato, yams, rice, tapioca, buckwheat, arrowroot	Wheat, oats, corn, barley millet, rye
Vegetables	All vegetables† except citrus fruits	Corn, peas (tomatoes)
Fruits	All fruits and juices† except citrus fruits, strawberries, tomatoes	Citrus fruits, strawberries, tomatoes
Sweeteners	Cane or beet sugar, maple syrup	Corn syrup, corn syrup solids
Oils	Safflower oil, coconut oil, olive oil, sesame oil	Butter, margarine, vegetable oils, soy oil, corn oil, peanut oil, nonspecific shortening or fats of animal origin
Other	Salt, pepper, all spices,† vanilla or lemon extract, baking soda and cream of tartar	Chocolate, coffee, tea, colas, and other soft drinks, alcoholic beverages Corn starch, baking powder with cornstarch

* From Krause, M.V., Mahan, L.K.: Food, Nutrition and Diet Therapy, 7th ed. Philadelphia, W.B. Saunders, 1984.
† Suggest limiting number to five to minimize dietary variables.
‡ Includes *any* products that contain these foods (see also Table 27–6).

age, Vivonex should not be used at full strength; rather, it should be increased gradually to two-thirds strength maximum. Vivonex at two-thirds strength provides a 20 kcal/oz formula, which is appropriate for infants in this age group. At this concentration, the infant needs an additional 1 teaspoon of oil daily and a multivitamin with iron. Thirty ounces of the two-thirds strength Vivonex (2 packages) per day must be consumed by the infant in order to meet the RDA. The older infant (6 months to 1 year) can tolerate more concentrated Vivonex (3 packages in 36 oz of water or 25 kcal/oz); 36 oz of this 25 kcal/oz formula along with 65 tsp of oil, 200 IU vitamin D, 5 mg vitamin C, and 40 mg calcium are needed daily to meet the RDA. The child 1 to 3 years of age can tolerate full-strength Vivonex (30 kcal/oz) and needs 50 oz (5 packages), 2.5 tsp of oil, and 80 IU vitamin D per day to meet the RDA, utilizing Vivonex as the only food source. Elemental diets also have been used as a staple for patients who have severe multiple food problems, but this is unusual. It is best accepted by infants who do not already have much experience with foods and have not formed definite ideas on

TABLE 27–2. Nutritional Considerations when Certain Foods are Avoided*

Food	Potentially Inadequate Nutrients	Suggested Supplementation
Milk	Vitamin D	Vitamin D
Milk and all milk products	Vitamin D, calcium, and riboflavin	Vitamin D, calcium
Animal flesh and proteins	Iron and zinc	Iron, zinc, and vitamin C to enhance non-heme-iron absorption
Wheat	Carbohydrate	Carbohydrate supplement or increased use of other grains
Citrus and many fruits	Vitamin C and folic acid	Vitamin C and folic acid, wheat germ, or increased use of beans

* From Mahan, L.K.: Nutrition and the Allergic Athlete. *In* Bierman, C.W., Pierson, W.E. (eds.): International Symposium on Special Problems and Management of Allergic Athletes. J. Allergy Clin. Immunol. 73:728–734, 1984.

what tastes good. In older children and adults with severe food allergies, it may be used to supplement a diet inadequate in protein due to restriction of animal proteins and grains to which they may be allergic.

The most severe form of the elimination diet is the fast. This is used to establish a symptom baseline for a short period (e.g., 48 hours in patients with daily hives) with which to compare symptoms, as foods are added back to the diet. *The fast is not recommended for children.* If extreme food elimination is warranted, an elemental diet is recommended.

An elimination diet requires the keeping of a record by the patient of the occurrence of symptoms and their severity concurrently with food elimination and timing of introduction of test foods. Table 27–4 is an example of a form that is useful for this recording purpose.

MODIFYING THE DIET IN THE MANAGEMENT OF FOOD ALLERGY

In most cases, dietary elimination involves two to four foods. However, it may require omission of several more foods which, when combined with the preferences or dislikes for foods, results in a nutritionally limited diet (Bierman et al., 1978). This limitation should be kept in mind, and necessary nutritional supplementation made. Table 27–2 lists the possible nutritional imbalances resulting from the elimination of certain foods.

Assessment of Nutritional Status — the ABC's

Anthropometry. Height, weight, and evaluation of growth are the crudest of measures, yet they are also easiest to obtain for overall nutri-

tional adequacy. A plateau or fall from the normal pattern of weight gain is a red flag for further evaluation. Interference with height gain is an index of more severe nutritional inadequacy and is even more deserving of attention and intervention. Triceps fat fold and upper arm circumference measurements and of arm muscle and fat area calculations are more specific measures of protein and fat stores and nutritional adequacy.

Biochemistry. Biochemical data such as hematocrit and hemoglobin values are good first measures in a nutritional evaluation. Biochemical data reflect nutritional status before clinical signs are apparent. Several texts, including Krause and Mahan (1984) list the usefulness of various biochemical measurements.

Clinical Signs. Clinical examinations with observation of signs of deficiency and history, which includes questions about diarrhea and vomiting are important. Other clinical signs, such as tongue, mouth, and skin changes, can be due to nutrient deficiency.

Some methods are touted as providing useful and accurate information on nutritional status but are *not* reliable. One such method is hair analysis. Only in a research setting when combined with data on serum and perhaps urine content, is hair analysis of any use and then only for a few nutrients. Commercial clinical laboratories engaged in hair analysis generally are neither accurate nor consistent; they are "unscientific, economically wasteful, and probably illegal" (Barret, 1985).

Diet. Dietary history with a careful, historical documentation of dietary intake can give good information on possible nutritional inadequacies. The 24-hour food recall is the easiest method in the office, but a 7-day prospective food record is the most accurate, although sometimes most difficult to obtain. An accurate

TABLE 27-3. Some Alternatives to Cow's Milk Formulas*

Formula	kcal/oz	Protein Source	Carbohydrate Source	Fat Source	Indication
INFANT FORMULAS					
Human milk	22	Lactalbumin, casein	Lactose	Human milk	Cow's milk protein allergy (CMPA), soy allergy
Isomil	20	Soy protein	Sucrose, corn syrup solids	Coconut oil, soy oil	CMPA, lactose intolerance, galactosemia
Prosobee	20	Soy protein	Corn syrup solids	Soy oil	CMPA, lactose intolerance galactosemia, postgastroenteritis
Soyalac	20	Soy protein	Soybean, sucrose, corn syrup	Soy oil	CMPA, lactose intolerance
Nutramigen	20	Casein hydrolysate	Modified tapioca, sucrose	Corn oil	CMPA, lactose intolerance, soy allergy, multiple food allergies, galactosemia
Pregestimil	22	Casein hydrolysate	Modified tapioca, corn syrup solids	Medium chain triglyceride (MCT) oil, corn oil	CMPA, soy allergy, multiple food allergies, disaccharidase
ELEMENTAL FORMULAS					
Flexical	30	Casein hydrolysate, amino acids	Tapioca starch, corn syrup solids	Soy oil, MCT oil	Multiple food allergies, disorders of digestion and absorption
Precision	30	Egg albumin, sodium caseinate	Glucose oligosaccharides, sucrose	Vegetable oil	Multiple food allergies, disorders of digestion and absorption
Vital	30	Partially hydrolyzed whey, soy and meat protein, free amino acids	Glucose oligosaccharides, glucose polysaccharides	MCT oil, safflower oil	Multiple food allergies, disorders of digestion and absorption
Vivonex	30	Amino acids	Glucose, glucose oligosaccharides	Safflower oil	Multiple food allergies, disorders of digestion and absorption

* From Krause, M.V., Mahan, L.K.: Food, Nutrition and Diet Therapy, 7th ed. Philadelphia, W.B. Saunders Co., 1984.

record can be computer analyzed and complete information on the nutritional content on the diet can be easily obtained.

NUTRIENT SUPPLEMENTATION

In some circumstances, so many nutritionally critical foods must be avoided that the diet becomes nutritionally inadequate. It is reemphasized that nutrient supplementation is necessary if the food avoidances are required for an extended period of time (see Table 27-2).

The most commonly supplemented nutrient is calcium. This can be used alone or in conjunction with vitamin D, the vitamin necessary for calcium absorption and uptake into bone. If a multiple vitamin supplement is used, vitamin D

TABLE 27–4. Diet and Symptom Diary

Name _____   Starting Date _____

Day #	1	2	3	4	5	6	7
Breakfast Morning snacks Drinks							
Symptoms							
Medicine							
Lunch Afternoon snacks Drinks							
Symptoms							
Medicine							
Dinner Evening snacks Drinks							
Symptoms							
Medicine							

is ordinarily provided and does not need to be added to a calcium supplement. Calcium can be taken as oyster shell calcium (this may not be a good idea in the patient with severe sensitivity to shellfish), dolomite (lime), bone meal, and calcium salt forms—calcium lactate, gluconate, ascorbate, and carbonate. There have been reports of lead in dolomite and bone meal (Roberts, 1983) and mercury in oyster shell calcium (Questions Readers Ask, Nutrition and the M.D., 1983); therefore, the safest form of calcium suplementation is probably as one of the salts. Tums consists of calcium carbonate (200 mg calcium in each tablet) and is probably the easiest and cheapest form of calcium supplementation. Calcium carbonate should be used with meals in order to facilitate ionization and absorption of the calcium. The 200 mg of calcium with each meal provides 600 mg calcium daily, close to the RDA of 800 mg/day for children and male adults. The RDA for adolescents is 1200 mg/day; an adolescent needs about two 200 mg calcium tablets with each meal. The RDA for calcium for premenopausal women is 1000 mg/day and 1500 mg/day for postmenopausal women; they would require 2 to 2.5 200 mg tablets with each meal. Several other calcium supplements are available (Table 27–5).

Attention to calcium and vitamin D intake

also should be part of the management of patients who require chronic steroid use for asthma. Long-term systemic steroid therapy may affect the metabolism of bone such that osteoporosis is increased (Chesney et al., 1979; Adinoff et al., 1983; Baylink, 1983; Brenner and Hollister, 1984). Whether this effect is related to vitamin D or to calcium metabolism or both has not been clarified. There is no information on possible similar effects in patients who use inhalational steroids for extended periods. In our opinion, patients, especially postmenopausal women, on daily or alternate day steroids

TABLE 27–5. Calcium Supplements

Supplement	Calcium (mg per tablet)
Tums	200
Tums-Ex	300
Vitafresh Natural Chewable Calcium	150
Neo-calglucon syrup	115*
Pac-Man Chewable Calcium Supplement	300
Stur-Dee Super Cal Chewable Dietary Supplement	500
Calcium Junior Chewable	300
Chewable Biocal	250
Mighty Mouse	150

* Milligrams per teaspoon.

should elicit attention concerning their calcium and vitamin D status, ensuring intake with supplementation if necessary to at least the RDA (Ried, 1986). The use of a vitamin D analog may also be appropriate, since it is suspected that vitamin D metabolism is altered by steroid use.

Another nutrient requiring attention is zinc. Children with severely limited diets have exhibited low serum zinc levels and poor growth (Hambidge et al., 1972). Zinc also is an important factor in immunity (Puri and Chandra, 1985). It is wise to ensure that the RDA (10 mg/day for children and 15 mg/day for adolescents and adults) is met.

CHOICES OF INFANT FORMULAS

For the infant who appears intolerant of cow's milk formula, the classic next step is to change the formula, often to soy. However, soy formula also is potentially allergenic. An alternative recommendation is a more elemental formula, such as Nutramigen or Pregestimil, which contains hydrolyzed casein as the protein source (Committee on Nutrition, American Academy of Pediatrics, 1983). For the extremely sensitive infant, an elemental formula, such as Vivonex, with appropriate supplementation as discussed previously may be necessary.

In the event that the infant appears intolerant of breast milk, weaning is not recommended as the initial step. Rather, commonly allergenic foods should be eliminated from the mother's diet; this should begin with a trial of cow's milk elimination, providing proper nutrient supplementation to the mother (Jakobsson and Lindberg, 1983).

Most children allergic to cow's milk also react to goat's milk, which therefore is not recommended as a cow's milk substitute. However, if used, the infant's diet should be supplemented with folic acid, vitamin C, and vitamin D, since these are not found in adequate amounts in goat's milk. This should continue until the diet includes a variety of foods, particularly dark green vegetables, orange juice, and whole grain cereals, and the child has sufficient sunlight exposure for vitamin D synthesis.

PRACTICALITIES OF FOOD AVOIDANCE

A given allergen can appear in different forms in processed foods and food mixtures. It is important to recognize how a food can appear on a label, what particular words refer to that food or its by-product. Table 27–6 lists various common allergenic "words" to look for when reading labels.

Table 27–7 gives some tips for substitutions of foods in cooking when milk, corn, eggs, chocolate, and wheat must be avoided. This is just a small sampling; many cookbooks on the subject are available. The most difficult food to avoid is wheat, since products of nonwheat items are difficult to make acceptable. Tips for cooking without wheat are given in Table 27–8. Referral to a dietitian for help with the diet can be invaluable to the patient.

The avoidance of specific foods usually can be managed by the family, but it may become a point of contention and manipulation, especially if the patient's (most commonly, a child's) reaction is not severe or life-threatening but merely bothersome. Relationships with peers can suffer if the child must avoid social functions because of a "special diet." The family should be as creative and flexible as possible in finding appropriate alternatives for the child so that normal social participation and psychosocial development is possible. Sharing of responsibility for planning and preparing the food is likely to elicit more cooperation from a child to participate in the diet.

MODIFYING THE DIET IN NONALLERGIC DISEASES

Dietary modification has been proposed as treatment for hyperactivity and behavior problems in children. Artificial colors and flavors, salicylates, sugar, mineral deficiencies, mineral excesses, and food "allergies" all have been proposed as culprits that can affect children's behavior adversely.

Artificial Colors and Flavors. The Feingold diet is free of artificial colors and flavors, salicylates, and the antioxidants butylated hydroxyanisole (BHA) and butylated hydroxytoluene (BHT). Feingold's theory that a large proportion of hyperactive children respond to the diet with improved behavior has not been confirmed in controlled studies (Conners et al., 1976; Harley et al., 1978). Controlled studies indicate that about 10 percent of hyperactive children may respond to this diet; this may be a placebo effect resulting simply from dietary change. It is common for any therapeutic change to engender new optimism in attitudes of family members, which is readily perceivable by the affected

TABLE 27–6. Food Selection in Food Allergy*

Restricted Foods	May be Listed on Label	Foods to Avoid	Substitutes
Milk	Casein Caseinate Whey Lactalbumim Sodium caseinate Lactose Nonfat milk solids Cream Calcium caseinate Nougat Half and half Curds Lactoglobulin	Cheese Cottage cheese Ice cream, yogurt Creamed soups and sauces Butter and many margarines Baked goods made with milk Some "nondairy" products Candy (creams and milk chocolate) Custards and puddings	Mocha mix Coffee Rich Soy formulas (Isomil, Prosobee) Tofu Milk-free baked goods Nut milk† Coconut milk Supplement for calcium and vitamin D
Egg	Albumin Egg whites Egg yolks Eggnog Mayonnaise Ovalbumin Ova mucoid	Many baked goods Egg noodles Custards, pudding Mayonnaise, some salad dressings Hollandaise sauce Meringue Many egg substitutes (Egg-beaters) Some batter fried foods	Egg-free baked goods‡ Spaghetti Rice Some egg substitutes‡ (read label)
Wheat	(Enriched) flour Wheat germ Wheat bran Wheat starch Gluten Food starch Vegetable starch Vegetable gum Bran Farina Graham flour Wheat gluten Whole wheat flour	Baked goods made with wheat flour Crackers Macaroni Spaghetti Noodles Gravies, thickened sauces Fried food coating Baking mixes Soy sauce Hot dogs with wheat filler Batter fried foods Some sausages	Wheat-free breads,‡ crackers (rice cakes, special breads) Certain cold cereals (corn, barley, rice) Oatmeal or cream of rice Corn pasta‡ Bean threads (oriental) Rice Corn tortillas Popcorn Wheat-free cereal, crumbs for "breading" Thickeners: cornstarch, rice flour, tapioca Flours: rye, rice, potato
Soy	Soy flour Soybean oil Vegetable oil Soy protein Soy protein isolate Textured vegetable protein (TVP) Soy lecithin Vegetable starch Vegetable gum Shoyu sauce	Soy sauce Teriyaki sauce Worcestershire sauce Tuna packed in vegetable oil Tofu Miso Baked goods or cereals that include soy Soy nuts Soy infant formulas (Isomil, Prosobee) Many margarines	Nut milk Coconut milk
Corn	Cornmeal Corn starch Corn oil Corn syrup (solids) Corn sweetener Corn alcohol Vegetable oil Vegetable starch Vegetable gum Food starch	Some baked goods Corn tortillas (chips, tacos) Popcorn Some cold cereals Corn syrup Pancake syrup Many candies Most baking powders Grits Hominy Maize	Wheat flour tortillas Thickeners: wheat, potato, rice Beet or cane sugar Maple syrup or honey Baking soda and cream of tartar (for leavening agent)

TABLE 27–6. *(Continued)*

Restricted Foods	May be Listed on Label	Foods to Avoid	Substitutes
Chocolate	Cocoa Cocoa butter	Candy Baked goods Colas	Carob products
Beef	Shortening Lard Gelatin	Soups Bouillon Beef gravies and sauces Hot dogs Cold cuts	Pure vegetable shortening Turkey hot dogs
Pork	Shortening Lard	Bacon Sausage Hot dogs Baked beans and soups with pork	All-beef hot dogs and cold cuts Vegetarian baked beans Pure vegetable shortening

* From Krause, M.V., Mahan, L.K.: Food, Nutrition and Diet Therapy, 7th ed. Philadelphia, W.B. Saunders Co., 1984.
† See Table 27–7.
‡ Products available from Ener-g Foods, 6901 Fox Avenue South, P.O. Box 84487, Seattle, Wash.

child; this in turn can cause an attitude and behavior change on the part of the child. Thus, when parents or teachers claim that the diet "works," it is by no means clear that the elimination of specific dietary elements or alterations in psychosocial interaction induced by the procedure of dietary manipulation are responsible for clinical changes claimed.

Sugar. Sugar (sucrose) has been proposed as a factor in hyperactive behavior based on the

TABLE 27–7. Cooking for the Allergic Person: Alternative Ingredients*

Milk
Use herbal tea or fruit juice in recipes calling for milk. They add a spicy fragrance to cookies, cakes, puddings, and breads.
Use soy, cashew, or almond milk for milk replacement. Combine 1 cup soy powder or ground cashew or almond powder with 3 cups water in a large saucepan. Whisk until well dissolved. Bring to a boil over high heat, stirring constantly. Lower heat and simmer for 3 minutes. Serve hot or cold. Makes 3 cups.

Corn
If a recipe calls for cornstarch, substitute equal amounts of arrowroot or potato starch or double the amount of whole wheat, soy, or barley flour.
Most baking powders include cornstarch. Make corn-free baking powder by combining ¼ tsp baking soda with ½ tsp cream of tartar. This is equivalent to 1 tsp baking powder.

Egg
In baking, you can achieve the emulsifying effect of 1 egg by combining 2 tbsp whole wheat flour, ½ tsp oil, ½ tsp baking powder, and 2 tbsp milk, water, or fruit juice. Egg substitutes are also available.

Chocolate
Use carob powder measure for measure when substituting for cocoa. As a substitute for 1 square of chocolate, use 3 tbsp carob powder plus 2 tbsp milk, water, buttter, or margarine.

Wheat
Wheat flour replacements and tips for cooking with wheat are listed in Table 27–8.

* Adapted from Krause, M.V., Mahan, L.K.: Food, Nutrition and Diet Therapy, 7th ed. Philadelphia, W.B. Saunders Co., 1984.

TABLE 27–8. Suggestions for Substitutions for Wheat Flour in Recipes*

One cup of wheat flour may be substituted in standard recipes by the following:

    1 cup corn flour
    ¾ cup coarse cornmeal
    1 scant cup fine cornmeal
    ⅝ cup potato flour
    ⅞ cup rice flour

There are some problems in the use of substitutes for wheat flour. The following suggestions will improve the eating quality of the final product:

1. Rice flour and cornmeal tend to have a grainy texture. A smoother texture may be obtained by mixing the rice flour or cornmeal with the liquid called for in the recipe, bringing this mixture to a boil and then cooling before adding to the other ingredients.

2. Soy flour must always be used in combination with another flour, not as the only flour in a recipe.

3. When using other than wheat flour in baking, longer and slower baking is required. This is particularly necessary when the product is made without milk and eggs.

4. When using coarse meals and flours in place of wheat flour, the amount of leavening must be increased. For each cup of coarse flour, use 2½ tsp. of baking powder.

5. Substitutes for wheat flour do not make a satisfactory yeast bread.

6. Muffins or biscuits, when made with other than wheat flour, are of better texture if baked in small sizes.

7. Dryness is a common characteristic of cakes made with flours other than wheat. Moisture may be preserved by (a) frosting, (b) storing in closed containers, or (c) adding a fruit, such as banana or applesauce, to the recipe.

* From Ohlson, M.A.: Experimental and Therapeutic Dietetics, 2nd ed. Minneapolis, Burgess Publishing Co., 1972.

theory that blood glucose level changes and hypoglycemia cause mood and behavior changes. These also have not been well substantiated (Wolraich, 1985). A small percentage of children do appear to respond to the omission of sugar from the diet with behavior changes, but these changes are attributable to placebo effect. One study showed that hyperactive boys become *less* active after sugar ingestion (Behar et al., 1984).

Megavitamins. There is no evidence for the effectiveness of megavitamin therapy in the treatment of hyperactivity, and its use is not justified in children (Committee on Nutrition, American Academy of Pediatrics, 1976; Haslam et al., 1984).

Hyperactivity is an extremely complex problem and should be evaluated with a thorough diagnosis followed by a team approach to treatment, which includes special education, counseling, parental support, behavior modification techniques, and probably nutritional guidance. Nutritional treatment in conjunction with other treatments may be useful, but it should not be the only one, just as medication should not be the only treatment.

Migraine Headaches and Food Allergy. Oligoantigenic diets (Egger et al., 1983), diets avoiding chocolate and tyramine-containing foods (Dalessio, 1972), and diets involving elimination based upon allergy tests (Mansfield et al., 1985) have been shown to reduce the prevalence and severity of migraine headaches. Further work is necessary to define the causal versus aggravating relationships between foods and migraines, the mechanisms by which foods induce migraines, and the means to define which patients may benefit from dietary therapy.

REFERENCES

Adinoff, A.D., Hollister, R.: Steroid-induced fractures and bone loss in patients with asthma. N. Engl. J. Med, 309:265–268, 1983.

Barret, S.: Commercial hair analysis: science or scam? J.A.M.A. 254:1041–1045, 1985.

Baylink, D.: Glucocorticoid-induced osteoporosis. N. Engl. J. Med. 309:306–308, 1983.

Behar, D., Rapoport, J.L., Adams, A.J., Berg, C.J., Cornblath, M.: Sugar challenge testing with children considered behaviorally "sugar reactive." Nutri. Behav. 1:279–288, 1984.

Bierman, C.W., Shapiro, G.G., Christie, D.L., Van Arsdel, P.P., Jr., Furukawa, C.T.A., Ward, B.H.: Allergy grand rounds: Eczema, rickets and food allergy. J. Allergy Clin. Immunol. 61:119–127, 1978.

Brenner, M., Hollister, R.: Osteoporosis in steroid-treated asthmatic children (abstract). J. Allergy Clin. Immunol. 73:137, 1984.

Chesney, R.W., Mazess, R.B., Hamstra, A.J., DeLuca, H.F., O'Reagan, S.: Reduction of serum 1,25-dihydroxyvitamin D_3 in children receiving glucocorticoids. Lancet 2:1123–1125, 1978.

Committee on Nutrition, American Academy of Pediatrics: Soy-protein formulas: recommendations for use in infant feeding. Pediatrics 72:359–363, 1983.

Committee on Nutrition, American Academy of Pediatrics: Megavitamin therapy for childhood psychosis and learning disabilities. Pediatrics 58:910–912, 1976.

Conners, C.K., Goyette, C.H., Southwick, D.A., Lees, J.M., Andrulonis, P.A.: Food additives and hyperkinesis: a controlled double-blind experiment. Pediatrics 58:154–166, 1976.

Dalessio, D.J.: Dietary migraine. Am. Fam. Phys. 6:60–65, 1972.

Egger, J., Wilson, J., Carter, C.M., Turner, M.W., Soothill, J.F.: Is migraine food allergy? A double-blind controlled trial of oligoantigenic diet treatment. Lancet 2:865–869, 1983.

Hambidge, K.M., Hambidge, C., Jacobs, M., Baum, J.D.: Low levels of zinc in hair, anorexia, poor growth and hypogeusia in children. Pediatr. Res. 6:868–874, 1972.

Harley, J.P., Roy, R.S., Tomasi, L., Eichman, P.L., Matthews, C.G., Chun, R., Cheeland, C.S., Traisman, E.: Hyperkinesis and food additives: testing the Feingold hypothesis. Pediatrics 61:818–828, 1978.

Haslam, R.H.A., Dalby, J.T., Rademaker, A.W.: Effects of megavitamin therapy in children with attention deficit disorders. Pediatrics 74:103–111, 1984.

Jakobsson, I., Lindberg, T.: Cow's milk proteins cause infantile colic in breast-fed infants: A double-blind crossover study. Pediatrics 71:268–271, 1983.

Krause, M.V., Mahan, L.K.: Food, Nutrition and Diet Therapy, 7th ed. Philadelphia, W.B. Saunders Co., 1984.

Mansfield, L.E., Vaughn, T.R., Waller, S.F., Haverly, R.W., Ting, S.: Food allergy and adult migraine: Double-blind and mediator confirmation of an allergic etiology. Ann. Allergy 55:126–129, 1985.

Megavitamins and the hyperactive child. Nutr. Rev. 43:105–107, 1985.

Puri, S., Chandra, R.K.: Nutritional regulation of host resistance and predictive value of immunologic tests in assessment of outcome. Pediatr. Clin. N. Am. 32:499–516, 1985.

Questions Readers Ask, Nutrition and the M.D. IX(8):6, 1983.

Reid, I.R., Ibbertson, H.K.: Calcium supplements in the prevention of steroid-induced osteoporosis. Am. J. Clin. Nutr. 44:287–290, 1986.

Roberts, H.J.: Potential toxicity due to dolomite and bone meal. So. Med. J. 76:556–559, 1983.

Wolraich, M., Milich, R., Stumbo, P., Schultz, F.: Effects of sucrose ingestion on the behavior of hyperactive boys. J. Pediatr. 106:675–682, 1985.

MANAGEMENT OF SKIN DISEASES

28

Principles of Diagnosis and Treatment of Skin Disorders

GUINTER KAHN, M.D.

ANATOMY AND PHYSIOLOGY OF THE SKIN

The skin is composed of three distinct structural compartments; the epidermis, dermis, and subcutaneous tissue.

Epidermis. The outermost portion of the epidermis is composed of a horny compaction of dead, keratinized cells called the stratum corneum. It varies greatly in thickness (15 to 700 μ), forms the major barrier that resists penetration, and provides for internal homeostasis. The thicker the stratum corneum, the better the protection. Teleologically, a thick stratum corneum at the palms and soles allows for frequent contact with foreign material, minimizing possible trauma and irritation.

Epidermal cells originate as a single band of columnar cells called the stratum basale, which rests primarily on the basement membrane (Fig. 28–1). This basal layer acts to rejuvenate the epidermis and to produce the cells above it, called prickle cells, which move upward and accumulate large granules to form a thin granular layer. The granules gradually disappear, and the cells flatten to become the compact layer of keratin called the stratum corneum. About 14 days are required for the migration of a cell from the basal layer to the stratum corneum; approximately 14 more days are required for the cell to traverse upward through the stratum corneum to be shed. The combination of the bottom, forming layer (stratum basale) and the upper, shielding layer (stratum corneum) provides the dermis with a self-regenerating, protective cover. Skin diseases usually disrupt this cover, often altering the rate of epidermal regeneration and percutaneous absorption (persorption).

Persorption of chemicals through the epidermis occurs to an extreme degree in premature infants, and less in infants, children, and adults. Most compounds placed on the skin of premature infants can be found in the urine and saliva only minutes later. Compounds are absorbed faster through the skin when the stratum corneum (the prime barrier) is made more permeable by trauma, heat, or hydration. The use of occlusion to facilitate topical penetration of inflamed skin takes advantage of all three conditions.

Melanocytes also are found in the epidermis, interspersed among the basal columnar cells. They are derived from neural tissue and function to synthesize melanin, which pigments the skin. About one of every six cells in the basal layer is a melanocyte.

Langerhans cells are identified throughout the epidermis by enzymatic or immunologic histochemicals. The cells have a clear cytoplasm, devoid of tonofilaments, but contain a bulbous granule (tennis racquet–like) of unknown function. The cells have surface marker characteristics similar to macrophages, i.e., Fc and C3 receptors and Ia antigens, the only epidermal cells to do so. The Langerhans cells are considered to be epidermal macrophages because of their ability to present soluble proteins and haptens to sensitized T cells (Katz, 1985).

The basal layer has the pluripotential to replenish the epidermis and to produce appendant structures, such as sweat glands. An eccrine sweat gland consists of a coiled base that leads into a duct that traverses the dermis and epidermis. Eccrine sweating is stimulated by heat, exertion, nausea, fever, and drugs, such as alcohol, pilocarpine, and acetylcholine. It is reduced by cold, dehydration, decreased metabolism, and anticholinergic drugs. Apocrine sweating is stimulated by emotional factors and

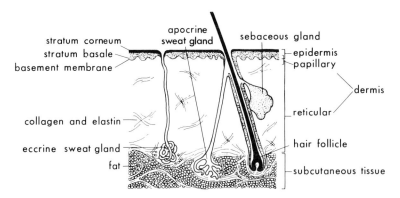

FIGURE 28-1. Diagram of the structure of the skin. (Modified from Kahn, G. (ed. and trans.): *Rassner's Atlas of Dermatology*. Baltimore, Urban and Schwarzenberg, 1978, p. 130.)

adrenergic drugs but not by heat. Apocrine sweat glands enter the pilosebaceous unit, as illustrated in Figure 28-1.

The basement membrane divides the epidermis from the dermis and holds the two layers together. It is this area in which local tissue edema can force the skin to separate and form bullae, a phenomenon that occurs easily in infants and children but less readily in older individuals.

Dermis. The dermis is a tough heterogeneous mixture of collagen, elastin, reticulin, and mucopolysaccharides. Cellular components include fibroblasts, mast cells, and histiocytes. Whereas the epidermis acts as a barrier to the outside world, the tough tissue of the dermis acts to support it and serves as a conduit to guide nerves and blood and lymphatic vessels to their end position in the uppermost (papillary) layer of the dermis, under the basement membrane. The dermis also serves to support the pilosebaceous unit consisting of an arrectores pilorum muscle, a hair, and its attendant sebaceous apparatus. Nerves of the skin are distributed in a random fashion except for direct innervation of hair follicles or sweat glands. Nerves do not innervate the sebaceous glands or the epidermis in general. Special end organs in the upper dermis allow exquisite tactile sensory perception. These cutaneous nerve endings, high in the dermis, receive elementary impulses indirectly via the epidermis and allow perception of heat, cold, touch, pain, pressure, and location.

Subcutaneous Tissue. Beneath the dermis, a layer of subcutaneous fat padding gives form to the exterior of the body and serves as a protective insulating buffer for the internal structures. The subcutaneous tissue consists of fat cells, fibrous tissue, nerves, blood vessels, occasional reticuloendothelial cells and transient white blood cells (Solomon et al., 1978).

DEVELOPMENTAL ASPECTS OF SKIN PHYSIOLOGY

Our knowledge about the changes that occur in the skin through infancy, childhood, and into adulthood is summarized in Table 28-1 (Montagna, 1965). Hormones have profound effects on individual components of the skin; those associated with sexual maturation have the most widely recognized effects. "Adolescent" hormonal effects begin at about the age of 8 years. The sebaceous unit enlarges and produces increased amounts of triglycerides. The apocrine apparatus grows and secretes glandular material, which is degraded by bacteria to form odoriferous end products. These changes frequently precede by years of appearance of secondary sexual characteristics. Sebum production and glandular size are decreased by estrogens and increased by androgens.

Cell proliferation and differentiation are regulated by intracellular levels of cyclic nucleotides, which are controlled in part by the actions of adrenergic agents and other chemical mediators normally accessible to the skin. Although all the structures with which they are associated have not been delineated, some specific kinds of receptors have been associated with nucleotide activation in the epidermis. Beta-adrenergic receptors predominate in the epidermis, whereas both alpha and beta receptors occur in the dermis. Alpha receptors are found only in dermal blood vessels. Cells involved with mediation of immune responses, including mast cells, basophils, lymphocytes, and polymorphonuclear leukocytes, can be found scattered in the dermis in varying numbers and proportions, depending upon the pathologic process involving the skin.

Cytokines of epidermal cells that may modulate immune as well as inflammatory reactions include thymic factors, prostaglandin E_2, leu-

TABLE 28–1. Summary of Age Related Skin Changes

Skin pH	About 6.5 for first 2 days of life; about 5 for the next 4 days; thereafter, about 4.5 (Solomon and Esterly, 1973).
Percutaneous absorption (persorption)	Premature newborns have substantially greater persorption than infants, children, and adults. No proven differences between infant and adult skin (Leyden et al., 1977). However, consideration must be given to the greater skin surface in proportion to the weight of infants compared with adults.
Contact irritant	No proven differences between infant (excluding premature infant) and adult skin (Leyden et al., 1977).
Blister formation	Occurs more easily on the skin of infants and children, the younger the child, the more readily blister formation occurs.
Melanocytes	Evenly distributed, not functioning until birth (e.g., light complexioned black newborn). Soon after birth, regional variation in distribution of melanocytes begins; pigment in nipples, face, and genitalia increases. Progressive loss of melanocytes occurs at a rate of about 11 percent per decade.
Hair	Hairs of newborn are fine (vellus type) and lightly pigmented. After birth they are replaced by coarser, pigmented (terminal type) hair. Groups of follicles (3 or more) per pilosebaceous unit do not occur until age 20. The number of hairs decreases progressively from birth to senescence; hair loss is not noted until 25 percent of the hair is missing.
Contact allergy	The ease of induction of contact sensitization gradually increases until the eighth year of life when adult reactivity is reached.
Sebaceous glands	They are well-developed at birth because of maternal androgens, involute during childhood, enlarge and become functional at 8 to 10 years, and continue to develop through adolescence. Increase in surface free fatty acids, triglycerides, and wax esters parallels increase in glandular activity (Strauss et al., 1976).
Apocrine glands	Enlarge during childhood, become functional at age 8 to 10. Axillary sweating begins a few years before puberty.
Eccrine glands	Nonfunctional at birth. Perspiration begins at 2 to 5 days; complete activity not achieved until age 2 to 3 years. Density of glands per cm² is greater in children than adults.
Nerve endings	There is a continuous reduction in the number of "touch" corpuscles (specialized Meissner and pacinian nerve endings) from birth to old age, whereas free nerve endings undergo no changes.
Collagen	Becomes increasingly mature (stable); it degenerates with age, but most rapidly from birth to age 2 years. Mucopolysaccharide concentration decreases with age, especially hyaluronic acid.

kotrienes, and interferon. The precise epidermal cell type producing these cytokines is not known. However, epidermal cell–derived thymocyte activating factor (ETAF), which is similar to interleukin-1 is produced by both Langerhans cells and keratinocytes. ETAF stimulates T-cell activation (Katz, 1985). A more detailed discussion of these cells, mediators, and their interrelationships is found throughout the text (Chapters 1 and 5).

DIAGNOSTIC PRINCIPLES

History and Physical Examination

A nondermatologist will feel more comfortable describing skin disorders by noting their size, shape, color, texture, tenderness, location, number, and odor. Definitions of commonly used dermatologic descriptive terms can found in Table 28–2 (Hurwitz, 1981). History taking is an underestimated art that can be extraordinarily helpful in dermatologic diagnosis. The dermatologic history should begin with variations of the following core questions:

1. What is the patient's complaint (lesion)?

TABLE 28–2. Common Dermatologic Lesions

Macule	Change in color that is level with the skin (it is visible but not palpable and less than 1 cm in diameter).
Patch	Macule larger than 1 cm in diameter.
Papule	Solid elevation less than 1 cm in diameter.
Nodule	Solid elevation more than 1 cm in diameter.
Wheal	Transitory (minutes to hours) solid elevation of the skin, synonymous with *hive* and *urtica*.
Vesicle	Clear fluid-filled elevation less than 1 cm in diameter; *blister* refers to similar lesions of any size.
Bulla	Clear fluid-filled elevation more than 1 cm in diameter, synonymous with *bleb*.
Pustule	Purulent vesicle that can become larger and form a *furuncle, abscess,* or *carbuncle; boil* is the general term.
Cyst	Sac of liquid or semisolid material.
Excoriation	Artifact produced by scratching or picking.
Fissure	Linear cleavage.
Scale	Exfoliation of dead epidermis.
Crust and scab	Coagulated, dried serum or blood on the skin.
Erosion	Superficial denudation.
Ulcer	Deep denudation or loss of tissue.
Scar	Fibrous replacement of skin.

2. When did it begin, and on what part of the body?

3. How has it changed?

4. What makes it better or worse?

5. What was the effect of any medication tried?

6. Who has recently treated it? (This question may tell you more about the patient than most personality screening tests. For example, if the patient is overly self-reliant and tends to treat himself or herself; if referral from or "around" the patient's primary physician; and if the patient is a "shopper.")

From this core information most patients will give peripheral details and are grateful for the invitation to talk freely. Now, look at the skin. The remainder of the conversation is secondary to the revelations of the initial history and of the physical findings. Here, the core knowledge of dermatology and allergy bears fruit. Family history may be important in atopy, acne, psoriasis, ichthyosis, bullous diseases, and many genodermatoses. Environmental history may reveal irritant eruption, the causes of which may vary from bubble gum to bubble baths, which may be secondary to hobbies or habits. Dermatitis from irritants is more common than dermatitis from allergens. Shoe allergy or contact dermatitis is more common than fungal infection on the feet of children. Prevalence of a disease is extremely important in dermatologic evaluation, e.g., it is common for pityriasis rosea to occur in small endemic clusters. Know which diseases itch and when (eg., scabies itch more at night), which do not usually itch (e.g., pityriasis rosea, psoriasis, and secondary syphilis), and which are transmissible (e.g., warts, molluscum contagiosum, scabies, and venereal diseases).

When taking the history and doing the physical examination, remember that infants and children differ from adults in that their skin is more reactive. Children more frequently have superficial bacterial infections; mucosal infections of herpes simplex and candidiasis (thrush); bullous reactions (e.g., congenital syphilis, mastocytosis); irritant reactions (contact allergy is less common); nevus development (pigmented, vascular); genodermatoses often characterized by masses, bullae, or dystrophic skin and adnexa; and eczematoid eruptions, which vary from seborrheic to candidal, to atopic, to irritant dermatitis.

Cross associations may be of key importance in history taking. For example, is there a background of diabetes in the patient with recurrent candidiasis? If the candidiasis is chronic and mucocutaneous, is there an associated endocrinopathy or immune deficiency? Is the skin infection recurrent? Is it accompanied by recurrent infections of other systems? Should one consider an immune deficiency or a deficiency in other host factors? Is there a family history of similar problems? After extracting all possible information from the history and physical examination, use the laboratory to complete the diagnostic evaluation.

Laboratory Methods

Potassium Hydroxide (KOH) Preparations for the Demonstration of Fungi, Parasites, and Ova. Scrape the lesion with a dull-edged scalpel blade. Place the material on a glass slide. Add a drop of 20 percent KOH. Apply a coverslip. To diagnose fungal diseases, heat gently over a flame until a bubble appears. The specimen is then ready for microscopic examination. If a fungus is suspected, similar scrapings should be placed onto Dermatophyte Test Media (Acuderm Labs, Inc.) or Sabouraud media for culture.

Bacterial Evaluation. Clean the skin with 70 percent alcohol for 2 minutes to remove resident organisms, but if crusted, apply a sterile compress to this area for a few minutes before debriding or lifting off a scale or blister covering. Expose the underlying exudative material for culture. For fluctuant lesions, the exudate is collected directly through a needle or on a sterile swab. Gram stain provides a direct method to determine if lesions contain pathogenic bacteria. Antibiotic sensitivity studies provide therapeutic guidelines. For deep infections (e.g., erysipelas), cleanse as described, inject preservative-free sterile saline into the most active area, then aspirate back into the syringe and onto the culture plate. Blood cultures and determination of serum factors that may reflect infection (e.g., DNase B for streptococcal infection) may be helpful. Request sheep blood agar media if beta-hemolytic streptococci are suspected or chocolate agar if gonorrhea is suspected.

Direct, 10-minute screening tests are available for streptococcal groups A and B, *Staphlococcus aureus, Haemophilus* sp., *Neisseria* sp., and other organisms. Most tests use latex particle agglutination, reacting with antigens in body or tissue fluids. This product technology is cost effective, i.e., about $2.00 per test, excluding the technician's time (Radetsky et al., 1985).

Viral tests. The most sensitive and specific method to diagnose herpes simplex is by viral culture. Obtain about 0.2 ml lesional fluid; in 24 to 72 hours cytopathic diagnosis will be available. The use of electron microscopy or animal testing rarely is required by practicing physicians. Tzanck test smear is a valuable tool that can help identify herpes simplex and zoster-varicella viruses. This procedure has a sensitivity of about 50 percent. Diagnostic information can be available in a few minutes following this simple technique: remove the blister top with a scalpel, scrape the floor of the blister, and spread the scrapings onto a clear glass slide, air dry, then stain with Giemsa material. Using a low power microscope, look for the giant cells of herpes simplex or zoster-varicella (Fig. 28–2).

Wood's Light Examination. Long wave ultraviolet light induces greenish fluorescence in hairs infected only by *Microsporum* species of fungus (not commonly a cause of scalp ringworm). *Lack of fluorescence, therefore, does not rule out tinea capitis.* Physicians tend to overuse Wood's light for fungal examination. It does not reveal the presence of common dermatophytes on the skin but does produce golden fluorescence, outlining the area of tinea versicolor infection. This is the only fungal infection of glabrous skin for which Wood's light is useful Bacterial infections caused by *Corynebacterium* organisms may fluoresce orange-pink. *Pseudomonas* metabolites fluoresce light green.

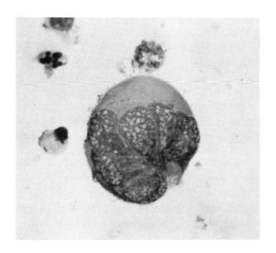

FIGURE 28–2. Multi-nucleated giant cell gently scraped from base of herpes simplex vesicle (magnified 480×). Note the adjacent white blood cells for size comparison.

Wood's light is useful in detecting the white fluorescence of vitiligo or pigment loss; also, the darkness of hypermelanotic lesions is intensified.

Tests for Dermographism. Neither pressure tests nor injections of cholinergic agents in the skin are sensitive tests. The application of an ice cube for 5 to 10 minutes to the skin of a patient suspected of having cold urticaria is a valuable diagnostic aid (Chapter 31).

Patch Test. At the appropriate concentration, suspected substances are applied under occlusion to the normal skin of the back for about 48 hours (Chapter 30).

Darkfield Examination. This examination and related blood studies for venereal disease are beyond the scope of this text. However, these diseases should be kept in mind in the differential diagnosis of diagnostically perplexing dermatologic problems.

Skin Biopsy. This may give or suggest the diagnosis, or it may limit the differential possibilities. Biopsy results may not be specific for infectious or papulosquamous processes or for most subacute or chronic dermatoses. Specific history is most helpful diagnostically for most tumors, for some ichthyoses, and for bullous diseases. Clinical correlation with histologic findings helps confirm the diagnosis or at least limits the differential diagnosis. The dermatopathologist can aid the clinician maximally only when detailed historical and physical findings and differential possibilities are made available, along with the biopsy material.

Direct and Indirect Immunofluorescent Tests. These tests are useful to detect immunoglobulins and complement in biopsy specimens and serum. They can be helpful in evaluating lupus erythematosus, dermatitis herpetiformis, linear IgA disease, pemphigus, bullous and cicatricial pemphigoid, and herpes gestationis.

THERAPEUTIC PRINCIPLES

The following discussion of therapy for skin diseases is intended as a general guideline. It omits the use of pastes, powders, and oils (which are of minimal value), gentian violet and iodochlorhydroxyquin (compounds which can stain and harm), and topical preparations containing sulfur (for which superior alternatives exist). Sunscreens and acne therapeutics are considered in other chapters.

1. Learn the normal course of the disease. For instance, many diseases of the newborn are

transient. Delay in treating nondescript papular erythematous lesions in the first week of life may be wise (Solomon and Esterly, 1973).

2. The more severe and acute the dermatitis, the more delicate and gentle should be the therapy (Weinberg et al., 1975).

3. If the condition is neither widespread nor serious, treat locally. Learn only a few topical remedies; know how to use them well.

4. Soaks and compresses with water alone help erosive, weeping, or acute dermatitis as much as water with added chemicals. Fewer side effects, less expense, and less inconvenience to the patient are benefits.

5. Towels make excellent dressings. Consider accessibility and cost to improve patient compliance.

6. Agents of unproven value, which are contraindicated because of adverse effects, include topical anesthetics, topical antihistamines, topical proteolytic enzymes, topical vitamins, boric acid, and hexachlorophene.

7. Soaps are useful cleansers but can irritate and dry the skin. The least harsh include Keri, Purpose, Neutrogena, Oilatum, and Dove. The harshest include Ivory, Lowila, Zest, and Irish Spring. Allergic sensitization to perfumes, antiseptics, and chemicals in soaps is rare.

8. Chlorhexidine gluconate in 4 percent alcohol (Hibiclens) is a recommended topical antiseptic because of its broad bactericidal spectrum and its ability to remain active on the skin. It is virtually free of side effects and is stainless and painless on open wounds. It is not approved for routine use on the full-term newborn at this time even though sufficient test data exist (Husak et al., 1981).

9. Learn to use two types of salves in dermatology as follows: a dry salve (cream) for oily, moist, and intertriginous surfaces, and an oily salve (grease) for dry surfaces. Eucerin is an inexpensive cream that is half aquaphor and half water. Others include Unibase, Plastibase, Polysorb, Hydrosorb, Keri, and Lubriderm. These creams can be made drier (less greasy) by adding water until they become a lotion. (Lotions are more drying than creams and are valuable for treating hairy surfaces).

10. Petrolatum is an inexpensive ointment. Others include Aquaphor, lard, Crisco, and Albolene. They can be made less greasy by adding Eucerin or other creams. Petrolatum is the standard ointment of dermatologic therapy. It is composed of long-chain hydrocarbons from petroleum. It does not cause contact allergy, and it provides a continuous (occlusive) cover.

To moisturize, soak the skin for several minutes in water, then cover the water-laden skin with petrolatum. A large variety of chemicals can be dispersed evenly in petrolatum for effective application to the skin.

For drying moist or intertriginous surfaces after application of a cream, air blown from any source is valuable. Creams are made from fatty solids by adding emollients that allow water to mix into the material, converting it into an opaque substance (cream). The amount of water in the fat determines how drying it will be. Creams are absorbed into the skin, making them cosmetically acceptable because they do not feel tacky or sticky. Their surface layer is discontinuous, i.e., they are not occlusive. Creams can become rancid unless preservatives are added. The more chemicals (emollients, preservatives) found in creams, the greater is the possibility for creams to be allergenic or irritant. In general, medications in creams are not as effective as medications in ointments. Nevertheless, medicated creams (e.g., steroids) outsell medicated ointments in the United States in the ratio of about 20 to 1. (The reverse is true in England where ointments are preferred.) In atopic dermatitis, ointments may be too occlusive.

11. Rubbing alcohol is an inexpensive antiseptic, but it stings on open wounds. Its drying effect can be altered by the addition of glycerin, 5 to 25 percent. Adding more than 10 percent glycerin to rubbing alcohol converts it into a moisturizing solution, because of the hygroscopic properties of glycerin. Other moisturizing lotions include Keri, Curel, and Cetaphil.

12. The following are examples of medications that can be added to the vehicles petrolatum, Eucerin, or alcohol with glycerin: 1 percent hydrocortisone to relieve inflammation; 1 percent phenol to relieve itching; and 2 to 6 percent salicylic acid to decrease scaling eruptions and acne.

Phenol in concentrated solutions can cause kidney disease. In the usual 0.5 to 2 percent concentrations, it rarely causes sensitization or side effects. When used on open surfaces, phenol may cause dizziness, and camphor may be used in its place. Salicylic acid rarely can sensitize and cause salicylism. If stronger concentrations are required, use them only on small areas.

13. Hydrocortisone and its derivatives are available in many strengths. Potent products enhance both beneficial and side effects. Twice daily application of topical corticosteroid prep-

arations appears optimal for most products. More frequent application may waste medicine and atrophy thin skin. Hydrocortisone salves may be strengthened by increasing hydrocortisone concentration, occluding the area with plastic wrap, or using stronger corticosteroid congeners. Application under plastic wrap enhances cortisone absorption by a factor of about ten, as does application under a warm, wet compress covered with plastic wrap. Hydrating and heating the stratum corneum reduces its barrier capability. Threfore, medication is best applied after a bath, while the skin is warm and moist. Occlusion with plastic wrap is intolerable to some children and dangerous to infants, because it can cause suffocation. A few patients with atopic dermatitis will not tolerate occlusion because of pruritus and infection. The plastic wrap should be removed in less than 8 hours, since infection may be generated after a longer period.

Corticosteroid salves and lotions are now available in so many forms and strengths that there is a detailed science for their optimal use (Cornell and Stoughton, 1984). The inexperienced individual can safely manage various diseases with 1 percent hydrocortisone. More potent steroids, such as betamethasone and triamcinolone (0.1 percent), may be tried for as long as 1 month. Formulations now available, however, have become sufficiently potent to produce systemic side effects. A physician inexperienced with strong agents should never recommend their use for generalized diseases on intertriginous areas or areas of thin skin (face). They should be employed only for short periods of time in other local areas. In general, the more potent topical preparations should be reserved for the armamentarium of those physicians with broad experience in the use of corticosteroids.

Local side effects of topical corticosteroids include the following (Hill and Rostenberg, 1978):

Sebaceous effects. Perioral dermatitis, rosacea-like dermatitis, steroid acne, aggravation of preexisting folliculitis, and granuloma gluteale infantum (large red nodules in the diaper area).

Atrophic effects. Cigarette paper–like wrinkling, delayed wound healing, and exacerbation of existing ulceration. Favored sites of atrophy include perianal, characterized by erythematous, smooth, shiny telangiectatic areas that are often pruritic and tender; digital, causing pencil sharp–like atrophy of the distal digiti; intertriginous, causing striae at anatomic sites of occlusion, purpura, ecchymosis, and telangiectasia.

Immune effects. Altered local response to dermatophyte infections, causing tinea incognito; conversion of ordinary scabies into the "Norwegian" type (Chapter 32).

Cosmetic effects. Hypertrichosis of the face; hypopigmentation.

Endocrine effects. The incidence of iatrogenic Cushing syndrome from topical corticosteroids has risen dramatically for the past 5 years. Even experienced physicians need to be reminded that 1 percent hydrocortisone under occlusion has the potential to induce the same side effects as the strongest known topical steroids applied with or without occlusion (Baden, 1978).

14. Hydroxyzine is the antihistamine of choice for pruritus or urticaria. Somnolence, its bothersome side effect, can be circumvented and used for sedation by giving the medication once daily, 2 hours before bedtime, and progressively increasing this single dose. Children usually tolerate large doses with minimal side effects. Recently, terfenadine (Seldane), an antihistamine that does not induce drowsiness, was introduced in the United States. This and similar long-lasting, H-blocking agents are available elsewhere in the world, some of which also are becoming available in the United States. These antihistamines are useful for patients when sedation is a problem (Kahn, 1987).

15. If an antibiotic is indicated for deep skin infection, it should be used systemically because topical therapy contributes little to healing and may be sensitizing. Autoinoculation and superficial pyoderma are curtailed by soaks, antibacterial soaps (chlorhexidine gluconate), and topical antibiotics. Mupirocin (pseudomonic acid) is a new and unique topical antibiotic marketed as Bactroban that is not related to other antibiotics, not irritating or sensitizing, and not prone to resistance (exception, *Pseudomonas*). Apply it three times daily for a week (White et al., 1985). Topical antibiotics applied to areas of minor skin trauma prevent streptococcal pyoderma for those at risk (Maddox et al., 1985).

REFERENCES

Baden, H.: Hydrocortisone vs. high-potency corticosteroid ointments. Arch. Dermatol. 114:798–99, 1978.

Cornell, R.C., Stoughton, R.B.: The use of topical steroids in psoriasis. Dermatol. Clin. 2:397–409, 1984.

Hajime, I., Adachi., Halprin, K.M., et al.: Cyclic AMP accumulation in psoriatic skin: differential responses to histamine, AMP, and epinephrine by the uninvolved and involved epidermis. J. Invest. Derm. 70:250–53, 1978.

Hill, C.J.H., Rostenberg, A.: Adverse effects from topical steroids. Cutis 21:624–28, 1978.

Hurwitz, S.: Clinical Pediatric Dermatology. Philadelphia, W.B. Saunders Co., 1981.

Husak, M., Wiltshire, J., Carr, H.: Effects of Hibiclens bathing on neonatal bacterial colonization (Abstract). 21st Intersci. Conf. Chicago, 714, 1981.

Kahn, G.: Techniques in Therapeutics. In Schachner, L.A., Hansen, R.L.: Pediatric Dermatology. New York, Churchill Livingstone, Inc., 1987.

Katz, S.I.: The skin as an immunologic organ. J. Am. Acad. Dermatol. 13:530–536, 1985.

Leyden, J.J., Katz, S., Stewart, R., Kligman, A.M.: Urinary ammonia and ammonia-producing microorganisms in infants with and without diaper dermatitis. Arch. Dermatol. 113:1678–80, 1977.

Maddox, J.S., Ware, J.C., Dillon, H.C.: The natural history of streptococcal skin infection: Prevention with topical antibiotics. J. Am. Acad. Dermatol. 13:207–212, 1985.

Montagna, W.: Advances in Biology of the Skin, vol. 6. New York, Pergamon Press, 1965.

Radetsky, M., Wheeler, R.C., Roe, M.A., et al.: Comparative evaluation of kits for rapid diagnosis of group A streptococcal disease. Pediatr. Infect. Dis. 4:274–281, 1985.

Solomon, L.S., Esterly, N.B.: Neonatal Dermatology. Philadelphia, W.B. Saunders Co., 1973.

Solomon, L.S., Esterly, N.B., Loeffel, E.D.: Adolescent Dermatology. Philadelphia, W.B. Saunders Co., 1978.

Strauss, J., Pochi, P.E., Downing, D.T.: The sebaceous glands. Twenty-five years of progress. J. Invest. Dermatol. 67:90, 1976.

Weinberg, S., Leider, M. Shapiro, L.: Color Atlas of Pediatric Dermatology. New York, McGraw-Hill Co., 1975.

White, J., Davies, B.I., Go, M.J., et al.: Pseudomonic acid, a new antibiotic for topical therapy. J. Am. Acad. Dermatol. 12:1026–1031, 1985.

29

Atopic Dermatitis

ALVIN H. JACOBS, M.D.
ALAN B. GOLDSOBEL, M.D.

Atopic dermatitis (AD) is a pruritic skin disease of characteristic distribution. It occurs usually in individuals with a personal or family history of allergic diseases and often is associated with xerosis, tendency to eczematization, abnormal function of the cutaneous vasculature, and immune aberrations. AD is characterized by extreme pruritus and persistent, often frantic, scratching, which induces papulation, excoriations, bleeding, oozing, crusting, secondary infection, and ultimately thickening or lichenification. Although the dermatitis can occur on any area of the body, there are typical locations of involvement that vary according to age.

All patients with AD manifest findings related to "skin susceptibility" to development of dermatitis as follows: sweat retention; decreased sebum production; abnormal vascular responses, such as white dermatographism; and decreased itching threshold, with increased itching from heat, irritation, psychologic tension, and infection. Pruritus, which induces scratching, seems to be the common factor through which allergic, irritant, and other factors contribute to the development of the disorder. The resulting pruritus is an essential ingredient in the pathogenesis of the dermatitis. In fact, "atopic dermatitis is not a rash that itches, but rather an itch that rashes."

INCIDENCE

Halpern and associates (1973) noted a 4.3 percent incidence of AD in 1753 children from birth through 7 years of age in the United States; similar studies in Great Britain have revealed an incidence of approximately 3 percent in infants and an incidence of about 1 percent in school children. The incidence of the disorder in adults is not clear, although Sulzberger (1955) estimated that AD resulted in 3 to 5 percent of all discharges for disease from the military services of the United States during World War II. There is no racial predilection. The disorder is more prevalent in city dwellers and more common in industrialized areas. Sixty percent of children with AD develop the disorder by 1 year of age, although it is rare for it to develop before 2 months of age. An additional 30 percent develop AD before 5 years of age; the remainder develop AD later in childhood or adulthood.

HEREDITY

AD runs in families, but despite its common occurence, the mode of inheritance is not established. Environmental factors influence expression and make family studies difficult. Furthermore, there is no one definitive clinical or laboratory marker for the disease so that criteria for the presence or absence of the disease rest on clinical impressions. The common relationships among respiratory allergies, physiologic aberrations that result in AD, and ichthyosis vulgaris suggest a genetic linkage. In this regard, it is of interest that about 50 percent of patients with autosomal dominant ichthyosis vulgaris also are atopic and have allergic diseases. Rajka (1975) reviewed the genetic factors in AD and concluded that it has a polygenic inheritance and that both exogenous and endogenous factors influence the expressivity of the gene effect.

Numerous studies examining human leukocyte antigen (HLA) associations with AD have failed to show any consistent patterns.

PATHOGENESIS

The pathogenetic basis of AD is unclear, but speculation in recent years has centered on three areas as follows: abnormal skin physiology and biochemistry, alteration in cyclic nucleotide metabolism, and specific immune abnormalities.

385

Physiologic Aberrations

Abnormal Sweat Responses. Any stimulation of sweating initiates pruritus in AD. Sweat duct obstruction leading to sweat retention and resultant escape of sweat into the dermis has been postulated as the mechanism. Sulzberger et al. (1953) described the sweat retention syndrome in which the sweat retention was associated with horny plugging of the sweat pores. They demonstrated that human sweat injected into the dermis of volunteers induced itching, particularly in atopic subjects. Sweat pore obstruction is contributed to not only by the hyperkeratosis but also by the damage to the stratum corneum from scratching and secondary infection. Application of oily or greasy preparations also contribute to the poral occlusion.

Sebaceous Gland Activity. In patients with AD, sebaceous gland activity is decreased. A decrease in sebum production could allow greater evaporation of moisture from the skin and contribute to xerosis. An increase in the proportion of cholesterol, both free and esterified, in the sebum of patients with AD and a relative deficiency of unsaturated fatty acids in the surface lipid has been found.

Xerosis. Patients with AD have dry skin, more marked on the extensor surfaces of the body than the flexor surfaces. Blank (1952) in a classic study demonstrated the importance of water in preserving the pliability and softness of the stratum corneum. The water content of this horny layer must be at least 10 percent for it to remain soft and flexible. When the moisture falls below this concentration, the keratin becomes progressively less flexible, rough, brittle, and eventually cracked. Under normal conditions, the skin contains about 10 to 30 percent water. The stratum corneum dries and becomes brittle if the relative humidity falls below 60 percent. The water content of the stratum corneum, which comes from deeper tissues by upward diffusion, is conserved by the presence of water soluble substances, consisting of a mixture of amino acids, organic acids, urea, and inorganic ions. Collectively these water soluble substances have been described as the "natural moisturizing factor." They are maintained in the stratum corneum by being sandwiched between layers of lipoprotein complex. The patient with AD presumably has a defect in this complex, so that washing or soaking in water dissolves out the natural moisturizing factor, leaving the skin drier after bathing than before.

Susceptibility to Infection. Patients with AD have an increased susceptibility to cutaneous viral and fungal infection; thus, warts and molluscum contagiosum are common. Herpes simplex tends to become generalized, resulting in eczema herpeticum (see Complications). Of greater importance is the apparent inability of the atopic skin to prevent colonization with *Staphylococcus aureus.* Leyden et al. (1974) isolated *S. aureus* from 91 percent of chronic lichenified plaques of patients with AD and from 100 percent of acute exudative lesions. Aly et al. (1977) confirmed these findings and also isolated *S. aureus* from the normal appearing skin of 76 percent of patients with AD. In contrast, persons without AD rarely have *S. aureus* on the skin surface.

In view of the staphylococcal colonization of patients with AD, it is of interest that Abramson et al. (1982) found that the elevated IgE level in atopic patients is antistaphylococcal. They speculate that interaction of staphylococcal antigens from bacteria on the skin with antistaphylococcal IgE antibodies on mast cells could induce mast cells to release histamine, evoke itch, and thus aggravate dermatitis.

Abnormal Vascular Responses. A striking abnormal vascular characteristic of the atopic individual is the marked tendency toward paradoxical vasoconstriction. The central pallor characteristic of the atopic facies probably is due to vasoconstriction. Stroking the skin of these patients with a blunt instrument results in the prompt appearance of a white spreading line. This response occurs on uninvolved as well as involved skin and is due to vasoconstriction. Stroking the skin of a normal person results in either a red line or the full triple response of Lewis, with a flare and wheal. Injection of acetylcholine or methacholine intracutaneously in the nonatopic individual will produce a flare, representing axon reflex vasodilatation beyond the injection wheal. In the atopic patient, this flare is replaced within 2 to 5 minutes by a blanched zone, often with pseudopods (delayed blanch reaction) (Winkelmann, 1966). This reaction occurs in 76 percent of patients with AD and is most likely due to vasoconstriction (Lobitz and Campbell, 1953; Reed et al., 1976). It is probable that the changes in acral skin temperatures in patients with AD also are related to a vasoconstrictive tendency. Atopic subjects demonstrate lower basal temperatures of the hands and feet. There is also a more rapid cooling and a slower warming in cold and warm rooms, respectively (Winkelmann, 1966).

Chemical Mediators. Elevated acetylcholine concentrations in blood and skin parallel disease severity. Norepinephrine stores in the skin and blood levels of kininogens also are increased in AD (Michaelsson, 1969). Intracutaneous administration of serotonin, kallikrein, and histamine will induce blanching or only slight erythema, compared with the marked erythema that occurs in normal skin. Prostaglandin E administration induces a delayed vasodilatory response (Juhlin and Michaelsson, 1969), though there is a normal response to intradermally injected saline and epinephrine.

Some patients with AD have increased levels of histamine in both uninvolved and involved skin. Numbers of mast cells may be normal or increased in involved skin (Mihm et al., 1976). Intramuscular injection of histamine produces a greater than normal increase in skin temperature; an intracutaneous injection produces less edema than normal. Abnormal histamine levels and altered responsiveness to histamine may be of particular relevance to the increased pruritus in AD, since the sensation of itching appears to be mediated by certain pain fibers, and there is evidence that histamine is a chemical mediator of cutaneous pain (Rosenthal, 1977).

CYCLIC NUCLEOTIDE ABNORMALITIES

Szentivanyi (1968) proposed that partial blockade of the beta-adrenergic receptor system is the constitutional basis for asthma and possibly other atopic disease. Various clinical observations in patients with AD are consistent with this hypothesis. Increased sensitivity of the sweat glands to cholinergic stimulation and heightened responses to alpha-adrenergic stimulation reported in AD could reflect decreased beta-adrenergic activity. Patients with AD pretreated with propranolol, a beta receptor blocking agent, do not have the expected increased sweat response to locally injected acetylcholine, suggesting that they already have maximal beta-adrenergic blockade (Hemels, 1970).

Numerous investigators have reported impaired *in vitro* beta-adrenergic function in peripheral blood leukocytes of patients with AD as well as other atopic disorders. This subsensitivity to beta-adrenergic agents was attributed to beta receptor blockade possibly due to decreased numbers or affinity of beta receptors on the cell surfaces or to autoantibodies to the beta receptor. More recent radioligand studies have not shown evidence of reduced receptor numbers or affinity, and autoantibodies have been found in small percentages of atopic individuals as well as in normals. Patients with AD have been shown to have abnormally low cAMP levels after incubation with beta-adrenergic agents but not with prostaglandin E_1, suggesting a specific beta receptor defect (Reed et al., 1976). Many workers have investigated the role of cyclic nucleotide abnormalities in AD and have shown that mononuclear leukocytes from patients with AD demonstrate depressed cAMP responses after *in vitro* exposure to isoproterenol as well as prostaglandin E_1 and histamine (Hanifin 1984; Giustina et al., 1984; Heskel et al., 1984). These data suggest a defect not limited to the beta receptor. They showed that leukocytes of nonatopic individuals could adopt this abnormal atopic pattern by "desensitization" with exposure to low concentrations of these same agents and demonstrated that desensitization with depressed cAMP response is associated with increased leukocyte cAMP-phosphodiesterase (PDE) activity and increased metabolism of cAMP. PDE activity is higher in patients with active or inactive AD and allergic rhinitis, but not in normal individuals or nonatopic patients with allergic contact dermatitis. It was suggested, therefore, that this finding in atopic individuals may be due to *in vivo* desensitization by increased blood and tissue levels of histamine. *In vitro* leukocyte histamine release is higher in patients with AD and directly correlates with elevated PDE activity, with resultant decreased cAMP inhibitory influence. These investigators also demonstrated a strong correlation between IgE production and PDE activity in human leukocytes. PDE activity is elevated in cord blood leukocytes of newborns of atopic mothers or fathers (Heskel et al., 1984); children appear to be more at risk for developing AD or other atopic disease. These studies suggest that elevated PDE activity in patients with AD may reflect an underlying basic genetic defect, which may be a marker of disease activity but also may contribute to the pathogenesis of AD.

Immune Mechanisms

IgE Antibody and AD. Seventy percent of patients with AD have or will develop allergic respiratory disease, and a similar percentage have a positive family history of atopic disease (Rajka, 1975). These respiratory allergies usually become clinically apparent after development of skin disease. There also is an unexplained tendency for AD and asthma to alternate in their course (Hanifin, 1984).

Total serum IgE levels are elevated in approximately 50 to 80 percent of patients with AD and are usually higher than in other atopic disorders. Although studies are conflicting, the severity of the skin involvement generally is proportional to the IgE level. There also is variable data as to whether or not allergic respiratory disease in conjunction with AD causes higher serum IgE levels. Levels as high as 30,000 IU/ml or higher may be seen in AD patients with or without allergic respiratory disease.

Immediate hypersensitivity skin test and serologic test results for IgE antibodies frequently are positive; the IgE has been shown to be directed against a wide variety of inhalant and food antigens (Hoffman et al., 1975; Chapman et al., 1983; Sampson, 1983). As noted previously, Abramson et al. (1982) have shown that AD patients also have high levels of IgE antibodies directed against *Staphylococcus aureus.* Early studies suggested that correlation of specific IgE antibodies present, comparing allergy skin test results with RAST results, was not as great in patients with AD as in patients with respiratory allergies. Possible reasons for this finding include inflammatory skin involvement, with subsequent difficulty interpreting allergy test results, and high serum IgE levels; the latter possibly leads to nonspecific binding to antigens coupled to solid media in radioallergosorbent tests (RAST) or other serologic IgE antibody tests with false positive results. More recent studies have taken these methodologic factors into account, using a double antibody-antigen binding technique to measure antigen specific IgE. Good correlation has been shown between prick skin test and RAST results for both food and inhalant antigens (see subsequent discussion). Other than studies of food antigens in which a causative role has been established in some patients with AD, adequate studies clearly defining the clinical significance of specific IgE antibodies present in patients with AD in contrast to respiratory allergic disease are lacking.

The specific role of IgE in AD, therefore, remains unclear. Consideration of the possible role of IgE in AD includes the following (Hanifin, 1984): (1) 20 percent of patients with typical flexural eczema have normal serum IgE levels; (2) patients have been described with typical flexural eczema, agammaglobulinemia, and no

skin test reactivity; (3) patients have high serum IgE levels in parasitoses and in various skin conditions (e.g., pemphigoid, mycosis fungoides, psoriasis, alopecia areata, pityriasis rubra pilaris), who have no clinical evidence for AD; and (4) patients have persistent high IgE levels when AD is in remission. On the other hand, IgE levels can be shown to be elevated only in approximately 60 to 70 percent of individuals with other atopic disease (e.g., allergic rhinitis, and allergic asthma), whereas 20 percent of an apparently nonatopic population may have elevated IgE levels (Johansson, 1982). IgE is produced by plasma cells predominantly located in lymphoid tissue associated with the respiratory and gastrointestinal tracts, with the serum level representing that which has diffused or is transported into the blood stream. As such, quantitative levels and measurement of antigen-specific IgE by serum determination or by skin tests may not accurately reflect immunopathogenetic processes in selected tissues. High persisting levels of IgE in AD in remission may be partially directed against *S. aureus*, which is frequently cultured from uninvolved skin in AD (Aly et al., 1977).

The regulation of IgE synthesis appears to be more highly T cell dependent than that of other immunoglobulins. This dependence was first suggested by animal experiments, but appears to apply to humans as well (Chapter 6). It would appear that increased serum IgE levels in AD and other hyper-IgE states are closely related to T cell immunoregulation.

There has been a resurgence of interest in the identification of specific antigens contributing to the skin lesions of AD. Sampson and co-workers (1983, 1984) performed studies correlating immediate food hypersensitivity with the pathogenesis of AD. Because of patient, family, and physician biases, double-blind placebo-controlled food challenges (DBPCFC) were employed using up to 8 to 10 gm of dried food in opaque capsules, juice, or broth. In a select population of children referred because of severe AD, histories of possible food hypersensitivity, and very high serum IgE levels (mean 8500 IU/ml), about half experienced at least one positive DBPCFC. Of those patients responding, 57 percent responded to only one antigen, 32 percent to two, and only 9 percent responded to three antigens, thus dispelling the notion of common multiple food sensitivities in AD. All reactions to DBPCFC occurred within 10 to 90 minutes, with a majority exhibiting cutaneous symptoms, predominantly pruritus. Gastrointestinal and respiratory symptoms also were frequent. Egg sensitivity was most common, with 42 percent of challenges being positive. Egg, along with peanut, milk, soy, wheat, and fish, contributed to 90 percent of all positive challenges. A personal or parental history of adverse reaction to a particular food was of little value in predicting a positive DBPCFC. Prick skin test reactions were found to be valuable for excluding immediate hypersensitivity reactions to foods. It was very rare for a patient with a negative prick skin test reaction to have a positive DBPCFC; the negative predictive accuracy was approximately 96 percent. Prick skin tests have a relatively poor positive predictive accuracy (approximately 40 percent), and positive test reactions are only suggestive of what foods should be considered for challenge. RAST alone or combined with the prick skin test had no advantage over the prick skin test alone.

Other investigators have shown a beneficial effect of an antigen avoidance diet in children with atopic dermatitis (Juto et al., 1978; Graham et al., 1984), including a double-blind, cross-over trial of egg and cow's milk elimination (Atherton et al., 1978). In a later study, however, there was no correlation between a positive prick test reaction and a response to the trial diet. Similar studies of DBPCFC in food-allergic adults also have been performed with somewhat similar results. Sampson and Jolie (1984) demonstrated increased plasma histamine concentrations after positive food challenges, implicating mast cell or basophil release of chemical mediators in the patients studied.

Platts-Mills and coworkers (Platts-Mills et al., 1983; Mitchell et al., 1982 and 1984; Chapman et al., 1983) investigated the role of inhalant or contact allergens in patients with AD. Patch tests were performed over abraded skin in AD patients with large amounts of antigen P_1, the major allergen of the house dust mite, *Dermatophagoides pteronyssinus*. After 48 hours, in patients with positive immediate skin test reactions, eczematoid reactions developed. These reactions possessed histologic characteristics of cutaneous basophil hypersensitivity, considered to be a form of delayed hypersensitivity, but which also may represent an IgE-mediated late phase reaction (Gleich, 1982). A similar response in AD patients also has been reported with intradermal injection of staphylococcal antigens (Henocq, 1981). Biopsy specimens of these reactions reveal a dermal infiltrate, with predominantly basophils and eosinophils as well as mononuclear cells and neutrophils. Although this finding is not identical to that seen in classic AD, with repeated cutaneous application of antigen P_1, a histologic reaction occurs more closely resembling that of AD. In such patients, high levels of specific IgE and IgG to antigen P_1, as well as specific *in vitro* T cell proliferation to antigen P_1 could be demonstrated. The kind of immune reactions demonstrated, as well as reports of clinical improvement of AD with house dust environmental control measures (believed to possibly contribute to the well-recognized improvement of AD patients admitted to relatively "dust mite free" hospital rooms), indicates that further investigation of the role of inhalant and contact allergens in the pathogenesis of AD is warranted.

Other Abnormalities of Humoral Immunity. Serum levels of IgG, IgM, and IgA generally are normal in patients with AD. IgG and IgM levels occasionally are elevated presumably secondary to chronic skin infections. IgD levels have been reported to be decreased in some adults with AD. Transient IgA deficiency at 3 months of age has been reported to be associated with the subsequent development of AD and other atopic disease in children of atopic parents, but this has not been established satisfactorily. Elevated serum immune complexes of IgG, IgA, and IgE have been demonstrated in patients with AD, and some investigators have shown the antigen in these complexes to be directed against foods. It is speculated that these immune complexes may bind complement with subsequent release of mediators from cutaneous and other mast cells, contributing to the pathogenesis of AD. Serum C3 levels have been found to be increased in infants with AD less than 2 years old.

Cell-Mediated Immunity. Numerous clinical observations suggest that patients with AD have defects in cell-mediated immunity. AD patients as a group have increased susceptibilities to cutaneous infections with viruses (herpes simplex, vaccinia, Coxsackie virus A16, verruca vulgaris, and molluscum contagiosum), and dermatophytes (particularly *Trichophyton rubrum*). They exhibit a decreased incidence of allergic contact dermatitis and have a high failure rate of cutaneous sensitization to dinitrochlorobenzene and *Rhus* extract. They have also diminished delayed hypersensitivity skin test responses to microbial antigens, such as *Trichophyton*, *Candida*, and streptokinase-streptodornase, even with documented previous infections. However, such patients have not been observed to have frequent mucosal or systemic infections with viruses, fungi, or protozoa as seen in patients with severe cell-mediated immune defects. *In vitro* evaluation of this cutaneous anergy has revealed a disassociation between delayed cutaneous hypersensitivity and lymphocyte transformation (Elliot and Hanifin, 1979a). Although numerous investigators have shown AD patients to have diminished T cell blastogenesis to various mitogens and antigens that usually correlates with disease severity, Elliot and Hanifin (1979a) demonstrated that more severely involved AD patients have diminished lymphocyte responsiveness: patients with milder disease demonstrate cutaneous anergy despite normal *in vitro* lymphocyte transformation to *Candida* and streptokinase-streptodornase. *In vitro* diminished responsiveness to phytohemagglutinin (PHA) in severely affected AD patients can be reversed by preincubation mononuclear cells for 4 days before adding PHA (Elliot and Hanifin, 1979b). This normalized *in vitro* response was thought possibly to be the result of maturation of T helper cells. The dissociation between defects of *in vitro* immune responses and clinically observed defects in cell-mediated immunity remains to be explained.

Numerous studies have shown decreased numbers of suppressor cells (T8+ cells) in the blood and in inflamed skin of patients with AD, as well as decreased functional activity ascribed to T suppressor cells.

In a prospective study, infants 1 to 2 months of age who subsequently developed AD were found to have decreased numbers of T8+ cells as well as diminished functional suppressor cell activity compared with age-matched normal infants (Chandra and Baker, 1983), suggesting that this immune abnormality is not a phenomenon secondary to the disorder and is consistent with the idea that it may have some role in its pathogenesis. Other recent experiments suggest that there may be defective T4+ helper/inducer cells as well and, in particular, a deficiency of a subset of inducer cells that are considered to represent an inducer circuit for the activation of T8+ suppressor/cytotoxic cells (Leung et al., 1983). This may better explain some of the observed functional T cell defects and abnormal suppressor cell activity seen in AD.

Investigations of natural killer (NK) cytotoxicity in AD have varied, showing decreased, increased, and normal cytotoxicity against K562 human myeloid leukemia cells. But one report has shown that patients with AD have circulating NK–like cells that are cytotoxic to autologous fibroblasts, suggesting that NK and cell-mediated mechanisms may contribute to the pathogenesis of this skin disease (Leung et al., 1982). This may represent an autoimmune-like phenomenon, and damaged fibroblasts may contribute to some of the abnormalities of the mechanical properties of the skin seen in patients with AD.

Abnormal Phagocyte Movement. Numerous investigators have reported defective *in vitro* chemotaxis of monocytes and neutrophils in patients with AD (Rogge and Hanifin, 1976; Fischer et al., 1977; Snyderman et al., 1977; Furukawa and Altman, 1978). This defect appears to correlate with cutaneous infection and severity but not serum IgE levels (Dahl et al., 1978). Chemotaxis has been shown to improve promptly when cutaneous infection is controlled with systemic antibiotics. The defect is particularly striking, since patients without AD but with cutaneous bacterial infection have hyperactive chemotactic responses (Hill et al., 1974). There appears to be a plasma factor in patients with severe AD that inhibits monocyte and neutrophil chemotaxis of normal cells (Hanifin and Rogge, 1977). The amount of plasma inhibitor also correlates with clinical severity of AD. The identity of this inhibitor currently is unknown, but speculation that it may be histamine is based on the fact that it can suppress the chemotactic response of neutrophils. Blocking the H2 receptor of neutrophils can abrogate this depression of chemotaxis (Seligmann et al., 1983).

Association with Immunodeficiency Disorders. Children with certain immunodeficiency disorders may have an eczematoid rash indistinguishable from AD. These include the Wiskott-Aldrich syndrome (WAS), ataxia-telangiectasia, and rarely Nezelof syndrome, DiGeorge syndrome, and other hypogammaglobulinemic or agammaglobulinemic disorders. Other characteristics suggesting similar immunoregulatory defects in AD and immunodeficiency states are the partial cell-mediated immune defects, elevated IgE levels, and occasional defective monocyte chemotaxis seen in WAS. Observations in bone marrow transplantation for immune reconstitution in WAS imply that clinical resolution of the eczema is related to T cell rather than B cell function.

The rash seen with the hyper-IgE syndrome is eczematoid, but the distribution and characteristics are not similar to classic AD. Differentiation in young children may be difficult. Many other clinical and laboratory similarities are seen, as these patients also have cutaneous infections with *S. aureus* and elevated levels of antistaphylococcal IgE antibodies. However, hyper-IgE patients demonstrate more deep-seated and systemic infections with *S. aureus*, including cutaneous and lung abcesses with pneumatoceles. These patients characteristically do not demonstrate clinical allergic disease despite extremely elevated IgE levels in the range of 2000 to 50,000 IU/ml. Nevertheless, T cell immunoregulatory defects contributing to elevated IgE levels and abnormal leukocyte chemotaxis are similar to those seen in AD. Study of any hyper-IgE state is likely to contribute to an understanding of the basis of immune aberrations in AD.

HISTOLOGIC FEATURES

Two basic lesions occur in AD, and these are classified as vesicular and lichenified on the basis of their gross appearance (Mihm et al., 1976). Vesicular lesions are confined mostly to the epidermis and consist histologically of intercellular edema (spongiosis) with vesicle formation, epidermal hyperplasia, and inflammatory cell infiltration with lymphocytes and macrophages. Only an occasional neutrophil, eosinophil, and basophil are seen. Mast cells are not increased in number, though they appear to be hypogranulated. The superficial venous plexus is altered, with hypertrophy of endothelial cells and reduplication and thickening of vascular basement membranes. The stratum corneum is markedly thickened, with retention of cellular debris.

Histologic examination of lichenified lesions reveals irregular hyperplasia of the epidermis with minimal intercellular edema, and marked thickening of the papillary dermis with increased numbers of lymphocytes and monocytes or macrophages. Mast cells are increased in number but do not appear to be degranulated. Changes of the superficial venous plexus are similar to those of vesicular lesions but are more prominent and also involve the venules in the reticular dermis. Dermal nerves are abnormal, exhibiting demyelination, fibrosis, and occasional vacuolated areas, which contain lipids. Similar but less marked abnormalities of the superficial venous plexus and venules occur in clinically normal skin of AD patients, but

epidermal hyperplasia, intercellular edema, and cellular infiltrates are minimal.

CLINICAL MANIFESTATIONS

The primary lesions of AD are not obvious. Much of what is thought of as the typical appearance of the disorder actually is the result of secondary phenomena. *The most important primary "lesion" is pruritus.*

In addition, dryness of the skin, due to retention of insufficient amounts of water in the stratum corneum, is an important primary feature of the disorder and contributes to pruritus. Another common primary feature of atopic skin is the presence of "goose bumps" (cutis anserina) over much of the skin of the trunk and proximal portions of the limbs (Fig. 29-1). These are tiny papules at all hair follicle orifices. In some areas, particularly the flanks and dorsa of the upper arms, these papules become larger and hyperkeratotic (keratosis pilaris). Where these papules are scratched or rubbed, they become confluent and develop into plaques of poorly marginated, thickened skin. This process is called lichenification (Fig. 29–2).

Most of the appearance commonly referred to as eczema is secondary, due to trauma to the skin resulting from scratching and rubbing with an almost inevitable secondary infection. Thus, the crusted, oozing skin so often seen in the infant or young child with AD is scratched, infected skin (eczematized-impetiginized).

Since the character of the eruption and its distribution vary at different ages, this discussion is divided into the infantile stage (up to 2

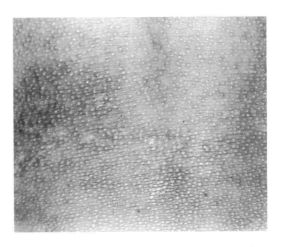

FIGURE 29–1. Typical "goose bumps" of atopic skin.

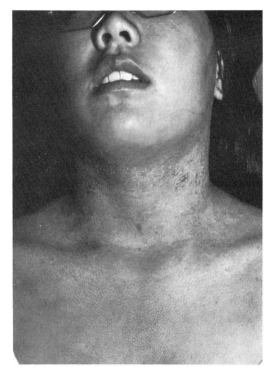

FIGURE 29-2. This adolescent girl with chronic atopic dermatitis shows excoriation and lichenification of the neck. Also note the apparent follicular prominence ("goose bumps"), which is characteristic of the atopic skin.

years), the childhood stage (2 to 12 years), and the adolescent and adult stage (12 years and older). This division is somewhat arbitrary since characteristics of the three stages may overlap.

Infantile Stage. AD rarely begins earlier than 8 weeks of age, though seborrheic dermatitis may preceed and coexist with it (Fig. 29-3 and Fig. 29-4). Lesions generally first appear on the cheeks, characterized by erythema that is dry and chapped in appearance, but they usually progress to vesiculation, oozing, and crusting, due to secondary infection. This infection is almost invariably *Staphylococcus aureus*. The lesions may involve progressively the forehead, scalp, trunk, and postauricular areas. As the infant reaches the crawling stage, the eruption frequently involves the extensor surfaces of the extremities. Although involvement of the flexural creases may occur in infancy, this is much more likely to occur later.

Itching usually is intense, causing the infant to be irritable and interfering with sleep. The eruption in the infantile stage tends to improve gradually, but the common opinion that it clears by 18 months to 2 years is overly optimistic.

Childhood Stage. The childhood stage can follow the infantile stage without interruption, or it can appear after a variable period of more or less complete remission (Fig. 29-5, Fig. 29-6, and Fig. 29-7). This phase of the disease may be less inflammatory and characterized more by dryness of the skin. It is in this childhood stage that the small, more or less skin-colored papules at the follicular orifices become more apparent. In areas where considerable scratching occurs, papules tend to become larger, somewhat crusted, and confluent, producing lichenified plaques with surrounding discrete papules. The flexor areas, particularly those of the antecubital (see Fig. 29-6) and popliteal

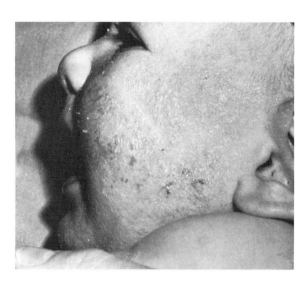

FIGURE 29-3. Eight-month-old infant with atopic dermatitis; note excoriations.

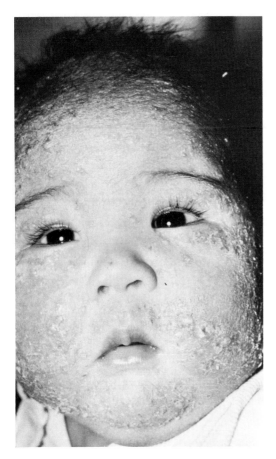

FIGURE 29–4. Nine-month-old infant with impetiginized atopic dermatitis.

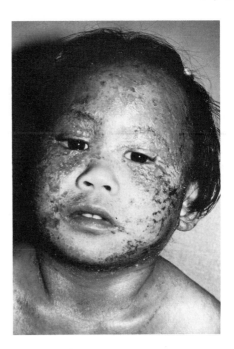

FIGURE 29–5. Three-year-old with severe atopic dermatitis. The extensive deep excoriations are evidence of this child's misery.

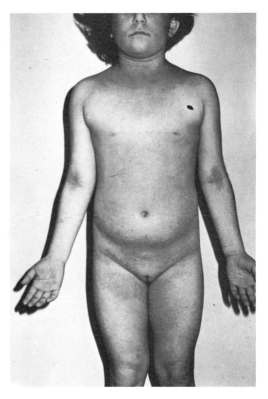

FIGURE 29–6. This 9-year-old girl shows generalized erythema with the typical flexural involvement of atopic dermatitis.

fossae (see Fig. 29–7) as well as the flanks and back of the neck, are favored locations in this stage. The face is less likely to be involved during childhood. School-age children often have predispositions to eczematous dermatitis either over the dorsa of the feet, where it masquerades as allergic contact dermatitis from footwear, or on the soles of the feet, where it frequently is called "athlete's foot" (Fig. 29–8). In the childhood stage, it still is possible for the intense scratching to introduce staphylococci with resulting eczematization. Again, complete remission can occur at any time during this stage, or the eruption can merge imperceptibly with the succeeding adolescent and adult phase.

Adolescent and Adult Stage. During this stage, AD may be manifest in general in two different forms. The most common expression of the disease during adolescence and adult life is rather a mild disorder. Patients continue to have dry skin with the continued presence of

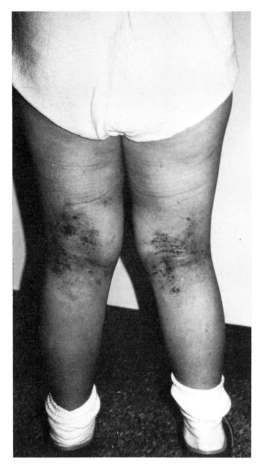

FIGURE 29–7. Excoriated, eczematized popliteal fossae in a typical atopic child.

prominent follicular papules and the presence of mild degrees of lichenification, especially in the popliteal or antecubital fossae (Fig. 29 – 9) or both. Older patients with AD are not as constantly itchy as are younger patients, but itching and scratching occur easily under the influence of various types of stress. When this occurs, scratching results in some degree of oozing and crusting. Often, an adult will seem to have "outgrown" dermatitis, although dry skin persists. At some later time, localized eczema may develop, especially of the hands (Fig. 29 – 10) and feet (see Fig. 29 – 8).

Less often, this stage of AD appears as a much more severe disorder. The skin is extremely dry and scaly with large, poorly marginated lichenified plaques in all flexural areas. There is widespread excoriation, which results in secondary infection, giving rise to exudation and crusting. The pruritus often is intolerable, causing severe emotional disturbances. The front and sides of the neck, the eyelids, forehead, scalp, anterior chest, wrists, dorsa of the fingers and toes, and dorsa of the feet are common sites of involvement. Occasionally, a generalized erythroderma ensues, and regional adenopathy can be found, particularly if the process is chronic and severe.

COMPLICATIONS

Skin Infection. In all types of atopic dermatitis, the most important complication is superimposed infection (Fig. 29 – 11). *Staphylococcus aureus* colonizes the skin of almost all patients and frequently plays an important role in the exacerbation of the dermatitis. Staphylococcal

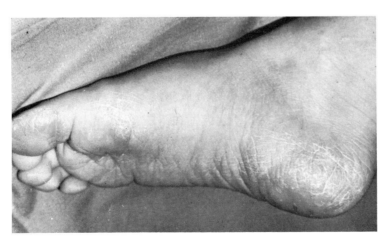

FIGURE 29–8. So-called athlete's foot in childhood is more commonly due to atopic dermatitis than to tinea pedis.

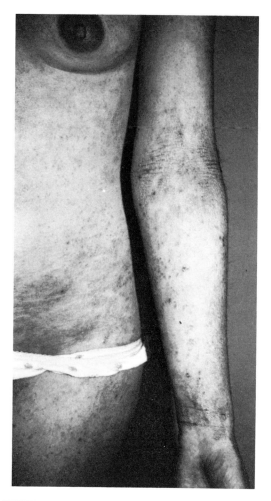

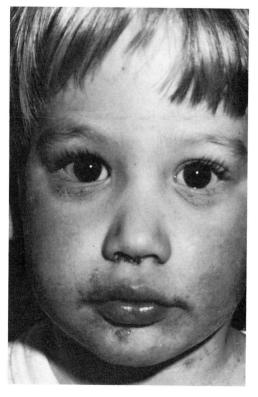

FIGURE 29–11. This child demonstrates two common features of atopic dermatitis. First, because of allergic conjunctivitis, he rubs his eyes and has developed lichenification of his lower lids. Second, as a complication of his allergic rhinitis, he has developed impetigo in the nostril that is already spreading to other areas of this susceptible skin.

FIGURE 29–9. Adolescent girl with chronic atopic dermatitis, showing excoriation and lichenification.

FIGURE 29–10. Involvement of the hands is very common in atopic children beyond infancy.

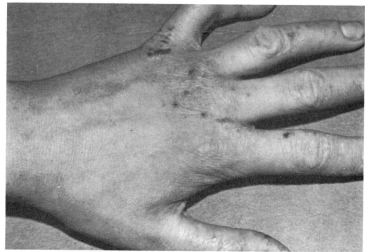

pustules accompany severe exacerbations of AD (Hanifin and Rogge, 1977). However, even lichenified, crusted, and fissured lesions are heavily colonized by these organisms (Leyden et al., 1974; Aly et al., 1977).

Patients with AD are also highly susceptible to cutaneous viral infections, the most serious of these being herpes simplex and vaccinia viruses. Eczema vaccinatum was estimated to occur once in 8.7 to 50 million vaccinia innoculations but is no longer a problem with discontinuation of smallpox vaccination. Clinical manifestations of eczema vaccinatum are indistinguishable from eczema herpeticum (Kaposi varicelliform eruption) (Fig. 29–12). Both are characterized by groups of umbilicated vesicles and pustules, predominantly involving sites of both active and quiescent dermatitis. Eczema herpeticum is responsive to intravenous acyclovir, although milder cases may merely require topical therapy, such as frequent cool wet compresses. Less important but quite common are other viral skin infections, such as molluscum contagiosum and warts.

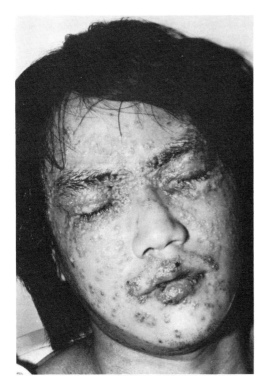

FIGURE 29–12. This young man with chronic atopic dermatitis has developed eczema herpeticum after contact with a friend's "cold sore."

Eye Complications. The incidence of cataract complicating AD has been reported to be about 8 percent but must be much less than this if mild cases of dermatitis are taken into consideration (Roth and Kierland, 1964). The cataracts usually are bilateral and occur many years after the onset of dermatitis. The typical cataract is characterized by anterior radiating lines or posterior cortical white plaques. Cataracts tend to mature rapidly, and extraction may be necessary.

Systemic administration of corticosteroids for various diseases has been associated with development of posterior subcapsular cataracts. The dose and duration of therapy are key factors. Production of lens' changes may take many years (Oglesby et al., 1961).

Keratoconus (conical cornea) is a rare occurrence in many eczematous skin disorders and probably results from constant eye rubbing (Copeman, 1965).

DIFFERENTIAL DIAGNOSIS

In infancy, the distinction between AD and seborrheic dermatitis can be difficult (Table 29–1), although the two may coexist. The pruritus of the atopic patient is severe and constant, whereas seborrheic dermatitis ordinarily is nonpruritic. The latter usually appears between 2 and 4 weeks of age; AD rarely is evident before 2 months of age. The usual findings in infantile seborrheic dermatitis are the thickened, yellow, and greasy-feeling scales; the dermatitis of the postauricular folds; and the fissuring and erythema of the intertriginous areas (Fig. 29–13; Fig 29–14; and Fig. 29–15). In contrast to AD, seborrheic patches are sharply demarcated and tend to be paler in the center. The lesions of AD show the most intense redness centrally. Seborrheic dermatitis in infancy is commonly and secondarily infected with *Candida albicans*. The adult form of seborrheic dermatitis rarely is confused with AD.

Contact dermatitis is relatively uncommon in infants, but becomes increasingly frequent in older children and adults. Atopic stigmata are absent, and positive reactions can be obtained with appropriate patch tests. There is less tendency for lichenification in contact dermatitis. Itching, although severe during an acute episode, is less prominent in the chronic stage.

TABLE 29–1. Features Distinguishing Seborrheic and Atopic Dermatitis in Infancy

	Seborrheic Dermatitis	**Atopic Dermatitis**
Family history	Usually none	History of atopic disorders
Age of onset	Usually under 2 months	Usually over 2 months
Distribution	Scalp; any flexures, especially genitoanal; in older child, eyebrows, eyelids	Cheeks, forehead, extensor surfaces of limbs (flexural involvement in older patients)
Lesions	Erythema with greasy, yellowish scales. Sharply demarcated flexural lesions	Erythema, papules, vesicles No scales (may be *crusted*) Tapering
Pruritus	Minimal	Severe (a hallmark of the disease)
Laboratory findings	Eosinophilia absent; negative skin test reactions	Eosinophilia; positive skin test reactions (especially for egg white) frequent
Prognosis	Usually clears in 3 to 4 weeks, up to 2 months. No associated defects	Prolonged course. High incidence of associated allergic rhinitis and asthma

Nummular dermatitis is a distinctive disorder characterized by coin-shaped lesions that develop on dry skin, especially in winter. Although in the past nummular eczema has been thought to be a manifestation of AD, recent

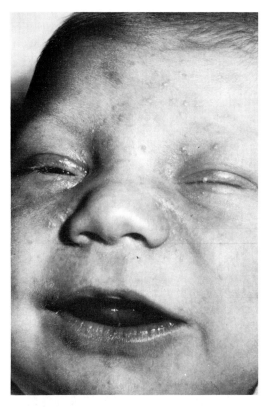

FIGURE 29–13. This infant has seborrheic dermatitis. There is erythema and scaling but no evidence of excoriation. The scale is yellow and greasy.

studies have shown that IgE levels are normal and suggest that nummular eczema is a manifestation of dry skin. However, in childhood, coin-shaped lesions often are seen in secondarily infected AD.

Psoriasis occasionally is confused with AD. The fully developed lesion of psoriasis is a red maculopapule with a loosely adherent silvery scale. Psoriatic lesions are well defined, with sharply delineated edges. The lesions of atopic dermatitis are not sharply demarcated. A valuable clue in the diagnosis of psoriasis is the frequent presence of nail dysplasia, with punctate pitting of the nail plate.

Scabies in infants and small children is commonly complicated by eczematous changes and may be easily confused with AD. The diagnosis of scabies is made by the characteristic distribution of lesions, the pathognomonic burrow, positive identification of the mite on microscopic examination of skin scrapings, and presence of infestation among other family members.

Chronic dermatitis of the hands and feet often occurs as an adult manifestation of AD and must be differentiated from dyshidrotic eczema, contact dermatitis, psoriasis, and tinea pedis.

A variety of metabolic, immunodeficiency, and congenital skin disorders have associated eruptions that resemble AD. These include phenylketonuria, Hartnup syndrome, Hurler syndrome, Wiskott-Aldrich syndrome, ataxia-telangiectasia, severe combined immunodeficiency, X-linked agammaglobulinemia, acrodermatitis enteropathica, and histiocytosis X.

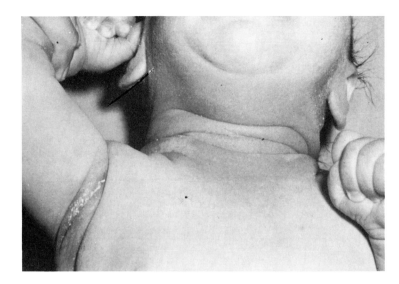

FIGURE 29-14. The typical intertrigo of seborrheic dermatitis in infancy. It is non-pruritic.

CLINICAL EVALUATION OF THE PATIENT WITH ATOPIC DERMATITIS

History and Physical Examination

The diagnosis of AD can be made with reasonable certainty from history and physical examination.

History. Since AD, asthma, or allergic rhinitis is present in a high percentage of relatives of patients with AD, a detailed family history should be recorded. The way in which dermatitis developed, when it became most severe, its current distribution, and symptomatology should be established. Details of treatment also are important. What topical medication, skin care, and systemic therapy have been prescribed? Did these medications clear the dermatitis or make it worse? Patients should be encouraged to bring in all medications so that their content can be determined. Not infrequently the dermatitis may have been worsened by treatment with topical medications, containing such substances as organic iodides, antibiotics, antihistamines, and anesthetics.

A possible relationship to dietary or environmental factors may provide important information. For example, in the infant, the relationship of the onset of exacerbation of dermatitis to the type of milk or solid foods in the diet may suggest allergy, whereas specifics of diet alterations

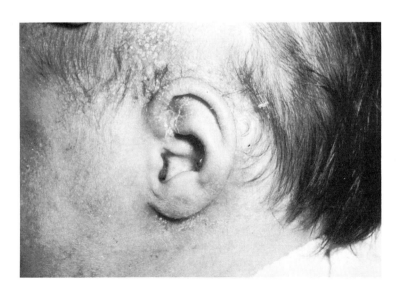

FIGURE 29-15. Greasy scale in the external ear and scalp of an infant with seborrheic dermatitis.

or restrictions may suggest clues to possible iatrogenic dietary deficiencies. The older individual may relate flares of dermatitis to specific items of food, but it is necessary to evaluate carefully the accuracy of these observations. In the studies by Sampson, a poor correlation between personal history of a reaction to a specific food and a positive double-blind food challenge was shown. The onset or exacerbation of dermatitis coincident with a move to a different house, installation of a new carpet, or acquisition of a new pet will suggest environmental factors. It is important to identify not only possible allergens in the environment but also materials, such as wool carpets or bubble baths, which may irritate the skin and intensify the pruritus.

It is important to determine the frequency and type of bathing. Adolescent and adult patients will commonly take frequent hot baths or showers, since the pruritus is relieved in hot water. However, on questioning, they will all admit that they itch worse after the bath or shower.

Physical Examination. Performing a physical examination on a small child with generalized dermatitis often is a trial for the physician. Frequently, the child is unhappy, irritable, resists examination, cries incessantly, and scratches paroxysmally when the clothing is removed. Height and weight measurements are important, since children may show growth retardation apparently associated with the disease or with therapy, including dietary restrictions. On first inspection, the presence of atopic

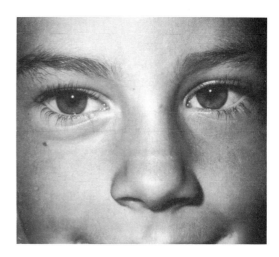

FIGURE 29-17. Transverse nasal crease resulting from the "allergic salute."

facies should be noted (Fig. 29-16). These consist of central facial pallor, blue shadows under the eyes ("allergic shiners"), and a distinct single or double pleat on the lower eyelids (Morgan lines). There also may be a transverse line on the nose, which results from the constant rubbing and pushing upward of the tip of the nose ("allergic salute") (Fig. 29-17).

The distribution of the dermatitis may provide a clue to causative factors; open weeping areas or pustules may be signs of skin infection. A diagram of involved areas is useful. The degree of dryness present in the skin that is not actually inflamed should be noted. The response of the skin to stroking with a blunt instrument, such as a tongue blade, also can be determined during the examination. Since AD frequently coexists with respiratory allergy, the ears should be examined by pneumatic otoscopy, the membranes of the nose should be examined for signs of nasal allergy, and the lungs should be examined for wheezing. If spleen or liver is palpable, it should be noted; the temperature of extremities relative to the environmental temperature should be noted. Observe also the length of the nails. In extensive dermatitis, generalized adenopathy is not unusual.

LABORATORY STUDIES

There are no laboratory tests that establish a diagnosis of AD. Increased levels of circulating eosinophils frequently are present, though the degree of eosinophilia does not appear to corre-

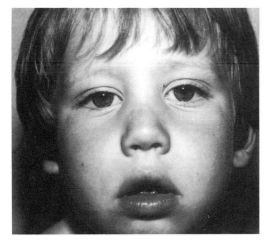

FIGURE 29-16. Allergic facies. Note central facial pallor, open mouth with exaggerated bow shape, allergic "shiners," and Morgan lines.

late with either severity of dermatitis or presence of other atopic manifestations.

A hematocrit value is important to rule out iron deficiency anemia secondary to dietary restrictions. A blood smear also should be examined to verify adequate platelets. A white blood count and differential for number of lymphocytes is appropriate. A nasal smear for eosinophils may suggest associated allergic rhinitis. Although skin infection in AD is almost invariably due to *Staphylococcus aureus,* one may wish to take cultures for antibiotic sensitivity tests. Skin responses to various pharmacologic agents and tests for immune abnormalities are detailed elsewhere, but such tests rarely are of practical use in diagnosis or treatment. Histologic examination of the skin rarely is necessary for diagnosis of AD.

Although the validity of inhalant allergen skin tests in implicating causative factors in AD is controversial, they may provide useful information in some patients. Prick skin tests with food antigens have been shown to have excellent negative predictive accuracy. Positive skin test reactions only identify which foods should be considered for challenge or elimination (in the absence of a definitive history implicating a specific food). A food challenge should not be performed in patients with histories of anaphylactic reactions to that food. Opaque capsules containing predetermined amounts of dried foods are commercially available for blind challenges. In children who have been placed on severely restricted and sometimes nutritionally inadequate diets, negative food skin test reactions are useful in persuading anxious parents to liberalize the child's diet. In children with coexisting respiratory allergy, allergy testing is useful in identifying factors that are important in allergic rhinitis or asthma.

TREATMENT

General Management

The physician is advised to spend considerable time with the patient in order to convey a clear explanation of the nature of atopic dermatitis and the multitude of factors that contribute to it that the patient understands. During this initial discussion, the alert physician will make an effort to detect evidence of emotional factors that might be contributing to the problem. Latent hostility, emotional lability, and maternal overprotection often exist. The constant pruri-

tus, its disturbance of sleep of both patient and family, its impact on behavior and attention span, and its cosmetic impact all may induce psychosomatic symptoms. Further, emotional tension may increase pruritus. It is important for the physician to give friendly, sympathetic support to the parents and patient, with assurance that with appropriate care the dermatitis will not result in permanent disfigurement. The adult with severe generalized dermatitis often needs psychiatric help.

Control of Infection. When first seen, most patients with AD have secondary infections, usually due to *Staphylococcus aureus*. In fact, even when not obviously infected, patients usually are heavily colonized with this organism, which contributes to the pruritus. For this reason, most patients require systemic antibiotic therapy. Erythromycin is the drug of choice, although occasionally resistant staphylococci will necessitate the use of cloxacillin or dicloxacillin. These drugs should be given in full therapeutic doses and continued until improvement is evident, even if this takes several weeks. Patients subject to frequent relapses may require long-term maintenance therapy with the antibiotic, given at one half the therapeutic dose and finally at one fourth the therapeutic dose for many months if necessary. Topical antibiotics are ineffective and many are potentially sensitizing.

Antipruritic Medication. The antipruritic action of antihistamines is beneficial in therapy and long-term use may be necessary in management of AD. Their clinical effectiveness appears to be related in part to sedation and in part to specific antipruritic effect. Hydroxyzine appears to be the most effective. One recommendation is to begin with 10 mg every 6 hours, increasing the dose 5 mg every 3 to 5 days until itching is minimized or intolerable side effects (e.g., sleepiness, lethargy) occur. Since patients with AD itch more at night, it is advisable to double or even triple the bedtime dose. In fact, in some patients, it is possible to minimize side effects with acceptable therapeutic effects, with a single, moderate to large dose at night. Children tolerate this drug better than adults. If increased doses of hydroxyzine do not give sufficient nighttime relief, diphenhydramine (Benadryl) in doses of 25 to 50 mg can be added at bedtime because of its greater sedative effect. It is important to emphasize that antihistamines must be prescribed on a regular basis to help or control pruritus, thus interrupting the itch-scratch cycle. Antihistamines never should be applied topically because of the risk of sensitization and secondary contact dermatitis.

Environmental Control. Specific irritants and allergens should be eliminated from the house. The patient allergic to house dust or animal danders can develop an exacerbation of dermatitis from direct contact with these substances. Details of environmental control are discussed in Chapter 18. Irritating and rough clothing, especially woolens, should be avoided, as should occlusive synthetic-fabric clothing. Cotton and some softer synthetics are preferable for the atopic patient. Cold weather, hot humid weather, and rapid temperature changes also may increase itching. New clothing and sheets should be washed prior to use to remove sizing and other chemicals with which they may have been treated. Harsh enzymatic detergents and fabric softeners should be avoided, and clothes rinsed thoroughly.

Sweating. Another important factor in the production of pruritus is any increased stimulation to sweating. Atopic dermatitis is associated with a degree of sweat retention that will produce itching. Therefore, excessive clothing, high environmental temperature, and physical activity predispose the patient to sweat retention pruritus.

Diet. Dietary management may be useful in patients with AD, particularly those with severe involvement, as discussed previously. Properly controlled food challenges may be difficult to perform in the physician's office. Elimination diets may be helpful, but efficacy is often difficult to gauge, because of physician, patient, and parent biases. When feasible, food challenges are suggested.

Hyposensitization. There is little evidence that allergen immunotherapy is helpful in controlling AD, although it may benefit the patients who has coexisting respiratory allergy. When used for this purpose in a patient with AD, it should be administered cautiously since it may exacerbate the dermatitis if the antigen concentration is increased too rapidly.

Systemic Corticosteroids. Oral or intramuscular corticosteroids should be avoided in the treatment of AD. On rare occasions, a burst of systemic steroid may be necessary for initial control of a very severe dermatitis while instituting proper general and topical therapy. However, it should be kept in mind that the dermatitis often flares when the steroid is stopped.

Topical Therapy

Acute Phase. When AD is seen in the acute phase, with inflammation, oozing, and crusting, it is important to recognize that secondary infection usually is present and that systemic antibiotic therapy must be instituted promptly. Reduction of inflammation and removal of crust and exudate are best done with intermittent, cool, wet, and open dressings applied over the inflamed skin. This practice reduces inflammation, decreases pruritus, and aids in the removal of crust and exudate. Two or three layers of gauze, Kerlix, or linen are thoroughly moistened with Burow solution and loosely applied to the involved areas for 15 to 30 minutes, 4 times daily. The dressings are dipped in the solution every 10 minutes during application to prevent drying and sticking. Burow solution (aluminum acetate, 1:40) is prepared by dissolving one tablet or packet of Domeboro in a quart of cool tap water. Therapy with wet compresses should not be used for more than 3 days.

Subacute and Chronic Phase. The prime feature of treatment in this phase is the complete avoidance of bathing with water. The dry skin of AD is due to a lack of sufficient water in the stratum corneum. The drier the skin, the greater the pruritus. Washing with water removes the water-soluble substances that retain water in the horny layer, resulting in increased dryness and itchiness after bathing. The treatment program is carried out as follows:

1. There should be *no* bathing with either soap or water. The only exception to this no-bathing rule is the use of a moist washcloth to cleanse the groin and axillary areas if necessary.

2. The entire skin surface is cleansed at least twice daily with a nonlipid cleansing lotion, consisting primarily of cetyl alcohol, sodium laurel sulfate, propylene glycol, and water (Cetaphil). The lotion is applied liberally and rubbed in until it foams. It is then gently wiped off, leaving a film, which aids in the retention of water in the horny layer without causing poral occlusion.

3. No oily or greasy lubricants or topical preparations are allowed. They are occlusive and increase sweat retention, thus intensifying pruritus. Avoid tar preparations; they can be irritating and may cause folliculitis and promote infection.

4. Inflamed or pruritic areas of the skin are treated with topical application of corticoste-

roid creams not ointments. In adults, one may begin use with a mid-strength steroid, such as triamcinalone (Kenalog or Aristocort), but in infants and small children, it is best to begin use with 1-percent hydrocortisone. These may be applied even three or four times daily at first. All acutely inflamed areas should clear promptly with the topical steroid preparation provided all aspects of management are adhered to. If these areas fail to clear, infection or noncompliance may be the cause.

5. After acutely inflamed areas have responded, improvement can be maintained by adhering to the no-bathing routine and Cetaphil cleansing. Topical steroids are then needed only occasionally (usually twice daily) when there is a brief flare of the dermatitis. When the skin has remained clear of eruption for several months, a brief cool bath is allowed once or twice monthly, always followed by a liberal application of the lipid-free lotion. Most patients can tolerate a brief, lukewarm bath as often as once weekly after their skin has remained clear for several more months. Cetaphil lotion must be continued daily and indefinitely for cleansing and lubricating. An occasional patient whose dermatitis has cleared but whose skin remains excessively dry, in spite of the use of Cetaphil, may use a relatively nongreasy emollient, such as Carmol-10.

Many dermatologists continue to adhere to the older method of hydrating the skin by frequent bathing followed by liberal application of heavy emollients, such as petrolatum. Even though this method ignores the drying effect of water bathing and the sweat retention contributed to by the lubricants, it is apparently successful in many cases. This effectiveness may be observed particularly in dry climates in which frequent (at least daily) baths followed by the use of emollient creams for hydration or, if the dermatitis is active, corticosteroid creams are successful.

PROPHYLAXIS

Prospective studies have been performed that examine the predictive value of cord blood IgE in newborns of atopic parents (Businco et al., 1983). Cord IgE levels were significantly higher in those infants who subsequently developed atopic disease, including AD. Dietary factors seemed to influence the development of atopy in these infants with elevated cord IgE. Of those infants with cord blood IgE levels over 0.8 IU/ml, 90 percent who were fed cow's milk developed atopic manifestations as compared with 37.5 percent who were exclusively breast-fed.

As with many other areas of research on AD, studies examining the dietary prophylaxis of the development of AD and atopic disease are conflicting and controversial (Chapter 21). A possible pathogenetic mechanism, explaining the improvement or prophylaxis of AD (when it occurs) with antigen avoidance, is the demonstration of increased intestinal permeability to macromolecules in AD. The number of different solid foods given in the first 4 months of life also seems to predispose the child to the subsequent development of AD. In the absence of conclusive information, it is prudent to consider breast-feeding with a controlled maternal diet and delayed introduction of solid foods in high risk infants, for the prophylaxis of AD and other allergic diseases.

PROGNOSIS

It is a common misconception that most affected children will outgrow dermatitis by 2 or 3 years of age. For many patients, this is a lifelong disease. *At least 50 percent of children with AD at age 2 years will have dermatitis into adulthood.* Most adults whose disease started in early childhood will have relatively mild expressions of their problems, such as hand or foot dermatitis or merely dry skin that itches easily, which may result in minor flares in response to stress. Those adults with persistent severe generalized dermatitis usually require psychiatric attention. Atopic dermatitis also is a harbinger of upper or lower respiratory atopic disease or both in as many as 75 percent of cases.

REFERENCES

Abramson, J.S., Dahl, M.V., Walsh, G: Antistaphylococcal IgE in patients with atopic dermatitis. J. Am. Acad. Dermatol. 7:105, 1982.

Aly, R., Maibach, H.I., Shinefield, H.R.: Microbial flora of atopic dermatitis. Arch. Dermatol. 113:780, 1977.

Atherton, D.S., Soothill, J.F., Sewell, M., Wells, R.S., Chilvers, C.E.C.: A double-blind controlled crossover trial of an antigen-avoidance diet in atopic eczema. Lancet 1:401, 1978.

Blank, I.H.: Factors which influence the water content of stratum corneum. J. Invest. Dermatol. 18:433, 1952.

Businco, L., Marchetti, F., Pellegrini, G., Perlini, R.: Predictive value of cord blood IgE levels in "at-risk" newborn babies and influence of feeding type. Clin. Allergy 13:503, 1983.

Chandra, R.K., Baker, M.: Numerical and functional deficiency of suppressor T cells precedes development of atopic eczema. Lancet 2:1393, 1983.

Chapman, M.D., Rowntree, S., Mitchell E.B., Di Prisco de Fuenmajor, M.C., Platts-Mills, T.A.E.: Quantitative assessments of IgG and IgE antibodies to inhalant allergens in patients with atopic dermatitis. J. Allergy Clin. Immunol. 72:27, 1983.

Cooper, K.D., Wuepper, K.D., Hanifin, J.M.: T cell subset enumeration and functional analysis in atopic dermatitis. Clin. Res. 28:566, 1980.

Copeman, P.W.M.: Eczema and keratoconus. Brit. Med. J. 2:977, 1965.

Cormia, F.E.: The basis of itching. J. Pediatr. 66:207, 1965.

Dahl, M.V., Cates, K.L., Quie, P.G.: Neutrophil chemotaxis in patients with atopic dermatitis without infection. Arch. Dermatol. 114:544, 1978.

Elliott, S.T., Hanifin, J.M.: Delayed cutaneous hypersensitivity and lymphocyte transformation. Arch. Dermatol. 115:36, 1979a.

Elliott, S.T., Hanifin, J.M.: Lymphocyte response to phytohemagglutinin in atopic dermatitis. Arch. Dermatol. 115:1424, 1979b.

Fischer, T.J., Rachelefsky, G.S., Gard, S.E., Stiehm, E.R.: Defective monocyte chemotaxis in atopic dermatitis. Ann. Allergy 38:308, 1977.

Furukawa, C.T., Altman, L.C.: Defective monocyte and polymorphonuclear leukocyte chemotaxis in atopic disease. J. Allergy Clin. Immunol. 61:288, 1978.

Giustina, T.A., Chan, S.C., Thiel, M.L., Baker, J.W., Hanifin, J.M.: Increased leukocyte sensitivity to phosphodiesterase inhibitors in atopic dermatitis: Tachyphylaxis after theophylline therapy. J. Allergy Clin. Immunol. 74:252, 1984.

Gleich, G.R.: The late phase of the immunoglublin in E-mediated reaction: a link between anaphylaxis and common allergic disease? J. Allergy Clin. Immunol. 70:160, 1982.

Graham, P., Hall-Smith, S.P., Harris, J.F.M., Price, M.L.: A study of hypoallergenic diets and oral sodium cromoglycate in the management of atopic eczema. Brit. J. Dermatol. 110:457, 1984.

Halpern, S.R., Sellars, W.A., Johnson, R.B., Anderson, D., Saperstein, W., Reisch, J.D.: Development of childhood allergy in infants fed breast, soy or cow's milk. J. Allergy Clin. Immunol. 51:139, 1973.

Hanifin, J.M.: Atopic Dermatitis. J. Allergy Clin. Immunol. 73:211, 1984.

Hanifin, J.M., Rogge, J.L.: Staphylococcal infections in patients with atopic dermatitis. Arch. Dermatol. 113:1383, 1977.

Hemels, H.: The effect of propranolol on the acetylcholine-induced sweat response in atopic and non-atopic subjects. Brit. J. Dermatol. 83:313, 1970.

Henocq, E., Gaillard, J.: Cutaneous basophil hypersensitivity in atopic dermatitis. Clin. Allergy 11:13, 1981.

Heskel, N.S., Chan, S.C., Thiel, M.L., Stevens, S.R., Casperson, L.S., Hanifin, J.M.: Elevated umbilical cord leukocyte cyclic adenosine monophosphate-phosphodiesterase activity in children with atopic parents. J. Am. Acad. Dermatol. 11:422, 1984.

Hill, H.R., Kaplan, E.L., Dajani, A.S., Wannamaker, L.W., Quie, P.G.: Leukotactic activity and nitroblue tetrazolium dye reduction by neutrophil granulocytes from patients with streptococcal skin infection. J. Infect. Dis. 129:322, 1974.

Hoffman, D.R., Yamamoto, F.Y., Geller, B., Haddad, Z.: Specific IgE antibodies in atopic eczema. J. Allergy Clin. Immunol. 55:256, 1975.

Johansson, S.G.O., Bennich, H.H.: The clinical impact of the discovery of IgE. Ann. Allergy 48:325, 1982.

Juhlin, L., Michaelsson, G.: Cutaneous vascular reactions to prostaglandins in healthy subjects and in patients with urticaria and atopic dermatitis. Acta Derm. Venereol. 49:251, 1969.

Juto, P., Engberg, S., Winberg, J.: Treatment of infantile atopic dermatitis with a strict elimination diet. Clin. Allergy 8:493, 1978.

Leung, D.V.M., Parkman, R., Feller, J., Wood, N., Geha, R.S.: Cell-mediated cytotoxicity against skin fibroblasts in atopic dermatitis. J. Immunol. 128:1736, 1982.

Leung, D., Saryan, J.A., Frankel, R., Lareau, M., Geha, R.S.: Impairment of the autologous mixed lymphocyte reaction in atopic dermatitis. J. Clin. Invest. 73:1482, 1983.

Leyden, J.J., Marples, R.R., Kligman, A.M.: Staphylococcus aureus in the lesions of atopic dermatitis. Brit. J. Dermatol. 90:525, 1974.

Lobitz, W.C., Campbell, C.J.: Physiologic studies in atopic dermatitis. I. The local cutaneous response to intradermally injected acteyl choline and epinephrine. Arch. Dermatol. Syph. 67:575, 1953.

Michaelsson, G.: Cutaneous reactions to kallikrein and prostaglandins in healthy and diseased skin. Thesis. Uppsala, Soderstrom and Finn, 1969.

Mihm, M.C., Soten, N.A., Dvorak, H.F., Austen, F.K.: The structure of normal skin and the morphology of atopic eczema. J. Invest. Dermatol. 67:305, 1976.

Mitchell, E.B., Chapman, M.D., Pope, F.M., Crow, J., Jouhal, S.S., Platts-Mills, T.: Basophils in allergen-induced patch test sites in atopic dermatitis. Lancet 1:127, 1982.

Mitchell, E.B., Crow, J., Rowntree, S., Webster, A., Platts-Mills, T.: Cutaneous basophil hypersensitivity to inhalant allergens in atopic dermatitis patients: Elicitation of delayed responses containing basophils following local transfer of immune serum but not IgE antibody. J. Invest. Dermatol. 83:290, 1984.

Oglesby, R.B., Black, R.L., vonSallmann, L., Bunim, J.J.: Cataracts in patients with rheumatic diseases treated with corticosteroids. Arch. Ophtholmol. 66:625, 1961.

Platts-Mills, T.A.E., Mitchell, E.B., Rowntree, I., Chapman, M.D., Wilkins, S.K.: The role of dust mite allergens in atopic dermatitis. Clin. Exp. Dermatol. 8:233, 1983.

Rajka, G.: Atopic Dermatitis. Major Problems in Dermatology, vol. 3. Philadelphia, W.B. Saunders Co., 1975.

Reed, C.E., Busse, W.W., Lee, T.P.: Adrenergic mechanisms and the adenylcylcase system in atopic dermatitis. J. Invest. Dermatol. 67:333, 1976.

Rogge, J.L., Hanifin, J.M.: Immunodeficiencies in severe atopic dermatitis. Arch. Dermatol. 112:1391, 1976.

Rosenthal, S.R.: Histamine as the chemical mediator for cutaneous pain. J. Invest. Dermatol. 69:47, 1977.

Roth, H.L., Kierland, R.R.: The natural history of atopic dermatitis. Arch. Dermatol. 89:209, 1964.

Sampson, H.A.: The role of immediate food hypersensitivity in the pathogenesis of atopic dermatitis. J. Allergy Clin. Immunol. 71:473, 1983.

Sampson, H.A., Albergo, R.: Comparison of results of skin tests, RAST, and double-blind, placebo-controlled food challenges in children with atopic dermatitis. J. Allergy Clin. Immunol. 74:26, 1984.

Sampson, H.A., Jolie, P.L.: Increased plasma histamine concentrations after food challenges in children with atopic dermatitis. N. Engl. J. Med. 311:372, 1984.

Seligmann, B., Fletcher, M.P., Gallin, J.I.: Histamine modulators of human neutrophil oxidative metabolism, locomotion, degranulation, and membrane potential changes. J. Immunol. 130:1902, 1983.

Snyderman, R., Robers, E., Buckley, R.H.: Abnormalities of leukotaxis in atopic dermatitis. J. Allergy Clin. Immunol. 60:121, 1977.

Sulzberger, M.B.: Atopic dermatitis: Its clinical and histologic picture. *In* Baer, R.L. (ed.), Atopic Dermatitis. New York, New York University Press, 1955.

Sulzberger, M.B., Hermann, F.B., Borota, A.: Studies of sweating. VI. Urticariogenic properties of human sweat. J. Invest. Dermatol. 21:293, 1953.

Szentivanyi, A.: The beta-adrenergic theory of the atopic abnormality in bronchial asthma. J. Allergy 42:203, 1968.

Wheatley, V.R.: Secretions of the skin in eczema. J. Pediatr. 66:200, 1965.

Winkelmann, R.K.: Nonallergic factors in atopic dermatitis. J. Allergy 37:29, 1966.

30

Contact Dermatitis
FRANK PARKER M.D.

PATHOGENESIS

Contact dermatitis is an inflammatory reaction of the skin induced by external substances coming in contact with the skin. When an agent causes contact dermatitis, reactions occur as a result of one of two processes. If the substance injures the skin by direct toxic action (e.g., damage from strong alkali and acids), an "irritant contact dermatitis" results. In contrast the second process, "allergic contact dermatitis," is an acquired immune reaction that results from contact with allergens that are abundant in the environment. The immune reaction is cell mediated (delayed-type hypersensitivity); small molecular componds (usually 500 daltons molecular weight) that act as haptens penetrate the stratum corneum and then combine or conjugate with autologous proteins of the skin to form a complete antigen. In order to induce an allergic reaction, the antigen is processed by epidermal Langerhans cells, which are dendritic, functionally immunocompetent, Ia-bearing macrophages with Fc-IgG and C3 receptors on their surface. It then is presented, in suitable form, on the surfaces of the Langerhans cells that bear immune response associated surface antigens (HLA-DR) for which T lymphocytes have specific surface receptors complementary to the physiochemical features of the antigen (Stingl, 1980). To trigger the process of sensitization, only a few T lymphocytes, bearing receptors that are complementary to the contact antigen and receptors for the HLA-DR antigen on the Langerhans cell membrane, need to be present at the exposed skin site. After this specific interaction, the activation and amplification of the sensitization process are controlled by the release of several substances from Langerhans and epidermal keratinocytic cells, including interleukin-1 (lymphocyte-activating factor) and interleukin-2 (lymphocyte-proliferating factor, which causes activated T lymphocytes to proliferate).

T lymphocytes, "induced" by exposure to a contact antigen, migrate from the epidermis to local lymph nodes. These T lymphocytes undergo further proliferation in the paracortical region of the nodes, generating large numbers of specific sensitized T effector and memory cells. Descendants of these lymphocytes enter the blood and are carried to all parts of the lymphoid system. Repeat contact with the sensitizer, no matter where it is applied to the skin, results in the movement of sensitized lymphocytes from the circulation into the area of contact, inducing an inflammatory reaction, generally 48 hours after the exposure (delayed-type hypersensitivity reaction). Thus, this process almost invariably results in the entire skin becoming hypersensitive to the contact allergen.

The importance of Langerhans cells in the sensitization process can be seen from the correlation of the ability to induce contact allergic sensitization in various areas of skin with the density of Langerhans present; in addition, ultraviolet light both alters the function of Langerhans cells and inhibits the induction of contact hypersensitivity (Bergstresser, 1980; Okamoto, 1981).

CLINICAL FEATURES AND PATHOLOGY

Though allergic sensitization can develop as soon as 7 to 10 days after first contact with an allergen, frequently it does not develop for many years. Once allergy develops and as long as it persists, subsequent encounters with the sensitizer produce dermatitis within 24 to 72 hours at any place on the skin where contact occurs. Contact allergies, once induced, tend to persist indefinitely.

It is difficult to differentiate allergic contact dermatitis from irritant dermatitis clinically and pathologically (Rostenberg, 1957). However, several features may help to distinguish between irritant and allergic contact reactions, as outlined in Table 30–1. Everyone exposed to an irritating substance in sufficient concentration will develop irritant dermatitis, whereas only a small percentage of individuals exposed to an antigen will develop allergic dermatitis. Irritant reactions are localized to the precise area of contact. Moreover, an erythematous or bullous eruption appears within a few hours of contact

TABLE 30-1. Factors Helping to Distinguish Between Irritant and Allergic Contact Dermatitis

	Irritant	Allergic
Number of patients affected	Many who come in contact	Few who come in contact
Extent of dermatitis	Localized closely to areas of contact	Spread of dermatitis beyond exact areas of contact
Time of reaction after contact	Within a few hours of exposure, depending on strength of irritant	24 to 72 hours after exposure
Skin reaction	Red, scaling—if very acute, bullous; often painful; may itch	Often red and vesicular; *itches*

with an irritant, whereas an allergic contact reaction characteristically appears 24 to 72 hours after exposure.

The acute phase of contact dermatitis, whether allergic or irritant, is characterized by redness, swelling, and formation of papules due to vascular dilatation, perivascular infiltration of lymphocytes, and dermal edema. As the inflammatory reaction proceeds, intra-epidermal edema (spongiosis) occurs, leading to vesicle formation. With disruption of vesicles, the skin weeps, oozes, and crusts (Fig. 30–1). Pruritus is an invariable and intolerable associated symptom, particularly of an allergic contact reaction. As the dermatitis becomes chronic, the skin undergoes lichenification (leathery thickening with accentuation of skin lines) and develops fissures and scales (Fig. 30–2).

Initially, allergic contact dermatitis is confined to the site of allergen contact, and its unique distribution pattern often suggests the diagnosis of contact reaction (See Fig. 30–2).

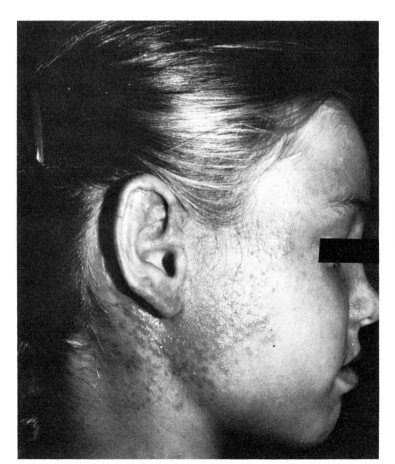

FIGURE 30-1. An acute, weeping allergic contact dermatitis caused by applications of a cream containing neomycin for otitis externa.

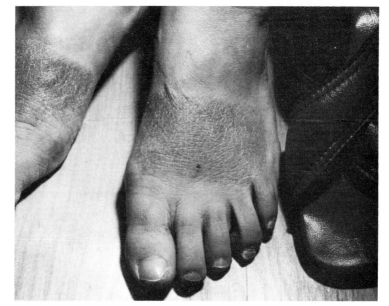

FIGURE 30-2. Chronic eczema, with lichenification of the skin. Note the sharp borders to the skin reaction, outlining the areas where sandal straps came in contact with the skin. This is an allergic contact dermatitis to paraphenylenediamine used in the leather.

Thus, reactions on ears, particularly the helix, may be due to shampoos or hair sprays. Otitis externa may be caused by sensitizing medications applied to the ear canals, particularly neomycin (Jensen et al., 1966) (see Fig. 30-1). Often, the piercing of ear lobes is a precipitating factor in nickel sensitivity. The penis and scrotum may react to sensitizers (e.g., poison oak) conveyed to these areas by the hands. The vulvar and perivulvar areas may be sites of reaction to sensitizers in bubble baths. Reactions on the feet may be mediated by sensitivity to rubber-containing substances, dyes, or metals used in the manufacture of shoes (see Fig. 30-2). In severe cases, the dermatitis initially localized to areas of allergen contact will disseminate over wide areas of the body (so-called autoeczematization), so that the dermatitis may not conform precisely to areas of the first allergen contact (Parish et al., 1965).

Occasionally, contact dermatitis may have a clinical appearance different from that described (Fregert, 1974). Certain rubber-containing chemicals can cause purpura-like dermatitis. Zirconium and beryllium can cause granulomatous dermatitis. Certain contactants, particularly neomycin and nickel, have been reported to produce a "dermal" contact reaction in which the eczematous element is absent, but an edematous, urticaria-like inflammation occurs.

Some of the most common sensitizers causing allergic contact dermatitis are noted in Table 30-2. These allergens cause allergic contact dermatitis in patients of all ages. Certain topical medications that produce sensitization in adults, such as mercury, benzocaine, and antihistamine, also produce dermatitis in children. Often, concentrations of medications that are

TABLE 30-2. The Most Common Sensitizers

Rhus
   Poison ivy, oak, sumac
Para-phenylenediamine
   A chemical used in hair and fur dyes, leather processing, rubber vulcanizing, and printing inks which cross reacts with "azo" and aniline dyes, "caine" preparations, and sulfonamides
Nickel compounds
   Earrings, zippers, metal clips
Rubber compounds
   Mercaptobenzothiazole (in shoes)
Ethylenediamine
   Commonly used as a preservative in various cream medications, such as antihistaminic creams and ophthalmic solutions
Dichromates
   Used in textile inks, paints, and leather processing in shoes*
Perfumes
   Fragrances in cosmetics, detergents, fabric softeners, toothpastes
Balsam of Peru
   Balmex baby powder, emollient, lotion; Diaprex ointment
Neomycin
   Antibiotic in powder or ointment (Mycolog)
Other
   Thiomerosal (Merthiolate) and Merbromin (Mercurochrome)

* Fisher, A. A.: Contact Dermatitis, 3rd ed., Philadelphia, Lea & Febiger, 1986.

not sensitizing in adults produce dermatitis in children.

Many household substances, including polishes, waxes, solvents, detergents, disinfectants, and insecticides, are potent irritants. Highly perfumed oils, soaps, and powders also can cause dermatitis, especially in body folds where these preparations may accumulate. For this reason, the use of nonperfumed oils, powders, and soaps free of antiseptics is recommended for infants and obese children and adults. When an infant begins to crawl, dermatitis of the legs, knees, and elbows can develop as a result of exposure to floor wax or polish, rough rug fabrics, and dust. Coveralls prevent these reactions.

TYPES OF CONTACT DERMATITIS

Diaper Dermatitis

Diaper dermatitis, the most common form of dermatitis in infancy, appears as erythema or, in severe cases, as papulovesicular areas or even eroded bullae over the external genitalia and buttocks that become secondarily infected. This dermatitis often spares the creases. The eruption can spread to include the lower half of the abdomen and thighs. In male infants, the reaction may occur as a urethral-meatal ulcer, causing painful urination. Diaper dermatitis is produced by prolonged contact with urine, feces, residual antiseptics, soaps, or detergents in the diapers. Many workers have implicated ammonia produced by bacteria in the urine and stool as the irritative substance, but this mechanism of diaper rash has probably been overemphasized (Jacobs, 1978).

The management of diaper dermatitis includes frequent changes of diapers, with careful cleaning with mild soap and water to rid the skin of urine and feces. Occlusive plastic clothing materials over diapers should be avoided. The new types of diapers with inner linings of synthetic hydrophobic fibers that allow passage of urine to the outer cotton layers keep the skin relatively dry and free of urine. When the diaper area is severely inflamed, the skin can be cleaned with mineral or olive oil rather than soap and water. Topical steroids, such as 1 percent hydrocortisone cream several times a day, and frequent use of a thick protective paste, such as zinc oxide ointment, will decrease the inflammatory response and protect the inflamed skin from direct contact with urine and feces. Occasionally, if 1 percent hydrocortisone cream does not cause improvement in the dermatitis, stronger fluorinated topical steroid preparations can be used 2 to 3 times a day for short periods of time (5 to 7 days). Longer use may cause severe dermal atrophy and stria formation and possibly may cause systemic effects by steroid absorption through the inflamed skin.

Other causes of diaper dermatitis include moniliasis, seborrheic dermatitis, impetigo, atopic dermatitis, and psoriasis. In general, when the eruption involves sites of the most intimate contact with the diaper, such as the convexities of the buttocks, medial thighs, and perineum, with sparing of the folds, contact dermatitis is the likely cause. In infancy, irritant dermatitis is most common, whereas contact allergy becomes more likely later. Sharply demarcated rashes in the folds suggest intertrigo due to sweat retention, heat, and moisture, often with secondary bacterial infection. Seborrheic dermatitis often manifests in this way and can be diagnosed if "cradle cap" is found, together with an erythematous rash in the axillae, neck folds, and retroauricular areas. If satellite, erythematous-based pustules are seen studding the borders of the lesions in the folds, *Candida* infection is likely. A band of erythema at the margins of the diapers, so-called tide mark dermatitis, is characteristic of an irritant reaction to recurring wetting and drying at the borders of the diapers. Large vesicles and bullae in the diaper area often are due to bullous impetigo.

Foot Dermatitis

Dermatitis of the feet may be caused by allergic sensitization to material in the shoes, particularly rubber (monobenzyl ether of hydroquinone, an antioxidant; tetramethylthiuram, an accelerator), leather (potassium dichromate and formaldehyde, tanning agents; paraphenylenediamine, dying agent), or metal (nickel sulfate) in the toes of some shoes. Most frequently, shoe dermatitis begins on the dorsal aspect of the big toe with eventual extension to other toes and then onto the feet, with sparing of the interdigital webs, instep, and flexural creases of the toes. Usually the dermatitis is symmetric (see Fig. 30–2).

In children, eczematous reactions on the feet often are not allergic contact reactions but are related to friction from tight-fitting shoes or to excessive perspiration, in which case the eruption often is on the toes and interweb areas, owing to maceration from unabsorbed sweat (Fisher, 1986; Gibson, 1963). Another common eczematous reaction of the feet in children is chronic scaling and fissuring over the soles of the feet and toes, related to atopic dermatitis. The so-called juvenile plantar dermatosis is a distinctive symmetric fissuring dermatitis that affects the weight-bearing surfaces of the feet in prepubertal children. Most of these patients are hyperhidrotic, and some are atopic without evidence of contact allergy. The thick stratum corneum of the affected areas cracks and fissures as a result of wetting (hyperhidrosis in enclosed shoe wear) and drying. Topical corticosteroids and a change to natural fiber socks and cooler shoes give good control (Steck, 1983). Although tinea pedis can mimic eczematous reactions, fungal infections of the feet are unusual in young, prepubertal children.

Contact dermatitis of the feet must be diagnosed by appropriate patch tests. If identified, the allergens may be avoided by wearing cotton liners, surgitubes, or Kellenex inside shoes or square toe socks.* If this mechanical protection does not help, special made-to-order shoes, free of the specific allergens, can be purchased.† Allergic contact dermatitis of the feet will respond to topical fluorinated steroid ointments several times a day, with occlusive plastic wrapping at night. This increases the humidity under the wraps, accelerating the penetration of topical steroids. Frequent use of emollients between the steroid applications prevents dryness and fissuring.

Since hyperhidrosis often predisposes the patient to the development of "shoe dermatitis," the control of hyperhidrosis in occlusive shoe wear may minimize dermatitis. Zeasorb powder (Stiefel) dusted into shoes and stockings may lessen perspiration. Drysol (Person & Covey), which is 20 percent aluminum chloride in ethyl alcohol, also can be effective in treating excess sweating by applying the solution every evening overnight. Tea (tannic acid) foot baths are another approach to hyperhidrosis, which also serve to calm acute dermatitis; four tea bags boiled in 1 quart of water for 10 minutes provide a solution in which to soak the feet for 30 minutes a day.

*True Last, J.W. Landenberger and Co., 3800 Castor Avenue, Philadelphia, Pennsylvania 19124.
†Foot-So-Port Shoe Company, Oconomowoc, Wisconsin 53006 or Julius Alfshul, Inc., 117–125 Graltan Street, Brooklyn, New York 11237.

Clothing Dermatitis

Contact dermatitis in children can be caused by woolen clothing or rough cuffs and collars, which, when wet, readily irritate the skin. Residues of soap and detergents in laundered clothes also can cause irritant dermatitis. A variety of substances in clothing can intiate contact dermatitis. Untreated natural and synthetic fabrics and fibers used in the manufacture of clothing seldom cause skin problems, but a variety of chemicals, such as durable-press finishes, dyes, rubber additives, chromates, nickel, and glues, added to these fibers during their manufacture and assembly into garments are the likely etiologic agents. The distribution of allergic contact dermatitis from clothing conforms to a pattern that coincides with the places on the skin where the garment fits most snugly. Variations in styling of men's and women's clothing explain differences seen in distribution. Men more likely have a neck dermatitis from stiffened dress shirt collars. Women who have durable press or dye dermatitis develop reactions of the anterior and posterior axillary folds from dress or shirt fabrics. Pants cause dermatitis on the inner and anterior thighs and the popliteal fossae.

It should also be recalled that poison oak and ivy oleoresins may cling to clothing and retain their dermatitis-producing potential for many days. Therefore, each time the clothing is worn it may begin a new bout of contact dermatitis. Washing the clothes will remove the oleoresins.

Diagnosing dermatitis due to clothing depends upon recognizing the distribution of the dermatitis that conforms to wearing apparel and upon patch testing to the various likely substances that cause such reactions. Patch testing with a piece of the suspect fabric may be most accurate, especially if the fabric is soaked in water 10 minutes before applying to the skin for 48 hours. Once it is determined that dermatitis is produced by specific wearing apparel, these clothes should be avoided. New clothing made of 100 percent polyester, acrylic, or cotton usually is well tolerated. The additional use of topical steroids and emollients will bring the dermatitis readily under control.

Soap and Detergent Dermatitis

Subacute primary irritant dermatitis is often brought about by frequent use of soap and water, prolonged bubble baths, use of excessive amounts of bubble bath concentrations, too frequent bathing, or a combination of these factors. Children with atopic dermatitis who normally tend to have xerotic skin often are severely affected. The commonest cause of chronic hand dermatitis is seen in housewives or persons involved in professions requiring constant exposure to water and soaps or detergents. This dermatitis is characterized usually by dryness, fissuring, and thickening of the skin rather than by vesicles. So-called housewife's eczema is an example of this problem, but medical personnel, dentists, bartenders, dishwashers, and canners may experience similar irritant hand dermatitis. Atopic eczema per se may involve the hands, but these so affected individuals are particularly susceptible to the drying effects of soaps and water. It is estimated that 65 percent of atopic individuals who do "wet work" develop dermatitis of the hands (Lammintausta, 1981). They should use soaps containing added oils, as well as emollients frequently, to treat this form of dermatitis.

Cosmetic and Medication Dermatitis

In addition to the dermatitis acquired by adults through direct contact with cosmetics, infants and children may acquire dermatitis through contact with cosmetics worn by the mother and other attendants or applied in plays. Adolescent girls, particularly, may experiment with a broad range of cosmetics. Perfume, lipstick, nail polish, and hair dye all can cause allergic reactions, which can be identified with patch tests to the various suspected substances. The physician should alert the patient with suspected contact allergy to cosmetics about the allergenic substances that may be found in them, such as preservatives, benzophenones, propylene glycol, fragrances, and dyes. Patch tests to confirm these suspicions should be done, and the patient with positive reactions should then avoid cosmetics with the specific substances in them. Often, these substances are listed on the cosmetics; the trend is toward requiring manufacturers to list the various substances in each cosmetic. If ingredients are not listed, it may be necessary to write to specific manufacturers to determine if offending materials are used in their cosmetic lines. Aside from para-phenylenediamine hair dyes, preparations that contain formaldehyde or its resins, and cosmetics that contain parabens or photosensitizers, the bulk of cosmetics in general use are "hypoallergic," since the products have been carefully screened before being marketed.

The application of various over-the-counter and prescription topical medications to cuts, scratches, bites, or sunburns can induce allergic contact dermatitis. Common offending substances in these topical preparations include various "caine" substances (benzocaine, surfacaine, metycaine), antihistamines (tripelennamine, diphenhydramine, antazoline), antibiotics (especially penicillin, streptomycin, neomycin), and ethylenediamine (Table 30–2).

Local anesthetics, especially benzocaine, found in a variety of anti-itch, anti-sunburn, and anti-poison oak preparations are particularly potent sensitizers and readily cross react with para-phenylenediamine (hair dye), sulfonamides, and "azo" dyes, as well as with para-aminobenzoic acid (PABA) found in sunscreens. Xylocaine (lidocaine) and Carbocaine (mepivacaine) are not related to the other "caines" and do not commonly cause contact dermatitis.

Topical antihistamines also cause allergic dermatitis, whereas oral antihistamines seldom cause sensitization. However, if the patient was previously sensitized topically, oral antihistamines may cause a generalized skin reaction. The common use of calamine lotion with diphenhydramine added (Caladryl) is to be condemned, as this may cause contact allergic reactions. The antihistamines antazoline, promethazine, and tripelennamine are ethylenediamine derivatives and are active topical sensitizers.

Ethylenediamine is one of the most common skin sensitizers in the United States. It is present in many ophthalmic solutions and may be a common cause of contact dermatitis of the eyelids. Ethylenediamine cross reacts with aminophylline (a combination of theophylline and ethylenediamine). The administration of aminophylline to patients previously topically sensitized to ethylenediamine causes generalized dermatitis, though these patients tolerate theophylline without reactions.

Topical antibiotics, particularly penicillin, neomycin, and streptomycin, are potent sensitizers (Rees, 1964). Penicillin and streptomycin never should be used topically. Neomycin is present in a host of creams, ointments, and other topical medications as well as in some cosmetics (Epstein, 1958). Once a person is topically sensitized to neomycin, systemic administration of streptomycin or kanamycin—both of which cross react with neomycin—may cause generalized dermatitis (Epstein and Wenzel, 1962). Neomycin commonly induces sensitization when applied for otitis externa (see Fig. 30–1) or for conditions in which the skin is inflamed and damaged (e.g., stasis dermatitis). Erythromycin rarely induces topical sensitization and can be used safely on the skin.

Propylene glycol is commonly used as a vehicle for topical therapeutics, cosmetics, and various hand and body lotions. In recent years, new vehicles based on fatty alcohol-propylene glycol combinations have been developed for topical corticosteroids (especially creams). In certain preparations, the amount of propylene glycol may be as high as 70 percent. Further, propylene glycol has been used as the only base for some antiperspirants. Both irritant and allergic contact reactions occur in response to propylene glycol; allergic reactions to potent topical steroid creams have been reported. A confusing clinical picture may result in that a patient with underlying eczema (such as atopic dermatitis) becomes worse with the application of steroid creams. Steroid ointments have less propylene glycol than the creams and tend not to be sensitizers. Otic preparations (VoSol Otic) and even K-Y Jelly contain propylene glycol and have been frequent causes of allergic contact dermatitis. The physician should always inquire as to what the patient or the patient's parents have been applying to any primary dermatitis.

Plant Dermatitis

Poison ivy, sumac, and oak are common causes of allergic contact dermatitis in children.

Poison ivy (*Rhus*) dermatitis is a summer disease caused by contact with the oleoresin of the plant. Frequently pets, particularly long-haired dogs, contact the plant and transmit the oleoresin to a child. Ingestion of poison oak oleoresin or marked cutaneous involvement may induce acute nephritis. Often the streaks of dermatitis where the plant has rubbed against the skin suggest the diagnosis (Fig. 30–3).

Other plants, such as chrysanthemum, pyrethrum and ragweed, as well as products of plants (e.g., turpentine, an oleoresin of pine; terpene, a limorene of lemon or lemon oil; and resins and balsams, of balsam of Peru, which contain cinnamic acid, a common sensitizer) cause allergic contact dermatitis. The Compositae family of plants (ragweed, chrysanthemum, pansy, sunflower) and liverworts contain sesquiterpene lactones, which are potent allergic sensitizers capable of causing widespread intense dermatitis of the hands, arms, and face mimicking photodermatitis.

Vicks Vaporub contains several plant substances (oil of turpentine, oil of eucalyptus, and oil of cedar) that may irritate or sensitize skin.

Topical steroids usually will control plant dermatitis, but in severe and extensive cases, a short course of oral steroids may be necessary.

Perioral Dermatitis

In children, the lips and adjacent skin are commonly irritated. Often this is caused by a habit of licking. Saliva trapped between the thumb and mouth of a thumb-sucking child may produce dermatitis of the lips and cheeks.

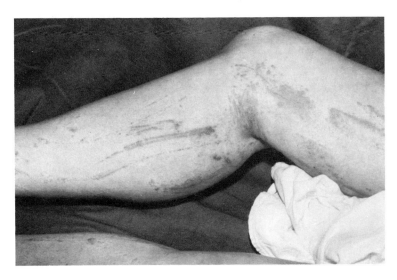

FIGURE 30–3. An acute contact dermatitis on the legs. Note the "lines" of erythema and vesicles where the leaves of a poison ivy plant brushed along the legs of this sensitive individual.

Similarly, children who are salivating because of tooth formation and eruption may suffer facial dermatitis. Children whose eating habits permit foods, such as spinach, carrots, and citrus fruits, to remain on the cheeks may suffer perioral dermatitis due to the irritation by the foods' juices. This dermatitis may closely resemble atopic eczema. Rubber-sensitive children may acquire perioral dermatitis from chewing rubber pencil erasers or rubber bands.

Topical 1-percent hydrocortisone cream and adherent pastes, such as zinc oxide, will clear the dermatitis and serve as a protective barrier to saliva or irritating fluids.

Atopic Dermatitis and Contact Dermatitis

Rarely, atopic infants who are allergic to eggs or fish acquire marked edema, urticaria, and flare of the atopic eczema of the skin or oral mucosa from contact with eggs or fish. Although children with atopic dermatitis are no more likely to develop contact dermatitis to potential sensitizers than other children (indeed, there is some evidence that such children are less readily sensitized to topical substances), they often develop contact allergic reactions because of frequent exposure to topical medications during their long courses of therapy. It is important that physicians who care for these patients not administer potential sensitizers. Patients and parents must be warned about the use of proprietary medications that contain substances which carry a high risk of sensitization. They especially should avoid the use of topical antibiotics (e.g., neomycin), antifungals, particularly nystatin (Mycolog) cream, antihistaminics, ethylenediamine, and propylene glycol–containing medications.

DIAGNOSIS AND TREATMENT

Patch Testing

The patch test is indispensable in proving the cause of allergic contact dermatitis. However, it should not be performed when the dermatitis is acute or extensive. This test may cause an exacerbation of the dermatitis. Systemic corticosteroid therapy, even in doses sufficient to suppress the dermatitis, will not completely suppress a strongly positive patch test reaction. Patients can be patch tested reliably while receiving oral steroids (O'Quinn and Isbell, 1969). Similarly, oral antihistaminics do not significantly influence the patch test reaction. However, topical corticosteroids can be suppressive and should be avoided in the area of patch testing for several days before testing.

Patch testing is performed by applying standard and suspected antigens on adhesive strips

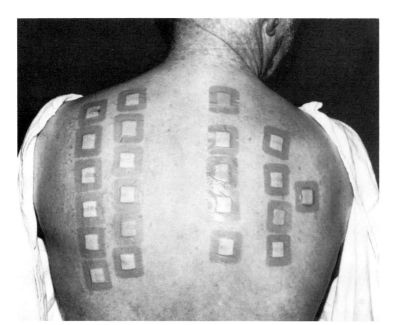

FIGURE 30–4. A series of patch tests in place over the upper back.

to the back, where they should be kept in place for 48 hours (Fig. 30–4). Tests are then read 20 minutes after removing the patches. As a rule, the site of a positive reaction itches and appears as vesicles on an edematous red base, exactly outlining the area covered by the allergen (Fig. 30–5). When there is a questionable reaction, such as mild erythema, it is worthwhile reexamining the site 72 to 96 hours later (Fisher, 1986). Redness that persists or increases probably signifies an allergic reaction. Erythema that fades in 24 hours is most likely not due to an allergic reaction. The following grading system is conventional:

No erythema	0
Erythema	1+
Erythema and papules	2+
Erythema, papules, and vesicles	3+
Marked edema and vesicles	4+

Positive patch test reactions may be due to irritants, but in general, irritants burn rather than itch; they induce a skin reaction sooner than do sensitizers. Strong irritants can cause a reaction in a few hours. A primary irritant reaction tends to remain confined to the site of application and fades rapidly after the site has been uncovered, whereas an allergic reaction tends to spread beyond the site, persists, and even becomes more intense for several days after the patch is removed.

Treatment of Contact Dermatitis

After the diagnosis of acute contact dermatitis is made by patch testing, the offending antigen and any substances that cross react with the antigen should be removed from the patient's environment.

The dermatitis is treated to control the inflammation and itching. Topical steroids and, in cases of severe widespread reactions, oral steroids are begun immediately. In addition, application of cool wet compresses (plain water or Burow solution, 1 : 20 dilution) for 10 to 15 minutes, three times a day in the acute, vesicular, oozing, and weeping stages of the dermatitis rapidly dries up the vesicles and oozing, relieves the itching, and debrides and cleans the skin surface. In the chronic phase, when the dermatitis is dry, lichenified, and fissured, application of topical steroid ointments and emollients between steroid applications will resolve the inflammation and alleviate the dryness.

Oral antipruritic medications, such as hy-

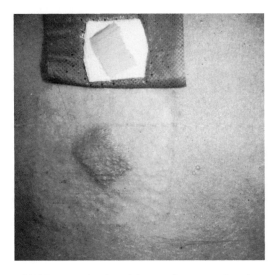

FIGURE 30–5. A 3+ positive patch test reaction showing erythema, papules, and vesicles of the skin, precisely mimicking the eczematous reaction.

droxyzine, cyproheptadine, and diphenhydramine hydrochloride, all are useful in helping control the intolerable itching associated with the dermatitis. Secondary infection (impetiginization) of the dermatitis is a common finding; if present, it should be treated with appropriate systemic antibiotics.

REFERENCES

Bergstresser, P.R., Toews, G.B., Gilliam, J.N., Streilein, J.W.: Unusual numbers and distributions of Langerhans cells in skin with unique immunologic properties. J. Invest. Dermatol. 74:312–314, 1980.

Epstein, S.: Dermal contact dermatitis from neomycin. Ann. Allergy 16:268–280, 1958.

Epstein, S., Wenzel, F.J.: Cross sensitivity to various "mycins." Arch. Dermatol. 86:183–194, 1962.

Fisher, A.A.: Contact Dermatitis, 3rd ed., Philadelphia, Lea & Febiger, 1986.

Fisher, A.A., et al.: Allergic contact dermatitis due to ingredients of vehicles. Arch. Dermatol. 104:286–290, 1971.

Fregert, S.: Manual of Contact Dermatitis. Scandinavian University Books, Munksgard, Copenhagen, 1974.

Gibson, W.B.: Sweaty sock dermatitis. Clin Pediatri. 2:175–177, 1963.

Jacobs, A.H.: Eruptions in the diaper area. Pediatri. Clin North Am. 25:209–224, 1978.

Jensen, C.O., Allen, H.J., Mordecai, L.R.: Neomycin contact dermatitis superimposed on otitis externa. J.A.M.A. 195:175–179, 1966.

Lammintausta, K., Kalimo, K.: Atopy and hand dermatitis in hospital wet work. Contact Dermatitis 7:301–308, 1981.

Okamoto, H., Horio, T.: The effect of .8-methoxypsoralen and long-wave ultraviolet light on Langerhans cell. J. Invest. Dermatol. 77:345–346, 1981.

O'Quinn, S.E., Isbell, K.H.: Influence of oral prednisone on eczematous patch test reactions. Arch. Dermatol. 99:380–389, 1969.

Parish, W.E., Rook, A.J., Champion, R.H.: A study of autoallergy in generalized eczema. Brit. J. Dermatol. 77:479–526, 1965.

Rees, R.B.: Cutaneous reactions to antibiotics. J.A.M.A. 189:685–686, 1964.

Rostenberg, A., Jr.: Primary irritant and allergic eczematous reactions. Arch. Dermatol. 75:547–558, 1957.

Steck, W.D.: Juvenile plantar dermatosis: the "wet and dry foot syndrome." Cleve. Clin. Q. 50:145–149, 1983.

Stingl, G.: New aspects of Langerhans cell function. Internatl. J. Dermatol. 19:189–213, 1980.

31

Urticaria and Angioedema

ALAN SCHOCKET, M.D.

Urticaria (hives) and angioedema are common medical problems that occur at some time in about 20 percent of the population. Although rarely life-threatening, they often are distressing problems for both patient and physician. It is helpful for the physician to be familiar with the clinical features, pathogenesis, etiology, and differential diagnosis to enable an organized approach to evaluation and management (Julin, 1981; Mathews, 1983). An essential part of the management is patient education both to enlist the patient's aid as an observer in the search of an etiology and to take an active and enlightened role in management.

CLINICAL FEATURES

Distribution, Duration, and Appearance

Urticarial lesions most commonly appear on the trunk but may appear on any part of the body. There frequently is a central area of superficial edema, i.e., a wheal of 1 to 2 cm in diameter, which may coalesce and become extremely large ("giant urticaria"). This is surrounded by a variable amount of erythema termed the "flare" which may be flat or have a raised border. Hives are almost always pruritic and may be intensely so. Individual hives may last 2 to 3 hours but not longer than 48 hours. Lesions lasting over 48 hours may represent papular urticaria secondary to insect bites, urticarial vasculitis, or another dermatologic condition, such as erythema multiforme. Most patients usually have only one or two acute episodes of urticaria during their lifetimes. However, a small percent develop daily chronic hives, lasting months to years, a form termed chronic urticaria. Forty percent of patients have urticaria alone, 50 percent have associated an-

gioedema and about 10 percent have only angioedema (Warin and Champion, 1974). Angioedema is a deeper, less circumscribed swelling, which more frequently affects areas of loose connective tissue with numerous mast cells, such as the face, eyelids, lips, tongue, and extremities. It is rarely pruritic but may be painful, burning, or paresthetic. The time course of angioedema is similar to urticaria.

CLASSIFICATION

Urticaria can be divided into three main types (acute, chronic, and physical), each of which has different etiologic, prognostic, and therapeutic implications.

Acute urticaria. This is the most frequent type. Most patients have a single to a few individual episodes. In general, younger age groups usually are affected. It frequently is seen in children and more frequently in the atopic population. There is often a specific cause, although in a single or sporadic episode, a cause may not be readily identifiable. For example, hives that develop a short time after a meal could represent a reaction to any number or combination of ingestants. For a single episode, which may never recur, extensive evaluation is hardly worthwhile. If, on the other hand, the episode is serious or associated with a systemic anaphylactic reaction, a more intensive evaluation may be indicated.

Chronic urticaria. This is defined as persistent or recurrent urticaria lasting longer than 6 weeks. It is less common than acute urticaria and is seen more frequently in older patients with a peak incidence from 40 to 60 years. Children also are affected, however (Harris et al., 1983). The incidence is higher in females than males, and the classic patient is a middle-aged female. There is no association with other atopic diseases. In most studies of chronic urticaria, a specific cause is identified in less than 20 percent of cases. Therefore, continual prolonged suppressive therapy with antihistamines or other drugs usually is required. Episodes may last from months to years and often remit as mysteriously as they appear. Although chronic urticaria usually is a cutaneous disease alone, symptoms involving other systems may be seen as follows: gastrointestinal (nausea, vomiting,

415

cramps, diarrhea), pulmonary (dyspnea), musculoskeletal (myalgias, arthralgias), and nervous (headache). Malaise, fever, and elevated sedimentation rates also occur.

Physical urticaria. Physical urticaria includes a variety of syndromes induced by application of physical stimuli, which include pressure, exercise, and extremes of temperature. The hives may be confined to the area of stimulus, such as in dermographism and cold urticaria, or may occur diffusely, as in exercise-induced or cholinergic urticaria. In most cases, urticaria develops within one-half hour after the stimulus, although in rarer types, such as delayed pressure urticaria, vibratory angioedema, and familial cold urticaria, the lesions develop several hours after exposure. In some cases of physical urticaria, such as cold and exercise-induced urticaria, the exposure may be so extensive that anaphylaxis may result (Kaplan et al., 1981). Individual types of physical urticaria are discussed in more detail at the end of this chapter.

DIFFERENTIAL DIAGNOSIS

There are several other cutaneous disorders that should be considered in the evaluation of the patient with urticaria and angioedema.

Papular urticaria is caused by insect bites (mosquitoes, gnats, ants). It resembles hives in its appearance, especially with the associated pruritus, but is not considered true urticaria. There frequently is more local inflammation, and the lesions persist longer and are often distributed on the lower legs. *Erythema multiforme* may resemble urticaria in its earlier stages. The lesions last longer, resemble a target (erythema with surrounding pallor), may become bullous, and often involve the palms and soles. It usually is a self-limited disease and is treated symptomatically with topical corticosteroids and antihistamines for itching. Severe involvement, such as Stevens-Johnson syndrome, may require systemic corticosteroids. *Scabies* is caused by infestation with mites, resulting in erythematous papules that are extremely pruritic, especially at night. Characteristic distribution includes the webs of the fingers, flexor aspects of the wrists, axillae, buttocks, scrotum, and breasts. Involvement may be more extensive in children. Some patients may develop secondary urticaria. Treatment (e.g., Kwell, Eurax) is directed at eliminating the mite infestation. *Cellulitis* can mimic angioedema al-

TABLE 31–1. Types and Causes of Pruritus

Local
  Pruritus ani, pruritus vulvae
  Neurodermatitis
  Herpes zoster
Generalized
  Xerosis (dry skin)
  Endocrine dysfunction: hyper- and hypothyroidism, diabetes mellitus, hyperparathyoidism
  Biliary obstruction, cholestasis
  Uremia
  Neoplasm: lymphoreticular, polycythemia vera, carcinoma, carcinoid syndrome
  Pregnancy
  Parasitic infestations
  Allergic reactions
  (?) Psychogenic

though the presence of fever, leukocytosis, pain, and erythema points to this diagnosis. In contrast to angioedema, the lesion gradually worsens without therapy. If this diagnosis is uncertain but still considered, antibiotics should be employed. *Hereditary angioneurotic edema* (HAE, C1 esterase inhibitor deficiency) is a rare disorder, which may cause localized edema (vide infra). In contrast to other forms of angioedema in which the onset to the peak of swelling usually is rapid, in HAE progression is more gradual, reaching its peak over several hours. The presence of hives virtually excludes the diagnosis of HAE. *Edema* secondary to cardiac, renal, or hepatic disease commonly is symmetric, dependent, pitting, nontender, and nonpruritic. The diagnosis usually is apparent from physical examination and laboratory results. *Other* uncommon possibilities include lymphedema, superior mediastinal syndrome, and periorbital edema associated with trichinosis; all usually persist longer than angioedema. Rare diseases include Melkersson-Rosenthal syndrome (lip swelling, fissured tongue, recurrent facial palsies) and Muckle-Wells syndrome (urticaria, deafness, renal amyloidosis). *Pruritus* alone should be included in the differential diagnosis of urticaria. The list of causes is extensive (Table 31–1). Generalized pruritus may be a manifestation of a systemic disease (Gilchrest, 1982). In severe cases, an extensive evaluation may be warranted.

PATHOPHYSIOLOGY

Histology. The histology of the urticarial lesion is not distinctive. The dermis is edematous with separation of the collagen bundles in the superficial dermis, flattening of the rete pegs, and widening of the dermal papillae. There may be small vessel dilatation, with minimal perivascular infiltrates of round cells or eosinophils. An increase in cutaneous mast cells in chronic urticaria has been reported (Natbony et al., 1983). In some patients with chronic urticaria, a more intense perivascular cellular infiltrate can be seen (Phanuphak et al., 1980), and findings consistent with vasculitis have been described (Monroe, 1981). The lesion of angioedema is similar to urticaria but involves the deeper area of the dermis and subcutaneous tissue.

Mediators. The wheal and flare (hive), which develop spontaneously, can be reproduced in normal skin by intracutaneous injection of histamine. This phenomenon was first described as the "triple response" (wheal, flare, and axon reflex) in the early 1900's by Sir Thomas Lewis (1927). Normally histamine, along with other vasoactive peptides and precursors, is stored in granules within mast cells in various tissues including the skin and in basophils found predominately in the circulation (Wasserman, 1983). With activation of these cells, histamine and other mediators are released from these granules into the surrounding tissue or plasma. These mediators induce increased capillary permeability (the wheal or swelling), vasodilatation (erythema or "the flare"), and irritation of nerve endings (pruritus), resulting in the clinical hive or angioedema.

Mechanisms of mast cell activation. There are three major mechanisms for activation of the mast cell. Immune activation occurs through interaction of antigen with IgE antibody on the surface of the mast cell. When two or more IgE molecules are bridged by the corresponding specific antigen, mediator release occurs. This mechanism is seen in urticarial reactions to drugs, such as penicillin; foods, such as peanuts; and grass (causing contact urticaria). Previous exposure and sensitization to the antigen and IgE production are required. Immune release via the action of *complement activation components C3a and C5a* (anaphylatoxins) also occurs. These complement components are capable of directly activating mast cells. Examples of this reaction include hives occurring during a serum sickness reaction and hives associated with systemic lupus erythematosus. In both cases, complement is activated by circulating immune complexes, which then ac-

tivates mast cells nonspecifically. IgE usually is not involved. Certain compounds also can act *nonspecifically* on mast cells (Paton, 1957). This can occur in all individuals, if exposed to sufficient amounts of such agents. However, patients with increased numbers of mast cells (mastocytosis, urticaria pigmentosa) may be particularly susceptible (Sutter et al., 1967). Examples of compounds capable of this reaction include drugs, such as narcotics, curari, and polymixin B; detergents such as compound 48/80; certain foods, such as strawberries and shellfish; and endogenous peptides, such as endorphins, substance P, and vasoactive intestinal peptide (Foreman and Jordan, 1983).

Etiology. In all forms of urticaria, the underlying cause may be difficult to identify. In acute urticaria, the patient often makes the cause-effect association without having to consult a physician. Unless the reaction is severe, an extensive evaluation in acute urticaria is neither useful nor cost effective, since it is likely that the hives will not recur. In chronic urticaria, however, the necessity for maintenance suppressive therapy with its side effects justifies a more aggressive attempt to find an avoidable or treatable etiology. Unfortunately, even with extensive evaluation, the etiology is determined in a minority of patients with chronic urticaria. A thorough history and physical examination are the cornerstones of a systematic evaluation of possible etiologies of all forms of urticaria. The following is a list of categories of etiologic factors to be considered in the evaluation of patients with urticaria (Table 31–2).

Drugs are the most common identifiable cause of urticaria. Drug-induced urticaria can be produced by any one of the various mechanisms described. Penicillin, the most common and best studied drug, can produce a full blown anaphylactic reaction or urticaria within min-

TABLE 31–2. Possible Causes of Urticaria and Angioedema

Drugs
Foods and Food Additives
Infections
Insect Bites and stings
Contactants
Inhalants
Systemic diseases
   Endocrine
   Collagen-vascular
   Malignancy
Hereditary angioneurotic edema (HAE)
Physical urticaria

utes of administration via an IgE-mediated allergic mechanism. Urticaria also can be a part of a later onset (hours to days) penicillin-induced serum sickness syndrome. This may develop days after discontinuation of therapy. When dairy cows were routinely treated with penicillin to prevent mastitis, penicillin in milk was a rare cause of chronic urticaria in sensitive patients. This should not be a problem now, since the treatment of dairy cattle with penicillin is illegal is most states. Other notable drugs that induce allergic reactions include hormones (insulin, ACTH, growth hormone) and larger heterologous proteins (horse serum, antitoxins). Almost any drug, however, is capable of inducing urticaria. As noted, drugs capable of directly activating mast cells include narcotics (codeine, morphine), curari, polymixin B, thiamine, and radiocontrast dye. Some drugs, such as nonsteroidal anti-inflammatory drugs (NSAIDS), do not release mediators but will cause exacerbations in 20 to 30 percent of patients with chronic urticaria (Doeglas, 1975). The mechanism is unknown. Adrenergic antagonists such as propranalol also may exacerbate urticaria and potentiate anaphylaxis (Jacobs et al., 1981). These drugs should be avoided, if possible, in patients with chronic urticaria.

The evaluation of patients for drug sensitivity should begin with a complete history specifically addressing previous drug reactions, including any possible cross sensitivity to drugs recently used. Sulfa sensitivity, for example, may involve sensitivity to certain diuretics and oral hypoglycemic agents, which are sulfa derivatives. Unless addressed directly, patients often do not consider proprietary formulations including vitamins, laxatives, aspirin, and hormones (thyroid or oral contraceptives) as drugs. With a few exceptions (penicillin, insulin, hormones), skin testing for drugs is unsatisfactory. Observation of remission of symptoms on discontinuation of medications, and substituting an alternative structurally unrelated medication if necessary provides useful information. Rechallenge may be informative, but is too dangerous in many cases. In sensitive patients in whom readministration of the drug is necessary, desensitization may be required (Chapter 53).

Foods and food additives are other commonly encountered causes of urticaria, especially acute urticaria, seen more frequently in children and atopic individuals. Reactions usually are IgE-mediated. The most common foods implicated are peanuts, nuts, seafood, dairy products, soybeans, and fruits. The occurrence of mouth itching or gastrointestinal symptoms after ingestion of a food suggests sensitivity to a specific ingestant.

As with drugs, some foods are capable of releasing mediators from mast cells nonspecifically. Consumed in sufficient quantities, foods such as tomatoes, strawberries, and shellfish can induce urticaria in some patients without "allergic" sensitivities. Attention recently has been focused on the causative role of yeasts and food additives in urticaria. Several anecdotal reports and uncontrolled studies have implicated various preservatives (benzoates, sulfites, BHA, BHT), food dyes (tartrazine, coal-tar derivatives), yeasts (*Candida*, baker's), natural substances (salicylates), and flavorings (MSG, saccharin) as causes of acute and chronic urticaria (Michaelsson and Juhlin, 1973; Doeglas, 1975). There is no doubt that this occurs, but probably less frequently than has been suggested. To establish cause, provocation tests are necessary (Genton et al., 1985).

The diagnosis of food sensitivity can often be made by the patient in the most obvious cases of sensitivity. On the other hand, the diagnosis may not be substantiated even by challenge, despite a good history. Problems arise when a reaction is delayed, occurs after ingestion of a meal of several foods at once, or requires a concomitant factor, such as exercise or pressure stimulus (dermographism, delayed pressure urticaria). These often are the situations in which direct challenge with a suspected substance is negative. To evaluate a patient for food sensitivity, several different approaches may be required. If reactions occur less than 2 to 3 times weekly, keeping a food diary is cost effective and at least focuses the patient on foods. Unfortunately, it only occasionally identifies the offending food. For more frequent or daily symptoms, elimination diets, artificial nutrients (e.g., Vivonex, Nutramigen), or fasting from 3 days to 1 week will provide useful information. If the symptoms do not resolve over the period of elimination (at least 3 to 7 days) an ingestant sensitivity can be virtually excluded. If symptoms resolve, challenges with the suspected foods determined by history, skin tests, or radioallergosorbent test (RAST) should be undertaken. Open food challenges are useful screening tests, but a double-blind challenge format, with a placebo control to eliminate bias, is the most definitive diagnostic method. Food skin testing (prick or scratch) sometimes is helpful in identifying an unsuspected food sensitivity, but positive reactions require confirmation by challenge. If a food or ingestant is identified, the most effective therapy is avoidance. In patients with multiple food or additive sensitivities, a severe elimination diet may cause nutritional deficiencies, especially in children. For this reason, sensitivities should be well-documented and consultation with a dietitian, if necessary, should be sought in order to ensure a nutritionally adequate diet. Other treatments, such as rotating diets, sublingual drops, and injection therapy, have no scientific basis and should not be used until efficacy has been established convincingly.

Infectious causes are common especially for acute or self-limited urticaria. The underlying mechanisms are not clear, although some episodes are related to a serum sickness–like syndrome, such as that seen in the prodromes of hepatitis B (Alpert et al., 1971) and infectious mononucleosis (Africk and Halprin, 1969). Some reports have related chronic urticaria to occult chronic bacterial infections, such as abcesses (dental) or vaginal infections, but these are uncommon. Other acute and chronic infections associated with urticaria include ECHO, coxsackie virus, cytomegalovirus, infectious mononucleosis, and hepatitis. Urticaria has been associated with nonspecific febrile illnesses, pharyngitis, and kidney infection. Although an association between chronic urticaria and infection with helminths (*Ascaris, Trichinella, Schistosoma*) and protozoa (amoeba, *Giardia, Trichomonas,* malaria) has been described, it is rare even in endemic areas (Pasricha et al., 1972). The presence of eosinophilia and elevated IgE level suggests this possibility and warrants at least an analysis of a stool sample for ova and parasites and possibly further serologic or skin testing.

Insect bites and stings are causes of acute urticaria. Urticarial reactions can be part of a systemic reaction to Hymenoptera (insect) stings and are warnings of potential fatal anaphylactic reactions on subsequent stings. Appropriate evaluation with skin tests with the possibility of immunotherapy for reactors and, at the very least, an emergency kit that includes a syringe preloaded with epinephrine (Ana-Kit, Epi-Pen) should be prescribed. As previously mentioned, papular urticaria (mosquito, gnat bites) and pruritic rash of scabies are part of the differential diagnosis of hives.

Contact urticaria is seen in highly sensitive individuals. Patients very sensitive to inhalants, such as animal dander or grass pollen, can develop local urticaria on contact with the antigen. Industrial chemicals, medications, and cosmetics also can cause contact urticaria. A positive response on patch testing with the appropriate antigen is diagnostic (Fisher, 1982).

Psychogenic urticaria is a questionable entity. Although chronic urticaria can induce anxiety and depression and emotional factors may exacerbate hives, there are no well-documented cases of urticaria due to psychogenic factors alone. Psychotherapy may be useful for some patients but is not likely to be curative.

Inhalant urticaria has been described, but poorly documented. This syndrome might be a result of a reduction in the threshold by which release of mast cell products can be induced ("priming effect") during inhalant allergy (hay fever) season. However, urticaria can result from direct contact with factors causing inhalant allergies, e.g., the grass sensitive patient who walks through a field of tall grass.

Underlying systemic disease can be associated with the occurrence of urticaria, especially chronic urticaria. In addition to infection, major disease categories include connective tissue disease, endocrine dysfunction, and malignancy. Some cases involve complement activation by immune complexes, but in most, mechanisms by which urticaria is induced are unknown. Seven percent of patients with systemic lupus erythematosus develop hives. Urticaria also is seen in rheumatoid arthritis. The syndrome of "urticarial vasculitis" is part of the differential diagnosis of chronic urticaria with systemic symptoms, especially when individual hives persist over 48 hours. In these so-affected patients, skin biopsy specimens reveal vasculitis involving post-capillary venules similar to those in Henoch-Shöenlein purpura (Soter, 1977). Other manifestations of this syndrome include fever, arthralgias, arthritis, elevated sedimentation rate, nephritis (rarely), and hypocomplementemia (occasionally) (Monroe, 1981). Some patients have precipitins to Clq, the first component of complement (Zeiss et al., 1980). Patients with severe disease often require corticosteroid therapy, although reports describe successful results with NSAID, hydroxychloroquine (Plaquenil) (Lopez et al., 1984), and dapsone. A skin biopsy is required to establish the diagnosis.

Endocrine disorders associated with urticaria include hyper- and hypothyroidism, thyroiditis, diabetes, and hyperparathyroidism. Treatment of the underlying disease usually produces resolution of the hives. Exacerbation of chronic urticaria with menses and pregnancy also has been described, and allergic sensitivity to progesterone has been reported (Meggs et al., 1984).

Concern over the presence of an occult malignancy in patients with chronic urticaria often leads to an extensive, unrewarding work-up. This association is uncommon but has been reported with polycythemia vera, chronic myelogenous leukemia, mastocytosis, lymphoreticular malignancies, and carcinomas. This development of a wheal and flare after stroking a pigmented skin macule (Darier sign) indicates urticaria pigmentosa, a benign disease seen mainly in children (Dennis, 1963). Episodes of severe flushing and hypotension with or without urticaria suggest systemic mastocytosis. In this disease, episodes can also be induced by administration of nonspecific histamine-releasing drugs, such as narcotics and curari (Sutter et al., 1967).

Hereditary angioneurotic edema (HAE) is a rare autosomal dominant disease resulting from a deficiency of the inhibitor of complement activation, C1 esterase inhibitor (C1-INA). This inhibitor also is important as a regulatory protein in the clotting, fibrinolytic, and inflammatory systems. Eighty-five percent of patients have inadequate levels of C1-INH; the remaining 15 percent have normal or elevated levels of a nonfunctional protein (Frank et al., 1976). There also are case reports of acquired C1-INH deficiency associated with malignancy. Although this disease often is considered in the differential diagnosis of chronic urticaria, *urticaria is not a feature of this disease*, and its presence virtually excludes the diagnosis of HAE. Two thirds of patients with HAE develop symptoms before age 13, but onset after age 50 has been reported.

Clinically, attacks are characterized by the gradual onset of swelling in any area of the body, frequently sites of trauma or infection. Suffocation can be caused by laryngeal swelling; this is the most common cause of premature death in these patients. Laryngeal involvement is heralded by hoarseness, and tracheostomy may be lifesaving. Visceral involvement with edema of the bowel has led to unnecessary laparotomy. Attacks are self-limited, lasting 2 to 3 days, unaccompanied by fever or leukocytosis, and unaffected by corticosteroids, epinephrine, or antihistamines. Definitive diagnosis is made by measuring C1-INH levels. Since C4 levels are consistently depressed, even between attacks, measurement of C4 is a good screening test. Finding of a normal level essentially eliminates the diagnosis of HAE. Treatment of acute attacks is symptomatic and supportive. In patients with infrequent mild attacks, prophylaxis for surgical or dental procedures with 2 units of fresh frozen plasma or the antifibrinolytic agent epsilon-aminocaproic acid (EACA) is adequate. In patients with severe or frequent attacks, long-term prophylactic therapy is recommended. Androgenic agents (danazol, stanozolol) alter regulator genes resulting in increased C1-INH production, reducing or eliminating attacks. Side effects from these agents include masculinization in females and children. In prepuberal children, chronic therapy with EACA is an effective alternative, although C1-INH levels are unaffected (Brickman and Hosea, 1983).

DIAGNOSIS

A complete history with special attention to the etiologic factors previously described is the most important diagnostic tool in the evaluation of the patient with urticaria. A thorough physical examination may uncover an underlying systemic disease or physical urticaria. In general, extensive, routine laboratory screening for the urticaria patient is not cost effective (Jacobson et al., 1980). The laboratory data and x-ray findings should be utilized, however, for follow-up of abnormalities on history and physical examination. If the patient is refractory to routine antihistamine therapy, more extensive evaluation may be undertaken. Immunologic testing and skin biopsy rarely are helpful in the absence of a history suggestive of connective tissue disease or vasculitis (Phanuphak et al., 1980). Diet manipulation, challenges, and skin testing are useful in selected cases.

THERAPY

Treatment of urticaria depends upon severity of symptoms. Scattered or mild hives are self-limited and usually require no treatment, or at most a mild antihistamine, such as diphenhydramine, 25 to 50 mg, or chlorpheniramine, 4 mg, P.O. every 4 to 6 hours. If the urticaria is generalized and severe with angioedema, it should be treated in a similar fashion to an anaphylactic reaction. In addition to the antihistamines, the mainstay of therapy in this case is subcutaneous epinephrine (1:1000 starting with 0.1 to 0.2 ml) or subcutaneous terbutaline (0.25 ml), readministering the drug every 15 minutes until symptoms improve or side effects become unacceptable. Subcutaneous injection of epinephrine suspension (Sus-Phrine) can be used for prolonged therapy, although oral ephedrine, 25 mg every 6 hours, or terbutaline, 2.5 to 5 mg every 8 hours, for three to four doses, may prevent recurrence. Unless the response to the initial adrenergic and antihistamine drugs is inadequate, corticosteroid therapy is not necessary since the onset of steroid action is delayed for several hours. If the episode is severe with associated angioedema or part of an anaphylactic reaction, the patient should be encouraged to carry and trained to use injectable epinephrine (e.g. Ana-Kit, Epi-Pen).

For management of chronic urticaria, when an etiology can be determined, avoidance of the agent and treatment of the underlying condition often is sufficient therapy. In the majority of cases, however, a cause cannot be identified.

Since the cause of *chronic urticaria* is not uncovered in 80 percent of patients, chronic symptomatic suppressive therapy ordinarily is necessary (Table 31–3). Antihistamines are the mainstay of therapy. They are most effective when a constant blood level is maintained by around-the-clock administration of shorter acting preparations or once daily administration of longer acting preparations. The major side effect, which often leads to noncompliance, is

somnolence. This can be minimized by taking a long acting antihistamine at bedtime. Hydroxyzine, 25 mg 2 or 3 times a day for adults or 5 to 10 mg 3 times a day for children, is a good starting regimen. If longer acting, more potent preparations are required, the tricyclic antidepressants are effective, especially doxepin starting with 10 mg at bedtime. The newer "nonsedating" antihistamines (e.g., terfenadine) have fewer side effects, but also are less potent. If hives continue despite adequate antihistamine therapy, sympathomimetic preparations (ephedrine, 25 mg, 3 to 4 times a day or terbutaline, 2.5 to 5 mg, 3 a times a day) are added. In adults, an H_2 antihistamine (cimetidine, 300 to 400 mg, 3 times a day, or ranitidine, 5 mg, 2 to 3 times a day) is added (Harvey et al., 1981). In some cases of delayed pressure urticaria (Sussman et al., 1982) and urticarial vasculitis (Milins, 1980), addition of a NSAID (indomethacin, 25 mg, 3 times a day) may be effective. Corticosteroids are a last resort to be used only after other agents fail. It is not unusual for patients with resistant urticaria to require high amounts of steroids administered in split daily doses, which cause maximal side effects.

The goal of symptomatic therapy is to keep the patient comfortable until the urticaria remits. About half of all urticaria patients have a single episode or short self-limited course. Most of the remaining half will have active disease, lasting 3 to 6 months. In 20 percent of these, the disease lasts 1 to 2 years; rarely, the

TABLE 31–3. Drug Therapy for Chronic Urticaria

Drug	Brand Name	Dosage for Adult	Dosage for Children
ANTIHISTAMINES			
H_1			
Hydroxyzine	Atarax Vistaril	25 mg TID to QID or 25 to 50 mg HS	Under 6: up to 10 mg QID (elixir 1 tsp = 10 mg) Over 6: 25 mg TID to QID (if necessary)
Cyproheptadine	Periactin	4 mg QID	0.25 mg/kg/day: 2 mg BID to TID (syrup 1 tsp = 2 mg)
Doxepin	Sinequan Adapin	10 to 25 mg HS 25 mg BID to TID (liquid 10 mg/ml)	Not recommended under 12 by the manufacturer
Terfenadine	Seldane	60 mg BID or TID	Not recommended under 12 by the manufacturer
H_2			
Cimetidine	Tagamet	300 to 400 mg TID	Not recommended under 12 by the manufacturer
Ranitidine	Zantac	150 mg BID	Not recommended under 12 by the manufacturer
SYMPATHOMIMETICS			
Ephedrine		25 mg TID to QID	10 to 25 mg TID
Terbutaline	Brethine Bricanyl	2.5 to 5 mg TID	Not recommended under 12 by the manufacturer

disease lasts for up to ten years (Champion et al., 1969).

PHYSICAL URTICARIA

By definition, physical urticaria is produced by a specific "physical" stimulus. Urticaria usually develops within 30 minutes of exposure to the stimulus; consequently, many patients are able to make an association between cause and effect. Physical urticaria is relatively common, affecting 15 percent of all urticaria patients. Young adults are most often affected. The reaction often can be predictably reproduced, and release of mediators can be demonstrated. Mechanisms of the reactions for the most part, however, still are poorly understood. Some forms of physical reactivity can be passively transferred with IgE in certain patients (Jorizzo and Smith, 1982). Some patients require more than a single stimulus to produce a reaction, which complicates evaluation. For example, with penicillin-induced dermographism and food-related, exercise-induced urticaria the reaction does not occur if one of the stimuli is absent.

Dermographism (factitious urticaria) is the most common type of physical urticaria, occurring in up to 5 percent of the population. It is defined as the production of greater than a 2 mm wheal on linear application of pressure ($>$4900 gm/cm²) to the skin by a key or tongue blade. In a small proportion of these patients, the local reaction is pruritic and is termed *symptomatic dermographism*. This is a more bothersome type of dermographism. It occurs more frequently in females and is not age related. Occasionally, dermographism develops following penicillin reactions, multiple insects bites, scabies, or other systemic allergic reactions, and sometimes persists for years afterward. It also is associated with endocrine disorders (diabetes, thyroid disease) and other forms of physical urticaria.

There are other distinct forms of pressure-induced lesions. In patients with chronic urticaria, hives often develop in areas of pressure (belt lines, bra straps) in the absence of demonstrable dermographism. Delayed pressure urticaria (DPU) is another syndrome that was originally described as a rare familial disorder. More recently it has been reported in some patients with chronic urticaria (Sussman et al., 1982). Lesions are erythematous, swollen, and painful. They develop 4 to 6 hours following a pressure stimulus (15 lb for 15 minutes over the shoulder). DPU is often mistaken for angioedema until a good history is obtained. Although IgE has not been implicated in DPU, the syndrome has been associated with specific food ingestion (Davis et al., 1984). A clue in this subgroup of DPU patients is the delayed reactions to food skin tests, with or without immediate wheal and flare. Some of these cases remit on avoidance of the particular food or foods. Treatment of DPU is difficult since in most patients, the DPU component is unresponsive to antihistamines. Some patients respond to NSAIDs, which should be tried in addition to antihistamine regimens. Over 50 percent of patients require daily steroids, i.e., prednisone, in doses up to 30 to 40 mg. Patients with symptomatic dermographism alone usually respond very well to hydroxyzine (10 mg to 25 mg at bedtime or up to 3 times a day) or doxepin (10 mg to 25 mg at bedtime). Hereditary vibratory urticaria is a variant of DPU.

Exercise syndromes include cholinergic urticaria and exercise-induced urticaria/anaphylaxis. Cholinergic urticaria is induced by exercise; "core heating," such as a hot bath (not local heat); sweating; and emotional stress. The characteristic urticarial lesions that develop are small, punctate, highly pruritic wheals surrounded by extensive erythema. These lesions may coalesce, however, forming more classic hives. Patients frequently have mild reversible obstructive changes on pulmonary function testing, and rarely some develop full-blown anaphylaxis (Kaplan, 1981). One diagnostic test is the intradermal injection of 0.1 mg of methacholine. A positive response requires the development of satellite wheals in addition to the wheal produced at the injection site. Although therapy with most antihistamines usually is effective, hydroxyzine (in doses of 100 to 200 mg daily) is the drug of choice.

Exercise-induced anaphylaxis/urticaria syndrome has been subclassified into two types (Sheffer et al., 1983). The first type, similar to cholinergic urticaria but without the classic skin lesions, pulmonary abnormalities, and positive methacholine skin test reaction, occurs predictably following each episode of exercise beyond a certain work level. These patients require around-the-clock antihistamines or treatment prior to exercise. Some respond to desensitization with warm baths or exercise and do well on a regular daily exercise program (Black, 1982). The other type of exercise-induced urticaria is much less predictable and often occurs without warning in someone who exercises regularly. In some cases, a second factor such as ingestion of specific foods or drugs has been implicated (Maulitz et al., 1979; Kushimoto and Toshiyuki, 1985). Despite the absence of reaction to either food or exercise alone, when the patient exercises within 8 to 12 hours of ingestion of the food, a reaction occurs. This is more frequent than is appreciated, especially in patients with sporadic allergic reactions, historically related to specific stimuli but not reproducible on rechallenge. Many of these patients have positive skin test or RAST reactions to suspected or unsuspected foods. Avoidance of the identified ingestant for at least 12 hours prior to exercise is necessary and the best form of management. In the absence of an identifiable factor, fasting for 8 to 12 hours prior to exercise may eliminate reactions. With severe reactions, exercising with a friend and carrying injectable epinephrine (e.g., Ana-Kit, EpiPen) are recommended.

Temperature-related physical urticaria includes *cold*- and *heat*-induced urticaria. Heat-induced urticaria usually falls under the category of cholinergic urticaria although patients have been described in whom urticaria could be produced by the local application of a hot stimulus such as hot water. Cold urticaria is more common and may be life-threatening. Sudden death from massive mediator release has been noted in patients with this disease who dove into a cold swimming pool, lake, or ocean. Acquired cold urticaria may develop following insect stings, viral infections, drug reactions, or even childbirth. It also is seen in association with cryoglobulinemia, cryofibrinogenemia, cold agglutinin disease, or paroxysmal nocturnal hemoglobinuria; these should be excluded in the initial work-up. Familial cold urticaria is a rare disease characterized by the delayed onset (4 to 8 hours) of a rash (classically *nonurticarial*), following generalized cold exposure.

Solar urticaria is rare and occurs usually within 30 minutes of sun exposure (Ravits et al., 1982). It sometimes results from drug ingestion (sulfonamides, tetracycline), sunburn, insect stings, infection, and underlying systemic disease such as systemic lupus erythematosus or porphyria. There are six types, depending on the wavelength of light to which the patient reacts. The most common is sensitivity to ultraviolet light (385 to 320 nm). Sunscreen often is effective therapy.

Aquagenic urticaria results from contact with water. Some patients have more than one concomitant physical urticaria, for example, combined cholinergic and aquagenic urticaria (Davis et al., 1981). Diagnosis can be very difficult, especially in these patients, unless careful challenges are performed. It is apparent that only with the identification of the urticarial stimulus or stimuli can the physician design an effective avoidance program.

REFERENCES

Alfrick, J.A., Harprin, K.M.: Infectious mononucleosis presenting as urticaria. J.A.M.A. 209:1524 1969.

Alpert, E., Isselbacher, K.J., Schur, P.H.: The pathogenesis of arthritis associated with viral hepatitis. N. Engl. J. Med. 285:185, 1971.

Black, A.K.: New approaches in treatment of physical urticarias. Clin Exp. Dermatol 7:301, 1982.

Brickman, C.N.M., Hosea, S.W.: Hereditary angioedema. Intern. J. Dermatol. 22: 141, 1983.

Champion, R.N., Roberts, S.O.B., Carpenter, R.G. Roger, J.: Urticaria and angioedema: A review of 554 cases. Brit. J. Dermatol. 81:588, 1969.

Davis, K.C., Mekori, Y.A., Kohler, P.F., Schocket, A.L.: Late cutaneous reactions in patients wiith delayed pressure urticaria (Abstract). J. Allergy Clin. Immunol. 73:183, 1984.

Davis, R.S., Remingio, L.S., Schocket, A.L., Bock, S.A.: Evaluation of a patient with both aquagenic and cholinergic urticaria. J. Allergy Clin. Immunol. 68:479, 1981.

Dennis, D.J.: The mastocytosis syndrome: Clinical and biological studies. Ann. Int. Med. 59:194, 1963.

Doeglas, H.M.: Reactions to aspirin and food additives in patients with chronic urticaria, including the physical urticarias. Brit. J. Dermatol. 93:135, 1975.

Fisher, A.A.: Contact urticaria due to medicaments, chemicals and foods. Cutis 30:171, 1982.

Foreman, J., Jordan, C.: Histamine release and vascular changes induced by neuropeptides. Agent. Act. 13:103, 1983.

Frank, M.M., Gelfand, J.A., Atkinson, J.P.: Hereditary angioedema: the clinical syndrome and its management. Ann. Int. Med. 84:580, 1976.

Genton, C., Frei, P.C., Pecoud, A.: Value of oral provocation tests to aspirin and food additives in the routine investigation of asthma and chronic urticaria. J. Allergy Clin. Immunol. 76:40, 1985.

Gilchrest, B.A.: Pruritus: Pathogenesis, therapy and significance in systemic disease states. Arch. Intern. Med. 142: 101, 1982.

Harris, A., Twarog, F.J., Geha, R.S.: Chronic urticaria in children: Course and Etiology. Ann. Allergy. 51:161, 1983.

Harvey, R.P., Wegs, J., Schocket, A.L.: A controlled trial of therapy in chronic urticaria. J. Allergy Clin. Immunol. 68:262, 1981.

Jacobs, R.L., Rake, G.W., Jr., Fournier, D.C., Chilton, R.J., Culver, W.G., Beckmann, C.H.: Potentiated anaphylaxis in patients with drug-induced beta-adrenergic blockade. J. Allergy Clin. Immunol. 68:125, 1981.

Jacobson, K.W., Branch, L.B., Nelson, H.S.: Laboratory tests in chronic urticaria. J.A.M.A. 243:1644, 1980.

Jorizzo, J.L., Smith, E.B.: The physical urticarias. Arch. Dermatol. 118:194, 1982

Juhlin, L.: Recurrent urticaria: clinical investigation of 330 patients. Brit. J. Dermatol. 104:369, 1981.

Kaplan, A.P., Natbony, S.F., Tarvil, A.P., Frudster, L.F., Foster, M.: Exercise-induced anaphylaxis as a manifestation of cholinergic urticaria. J. Allergy Clin. Immunol. 68:319, 1981.

Kushimoto, H., Toshiyuki, A.: Masked type 1 wheat allergy. Arch. Dermatol. 121:355, 1985.

Lewis, T.: The blood vessels of the human and their responses. London, Shawn and Sons, Ltd., 1927.

Lopez, L.R., Davis, K.C., Kohler, P.F., Schocket, A.L.: The hypocomplemetemic urticarial-vasculitis syndrome: Therapeutic response to hydroxychloroquine. J. Allergy Clin. Immunol. 73:600, 1984.

Mathews, K.P.: Urticaria and angioedema. J. Allergy Clin. Immunol. 72:1, 1983.

Maulitz, R.M., Pratt, D.S., Schocket, A.L.: Exercise-induced anaphylaxic reaction to shellfish. J. Allergy Clin. Immunol. 63:433, 1979.

Meggs, W.J., Pescovitz, O.H., Metcalfe, D., Loriaux, D.L., Cutler, G., Kaliner, M.: Progesterone sensitivity as a cause of recurrent anaphylaxis. N. Eng. J. Med. 311:1236, 1984.

Michaelsson, G., Juhlin, L.: Urticaria induced by preservatives and dye additives in food and drugs. Brit. J. Dermatol. 88:525, 1973.

Milins, J.L., Randle, H.W., Solley, G.O., Dicken, C.H.: The therapeutic response of urticarial vasculitis to indomethacin. J. Am. Acad. Dermatol. 3:349, 1980.

Monroe, E.W.: Urticarial vasculitis: An updated review: J. Am. Acad. Dermatol. 5:88, 1981.

Natbony, S.F., Phillips, M.E., Elias, J.M., Godfrey, H.P.,

Kaplan, A.P.: Histologic studies of chronic idiopathic urticaria. J. Allergy Clin. Immunol. 71:177, 1983.

Pasricha, J.S., Pasricha, A., Prakash, O.M.: Role of gastrointestinal parasites in urticaria. Ann. Allergy 30:348, 1972.

Paton, W.D.M.: Histamine release by compounds of simple chemical structure. Pharmacol. Rev. 9:269, 1957.

Phanuphak, P., Kohler, P.H., Stanford, R.E., Schocket, A.L., Carr, R.I., Claman, H.N.: Vasculitis in chronic urticaria. J. Allergy Clin. Immunol. 65:436, 1980.

Ravits, M., Armstrong, R.B., Harber, L. C.: Solar urticaria: Clinical features and wavelength dependence. Arch. Dermatol. 118:288, 1982.

Sheffer, A.L., Soter, N.A., McFadden, E.R., Austen, K.F.: Exercise-induced anaphylaxis: a distinct form of physical allergy. J. Allergy Clin. Immunol. 71:311, 1983.

Soter, N.A.: Chronic urticaria as a manifestation of necrotizing vasculitis. N. Eng. J. Med. 296:1440, 1977.

Sussman, G.L. Harvey, R.P., Schocket, A.L.: Delayed pressure urticaria. J. Allergy Clin. Immunol. 70:337, 1982.

Sutter, M.C., Beaulieu, G., Birt, A.R.: Histamine liberation by codeine and polymyxin B in urticaria pigmentosa. Arch. Dermatol. 86:217, 1962.

Warin, R.P., Champion, R.H.: Urticaria. Philadelphia, W.B. Saunders Co., 1974.

Wasserman, S.I.: Mediators of immediate hypersensitivity. J. Allergy Clin. Immunol. 72:101, 1983.

Zeiss, C.R., Burch, F.X., Marder, R.J., Rurney, N.L., Schmid, F.R., Gewurz, H.: A hypocomplementemic vasculitic urticarial syndrome. Report of four new cases and definition of the disease. Am. J. Med. 68:867, 1980.

32

Other Skin Disorders
DON WARREN PRINTZ, M.D.

In this chapter, common congenital and hereditary disorders of the skin, infectious dermatoses, and other skin disorders with features that sometimes raise the question of "allergy" are reviewed. Immune mechanisms have been implicated in the pathogenesis of some disorders. A more comprehensive review of these disorders can be found from the general references at the end of this chapter.

INFECTIOUS DERMATOSES

Fungal

Superficial Fungal Infections. Only three genera of fungi, *Tricophyton, Microsporum,* and *Epidermophyton,* account for virtually all superficial fungal disease from childhood to adulthood in North America. An interesting epidemiologic change has taken place in tinea capitis over the past 35 years. Whereas, formerly, almost all epidemic tinea capitis was caused by *M. audouinii,* in the past 35 years, this organism has been virtually replaced completely by *T. tonsurans.* This trend was first observed in the Southwestern United States and has now reached Canada. It is important to note that unlike *M. audouinii, T. tonsurans* exhibits no consistently reliable fluorescence under Wood's light examination, mandating the use of KOH preparations and culture for diagnostic confirmation. Furthermore, alopecia, which is sometimes cicatricial, can sometimes occur in *T. tonsurans* infections without the characteristic short broken-off hairs seen in *M. audouinii* infections. Thus, *T. tonsurans* infection should always be considered in a patient with otherwise unexplained hair loss.

Tinea capitis occurs almost exclusively before puberty, and it has been suggested that free fatty acids in sebum, which are first secreted at puberty, have an inhibitory effect on these fungi. Moreover, *T. tonsurans* is more likely to be involved in kerion formation in which a boggy, pustular faintly fluctuant lesion develops in the scalp. The lesion may be over 5 cm in diameter. It is important that the clinician realize that this lesion represents a delayed hypersensitivity reaction to the fungus. Because of its etiology, there is no response to antibiotics despite the purulence observed in this lesion. A brief course of systemic corticosteroids (e.g., prednisone, 0.9 mg/kg/day in 3 divided doses) may be necessary for prompt resolution of the lesion. Kerions often form shortly after the initiation of systemic antifungal therapy. Delayed hypersensitivity reactions also are seen in tinea corporis. Jones et al. (1974) demonstrated a correlation between severity of disease and response to intradermal skin tests with purified *Tricophyton* antigen. In 1973, Jones showed a greater frequency of dermatophyte infections in individuals with atopic dermatitis.

Superficial fungal infections of the face are almost completely confined to patients in the pediatric age group. Often, the characteristic lesions on the malar areas are the result of holding infected household pets against the face.

Treatment of the superficial dermatophytic infections (except for tinea capitis) usually can be accomplished with use of topical therapy alone; the agents econazole nitrate and ciclopirox olamine applied twice daily are agents of choice. Tinea capitis requires systemic therapy. Griseofulvin (ultramicrosize) must be administered twice daily (10 mg/kg divided into 2 doses) for at least 3 weeks. Since it is fat soluble, it should be administered with milk or peanut butter. Because of the high cost of the suspension, crushing the tablets in peanut butter is an economic and a practical method of giving the medication to younger children. From an epidemiologic standpoint, the concomitant use of selenium sulfide shampoos twice weekly (Selsun prescription, not Selsun Blue) renders the patient noninfectious much more rapidly than griseofulvin alone because of its sporicidal effect.

Candidosis. Candidosis may affect patients of all ages. Except in congenital candidosis, it appears as characteristic beef-red, faintly glistening and macerated, sharply demarcated lesions with satellite lesions separated from the main body of the eruption. Thrush is a uniform

425

finding in neonatal candidosis, which appears in the second week after birth. In adolescent males, the scrotum is characteristically affected in candidosis and spared in tinea cruris. Diaper dermatitis complicated by *Candida* is a classic presentation. By contrast, congenital candidosis is present at birth or within 12 hours after delivery, presenting as a vesiculopustular eruption chiefly on the extremities; it rapidly desquamates, resulting in collarette scaling and diffuse erythroderma.

Using murine models, Ray (1985) has demonstrated the remarkable ability of *Candida* to adhere to the stratum corneum. In this system, the organism secretes an acid protease, which is keratolytic. The process is associated with the elaboration of a mucoid "cohesin," which is present within 10 minutes after experimental inoculation. Ray also demonstrated that cell wall extracts from *Candida* can activate complement by the alternative pathway. In addition, complement activation evokes neutrophil chemotaxis and promotes opsonization and subsequent phagocytosis of the organism.

Host defenses rest chiefly on cell-mediated immunity; when T-cell mechanisms are deranged, chronic *Candida* infections are frequent. Immunoglobulins, including IgG, IgA, IgM, and IgE, are produced in response to the organism but have no effect on the *in vitro* growth of homogenized organisms. Clinically, patients with immunoglobulin deficiencies do not appear to be unusually susceptible to *Candida* infections. Conversely, patients with chronic candidosis with T-cell aberrations may have high immunoglobulin levels that are not protective.

Treatment involves topical agents, such as econazole nitrate and clotrimazole, applied twice daily. Oral nystatin suspension, $\frac{1}{2}$ teaspoonful administered every 2 hours while the patient is awake, is useful in treating thrush. Since 80 percent of nystatin is hydrolyzed by the low pH of the gastric contents, its systemic effect in the doses usually employed is questionable.

Local factors are critical in successful management. The affected areas must be kept as dry as possible. In infants, this is accomplished through avoidance of disposable diapers and use of cloth diapers without rubber pants. When the acute phase subsides, the use of methylcellulose containing powder (ZeaSorb) can be an effective preventive measure because of its greater absorbency than pure talc.

Viral

Herpes Simplex. Grouped vesicles arising on an erythematous base should bring to mind the diagnosis of herpes simplex virus (HSV) in patients of any age. However, only 70 percent of neonates infected with HSV will exhibit the characteristic skin eruptions. Any history of maternal genital HSV infection should raise the clinician's index of suspicion in case of abnormal neonatal development. The virus is easily cultured from mucous membranes as well as skin. The Tzanck smear is reliable for a quick diagnosis if vesicles are present.

In the majority of children and adults, primary HSV infections of the facial-oral type are asymptomatic. Primary inoculations in older adolescents or adults at either facial or genital locations are usually quite painful and accompanied by fever to 105°F and localized adenopathy. The primary inoculation of the finger, or herpetic whitlow, is an occupational hazard in dental and nursing personnel who must handle tracheobronchial secretions.

Recurrent herpetic infections, triggered by a wide variety of factors, need no longer be the bane of existence for so many patients. Acyclovir, 18 mg/kg/day in 5 divided doses for 5 days, given early in the course of the recurrence (during the prodromal phase if possible) not only speeds the resolution of the current eruption, but after repeated courses seems to prolong the recurrence-free interval. Although not effecting a cure, the treatment helps relieve pain and discomfort and may prevent recurrence.

Varicella and Zoster. These two diseases are caused by members of the herpesvirus group. Herpes simplex types 1 and 2, cytomegalovirus, and Epstein-Barr virus of infectious mononucleosis are all members of the group.

Varicella, the most contagious of the "childhood" diseases, usually begins on the face and scalp and spreads rapidly to the extremities and trunk. The lesions quickly pass through several morphologic stages, beginning as erythematous macules that rapidly evolve into vesicles, pustules, and crusts. The entire process may take less than 24 hours. Lesions occur in varying stages of development in "crops," unlike variola, and resolve over 8 to 9 days. Varicella in children usually requires only supportive treatment, such as bland lotion.

Herpes zoster, caused by varicella virus, is a result of reactivation of latent virus, which resides in sensory ganglia. Unknown factors activate the virus, which then spreads antidromically down the sensory nerve, producing discomfort even before the characteristic grouped vesicles, arising on an erythematous base and arranged in dermatomal fashion, appear.

The immunology of varicella-zoster is complex. Although IgA, IgM, and IgG antibodies occur within a few days of visible varicellar lesions, with low levels of IgG persisting throughout life, children with agammaglobulinemia do not experience severe or recurrent varicella. On the other hand, children and immunosuppressed adults with deficient cell-mediated immunity develop severe or long-lasting varicella-zoster. Interestingly, varicella-zoster immuneglobulin greatly modifies the course of the disease in such patients and may be lifesaving.

Unfortunately, acyclovir is of limited value for treatment of herpes zoster. The standard dosage (200 mg, 5 times daily) of acyclovir is not particularly effective; attempts to double and triple the oral dose afford some relief, but this regimen usually is limited by gastrointestinal side effects. Parenteral treatment of immunocompromised patients has been successful. In patients affected with zoster 70 years of age or older, the administration of prednisone 20 mg, t.i.d. for 6 days, followed by 20 mg, every other day for 2 weeks, along with the application of potent topical steroids (clobetasol 0.05 percent b.i.d.) has been shown to limit the incidence of postherpetic neuralgia greatly. The application of firm pressure, such as an elastic bandage, to the trunk area overnight offers the patient considerable comfort without resorting to potentially addictive analgesics for this long-term complication.

Warts. Warts come in all shapes and sizes, can occur anywhere there is stratified squamous epithelium, and are the bane of existence of countless patients, especially those suffering from painful plantar warts. The etiology is the papilloma virus, a DNA-containing virus that can be separated into numerous types, each demonstrating a striking site specificity. Types 6 and 11 have been associated with urogenital tumors, including verrucous carcinoma; types 16 and 18 may be the major causes of carcinoma of the cervix and urogenital Bowen disease.

Immunity against this virus seems to depend on cell-mediated pathways. Patients with acquired immune deficiency syndrome (AIDS) frequently have large numbers of flat warts, particularly in the bearded area. Warts are common in immunosuppressed patients and are notoriously difficult to treat in these patients as well as patients with advanced Hodgkin's disease.

A variety of treatment methods are available. Cryotherapy for multiple, relatively flat warts leaves no scarring and is almost painless under nitrous oxide analgesia. Verrusol, a compound containing podophyllin, cantharidin, and salicylic acid, is particularly useful for periungual and subungual warts. Electrodesiccation, excision, curettage, and final electrofulguration have a very high rate of success, although they leave small scars and require the use of intralesional anesthesia. Laser treatment is quite similar in this regard. Podophyllin (25 percent) in a compound tincture of benzoin is useful for treatment of genital warts. The compound should not be left *in situ* more than 4 hours at the initial treatment; the time should be increased at weekly intervals. X-ray therapy is now infrequently employed. Duofilm, a salicylic acid-lactic acid compound in an acetone base, is especially useful for small new warts. Since the incubation period of warts can be at least 6 months, patients should be alerted to look for new lesions, especially near lesions that have been removed. Duofilm offers a painless way to remove these new lesions.

Molluscum Contagiosum. This is an extremely common viral disease of children. The typical lesion is an umbilicated flesh-colored papule, 1 to 5 mm in diameter. Although "giant" molluscous bodies measuring up to 2 cm occur, these are more common in adults. The molluscum contagiosum virus is a member of the poxvirus group. The disease is transmissible both from person to person and autoinoculation. It is not uncommon for patients to present with 50 or more lesions.

The lesions are readily treated by simple curettage. Nitrous oxide analgesia greatly simplifies this procedure for both physician and patient when there are multiple lesions. The use of Keralyt, a 7-percent salicylic acid gel, twice daily for 2 weeks before the curettage of multiple lesions, makes the procedure much less painful. Several treatment sessions at monthly intervals are usually necessary to remove newly developing lesions.

Hand, Foot, and Mouth Syndrome. A number of rashes can be confused with allergy. One of the more dramatic is that of hand, foot, and mouth syndrome. It consists of an exanthem-enanthem syndrome, consisting of papulovesicles on the hands and feet associated with oral ulceration especially on the tongue. Usually the cutaneous papulovesicles arise on an erythematous base, and the vesicle is gray rather than clear. The etiologic agent is coxsackie virus A-16 and possibly other enteroviruses. The incubation period is 3 to 6 days, and the clinical manifestations are self-limited, running a course from 5 to 7 days (AAP, 1986).

Immunologically, serum-neutralizing antiviral antibody is present transiently, and complement-fixing antibodies are present during the convalescent stage. There is no specific treatment.

Bacteria

Bacterial Infections of the Skin (Pyoderma). A few years ago, virtually every adult patient presenting with impetigo or similar skin infections had direct contact with children. It was an occupational hazard in nursery school workers, baby sitters, and certainly pediatricians and their staffs. Now these superficial pyodermas seem to occur spontaneously in adults and children. Also, mosquitoes and other biting insects can serve as vectors for transmission of staphylococcal and streptococcal infections, especially during late summer.

More ominously, methicillin-resistant staphylococcal pyodermas are being seen with increasing frequency in patients referred to tertiary centers. Erythromycin-resistant strains are observed with increasing frequency in the general population. Since penicillins do not reach the uppermost layers of the skin as well as erythromycin and cephalosporins, the clinician's armamentarium is somewhat reduced. It should be emphasized that studies over the past 20 years have demonstrated the inadequacy of topical therapy for impetigo and other pyodermas. The long-term use of Hibiclens (chlorhexidine gluconate) in any family who is prone to recurrent pyodermas may be of great help.

Staphylococcal Scalded Skin Syndrome (SSSS). Formerly known as Ritter disease, SSSS is principally a disease of infants; children under the age 5 years are occasionally affected. Following a brief macular erythematous phase, the disease quickly progresses to an intensely erythematous eruption almost always with facial involvement. At this time the skin is extremely tender. Perinasal and perioral vesicles and bullae usually herald the development of the subsequent phase in which sheets of the epidermis are shed, leaving eroded, weeping lesions that are burn-like in appearance. There is little or no mucous membrane involvement, which serves to differentiate SSSS from the Stevens-Johnson syndrome. In case of doubt, histology reveals a characteristic separation at the granular-cell layer of the epidermis. The etiology is an infection with *Staphylococcus* group 2, phage type 71, which produces a potent epidermolytic toxin. Treatment is with dicloxacillin, 18 mg/kg/day in 4 divided doses.

Lyme Disease. Lyme disease is a complex consisting of characteristic skin lesions (erythema chronicum migrans), mono- or oligo-articular arthritis of the large joints, and various constitutional symptoms. It is caused by a spirochete, *Borellia burgdorfii*, and is transmitted by the bite of a tick of the genus *Ixodes*. Most cases have occurred in the Northeastern United States, although sporadic cases have been reported elsewhere in the United States and in Europe.

The characteristic erythema is extremely prolonged and may spread to involve wide areas. There is no scale; the erythema is deep, producing a blue tinge, and there is tendency toward central clearing. Specific serum IgM antibodies are present in the first few weeks of the disease; IgG antibodies can be demonstrated later. Response to penicillin therapy, orally 500 mg 4 times daily for 1 week, is dramatic. Untreated, the disease may persist for years.

Mites and Insects

Scabies. The most frequently encountered mite infection in North America is that caused by *Sarcoptes scabiei*. Sites of predilection are the interdigital spaces and the genitalia. So-called Norwegian scabies, in institutionalized patients, often occurs with large erythematous papular lesions on the palms and soles. Mites involved in these cases number in the dozens rather than only a few.

Lindane currently is the treatment of choice. The medication is applied over the entire body surface from the neck down and left on for an absolute minimum of 12 hours. The alternate drug, crotamiton, has the advantage of being intrinsically antipruritic but less effective in the experience of most clinicians. The lindane conundrum has been well discussed by Rasmussen (1981), who observed that (1) most cases of neurotoxicity have been associated with gross misuse of the drug and (2) the skin of children over 1 year of age absorbs much less of the medication. At the time of this writing, lindane remains fully effective in its scabicidal properties. However, the total resistance of *Pediculus humanus var. capitis* among Indian tribes in the San Blas Islands of Panama may bode ill for the future of lindane in other infestations; newer and safer therapeutic agents are in the testing stage.

Papular Urticaria. Despite the name, this entity is in reality a delayed hypersensitivity reaction to arthropod bites, usually to that of the flea harbored by domestic animals. It manifests itself in an early age group, usually those under age 7. The changing immune response to insect bites, such as mosquitoes, with age can be seen in Table 32–1.

In intensely mosquito-infested areas, most adults are in the final stage of this scenario. Prevention of papular urticaria consists of the use of effective insect repellents. Treatment is application of a potent corticosteroid, such as clobetasol, on the papules b.i.d. for 5 days.

Kawasaki Disease

The formal name for this entity is mucocutaneous lymph node syndrome. However, the disease can occur without appreciable lymphadenopathy. The disease is diagnosed using the following clinical criteria: (1) fever of abrupt onset, persisting at least 5 days and unresponsive to treatment; (2) conjunctival injection without exudation; (3) oral changes, including fissuring cheilitis, "strawberry tongue," and diffuse erythema of the oropharynx; (4) erythema of the palms and soles, progressing to acral induration and distal desquamation of the digits; (5) a polymorphous exanthem of the trunk, which may resemble erythema multiforme; and (6) adenopathy, principally cervical

TABLE 32–1. Temporal Differences in Immune Responses to Insect Bites

Stage	Wheal	Papule
No exposure	0	0
Early exposure	+	0
Typical response in midlife	+	+
Delayed hypersensitivity	0	+
Full immunity	0	0

(1.5 cm or more in diameter). Virtually all patients are under 10 years of age, and the majority are under the age of 5. The etiology remains unknown; a host of infectious agents has been suspect.

Laboratory findings are nonspecific. Elevation of IgE level has been reported during the first 2 weeks of illness, followed by a subsequent decline. Thrombocytosis during the second week of the disease is a consistent finding. Complications include aneurysms of the coronary arteries, thrombosis of which may prove fatal. Low-dose salicylate therapy, especially during the thrombocytic phase of the disease, has been widely advocated in an effort to minimize the cardiac complications.

BULLOUS DERMATOSES AND VASCULITIDES

Erythema Multiforme. Erythema multiforme is a cutaneous reaction pattern to a variety of etiologic factors rather than a separate disease entity. It varies in severity from a few transient skin lesions to fatal Stevens-Johnson syndrome. The most common infectious etiologic factors are herpes simplex, *Streptococcus,* and *Mycoplasma pneumoniae.* The most common drugs implicated in erythema multiforme are penicillin and the sulfonamides. Many episodes are idiopathic.

The characteristic lesion of erythema multiforme is the "iris" or "target" lesion, often observed on the palms, soles, and mucous membranes; unlike urticaria, the lesions persist for days or weeks. Such lesions exhibit a dusky red central maculopapule surrounded by erythematous concentric rings. In more severe forms of the disease, hemorrhagic mucosal erosions, affecting virtually every body orifice, may be present; these are accompanied by severe constitutional symptoms, high fever, and renal, cardiac, or pulmonary involvement. The cutaneous manifestations also may include bullae, with the entire clinical picture virtually indistinguishable from toxic epidermal necrolysis. Immunohistology reveals granular deposits of immunoglobulin (IgM) and complement (C3) in superficial dermal blood vessels, provided a fresh lesion is biopsied. Treatment of mild cases of erythema multiforme is supportive. Patients with severe cases of Stevens-Johnson syndrome are managed essentially as patients with severe burns. The use of corticosteroids remains controversial. Although controlled studies are lacking, many clinicians employ pharmacologic doses of corticosteroids early in the disease. There is some retrospective evidence that corticosteroids may delay recovery, and some dermatologists believe they should not be used at all in this syndrome.

Erythema Nodosum. Erythema nodosum is a vasculitis caused by various etiologic factors, as follows:

1. Streptococcal infection
2. Herpes simplex infection
3. Tuberculosis
4. Drugs (sulfonamides, penicillin, salicylates)
5. Coccidioidomycosis
6. Rare diseases (leprosy, lymphogranuloma venereum)

The disease manifests as tender nodules, particularly on the shins. Biopsy adds little to the clinical diagnosis. Treatment with prednisone, 1 mg/kg/day divided into 3 doses for 6 days, is dramatic in reducing signs and symptoms.

Linear IgA Bullous Disease of Childhood. Until the development of immunofluorescent microscopy, this entity masqueraded under a variety of clinical names and classifications. Weston (1985) observes that this may be the most common nonhereditary bullous disease of childhood.

The vesicles and bullae in this disease are pleomorphic, ranging from pinhead-sized grouped lesions that mimic dermatitis herpetiformis, to large tense round or oval lesions, containing clear or hemorrhagic fluid. Distribution also is variable, although usually there is prominent involvement of the buttocks and inguinal region. Itching ranges from intense to total absence.

Direct immunofluorescence reveals linear IgA and C3 deposits in the basement membrane zone in both lesional and perilesional skin. Indirect immunofluorescence has revealed circulating antibasement membrane zone antibodies, also in the IgA class. Treatment is with sulfapyridine (3 mg/kg) or dapsone (1.5 mg/kg). Gluten-free diets are ineffective.

Vasculitis. Vasculitis is an immune complex disease characterized by the presence of immunoreactive products (immunoglobulins, complement), circulating immune complexes, and neutrophils with varying degrees of leucocytoclasia. The immune complexes bind to blood vessel walls, and complement binding occurs, which is followed by erythrocytic diapedesis.

In Henoch-Schönlein (anaphylactoid) purpura, such changes occur in the capillaries and post-capillary venules. Immunofluorescent studies of skin biopsy specimens reveal the presence of IgA in the vessel walls. In addition, serum levels of IgA may be elevated. IgA deposition also may be observed in renal biopsy specimens. The clinical picture of an initially erythematous macular eruption that blanches on pressure evolving into a nonblanching purpuric lesion correlates with the extravasation of erythrocytes, as the lesion matures.

Some classifications of vasculitis would broaden the aforementioned criteria to include the lymphocytic infiltrative disorders, such as pityriasis lichenoides et varioliformis acuta that similarly exhibits erythrocytic diapedesis and the presence of C3 and IgM in dermal blood vessel walls. Neutrophils characteristically are absent. Individual lesions heal within a few weeks, often with smallpox-like scarring which reflects the severity of the vasculitic process.

Epidermolysis Bullosa. This constellation of diseases comprises nine major groups and some subgroups based on the site of skin cleavage involved. Recent advances in electron microscopy have provided the tools for organizing this group of diseases in this manner. The disorders will be considered briefly here, and the reader is referred to Cooper et al. (1987) for more extensive discussion. As these investigators state, "Epidermolysis bullosa (EB) is the term applied to a group of disorders whose common primary feature is the formation of blisters following trivial trauma."

As mentioned, a convenient way of classifying these disorders is to group them according to the level of skin cleavage: (1) the nondystrophic diseases, in which the site of cleavage is in the epidermis (these are the only truly *epidermolytic* diseases in the epidermolysis bullosa group); (2) the atrophic diseases, in which the site of cleavage is at the dermoepidermal junction; and (3) the dystrophic diseases, which are dermolytic in nature.

The dystrophic diseases follow an autosomal dominant pattern of inheritance. Thus, families are generally affected by and familiar with many aspects of the disease; genetic counseling is mandatory. Epidermolysis bullosa simplex may be generalized or localized. The generalized disease tends to flare in warm weather and heals without scarring. The localized form, known as Weber-Cockayne disease, may become manifest only later in life, with blisters forming on the hands and feet following vigorous physical exercise, such as long hiking. Treatment of both conditions, which heal spontaneously, is based on removing the offending agents; heat, friction, and physical trauma. Saline soaks and topical antibiotics may be helpful in resolving the lesions.

The atrophic diseases, with cleavage occurring at the dermoepidermal junction, are inherited in an autosomal recessive pattern. The blisters may be extensive at birth, and generally heal without scarring, but with some residual atrophy. However, the prognosis is grave for patients affected by some variants, with mortality greater than 50 percent in the first 2 years of life, often accompanied by pyloric atresia and refractory anemia. Those patients with these diseases generally require care at specialized medical centers by trained personnel.

Acquired epidermolysis bullosa is a nonhereditary adult-onset disease characterized by bullae forming over the joints after only minor trauma, accompanied by atrophic scarring and nail dystrophy. It has nothing in common with the inherited forms of the disease except for the clinical similarity. This is an autoimmune disorder, with direct immunofluorescence studies demonstrating a linear deposition of IgG along the basement membrane zone. IgG in the upper dermis is demonstrated through immunoelectron microscopy of perilesional skin. Light microscopic examination findings are identical to the findings in bullous pemphigoid and porphyria cutanea tarda.

ACNE

Acne Vulgaris. Acne is virtually a universal occurrence at some time in every adolescent's life, varying in severity from a few evanescent lesions to severe cystic and pustular forms resulting in both cutaneous and psychologic scars.

Acne has a multifactorial etiology, as follows: (1) the effects of androgens on the maturation of the epidermal cells in the infundibulum of the pilosebaceous apparatus cause cellular adherence rather than orderly desquamation and thus begin comedo formation; (2) the effects of *Propionibacterium acnes*, an anaerobic diphtheroid, increase the content of free fatty acids in sebum and induce an inflammatory response either directly or indirectly through metabolic products; (3) the effects of plugging of the pilosebaceous-follicular orifice result in the accumulation of neutrophils, complement, immunoglobulins (IgG, IgM, IgA), and other mediators of inflammation with development

of pustular cysts which often rupture. This frequently produces permanent scarring as the inflammatory process resolves. In addition, *P. acnes* probably activates the T-cell system. Intradermally injected heat-killed organisms evoked a delayed hypersensitivity reaction in patients with acne.

The foundation for acne therapy is composed of antimicrobial agents and retinoids. Topical agents, such as benzoyl peroxide and clindamycin, and systemic antibiotics, such as tetracycline and erythromycin, are efficacious in eradicating *P. acnes*. These antibiotics, which also inhibit leukocyte migration, are more effective clinically than the penicillins, although *P. acnes* is sensitive to both groups of antibiotics.

The retinoids, either tretinoin (Retin-A) topically or 13-cis retinoic acid (Accutane) systemically, restore the epithelial maturation in the follicular infundibulum to its normal state, promoting orderly desquamation and preventing comedo formation. Accutane additionally reduces sebum production by 98 percent or more within 2 weeks after initiation of therapy. At least 25 percent of patients treated with Accutane for 4 months continue to exhibit decreased sebum production at least 1 year after cessation of the drug. Although this may be a desirable factor in the long-term effectiveness of the drug, the accompanying xerotic cheilitis and xerophthalmia causing difficulty in the wearing of hard contact lenses are long-term side effects that must be balanced against the benefits of the drug. In my experience, at least 70 percent of patients treated with full 4-month courses of Accutane must be maintained on topical tretinoin, or they must receive repeat courses of Accutane within 6 months after completing the initial course of the drug in order to maintain acceptable clinical clarity. The other side effects of Accutane, such as elevation of serum triglyceride levels with concomitant elevation of low density lipoprotein levels and decrease of high density lipoprotein levels, colitis, vertebral skeletal abnormalities, and teratogenicity, mandate that it be reserved for those patients who do not respond to other therapeutic modalities.

Acne Rosacea. Rosacea is distinctly unusual in the pediatric age group, but common in adults. It is characterized by multiple closed comedos on the central portion of the face accompanied by rhinophyma.

The treatment of choice is tetracycline, 250 mg t.i.d., but resistant cases often respond to topical sulfacetamide (Sulfacet lotion), applied b.i.d. The lotion is believed to kill *Demodex folliculorum,* an ectoparasite found in profusion in the dilated pilosebaceous apparatus in rosacea.

The most dramatic resolution of rhinophyma is with isotretinoin (Accutane) in a dosage of 1 mg/kg daily for 6 weeks. It is not unusual to see the size of the nose decrease 50 percent in this period of time. The therapy may be continued for 4 months if necessary.

ALOPECIA

Alopecia Areata. The dense perifollicular accumulation of lymphocytes at the base of the hair shaft has been cited as the rationale that this is an autoimmune disease. The treatment of alopecia areata by the deliberate development of delayed hypersensitivity, allegedly to bring in "normal" lymphocytes and reverse the "abnormal" process, is certainly in question, not only for its efficacy but its rationale. It must be remembered that purely irritant therapy (application of phenol, ultraviolet light) was employed decades ago with gratifying results.

The etiology of this disease remains controversial. Empiric treatment of the typical well-circumscribed nummular areas of alopecia with intralesional corticosteroids (5 mg/ml triamcinolone with lidocaine, up to 20 mg/ml) and systemic corticosteroids (prednisone, 20 mg every second day for 2 to 3 months) is employed in extensive alopecia, particularly that which begins on the occipital or marginal (ophiasis) scalp areas. This therapy is accompanied by the use of potent topical corticosteroids (clobetasol, 0.05 percent b.i.d.) even to the point of atrophy to induce hair regrowth. The mutagenic effects of dinitrochlorobenzene (DNCB) have been a problem with long-term use (up to 5 years) (Muller, 1985).

If alopecia begins in the occiput or scalp margins, begin therapy quickly, even if only with topical clobetasole. Bald patients may not appreciate therapeutic nihilism.

Trichotillomania. An irregular pattern of hair loss, with varying lengths of regrowing hair should suggest the diagnosis of self-induced alopecia. Unlike factitial dermatitis, in which skin lesions are consciously produced with intent to deceive, the patient with trichotillomania may be almost unaware of hair plucking. Absent-mindedly twisting the hair while reading or watching television is a common history. The clinician can play a valuable role in explaining to both patient and parent the nature of the disease and that it may be an expression of a deep-seated need for better family communication. Counseling, not drugs, is the treatment of choice. The physician's prime duty is to allay feelings of guilt by any party.

OTHER DISORDERS

Miliaria. Miliaria crystallina, in which multiple tiny nonerythematous vesicles develop, is seen frequently in premature infants. It resolves in 1 to 3 days without treatment. Full-term and older infants develop sweat gland blockage at the midepidermis with rupture of the duct and resultant inflammation. Almost inevitably these children are in an overheated environment (miliaria rubra). Loosening or use of less clothing and blankets results in clearing. Bland shake lotions, such as milk of bismuth (NF), may dry the skin and afford faster clearing. The very brief use of corticosteroid *lotion* (Cordran Lotion t.i.d. not to exceed 4 days) will resolve the erythema almost immediately and provide some drying simultaneously.

Infants and older children can be spared all manifestations of miliaria rubra if they are in an air-conditioned environment for only 8 hours of 24. This preventive practice is effective even in tropical areas; the United States Armed Forces installed air-conditioned barracks to avoid the serious morbidity associated with tropical miliaria.

Keratosis Pilaris. Keratosis pilaris is a familial hyperkeratosis of follicular orifices, with the plugging of the infundibulum of the hair follicle. It is thought to be inherited as an autosomal dominant disorder. It commonly appears in early childhood and persists through adolescence. The characteristic "goose-flesh" appearance is seen predominantly on the extensor surfaces of the arms and thighs, although it can appear on the face and eyebrows. Individual lesions are red papules with a dry, central scale. Treatment consists of avoiding tight clothes; using topical keratolytic agents, such as retinoic acids, alpha-hydroxy acids, or salicylic acid; and skin hydration by standard dermatologic hydration and lubrication techniques.

Nummular Eczema. Sharply demarcated, excoriated, weeping, and occasionally crusted coin-shaped lesions (Latin nummulus, coin) are the hallmarks of this disorder. Many etiologic factors have been proposed, but the cause remains unknown. Basically, an itch-scratch cycle is developed. Many of the lesions persist for long periods because of unconscious rubbing and scratching of the lesions. Since Serum IgE levels are normal (Krueger et al., 1973), it is not surprising that antihistamines have little or no effect. The very brief short-term use, not to exceed 5 days, of a potent corticosteroid (clobetasone t.i.d.) is most effective in breaking the excoriation cycle. If the eruption is accompanied by xerosis, the use of superfatted soap and stratum corneum hydrating agents (Complex 15, UltraMide) applied to the moist skin after bathing may be invaluable in preventing recurrence.

Pityriasis Rosea (PR). A member of the maculopapulosquamous group of diseases, this viral skin infection is frequently seen in the older pediatric and adolescent age groups. Clustering of cases, demonstration of picornavirus-like particles from the lesions by electron microscopy, recovery of a virus of the picornavirus series from tissue inoculation, and rapid improvement of the disease following injection of convalescent plasma are all indirect evidence of a viral etiology. Anticytoplasmic IgM antibodies to keratinocytes in 100 percent of patients with PR also have been demonstrated.

The initial "sentinel" lesion characteristically appears 5 to 21 days prior to the onset of the generalized eruption and is usually larger and more irregularly shaped than the subsequent lesions. Because of its peripheral scaling and accentuation of peripheral erythema, it often is misdiagnosed as tinea circinata.

The definitive eruption consists of an oval-shaped, erythematous, peripherally scaling primary lesion, with the long axis arranged parallel to the lines of skin cleavage, producing the typical "Christmas-tree" pattern. The face and distal extremities characteristically are spared, although an "inverse" form of the disease occurs that affects these areas only. The eruption varies from asymptomatic to moderately pruritic; itching is often triggered by a hot bath or shower.

Untreated, the disease varies, as a rule, from 4 to 10 weeks although persistence for as long as 6 to 8 months occasionally may occur. A brief regimen of systemic steroids (0.2 to 0.5 mg/kg t.i.d., 5 days) and topical steroid lotions (Cordran Lotion t.i.d., 7 days) greatly shortens the course of the disease and alleviates itching.

Psoriasis. The majority of psoriasis patients develop the disease in adult life. However, it can occur in childhood also. Several principles in the pediatric and adolescent age groups are significant, the earlier the onset: (1) the greater the probability of a positive family history of psoriasis, (2) the greater the likelihood of more severe and extensive involvement in adult life, and (3) the more resistance to treatment of the adult disease.

Psoriasis, one disease of the maculopapulosquamous group, consists of the development of sharply demarcated plaques surmounted by a silvery, thick scale. The extensor surfaces generally show the greatest involvement, especially at sites of minor trauma, such as the elbows and knees. The scalp is another frequent site of involvement; there may be an overlap with seborrheic dermatitis in the adolescent age group that exacerbates the disease.

The Koebner phenomenon, the production of isomorphic lesions at sites of trauma, is triggered not only by physical trauma but also the trauma of other dermatologic disease. For example, the psoriatic patient who develops pityriasis rosea or poison ivy may be expected to develop lesions of psoriasis at these affected areas after several weeks. The astute clinician can forewarn the patient to begin antipsoriatic therapy as soon as such new lesions develop (or to employ general measures, such as sunbathing, to act as preventives).

Treatment of psoriasis in the view of the nondermatologist seems a reversion to the days of alchemy, employing as it does elements of earth (tar), air (climatologic therapy), fire (ultraviolet radiation), and water (emollient baths) causing the clinician considerable distress. Somewhat simpler methods are available, however. The highly potent topical corticosteroid clobetasole (0.05 percent), recently released in the United States as Temovate, affords spectacular results in clearing psoriatic patients with the following caveats:

1. Never give the patient more that 1 week's supply.
2. Never apply the medication to over 50 percent of the body surface.

The drug causes rapid steroid atrophy if applied longer than 10 to 14 days and suppresses the pituitary-adrenal axis if applied over wide areas. It should be used to control acute disease flares, with long-term treatment then substituted, using 1 percent hydrocortisone ointment b.i.d. or 0.025-percent triamcinolone ointment b.i.d.

Other agents all have serious toxic drawbacks in the pediatric-adolescent age groups, except for the cosmetically offensive products that patients universally despise, such as tar baths and tar-containing topicals, Baker's P & S Liquid, and P & S Plus Tar Gel. These effectively remove scalp scaling at the cost of soiled pillowcases, and all have the elegance of a mange cure. The total body, occlusive "wet suits" to facilitate topical therapy at night trap so much body heat that their use is questionable.

Other therapeutic agents available but not recommended are methotrexate, which should not be used as a gambit to lifetime therapy; PUVA, which causes squamous cell carcinomas after 5 to 8 years of use. Etretinate, a retinoid of greatest value in pustular psoriasis released in 1987, has the amazing serum half-life of 3 months and causes frightening teratogenicity. Anthralin and its derivatives can be disastrous if a patient rubs the medications into the eyes at night. Systemic corticosteroids should not be considered, as frightful flares occur when weaning is attempted.

In summary, if psoriasis doesn't respond to a brief course of topical therapy as outlined, along with judicious sunlight, you're in trouble. Refer the patient to a dermatologist.

Urticaria Pigmentosa. This is the most common of the mastocytosis group of diseases. Inevitably, it occurs before the age of 2 years. Vesiculobullous lesions are common in the initial stages of the eruption. The lesions tend to occur in crops, later subsiding to papular or macular pigmented lesions. Darier sign, the production of a wheal by vigorous stroking of a lesion, is virtually diagnostic. Dermographism also may be present.

Prognosis is excellent, with spontaneous resolution occurring almost universally by late adolescence. If symptomatic (pruritus or overanxious parents), an H_1 blocker may be used to prevent whealing.

Sun Sensitivities. The sun exposure clock begins running at birth. With the widespread consumption of vitamin D–fortified milk, the only rational indication for sun exposure is gone. All other effects, from skin cancer to aging, are deleterious and may be prevented with sunscreens with a sun protective factor (SPF) of 15.

Ultraviolet, midrange, UVB(280–320 nM), generally is responsible for sunburn and skin cancer. The longer wavelengths of UVA (320–344 nM) are responsible for most other sun sensitivity diseases, including melanoma, erythropoietic protoporphyria, prophyria cutanea tarda, berloque dermatitis, polymorphous light eruption, discoid and systemic lupus erythematosus, and poikiloderma, to name but a few. So affected patients require opaque blocking agents, such as RV Paque (Elder) for protection. The longer wavelengths of UVA also elicit the development of aggressive squamous cell carcinomas and, because of their deeper penetration in the skin, actually irradiate the blood circulating through the skin during the time of exposure. This effect, coupled by the death of the Langerhans cells with any appreciable length of UVA or UVB exposure, is a potentially ominous situation, considering the Langerhans cells' presumptive role of detecting foreign antigens including malignancies. The rate of internal malignancy in patients who receive psoralen and UVA (PUVA) treatment for psoriasis for 6 years or more is increased, as is the rate of occurrence of aggressive squamous cell carcinoma. To paraphrase Thomas Jefferson, he does best who is irradiated least.

DISORDERS OF PIGMENTATION

Vitiligo. Vitiligo is an acquired idiopathic depigmentation, with borders sharply circumscribed by normal or hyperpigmented skin. The most frequently affected sites are the face, neck, sternal area, arms, and dorsal surface of the hands; but the condition may be generalized. It is thought to be due to an autoimmune mechanism. Antibodies to melanin-producing cells have been detected.

There is some association between vitiligo and hyperthyroidism, adrenocortical insufficiency, pernicious anemia, and diabetes. There also is a reportedly increased frequency of vitiligo associated with IgA deficiency syndromes, as well as an increased association with combined occurrence of antithyroid antibodies and the HL-A I3 haplotype. Histologically, there is a complete absence of dopa-positive melanocytes. Pruritus may occur after sunburn of vitiliginous areas but also can occur without sun exposure. Treatment is mainly supportive, but intralesional steroids, oral psoralens, artificial keratin staining, and tattooing all have been used with varying success.

Leukoderma. The acquired hypopigmentation of skin that is produced by specific substances or is secondary to dermatitis is known as leukoderma. This has been shown in association with occupational dermatitis (e.g., from rubber garments as well as phenolic detergent germicides). These forms are rarely seen in children. The postinflammatory form of leukoderma is seen with a variety of inflammatory skin diseases, including pityriasis rosea, herpes zoster, psoriasis, atopic dermatitis, secondary syphilis, and morphea. Resolution consists of removing the offending substance and treating the underlying dermatosis. Leukoderma usually is reversible.

Pityriasis Alba. Pityriasis alba appears in children and adolescents as hypopigmented, scaly, oval patches, usually on the face, upper arms, neck, and shoulders. Histologically, a mild dermatitis is seen. Pruritus, when it occurs, usually is mild. Treatment consists of hydration and lubrication techniques or application of topical low potency steroids.

Incontinentia Pigmenti. This uncommon dermatosis usually affects female infants. When it does affect males, it tends to be lethal. There are three characteristic stages of the disorder; vesiculobullous, verrucous or papillomatous, and hyperpigmented. The lesions tend to be arranged in a linear or grouped fashion, mainly on the flexor surfaces of the extremities and the lateral trunk. Eosinophil counts are elevated in most cases. Other ectodermal defects include skin, hair, and dental; neurologic and ocular defects are found in 30 percent of patients with this disorder. Abnormalities in skin pigmentation tend to disappear by adulthood.

There is no known treatment. Genetic counseling is important in families with this disorder.

REFERENCES

AAP (American Academy of Pediatrics): Report of Committee on Infectious Disease, 170:149, 1986.

Cooper T.W., Bauer E.A., Briggaman R.A.: The Mechano Bullous Diseases (Epidermolysis Bullosa). *In* Fitzpatrick T.B., Eisen A.Z., Wolff K., Freedberg I.M., Austin K.F., (eds.), *Dermatology in General Medicine.* New York, McGraw-Hill, 1987.

Krueger G.G., Kahn G., Weston W.L., Mandez M.J.: IgE levels in nummular eczema and ichthyosis. Arch Derm 107:56–58, 1973.

Jones H.E., Reinhardt J.H., Rinaldi M.G.: A clinical, mycological and immunological survey for dermatophytosis. Arch Derm 108:61–65, 1973.

Jones H.E., Reinhardt J.H., Rinaldi M.G.: Model dermatophytosis in naturally infected subjects. Arch Derm 110:369–374, 1974.

Muller S.: Dinitrochlorobenzene in treatment of alopecia areata. Paul O'Leary Seminar, Mayo Clinic, September, 1985.

Ray T.L.: Candidosis, In Stone E. (ed.), *Dermatologic Immunity and Allergy.* St. Louis, C.V. Mosby Co., 1985.

Rasmussen J.E.: The problem of lindane. J Am Acad Dermatol 5:507–516, 1981.

Weston W.L.: *Practical Pediatric Dermatology.* Boston, Little, Brown & Company, 1985.

MANAGEMENT OF UPPER RESPIRATORY TRACT DISEASES

33

Principles of Diagnosis and Treatment of Upper Respiratory Tract Diseases

CHARLES D. BLUESTONE, M.D.
TIMOTHY P. MCBRIDE, M.D.

The Nose and Paranasal Sinuses

TIMOTHY P. McBRIDE, M.D.

NOSE

Anatomy and Physiology

The nose is a complex structure that performs multiple functions. Under most circumstances, it is the body's airway of choice. It humidifies inspired air and alters temperature. It has cyclic resistance patterns that are integrated into the overall pulmonary functions via neural reflexes. In addition, it contains specialized nerve endings that provide the sense of smell.

Nasal Skeleton

It is simplest to think of the nose as a protruding, exposed midface structure that is susceptible to blunt trauma. Anatomically, it is composed of four parts; the bony pyramid, the upper lateral cartilages, the lower lateral cartilages, and the septum (Fig. 33A–1).

An area of importance is the nasal valve region. It is the area of greatest resistance to airflow and thus may be considered a choke point for control purposes. It lies between the upper lateral and lower lateral cartilages. The stiffness of the nasal cartilages is of absolute importance to prevent inspiratory collapse of the nasal soft tissues.

The septum, which divides the nose into two compartments, is composed of the quadrangular cartilage and vomer. The columella is the portion of the quadrangular cartilage which is draped with skin and divides the right and left nostril.

Internal Nose

The walls and floor of the nose are rigid. The roof is arched upwards from the nasal tip to the cribriform plate, but the floor is level. Internally, the nose opens posteriorly into the pharynx through two oral choanae. The shape and location of structures within the nose serve to modify and direct airflow.

The septum in its posterior portion becomes boney. It is composed of the perpendicular plate of the ethmoid superiorly, the vomer and rostrum of the sphenoid bone posteriorly, and the crests of the maxillary and palatine bones inferiorly. Various deformities including fractures, spurs, and congenital abnormalities of any portion of the septum may result in restricted airflow or nasal obstruction.

There are three turbinates that are attached to each lateral nasal wall (Fig. 33A–2). The inferior turbinate is the largest, most prominent, and most easily seen on intranasal examination. The inferior turbinate has a boney skeleton. The middle and superior turbinate are extensions of the ethmoid bone.

It is important to realize that all of the paranasal sinus secretions must drain into the nose. The sinuses are connected to the nose by small

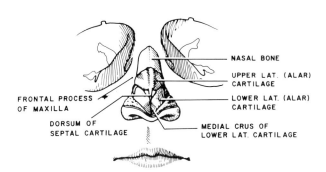

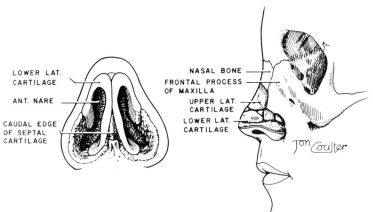

FIGURE 33A–1. Structural framework of the nose.

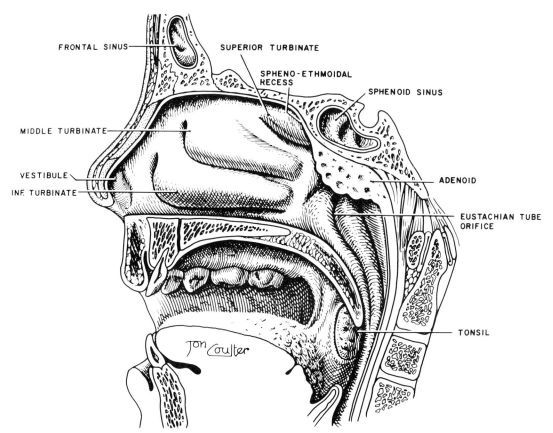

FIGURE 33A–2. The lateral wall of the nose.

ostia, which lie hidden between the turbinates. Various degrees of nasal inflammation may narrow any of these ostia and predispose the patient to sinus blockage and possible infection. The ostia are grouped into three meati; the superior, the middle, and the inferior. The middle meatus, which lies between the middle and inferior turbinate, is the most important. The middle meatus ostia from anterior to posterior drain sequentially the frontal sinus, the maxillary sinus, and the anterior ethmoid cells. The superior meatus, under the superior turbinate, drains the posterior ethmoid cells. The inferior meatus, which lies under the midportion of the inferior turbinate, does not drain a sinus but rather is the orifice for the nasolacrimal duct. This is essential for draining the large volume of normal tears from the eye.

The bones and cartilage that form the framework of the nose are covered by periosteum or perichondrium. Inside the nose, the covering is thick, richly vascular mucous membrane. This highly specialized membrane is continuous with a similar mucous membrane lining the paranasal sinuses, eustachian tube middle ear, mastoid air cells, and tracheobronchial tree.

Mucous Membrane

The respiratory epithelium is composed mostly of pseudostratified columnar cells surmounted by cilia. It is not uniform in structure at all levels of the respiratory tract. In fact, its microstructure seems to be adapted for the type of airstreams flowing over it. In the anterior third of the nose, especially on the rounded ends of the turbinates where the air is likely to be cold, dry, and unfiltered, the respiratory epithelium has no cilia, and the surface cells resemble squamous cells rather than columnar cells. The epithelium covering the medial aspect of the turbinates and adjacent septum is composed of long columnar cells with short, irregular surface cilia. Within the middle and inferior meatus where airflow is gentle, the epithelium is composed of short columnar cells with lengthy cilia. The sinuses, which usually receive only minute quantities of expired air, are lined by thin epithelium.

The dense vascularity and plethora of glands within the stroma of the submucosa of the nose warm and moisten inspired air. The glands are of the racemose type and contain both serous and mucous cells. In addition, varying numbers of goblet cells lying between surface columnar cells contribute to the secretion. The number of goblet cells is not constant but may vary with conditions that alter airflow patterns and possibly with inflammation or infection.

The cilia seem to function almost automatically. In fact, the contraction of the cilium can be observed even after most of the underlying cell has been removed. A single cilium will continue to stroke as long as a small amount of cytoplasm remains attached to it. The movements of the cilia in any given area of eipthelium appear to be synchronous and purposeful, stroking in unison without bumping or distorting each other. Each stroke has a powerful rapid phase in one direction, with the cilium straight and stiff, followed by a slower phase of recovery during which the cilium bends. In this way, secreted mucus is moved in one direction.

Ciliary motion can be influenced by the factors that follow (Ballantyne and Groves, 1971).

Drying. Adequate moisture is necessary for normal ciliary function. Prolonged breathing of excessively dry air, inadequate secretion by mucosal glands, or both can lead to drying and impairment of ciliary activity. Conditions such as deviation of the nasal septum, which deflects the inspired airstream, produce excessive local evaporation, increased viscosity of the nasal mucus, stasis of the mucous blanket, and impaired ciliary activity.

Temperature. Ciliary activity is depressed by both low and high temperatures. Ciliary activity ceases at about 7 to 10°C and is depressed by temperatures above 35°C.

Acid-base Balance. Ciliary activity is depressed by low pH and stops completely at pH 6.4. It is increased by modest increases in pH.

Topical Medications. Epinephrine hydrochloride (1:10,000) applied to the ciliated cells for 20 minutes causes reversible inhibition of ciliary activity; with a 1:1000 solution this occurs in a much shorter time. However, ephedrine sulfate (0.5 percent solution) does not affect ciliary action.

Mucous Blanket

The so-called mucous blanket is a thin, sticky, continuous, highly viscid secretion that extends into all spaces within the nose, sinuses, eustachian tube, middle ear, mastoid, pharynx, and bronchial tree. The cilia propel it continuously along with particles that have been trapped by it. The pH remains at a relatively constant 7.0. The mucus in the sinuses moves through the ostia into the nose. The mucous blanket in the nose moves posteriorly through the choanae into the pharynx, where mucus is swallowed. Gastric secretions destroy bacteria and other minute particles that have been trapped by the mucus.

Blood, Nerve Supply, and Lymphatic Drainage

The sphenopalatine branch of the internal maxillary artery provides the arterial supply to the turbinates, meatus, and septum. The anterior and posterior ethmoid branches of the ophthalmic artery supply the ethmoid and frontal sinuses and the roof of the nose. A branch of the superior labial artery and the infraorbital and alveolar branches of the internal maxillary artery supply the maxillary sinus, while the pharyngeal branch of the internal maxillary artery is distributed to the sphenoid sinus.

The arterioles of the nasal respiratory mucosa are distinctive because they lack an internal elastic membrane, and the vascular endothelial basement membrane is continuous with the basement membrane of smooth muscle cells in the wall of the arteriole. In addition, the endothelial basement membrane is exceptionally porous. As a result, the subendothelial musculature of these vessels may be influenced more readily than other blood vessels by agents such as histamine and systemically administered vasoconstrictors (Mygind, 1978).

Within the lamina propria of the nasal mucosa are small, regular capillaries. Below the surface epithelium, the capillaries are larger and have fenestrations. The fenestrae are small areas in the endothelial lining where the endothelial cell consists only of a thin single membrane. This membrane and the porous basement membrane, reinforced by pericytes, constitute the only barrier between blood plasma and tissue fluid and provide for rapid passage of fluid through the vascular wall.

Veins within the nose form a cavernous plexus underneath the mucous membrane. The plexus is especially well developed over the middle and inferior turbinates and the lower portion of the septum where it forms erectile tissue. Venous drainage is principally through the ophthalmic, anterior facial and sphenopalatine veins. The venous system of the nose, paranasal sinuses, and orbit communicate freely through valveless veins. Venous stasis related to nasal congestion can cause dark circles or discoloration beneath the eyes known as "allergic shiners."

Lymphatic drainage of the nose is divided into an anterior and posterior network. The anterior network drains along the facial vessels toward nodes in the submaxillary glands. Most of the anterior nose, the vestibule, and the preturbinal area are drained by this system. The posterior network drains the major portion of the nose, and it forms three channels. The superior group, from the middle and superior turbinates and adjacent septum, form channels passing above the eustachian tube to drain into retropharyngeal nodes. The middle group, passing below the eustachian tube, serves the inferior turbinate, inferior meatus, and a portion of the floor and drains into the external jugular chain of lymph nodes. The inferior group, from the septum and part of the floor, drain through lymph nodes along the internal jugular vein.

The nerve supply to the nose is complex. The olfactory mucosa, located high in the nose is characterized by the presence of "special sense" receptor nerve cells in which the central processes unite to form small nerve fiber bundles that pass through the cribriform plate to enter the brain. These nerves constitute the neuronal pathway for the sense of smell. The anterior and posterior ethmoid nerves, branches of the ophthalmic division of the trigeminal nerve, supply pain, temperature, and touch sensations to the mucous membrane in the lateral wall anterior to the turbinates and meatus and the corresponding area of the septum. Nasal branches of the sphenopalatine ganglion, containing fibers of the maxillary division of the trigeminal nerve, supply pain, temperature, and touch sensations to much of the rest of the nasal mucosa.

The parasympathetic nerve supply is derived from the seventh cranial nerve. It leaves the facial nerve at the level of the geniculate ganglion in the temporal bone. These preganglionic fibers after following a tortuous course along the base of the skull finally synapse in the sphenopalatine ganglion. The postsynaptic fibers are distributed to the glandular epithelium of the nose and the blood vessel plexus. Stimulation of these fibers releases acetyl choline, which results in glandular secretion and transient vasodilatation.

The sympathetic nerve supply follows the carotid artery after leaving the stellate ganglion in the lower neck. It follows the arterial supply of the nose to the nasal surface and remains richly distributed around the blood vessels. Stimulation of these fibers releases norepinephrine, which causes vasoconstriction. The subepithelial cavernous sinusoids are kept partially constricted by continuous sympathetic stimulation. As the sinusoids account for a large part of nasal blood volume in the turbinates, changes in the autonomic innervation can rapidly cause changes in the thickness of the nasal mucosa and, in turn, can affect the degree of nasal patency (Mygind, 1978).

Both the secretory and contractile myoepithelial elements of the human nasal glands are under parasympathetic control in contrast to the salivary glands, which possess a dual autonomic nerve supply. Since secretion of the glands depends upon their blood supply, however, secretion of the nasal glands is indirectly affected by sympathetic nerve fibers through the innervation of blood vessels.

Glands

The glands of the lamina propria of the nasal mucosa consist of anterior serous glands and scattered seromucous glands. The openings of the serous glands are comparatively large, and the serous ducts often have an ampullated area near the area where the duct bends toward the surface. The seromucous glands are smaller and more numerous than the serous glands. Specialized cells in the seromucous glands contribute to the formation of secretions. Proteinaceous secretion is released from the glandular cells of the secretory tubules, then as the secretion passes through the mucous secretory tubules, large amounts of mucus are added. This combined primary secretion is collected in a duct that is able to modify and control the ion and water concentration of the final glandular secretion. In the ciliated collecting duct, goblet and ciliated cells form the mucociliary transport apparatus that assists in the expulsion of secretion from the gland opening.

Secretion

Nasal fluid is a mixture of nasal, sinus, and orbital secretions. The major components of the fluid are water (95 to 97 percent), mucin (2.5 to 3 percent), and electrolytes (1 to 2 percent). There also is a trace quantity of protein which are from transudated fluid or are partially synthesized in the mucosa (Mygind, 1978). The mucin forms long threads or fibrils, giving nasal secretion its viscoelastic properties. Electrolyte concentrations are similar to those in serum, with the exception of potassium, which is about three times higher in nasal secretions. With nasal hypersecretion resulting from respiratory infections, there is a decrease in sodium, chloride, calcium, and protein concentrations in the secretion. However, in the nasal secretion that results from allergen challenge, potassium concentration decreases and protein concentration increases, possibly owing to increased transudation from plasma induced by allergic mediators. The exact actions of the allergic mediators, which are multiple (Naclerio, 1983), are not well understood. There appears to be a difference between mediators of the allergic response and the mediators that cause nasal hypersecretion during a viral cold (Eggleston, 1984).

Immunity

Secretory IgA (dimer + secretory component) is the principal immunoglobulin found in nasal secretions. The dimeric IgA is found in plasma cells surrounding the exocrine glands in the lamina propria of the nasal and sinus mucosae. It is transformed to secretions by an active process. Secretory component that is produced in the glandular cells binds to the IgA to form secretory IgA. Secretory IgA covers the mucosal surface of the mucous membrane and acts to protect against invasion of microorganisms; it inhibits the adherence of microorganisms to the surface and neutralizes viruses.

Although IgG is an immunoglobulin found mostly in the blood, it does pass from blood to tissue fluid and, to a lesser degree, from tissue fluid to secretions. Inflammation increases the permeability of blood vessels and epithelium, allowing larger amounts of IgG antibodies to reach the surface of the mucous membrane. There normally are relatively few IgG-producing plasma cells in nasal mucosa; however, they increase in number with chronic nasal infection.

IgE is of great importance in allergic nasal disease (see Chapter 6). IgE binds to mast cells in the mucosa and submucosa. It is not linked with a secretory component, and it appears to be transported actively through the epithelium. When the antigen comes into contact with the mast cell–IgE complex, inflammatory mediators are released. These mediators include histamine; enzymes, such as TAMe; esterase; prostaglandin D_2; and leukotrienes (Creticos 1984; Naclerio 1983). The release of these mediators is associated with the onset of clinical symptoms.

Functions of the Nose

The major functions of the nose are olfaction and filtration, humidification, and warming of air for respiration. With ordinary tidal breathing, airflow is low in the nose and odors usually are not perceived unless they are strong. In order to sense an odor, air must be brought higher into the nose where olfactory receptors are located. This is accomplished by sniffing, that is, fixing the rib cage and abruptly moving the diaphragm down. Nasal polyps or any mechanical obstruction within the nose that alters airflow patterns can impair the sense of smell.

"Air conditioning" probably is the most important function of the nose. The turbinates serve to further direct the flow of air and create controlled air turbulence within the nose, which facilitates filtration, warming, and humidification of inspired air. The air is warmed by rapid heat transfer from blood in the capillary networks and venous sinuses.

The ability of the nose to cleanse air of particulate matter depends upon the nature of the particles. Allergic particles, such as pollen, dust, and dander, are partially filtered from inspired air in the nose. Size, shape, and density of the particles are important. In general, the larger and heavier the particles, the sooner they will be filtered from inspired air and deposited within the nose. Some particles from aggregations, and some hygroscopic dusts take on water, becoming larger until they reach an equilibrium determined by vapor saturation at the ambient body temperature (Hinchcliff and Harrison, 1976). Bacteria, although small, may form agglomerates or may be included in droplets. Viruses also can be enclosed in droplets. All of these then behave as larger particles and are trapped by the nasal mucous blanket. Factors such as particle inertia, density, and surface area, as well as velocity and turbulence of airflow, affect air filtration in the nose.

A large portion of foreign material in inspired air is deposited in the anterior third of the nose. After passing through the anterior nares, the flow rate of inspired air decreases as it is filtered through the hairs in the vestibule. The flow rate increases at the nasal valve region, then decreases in the preturbinal area as it strikes the anterior blunt ends of the inferior and middle turbinates. The shape of the turbinates induces turbulence and directs airflow backward instead of up. As the air flows posteriorly toward the choanae, it deposits particles. Additional deposition occurs even after air passes through the choanae into the pharnyx. Noxious gases contained in inspired air diffuse into the mucous blanket.

The Nose and Pulmonary Function

It is important to recognize that the nose is one integral unit functioning in concert with other portions of the respiratory system. Normal aeration of pulmonary alveoli depends upon the maintenance of an adequate resistance to the flow of air within the tracheobronchial tree. The nose furnishes from 50 to 70 percent of the total respiratory resistance. Nasopulmonary and nasobronchial reflexes increase bronchial tone in cases of nasal obstruction and also increase pulmonary resistance while decreasing compliance. Thus, nasal obstruction can increase pulmonary resistance and decrease compliance.

"Nasal Cycle"

The term nasal cycle refers to the alternating changes in patency of the right and left nasal cavities. Congestion and decongestion of the erectile tissues of the nasal mucosa of the lateral wall and septum occur in rhythmic sequence in most individuals. As one nasal chamber opens and mucosal glands secrete, the erectile tissues of the opposite chamber fill with blood, and secretions of the mucosal glands diminish. The cycle is controlled by peripheral autonomic centers in the sphenopalatine and stellate ganglia. The cycle seems to be most active during adolescence when hormonal factors may act on nasal erectile tissue. Head position and body posture can influence hydrostatic pressure of blood in the head and, in turn, influence the nasal cycle. Vasoconstrictor nose drops can interrupt this cycle temporarily.

Protective Mechanisms

The sneeze is a simple yet important nasal reflex. Irritation of the nasal mucosa causes sneezing and associated cardiorespiratory responses. Such irritation may be due to allergic, autonomic, and psychologic factors. Ciliary propulsion of mucus is a protective mechanism in that it aids in the expulsion of foreign matter. Noxious stimuli increase nasal secretions. Immunoglobulins in nasal secretions (primary IgA) can inactivate viruses. Lysozymes present in nasal secretions may aid in bacterial defense. When the mucociliary defenses fail and organisms invade the tunica propria or stroma of the mucosa, phagocytosis becomes important. Fibroblasts, ameboid wandering cells, undifferentiated mesenchymal cells, mast cells, and histiocytes also play roles in the removal of debris, pollen, bacteria, or other foreign material. Polymorphonuclear leukocytes are the active phagocytes in acute infection; histiocytes are active in subacute and chronic inflammation.

Examination of the Nose

Before examining the inside of the nose, the external nose should be inspected. The shape of the upper bony portion and lower cartilaginous portion should be noted. Palpation of the bony nasal dorsum can reveal deformities not apparent on inspection. Abnormal contour of the nasal alae, displacement of the septum, or retracted columella may contribute to nasal obstruction. A transverse crease across the lower third of the nose at the junction of the bulbous

soft portion and the more rigid bony dorsum suggests chronic nasal rubbing associated with allergic rhinitis. Persistent nasal obstruction with intranasal edema can cause broadening of the bony dorsum of the nose.

The internal nose is best examined with the aid of a nasal speculum to spread the nares with bright illumination reflected from a headlight or head mirror into the nose. A knowledge of normal anatomic landmarks is essential. Edematous, pale bluish turbinates often are seen in children with allergic rhinitis. Purulent discharge in the middle meatus is indicative of sinusitis (Fig. 33A–3). Nasal polyps in children are more likely to be associated with cystic fibrosis than with allergic diathesis. Since masses, such as meningoceles or encephaloceles, can be mistaken for benign polyps, biopsy should not be performed without thorough investigation. Small, superficial, unexplained, nonhealing lesions in the nasal mucosa warrant biopsy. However, when the total extent and origin of an intranasal mass cannot be judged adequately on intranasal examination, it is wise to obtain radiographic studies of facial bones and paranasal sinuses before proceeding to biopsy. These radiographic studies should include the standard sinus views and occasionally computerized tomographic scans. The development of nuclear magnetic resonance imaging may provide an additional method of sinus evaluation, particularly with respect to soft tissue analysis.

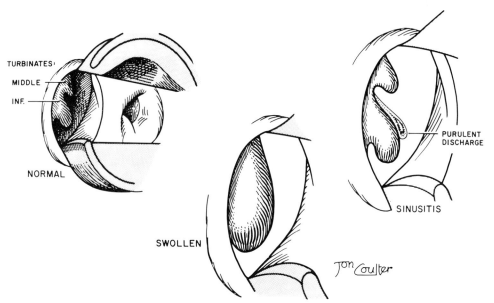

FIGURE 33A–3. Intranasal examination with speculum. Normal findings; swollen inferior turbinate (often associated with allergic rhinitis); and findings in sinusitis.

When there is significant swelling of the nasal mucosa, examination is not complete until a topical vasoconstrictor, such as phenylephrine hydrochloride or ephedrine sulfate, has been applied to shrink the mucous membrane and allow better visualization of the entire nasal chamber.

A flexible fiberoptic or a rod lens telescopic nasopharyngoscope is useful in close examination of the posterior nose and nasopharynx. Prior to insertion of the instrument and prior to nasal biopsy, it is advisable to use 5 percent lidocaine hydrochloride (Xylocaine) as a topical anesthetic. The small nasopharyngeal mirror inserted posterior to the soft palate gives a view of the choanae and eustachian tube orifices, but use of the mirror requires considerable skill and practice.

Nasal Smear Cytology

Since intranasal inspection may not always lead to a definitive diagnosis, it is sometimes helpful to obtain a specimen from the inside of the nose for cytologic study. A method for nasal cytologic examination is described in detail by Bryan and Bryan (1974). This is accomplished by gently passing a wire applicator thinly wrapped with cotton along the floor of the nose and up under the inferior turbinate three times in each side of the nose. The motion should be one of wiping rather than dabbing or blotting.

After each wiping, the contents on the probe are gently rolled, not smeared, onto a glass slide. Next, the slide is fixed by placing it in a solution of 95 percent alcohol and ether (reagent quality) for 5 minutes. Alternatively, a commercial spray fixative can be used. Wright-Geimsa stain is applied for approximately 30 seconds, then immediately flooded for 30 more seconds with a buffer of pH 6.4 to 6.8. The slide is then washed with distilled water. Deliberate understaining is advisable so that the stained epithelial cells do not obscure the mast cells.

Evaluation of the Nasal Cytogram

Cytologic examination of a nasal smear for accumulations of eosinophils is helpful in differentiating allergic disorders from other conditions such as viral or bacterial infections or tumors. More than 10 percent eosinophils in the specimen is considered abnormal, but more than one specimen may be necessary for interpretation (Mullarky et al., 1980).

Ciliated cells undergo distinctive destructive changes in the presence of rhinovirus infections (Fig. 33A–4), but this is not easily detected nor is it virus specific (Hendley, 1983). Biopsy of the nasal mucosa also is of little value. Biopsy specimens appear to show only a decreased number of ciliated cells during experimental rhinovirus infections and no evidence of massive destruction (Pederson, 1983). Quantification of poly-

RESPONSE OF NASAL EPITHELIAL CELLS TO VIRAL INFECTION

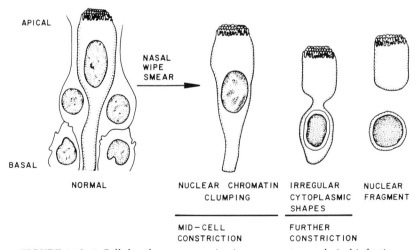

FIGURE 33A–4. Cellular changes occurring in response to nasal viral infection.

morphonulear neutrophils may be useful in distinguishing infection from allergy.

Rhinomanometry

Rhinomanometry is the measurement of nasal respiratory function. Several devices have been designed that are capable of measuring pressure, resistance, and volume of nasal airflow. Measurements can be made quickly and easily, and children usually tolerate the test procedures without becoming frightened. Analysis of rhinomanometric data has revealed that a fundamental function of the nose is to act as a servomechanism for matching the impedance of the upper respiratory tract to that of the lower. The nose is also involved in matching the impedance of the entire respiratory tract to alveolar ventilation, balancing a demand for oxygen with energy expended and modulating the mechanical efficiency of respiration (Williams, 1970). Although rhinomanometry was once considered purely a research tool, it now is useful in the following clinical situations: (1) it can be helpful in determining whether an obstruction is caused primarily by engorgement of nasal mucosa or by adenoidal hypertrophy, and (2) it can be utilized as a means for monitoring the effectiveness of medical or surgical measures in the treatment of chronic nasal obstruction.

PARANASAL SINUSES

General Considerations

The paranasal sinuses are a series of mucosa-linked pneumatic cavities that surround the nose and lie adjacent to the orbit (Fig. 33A–5). Some of the sinuses begin to develop during fetal life, others during early childhood. Pneumatic expansion continues throughout the childhood years until early adulthood. The mucoperiosteum lining of the sinuses contains cilia and mucous glands, though they are sparser than in the nasal mucosa. The sinus mucosa is covered with a layer of mucus that is propelled by the cilia toward the ostia. The mucosa is able to regenerate if portions are damaged by infection, injury, chemicals, or surgery. However, regenerated mucosa appears to be more susceptible to infection because it has fewer cilia and goblet cells than normal mucosa and may be scarred.

Functions

The function of the paranasal sinuses is not clear. They may have an olfactory function

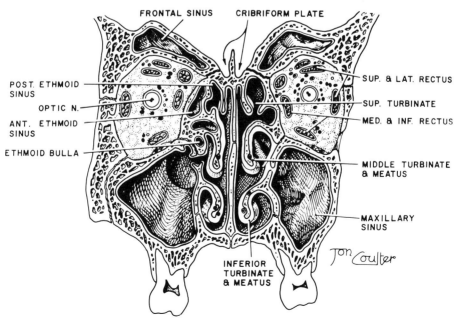

FIGURE 33A–5. Sagittal section through the nose showing the relationship of the sinuses to nasal landmarks (see text).

since inspired air is evenly distributed within them, a resonating function in voice production, and a protective function in producing mucus to moisten the nasal chambers. In addition, they lessen the weight of the skull.

Maxillary Sinus

The maxillary sinus is the first of the cavities to develop. A small ridge develops superior to the inferior turbinate and projects medially into the middle meatus at approximately 10 weeks of gestation. A mucosal evagination slowly extends laterally into the maxilla and expands. The maxillary sinus cavity, measuring approximately $7 \times 4 \times 4$ mm, is present at birth. As the facial structures grow anteroinferiorly away from the skull after birth, the maxillary sinus also expands in the same direction at the rate of 2 mm vertically and 3 mm anteroposteriorly each year. By the age of 12 years, the floor of the sinus lies on a horizontal level with the floor of the nasal chamber. Anatomically, the floor of the maxillary sinus is closely related to the maxillary teeth. As a tooth erupts, the space vacated by it becomes pneumatized by the expanding sinus lumen. Expansion is complete after the permanent teeth erupt, with a final volume of 14 to 15 cc.

Since the lumen of the sinus grows progressively from above downward, the younger the patient, the more likely that the floor of the sinus lies above the level of the floor of the nasal chamber. In young children, needles must be directed superiorly in order to enter the maxillary sinuses to irrigate them or to obtain secretions for cultures.

The ostium of the maxillary sinus is round or oval, approximately 4 mm in diameter, and lies in the middle meatus. Within the sinus, the ostium is located immediately below the orbital floor, at the highest point of the maxillary antrum. The position of the ostia is not conducive to gravity drainage in the upright position. Rather, the continual beating of the cilia sweeps the elaborated mucous blanket from the niches of the sinuses to the ostia without concern for gravity. This system can be severely disturbed during infection.

Ethmoid Sinuses

The ethmoid sinuses consist of a group of three to fifteen air cells within the ethmoid bone

on each side of the nose. These sinuses begin to develop during the fifth month of intrauterine life as numerous evaginations from the fetal nasal chamber. At first these evaginations are mere slits, but they develop rapidly, assuming a round or globular shape as they expand within the ethmoid bone. The air cells eventually abut each other, with thin bony walls between the mucosa-lined air cells. The expansion of the ethmoid group of cells usually continues until late puberty. The ethmoid cell block, sometimes termed the ethmoid labyrinth, is pyramidal in shape, being wider posteriorly (where it abuts the sphenoid bone) than anteriorly (where it meets the lacrimal bone). Even though growth of the air cells results in air sinuses that are of different size and shape, the ostium of each ethmoid sinus is at the site of the cell's initial evagination from the fetal nasal chamber.

The ostia of the ethmoidal sinuses are the smallest of all the paranasal sinuses, measuring only 1 to 2 mm in diameter. Perhaps it is the small luminal diameter that makes these ostia so susceptible to occlusion by mucosal edema or growth of polyploid granulation tissue. Usually the ostia of the anterior ethmoidal cells are even smaller than those of the posterior ones.

The lamina papyracea is the thin bony plate that separates the ethmoid sinus air cells from the orbit. Occasionally, natural dehiscences occur in this bone so that there is communication between the ethmoid sinus and the orbit.

Orbital cellulitis usually occurs between the ages of 6 and 9 years and is the most common complication of acute sinusitis (usually acute ethmoiditis) in children. The infection spreads from the ethmoid mucosa through a natural dehiscence, via the vascular foramina, or through a thrombophlebitis of veins communicating between the sinus and the orbit.

Frontal Sinus

The nasofrontal region is an evagination of the anterosuperior part of the middle meatus. At 3 to 4 months of fetal life, furrows develop in this region; during subsequent development there is gradual deepening of the furrows and formation of a single large pit or several small pits. These pits can be recognized at birth; as they continue to expand, their growth pushes one or two of them upward into the frontal bone. By 6 years, the sinus has grown sufficiently large to be radiographically visible in the frontal bone. On rare occasions, the frontal sinus develops as an extramural expansion of one of the ethmoid air cells. Sometimes the frontal sinus fails to develop altogether, and usually the right and left chambers are of unequal size.

When the sinus develops directly as an extension of the whole frontal recess, the ostium of the sinus drains directly into the anterior upper part of the middle meatus. When the frontal sinus originates from a frontal recess furrow or from one of the cells of the ethmoidal infundibulum, drainage is into the nose via a nasofrontal duct.

The proximity of the sinus to the bone marrow of the frontal bone permits spread of infection from the sinus into the marrow and blood stream. Consequently, abscesses in the frontal bone can complicate frontal sinusitis.

Sphenoid Sinus

The sphenoid sinus begins to develop in the fourth month of fetal life as a posterior evagination from the nasal capsule into the sphenoid bone. Usually, the sinus is round; however, it sometimes expands by diverticula off the main lumen into the various parts of the sphenoid bone. Hence, the greater wing of the sphenoid bone often contains a pneumatic extension, and the lesser wing sometimes also contains an extension.

The sinus is classified as nonpneumatic, presellar or sellar depending on the amount of bone surrounding the pituitary gland. This system is of use in planning the surgical removal of pituitary tumors. Large sellar sinuses will sometimes expand so widely that the internal carotid artery and nerves adjacent to the sinus lumen appear as ridges on the bony wall of the sinus. The optic, ophthalmic, and mandibular divisions of the trigeminal or vidian nerve may lie separated from the sinus mucosa by only a thin layer of bone.

The ostium of the sphenoid sinus usually is round and located one half to one third of the way up the face of the sphenoid sinus. It usually lies 2 to 5 mm from the dura and the same distance from the midline. It is hidden from view by the superior turbinate during anterior rhinoscopy.

Methods of Examination

The sinuses are examined primarily by palpation and transillumination. Transillumination is done with a high intensity, narrow beam or light source applied to the hard palate or front of the maxilla (maxillary sinuses), or to the inferior aspect of the supraorbital rim (frontal sinuses). Results of transillumination testing are often equivocal and of questionable clinical importance.

Tenderness on palpation of a sinus is a sign of acute sinusitis. Although it has been customary for an examiner to tap on the patient's forehead or malar eminence to elicit tenderness, children are sometimes frightened by the sudden pain that results from percussion of the wall of an inflamed sinus. Rather, it is better to exert increasing pressure gently at the sites depicted in Figure 33A – 6. It is helpful to ask the child to let you know if the pressure causes pain and, if so, whether the pain is greater on the left or right side.

Pain from sinus disease can be referred to areas adjacent to the involved sinus. Pain from inflammation and irritation of a maxillary sinus ostium can be referred to the infraorbital and temporal areas or to the maxillary premolar teeth. Pain from the frontal sinus can be perceived as coming from within the eye or in the area of the temporomandibular joint. Irritation of the frontonasal duct can cause pain in the premolar teeth. Pain from the sphenoid sinus can cause occipital pain, vertex pain, or a deep-seated headache.

Radiography

In adults with sinus disease, sinus radiographs may show changes ranging from mucosal thickening, variations in air-fluid levels, to partial or complete opacification of one or all sinuses. However, since radiographic findings must be correlated with clinical signs and symptoms, there is a wide variation in the radiographic appearance of normal sinuses, and many findings may be subtle. For example, it is difficult to decide when mucosal thickening is within normal limits and when it indicates response to infection or allergy.

In children, the interpretation of sinus radiographs becomes even more complicated since there is a variation between individuals in the rate at which sinuses develop. It can be difficult to differentiate pathologic opacification from poorly developed or late-to-develop sinuses. Further, the interpretation of abnormal sinus radiographs has become controversial. For instance, Caffey (1967) believed that opacified

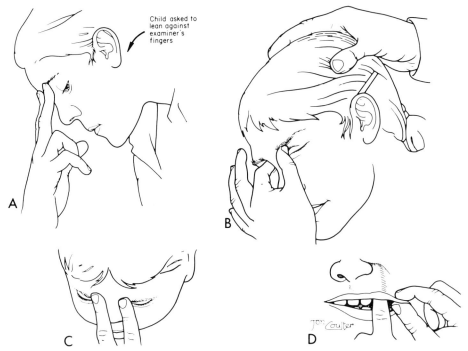

Child asked to lean against examiner's fingers

FIGURE 33A–6. Method of palpating paranasal sinuses. *A* and *B* = frontal sinuses; *C* = ethmoid sinuses; *D* = maxillary sinus.

sinuses on radiographs could result from redundant sinus mucosa or from fluid from tears. Shopfner and Rossi (1973) studied sinus radiographs from 329 children to define criteria for interpretation. In this series only half of the children who were diagnosed as having sinusitis on clinical grounds had radiographic evidence of sinusitis. Fifty-seven percent of children without clinical evidence of sinusitis had radiographic findings that were considered abnormal according to their criteria. Abnormal paranasal sinus films were present most commonly in children with upper respiratory infections without clinical evidence of sinusitis. Unfortunately, their study has been interpreted widely by pediatricians as demonstrating that sinus radiographs in children are of no value rather than that the significance of radiographic findings depends upon correlation with history and physical findings.

Another widespread misconception is that the paranasal sinuses cannot be visualized in very young children. Ethmoid sinuses can be visualized by radiography in children as young as 10 months. The three radiographic views that are most useful in evaluating paranasal sinus pathology in children are the posteroanterior (Caldwell) view, the occipitomental (Waters) view, and the lateral view. The pos-

teroanterior view demonstrates the frontal sinuses and the superior ethmoid cells. The occipitomental view best demonstrates developmental or pathologic changes in the maxillary sinus. The lateral view provides considerable information about all the paranasal sinuses. It demonstrates the thickness of the anterior wall and the anteroposterior depth of the frontal sinus and the anteroposterior depth of the sphenoid sinuses. Although the right and left maxillary sinuses are superimposed in a lateral view, the thickness of the walls of the maxillary sinuses and the relationship of the antral floor to the teeth is demonstrated. The nasopharynx, adenoids, tonsils (if enlarged), and palate are well visualized in the lateral views.

Radiographic findings that tend to substantiate a clinical diagnosis of allergic rhinosinusitis are thickening of paranasal sinus mucosa and sometimes polyps visible within the sinus.

Pathophysiology

Normal physiology of the paranasal sinuses is dependent upon several factors. These include the patency of the ostia, the function of the mucosal cilia, and the quality of the secretions. If any of these three conditions are altered, retention of secretions may occur. This in turn will lead to stasis and bacterial overgrowth.

It is estimated that 0.5 to 5 percent of upper respiratory infections are complicated by sinusitis. Adults average two to three colds per year and children somewhat more. It is unknown what percentage of episodes of sinusitis is due to allergic inflammation. Nevertheless, allergists have noted an increased frequency with which sinusitis complicates allergic disease (Shapiro, 1985).

The intranasal immune event leads to mucosal membrane edema and increased production of nasal secretions. This environment is thought to be very similar to that of a viral upper respiratory infection. While membrane edema occludes the ostia and leads to relative stasis, the pooling of sinus secretions may alter normal ciliary function. The secretions in turn form a rich culture medium for bacterial pathogens. Abnormal radiographs, including major changes such as clouding, are found in 20 percent of patients with allergic rhinitis (Mygind, 1978). This indicates some evidence for the pooling and stasis thought necessary for sinusitis.

There appears to be a relationship between sinusitis and airway hyperreactivity. When chronic asthmatics with abnormal sinus radiographs are treated for sinusitis, there is a decreased bronchial reactivity and a reduced use of bronchodilator drugs. This relationship holds true even when diagnostic maxillary puncture reveals no bacteria (Cummings, 1984). This information is of value in the decision to treat asymptomatic patients with abnormal sinus radiographs who have underlying airway disorders. Further investigations quantitating nasal and sinus relationships during the allergic inflammatory response would be of great value.

REFERENCES

Adams, L., Boies, L., Paparella, M.: Boies' Fundamentals of Otolaryngology, 5th ed. Philadelphia, W.B. Saunders Co., 1978.

Ballantyne, J., Groves, J.: Scott-Brown's Diseases of the Ear, Nose and Throat, 3rd ed. London, Butterworth and Co., 1971.

Bernstein, L. (ed.): Surgery of the nasal sinuses. Otolaryngol. Clin. North Am. 4:3–13, 1971.

Bryan, M.P., Bryan, W.T.K.: Cytologic diagnosis in allergic disorders. Otolaryngol. Clin. North Am. 7:637, 1974.

Caffey, J.: Pediatric X-Ray Diagnosis, 5th ed. Chicago, Year Book Publishers, Inc., 1967.

Creticos, P.S., Petus, P., Adlainson, F.N., Naclerio, R.M.,

Hayes, E.C., Norman, P.S., Lichtenstein, L.: Peptide leukotriene release after antigen challenge in patients sensitive to ragweed. N. Engl. J. Med. 310:1626, 1984.

Cummings, N.P., Lere, J.L., Wood, K.: Effect of treatment of sinusitis on asthma and bronchial reactivity; results of double blind study. J. Allergy Clin. Immunol. 73:143, 1984.

Dodd, G.D., Jing, B.: Radiology of the Nose, Paranasal Sinuses and Nasopharynx. Baltimore, Williams & Wilkins Co., 1977.

Eggleston, P., Hendley, J.O., Gwaltney, J.M.: Mediators of immediate hypersensitivity in nasal secretions during natural colds and rhinovirus infections. Acta Otolaryngol. (Stockholm) 4:25–35, 1984.

Hajek, M.: Pathology and Treatment of the Inflammatory Diseases of the Nasal Accessory Sinuses. St. Louis, C.V. Mosby Co., 1926.

Hendley, J.O.: Rhinovirus colds: Immunology and Pathogenesis. Eur. J. Respir. Dis. 340–343, 1983.

Hinchcliff, R., Harrison, D. (eds.): Scientific Foundations of Otolaryngology. Chicago, Yearbook Medical Publishers, 1976.

Mygind, N., Dirksen, A., Johnson, N.G., Weeke, B.: Perennial rhinitis: An analysis of stain testing, serum IgE, and blood and smear eosinophilia in 201 patients. Clin. Otolaryngol. 3:189–196, 1978.

Mygind, N.: Nasal Allergy. Oxford, Scientific Publications, 1978.

Mullarkey, M.F., Hill, J., Webb, D.R.: Allergic and nonallergic rhinitis: Their characterization with attention to the meaning of nasal eosinophilia, J. Allergy Clin. Immunol. 65:122–126, 1980.

Naclerio, R., Meier, H., Kagey-Sobotka, A., Adkinson, F.N., Meyers, D., Norman, P., Uchtenstein, L.: Mediator release after nasal airway challenge with allergen. Am. Rev. Respir. Dis. 128:597–602, 1983.

Pederson, M., Sakakura, Y., Winther, B., Brofeldt, S., Mygind, N.: Nasal mucociliary transport, numbers of ciliated cells, and beating patterns in naturally acquired common colds. Eur. J. Respir. Dis. 128:355–364, 1983.

Ritter, F.N.: The Paranasal Sinuses — Anatomy and Surgical Technique, 2nd ed. St. Louis, C.V. Mosby Co., 1978.

Shapiro, G.: Role of allergy in sinusitis. Pediatr. Infect. Dis. 4:555–563, 1985.

Shopfner, C., Rossi, J.: Roentgen evaluation of the paranasal sinuses in children. J. Radiol. 118:176, 1973.

Williams, H.L.: Report of Committee on Standardization of Definitions, Terms Symbols in Rhinomanometry of the American Academy of Ophthalmology and Otolaryngology (A.A.O.O.), Rochester, Minn., 1970.

The Ear

CHARLES D. BLUESTONE, M.D.

Allergic disorders can involve any of the mucous membrane–lined, air-containing spaces of the middle ear, mastoid, and nose as well as the paranasal sinuses. Knowledge of the anatomy and physiology of the ear provides the basis for an understanding of the pathophysiology of its involvement in allergic disorders of the upper respiratory tract.

Anatomically, the ear may be divided into five portions; the auricle (pinna), external canal, eardrum, tympanum (middle ear space), and the inner ear.

AURICLE

The auricle (or pinna) consists of a thin piece of yellow fibrocartilage covered with skin and connected with surrounding parts by ligaments and muscles. The skin is firmly adherent on the anterior surface and looser on the posterior surface. The lymphatics of the posterior surface drain to nodes at the mastoid tip, from the tragus and upper part of the anterior surface to parotid lymph nodes and from the inferior part to nodes immediately caudal to the lobule.

Contact dermatitis of the auricle frequently is due to cosmetics, hair sprays, hair dyes, and jewelry. Seborrheic dermatitis both in early infancy and in adolescence may involve the auricle as well as the scalp. In young children, ear discomfort associated with inadequate middle ear ventilation may induce scratching and excoriation of the auricles.

THE EXTERNAL AUDITORY CANAL

The external auditory canal is about 2.5 cm in length in adults and usually less than 2 cm in length in young children. It is S-shaped in that its general direction is upward and backward in the outer cartilaginous part, then slightly downward and forward more medially in the bony part that meets the eardrum. In newborn or young infants, the bony canal has not yet formed, and the eardrum lies in an almost horizontal position. As a result, the external canal is more or less collapsed upon the surface of the eardrum. Since the infant's ear canal is almost entirely composed of cartilage, it is relatively distensible. For this reason, in infants movement of the ear canal on tympanometry may appear to indicate good eardrum movement even when a middle ear effusion is present.

The external auditory canal is the only cul-de-sac in the human body lined by skin. The skin of the outer one third is closely adherent to the cartilage and contains tiny hairs, sebaceous glands, and ceruminous glands. Almost all the sebaceous glands open into the lumina of the hair follicles. The ceruminous glands are simple coiled tubular structures with cuboidal secretory cells surrounded by an outer myoepithelium. Contraction of the myoepithelium compresses the lumen of the tubule and expels the contents. The ceruminous glands lie in the deeper portion of the dermis, and the ducts from the glands reach the epidermis, emptying either into the lumen of a hair follicle or on the free epidermal surface.

Earwax (cerumen) is the product of both sebaceous and ceruminous glands and can be "wet" or "dry." The type of earwax that a person has is genetically inherited, the wet type being dominant. Though it has no antibacterial, antifungal, or insect repellent properties, cerumen provides protection for the eardrum by acting as a vehicle for the collection and removal of epithelial debris and contaminants. It also provides lubrication and prevents desiccation of the epidermis. The skin of the ear canal and caudal portion of the auricle may become macerated and edematous from chronic ear drainage. Since the cartilage of the auricle is continuous with the cartilaginous portion of the external ear canal, movement of the auricle or tragus results in severe pain in diffuse external otitis but usually not in otitis media. However, even in the child with severe external otitis, middle ear disease should be considered as an etiologic factor. The eardrum must be visualized and inspected for perforations despite an edematous, macerated or excoriated ear canal.

THE TYMPANIC MEMBRANE

The tympanic membrane (eardrum) is an elliptic disc composed of three layers; an outer layer of epidermis, a middle fibrous layer, and an inner mucous membrane layer. The eardrum is nearly conical in shape with its concave surface toward the external ear canal. The lateral (short) process of the malleus protrudes from the surface of the eardrum toward the ear canal. The smaller portion of the eardrum above the short process is called the Shrapnell membrane or the pars flaccida. The larger portion below the short process is the pars tensa. The eardrum forms the lateral wall of the middle ear space and is frequently involved in middle ear disease.

THE EUSTACHIAN TUBE

The eustachian tube connects the middle ear and mastoid air cells directly to the nasophar-

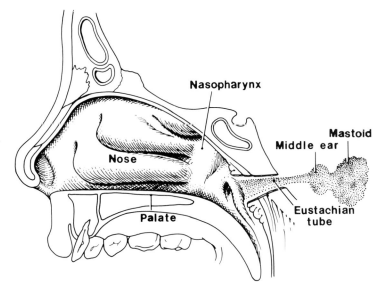

FIGURE 33B–1. Eustachian tube system.

ynx and indirectly to the nasal cavities and palate (Fig. 33B–1). In the adult, the anterior two thirds of the eustachian tube is cartilaginous and the posterior third bony, but in the infant, the bony portion is relatively longer. The lumen of the eustachian tube is shaped like two cones with the apex of each directed toward the middle. The aural orifice of the tube is oval in shape, measuring 5 mm high and 2 mm wide in the adult. The nasopharyngeal orifice in the adult is 8 to 9 mm in diameter, appearing as a vertical slit at right angles to the base of the skull; in the infant this opening is 4 to 5 mm and oblique, owing to the more horizontal position of the cartilage. The mucosal lining of the cartilaginous portion is similar to that of the nasopharynx and contains mucous glands. The mucosa in the protympanic portion of the eustachian tube is similar to that of the middle ear and contains both mucus-producing elements and cilia (Rood and Doyle, 1985).

Usually the eustachian tube is closed, but it opens during swallowing, yawning, and sneezing, permitting air pressure in the middle ear to equalize with atmospheric pressure. The tensor veli palatini is the only muscle related to active tubal opening (Cantekin et al., 1979; Honjo et al., 1979). No constrictor muscle of the tube has ever been demonstrated, and closure has been attributed to the relaxation of the tensor muscle with passive return of the tubal walls to a condition of approximation. The eustachian tube has at least three physiologic functions with respect to the middle ear as follows (Fig. 33B–2): (1) *ventilation* of the middle ear to equilibrate air

pressure in the middle ear with atmospheric pressure, (2) *protection* from nasopharyngeal sound pressure and secretions, and (3) *clearance* of secretions produced within the middle ear into the nasopharynx. Assessment of these functions has been helpful in understanding the physiology and pathophysiology of the eustachian tube, as well as in diagnosis and management of patients with middle ear disease.

Physiology of the Eustachian Tube

The normal eustachian tube is functionally obstructed or collapsed at rest (Fig. 33B–3). Intermittent active opening of the tube maintains near ambient pressures in the middle ear (Bluestone and Beery, 1976). When active opening of the eustachian tube is inefficient, functional collapse of the tube may persist and appears to be common in children who may have moderate to high negative middle ear pressures on tympanometry but normal eustachian tube function otherwise (Beery et al., 1975).

Eustachian tube function also may vary according to season (Beery et al., 1979). Serial studies on children with tympanostomy tubes revealed better eustachian tube function in the summer and fall than in the winter and spring. Considerably more research is needed to elicit in-depth knowledge of eustachian tube-middle ear physiology.

Physiology

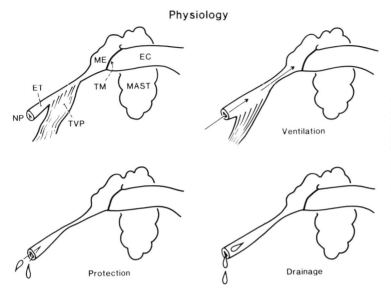

FIGURE 33B–2. Three physiologic functions of the eustachian tube in relation to the middle ear. *NP* = nasopharynx; *ET* = eustachian tube; *TVP* = tensor veli palatini muscle; *ME* = middle ear; *Mast* = mastoid; *TM* = tympanic membrane; *EC* = external canal.

Causes of Eustachian Tube Dysfunction

The eustachian tube can be obstructed by intrinsic or extrinsic factors. Congenital, traumatic, neoplastic, degenerative, metabolic, inflammatory, and idiopathic conditions can lead to eustachian tubal abnormalities (Bluestone and Klein, 1983).

Cranofacial anomalies, such as Down Crouzon Apert, and Turner syndromes, as well as cleft palate, are associated with middle ear dis-

PHYSIOLOGY OF PRESSURE REGULATION

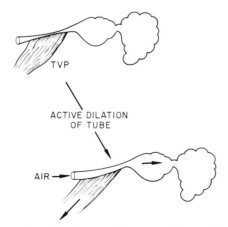

FIGURE 33B–3. Diagrammatic representation of physiologic ventilation of the middle ear during active opening of the eustachian tube by the tensor veli palatini muscle (TVP).

ease, probably because of abnormal tensor veli palatini muscle function.

Some children and adults with middle ear disease appear to have a congenital defect that results in excessive patency or functional obstruction of the tube, possibly owing to an abnormal relation between the eustachian tube and the tensor veli palatini muscle. This may account for racial differences in the prevalence and incidence of otitis media. Native Americans (Eskimos and American Indians) have a higher incidence of otitis media than whites, whereas blacks have an incidence of otitis media that is half that of whites. There is also some evidence that otitis media is more prevalent in certain families (Doyle, 1980).

Dentofacial abnormalities may be associated with abnormal eustachian tube function as well as with deviated nasal septum. In these conditions eustachian tube function may improve with correction of the defect.

Relationship of Eustachian Tube Dysfunction to Middle Ear Disease

Otitis media may result from eustachian tube obstruction, abnormal patency, or both (Bluestone et al., 1979). Either functional or mechanical factors may lead to eustachian tube obstruction. The eustachian tube may collapse functionally because of an increased tubal compliance, an abnormal active opening mechanism, or both. Functional eustachian tube obstruction is common in infants and younger

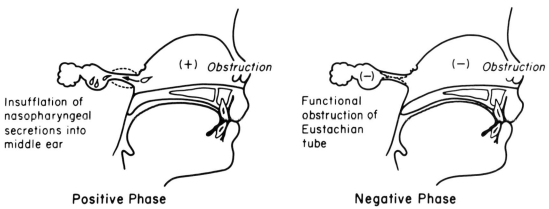

Positive Phase   **Negative Phase**

FIGURE 33B–4. Diagrammatic representation of the "Toynbee phenomenon."

children because of insufficient cartilaginous support of the eustachian tube and because of age-related anatomic features prior to puberty in the craniofacial base, predisposing to inefficient function of the tensor veli palatini muscle. Children with cleft palates have effusions due to functional obstruction (Bluestone, 1971; Doyle et al., 1980). Intrinsic or extrinsic factors may obstruct the eustachian tube mechanically. Intrinsic obstruction results most commonly from acute or chronic inflammation of the mucosal lining (due to infection or possibly allergy) but may also be associated with polyps or cholesteatoma (Bluestone et al., 1977, 1978). Extrinsic obstruction could result from increased extramural pressure, which occurs in the supine position, or peritubal compression from a tumor or possibly an adenoid mass (Bluestone et al., 1972b, 1975). Swallowing when the nose is obstructed induces positive nasopharyngeal pressure, which might insufflate infected secretions into the ear followed by a negative phase that could lead to further obstruction ("Toynbee phenomenon," Fig. 33B–4) (Bluestone et al., 1974, 1975).

In the extreme form of abnormal patency, the eustachian tube is open even at rest. A patulous tube allows air as well as nasopharyngeal secretions to flow from the nasopharynx into the middle ear readily and results in "reflux otitis media." A semipatulous eustachian tube may be obstructed functionally as a result of increased tubal compliance, and the middle ear may have negative pressure, effusion, or both. Nasopharyngeal secretions may be insufflated into the middle ear as a result of nose blowing, sneezing, crying, or closed-nose swallowing. Increased patency of the tube may be due to abnormal tube anatomy or to a decrease in the extramural pressure, such as occurs in weight loss.

ALLERGY AND EUSTACHIAN TUBE FUNCTION

The role of allergy in the etiology and pathogenesis of acute otitis media and otitis media with effusion may be one or more of the following mechanisms: (1) middle ear functioning as a target organ; (2) inflammatory swelling of the eustachian tube; (3) inflammatory obstruction of the nose; and (4) reflux, insufflation, or aspiration of bacteria-laden allergic nasopharyngeal secretions into the middle ear cavity (Fig. 33B–5). The last three mechanisms would be associated with abnormal function of the eustachian tube.

Even though there is a lack of convincing evidence that allergy plays a significant role in the etiology of otitis media, there may be a relation between upper respiratory tract allergy and eustachian tube dysfunction (Friedman et al., 1983). A prospective study of children with recurrent or chronic middle ear disease, who had evidence of functional obstruction of the eustachian tube, demonstrated more severe obstruction (mechanical) of the tube when an upper respiratory tract infection developed (Bluestone et al., 1977). A similar relationship has been reported between upper respiratory tract allergy and eustachian tube function. In a study of adult volunteers who had normal tympanic membranes, negative otologic histories, and normal eustachian tube functions prior to an intranasal challenge with an antigen to which they were sensitive, all developed partial eustachian tube obstructions following challenge

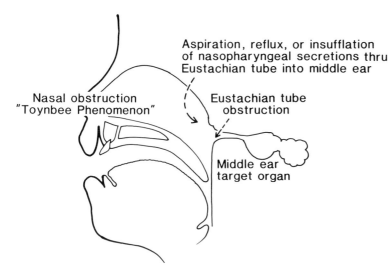

Aspiration, reflux, or insufflation of nasopharyngeal secretions thru Eustachian tube into middle ear

Nasal obstruction "Toynbee Phenomenon"

Eustachian tube obstruction

Middle ear target organ

FIGURE 33B–5. Allergy in the etiology and pathogenesis of otitis media.

(Friedman et al., 1983). However, otitis media did not develop in these subjects. Recently, animals that had been passively sensitized had eustachian tube dysfunction following intranasal challenge (Doyle et al., 1984 and 1985).

From these studies, the following sequence of events is postulated in patients who have allergy and otitis media. Most likely, a basic eustachian tube dysfunction is present that becomes compromised in the presence of upper respiratory tract allergy, which is similar to eustachian tube obstruction caused by upper respiratory tract infection. Upper respiratory tract allergy may cause some intrinsic mechanical obstruction in patients who have normal eustachian tube function, but their normal active opening mechanism, i.e., tensor veli palatini muscle pull, is able to overcome the obstruction. Therefore, patients who have functional obstruction due to poor muscular opening would be at highest risk for developing sufficient mechanical obstruction to induce middle ear disease. Since many children have difficulty in actively opening their eustachian tubes, they are a population at high risk. If the eustachian tube obstruction is minimal, the patient will have only signs and symptoms of *eustachian tube dysfunction*, such as otalgia, "popping" and "snapping" sounds in the ear, mild hearing loss, tinnitus, and even vertigo. Often these symptoms will fluctuate and appear only during the worst periods of the patient's allergic rhinitis.

Even though there is no evidence that allergic nasopharyngeal secretions can be *aspirated* into the middle ear, this concept seems reasonable. Acute otitis media resulting from the aspiration

of bacteria from the nasopharynx has been documented in animal models, which would lend credence to this pathogenic mechanism. Likewise, it is possible that nasopharyngeal secretions containing bacteria could be *refluxed* into the middle ear if the eustachian tube is abnormally patent, which could result in "reflux otitis media." Bacteria-laden nasopharyngeal secretions secondary to allergy also could be *insufflated* into the middle ear during nose blowing, jumping or diving into water when swimming, crying in an infant, or closed-nose swallowing, i.e., the Toynbee phenomenon.

Allergic rhinitis, which is severe enough to cause nasal obstruction, might cause middle ear disease due to the Toynbee phenomenon. If nasal obstruction exists, the nasopharyngeal pressure during closed-nose swallowing is first positive due to the elevation of the soft palate and closing off the velopharyngeal space; this is followed by negative pressure when the soft palate is in a lower position. These pressures are similar to pressure changes that occur in the lower pharynx during physiologic swallowing. If the eustachian tube opens during the positive phase of closed-nose swallowing, allergic nasopharyngeal secretions could be insufflated into the middle ear, resulting in otitis media. More likely, however, the eustachian tube is prevented from opening because of the high negative pressure developed in the nasopharynx during the second phase of closed-nose swallowing. This could cause eustachian tube obstruction and negative middle ear pressure, which would be manifested by signs and symptoms of eustachian tube dysfunction (fluctuating or sustained otalgia, hearing loss, tinnitus, or vertigo); atelectasis of the tympanic membrane-middle ear or otitis media could develop. "Locking" of the eustachian tube also could be possible, and it would be difficult for the patient to open the tube even after swallowing. Aspiration of allergic nasopharyngeal secretions in which bacteria were present could also be possible with this type of mechanism.

However, at present, there is no scientific proof in animals or humans that the Toynbee phenomenon is involved in the pathogenesis of otitis media, but the mechanism seems reasonable. Likewise, there is no conclusive evidence that upper respiratory tract allergy can cause otitis media when there is an associated eustachian tube dysfunction, but the study of adult volunteers which showed partial eustachian tube obstruction when they were challenged with antigen showed that the eustachian tube certainly may be involved by allergy. Even though conclusive proof of this relationship is lacking, it would appear that in the individual with upper respiratory allergy and eustachian tube dysfunction, otitis media could be a result of this combination. Future studies are needed to define the role of allergy in the pathophysiology of the eustachian tube and the pathogenesis of otitis media. Randomized clinical trials will be required to determine the efficacy of the currently popular forms of immunotherapy and allergy control in the prevention of otitis media.

PHYSICAL EXAMINATION OF THE EARS

The position of the patient for otoscopy depends upon age and ability to cooperate the clinical setting, and the preference of the examiner. Otoscopic evaluation of the neonate and young infant is best performed on an examining table. The parent or an assistant is necessary to restrain the baby since movement interferes with adequate evaluation. However, an infant or a young child can be evaluated while sitting on the parent's lap. When necessary, the child may be restrained by the parent, who can use one hand to hold both wrists against the child's abdomen, the other to hold the child's head firmly against the parent's chest, and the legs can be held between the thighs, if necessary. Cooperative children can be evaluated while sitting in a chair or on the edge of an examination table.

All obstructing cerumen must be removed from the canal so that the external canal and tympanic membrane can be adequately visualized. This usually can be accomplished with the aid of an otoscope with a surgical head and wire loop or a blunt cerumen curette or with gentle irrigation of the ear canal with warm water, employing a dental irrigator (Waterpic). Impacted cerumen can be softened by the instillation of a combination of glycerin and peroxide otic drops (equal parts mixture) and irrigated at a later date. However, if an immediate diagnosis is required, the cerumen should be skillfully cleaned under direct vision (otoscope or otomicroscope) without traumatizing the canal walls, since any bleeding will obscure the tympanic membrane. After thorough cleaning, the external canal should be inspected for signs of inflammation.

Proper assessment of the tympanic membrane and its mobility are accomplished by the use of the pneumatic otoscope in which the diagnostic head has an adequate seal. Precise otscopy is limited currently by certain deficiencies in the design of commercially available otoscopes. In many models, an airtight seal is difficult to obtain because of leaks within the otoscope head or between the stiff ear speculum and the external auditory canal. A small section of rubber tubing placed over the tip of the ear speculum aids in obtaining a seal with the ear canal. Many otolaryngologists prefer to use a Bruenings or Siegle otoscope with the magnifying lens, both of which are excellent to assess drum mobility since they have an almost airtight seal.

Inspection of the tympanic membrane should include the following; position, color, degree of translucency, and mobility. The assessment of the light reflex is of limited value in the evaluation of tympanic membrane–middle ear pathology. The normal eardrum should be in the neutral position, the short process of the malleus should be visible but not prominent. Mild retraction of the tympanic membrane usually indicates the presence of middle ear negative pressure, in which case the short process of the malleus and posterior mallear fold are prominent, and the manubrium of the malleus appears foreshortened. Severe retraction (atelectasis) of the tympanic membrane is characterized by a prominent posterior mallear fold and a short process of the malleus with a severely foreshortened manubrium. In such an ear, a horizontal line may be visible below the umbo of the malleus, which is the tympanic membrane resting on the promontory of the cochlea. However, the tympanic membrane may be severely retracted without the presence of high negative middle ear pressure when assessed by pneumatic otoscopy or tympanometry. This retraction presumably is due to previous high negative middle ear pressure with subsequent fixation of the ossicles and ligaments of the middle ear. Fullness of the tympanic membrane is apparent initially in the posterosuperior portion of the pars tensa and the pars flaccida since these two areas are the most highly compliant parts of the tympanic membrane (Khanna and Tonndorf, 1972). The short process of the malleus usually is obscured. The fullness may be due to increased air pressure, effusion, or both within the middle ear. In the most extreme condition, a bulging tympanic membrane involves the entire eardrum, in which instance the malleus usually is obscured.

The normal tympanic membrane has a ground-glass appearance; a blue or yellow color usually indicates a middle ear effusion visualized through a translucent tympanic membrane. A red tympanic membrane alone may not be indicative of a pathologic condition since the blood vessels of the drum may be engorged as the result of crying, sneezing, or blowing the nose. It is important to distinguish between translucency and opacity. The normal tympanic membrane should be translucent. The observer should be able to see through the drum to visualize the middle ear landmarks, i.e., the incudostapedial joint, promontory, round window niche, and chorda tympani nerve. If a middle ear effusion is present medial to a translucent drum, an air-fluid level or bubbles of air may be visible, which can be differentiated from scarring of the tympanic membrane by altering the position of the head or by visualizing movement of the fluid during pneumatic otoscopy. If sufficient negative pressure can be applied with the pneumatic otoscope, the line frequently seen when a severely retracted membrane touches the cochlear promontory will disappear, i.e., the drum will pull away from the promontory. Inability to visualize the middle ear structures indicates opacification of the drum, which usually is the result of thickening of the tympanic membrane, effusion, or both. Otoscopes should have the batteries replaced frequently to provide the maximum intensity of light to enable the examiner to "look through" the tympanic membrane.

Abnormalities of the tympanic membrane-middle ear are reflected in the pattern of tympanic membrane mobility when first positive and then negative pressure is applied to the external auditory canal with the pneumatic otoscope. This is achieved by first applying slight pressure on the rubber bulb (positive pressure) and then, after momentarily breaking the seal, releasing the bulb (negative pressure). At ambient middle ear pressure, the normal tympanic membrane moves inward with slight positive pressure in the ear canal and outward toward the examiner with slight negative pressure. The motion observed is proportionate to the applied pressure and is best visualized in the posterosuperior portion of the tympanic membrane. A middle ear effusion, high negative pressure, or both dampen the movement of the eardrum. If a monomeric membrane or atrophic scar—secondary to an old perforation—is present, mobility of the tympanic membrane can be more readily assessed by observing the movement of the flaccid area.

Figure 33B–6 shows the relationship between the assessment of mobility of the tympanic membrane with the pneumatic otoscope and the middle ear contents and pressure. As compared with the normal tympanic membrane when the middle ear contains only air at ambient pressure (Frame 1), a hypermobile eardrum (Frame 2) is seen most frequently in children whose membranes are atrophic or flaccid. The mobility of the tympanic membrane is greater than normal when even slight positive and negative external canal pressures are applied. Hypermobile tympanic membranes have been associated with subsequent loss of drum stiffness due to abnormal function of the eustachian tube (Elner et al., 1971), which probably is related to wide fluctuations in middle ear pressures. A middle ear effusion occurs rarely with hypermobile drums even when there is high negative middle ear pressure. Tympanic membrane mobility to both positive and negative pressure is decreased with ambient middle ear pressure if the drum is thickened as a result of tympanic membrane inflammation or scarring or if a partial middle ear effusion is present (Frame 3).

When the eardrum is maximally retracted because of negative middle ear pressure (Frames 4 to 6), it cannot be deflected further with positive ear canal pressure. However, applied negative pressure equivalent to that of the middle ear will permit the eardrum to return toward the neutral position (Frame 4). When the middle ear pressure is even lower, there may be only slight outward mobility of the tympanic membrane (Frame 5) because of the limited negative pressure that can be exerted through the otoscope.

	OTOSCOPY						MIDDLE EAR	
	TYMPANIC MEMBRANE POSITION*		EXTERNAL CANAL PRESSURE+				CONTENT	PRESSURE
			POSITIVE		NEGATIVE			
			LOW	HIGH	LOW	HIGH		
1.	NEUTRAL	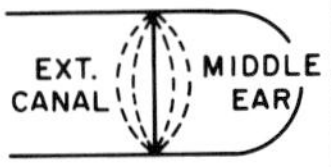	1+	2+	1+	2+	AIR	AMBIENT
2.	NEUTRAL	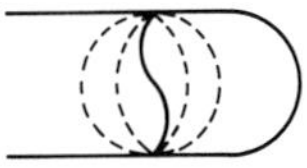	2+	3+	2+	3+	AIR	AMBIENT
3.	NEUTRAL	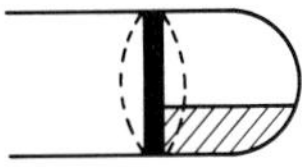	0	1+	0	1+	AIR OR AIR AND EFFUSION	AMBIENT
4.	RETRACTED	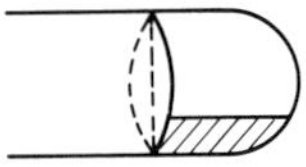	0	0	1+	2+	AIR OR AIR AND EFFUSION	LOW NEGATIVE
5.	RETRACTED	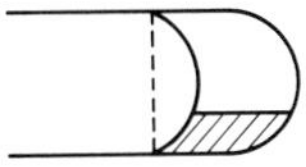	0	0	0	1+	AIR OR EFFUSION AND AIR	HIGH NEGATIVE
6.	RETRACTED	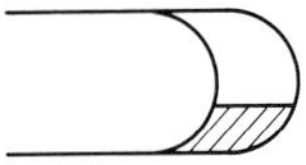	0	0	0	0	AIR OR EFFUSION OR BOTH	VERY HIGH NEGATIVE OR INDETERMINATE
7.	FULL	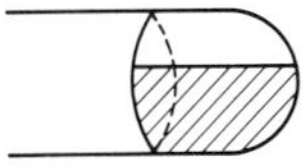	0	1+	0	0	AIR AND EFFUSION	POSITIVE OR INDETERMINATE
8.	BULGING	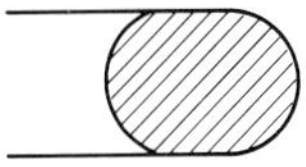	0	0	0	0	EFFUSION	POSITIVE OR INDETERMINATE

* POSITION AT REST (SOLID LINE) AND WITH APPLIED PRESSURE (DOTTED LINE)

+ DEGREE OF TYMPANIC MEMBRANE MOVEMENT AS VISUALIZED THROUGH THE OTOSCOPE; 0 = NONE, 1+ = SLIGHT, 2+ = MODERATE, 3+ = EXCESSIVE

FIGURE 33B–6. Pneumatic otoscopic findings related to middle ear contents and pressure (see text).

One must be careful not to assume that the return of the tympanic membrane to the resting retracted position is a normal response to positive pressure. If the eardrum is severely retracted with extremely high negative middle ear pressure or if there is middle ear effusion, or both, the examiner is not able to produce significant outward movement (Frame 6).

The tympanic membrane that exhibits fullness (Frame 7) will move to applied positive pressure but not to applied negative pressure if some air is present. This occurs commonly in the initial stage of acute otitis media with effusion. A full tympanic membrane with positive middle ear pressure without an effusion is seen frequently in neonates and young infants who are crying during the otoscopic examination and in older infants and children after sneezing, nose blowing, or swallowing when nose is obstructed. When the middle ear-mastoid air cell system is filled with an effusion and little or no air is present, the mobility of the bulging tympanic membrane (Frame 8) is severely decreased or absent to both applied positive and negative pressure.

Otomicroscopy. Many otolaryngologists employ the otomicroscope to improve the accuracy of diagnosis of otitis media and related conditions, since the microscope provides binocular vision and, therefore, depth perception, better light source, and greater magnification. For most conditions, microscopic examination is impractical and generally not necessary. However, when diagnosis by pneumatic otoscopy is in doubt, the otomicroscope is an invaluable aid.

LABORATORY TESTS

Impedance Testing

The electroacoustic impedance bridge (Fig. 33B–7), which measures three basic middle ear functions — tympanometry, middle ear muscle reflex, and static compliance — has provided an invaluable tool in identifying middle ear disease.

The electroacoustic impedance bridge provides an objective assessment of the mobility of the tympanic membrane and the dynamics of the ossicular chain, intra-aural muscles with their attachments, and middle ear cushion. Its design permits the introduction of a signal through one of three small openings in the probe tip, which is sealed in the external auditory canal. A portion of the signal is transmitted into and through the tympanic membrane and middle ear, and a portion is reflected into the ear canal and recorded by the microphone circuit of the ear probe. The reflected signal is related to the mechanical properties of the tympanic membrane. Air pressure within the ear canal is varied through the third aperture of the probe either manually or automatically. With this arrangement, impedance can be monitored at varying air pressures. The measurement of impedance changes at the tympanic membrane with a dynamic air pressure load is termed tympanometry, and when there is a static pressure load, static compliance can be measured. De-

tails of tympanometry and of the interpretation of tympanograms are discussed in Chapter 36.

Tests of Ventilatory Function

The ventilatory function of the eustachian tube can be assessed by manometry, sonometry, and tympanometry. Sonometry is only available for investigation in the laboratory, but the other two tests can be used in the clinical setting. The principles of these tests are discussed, although detailed description of techniques is beyond the scope of this text. In general, one set of tests is designed to examine eustachian tube function when the tympanic membrane contains a ventilating tube or perforation, while the other measures eustachian tube function when the membrane is intact.

Manometry. The simplest manometric technique consists of connecting the ear canal to a pressure monitoring device using a catheter with an airtight seal. The middle ear pressure can be measured directly if the drum contains ventilating tubes or a perforation (intratympanic manometry). Air pressure can be increased or decreased in the ear canal with a syringe or air pump connected to the catheter with a valve. Different levels of positive or negative middle ear pressures can be created, and the ability of the eustachian tube to equilibrate to ambient pressures can be tested directly as the subject swallows. A variation of this method, the "force-response test" (Cantekin et al., 1979b), is able to distinguish between inefficient active opening and structural abnormalities of the eustachian tube.

When the tympanic membrane is intact, middle ear pressure must be inferred from pressure changes in the ear canal (extratympanic manometry). These recordings are of little value

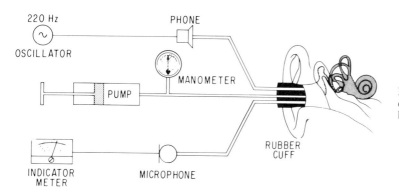

FIGURE 33B–7. Schematic design of electroacoustic impedance bridge.

for assessing tubal function because the small volumes displaced by changes in middle ear pressure are more than offset by changes in temperature and atmospheric pressure.

Inflation-Deflation Test. The inflation-deflation test measures the ventilatory function of the eustachian tube through a perforation of the drum or tympanostomy tube using a pump-manometer portion of an impedance bridge (Bluestone et al., 1972a) or a controlled syringe pump and manometer (Bluestone et al., 1977). The test consists of the application of enough positive pressure to the middle ear to force open the eustachian tube. The pressure remaining in the middle ear after passive opening and closing is termed the closing pressure. Further equilibration of pressure is by swallowing, which induces the tensor veli palatini muscle to contract (Rich, 1920; Cantekin et al., 1979a; Honjo et al., 1979) and permits air to flow down the tube. The pressure can be monitored on a strip chart recorder; the pressure remaining in the middle ear after passive and active function is termed the residual positive pressure. In the deflation tests, low negative pressure is applied to the middle ear and is equilibrated by active tubal opening. The pressure remaining in the middle ear after swallowing is termed the residual negative pressure. In certain instances, the ability of the tube to open actively in response to applied low positive pressure also is assessed. Failure to equilibrate the applied negative pressure during the test indicates locking of the eustachian tube during the test. This type of tube is considered to have increased compliance or is "floppy" in comparison with the tube with normal function.

Forced Response Test. A new technique has recently been developed to test eustachian tube function in subjects with *nonintact* tympanic membranes (Cantekin et al., 1979b). During this test, the middle ear is inflated at a constant flow rate, forcing the eustachian tube open. Following the forced opening of the tube, the pump will continue to deliver a constant airflow rate, maintaining a steady stream of air through the tube. Then the subject is instructed to swallow in order to assess the active dilation of the tube. This test enables the investigator to study the passive response of the eustachian tube as well as the active response due to the contractions of the tensor veli palatini muscle, which displaces the lateral walls from the cartilage-supported medial wall of the tube. Thus, the clinician can determine if tubal dysfunction is due to the material properties of the tube or to a defective active opening mechanism.

Microflow Displacement Tests. Determinations of eustachian tube function in individuals with intact tympanic membranes may be made by volume displacement measurements using microflow techniques. When the drum is moving, airflow is produced in the external ear canal. This flow is recorded by a flowmeter and then integrated to give quantitative measurements of volume displacement. Displacements as small as 1 μl have been recorded with up to 95 percent accuracy.

Indirect Methods Using Tympanometry

Eustachian tube function can be evaluated clinically in subjects with intact tympanic membranes using tympanometry to measure resulting middle ear pressures.

Resting middle ear function can be determined reliably. A single measurement of normal resting middle ear pressure does not necessarily indicate normal eustachian tube function, but a measurement of negative middle pressure is presumptive evidence of eustachian tube dysfunction.

Toynbee and Valsalva Tests. These procedures give a semiquantitative indication of the ability of the eustachian tube to equilibrate to positive and negative pressures in the middle ear (Bluestone, 1975). After a tympanogram, the subject is asked to perform a Toynbee maneuver, which should produce negative middle ear pressure. If it doesn't, the subject probably has tubal dysfunction. If it does, the subject is asked to swallow in an attempt to equilibrate the negative pressure. If with a single swallow equilibration is not complete, repeated swallows are performed, and the pressure remaining in the middle ear is termed the residual negative pressure. A similar test measures the ability of the eustachian tube to allow equilibration to positive middle ear pressure. One problem with these tests is the inability to control the degree of positive and negative pressure generated in each individual.

The Holmquist test involves using a device to create a negative pressure in the nasopharynx and to induce a pressure of -400 mm H_2O in the middle ear (Holmquist, 1969, 1972). Otherwise it is similar to the Toynbee test. However, it frequently results in false positive results (Siedentop et al., 1978).

The inflation-deflation test assesses the ability of the subject to equilibrate up to 200 mm H_2O negative or positive air pressure in the ear canal (Bluestone, 1975). After an initial tympanogram, a pressure of $+200$ mm H_2O is placed in the ear canal, which causes an inward deflection of the tympanic membrane and an increase in middle ear pressure (inflation). If the eustachian tube is normal, middle ear pressure should equilibrate with that in the nasopharynx. The deflation test is similar but uses negative middle ear pressure.

The patulous eustachian tube test compares the tympanogram while the patient is breathing normally with that while the patient holds his or her breath. A fluctuation in the tympanometric line that coincides with breathing indicates a patulous eustachian tube. These changes can be exaggerated by forced inspiration and expiration through one nostril or by the Toynbee maneuver.

Nine-Step Inflation-Deflation Tympanometric Test. Another method of assessing the function of the eustachian tube when the tympanic membrane is intact is called the nine-step inflation-deflation tympanometric test, al-

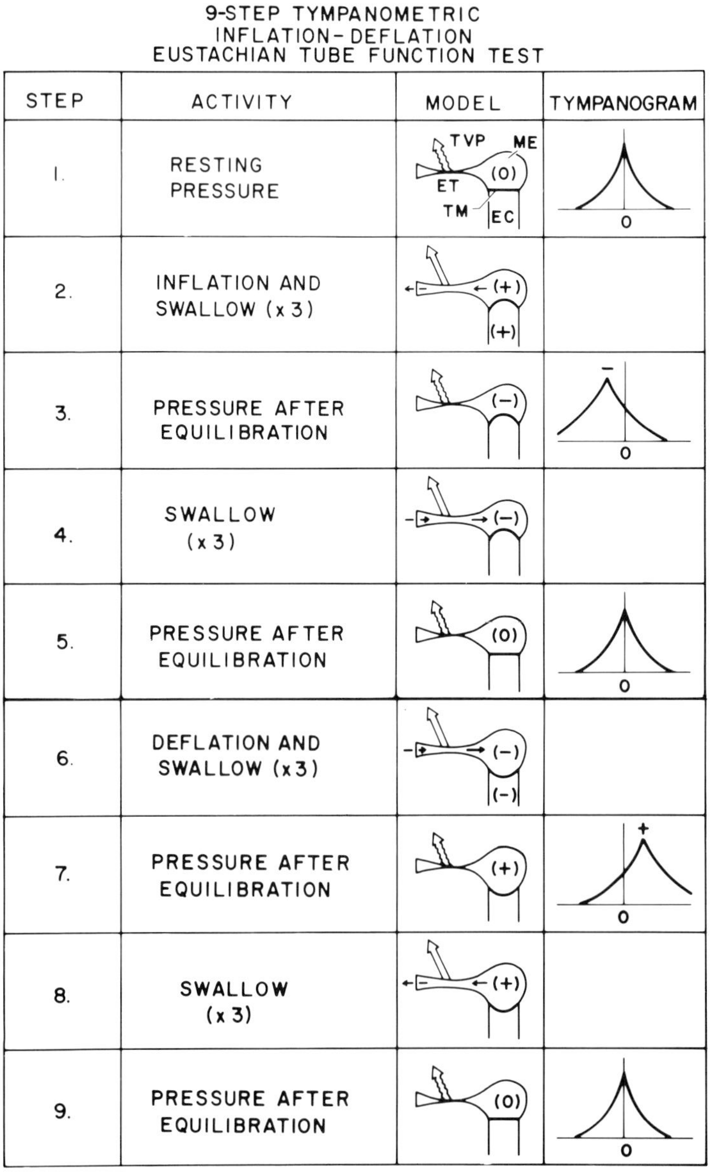

FIGURE 33B–8. Nine step eustachian tube function test that uses tympanometry.

though the applied middle ear pressures are very limited in magnitude (Fig. 33B–8). The middle ear must be free of effusion. The nine-step tympanometry procedure may be summarized as follows (Bluestone, 1975):

1. The tympanogram records resting middle ear pressure.

2. Ear canal pressure is increased to +200 mm H_2O, with a medial deflection of the tympanic membrane and a corresponding increase in middle ear pressure. The subject swallows to equilibrate middle ear overpressure.

3. While the subject then refrains from swallowing, ear canal pressure is returned to normal, thus establishing a slight negative middle ear pressure (as the tympanic membrane moves outward). The tympanogram documents the established middle ear underpressure.

4. The subject swallows in an attempt to equilibrate negative middle ear pressure. If equilibration is successful, airflow is from nasopharynx to middle ear.

5. The tympanogram records the extent of equilibration.

6. Ear canal pressure is decreased to −200 mm H_2O, causing a lateral deflection of the tympanic membrane and a corresponding decrease in middle ear pressure. The subject than swallows to equilibrate negative middle ear pressure; airflow is from the nasopharynx to the middle ear.

7. The subject refrains from swallowing while external ear canal pressure is returned to normal, thus establishing a slight positive pressure in the middle ear as the tympanic membrane moves medially. The tympanogram records the overpressure established.

8. The subject swallows to reduce overpressure. If equilibration is successful, airflow is from the middle ear to the nasopharynx.

9. The final tympanogram documents the extent of equilibration.

The test is simple to perform and can give useful information regarding eustachian tube function and should be part of the clinical evaluation of patients with suspected eustachian tube dysfunction. In general, most normal adults can perform all or some parts of this test, but even normal children have difficulty.

INDICATIONS FOR TESTING EUSTACHIAN TUBE FUNCTION

The most direct method to test eustachian tube function available to the clinician today is the inflation-deflation method through a perforation of the tympanic membrane or a tympanotomy tube. Since most patients have either functional obstruction or an abnormally patent tube, no other test procedures may be needed. However, if the tube appears to be totally blocked anatomically, then further testing must be performed. Most cases of mechanical obstruction are due to inflammation at the bony end of the eustachian tube, which usually will resolve with medical or surgical management. However, if no cause of pathologic conditions in the middle ear is obvious, roentgenographic studies should be performed to rule out the possibility of neoplasm of the nasopharynx. Computed tomography is most helpful in determining the site of obstruction.

Since resting middle ear pressure may provide an indirect measurement of eustachian tube function, serial tympanograms may be helpful in patients with symptoms such as fullness, snapping, or popping in the ear, fluctuating hearing loss, tinnitus, or vertigo.

REFERENCES

Beery, Q.C., Bluestone, C.D., Cantekin, E.I.: Otologic history, audiometry and tympanometry as a case finding procedure for school screening. Laryngoscope 85: 1976, 1975.

Beery, Q.C., Doyle, W.J., Cantekin, E.I., Bluestone, C.D.: Longitudinal assessment of ventilatory function of the eustachian tube in children. Laryngoscope 89:1446, 1979.

Bluestone, C.D.: Eustachian tube obstruction in the infant with the cleft palate. Ann. Otol. Rhinol. Laryngol. 80:1–30, 1971.

Bluestone, C.D.: Eustachian tube obstruction in the infant with middle ear effusion. Laryngoscope 82:1654, 1972a.

Bluestone, C.D.: Assessment of Eustachian Tube Function. Handbook of Clinical Impedance Audiometry. New York, American Electromedics Corp,. 1975.

Bluestone, C.D., Beery, Q.C.: Concepts on the pathogenesis of middle ear effusions. Ann. Otol. Rhinol. Laryngol. 85:182, 1976.

Bluestone, C.D., Beery, Q.C., Andrus, W.: Mechanics of the eustachian tube as it influences susceptibility to and persistence of middle ear effusions in children. Ann. Otol. Rhinol. Laryngol. 83:27, 1974.

Bluestone, C.D., Cantekin, E.I.: Design factors in the characterization and identification of otitis media and certain related conditions. Ann. Otol. Rhinol. Laryngol. 88:13, 1979.

Bluestone, C.D., Cantekin, E.I., Beery, Q.C.: Certain effects of adenoidectomy on eustachian tube ventilatory function. Laryngoscope 85:113, 1975.

Bluestone, C.D., Cantekin, E.I., Beery, Q.C.: Effect of inflammation on the ventilatory function of the eustachian tube. Laryngoscope 87:493, 1977.

Bluestone, C.D., Cantekin, E.I., Beery Q.C. Stool, S.E.:

Function of the eustachian tube related to surgical management of acquired aural cholesteatoma in children. Laryngoscope 87:1155, 1978.

Bluestone, C.D., Klein, J.O.: Otitis Media with Effusion, Atalectasis, and Eustachian Tube Dysfunction. In Pediatric Otolaryngology, Bluestone C.D., Stool, S.E. (eds.), Philadelphia, W.B. Saunders Co., 356–576, 1983.

Bluestone, C.D., Wittel, R., Paradise, J.L., Felder, H.: Eustachian tube function as related to adenoidectomy for otitis media. Trans. A.A.O.O. 76:1325, 1972b.

Cantekin, E.I., Bluestone, C.D., Saez, C., Doyle, W.J., Phillips, D.: Normal and abnormal middle ear ventilation. Ann. Otol. Rhinol. Laryngol. 86:1, 1977.

Cantekin, E.I., Doyle, W.J., Reichert, T.J., Phillips, D.C., Bluestone, C.D.: Dilation of the eustachian tube by electrical stimulation of the mandibular nerve. Ann. Otol. Rhinol. Laryngol. 88:40, 1979a.

Cantekin, E.I., Saez, C.A., Bluestone, C.D., Bern, S.A.: Airflow through the eustachian tube. Ann. Otol. Rhinol. Laryngol. 88:603, 1979b.

Clemis, J.D.: Identification of allergic factors in middle ear effusions. Ann. Otol. Rhinol. Laryngol. 85:234, 1976.

Doyle, W.J., Cantekin, E.I., Beery, Q.C., Bluestone, C.D.: Eustachian tube function in cleft palate children. Ann. Otol. Rhinol. Laryngol. 89:34–40, 1980.

Doyle, W.J., Friedman, R., Fireman, P., Bluestone, C.D.: Eustachian tube obstruction after provocative nasal antigen challenge. Arch. Otolaryngol. 110:508–511, 1984.

Doyle, W.J., Takahara, T., Fireman, P.: The role of allergy in the pathogenesis of otitis media with effusion. Arch. Otolaryngol. 111:502–506, 1985.

Draper, W.L.: Secretory otitis media. Larynscope 78:636, 1967.

Elner, A., Ingelstedt, S., Ivarsson, A.: The elastic properties of the tympanic membrane system. Acta Otolaryngol. 72:397, 1971.

Friedman, R.A., Doyle, W.J., Casselbrant, M.L., Bluestone, C.D., Fireman, P.: Immunologic-mediated eustachian tube obstruction: A double-blind crossover study. J. Allergy Clin. Immunol. 71:442–447, 1983.

Holmquist, J.: Eustachian tube function assessed with tympanometry. Acta Otolaryngol. 68:501, 1969.

Holmquist, J.: Tympanometry in testing auditory tubal function. Audiology 11:209, 1972.

Honjo, I., Okazaki, N., Kumazawam, T.: Experimental study of the eustachian tube function with regard to its related muscles. Acta Otolaryngol. 87:84, 1979.

Khanna, S.M., Tonndorf, J.: Tympanic membrane vibrations in cats studied by time-averaged holography. J. Acoust. Soc. Am. 51:1904, 1972.

Lim, D.J., Liu, Y.S., Schram, J., Birck, H.G.: Immunoglobulin E in chronic middle ear effusions. Ann. Otol. Rhinol. Laryngol. 85:119, 1976.

McGovern, J.P., Haywood, T.J., Fernandes, A.: Allergy and secretory otitis media. J.A.M.A. 200:134, 1967.

Mogi, G.: Secretory IgA and antibody activities in middle ear effusions. Ann. Otol. Rhinol. Laryngol. 85:97, 1976.

Rich, A.R.: A physiological study of the eustachian tube and its related muscles. Johns Hopkins Hosp. Bull. 31:206–214, 1920.

Rood, S.R., Doyle, W.J.: Anatomy — Introduction. In Eustachian Tube Function: Physiology and Role in Otitis Media — Workshop Report. Bluestone, C.D., Doyle, W.J., (eds.), Ann. Otol. Rhinol. Laryngol. 94:6–8, 1985.

Siedentop, K.H., Loewy, A., Corrigan, R.A., Osenar, S.B.: Eustachian tube function assessed with tympanometry. Ann. Otol. Rhinol. Laryngol. 87:163, 1978.

34

Diseases of the Nose
NIELS MYGIND, M.D.
HANS BISGAARD, M.D.

Rhinitis plays a major role in the morbidity of allergic diseases. This chapter discusses allergic and other noninfectious rhinitis and allied disorders. In addition to the chapter references listed, see Proctor and Andersen, 1982 for a more detailed discussion of nasal physiology. Also, comprehensive considerations of rhinitis can be found in monographs by Mygind (1979), Settipane (1984), Bierman (1984), Mygind and Weeke (1985), and Mygind et al. (1986). For more extensive evaluation of the interplay between upper and lower airways, a series of articles edited by Mygind and co-workers (1983) is recommended.

FUNCTIONAL ANATOMY OF THE NOSE

Because of the prominence of the turbinates, the nasal cavities are narrow, slit-like passages, 1 to 4 mm wide. The nose accounts for nearly 50 percent of the total airway resistance due to this special anatomy. This is critical to its major tasks of heating, humidification, and filtration of the inhaled air.

Air Conditioning

Air at room temperature, inhaled through the nose, is warmed to about 30°C by the time it reaches the pharynx and is almost saturated with water. Nasal factors important for air conditioning are (1) the large arterial blood flow in the arteriovenous anastomoses (about 50 percent of total flow); (2) the high secretory capacity of the nose (100,000 glands, the same number in infants and adults) (Tos, 1982); and (3) the large venous sinusoids that control the width of the nasal cavity by control of venous engorgement.

Filtration of Inhaled Air

The nose is an effective filter for inhaled air. Anatomic factors contribute to this function by promoting turbulence behind the narrow entrance to the cavity (1.5 cm from the nostril), increasing particle deposition and facilitating particle impingement against the mucous membrane through bending of the inhaled airstream. The efficacy of the nasal filter depends upon particle size. Few particles larger than 10 μm (pollen grains) will penetrate the nose, whereas most particles smaller than 2 μm will reach the lower airways.

The nose also acts as a "gas mask" by retaining inhaled, water-soluble gases (Andersen et al., 1974). Common pollutants that are potent irritants to the lower airway, such as formaldehyde and ozone, are largely removed by the nose.

Chronic rhinitis, which interferes with nasal breathing, is potentially harmful to individuals with hyperreactive airways when exposed to environmental pollutants. Exercise during oral breathing, which circumvents the humidification and heating of the nose, causes bronchoconstriction from airway cooling or water loss. This can be prevented in part by nasal breathing (Griffin et al., 1982).

Sympathetic Nerves

There is an abundance of adrenergic fibers around the blood vessels in the nose; sympathetic innervation of the glands is sparse and insignificant. Stimulation of the postganglionic adrenergic fibers releases norepinephrine, which acts both on alpha adrenoreceptors to induce vasoconstriction, and on beta adrenoceptors to produce slight vasodilatation. The dominant effect of adrenergic stimulation, therefore, is vasoconstriction.

Alpha adrenoreceptor agonists are used as nasal decongestants. Alpha adrenoceptor antagonists and drugs that inhibit the release of norepinephrine, such as antihypertensive agents and psychosedatives, increase nasal airway resistance. They are common causes of "dry nasal blockage." Beta-2 adrenergic drugs used as bronchodilators in asthma are weak vasodilators and do not cause an increase in nasal airway resistance when used orally for asthma.

Parasympathetic Nerves

Cholinergic fibers are found close to blood vessels and are particularly numerous around the glands (Fig. 34–1). Stimulation of these fibers releases acetylcholine from the postganglionic terminal. Release of acetylcholine results in glandular secretion and transient vasodilatation. Cholinoceptor antagonists, such as atropine, inhibit hypersecretion but not acetylcholine-induced nasal blockage. Recent studies have suggested that other substances, such as vasoactive intestinal polypeptide, also are of importance for the transmission of parasympathetic impulses, but their exact role in this process remains to be established (Anggard et al., 1983).

Reflexes

The efferent parasympathetic fibers, running in the vidian nerve, are part of a reflex arc with afferent sensory fibers in the trigeminal nerve (see Fig. 34–1). The sensory nerves in the nose are exposed constantly to stimulation from polluted and unconditioned inhaled air. It seems likely, therefore, that there is constant reflex activity in the nose which modulates secretory activity and nasal patency. In relation to teleology, these reflex-related changes can be seen as attempts to adapt the air conditioning function of the nose to the steadily changing demands of the environment.

Nasal sensory nerves contain the neuropeptide, substance P, which is a potent vasodilator and increases vascular permeability. Substance P may participate in the initiation of parasympathetic reflexes and play a role in local axon reflexes. In addition, nasal sensory nerves may release substance P that acts directly on the mucous membrane to induce vasodilatation and increase vascular permeability (Anggard et al., 1983).

Nasal Hyperreactivity

Everyone reacts to exposure to large amounts of dust, high levels of inhaled irritants, and ex-

INCREASED REFLEX ACTIVITY – HYPER-REACTIVITY

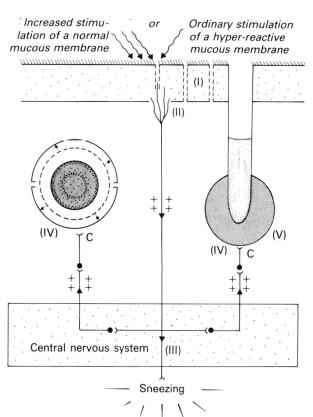

FIGURE 34–1. Nasal reflexes. The afferent sensory nerves to the nose run in the trigeminal nerve. The efferent parasympathetic fibers are derived from the facial nerve; the synapse between preganglionic and postganglionic fibers is located in the pterygopalatine ganglion. Most of the preganglionic fibers travel via the nerve of the pterygoid canal (the vidian nerve), which is accessible for surgery (vidian neurectomy). Parasympathetic stimulation of glands and blood vessels is mediated via cholinoceptors and receptors for vasoactive intestinal polypeptide (VIP). Ordinary inhaled air, due to its unphysiologic condition, slightly stimulates the sensory nerves in the nose. The resulting parasympathetic reflex activity causes a slight hypersecretion and insignificant vasodilatation, not noted by the normal subject. Ordinary daily stimuli can cause the same symptoms in hyperreactive mucous membranes, as does vigorous stimulation of normal mucosa. (From Mygind, N: *Essential Allergy*, Oxford, Blackwell Scientific Publications, Inc., 1985.)

treme temperature changes with nasal obstruction (Fig. 34–1). Patients with rhinitis also react on exposure to various common stimuli which are normally tolerated. This "nonspecific hyperreactivity" is characteristic for both allergic and nonallergic rhinitis. Thus, symptoms provoked by dust, odors associated with cooking, printing ink, or alcoholic beverages are not diagnostic of *allergic* sensitivity.

ETIOLOGY AND PATHOGENESIS OF RHINITIS

Allergic Rhinitis

The nose is constantly exposed to allergic particles, as it filters them from inhaled air. Accordingly, it is the site of more allergic symptoms and illnesses than any other organ.

Surface Mediator Cells. Several observations suggest that histamine and other chemical mediators are released from mediator cells near the epithelial surface, some of which are located in the nasal lumen. These mediator cells are predominantly mast cells but may include basophil leukocytes (Hastie et al., 1979; Okuda et al., 1983). At present, it is uncertain whether the human nose contains two types of mast cells as observed in animals; connective tissue mast cells and mucosal mast cells. This question is of clinical importance since the two populations of mast cells (e.g., in rat intestine) may respond differently to drugs. The number of mediator cells is increased in allergic rhinitis (Mygind, 1982a).

The immediate allergic reaction in the nose can be divided into three major steps as follows: (1) interaction between allergen and IgE antibody; (2) mediator release from mast cells that act directly on effector cells; and (3) induction of tissue changes through stimulation of reflexes (largely produced also through mediator release). The surface mediator cells hold key positions in this double amplification system, since they release histamine close to effector cells and to sensory nerve endings (Fig. 34–2).

Histamine. Histamine is the most important mediator of allergy in the nose. It acts in two different and complementary ways as follows:

ALL EFFECTS OF HISTAMINE

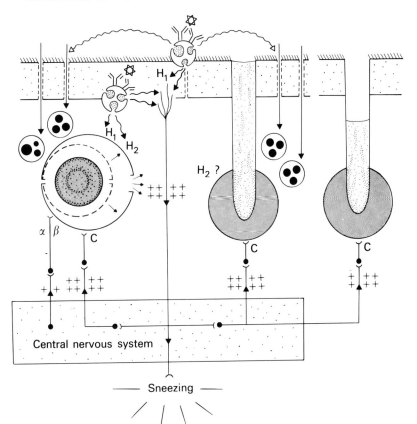

FIGURE 34–2. Simplified hypothesis of the pathogenesis of allergic rhinitis. Only the effects of histamine are included, since our knowledge of the significance of other biochemical mediators is still insufficient. Histamine is released from surface mediator cells, occurring in an increased number in symptomatic allergic rhinitis. Histamine acts in three different ways as follows: (1) most importantly, it stimulates sensory nerves (probably H_1 receptors), thereby causing sneezing, significant bilateral hypersecretion, and slight, short-lasting vasodilatation; (2) it acts directly on vascular receptors (H_1 and probably H_2), causing vasodilatation and edema formation; and, finally, (3) histamine increases epithelial permeability and possibly allergen penetration. (From Mygind, N: *Essential Allergy*, Oxford, Blackwell Scientific Publications, Inc., 1985.)

(1) directly on cellular histamine receptors, inducing vasodilatation and increasing capillary permeability to cause edema and persistent blockage, and (2) indirectly via reflexes, inducing sneezing and hypersecretion (Kirkegaard et al., 1983; Secher et al., 1982) (see Fig. 34–2.)

Other Mediators. The mast cells in the nose, as in other organs, release not only histamine but other mediators as well. These include ECF-A and arachidonic acid metabolites, such as leukotrienes and prostaglandins (see Chapter 5). These mast cell–derived mediators have been identified in nasal lavage fluid following allergen provocation, as have potent mediator substances such as kinins, which are not derived from mast cells (Naclerio et al., 1983; Creticos et al., 1984; Shaw et al., 1985). Some role for these mediators in allergic rhinitis is presumed but currently is largely unknown.

Late Occurring Symptoms. Nasal symptoms that occur rapidly after allergen exposure can be explained largely on the basis of histamine release. Other mediators and inflammatory reactions may be responsible for symptoms that occasionally occur hours following allergen provocation. In contrast to late bronchial reactions, however, it is difficult to identify late nasal reactions which are reproducible and readily definable as such (Richarson et al., 1979). On the other hand, allergen-induced increases in mucosal reactivity to similar and unrelated allergens are more easily demonstrated. What relation this primary effect of allergen exposure on the nose is to so-called late allergic reactions, which appear also to increase nonspecific tissue sensitivity, remains to be determined (Connell, 1969; Borum and Mygind, 1980). This effect is probably not due to histamine per se, since repeated histamine provocations in the nose do not increase mucosal reactivity.

Nonallergic Rhinitis

"Autonomic imbalance." Nasal air conditioning depends upon the function of blood vessels and glands which are under nervous system control. In some patients with chronic noninfectious rhinitis, neither an allergic etiology nor evidence of inflammation can be found (e.g., lack of eosinophils). Such patients often act as if they have hyperreactive nasal mucosa with exaggerated response to a large number of stimuli ordinarily tolerated. An imbalance in the autonomic nervous system, in popular terms, "maladjustment of the nasal air conditioner," is the only "explanation" we can offer for this subgroup of patients with nonallergic rhinitis *without eosinophils*. In another subgroup of patients with chronic noninfectious rhinitis, in which an allergic etiology can be excluded, nasal hyperreactivity is associated with and probably is caused by a chronic inflammatory reaction characterized by local eosinophilia. The etiology of this "eosinophilic-inflammatory" disease is unknown, but it may be the upper airway equivalent of nonallergic, so-called intrinsic asthma. This syndrome has been termed nonallergic rhinitis with eosinophilia or eosinophilic nonallergic rhinitis in the literature. Non-IgE mediated, mast cell–mediator release probably is involved in its pathogenesis. Specific provoking factors are seldom identified, but some patients react to acetylsalicylic acid, preservatives, and food dyes. These agents rarely are significant causes of the daily symptoms, however.

SEASONAL ALLERGIC RHINITIS

In temperate zones, pollen allergy causes seasonal allergic rhinitis and rhinoconjunctivitis. In subtropic and tropic areas, the pollen season and the disease are perennial. The term "hay fever" relates to the observation made more than 100 years ago that nasal symptoms develop on exposure to flowering hay fields, "fever" implying disease rather than pyrexia. Hay fever is the term commonly employed by physicians for pollen allergy and is common parlance for all types of allergic rhinitis.

Pollen

Pollen grains, as large particles, impinge against the eye and are trapped in the nasal filter. As very few pollen grains reach the lower airway, the exact mechanism of pollen asthma remained uncertain until recently when it was shown that pollen allergens can occur as submicronic aerosols in the atmosphere (Solomon, 1984). The most important sources of pollen allergens are trees, grasses, and weeds, which have pollen seasons in spring, summer, and early autumn, respectively.

Prevalence

The risk of developing hay fever depends on an inherited predisposition to make IgE antibody and on the degree of exposure to allergen with a high sensitizing capacity. Consequently, the prevalence rate for hay fever varies from one location to another, but worldwide it is the most common clinical expression of IgE-mediated allergic disease. Twenty million people have hay fever in the United States.

Although seasonal allergic rhinitis is a remarkably well-defined clinical disease, it is less so in epidemiologic terms. The clinician sees only the troubled patient, the "tip of the iceberg." Many allergic subjects have little or no bothersome symptoms and do not seek medical attention. This may explain why reported frequency figures vary from 2 to 20 percent. A reasonable average figure for cumulative prevalence of symptomatic hay fever probably is 10 percent. Many of these patients appear to be undertreated or not treated at all for what they believe is a "prolonged summer cold."

Natural History

Although the disease can start in middle age, most cases first appear in middle childhood and adolescence. The disease tends to worsen for the first two to three seasons, remains stationary for two to three decades, improves in middle age, and seldom is a problem in the elderly. Pollen counts can vary considerably from season to season, and it is therefore difficult to judge over a few seasons what is the spontaneous course of the disease or the result of therapy.

Hay fever patients have a 2- to 3-fold increased risk of developing perennial asthma, which occurs in at least 5 to 10 percent. In children, asthma more often precedes hay fever than follows it.

Symptoms

Rhinitis. Nasal itching results in serial sneezing (five to 20 sneezes), and nose rubbing. Rhinorrhea necessitates constant use of a handkerchief (the nose can produce 20 ml of secretions per hour). Congestion gives patients nasal voices and makes them feel "stuffy in the head," but congestion usually is less pronounced than in perennial rhinitis. Itching of

the soft palate indicates that the mucociliary system has transported allergens to the nasopharynx. Some patients get referred itching in the ears due to the common innervation of the pharyngeal mucosa and the ear (glossopharyngeal nerve).

Conjunctivitis. Itching of the eyes is characteristic of pollen allergy. It leads to eye rubbing, creating a vicious circle of eye irritation, ending with red and smarting eyes. For unknown reasons, some patients have predominantly eye symptoms, while others have nasal symptoms mainly (four of five).

Asthma. Some patients, especially those with severe rhinoconjunctivitis, develop lower respiratory tract symptoms in the pollen season. A dry cough and wheezing with slight chest tightness is frequent, but a severe asthma attack can occur. Patients with seasonal asthma may have increased bronchial reactivity year-round and increased risk of developing perennial asthma.

Diagnosis

History. The diagnosis of hay fever is seldom difficult. A patient will often suspect pollen allergy, especially when announcement of the daily pollen count has drawn his or her attention to the possibility.

Testing. Skin prick testing is usully sufficient to confirm the history. Reactivity to more than one allergen is the rule, and it is prudent to test for all allergens that might account for symptoms in that area during the problem season. Intradermal testing may be revealing for less profound sensitivity. Alternatively, serologic tests may be used (see Chapter 17).

Principles of Treatment

"A Normal Life." The quality of life can be severely impaired, and the goal of treatment is to allow the patient to live a normal life during his or her problem season.

Avoidance Not Possible. Allergen avoidance is not possible outdoors, because pollens are well mixed in the lower atmosphere. However, excessive exposure usually can be avoided by common sense measures. Patients should avoid close contact with wild and cultivated grass (hay), but can enjoy their gardens, as cutting grass (by a family member) reduces pollination from the lawn. Closing bedroom windows, at least in the evening and early mornings, should be advised; an air conditioning system increases protection when indoors.

Pharmacotherapy. Antihistamines have proved effective as a first line drug in the treatment of hay fever for many years. Numerous antihistaminic drugs are available. They may be divided into different groups based on chemical structure (see Chapter 19). They are in principle similar, but differ for the most part in potency, anticholinergic effect, and most importantly sedative effect. Chlorpheniramine, bromphenaramine, and clemastine are widely used, as they are among the preparations with the best ratio between therapeutic and adverse effects (see Chapter 19). Nonsedative antihistamines, such as astemizole and terfenadine, have been developed recently and marketed in some countries. Reduced penetration across the blood-brain barrier and higher affinity for peripheral than for central nervous system receptors are important to their lack of sedative effect. Astemizole (not yet available in the United States) binds to the H_1 receptor for weeks and is very long acting. It is suitable for basic maintenance therapy but not for immediate relief. Weight gain can be a problem, and the unusual duration of its receptor binding must be considered when fertile women are treated and before skin testing (Wihl et al., 1985). Terfenadine kinetics and usage are similar to the classic antihistamines (Editorial, 1983), but this drug seems to be less effective. Seasonal allergic rhinitis is one of the principal indications for the use of antihistamines. They have a good effect on itching in the eyes, nose, and throat; on sneezing; and on watery discharge; but little effect on nasal obstruction (Munch et al., 1983). Antihistamines, therefore, are often combined with vasoconstrictors for treatment of nasal congestion, especially for treatment of perennial rhinitis (see subsequent discussion). Antihistamines are competitive inhibitors of histamine action and are most effective if employed in anticipation of symptoms.

The corticosteroid sprays applied topically to the nasal mucosa are more effective than antihistamines in patients with nasal blockage. This form of therapy can control nasal symptoms in a large majority of hay fever patients, but caution is advised in the use for prolonged periods of time, especially in children. Local dryness and irritation may lead to bleeding, crusting, and scab formation, and subsequently, in the rare case, may conceivably result indirectly in nasal septal perforation. Consequently, it is essential to instruct patients thoroughly in proper use of corticosteroid sprays. Topical treatment may be employed alone or in conjunction with antihistamines. The lowest dose of steroid needed to control symptoms is advised. Initially, a topical nasal decongestant may be needed just prior to insufflation of the topical steroid spray to facilitate the penetration of the latter into the nose.

Cromolyn sodium in the nose is often preferred by pediatric physicians in particular but is less effective than steroid sprays. The drug, which acts by stabilizing the mast cells, is given every 3 to 4 hours. Cromolyn sodium, similar to topical steroid sprays, can be used with antihistamines and immunotherapy for additive effect. The drug is virtually nontoxic. Cromolyn sodium eye drops are safe and effective in both allergic conjunctivitis and vernal conjunctivitis.

It is important to inform the patient that steroid and cromolyn sprays, in contrast to decongestant sprays, must be used prophylactically and that immediate relief of symptoms will not occur. Treatment is started as soon as the patient experiences the first symptoms and continues during the entire pollen season. Education about the need to use medication regularly is important, since patients are inclined not to use drugs on symptom-free days.

Topical antihistamine-vasoconstrictor eye drops or cromolyn sodium can be used in place of or in addition to systemic medication for eye involvement.

When the treatment described is inadequate, a short course of systemic steroids (prednisone or prednisolone) can be added in adults. No more than a 7 to 10 day course is generally recommended. The steroid is added to any ongoing therapy. The use of short-acting steroids by the oral route is preferred over depot injections. This enables high dose and shorter term use of the drug, thus minimizing risk of unnecessary side effects associated with longer term use, and avoidance of the occasional local subcutaneous and muscle atrophy associated with depot steroid injections.

Immunotherapy. Immunotherapy should be considered if symptoms are severe or are not readily controlled by drugs, with little or no side effects to the patient; if exposure to the allergen is prolonged (months); if allergic asthma is involved; and if the patient has a preference for this type of therapy. Immunotherapy is not recommended for allergens that can be avoided (see Chapter 20).

PERENNIAL RHINITIS

Classification

Year-round rhinitis can be more troublesome than seasonal allergy, and nasal pathologic changes more pronounced. The clinical presentation has greater similarities to perennial nonallergic rhinitis than to seasonal allergic rhinitis. Therefore, perennial rhinitis often is considered as an entity regardless of etiology (Toogood, 1976; Church, 1980; Norman, 1983).

Allergic and nonallergic mechanisms often act in concert, and perennial rhinitis is seldom completely allergic or nonallergic. The mixed etiology makes a strict classification difficult. Perennial nonallergic rhinitis is a heterogeneous disorder, consisting of at least two subgroups. One is characterized by nasal eosinophilia, frequent occurrence of nasal polyps, asthma, and good response to pharmacotherapy. These characteristics are usually lacking in the other subgroup (Table 34–1). This subclassification is useful for comparison between

groups but not always pertinent to the individual. The term "vasomotor rhinitis" is, in Europe and to some extent in the United States, often used for noninfectious, nonallergic rhinitis.

Occurrence and Prevalence

About 2 to 4 percent of the general population suffer from chronic nasal diseases with daily symptoms and need regular medications. This figure is suspect, however, because of the vague definition of the disease and lack of epidemiologic studies. Allergic rhinitis often starts in childhood, while the first appearance of nonallergic rhinitis more often is in adulthood. The course of the disease is capricious, but severe persistent symptoms will usually portend a long course.

Etiology

House Dust Mite. The house dust mite is a common cause of perennial allergic rhinitis in

TABLE 34–1. Comparison of Different Types of Perennial Noninfectious Rhinitis*

Findings	Allergic Rhinitis	Nonallergic Rhinitis Eosinophilic Subgroup	Noneosinophilic Subgroup
Age at onset	Childhood	Childhood or adulthood	Childhood or adulthood
Symptoms			
Congestion	Moderate	Marked	Slight-moderate
Sneezing	Frequent	Occasional	Rare
Itching	Usual	Occasional	Uncommon or mild
Rhinorrhea	Profuse	Profuse	Profuse
Anosmia	Occasional	Frequent	Rare
Physical examination			
Swollen turbinates	Moderate-marked	Marked	Moderate
Character of secretions	Watery	Mucoid	Watery
Associated findings			
Predominant cell in secretion	Eosinophil	Eosinophil	Few neutrophils
Infection	Occasional	Frequent	Rare
Aspirin intolerance	Rare	Occasional	Rare
Concurrent diseases			
Conjunctivitis	Frequent	Rare	Absent
Asthma	Frequent	Frequent	Rare
Urticaria	Rare	Occasional	Rare
Sinus x-ray examination			
Mucosal thickening	Slight	May be marked	Slight
Fluid	Rare	Occasional	Rare
Response to therapy			
Antihistamines	Good	Fair	Poor
Decongestants	Limited	Limited	Poor
Corticosteroids	Excellent	Excellent	Poor to moderate
Cromolyn sodium	Good	Poor	Poor
Ipratropium	Limited	Fair	Good

* From Mygind N, Weeke B. Allergic and nonallergic rhinitis. *In* Middleton E Jr, Reed CE, Ellis EF (eds.), Allergy: Principles and Practice, 2nd ed. Saint Louis, C.V. Mosby Co., 1983.

most climates, where the humidity tends to exceed 50 percent. Often there is seasonal variation in symptoms. Allergen exposure is maximal in bed, but nasal obstruction in rhinitis is always maximal in the supine position. Symptoms of sneezing and rhinorrhea are most pronounced in the hours immediately after waking, regardless of etiology. Thus, the history is of limited help in making a specific diagnosis. However, symptoms provoked by making the bed and emptying the vacuum cleaner are suggestive of mite allergy. Occasionally, cockroaches or other insects have been reported to be significant allergens in house dust. Animal allergens are another major antigenic component in "house dust."

Molds. Symptoms provoked by molds also are perennial with seasonal variations, although they can be mainly seasonal. Mold allergy is a well-known cause of rhinitis in asthmatic children, but its role in nonasthmatic adults is less certain.

Animal Allergens. Allergy to animals is frequent, but most individuals have only occasional obvious symptoms. Animal allergy can cause daily symptoms and chronic disease when highly sensitive patients are exposed indirectly to animal allergens via other's clothes on a frequent basis and, of course, when they are exposed daily to animal danders, saliva, and other animal emanations at home. Patients with low-grade sensitivity may not realize that daily allergen exposure, without causing obvious immediate symptoms, can increase nonspecific nasal reactivity. Such patients may claim to be allergic to, for instance, red wine, which now provokes symptoms in the hyperreactive mucous membrane. Allergy to experimental animals (mice, rats, guinea pigs) is frequent (20 percent) among people exposed to them daily at work, and it can have serious professional consequences.

Foods. Foods, and alcoholic beverages in particular, frequently precipitate symptoms by nonallergic mechanisms. Ingested allergens also play a minor role as etiologic factors in children, however. Ragweed-allergic subjects often report itching in the throat from eating bananas and melons; birch-allergic patients often react to nuts, fresh apples, peaches, and other fruits, especially during their problem season. These sensitivities are unlikely to be important provoking factors for daily nasal symptoms. Acetylsalicylic acid, dyes, and preservatives also may provoke symptoms in an occasional patient, but rarely on a perennial basis.

Idiopathic. The etiology of rhinitis remains obscure in patients in whom allergic mechanisms cannot be implicated. The percentage of nonallergic patients varies considerably (20 to 80 percent), depending upon patient age, selection, diagnostic criteria, and country. It is better to explain to nonallergic patients that their nasal disease is "allergy-like" but is not actually allergic even if we do not know its true nature, rather than to label them "allergic" to an unknown allergen. Otherwise, a patient is more likely to spend time and money in an attempt to find the offending allergen in the hope of finding a cure for that "allergy." For the same reason, nasal polyps (which ordinarily are *not* due to allergy) should not be referred to as "allergic polyps" (see subsequent discussion).

History

Nasal symptoms may occur daily, periodically, or occasionally. They are similar to those of hay fever, but eye itching is less frequent and nasal obstruction more prominent. The patient should be questioned about the following: nasal itching, distinct from irritation of the nostril; sneezing attacks; eye itching, distinct from smarting and irritation; characterization of nasal discharge, whether dripping from the nostrils, easily blown out, or cleared with difficulty by sniffing and swallowing as "postnasal drip"; type of discharge — milky/colored (purulent) or clear and watery/mucoid (nonpurulent); nasal blockage, which can be bilateral, unilateral, or alternating from side to side; mouth breathing, especially at night, and its consequences which are sore throat, snoring, disturbed sleep, sleep apnea, and daytime fatigue; nasal voice; reduced sense of smell and "taste"; and symptoms referable to sinus or ear disease (see Chapters 35 and 36) and its effect on work.

Some patients complain mainly of sneezing and watery rhinorrhea ("sneezers"), while others have nasal blockage and mucoid secretion as dominant symptoms ("blockers"). A sneezer can be transformed to a blocker when polyps develop. The more chronic the disease, the more prominent the blockage. Other patients, especially the elderly, have watery rhinorrhea as the only symptom ("nose blowers").

Quantitative criteria are necessary to distinguish a minor disorder from a significant disease requiring further examination and therapy. The average number of sneezes, number of nose blowings, and daily duration of symptoms are useful measures of severity. Most reliable is a detailed recording of symptoms on a diary card over a 2-week period. The physician must evaluate symptoms within a framework of each individual's personality and coping styles. Some individuals have an unusual awareness of nasal symptoms and seem to complain disproportionately. Others (especially children) complain little or deny symptoms in the presence of impressive nasal obstruction, for example.

The family history, social environment, occupational history, and history of other atopic symptoms are important. They are detailed in Chapter 16.

Physical Examination

Examination of the nose begins with inspection of the face and the outer nose. Many children with long-standing allergic rhinitis can be recognized by their facial characteristics and mannerisms (Marks, 1967). There often is discoloration ("dark circles," "shiners") and edema ("bags") under the eyes. If nasal obstruction is severe, the typical open-mouthed "adenoidal face" may be observed ("allergic gaper"). This can predispose the child to a high-arched palate, overbite, and malocclusion (Shapiro and Shapiro, 1984). Frequent upward rubbing of the nose to alleviate itching, "the allergic salute," results in the development of a transverse "nasal crease" across the lower third of the nose.

A thorough examination of the nose should be carried out in all patients with chronic nasal symptoms. In most patients with perennial rhinitis the mucous membrane is somewhat swollen, wet, and pale bluish in color. This color is often considered "typical allergic," but it can have other causes. Children often have enormously swollen turbinates. The mucous membranes can be normal in adult patients and abnormal in symptom-free subjects. The presence of nasal polyps is suggestive of nonallergic rhinitis (eosinophilic subgroup).

Laboratory Tests

Nasal Cytology. Secretions for cytologic examination can be blown into a plastic sheet or, in young children, aspirated with a rubber bulb syringe. Alternatively, a wiped smear can be obtained by a tightly wound cotton swab. It is introduced 2 to 3 times into each side, and the mucosa scraped with a firm, rolling movement. As the cells are often unevenly distributed, it is important to get as much secretion as possible. The swab must reach into the posterior part of the nose; a smear taken from the anterior part will only contain squamous cells in watery discharge. An epithelial scrape biopsy obtained by a flexible plastic probe is a better standardized method used for cytologic examination. More than 10 percent eosinophils in the smear is considered abnormal, but the judgment of a trained microscopist is more valuable than an exact percent, as the cells often appear in clumps (Malmberg, 1979).

Nasal cytology is helpful in making a distinction between infectious and noninfectious rhinitis and in subclassification of perennial rhinitis (Mullarkey et al., 1980). However, the variation in nasal cytology is so great that a single smear seldom gives a conclusive result; two to three examinations may be required for classification of the disease.

Allergy Diagnosis. Allergy testing, preferably skin testing by the prick technique, should be considered in all patients with allergic rhinitis. It may be necessary in selected cases to confirm a positive skin test by radioallergosorbent test (RAST). Food allergy is a rare cause of isolated rhinitis, at least in adults. The importance of positive test results should be confirmed by blind challenge.

Serum IgE. Most of the adults and half of the children with rhinitis not associated with asthma or dermatitis do not have elevated serum IgE levels. It is important to realize that a normal serum IgE level does not exclude allergy (Mygind et al., 1978).

Blood Eosinophil Count. Blood eosinophilia can occur both in allergic and in nonallergic rhinitis (eosinophilic subgroup). In most patients with rhinitis without other disease present, normal values are the rule.

Radiographic Examination of Paranasal Sinuses. About 20 percent of perennial rhinitis patients have minor changes (marginal loss of translucency) in the maxillary sinuses, and another 20 percent, major changes (Mygind et al., 1978). Clouding of the ethmoidal cells, indicative of the beginning of polyp formation, is usually associated with bilateral clouding of the maxillary sinuses. A unilateral clouding or a fluid level suggests infections, and treatment is indicated. Note that a patient who has had a Caldwell-Luc operation will always have an opaque radiogram (see Chapter 35).

Principles of Treatment

Environmental Control. Allergen avoidance is the first to be recommended in animal, mold, or mite allergic subjects. In each case, changes in the bedroom alone may reduce symptoms. An elimination diet with a diet-symptom diary may be tried in selected cases (see Chapter 10).

Antihistamines. If avoidance cannot be complete, H_1 antihistamines are usually the next step. Generally, they are more effective in seasonal than in perennial allergic rhinitis. Also patients with nonallergic rhinitis, associated with sneezing, watery discharge, and nasal eosinophilia usually respond to antihistamines. They are of little help in patients with pronounced obstruction and nasal polyps.

Nasal Decongestants. Oral medication with alpha adrenoceptor agonists has less effect in the nose than topical treatment, but it can be used regularly without causing rhinitis medicamentosa. Oral vasoconstrictors are contraindicated in pregnancy and must be used with caution in children (risk of psychotic episodes), elderly (with prostatism), and in patients with heart disease or hypertension (Anggard and Malm, 1984). Topical vasoconstrictors can be given from a drop-bottle/pipette or from a nebulizer/pump spray. A plastic bottle nebulizer should be used cautiously in children; some parents will turn it upside down and empty the bottle into the child's nose and severe intoxication can result. Because of the risk of rebound congestion and development of rhinitis medicamentosa, topical decongestants should not be used for more than 4 days in a week. Strict instruction with strong warnings against overuse is the best way to prevent rhinitis medicamentosa.

Steroids. When antihistamines or vasoconstrictors are inadequate or cause side effects, a steroid spray can be considered either as an alternative or as additive therapy (Mygind, 1982b). Steroid sprays are effective on the same types of patients who respond to antihistamines and are more effective, especially in "blockers." Nasal eosinophilia usually predicates treatment success, whereas neutrophilia predicates treatment failure. Adequate mucosal distribution of the drug is important, and patients should be instructed to apply topical adrenergic agents initially to effect nasal decongestion and to facilitate penetration by the steroid agent. Up to 2 weeks of treatment with systemic steroid may be recommended initially in some adults with severe, chronic rhinitis in order to open the nasal airway.

Local therapy can be given as a freon-propelled aerosol of a micronized powder from a pressurized canister (beclomethasone diproprionate, budesonide) or as a solution from a metered-dose pump spray (flunisolide, beclomethasone diproprionate, triamcinolone). The pump spray gives the best intranasal drug distribution, but the pressurized canister is easier to use. Dryness in the anterior part of the nose and blood-stained crusts can occur. Dose reduction, temporary discontinuance, use of a bland ointment in the nostril, change to a pump spray, or change to cromolyn sodium can be helpful in these cases. A few cases of septal perforations have been reported, related possibly to direct steroid effect on the septum in the case of strong topical steroids. Recurrent dislodging of scab and mucous membrane, with progressive ulceration, leads to perforation in some cases.

Cromolyn Sodium. Most pediatricians reserve steroid sprays for patients with severe symptoms not controlled by cromolyn sodium. Cromolyn is most valuable in children and youngsters who usually have uncomplicated allergy. In adults, the degree of symptom amelioration more often is not as impressive. The following factors suggest the likelihood of a good response to the use of cromolyn: obvious allergic etiology; local eosinophilia; predominance of sneezing and rhinorrhea; absence of polyps; young age; and short duration of disease. It is a definite advantage of cromolyn sodium that it does not cause any side effects, even after long-term use.

Ipratropium Bromide. Perennial rhinitis without eosinophilia is largely refractory to therapy, but ipratropium nasal spray can reduce watery hypersecretion (not yet marketed in the United States) (Borum et al., 1979).

Immunotherapy. Immunotherapy often will be of help in mite allergic patients with severe symptoms and in pollen allergic patients. Its effectiveness in mold sensitivity is largely testimonial. Allergen injections can be effective in animal allergy, but treatment should be reserved only for those instances when allergen avoidance is not possible.

Surgery. Surgery plays a minor role in the treatment of allergic rhinitis but can be helpful in severe nonallergic rhinitis when medical treatment has failed. A persistently enlarged inferior turbinate can be cauterized, preferably with a diathermy needle in the submucosa. A surgical removal of the lower edge of the turbinate (partial turbinectomy) is more effective. This form of surgical treatment is rarely, if ever, recommended for children and then only after growth is complete.

Other Measures. When the skin in the nostril becomes macerated by rhinorrhea (vestibulitis), it can activate reflexes that result in the symptoms of rhinitis. In such cases, daily use of bland ointment in the nostril is useful. When secretions are viscid, repeated sniffings to remove "postnasal drip" will dry the mucous membrane and further aggravate the situation. Administration of normal saline sprays or drops is recommended for such patients in order to minimize the need for repeated sniffing, which easily becomes habitual. Patients who have a blocked nose during the night often are aided by elevation of the head of the bed to reduce the congestant effects of gravity on the nose.

NASAL POLYPS

Characteristics

A polyp is an edematously transformed mucous membrane. It is soft, pale yellow, and has a glistening surface. Polyps in the maxillary sinuses are rounded, while polyps in the nose are pear-shaped with a stalk. They originate in the upper part of the nose and the ethmoidal sinuses. Patients with recurrent multiple polyps have hyperplastic rhinosinusitis. Sinus radiographs invariably show clouding of ethmoidal and maxillary sinuses.

Etiology

Although polyps may be associated with any form of chronic rhinosinusitis, they are typically seen in perennial nonallergic rhinitis (eosinophilic subgroup) and in cystic fibrosis. Nasal polyps are often referred to as "allergic polyps," but allergy does not occur more frequently in patients with polyps than in the general population (Settipane and Chafee, 1977). Inhaled allergens will not reach the paranasal sinuses, and food allergy has not proved to be a significant cause of polyp formation. When there is a coincidental occurrence of allergy and polyps, allergen exposure may aggravate the polyposis. Thus, in a child who presents with nasal polyps, a sweat test should be considered as a greater priority than an allergy examination. Children with perennial allergy will often have markedly swollen mucous membranes but rarely develop polyposis.

Diagnosis

The diagnosis is easily made by rhinoscopy, but the use of a vasoconstrictor spray may be necessary. Nasal polyps are typically multiple and bilateral. Unilateral masses should alert the physician to other conditions, such as malignant tumors, papillomata, and meningoceles.

Clinical Presentation

Rhinitis. Nasal polyps, as a rule, develop in a patient who has suffered from perennial nonallergic rhinitis for some years. Nasal obstruction gradually develops and can become complete. Loss or impairment of the sense of smell and of "taste," is due to obstruction of the upper part of the nasal airway. This very annoying symptom, which mars the pleasure of eating and drinking, is more pronounced, persistent, and difficult to treat in rhinitis patients with polyps than in those without polyps. The disease can vary in severity from a single period of nasal blockage relieved by polypectomy, to constant daily symptoms requiring repeated surgery and continuous medication.

Sinusitis. Polyps may appear with polypoid hyperplasia of the maxillary mucous membrane, as discovered on radiography; ethmoidal cells also may be seen to be filled with polyps. Polyps increase the tendency to bacterial infection in the nose and paranasal sinuses, especially following a common cold. Symptoms of sinusitis with polyposis include persistent purulent discharge and pressure/pain over the cheeks (maxillary sinusitis) or the nasal bridge (ethmoidal sinusitis).

Asthma. Severe polyposis is associated with a high blood eosinophil count and is often associated with nonallergic asthma. A classic triad consisting of polyposis, nonallergic asthma, and intolerance to acetylsalicylic acid is described in Chapter 41.

Principles of Treatment

Polyps, as "fluid-filled bags," do not respond as well to medical treatment as do swollen mucous membranes, and surgical treatment often becomes necessary. In the patient with multiple polyps, a simple polypectomy, preferably with local analgesia, followed by a short course of systemic steroid treatment will facilitate a better inspection of the nasal cavities. Any remaining polyps can then be removed. Topical steroid treatment should be started in those patients who either have daily rhinitis symptoms or need polypectomy more than one to two times a year. Daily use of a steroid spray will both improve the symptoms and to some extent prevent the growth of polyps, and it can be used as initial therapy in the case of small polyps to delay or obviate the need for surgery.

Most patients can be managed by the combined use of polypectomy, short-term treatment with systemic steroids, and long-term treatment with local steroids. Antibiotics are helpful in periods of purulent rhinitis. A few cases, resistant to this treatment schedule, require ethmoidectomy with evacuation of as many ethmoidal cells as technically possible.

OTHER CAUSES OF NASAL SYMPTOMS

In childhood, allergic rhinitis is often unsuspected and mistaken for recurrent infections. Congenital choanal atresia can be a cause of unilateral nasal obstruction, with discharge, in infants (Table 34–2); a foreign body is much more common at that age. Enlarged adenoids are frequent causes of mouth breathing. Septal deviation is another well-known cause of nasal obstruction, often bilateral (S-shaped deviation). A nasal blockage, developing in an adult, cannot be ascribed to septal deviation, unless the patient has had trauma with a fracture. However, the mucosal swelling of rhinitis can make an asymptomatic septal deviation clinically significant. Nasal blockage also can be caused by oral antihypertensive and psychosedative drugs with alpha adrenoceptor antagonist properties. Cocaine sniffing produces chronic rhinorrhea and septal perforation.

Continuous use (abuse) of nasal vasoconstrictor sprays is a common cause of chronic irritation and of rebound congestion. Treatment of rhinitis medicamentosa ("nose-drop nose") consists of instructing the patient about the na-

TABLE 34–2. Other Causes of Nasal Symptoms

Mechanical factors

Septal deviation
Nasal polyps
Foreign body
Tumors of the nasopharynx
Tumors of the nose and sinuses
Meningocele
Choanal atresia

Infections

Viral infection
Bacterial infection
Adenoiditis
Sinusitis
Leprosy
Immunodeficiency
Kartagener syndrome

Miscellaneous

Rhinitis medicamentosa
Pregnancy
Antihypertensives
Wegener granulomatosis
Cystic fibrosis
Liquorrhea
Atrophic rhinitis

ture of the disease and discontinuing the topical vasoconstrictor. Oral decongestants, a steroid nasal spray especially useful to facilitate the elimination of the topical decongestant, and treatment of the underlying disease all may be required.

A persistent hormonal rhinosinusitis may develop in the last trimester in otherwise healthy women ("rhinitis of pregnancy"). Its severity parallels the blood estrogen level. This disorder is highly refractory to treatment, but most women are satisfied with assurance that the symptoms will disappear at delivery. It should be noted that oral vasoconstrictors are strictly contraindicated in pregnancy.

Malignant tumors in the nose and paranasal sinuses and Wegener granulomatosis usually start with nasal obstruction. An initial diagnosis of "rhinitis" is not uncommon in such cases. Radiographic examination of paranasal sinuses and rhinoscopy will usually suggest the correct diagnosis. Rhinoscopy, preferably with a fiberscope, is obligatory in patients with unilateral symptoms, hemorrhagic secretions, and pain.

REFERENCES

Andersen, I., Lundquist, G.R., Proctor, D.F.: Human response to controlled levels of sulfur dioxide. Arch. Environ. Health 28:31–9, 1974.

Anggard, A., Lundberg, J.M., Lundblad, L.: Nasal autonomic innervation with special reference to peptidergic nerves. Eur. J. Respir. Dis. 128:64, 1983. 143–9.

Anggard, A., Malm, L.: Orally administered drugs in disorders of the upper respiratory passages: a survey of clinical results. Clin. Otolaryngol. 9:43–49, 1984.

Bierman, C.W. (ed.): ENT Allergy. Clin. Rev. Allergy 2:169–441, 1984.

Borum, P., Larsen, E.S., Mygind, N.: Intranasal ipratropium: a new treatment for perennial rhinitis. Clin. Otolaryngol. 4:47, 1979.

Borum, P., Mygind, N.: Inhibition of the immediate allergic reaction in the nose by the beta-2 adrenostimulant fenoterol. J. Allergy Clin. Immunol. 66:25–32, 1980.

Church, J.A.: Allergic rhinitis. Clin. Pediatr. 19:655–659, 1980.

Cohan, R.H., Bloom, F.L., Rhoades, R.B., Wittig, H.J., Haugh, L.D.: Treatment of perennial allergic rhinitis with cromolyn sodium. J. Allergy Clin. Immunol. 58:121–128, 1976.

Connell, J.T.: Quantitative intranasal pollen challenge. J. Allergy Clin. Immunol. 43:33, 1969.

Creticos, P.S., Peters, P., Adkinson, F.N.J., Naclerio, R.M., Hayes, E.C., Norman, P.S., Lichtenstein, L.M.: Peptide leukotriene release after antigen challenge in patients sensitive to ragweed. N. Engl. J. Med. 310:1626, 1984.

Editorial: No sneezing—or dozing—seen with new H_1 blockers. J.A.M.A. 249:3151–3152, 1983.

Griffin, M.P., McFadden, E.R., Ingram, Jr, R.H.: Airway cooling in asthmatic and nonasthmatic subjects during nasal and oral breathing. J. Allergy Clin. Immunol. 69:354–359, 1982.

Hastie, R., Heroy, J.H., Levy, D.: Basophil leukocytes and mast cells in human nasal secretions and scrapings studied by light microscopy. Lab. Invest. 40:554, 1979.

Kirkegaard, J., Secher, C., Mygind, N.: Inhibition of the histamine-induced symptoms by the H_1 antihistamine chlorpheniramine maleate: demonstration of topical effect. Brit. J. Dis. Chest. 77:113–122, 1983.

Malmberg, H.: Symptoms of chronic and allergic rhinitis and occurrence of nasal secretion granulocytes in university students, school children and infants. Allergy 34:389–94, 1979.

Marks, M.B.: Physical signs of allergy of the respiratory tract in children. Ann. Allergy 25:310, 1967.

Mullarkey, M.F., Hill, J., Webb, D.R.: Allergic and nonallergic rhinitis: their characterization with attention to the meaning of nasal eosinophilia. J. Allergy Clin. Immunol. 65:122–126, 1980.

Munch, E.P., Søborg, M., Nørreslet, T.T., Mygind, N.: A comparative study of dexchlorpheniramine maleate sustained release tablets and budesonide nasal spray in seasonal allergic rhinitis. Allergy 38:517–524, 1983.

Mygind, N.: Nasal Allergy, 2nd ed. Oxford, Blackwell Scientific Publications, 1979.

Mygind, N.: Mediators of nasal allergy. J. Allergy Clin. Immunol. 70:149–159, 1982a.

Mygind, N.: Topical steroid treatment for allergic rhinitis and allied conditions. Clin. Otolaryngol. 7:343–352, 1982b.

Mygind, N.: Essential Allergy. Oxford, Blackwell Scientific Publications, 1985.

Mygind, N., Dirksen, A., Johnsen, N.J., Weeke, B.: Perennial rhinitis: an analysis of skin testing, serum IgE, and blood and smear eosinophilia in 201 patients. Clin. Otolaryngol. 3:189–196, 1978.

Mygind, N., Pipkorn, U., Weeke, B. (eds.). Allergic and Vasomotor Rhinitis: Pathophysiological Aspects. Copenhagen, Munksgaard, 1986.

Mygind, N., Rasmussen, F.V., Mølgarad, F., (eds.): Cellular and neurogenic mechanisms in nose and bronchi. Eur. J. Respir. Dis. 64:1–557, 1983.

Mygind, N., Weeke, B.: Allergic and nonallergic rhinitis. In Middleton, E. Jr., Reed, C.E., Ellis, E.F. (eds.), Allergy: Principles and Practice, 2nd ed. St. Louis, C.V. Mosby Co., 1983.

Mygind, N., Weeke, B. (eds.): Allergic and Vasomotor Rhinitis: Clinical Aspects. Copenhagen, Munksgaard, 1985.

Naclerio, R.M., Meier, H.L., Kagey-Sobotka, A., Adkinson, N.F., Jr., Meyers, D.A., Norman, P.S., Lichtenstein, L.M.: Mediator release after nasal airway challenge. Am. Rev. Respir. Dis. 128:597–602, 1983.

Norman, P.S.: Review of nasal therapy: update. J. Allergy Clin. Immunol. 72:421–432, 1983.

Okuda, M., Ohtsuka, H., Kawabori, S.: Basophil leukocytes and mast cells in the nose. Eur. J. Respir. Dis. 64:7–14, 1983.

Proctor, D.F., Andersen, I. (eds.): The Nose: Upper Airway Physiology and the Atmospheric Environment. Amsterdam, Elsevier Biomedical Press, 1982.

Richarson, H.B., Rajtora, D.W., Penick, G.D., et al.: Cutaneous and nasal allergic responses in ragweed hay fever: lack of clinical and histopatologic correlations with late phase reactions. J. Allergy Clin. Immunol. 64:67–77, 1979.

Secher, C., Kirkegaard, J., Borum, P., Mansson, A., Osterhammel, P., Mygind, N.: Significance of H_1 and H_2 receptors in the human nose: rationale for topical use of combined antihistamine preparations. J. Allergy Clin. Immunol. 70:211–215, 1982.

Settipane, G.A. (ed.): Rhinitis. Rhode Island, The New England and Regional Allergy Proceedings, 1984.

Settipane, G.A., Chafee, F.H.: Nasal polyps in asthma and rhinitis. J. Allergy Clin. Immunol. 59:17–21, 1977.

Shapiro, G.G., Shapiro, P.A.: Nasal airway obstruction and facial development. Clin. Rev. Allergy 2:225–235, 1984.

Shaw, R.J., Fritzharris, P., Cromwell, O., Wardlaw, A.J., Kay, A.B.: Allergen-induced release of sulphidopeptide leukotrienes (SRS-A) and LTB_4 in allergic rhinitis. Allergy 40:1–6, 1985.

Solomon, W.R.: Aerobiology of pollinosis. J. Allergy Clin. Immunol. 74:449–461, 1984.

Toogood, J.H.: Perennial rhinitis with negative allergy skin test. ORL Digest 38:7–14, 1976.

Tos, M.: Goblet Cells and Glands in the Nose and Paranasal Sinuses. In Proctor, D.F., Andersen, I. (eds.): The Nose: Upper Airway Physiology and Atmospheric Environment. Amsterdam, Elsevier Biomedical Press, 1982.

Wihl, J-A., Petersen, B.N., Petersen, L.N., Gundersen, G., Bresson, K., Mygind, N.: Effect of the non-sedative H_1 receptor antagonist, astemizole in perennial allergic and nonallergic rhinitis. J. Allergy Clin. Immunol. 75:720–727, 1985.

35

Disorders of Paranasal Sinuses

GARY S. RACHELEFSKY, M.D.
SHELDON L. SPECTOR, M.D.

Sinusitis, or inflammation of the paranasal sinuses, is a common problem in children and adults though its true incidence is unknown. Sinus disease is caused by inflammation, cysts, tumors, and foreign bodies. The major emphasis in this chapter is on infectious and allergic sinus disease. Acute sinusitis is defined as a condition present for less than 3 weeks, and chronic sinusitis for more than 3 weeks.

DEVELOPMENT AND FUNCTION OF THE PARANASAL SINUSES

The paranasal sinuses form as evaginations of the mucous membrane of the nasal meatuses and are lined by the same mucosa as the nose. The origin of the ethmoid and maxillary sinuses is apparent by the third to fourth month of fetal life. Frontal sinuses become recognizable anatomically by the sixth to twelfth month of extra-uterine life, while the sphenoid sinus appears later (Bernstein, 1971). Whereas the maxillary and ethmoid sinuses are evident by radiography in early infancy, the sphenoid sinuses appear by about the third year of life, and the frontal sinuses between the third and seventh years. Developmental variants include hypoplasia of frontal sinuses (common), with partial or complete absence of the sinuses. Occasionally, the maxillary antra are asymmetric, and they may be subdivided by septa and ridges into several small cavities. The ethmoid sinuses are a somewhat variable labyrinthine network of air spaces. Although they are grouped as anterior, middle, and posterior, there is considerable individual variation in structure (Caffey, 1972). Sinus abnormalities appear to be common in patients with cleft lips, and palates, and in association with midfacial hypoplasia (e.g., Treacher Collins syndrome).

The functions of the paranasal sinuses include lightening the weight of the skull, improving the resonance of the voice, warming and moisturizing inspired air in auxiliary heat exchange, olfactory function, insulating heat at the base of the skull, and protecting the area from trauma (Rohr and Spector, 1984).

PATHOPHYSIOLOGIC CONSIDERATIONS

Mucociliary Function

The paranasal sinuses are lined by pseudostratified ciliated epithelium and bathed in a mucus layer produced by mucosal glands and goblet cells. Projecting from the border of each columnar cell are cilia, the ends of which are in contact with the overlying mucus. Microorganisms and foreign particles that enter the sinuses are removed by the constant motion of the mucus layer, propelled by the underlying cilia. Mucus is carried to the ostium of the sinus in this manner, often against gravitational forces. (This is particularly prominent in the maxillary sinuses where the ostia are located superior to the body of the sinuses.)

Mucus secretions and saliva contain substances (including lysozymes) that decrease bacterial attachment, inhibit bacterial or viral replication, and destroy specific bacteria (Hoffman, 1966). Interferon in the nasal passages decreases the multiplication of viruses.

Secretory Immune System

The secretory immune system is the first line of defense against invading organisms. Local exposure of mucous membranes to antigens induces formation of secretory antibodies which provide protection against infecting organisms. Secretory IgA is the predominant immunoglobulin in secretions that bathe mucous membranes that possess antibody activity against viral agents (Tomasi and Bienenstock, 1968; Artenstein et al., 1964). Secretory IgA antibodies protect against parainfluenza virus and poliovirus (Hanson et al., 1971).

Secretory IgA antibodies against bacteria have been demonstrated to inhaled tetanus

476

toxoid (Hanson et al., 1971), inhaled diphtheria toxoid (Newcomb et al., 1969), and to parenterally administered *Salmonella typhi* vaccine (Tourville and Tomasi, 1969). Secretory antibody also has been shown to interfere with the attachment of oral streptococcal strains to buccal mucosal cells (Williams and Gibbons, 1972). Although secretory IgA antibodies appear to play an important role in protecting the upper respiratory tract against various kinds of infections, some individuals who lack IgA antibodies do not have increased numbers or increased severity of respiratory infections, possibly because of "compensatory" increases in quantities of IgG and IgM in the secretions.

Nonspecific Surface Defenses. Other mechanical mechanisms may act to clear organisms and debris from the nasal passages, such as the following: flowing of free fluid that helps to wash away organisms, moving air currents, coughing, sneezing, and possibly chewing.

Pathogens in Sinus Disease

The majority of studies on the etiology of sinusitis have involved adults, although adequate information is available for children. Isolation of pathogens has been accomplished by aspiration of the middle meatus (Bridger, 1980), by antral wash, by direct antral swabbing. In general, nasal cultures are of limited value in identifying organisms in the sinuses and do not correlate well with the aforementioned techniques.

The bacteriology of maxillary sinusitis has been studied most extensively because of its accessibility and frequency of involvement. There seems to be an unimpressive correlation between nasal and sinus cultures. Axelsson and Brorson (1973) found that nasal cultures from patients with acute maxillary sinusitis were either bacteriologically sterile or showed *Haemophilus influenzae*, pneumococcus, and *Staphylococcus aureus*, in that order. Aspirated sinus secretions contained a predominance of pneumococcus or *H. influenzae* or were sterile. Staphylococci were uniquely limited to the nose. These investigators found the same organisms in nasal and sinus cultures in 64 percent of their patients. Wald et al. (1984) evaluated 30 children between 1 and 16 years of age with acute maxillary sinusitis. Maxillary sinus aspirations were performed, with at least one sinus found to be infected in 23 of the 30 children. In 34 of 47 sinus aspirates, bacteria were cultured.

Streptococcus pneumoniae, H. influenzae (nontypable with two recoveries resistant to ampicillin), and *Branhamella catarrhalis* were the most common organisms recovered. There was no correlation between the bacterial species predominating in the nasopharynx and throat versus the sinuses. Viruses were recovered twice; a parainfluenza virus was recovered from one subject without an associated bacterial pathogen, and an adenovirus was recovered from another subject in association with *B. catarrhalis.*

Aspiration of fluid from the maxillary sinus is the most reliable means of identifying bacterial pathogens. Specimens obtained directly from sinuses in adults with acute sinusitis most commonly grow *H. influenzae, Streptococcus viridans,* and *Staphylococcus aureus* (Evans et al., 1975), though some may have anaerobic bacteria thought to be of dental origin. *H. influenzae* organisms either have not been typed or have been reported as nontypable.

Cultures from "chronic sinusitis" in adults have frequently contained anaerobic bacteria, such as alpha-hemolytic streptococci, *Bacteroides, Veillonella,* and *Corynebacterium* (Frederick and Braude, 1974). Spector and Farr (1984) compared the bacteriology of the middle meatus of the nose and the maxillary sinus at operation for chronic maxillary sinusitis. *Staphylococcus aureus, Staphylococcus albus,* and diphtheroids were cultured from the nose, whereas alpha-hemolytic streptococci and pneumococci were cultured from the sinuses, or the cultures were sterile. There was poor correlation between nasal and sinus organisms, with complete correlation present in only 9 percent of the cases.

In children, the role of anaerobes in chronic sinusitis has not been fully evaluated. Brook (1981a) aspirated secretions from the sinuses of 40 children (mean age, 11 years) with chronic disease defined as more than 30 days of illness. Of the 121 isolates, 24 grew aerobic and 97 grew anaerobic organisms. The predominant aerobic organisms were alpha-hemolytic streptococci, *S. aureus,* and *Hemophilus sp.;* the predominant anaerobic organisms were *Bacteroides sp.,* gram-positive cocci, and *Fusobacterium spp.* All the anaerobes recovered were sensitive to penicillin.

Though the normal maxillary sinus has been thought to be sterile, Brook (1981b) investigated the bacterial flora of noninflamed maxillary sinuses in 12 adults. Anaerobes were isolated from all 12, and in 7 both anaerobes and aerobes were isolated. The former included *Bacteroides sp.*, gram-positive cocci, and *Fusobacterium sp.* The aerobes included beta-hemolytic streptococci, alpha-hemolytic streptococci, *Streptococcus pneumoniae*, and *H. influenzae.* Therefore, results of this limited study suggest that there is a normal bacterial flora of the maxillary sinus cavity; further, it includes the same organisms that cause sinusitis.

The role of viral infections in acute sinusitis has not been studied in depth. Rhinoviruses and adenoviruses have been isolated from patients with chronic sinusitis (Spector et al., 1973). L-forms also have been isolated from patients with chronic sinusitis. An implied role for *Mycoplasma pneumoniae* in sinusitis remains to be explored. Sporadic cases of fungal sinusitis have been reported, but appropriate techniques for culturing fungi have not been employed in most studies.

In summary, aerobic organisms associated with acute and chronic sinusitis in children and adults appear to be similar and usually include *H. influenzae* and *Streptococcus pneumoniae.* Younger children may have beta-hemolytic streptococci. Anaerobic organisms are commonly observed with chronic sinusitis in adults. Further studies are needed in children with chronic sinusitis. Sinuses that appear opacified and have air-fluid levels or marked mucosal thickening, radiographically, are more likely to contain bacteria which can be cultured when they are aspirated than are sinuses with lesser pathology.

Factors that Predispose Individuals to Sinus Disease (Table 35–1)

It appears that some compromise of normal defense mechanisms may predispose to acute or chronic sinusitis. Defense mechanisms of paranasal sinuses may function effectively only when the sinus ostia are unobstructed. Respiratory infections cause nasal mucosal edema which occludes the sinus ostia and inhibits normal ciliary cleansing action. This leads to mucus retention and provides an environment for bacterial sinus infection. When viral infections or overuse of topical nasal decongestants are superimposed on obstruction due to allergy, sinus infection becomes even more likely. Nasal allergy is frequently associated with sinus disease, since the allergic reaction also increases mucus production and causes nasal mucosal edema. Another factor that can contribute to

TABLE 35–1. Conditions Predisposing Individuals to Sinusitis or Associated with Sinusitis

Viral upper respiratory tract infections	Swimming
	Trauma
Rhinitis	Facial fractures
Allergic, nonallergic	Oroantral fistula
Rhinitis medicamentosa	Barotrauma
Nasal obstruction	Idiosyncratic reactions
Choanal atresia	Aspirin
Septal deviations	Nonsteroidal anti-inflammatory agents
Foreign bodies	
Polyps	Tartrazine (yellow dye no. 5)
Hypertrophied adenoids (infected?)	Cystic fibrosis
Tumors	Immune disorders
Benign	Immotile cilia syndrome
Malignant	Down syndrome
Dental problems	

maxillary sinusitis is the proximity of these sinuses to the upper teeth; dental abscesses may contaminate the maxillary sinus, especially with anaerobes. Nasal polyps probably predispose individuals to sinusitis by obstructing the sinus ostia. Table 35–1 lists other causes of sinusitis, including systemic disorders. Swimming and diving can force pathogenic bacteria into paranasal sinuses.

CLINICAL PRESENTATION OF SINUSITIS

Acute Sinusitis

Symptoms. *Acute sinusitis may occur in early infancy.* In the young child, acute ethmoid sinusitis often is preceded by 2 to 3 days of an upper respiratory viral illness, which may seem to resolve. This transient improvement is followed by a persistent purulent or serous white to green rhinorrhea. Postnasal drainage commonly produces night coughing, which may be "barking" and associated with lower respiratory sounds (e.g., harsh "bronchitic" sounds, rhonchi). Younger children often have fever, whereas teenagers and adults complain of unpleasant smells and tastes, purulent nasal discharges, headaches, localized pain over the involved sinus (magnified with bending over), and coughing. Both older children and adults may complain of lethargy, malaise, and low grade fever. Some older children and adults may complain only of painful teeth or jaws. The pain is referred from the sinus cavities (see Chapter 56).

Signs. Physical signs of sinusitis differ by age. Rhinorrhea is found in most patients. There may be slight flushing of the cheek with swelling of the lower eyelid in maxillary disease and the upper eyelid in frontal sinusitis. Ethmoiditis may lead to orbital cellulitis or abscess. Pressure over the involved sinuses may be painful. The nasal mucosa is erythematous and swollen. If the edematous nasal mucosa shrinks with a topical vasoconstrictor, the physician may see a localized area of erythematous and swollen membranes with a thick mucopurulent discharge in the area of the ostium of the involved sinus. The pharynx may be coated with thick purulent material, which forms a blanket over its posterior wall.

Chronic Sinusitis

Children and adults with chronic sinusitis often present with symptoms such as cough, especially at night, and nasal discharge or persistent postnasal drainage or both. The postnasal drainage will not always be purulent. The cough is often refractory to conventional therapy. These patients may complain of sore throat, nasal congestion, sniffing, earache, fatigue, and irritability. The younger child may have impetiginous lesions around the external nostrils, and at least half may have recurrent otitis media or middle ear dysfunction. Headache (worse in the morning) is more common in adults than children. The older child and adult may often complain of anosmia (impairment of the sense of smell). Fever, laryngitis, and epistaxis are uncommon in both groups. In children and adolescents the illness may be associated with weight loss and extensive school absenteeism. Paroxysmal nocturnal coughing may lead to vomiting.

The nasal mucosa is usually swollen and inflamed. Mucopurulent material may be seen coming from the ostium of the infected sinus. Nasal secretions may range from a clear watery discharge to a greenish, thick, purulent discharge or may be absent. Often these secretions will coat the upper surface of the palate, descending along the lateral pharyngeal gutter onto the posterior pharyngeal wall. The central and lateral pharyngeal lymphoid tissue often is swollen. Rhinoscopy reveals enlarged and sometimes infected adenoids. Infected teeth rarely are responsible for sinusitis in children, in contrast to adults; an abscess from a deciduous tooth usually drains into the buccal cavity, whereas in adults a periodontal abscess drains into the adjacent antral sinuses.

At times, neither adults nor children exhibit signs or symptoms directly related to the nose or sinuses and exhibit only secondary complications. These include bronchitis (Rohr et al., 1984), laryngitis, otitis media, and dental infections (Lindahl et al., 1982). (For more detailed discussion, see the following: Rachelefsky et al., 1982 and 1984; Rachelefsky, 1984; Spector and Farr, 1984.) Nasal polyps should alert the physician to sinusitis because of their frequent association with chronic sinusitis.

DIAGNOSTIC CONSIDERATIONS

In an inflammatory disease of the sinuses, diagnosis requires more than history and physical examination, especially if the condition is chronic. The diagnostic aids commonly used are cytologic examination of nasal secretions, x-ray examination, transillumination, rhinoscopy, ultrasonography, and antral lavage. The peripheral white blood cell count and differential, and the erythrocyte sedimentation rate are of value especially in the patient with acute sinusitis.

A valuable laboratory tool is the cytologic examination of fresh nasal secretions. A large number of polymorphonuclear cells, especially with intracellular bacteria, are frequent findings in patients with sinusitis. Although polymorphonucleocytes may predominate during viral upper respiratory infection, their presence in large numbers in a profuse rhinorrhea of several weeks' duration suggests sinusitis.

There are four standard views used in the radiographic evaluation of the paranasal sinuses; occipitomental (Waters), occiput frontal (Caldwell), lateral, and submentovertical. For acute disease one should obtain at least a Waters (maxillary) and a Caldwell (ethmoid) view. Many radiologists have stated that there are many normal children with abnormal sinus x-ray findings. However, in a recent study, Kovatch et al. (1984) evaluated 112 unselected children by history and physical examination; the results of these examinations were compared with frequency of abnormal maxillary sinus radiographs. The investigators concluded that crying was not associated with abnormal radiographs and that, in children more than 1 year of age, abnormal maxillary sinus radiographs are infrequent and are related to recent inflammation (infection or allergy or both) of the upper respiratory tract.

The diagnostic radiographs of sinusitis in one or more sinuses show opacification, air fluid level, marked membrane thickening, or filling of more than 50 percent of maxillary space. There is a high correlation of culture-proven infection from antral irrigations with these radiographic findings. Sinus opacification may occur from bacterial infection, severe allergic mucosal edema with or without secretions, or acute viral respiratory infection. Although there may be active infection with less prominent mucous membrane thickening, the correlation with culture evidence for infection is weaker. In these instances, the total clinical picture and clinical judgment should dictate therapy. In a patient with recurrent sinusitis, repeated sinus radiographs are not necessary if the clinical picture makes the diagnosis obvious. However, it is helpful to repeat the radiograph in the patient with recurrent or persistent sinusitis after medical treatment to be certain that the sinuses are clear. A Waters view alone may suffice with maxillary disease. Although transillumination of the frontal paranasal sinuses may have predictive value, the technique has limited usefulness as a diagnostic tool and is not an adequate substitute for radiography (Spector et al., 1981).

Rhinoscopy (and ultrasonography) are useful when radiography is refused or medically contraindicated as in pregnancy. Rhinoscopy can be utilized to view directly purulent drainage from the ostia of the paranasal sinuses. Ultrasonography, although highly specific, is relatively insensitive and therefore is not very useful as a diagnostic tool (Shapiro et al., 1986). However, it may be employed serially to follow a patient who has been diagnosed with sinusitis (Rohr et al., 1984). Computer-analyzed tomography and antral lavage may be useful in certain situations (Unger et al., 1984).

TREATMENT OF SINUSITIS

Medical Management

Treatment of sinus disease should be aimed at promoting drainage, controlling infection, and providing symptomatic relief. While definitive studies of optimal duration of antibiotic therapy have not been carried out, clinical experience suggests that a 2-week course is adequate for most but not all patients.

Acute sinusitis is best treated with amoxicil-lin, cefaclor, or amoxicillin-clavulanic acid for 14 days. At present, the drug other than cefaclor to use in the penicillin-allergic child under 9 years of age includes trimethoprim-sulfamethoxazole plus erythromycin. In the seriously ill patient, hospitalization should be considered. Therapy for beta-lactamase producing staphylococci should be ampicillin and oxacillin or ampicillin and chloramphenicol (see also Chapter 23).

Drainage from sinus cavities may be enhanced by administering nasal decongestant drops or sprays, which should be used at low concentrations and for no more than 3 to 5 days. The use of topical or oral decongestants has not been evaluated adequately for efficacy in the treatment of acute sinusitis. Antihistamines alone or in combination with decongestants can be prescribed empirically in an attempt to shrink nasal mucosa and promote drainage. For some patients, humidification of the environment and application of moist heat to the face several times a day may be helpful to prevent drying of the mucosa. Surgical drainage rarely is necessary. Rachelefsky and coworkers (1982b) evaluated the role of antimicrobial agents in the treatment of chronic maxillary sinusitis in allergic children. Eighty-four children were treated in a double-blind protocol with amoxicillin, erythromycin, or trimethoprim-sulfamethoxazole. Radiographic and clinical responses were best with amoxicillin, but trimethoprim-sulfamethoxazole was an adequate alternative. Erythromycin was not any better than an antihistamine with decongestant. In situations in which 2 weeks of therapy result in temporary cessation of symptoms, 4 weeks of further therapy should be used if the patient experiences a relapse.

If the patient fails to have complete resolution of symptoms after completing the first 14-day antibiotic course, a second 4-week antibiotic course should be used. This can be cefaclor (if not used initially), amoxicillin-clavulanic acid, a combination of erythromycin and trimethoprim-sulfamethoxazole, or a combination of erythromycin and sulfasoxazole acetyl. If significant clinical disease continues, an otolaryngologic consultation should be obtained. Antral lavage sometimes will reveal anaerobic organisms whose antibiotic sensitivities should be determined (Brook, 1983). Therapy of chronically opacified maxillary sinuses, especially in cases of persistent symptoms, with associated chronic otitis media, difficult to control asthma, or chronic sinus pain may require antral irrigation. The effectiveness of long-term prophylactic antibiotics, topical cromolyn sodium, and cortiosteroids is unknown.

Surgical Management

Maxillary sinus irrigation is performed to clear purulent secretions and to obtain bacterial cultures. In children, the maxillary sinus is the only one that is usually approached. Irrigation often results in a cloudy exudate which contains polymorphonuclear leukocytes and bacteria. This procedure may result in complications. The needle may fail to enter the sinus cavity, may enter the orbit and produce pain in the cheek or eye, or may cause local emphysema or air embolus.

Nasal antrostomy (nasal antral window) is a surgical procedure that creates an opening in the medial wall of the maxillary sinus, usually in the inferior meatus. This procedure creates an additional route of drainage for the sinus secretions, one which also takes advantage of gravitational factors that may aid in sinus drainings, particularly when there is mucociliary drainage. Nasal antrostomy is considered in patients with recurrent sinus infections secondary to stenosis of the natural ostium, either from prior sinus infections or from obstructions by swollen mucous membranes or nasal polyps. Bleeding is the major complication, although adhesions may develop. Nasal antrostomy is usually not necessary in children. When such a drainage procedure is medically indicated, either the enlargement of the natural ostium or creation of an accessory ostium using the middle meatus is the preferred operation.

Though avoided in children because of its potentially deleterious effect on facial growth and dentition, a Caldwell-Luc operation is often used in adults. Postoperative problems include recurrent sinusitis, numbness, nasal synechiae, and persistent facial and dental complications.

The Montgomery procedure for the frontal sinuses or the equivalent for the maxillary sinuses is sometimes indicated for adults with healthy fibrous tissue. It consists of a fatty implant into the sinus cavity in order to replace the diseased sinus mucosa that has been scraped clean (English, 1983).

COMPLICATIONS OF SINUSITIS

Sinus infections have been associated with lower respiratory tract infections and asthma (Quinn and Meyer, 1929; McCavrin, 1935). Infection may also spread from the tracheobronchial tree to the paranasal sinuses (Hogg, 1950). Radiopaque contrast material used for bronchograms can be seen in the paranasal sinuses soon after instillation.

Though a relationship between sinusitis and asthma has been reported, a double-blind, placebo-controlled study has not been performed. Nevertheless, our clinical experience suggests that patients with sinusitis and difficult to control asthma may benefit from medical treatment with appropriate antibiotics or surgical therapy. Rare complications of sinusitis may include orbital cellulitis, orbital abscess, intracranial involvement (meningitis, cavernous sinus thrombosis, brain abscess, and subdural empyema), and osteomyelitis. Obviously, an appropriately designed placebo-controlled study is needed to clarify this controversial subject.

REFERENCES

Artenstein, M.S., Bellanti, J.A., Buescher, E.L.: Identification of antiviral substances in nasal secretions. Proc. Soc. Exper. Biol. Med. 117:558–568, 1964.

Axelsson, A., Brorson, J.E.: The correlation between bacteriological findings in the nose and maxillary sinus in acute maxillary sinusitis. Laryngoscope 83:2003, 1973.

Bernstein, L.: Pediatric sinus problems. Otolaryngol. Clin. North. Am. 4:127, 1971.

Bridger, R.C.: Sinusitis: an improved regimen of investigation for the clinical laboratory. J. Clin. Pathol. 33:276–281, 1980.

Brook, I.: Bacteriologic features of chronic sinusitis in children. J.A.M.A. 246:967, 1981a.

Brook, I.: Aerobic and anaerobic bacterial flora of normal maxillary sinuses. Laryngoscope 91:372, 1981b.

Brook, I.: Treatment of anaerobic infections in children with metronidazole. Dev. Pharmacol. Ther. 6:187–198, 1983.

Caffey, J.: Pediatric X-ray Diagnosis. Chicago, Year Book Medical Publishers, 1972.

English, G.: Nasal polyps and sinusitis. *In* Middleton, E. Jr., Reed, C.E., Ellis, E.F. (eds.), Allergy: Principles and Practice. St. Louis, C.V. Mosby Co., 1983.

Evans, E.O., Sydnor, J.B., Moore, W.E.C., Moore, G.R., Manwaring, J.L., Brill, A.H., Jackson, R.T., Hanna, S., Skaar, J.S., Holdeman, L.V., Fitz-Hugh, G.S., Sande, M.A., Gwaltney, J.M.: Sinusitis in the maxillary antrum. N. Engl. J. Med. 292:735, 1975.

Frederick, J., Braude, A.I.: Anaerobic infection of the paranasal sinuses. N. Engl. J. Med. 290:135, 1974.

Hanson, C.A., Borssen, R., Holmgren, J., Jodal, U., Johansson, B.G., Kaijser B.: Secretory IgA. *In* Kagan, B., Stiehm, E.R. (eds.), Immunologic Incompetence. Chicago, Year Book Medical Publishers, 1971.

Hoffman, H.: Oral microbiology. Adv. Appl. Microbiol. 8:195, 1966.

Hogg, J.C.: Discussion on the role of sinusitis in bronchiectasis. Proc. R. Soc. Med. 43:1089, 1950.

Kovatch, A.L., Wald, E.R., Ledesma-Medina, J., Chiponis, D., Bedingfield, B.: Maxillary sinus radiographs in children with nonrespiratory complaints. Pediatrics 73:306–308, 1984.

Lindahl, L., Melen, I., Ekedahl, C., Holm, S.E.: Chronic maxillary sinusitis: Differential diagnosis and genesis. Acta Otolaryngol. 93:147–150, 1982.

McCavrin, J.G.: A review of the interrelationship of paranasal sinus disease and certain chest conditions, with special consideration of bronchiectasis and asthma. Ann. Otol. Rhinol. Laryngol. 44:344–353, 1935.

Newcomb, R.W., Ishizaka, K., DeVald, B.L.: Human IgG and IgA diphtheria antitoxins in serum nasal fluids and saliva. J. Immunol. 103:215, 1969.

Quinn, L.H., Meyer, O.O.: The relationship of sinusitis and bronchiectasis and asthma. Arch. Otolaryngol. 10:152–165, 1929.

Rachelefsky, G.S., Katz, R.M., Siegel, S.C.: Diseases of Paranasal Sinuses in Children. *In* Gluck, L. (ed.), Current Problems in Pediatrics. Chicago, Year Book Medical Publishers, 1982a.

Rachelefsky, G.S., Katz, R.M., Siegel, S.C.: Chronic sinusitis in children with respiratory allergy: The role of antimicrobials. J. Allergy Clin. Immunol. 69:382–387, 1982b.

Rachelefsky, G.S.: Sinusitis in children—Diagnosis and management. Clin. Rev. Allergy 2:397–408, 1984.

Rachelefsky, G.S., Katz, R.M., Siegel, S.C.: Chronic sinus disease with associated reactive airway disease in children. Pediatrics 73:526–529, 1984.

Rohr, A.S., Spector, S.L.: Paranasal sinus anatomy and pathophysiology. Clin. Rev. Allergy 2:387–395, 1984.

Rohr, A.S., Spector, S.L., Katz, R.M., Rachelefsky, G.S.: Comparison of x-ray and ultrasound in the diagnosis of maxillary sinusitis. Ann. Allergy 52:233, 1984.

Shapiro, G.G., Furukawa, C.T., Pierson, W.E., Gilbertson, E., Bierman, C.W.: Blinded comparison of maxillary sinus radiography and ultrasound for diagnosis of sinusitis. J. Allergy Immunol. 77:59–64, 1986.

Slavin, R.G., Cannon, R.E., Friedman, W.H., Palitang, E., Sundaram, M.: Sinusitis and bronchial asthma. J. Allergy Clin. Immunol. 66:250–257, 1980.

Spector, S.L., English, G., McIntosh, K., Farr, R.S.: Adenovirus in the sinuses of an asthmatic with apparent selective antibody deficiencies. Am. J. Med. 55:277–231, 1973.

Spector, S.L., Farr, R.S.: The interface between allergy and otolaryngology. *In* English, G. (ed.), Otolaryngology, vol. 2. New York, Harper & Row, 1984.

Spector, S.L., Lotan, A., English, G., Philpot, I.: Comparison between transillumination and the roentgenogram in diagnosing paranasal sinus disease. J. Allergy Clin. Immunol. 67:22–26, 1981.

Tomasi, T.B., Bienenstock, J.: Secretory immunoglobulins. Adv. Immunol. 9:1, 1968.

Tourville, D.R., Tomasi, T.B.: Selective transport of gamma A. Proc. Soc. Exper. Biol. Med. 132:475, 1969.

Unger, J.M., Shaffer, K., Duncavage, J.A.: Computed tomography in nasal and paranasal sinus disease. Laryngoscope 94:1319–1324, 1984.

Wald, E.R., Reilly, J.S., Casselbrant, M., Ledesma-Medina, J., Milmoe, G.J., Bluestone, C.D., Chiponis, D.: Treatment of acute maxillary sinusitis in childhood: A comparative study of amoxicillin and cefaclor. J. Pediatr. 104:297, 1984.

Williams, R.C., Gibbons, R.J.: Inhibition of bacterial adherence by secretory immunoglobulin A. A mechanism of antigen disposal. Science 177:697, 1972.

36

Diseases of the Ear

JAMES DONALDSON, M.D.
C. WARREN BIERMAN, M.D.

Otitis media with effusion (OME), an inflammatory disease of the mucoperiosteal lining of the eustachian tube, middle ear, and mastoid air cells affects large numbers of children. Approximately 10 million children are treated each year for this condition in the United States alone (Cotton and Zalzal, 1986), and it is the most common reason for surgery in children in England and Wales (Black, 1985) and in the United States (Gates et al., 1986). This disease is associated with an accumulation of fluid in the middle ear and is the most common cause of acquired hearing loss in children today. Although it occurs most often in preschool aged children, it causes substantial morbidity and may be a frequent handicap of younger school aged children. OME can occur at any age, however, and even older adults can have middle ear effusions that cause intermittent hearing losses and interfere with effective communication. To date, the incidence of such problems in the adult population has not been studied systematically. Table 36–1 indicates the differences between OME in children and adults.

Some investigators believe that this disorder may represent the most common precursor of chronic irreversible otitis media in older children and younger adults (Bernstein, 1984). Even when the disease is self limited, it can result in adverse effects of speech development and cognition, especially in the young child (Holm and Kunze, 1969), although the degree to which this occurs is controversial (Roberts et al., 1986). It can be especially devastating when superimposed on an underlying sensorineural hearing loss (Milner et al., 1985).

The term suppurative otitis media is considered to be synonymous with acute otitis media (AOM); OME is generally referred to as nonsuppurative otitis media or "glue ear." Though controversial, "serous," "mucoid," and "purulent" otitis are believed by some to reflect stages of variations of disease which may coexist (Cotton and Zalzal, 1986). These disease states are thought to be secondary to eustachian tube dysfunction (ETD) or to other causes of middle ear dysfunction (MED). The terms otitis media with effusion (OME) and middle ear dysfunction (MED), proposed by several international symposia on otitis media, will be employed throughout this chapter.

MIDDLE EAR DYSFUNCTION

OME is the result of many factors acting on the middle ear, the eustachian tube, or both (Teele et al., 1980). Animal experiments have demonstrated that with obstruction of the eustachian tube, oxygen in the middle ear and mastoid air cells is absorbed by mucosal capillaries, producing negative middle ear pressure. The middle ear mucosa becomes thickened and edematous; a transudate forms from the subepithelial fluid leaking from blood vessels. This transudate ruptures the basement membrane, distorting nonciliated cells as it traverses these cells to enter the middle ear space (Paparella et al., 1970).

With prolonged eustachian tube obstruction, middle ear fluid develops which contains varying amounts of mucus, cellular remnants, and neutrophils. The mucosa becomes hyperplastic, with a change to stratified respiratory epithelium; the goblet cells proliferate; the mucosa invaginates to form submucosal cysts; and the glands and subepithelial vessels proliferate (Cotton et al., 1984). Inflammatory cells then infiltrate in large numbers. As a result, immunocompetent cells, especially macrophages and lymphocytes, enter the middle ear and create a distinct system of local immunity, as shown in Figure 36–1 (Bernstein, 1985; Tos, 1984).

Negative middle ear pressure impedes sound transmission in the middle ear; middle ear effusion can cause a 20 to 50 decibel hearing loss which affects lower frequencies to a greater extent than higher ones. If normal eustachian tube function does not return and the aforementioned cycle continues, damage from the inflammatory process eventually can result in a permanent change in middle ear and mastoid mucosae, with associated bone resorption.

483

TABLE 36–1. Differences Between OME in Adults and Children*

Characteristic	Adult	Child
Silent or asymptomatic	Unusual	Common
Ear involved	Unilateral (often)	Bilateral (84 percent)
Enlarged adenoids	Rare	Common
Tympanic membrane transparency maintained	Frequent	Rare
Symptoms of vertigo	Occasional	Rare
Associated neoplasia	Occasional	Rare

* Adapted from Bernstein, J.M., et al.: Immunologic ear disease. Clin. Rev. Allergy 2:349–375, 1984.

Etiology of Middle Ear Dysfunction

MED may result from abnormal eustachian tube function; infection; allergy; diseases of adenoids or sinuses or both; and genetic diseases, such as immotile cilia syndrome. ETD, acute otitis media, and upper respiratory allergy are conditions most frequently associated with MED and OME.

ETD can result from abnormal patency or ob-

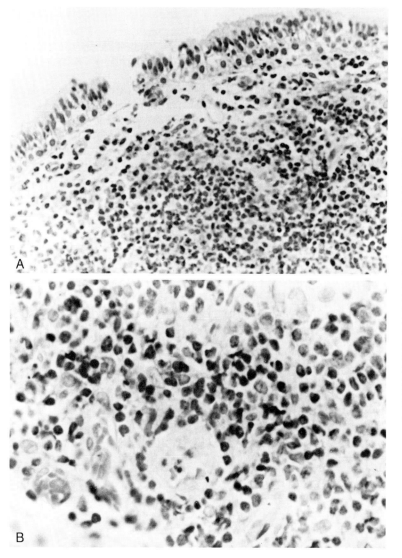

FIGURE 36–1. A, High power photomicrograph of pseudostratified ciliated epithelium characteristic of respiratory mucosa from the middle ear mucosa of a child with otitis media with effusion. There are dilatated capillaries and multiple mononuclear cells, particularly plasma cells in the lamina propria. H&E($\times$ 225). B, High power photomicrograph of the lamina propria of middle ear mucosa in chronic otitis media with effusion. A dilated capillary is surrounded by mononuclear cells. This histologic picture is often seen in chronic otitis media with effusion and is consistent with a cell-mediated immune reaction. H&E ($\times$ 450). (Reproduced by permission from Bernstein, J.M.: Recent advances in otitis media with effusion. Ann. Allergy 55:547, 549, 1985.)

struction of the eustachian tube. An abnormally patent tube permits reflux of nasopharyngeal secretions into the middle ear, which induces infectious or noninfectious inflammation (see Chapter 33). Eustachian tube obstruction prevents ventilation of the middle ear and leads to creation of negative middle ear pressure and the process which results in OME. It can result from intrinsic factors, such as mucosal edema from inflammation due to viral or bacterial infections; chronic exposure to irritants, such as cigarette smoke; nasal allergy or congenital or acquired abnormalities in structure or function of involved tissues, such as cystic fibrosis, Down syndrome, cleft palate, immotile cilia syndrome, and immunodeficiency. Viral or bacterial infections can be primary or secondary to poor drainage of middle ear secretions, with stasis and bacterial growth.

The etiologic factors thought to be of major importance in adults are noted in Table 36–2.

The role of infection in the pathophysiology of OME is not clear at present. Acute otitis media (AOM), an extraordinarily common infection in children, has its highest incidence between 6 and 24 months of age (Teele et al., 1980). Subsequently, the incidence falls until the age of 5 to 6 years when a second peak coincides with school entrance, possibly caused by an increased incidence of viral respiratory tract infections. Boys develop acute and recurrent otitis media more commonly than girls. AOM also occurs more frequently in some racial groups, especially in Eskimos and American Indians, and in whites more commonly than in blacks.

In a prospective study of 2500 children, 47 percent had a first episode of AOM by 1 year, and 71 percent had had at least one episode by 3 years. By 3 years, one third of the group had had three or more episodes of AOM, and 10 percent developed OME for as long as 3 months after their initial infection in spite of prompt and appropriate therapy (Teele et al., 1983). Lim (1982) has noted that there is a striking similarity between the incidence of AOM and OME, though the peak incidence of OME occurred after that of AOM. Thus, there is strong circumstantial evidence that AOM in some way predisposes patients or is pathogenetically related to OME, at least in some patients.

The most common bacteria cultured from the middle ear in acute otitis media are *Streptococcus pneumoniae*, particularly types 14 and 19; *Haemophilus influenzae* (non-type B), usually biotypes 2 and 3; *Branhamella catarrhalis;* and coagulase-negative *Staphylococcus* (Bernstein, 1985).

The role of these organisms in the pathogenesis of OME, however, is not clear. In most studies, these organisms are cultured far less frequently from OME effusions than from AOM. Some workers have cultured one type of organism from 25 to 30 percent of effusions (Liu et al., 1976; Klein, 1980), whereas others have found bacteria in 8 percent or less (Maw and Speller, 1985). Viral cultures of effusions have been negative for *Mycoplasma*, respiratory syncytial virus (RSV), parainfluenza virus, and adenovirus (Parker et al., 1985). Increased levels of complement components, especially those associated with the alternative pathway, are

TABLE 36–2. Classification of OME in Adults*

Inflammatory	**Traumatic/Structural**
Infectious (after upper respiratory infection, acute otitis, sinusitis, cilia dyskinesis, immune deficiency, tuberculosis)	Barometric
	Cerebrospinal fluid or perilymphatic otorrhea
Allergic rhinitis (perennial and seasonal)	Blunt (basilar skull fracture)
Eosinophilic nonallergic rhinitis	Destructive (cholesteatoma, tumor)
Aspirin sensitivity	Post-surgical
Nasal polyps	Congenital (dura defects)
Systemic immunologic disorders (Wegener granulomatosis, polyarteritis, sarcoid, Sjögren syndrome)	
Neoplastic	**Miscellaneous**
Benign (branchial cyst)	Obesity
Malignant	Palatal paralysis due to central nervous system disorders
Epithelial (squamous cell carcinoma, adenocarcinoma, adenoid cyst, melanoma, and so forth)	Hypothyroidism
Mesenchymal (rhabdomyosarcoma, chordoma)	
Reticuloendothelial (lymphoma, leukemia)	

* From Bernstein J.M., et al.: Immunologic ear disease. Clin. Rev. Allergy 2:349–375, 1984.

present in middle ear effusions and suggest an active inflammatory process. Unfortunately, there is little correlation between the presence of levels of complement components and the clinical courses of patients with OME (Parker et al., 1985).

The relationship between viral infections of the nasopharynx and bacterial infections of the middle ear has been suggested clinically and in animal models (Giebink et al., 1980). Bernstein (1985) has proposed a mechanism by which RSV, known to induce an IgE response in some children, may induce edema of the eustachian tube, impaired ciliary function, and OME or AOM or both.

Upper respiratory allergy is recognized increasingly as a factor that may contribute substantially to OME, MED, or both. Circumstantial evidence suggests that it may act directly on the middle ear to induce mucociliary dysfunction and effusion in a small proportion of patients or, more commonly, on the eustachian tube to induce proliferation of lymphoid tissue or peritubal edema, which impairs lymphatic drainage and obstructs the tube at its pharyngeal outlet. Allergy also could act indirectly by causing nasal obstruction and nasopharyngeal pressure differences which could induce reflux of pharyngeal secretions into the middle ear by the Toynbee phenomena (Cotton et al., 1984; Kraemer et al., 1984).

Evidence implicating allergy as a risk factor in OME has originated in three types of studies as follows: (1) epidemiologic studies of children with OME referred for insertion of tympanotomy tubes, (2) studies of children with atopic disease referred to specialized clinics for evaluation, and (3) double-blind placebo-controlled nasal insufflation challenge studies with allergens or histamine or both.

Kraemer and colleagues (1984) studied 76 children with chronic middle ear effusions who were referred for tympanotomy tube insertion, comparing them with 76 children who were admitted to hospitals for other elective surgery. Three major factors increased the risk of middle ear effusion as follows: (1) exposure to environmental cigarette smoke, (2) nasal congestion, and (3) atopic disease. When exposed to two or more cigarette smokers, children had a nearly three-fold increased risk of persistent middle ear effusions. This risk increased nearly four-fold when they were exposed to smoke from more than three packs of cigarettes per day. Persistent rhinitis, which occurred more frequently in children with OME, increased the

risk three to five fold. Atopic diseases (asthma, allergic rhinitis, atopic dermatitis) occurred twice as frequently in children with OME. Chronic atopic symptoms of any kind (at least 15 days/month) caused the risk of OME to rise nearly four fold. When the three factors coexisted, the risk increased six fold.

In 488 consecutive new patients referred to a pediatric allergy practice for evaluation, 57 percent had asthma, 95 percent allergic rhinitis, and 16 percent atopic dermatitis. All patients were tested with impedance audiometry. Forty-nine percent had middle ear dysfunction with type B (flat) or type C_2 (> 199 mm H_2O peak pressure) tympanograms. The peak age for MED in this group occurred between 2 and 6 years (Fig. 36–2). However, if the incidence of MED or OME is related to the total number of patients in each age group, these allergic patients appeared to be at an almost equal risk of MED, irrespective of age (Marshall et al., 1984).

In a 3-year study, Bernstein and coworkers (1985) evaluated 100 children with OME for respiratory allergy. Thirty five were diagnosed as having allergic rhinitis. Sixteen of these children had elevated serum IgE levels; all 16 had IgE levels in their nasal secretions which were higher than corresponding serum IgE levels. In addition, eight children had elevated IgE levels in middle ear fluid, which were substantially higher than corresponding serum IgE levels. Thus, children with allergic rhinitis have local IgE synthesis in the nose, and some also may have local IgE synthesis in the middle ear. The investigators interpreted these data as indicating that nasal allergy was present in a substantial number (35 percent) of children with OME; and in a small proportion (8 of 35), the middle ear appeared to be the primary target organ, whereas in the others the eustachian tube was the presumed target organ.

Direct evidence of eustachian tube involve-

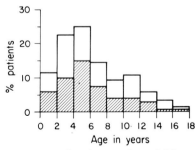

FIGURE 36–2. Age distribution of 488 children referred for evaluation of allergic disease. Shaded areas indicate those with middle ear disease (MED or OME).

ment in OME comes from nasal challenge studies in both human and subhuman primates. Walker and colleagues (1985) challenged atopic and nonatopic subjects with nasal histamine insufflation. Nine of the 12 atopic subjects developed eustachian tube obstruction as well as increased nasal resistance. By contrast, none of the ten nonatopic subjects studied showed eustachian tube involvement even though all subjects showed increased nasal resistance after challenge, suggesting that the eustachian tubes of atopic patients are more likely to react to histamine than those of normal subjects. Friedman et al. (1983), employing double-blind intranasal pollen challenges in subjects with allergic rhinitis, induced both allergic rhinitis and eustachian tubal obstruction with pollen but not with placebo preparations. In some subjects, ETD persisted for several days. However, the amount of pollen administered was far greater than would have been encountered with normal exposure. Also, in this study, there was no evidence of OME.

Other antigens, such as house dust mite, ragweed, and grass pollen, have induced similar changes in atopic subjects. This effect was found to be allergen specific and not of an irritative nature (Doyle et al., 1984; Skonker et al., 1985), since the effects of these allergens could be blocked by pretreatment with specific drugs, such as antihistamines, topical intranasal corticosteroids, and cromolyn sodium (Fireman et al., 1983).

Rhesus monkeys passively sensitized to ragweed develop allergic rhinitis and eustachian tube dysfunction when challenged with aerosolized ragweed pollen. In these sensitized animals, active tubal function was impaired markedly after challenge though passive resistance increased only slightly. This finding suggests that the primary site of IgE-mediated ETD is in the nasopharynx where there is impairment of the muscle assisted opening of the eustachian tube (Fireman, 1985).

Complications of Prolonged Middle Ear Dysfunction

One of several hypotheses suggests that MED with persistent negative middle ear pressure may predispose an individual to cholesteatoma formation. Some workers believe that prolonged negative middle ear pressure induces formation of a retraction pocket in the attic or posterior-superior quadrant; as the squamous debris from the outer layer of the tympanic membrane builds up in the pocket, it forms a cholesteatoma that acts as a "tumor" that can invade the middle ear. As the pocket deepens, the cholesteatoma may invade the mastoid air cells and destroy the ossicles (Cotton et al., 1984).

Prolonged MED also can lead to squamous metaplasia of the middle ear mucosa and form an expanding keratin cyst. In addition, prolonged negative middle ear pressure can lead to atelectasis of the middle ear. The atelectatic tympanic membrane may adhere to the ossicles and medial wall of the middle ear and form an irreversible adhesive otitis media (Cotton et al., 1984).

Clinical Evaluation

Figure 36–3 is a flow diagram of the therapeutic approach to the patient with OME. The goal of medical management is to restore normal middle ear and eustachian tube function by controlling extrinsic and intrinsic factors that predispose the patient to disease or prolong disease.

History

A comprehensive clinical history is essential to the proper diagnosis and management of middle ear disease. The importance of a thorough history cannot be overemphasized. The origin, course, progression, and treatment of disease should be documented. A thorough environmental history is necessary to identify allergic or irritant factors in the home, school, or work environment that may predispose the patient to nasal congestion. A history of exposure to irritants, such as cigarette smoke, or allergens, such as house dust, molds, or pets in the home, school, or work environment, will aid in selection of allergy tests as well as provide information necessary to modify the patient's environment. Symptoms suggesting adenoidal hypertrophy, such as snoring and nasal obstruction, should be identified.

Physical Examination

Pneumatic otoscopy should be employed to examine tympanic membrane structure and function. A proper otoscopic examination re-

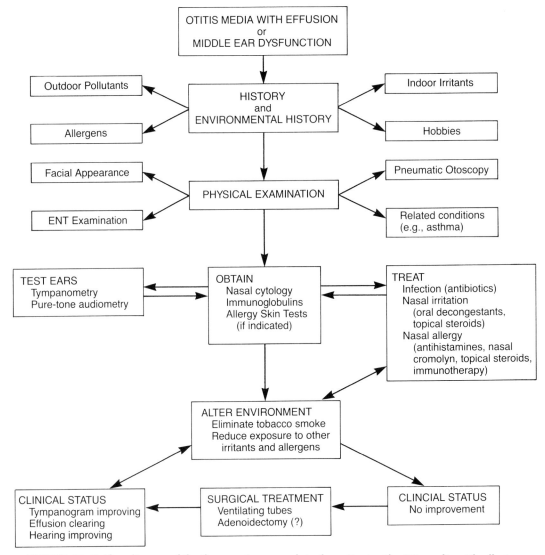

FIGURE 36–3. Flow diagram of the therapeutic approach to the patient with otitis media with effusion.

quires an optimal light, an airtight otoscope head, and a speculum large enough to seal the ear canal (Fig. 36–4). The position, color, translucency, and mobility of the tympanic membrane is noted. A normal tympanic membrane should be translucent and should permit a view of the middle ear landmarks. A reddish tympanic membrane alone may not indicate pathology, as the blood vessels to the drum may be engorged by crying, sneezing, or blowing the nose. Mild retraction of the tympanic membrane usually indicates negative middle ear pressure, effusion, or both. Severe retraction of the tympanic membrane is characterized by a prominent lateral process of the malleus and

abnormally acute angulation of the malleus handle (Bluestone, 1982). Only 15 percent of patients with middle ear effusions present with an air fluid level or bubbles of air mixed with liquid and a bluish or yellowish hue to the drum; however, an effusion affects the mobility of the tympanic membrane when negative pressure is applied to the external auditory canal. A partial effusion or significant negative middle ear pressure requires a strong negative pressure to move the tympanic membrane. When total effusion is present, the drum cannot be moved even with moderate negative pressure. However, when strong negative pressure is applied in the presence of a large amount of

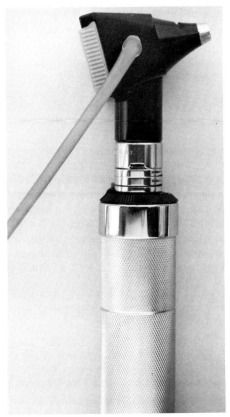

FIGURE 36–4. Modification of closed-head otoscope for pneumatic otoscopy with pipette tubing (see text).

viscid fluid, the drum may appear to "crinkle," which may be mistakenly identified as mobility.

The nose should be examined carefully for signs of chronic rhinitis, obstruction, and allergic disease. Mouth breathing and hyponasal speech can indicate nasal obstruction. A submucous cleft palate or bifid uvula often is associated with ETD. Nasal examination may reveal edema of the turbinates, nasal septal deviation, or nasal polyps. Nasal polyps in children are associated frequently with cystic fibrosis and, in adolescents or adults, are associated with chronic sinus disease more consistently than with "allergy" (Settipane and Chafee, 1977).

Laboratory Examination

Once the clinical diagnosis of OME has been made, hearing function should be tested and allergy tests conducted, if the patient appears to manifest respiratory allergy.

Impedance Audiometry or Tympanometry. *Impedance audiometry* or tympanometry has been developed to test middle ear function and can be performed easily in a physician's office (Sly et al., 1980). It is important to understand that this is not a hearing test but merely a test of some aspects of middle ear physiology. It is a useful screening test but has limited application for experienced clinicians, with respect to the medical management of OME. *It is not a substitute for a test of hearing.* It can be used to evaluate middle ear function in children too young to respond to pure tone audiometry. Because impedance audiometry is noninvasive and does not require the child to respond, it can be performed readily on a child as young as 12 months of age (Tos, 1979). It is also particularly useful in uncooperative children whose ear canals are incompletely occluded by cerumen. Very useful information can be obtained with minimal manipulation.

Tympanometry can determine the pressure of air in the middle ear, the mobility of the tympanic membrane and of the ossicles, and can relate information that indicates the presence of middle ear fluid. Tympanometry is performed by inserting a probe containing three microchannels in a rubber ear plug that seals the ear canal. One microchannel transmits a sound at 200 hertz (Hz); another contains a sensitive microphone that picks up the reflection of the signal; and the third regulates pressure in the ear canal.

Most instruments can alter ear canal pressure from +200 to −400 mm H_2O. As tympanic membrane compliance is greatest when air pressure on both sides of the drum is equal, peak sound conductance normally occurs between 0 and −100 mm. This is referred to as an A curve. As middle ear pressure decreases, the peak shifts to the negative pressure zone. As middle ear pressure becomes increasingly negative, the tympanogram peak becomes flatter and wider and a C curve is seen. A more recent classification divides the C curve into C_1 (−100 to −199 mm H_2O) and C_2 (> 199 mm H_2O with a definite peak) curves, which represent the phases that children pass through when they are developing a B curve or when the process producing a B curve is resolving. The A and C_1 curves appear most stable, whereas the C_2 curve is the least stable (Birch and Elbrond, 1985). A flat curve with no recognizable peak (B curve) usually is indicative of fluid. Fluid also may be present with other curve configurations (see Chapter 17).

Pure tone audiometry can be used in the physician's office or clinic as a screening test. It is performed by testing hearing at four sound frequencies (500, 1000, 2000, and 4000 Hz) at three sound intensities (20 or 25, 40, and 60 decibels). More accurate thresholds are obtained when tests are performed in a sound-proof room. Hearing is tested utilizing octaves from 125 Hz to 8000 Hz, and the threshold of hearing is determined for each tone. This is performed for both air and bone conduction. Bone conduction bypasses the middle ear, and the sound is carried directly to the inner ear.

This procedure permits determination of how much hearing loss is caused by disease in the middle ear, in the organ of Corti, or in the auditory nerve. OME is associated with a low-frequency hearing loss and often is associated with a conductive hearing loss in the "speech" frequencies. By contrast, sensorineural disease is associated frequently with a high frequency hearing loss.

Morphology of Nasal Secretions. In the child with OME, eosinophils in nasal secretions usually suggest nasal allergy. However, in the adolescent or adult in particular, eosinophils also may be associated with eosinophilic nonallergic rhinitis, a condition uncommon in children (Jacobs et al., 1981). The absence of eosinophils does not rule out allergy. For example, the patient with allergic rhinitis who has a superimposed upper respiratory tract infection may have a predominance of polymorphonuclear leukocytes, and mononuclear cells and eosinophils may appear only after the upper respiratory infection has cleared.

Quantitative Immunoglobulin Serum Levels. Serum levels of IgG, IgM, and IgA can be useful in diagnosing disease in patients with recurrent ear infections due to hypogammaglobulinemia or dysgammaglobulinemia. An elevated serum IgE level may point to respiratory allergy. However, IgE levels can be normal in patients with significant respiratory allergy, especially in the absence of concomitant atopic eczema and asthma (see Chapter 17).

Allergy Skin Tests. Skin tests should be limited to factors suggested by the history as possible allergens. These bioassays are highly sensitive, cost effective, and safe in experienced hands as indicators of immediate type I hypersensitivity. Serologic tests, e.g., radioallergosorbent test (RAST) can detect specific IgE antibodies but are less sensitive and less effective than skin tests (see Chapter 17).

Medical Management of OME

Strategy for the medical management of the patient with OME includes four distinct procedures. First, it is important to identify and avoid allergic and irritant factors in the environment that predispose the patient to OME. Second, various medications, such as antibiotics, antihistamines, oral decongestants, and corticosteroids, may be indicated to clear infection, alleviate inflammation, and reduce secondary obstruction. Third, immunotherapy (desensitization, hyposensitization) may be indicated in atopic children who cannot avoid specific airborne allergens. Fourth, inflation with a Mathes inflator (Fig. 36–5) may open a tube that is functioning poorly, may ventilate the middle ear, and may rid the middle ear of fluid.

ENVIRONMENTAL CONTROL

Irritants and allergens to which the child may be allergic should be avoided if possible. Parents should be instructed about the specific procedures for avoidance of such household allergens as house dust mites, household molds, and animal danders (see Chapter 18). Particularly important for the OME patient is the avoidance of tobacco smoke. Parents and babysitters must not smoke in the home, automobile, or any place where the patient might be in a confined space. If the child is exposed to cigarette smoke in a day care center, an alternative day care facility should be sought.

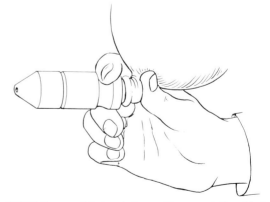

FIGURE 36–5. Mathes inflator. Using an inflated balloon as a pressure source, air is introduced into the nose during swallowing.

ANTIMICROBIAL MEDICATION

If a bacterial infection is present in the middle ear, nose, or paranasal sinuses, it should be treated with appropriate antibiotics. Acute middle ear infection usually is obvious and easy to diagnose. However, in OME without obvious local or systemic signs of infection it is not possible on physical examination to predict the presence of pathogenic bacteria. As symptomatic middle ear effusions may yield pathogenic bacteria upon tympanocentesis and culture, a treatment course of at least 10 days is recommended as minimal for patients with OME, especially if there is coexistent paranasal sinusitis (Wald et al., 1981; Rachelefsky et al., 1982; Gates et al., 1986).

Amoxicillin or ampicillin is the drug of choice for initial treatment because of activity against *Streptococcus pneumoniae* and most *Haemophilus influenzae*. Other acceptable alternatives include trimethoprim-sulfamethoxazole, cefaclor, and combinations of a sulfonamide with oral erythromycin, penicillin G or V, clindamycin, or benzathine penicillin G (IM).

Currently recommended doses for treatment include the following:

1. Ampicillin, 50 to 100 mg/kg/24 hours, in 4 divided doses for 10 days.
2. Amoxicillin, 40 mg/kg/24 hours, in 3 divided doses for 10 days.
3. Combination of oral erythromycin, 40 mg/kg/24 hours, and sulfisoxazole, 120 mg/kg/24 hours, in 4 divided doses for 10 days.
4. Trimethoprim-sulfamethoxazole, 8 mg/kg/24 hours trimethoprim and 40 mg/kg/24 hours sulfamethoxazole, in 2 divided doses for 10 days.
5. Cefaclor, 20 mg/kg/24 hours, in 3 divided doses for 10 days.
6. Amoxicillin-clavulanate potassium, 40 mg/kg/24 hours in 3 divided doses (based on amoxicillin component).

When a patient does not respond to initial therapy with ampicillin or amoxicillin, infection with *Staphylococcus aureus*, a resistant strain of *Haemophilus influenzae* or *Branhamella catarrhalis*, or an uncommon organism should be considered, and the patient administered one of the alternative regimens outlined. Other causes of failure to respond to an antibiotic include viral or other nonbacterial infection, focus of infection outside the ear, immune deficiency, anatomic defect, presence of foreign body, in-

adequate compliance, improper dosage of the chemotherapeutic agent, inadequate diffusion to infection site, and deterioration of the agent.

Recommendations for prophylaxis of recurrent bouts of AOM include amoxicillin, 20 mg/kg every 24 hours in 1 dose, or sulfonamide, 50 mg/kg every 24 hours in 2 divided doses. This prophylactic regimen should be continued for 6 months, during which time the child should be seen monthly. A double-blind-placebo-controlled study, however, suggests that sulfisoxazole is less effective than tympanotomy tube insertion in prophylaxis of recurrent episodes of AOM (Gonzalez et al., 1986).

ANTIHISTAMINE/DECONGESTANT THERAPY

The use of antihistamine/decongestant preparations has become controversial in pediatrics. A double-blind study of these agents versus placebos in children with upper respiratory infections showed that these agents did not protect children from AOM (Haugeto et al., 1981).

A study by Cantekin and coworkers (Cantekin et al., 1983) showed that these drugs were no more effective than placebos in treating middle ear effusions. However, this study eliminated patients with asthma and included only about 4 percent of patients in each group with allergic rhinitis. Therefore, it excluded specifically the atopic population that might have benefited most from this treatment.

Pierson et al. (1982) studied a series of allergic children who had ETD but no effusion by a double-blind placebo-controlled administration of triprolidine and pseudoephedrine. The mean peak pressure on entry into the study was -236.6 mm H_2O, and the mean gradient was 0.271. All four groups of patients improved significantly in relation to peak pressure over the study period of 4 weeks. However, only triprolidine-pseudoephedrine treated patients showed a significant pressure-gradient improvement ($P = 0.04$).

Antihistamine/decongestant drugs may be useful in allergic patients who have MED. Whether such drugs are of any value in patients with OME has not been established.

ANTIBIOTICS

The effectiveness of prolonged antibiotic therapy for otitis media with effusion is not clear. Most studies have consisted of open trials (Healy, 1984; Marker et al., 1981, Giebink et al., 1986). Some patients show benefit for prolonged antimicrobial therapy (trimethoprim-sulfamethoxazole, cefaclor, or erythromycin-sulfisoxazole) and some do not. A double-blind controlled trial of prolonged antibiotic therapy in atopic children has yet to be carried out.

TOPICAL NASAL STEROIDS

Shapiro and coworkers (1982) have studied the effectiveness of topical dexamethasone and flunisolide nasal sprays in children with OME. When dexamethasone was compared with placebo, there was a significant improvement in eustachian tubal function at the end of the first week in patients treated with the active drug. Fasting, 8:00 a.m. cortisol levels were similar for the two groups, suggesting that 3 weeks of topical dexamethasone did not interfere with adrenal function.

Similar findings were noted in a study of nasal flunisolide (Shapiro et al., 1982). Children 2 to 12 years of age with allergic rhinitis, who had type C tympanograms with middle ear pressure of -199 mm H_2O or greater in one or both ears, were treated with nasal flunisolide or placebo. Adrenal function was tested, utilizing cosyntropin on entry and after 4 weeks of treatment. Both patient groups also improved with time in this study. Flunisolide-treated patients improved more rapidly than placebo-treated patients. There were no differences between the initial and final cosyntropin test results in either group, indicating that a 4-week course of topical nasal flunisolide was both safe and effective in children. No similar studies have been carried out in adults.

SYSTEMIC CORTICOSTEROIDS

Systemic corticosteroids have been recommended for OME, but most studies showing efficacy have been poorly controlled and all have been short term. The only controlled study did not examine hypothalamic-pituitary-adrenal axis effects (Schwartz et al., 1980). Until a well-designed study examines both safety and efficacy, one should use systemic steroids for OME cautiously.

Macknin and Jones (1985) evaluated a tapering dosage of dexamethasone in 22 patients with improvement in 45 percent of those treated compared with 22 percent of controls. Woodhead et al. (1986) found no benefit for prednisone in persistent OME in patients on prophylactic antibiotic therapy. Other studies have found no difference between antibiotic and prednisone treated patients after four weeks of therapy (Giebink et al., 1986).

The effectiveness of the combination of antimicrobial therapy and steroids has been studied by several workers (Berman et al., 1987; Heisse, 1963; Shea, 1971; Persico et al., 1978). In general, they report benefit for these combinations. However, more studies have examined potential adverse effects of adrenal suppression of systemic steroids. In one 8 a.m. cortisol levels were studied in a small subpopulation (6 of 47 patients), and an abnormal level was found in one that returned to normal 3 days later. Any future studies should address this problem.

TOPICAL CROMOLYN

Topical intranasal cromolyn sodium solution has recently been introduced in the United States. Whereas it appears to help reduce nasal symptoms in children with hay fever, there are no data concerning its effects on middle ear function.

Surgical Management of Chronic OME

Strategy for surgical management of the patient with OME has included tonsillectomy, adenoidectomy, myringotomy, and ventilating tube insertion. These procedures have been used singly and in combination. Although results of controlled studies have varied, some conclusions can be drawn.

THE ROLE OF TONSILLECTOMY

Maw and Herod (1986) studied 150 children between 2 and 9 years of age who had OME with a mean duration of hearing loss of 18 months. They were randomly allocated among adenotonsillectomy, adenoidectomy, and neither. Additionally, one ear had a myringotomy with a ventilating tube, and the other was only examined. When studied after 1 year, those patients who had adenotonsillectomy or adenoidectomy had fewer middle ear effusions than did those who had neither. Adenotonsillectomy was no more effective than adenoidectomy alone. From this study and others, it would appear that there is little if any role for tonsillectomy in prophylaxis or treatment of middle ear disease.

THE ROLE OF ADENOIDECTOMY

After appropriate medical management, Roydhouse (1980) eliminated responding patients and randomized 100 children (ages 3.2 to 14.0 years) into bilateral myringotomies with ventilating tube insertion with and without adenoidectomy. Patients were followed over a 6-year period. There was no significant difference between the two groups. For those patients who did not have adenoidectomy, the relapse rate was independent of the size of the adenoids.

Black, Crowther, and Freeland (1986) studied children between ages 4 and 10 years. They were randomly divided into two groups. Half the patients had adenoidectomies and half did not. Both groups were further randomized so that half underwent bilateral myringotomy with unilateral ventilating tube and half underwent unilateral myringotomy with ventilating tube insertion. The study is planned to provide a 5-year follow-up. When studied at 6 weeks, the group that had adenoidectomy could hear better (when tested audiometrically) than could the group without adenoidectomy. At 6 months and at 1 year, however, there was no difference in hearing between the two groups. In the study by Maw and Herod (1986), however, patients' having either adenoidectomy or adenotonsillectomy required fewer tube reinsertions during the following 12 months than did patients' having only myringotomy and tube insertions. Thus, there is at least some evidence that adenoidectomy can be beneficial in the treatment of chronic OME, but therapeutic effectiveness of this procedure for chronic OME is arguable.

THE USE OF MIDDLE EAR VENTILATING TUBES

Maw and Herod (1986) found that myringotomy with insertion of ventilating tubes was associated with improved hearing at both 6 and 12 months compared with patients who were only observed during this period. This beneficial effect occurred whether or not adenoidectomy or adenotonsillectomy was performed. Bonding and Tos (1985) reported similar findings in a prospective study of 193 children. However, ventilating tubes yielded significantly better hearing results for only as long as the tube was in place and patent.

Wacker and Howe (1986) used middle ear cilia activity to determine whether or not a tube is necessary after fluid has been removed. They found that patients with actively beating cilia rarely required ventilation with a tube.

In a retrospective study of 630 patients who had myringotomy with ventilating tube placement, Curley (1986) found that the grommet remained in place for an average of 8.6 months and that it was not blocked for 8.2 months. It was of interest that the youngest group (< 3 years) did not have the greatest number of admissions for repeat procedures.

Milner et al. (1985) have emphasized the importance of more aggressive treatment of OME in a child who has an underlying sensorineural hearing loss, because of the greater interference of additional hearing loss on the child's communication.

Ventilating tubes are essentially devices that maintain the patency of a perforation and consequently keep the middle ear ventilated in instances when the eustachian tube fails to accomplish this. Gebhart (1981) has shown that tubes also are effective in reducing the incidence of otitis media in children who are "otitis prone."

Ventilating tubes are available in a variety of shapes and materials. Basically, there are short-acting and long-acting tubes (Fig. 36–6). Short-acting tubes usually are double flanged, with one flange medial to the tympanic membrane to impede extrusion and one flange lateral to the tympanic membrane to prevent the tube from falling into the ear. A long-acting tube usually has a larger medial flange or a "T," which delays extrusion for a greater period of time. The tubes may be fashioned from silicone, Teflon, polyethylene, vinyl, stainless steel, or titanium. They may be transparent, metallic, or colored blue or green for easier identification. The larger the diameter of the medial flange or

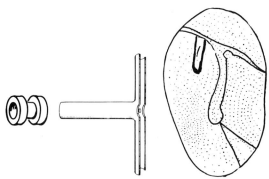

FIGURE 36–6. Examples of middle ear ventilating tubes. They are drawn to the same scale as the tympanic membrane.

"T," the longer the tube tends to remain in place. The chances that a perforation will persist after tube extrusion or removal are directly related to the length of time the tube is in place. For this reason, many surgeons use short-acting tubes initially and reserve long-acting tubes for patients requiring reinsertions. Many surgeons suggest that patients use eardrops in each external auditory canal for 5 days after tubes are placed. The drops appear to decrease the incidence of otorrhea immediately after surgery and to decrease the chance that the tube lumen will become occluded by blood. Although some surgeons use potentially ototoxic drops, such as those containing neomycin, there does not appear to be any evidence that these drops pass through the ventilating tube or damage the inner ear.

When tubes are in place, patients usually are advised to keep water out of their ears. This is best accomplished by occlusion of the meatus with ear plugs (custom molded acrylic, wax, silicone putty, and so forth) when bathing or swimming, but no completely dependable method of occlusion has been devised. Patients with ventilating tubes are asked to refrain from nose blowing during upper respiratory infections, since infected material is more likely to go via the eustachian tube to the tympanum when a tube is in place than when the membrane is intact.

The main complications of ventilating tubes are otorrhea, persistence of a perforation in the tympanic membrane after the tube is removed, and rarely the development of cholesteatoma, following removal of the tube. Tos et al. (1983) demonstrated increasing frequency of tympanosclerosis in intubated ears when compared with control ears after 1 to 3 years. This type of scarring does not appear to have any effect on hearing.

Most ventilating tubes extrude spontaneously. When short-acting tubes have not extruded after 1 year or long-acting tubes have not extruded after 2 years, they usually are removed. It is necessary to consider tympanometry, physical findings, and clinical course in deciding when to remove ventilating tubes. Removal is particularly desirable in the spring to permit the tympanic membrane to heal, allowing the patient to swim during the summer.

DISEASES OF THE EXTERNAL AUDITORY CANAL

Cerumen often must be removed because it occludes the ear canal and interferes with hearing or because it obstructs the physician's view of the tympanic membrane. This usually can be accomplished with a cerumen spoon (Fig. 36–7). If the cerumen is soft and the tympanic membrane is intact, it may be removed by irrigation with water at body temperature, using a syringe or water pic. At times it is necessary to soften the cerumen with carbamide peroxide (Debrox) prior to irrigation.

Foreign bodies in the ear frequently present a difficult challenge. It is important to avoid forcing the foreign body further into the ear canal. Frequently a small right-angled instrument can be passed beyond the foreign body, rotated, and then removed, bringing the foreign body with it.

Otitis externa may represent an acute circumscribed furunculosis or a diffuse dermatitis of the external auditory canal. The most common organisms of diffuse otitis externa are *Pseudomonas spp.,* which respond well to cleaning the ear canal with suction and using acidifying drops, such as acetic acid (VoSol, 5 drops q.i.d.) or antibiotic steroid drops. The combination drops cause more rapid resolution of the problem, but since they usually contain neomycin, occasional contact sensitization results. An ear wick (Fig. 36–8) may be used to keep the

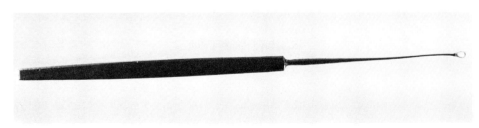

FIGURE 36–7. Shapleigh cerumen spoon. This model has fine serrations which help manipulate the cerumen, together with a narrow shaft to allow maximum visibility and manipulation.

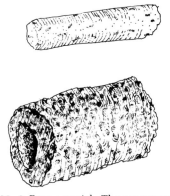

FIGURE 36–8. Pope ear wick. The compressed wick is inserted into the external auditory canal and moistened. It then expands to fill the canal holding medication against the entire circumference.

drops in contact with the skin of the ear canal. The ear wick is removed in 3 to 6 days, and the canal should be thoroughly cleaned with suction or irrigation.

Patients susceptible to otitis externa may prevent it by using rubbing alcohol (4 drops in each ear) after swimming. It is preferable that they not use ear plugs, which may cause abrasion and initiate external otitis.

DISEASES OF THE INNER EAR

Tinnitus

Objective tinnitus can be perceived by the examiner using a stethoscope over the ear. The main causes of objective tinnitus are vascular changes, vascular anomalies, or a tic of the tensor tympani muscle. Medial movement of the tympanic membrane by contraction of the tensor tympani can be observed with an otoscope.

Subjective tinnitus usually indicates damage to the hair cells of the inner ear and may be the result of head or noise trauma, infection, advanced age, toxins, or drugs (e.g., aspirin, aminoglycosides, and quinine) on the cells.

Ménière Disease

Ménière disease consists of episodes of vertigo, hearing loss, and roaring tinnitus. Occasionally, there may be a sensation of pressure in the ear. Symptoms occur abruptly, and vertigo may be intense (Schuknecht, 1981). The disease is most often diagnosed in adults but is diag-

nosed increasingly in children and occasionally in infants.

The pathogenesis of this disease is hydrops of the endolymphatic system, with progressive accumulation of endolymph and eventual rupture of the endolymphatic system. This permits entry of potassium into the perilymphatic system where it is toxic to hair cells (Bernstein et al., 1984). The basic pathology is believed by some to result from an autoimmune disease in which antibody is directed against type II collagen of the lamina propria of the endolymphatic system (Yoo et al., 1982).

Medical therapy with diuretics, low salt diet, caffeine elimination, and stress reduction is usually effective. Surgical therapy that ranges from selective destruction of the balance mechanism to total destruction of the labyrinth is occasionally necessary. While destructive surgery is effective in eliminating the episodic vertigo, it totally destroys the hearing in the involved ear. Alternatively, the selective sectioning of the vestibular nerve can eradicate the vertigo and spare the remaining hearing.

Labyrinthitis

Labyrinthitis is characterized by true vertigo, which usually comes on suddenly and lasts for hours or days. It may be associated with nausea and vomiting. The symptoms are aggravated by motion. Most often labyrinthitis is caused by a virus and is self limited. Treatment consists of maintaining hydration and electrolytes and suppressing the vertiginous symptoms. The most effective labyrinthine suppressant is diazepam (Valium).

In the presence of acute or chronic ear disease, bacteria may enter the inner ear causing a true bacterial labyrinthitis. When this occurs, hearing in the ear is lost for both air and bone conduction. Appropriate antibiotic therapy is necessary to prevent intracranial complications.

Paroxysmal Positional Vertigo

Paroxysmal positional vertigo (PPV), also known as cupulolithiasis, is characterized by the onset of vertigo whenever the head is parallel to the floor and the involved ear is down. This may occur while in bed, while painting a ceiling, while working on plumbing under a sink, and so forth. The vertigo is characterized by latency, fatigue, and rebound. PPV appears to be associated with hypertension, viral episodes, head trauma, and ear surgery. Presumably, otoliths in the inner ear become freely floating in endolymph and cause symptoms, when the affected ear is down, until they are reabsorbed. Symptoms rarely last more than 6 weeks. In persistent cases, a singular neurectomy may be necessary.

REFERENCES

Bennett, F.C., Furukawa, C.T.: Effect of conductive hearing loss on speech, language and learning development. Clin. Rev. Allergy 2:377–386, 1984.

Berman, S., Grose, K., Zerbe, G.O.: Medical management of chronic middle ear effusion: results on a clinical trial of prednisone combined with trimethoprim-sulfamethoxazole. (In press.)

Bernstein, J.M.: Immunologic reactivity in otitis media with effusion. Clin. Rev. Allergy 2:303–318, 1984.

Bernstein, J.M.: Recent advances in otitis media with effusion. Ann. Allergy 55:544–551, 1985.

Bernstein, J.M., Lee, J., Conboy, K., Ellis, E., Li, P.: Further observations on the role of IgE-mediated hypersensitivity in recurrent otitis media with effusion. Otolaryngol. Head Neck Surg. 93:611–615, 1985.

Bernstein, J.M., Schatz, M., Zeiger, R.: Immunologic ear disease in adults. Clin. Rev. Allergy 2:349–375, 1984.

Birch, L., Elbrond, O.: Daily impedance audiometric screening of children in a day-care institution. Scand. Audiol. 14:5–8, 1985.

Black, N.: Causes of glue ear. An historical review of theories and evidence. J. Laryngol. Otol. 99:953–966, 1985.

Black, N., Crowther, J., and Freeland, A.: The effectiveness of adenoidectomy in the treatment of glue ear: a randomized controlled trial. Clin Otolaryngol. 11:149–55, 1986.

Bluestone, C.D.: Diagnosis of chronic otitis media with effusion. Pediatr. Infect. Dis. 1:539–569, 1982.

Bonding, P., Tos, M.: Gormmets versus paracentesis in secretory otitis media. A prospective, controlled study. Am. J. Otolaryngol. 6:455–460, 1985.

Cantekin, E.I., Mandel, E.M., Bluestone, C.D., et al.: Lack of efficacy of a decongestant-antihistamine combination for otitis media with effusion in children. N. Engl. J. Med. 308:297, 1983.

Cotton, R.T., Bierman, C.W., Zalzal, G.H.: Serous otitis in children: medical and surgical aspects, diagnosis and management. Clin. Rev. Allergy 2:329–348, 1984.

Cotton, R.T., Zalzal, G.H.: Keeping otitis media and its sequelae at bay. J. Resp. Dis. 7:108–122, 1986.

Curley, J.: Grommet insertion: some basic questions answered. Clin Otolaryngol. 11:1–4, 1986.

Doyle, W.J., Friedman, R., Fireman, P., Bluestone, C.D.: Eustachian tube obstruction after provocative antigen challenge. Arch. Otolaryngol. 110:508, 1984.

Doyle, W.J., Ingraham, A., Fireman, P.: Histamine-induced eustachian tube obstruction in monkeys. J. Allergy Clin. Immunol. (In press.)

Fireman, P.: Eustachian tube obstruction and allergy: A role in otitis media with effusion? J. Allergy Clin. Immunol. 76:137–140, 1985.

Fireman, P., Ackerman, M., Friedman, R., Doyle, W.J., Bluestone, C.: Effect of drugs on provocative antigen-induced eustachian tube obstruction (ETO). J. Allergy Clin. Immunol. 71:155, 1983.

Friedman, R.A., Doyle, W.J., Casselbrant, M.L., Bluestone, C.D., Fireman, P.: Immunologic-mediated eustachian tube obstruction: a double-blind crossover study. J. Allergy Clin. Immunol. 71:442, 1983.

Gates, G., Wachtendorf, C., Holt, G., Hearne, E.: Medical treatment of chronic otitis media with effusion. Otolaryngol. Head Neck Surg. 94:350–354, 1986.

Gebhart, D.: Tympanostomy tubes in the otitis media prone child. Laryngoscope 91:849–866, 1981.

Giebink, G.S., Berzins, I.K., Quie, P.G.: Animal models for studying pneumococcal otitis media and pneumococcal vaccine efficacy. Ann. Otol. Rhinol. Laryngol. 89:339–343, 1980.

Giebink, G.S., Le, C.T., Batalden, P.B., et al.: Antimicrobial and anti-inflammatory treatment of chronic otitis media with effusion. Pediatr. Res. 20:310, 1986.

Gonzalez, C., Arnold, J.E., Erhardt, J.B., Woody, E.A., Pratt, S.R., Getts, A., Kueser, T.J., Kolmer, J.W., Sachs, M., Wood, F.L.: Prevention of recurrent acute otitis media: chemoprophylaxis versus tympanotomy tubes. Laryngoscope 96:1330–1334, 1986.

Haugeto, O.K., Schroder, K.E., Mair, I.W.S.: Secretory otitis media, oral decongestant and antihistamine. J. Otolaryngol. 10:359–362, 1981.

Healy, G.B.: Antimicrobial therapy for chronic otitis media with effusion. In Lim, D.G. (ed.), Recent Advances in Otitis Media with Effusion. Philadelphia, B.C. Decker, Inc., 1984.

Heisse, J.W.: Secretory otitis media: Treatment wih depomethylprednisolone. Laryngoscope 73:54–59, 1963.

Holm, V.A., Kunze, L.H.: Effect of chronic otitis media on language and speech development. Pediatrics 43:833, 1969.

Jacobs, R.L., Freedman, P.M., Boswell, R.N.: Non-allergic rhinitis with eosinophilia (Nares syndrome). J. Allergy Clin. Immunol. 67:253–262, 1981.

Klein, J.O.: Microbiology of otitis media. Ann. Otol. Rhinol. Laryngol. 89:98–101, 1980.

Kraemer, M.J., Marshall, S.G., Richardson, M.A.: Etiologic factors in the development of chronic middle ear effusions. Clin. Rev. Allergy 2:319–328, 1984.

Lim, D.J., DeMaria, T.F.: Pathogenesis of otitis media. Bacteriology and immunology. (Panel discussion:) Laryngoscope 92:278–286, 1982.

Liu, Y.S., Lim, D.J., Lang, R., Birck, H.G.: Microorganisms in chronic otitis media with effusion. Ann. Otol. Rhinol. Laryngol. 85:245, 1976.

Macknin, M.L., Jones, P.K.: Oral dexamethasone for treatment of persistent middle ear effusion. Pediatrics 75:329–335, 1985.

Marks, M.J., Mills, R.P., Shakien, O.H.: A controlled trial of co-trimoxazole therapy in serous otitis media. J. Laryngol. Otolaryngol. 95:1003–1009, 1981.

Marshall, S.G., Bierman, C.W., Shapiro, G.G.: Otitis media with effusion in childhood. Ann. Allergy 53:370–378, 1984.

Maw, A. and Herod, F. Otoscopic, impedance, and audiometric findings in glue ear treated by adenoidectomy and tonsillectomy, a prospective randomized study. Lancet 21:1399–1402, 1986.

Maw, A.R., Speller, D.G.: Are the tonsils and adenoids a reservoir of infection in otitis media with effusion (glue ear)? Clin. Otolaryngol. 10:265–269, 1985.

Milner, R.M., Weller, C.R., Brenman, A.K.: Management of the hearing impaired child with serous otitis media. Int. J. Pediatr. Otorhinolaryngol. 9:233–239, 1985.

Paparella, M.M., Hiraide, F., Juhn, S.K., Kaneko, Y.: Cellular events involved in middle ear fluid production. Ann. Otol. 79:766, 1970.

Parker, M.J., Leopold, D.A., Stitzel, A.E., Welch, T.R., Weiner, L.B., Spitzer, R.E.: Components of the alternative pathway of complement in otitis media with effusion. Otolaryngol. Head Neck Surg. 93:607–611, 1985.

Persico, M., Podoshin, L., Fradis, M.: Otitis media with effusion: A steroid and antibiotic therapeutic trial before surgery. Ann. Otol. Rhinol. Laryngol. 87:191–196, 1978.

Pierson, W.E., Kraemer, M.J., Perkins, G.J., Bierman, C.W.: Antihistamine and decongestant therapy for eustachian tube dysfunction in allergic children. J. Allergy Clin. Immunol. 69:143, 1982.

Rachelefsky, G.S., Katz, R.M., Siegel, S.C.: Chronic sinusitis in 754 children with respiratory allergy: The role of antimicrobials. J. Allergy Clin. Immunol. 69:382–387, 1982.

Rees, T.S., Bierman, C.W., Shapiro, G.G., Furukawa, C.T., Pierson, W.E.: Double-blind evaluation of nasal flunisolide for modifying eustachian tube dysfunction in allergic children. J. Allergy Clin. Immunol. 69:149, 1982.

Roberts, J.E., Sanyal, M.A., Burchinal, M.R., Collier, A.M., Ramey, C.T., Henderson, F.W.: Otitis media in early childhood and its relationship to later verbal and academic performance. Pediatrics 78:423–430, 1986.

Roydhouse, N.: Adenoidectomy for otitis media with mucoid effusion. Ann. Otol. Rhinol. Laryngol. 89:312–315, 1980.

Schuknecht, H.: The pathophysiology of Ménière's disease, pathogenesis, diagnosis and treatment. In Vosteen, K.H. (ed.), Ménière's Disease. New York, Thieme-Stratton, 1981.

Schwartz, R.H., Puglese, J., Schwartz, D.M.: Use of a short course of prednisone for treating middle ear effusion. A double-blind crossover study. Ann. Otol. Rhinol. Laryngol. 89:296–300, 1980.

Settipane, G.A., Chafee, F.H.: Nasal polyps in asthma and rhinitis. J. Allergy Clin. Immunol. 59:17–23, 1977.

Shapiro, G.G., Bierman, C.W., Furukawa, C.T., Pierson, W.E., Berman, R., Donaldson, J., Rees, T.: Treatment of persistent eustachian tube dysfunction in children with aerosolized nasal dexamethasone phosphate versus placebo. Ann. Allergy 49:81, 1982.

Shea, J.J.: Autoinflation treatment of serous otitis media in children. J. Laryngol. 85:1254–1258, 1971.

Skonker, D., Chamovitz, A., Doyle, W.J., Bluestone, C., Fireman, P.: Eustachian tube obstruction (ETO). J. Allergy Clin. Immunol. 71:155, 1983.

Sly, R.M., Zambie, M.F., Fernandes, D.A., Frazer, M.: Tympanometry in kindergarten children. Ann. Allergy 44:1–7, 1980.

Teele, D.W., Klein, J.O., Rosner, B.A.: The greater Boston otitis media study group: Middle ear disease and the practice of pediatrics. J.A.M.A. 249:1026, 1983.

Teele, D.W., Klein, J.O., Rosner, B.A.: Epidemiology of otitis media in children. Ann. Otol. Rhinol. Laryngol. 89:5, 1980.

Tos, M.: Pathology of acute otitis media and chronic secretory otitis media. Clin. Rev. Allergy 2:285–302, 1984.

Tos, M., Bonding, P., Poulsen, G.: Tympanosclerosis of the drum in secretory otitis after insertion of grommets. J. Laryngol. Otol. 97:489–496, 1983.

Tos, M., Poulsen, G., Hanike, A.B.: Screening tympanometry during the first year of life. Acta Otolaryngol. (Stockh.) 88:388–394, 1979.

Wacker, D.F., Howe, M.L.: Middle ear cilia activity as a determinant of typanotomy tube replacement. Otolaryngol. Head Neck Surg. 95:434–437, 1986.

Wald, E.R., Milmoe, G.J., Bowen, A.D., Ledesma-Medina, J., Salamon, N., Bluestone, C.E.: Acute maxillary sinusitis in children. N. Engl. J. Med. 304:749–754, 1981.

Walker, S.B., Shapiro, G.G., Bierman, C.W., Morgan, M.S., Marshall, S.G., Furukawa, C.T., Pierson, W.E.: Induction of eustachian tube dysfunction with histamine nasal provocation. J. Allergy Clin. Immunol. 76:158–162, 1985.

Woodhead, J.C., Milavetz, G., Dusdieker, L.B., et al.: Prednisone treatment of otitis media with effusion. Am. J. Dis. Child. 140:318, 1986.

Yoo, T.J., Stuart, J.M., Kang, A.H., et al.: Type II collagen autoimmunity in otosclerosis and Ménière's disease. Science 217:1153–1155, 1982.

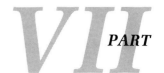

MANAGEMENT OF LOWER RESPIRATORY TRACT DISEASES

37

Principles of Diagnosis and Treatment of Lower Respiratory Tract Disease

F. ESTELLE R. SIMONS, M.D.
VICTOR CHERNICK, M.D.

DEVELOPMENT OF THE RESPIRATORY TRACT

Laryngeal structures, including the epiglottis, develop as an outgrowth from the floor of the pharynx, with contributions from the fourth and sixth branchial arches. They are well defined by the twelfth week of gestation. The position of the larynx changes with increasing age, with the position in the adult being approximately two vertebral bodies lower than in the infant.

Before birth, the lung passes through the four following stages of development, with gradual transition between stages: (1) an embryonic phase from 0–5 weeks, culminating in the presence of lobar buds; (2) a pseudoglandular stage from 5–16 weeks, during which the buds divide by irregular dichotomous branching until all the conducting airways in the tracheobronchial tree are formed; (3) a canalicular phase from 16–24 weeks characterized by proliferation of mesenchyme, development of blood supply, and thinning of the epithelium; and (4) a terminal sac phase from 24 weeks onwards, during which terminal bronchioles give rise to nonalveolar respiratory bronchioles that termi-

nate in pairs of delicate clusters of thin-walled saccules (Inselman and Mellins, 1981). At birth, only rudimentary alveoli are present. In the early months of postnatal life, peripheral bronchioles enlarge and alveoli appear in a centripetal direction. Alveolar multiplication is rapid in the first year of life and probably continues until at least 8 years. The size of the alveoli continues to increase until adulthood. Alveolar surface area doubles by age 18 months and trebles by age 3 years, so it is evident that there is a smaller reserve for gas exchange in the very young child. In the mature adult lung, the number of alveoli varies from 200 million to 600 million.

Conducting airways increase in size, but not in number, from the sixteenth or seventeenth week of gestation to adulthood. Postnatal lung growth involves the terminal respiratory unit to a greater extent than the bronchial tree.

In infants and young children, there are fewer and smaller interalveolar communications (pores of Kohn), fewer communications from bronchi to alveoli (Lambert canals), and fewer openings between alveolar ducts of different acini (portions of the lung supplied by the terminal bronchioles). Mechanical obstruction from edema, mucus, and cellular infiltrates has a greater adverse effect in the infant and young child because of disproportionately narrow peripheral airways, increased peripheral resistance to airflow, and poorly developed collateral ventilation.

The relative amount of smooth muscle in the wall of peripheral airways increases throughout childhood. There also is a decrease in the proportion of mucous glands from birth through adulthood.

As the anatomy and the mechanical properties of the lung change progressively through infancy and childhood, the manifestations of nonprogressive pulmonary diseases also change, generally becoming milder with increasing age. On the other hand, there is growing evidence that acute respiratory illness in childhood may be an important antecedent risk factor for chronic respiratory disease in later years (Strope and Stempel, 1984).

ANATOMY OF THE RESPIRATORY TRACT

Gross Anatomy. The larynx consists of four major cartilages (the cricoid ring, the thyroid cartilage, and the arytenoids) and various accessory cartilages (the epiglottic cartilage at the base of the tongue and the paired cuneiform and corniculate cartilages), all united by various ligaments, membranes, and muscles. The larynx safeguards the lower airway from aspiration of foreign substances and also is important in phonation, coughing, respiration, and deglutition. The epiglottis deflects food boluses from the airway and shields the false vocal cords.

The structural rigidity of the conducting airways is maintained by cartilaginous plates, which contribute to airway patency, especially during expiration. In the trachea and main bronchi, these plates are horseshoe shaped; in the lobar and segmental bronchi, they are arranged in a jigsaw pattern; and distally they are replaced entirely by bronchial smooth muscle.

Gross anatomic relationships of lung lobes and segments are relatively constant from patient to patient. (Fig. 37–1). The proportion of total lung weight represented by each lobe changes little with age. During physical examination of the chest, the physician should be aware of the surface anatomy of the lobes and segments in order to accurately localize pulmonary pathology (Waring, 1983).

The entire right ventricular output enters the lung via the pulmonary arteries, and the blood reaches the gas exchange unit via one of the pulmonary arterial branches. The bronchial arteries supply oxygenated systemic blood to the bronchi, bronchioles, blood vessels, nerves, lymphatic system, and visceral pleura. The lung contains an extensive interconnecting network of lymphatic vessels.

The principal muscle of respiration is the diaphragm, although intercostal, abdominal, scalene, and sternocleidomastoid muscles may also be considered to be respiratory muscles. The ratio of high oxidative, fatigue resistant muscle fibers to fatigable fibers varies with age; infants have a higher proportion of fatigable fibers.

Microscopic Anatomy. In the epithelium of the pulmonary airways, ciliated columnar cells and goblet cells predominate. The ciliated cells line the respiratory tract from the middle nares to the region of the bronchioles, apart from squamous epithelium in the pharynx and larynx. Ciliated cells have broad luminal surfaces covered with microvilli and about 250 to 300 cilia per cell. Most of the cilium shaft is bathed in a watery high-shear fluid, but the tip of the cilium penetrates the mucous layer, which is a

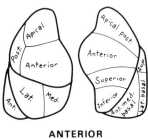

ANTERIOR

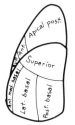

POSTERIOR

FIGURE 37–1. Pulmonary lobes and segments.

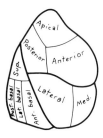

RIGHT LATERAL

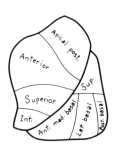

LEFT LATERAL

low-shear gel. By coordinated rhythmic movement, mucus is propelled by the cilia towards the oropharynx. Goblet cells lack cilia and may be tall and slender when not secreting glycoproteins (mucus).

Respiratory tract epithelium also contains endocrine-like cells, possibly of more than one type. Some endocrine cells resembling the intestinal Kulchitsky or K cells are found more frequently in subsegmental bronchi and are more readily identified in the lungs of fetuses and neonates than in adults. Some endocrine cells occur in groups called neuroepithelial bodies, located chiefly at or near bifurcation points of the intrapulmonary airways. Functions attributed to the endocrine-like cells, mediated via the vasoactive amines and peptides contained in the cell granules, include regulation of bronchial smooth muscle tone and control of pulmonary circulation, via the vasoactive amines and peptides contained in the cell granules.

Nonciliated cells (Clara cells), found in the epithelium of the terminal bronchioles, contribute to the watery, periciliary fluid and to the hypophase, i.e., the thick basal layer underlying the molecular film surface – active material in the alveoli. Also, Clara cells are metabolically active and act as progenitor cells for the bronchiolar epithelium.

Underlying the epithelium is a basement membrane that appears as a well defined homogenous hyaline structure by light microscopy but consists of electron-dense bands and interwoven fibrillar structures and translucent zones when viewed by electron microscopy. The submucosa is composed of loose connective tissue rich in capillaries and lymphatics. The lamina propria contains bronchial mucosal glands, compound tuboacinar structures connected to the lumen by a short excreting duct. Mast cells, located in the lamina propria, in the alveolar walls, around small blood vessels, and in the pleura, are target cells in immediate hypersensitivity reactions and are filled with metachromatic electron-dense granules that contain heparin and various vasoactive amines and enzymes.

Smooth muscle is present as a spiraling network throughout the tracheobronchial tree, including alveolar walls where interstitial cells contain contractile elements.

Alveoli are lined by a continuous layer of epithelial cells. Type I epithelial cells have long thin cytoplasmic extensions and few cytoplasmic organelles. They are incapable of mitotic division, have no known metabolic activity, and are vulnerable to the toxic effects of high oxygen concentrations and inhaled irritants. Regeneration of this cell type occurs by division of type II cells and subsequent transformation to type I cells. Type II pneumocytes have abundant endoplasmic reticulum, cytoplasm rich in mitochondria, and lamellar bodies, in which surfactant, the alveolar stabilizing substance that reduces surface tension, is stored. Type II cells proliferate if the alveoli are injured. Blood gas exchange is assumed to take place in the thinnest part of the alveolar unit, where the barrier consists of a type I pneumocyte, endothelial cell, and basement membranes (Gail and Lenfant, 1983).

BASIC CONCEPTS IN PULMONARY PHYSIOLOGY

General Considerations. Classically, human tracheobronchial smooth muscle is said to be controlled directly by the parasympathetic and the sympathetic nervous systems. Stimulation of parasympathetic fibers releases acetylcholine and causes constriction, whereas stimulation of sympathetic fibers results in relaxation, either by direct action on beta adrenergic receptors of smooth muscle or by indirect action through alpha adrenergic receptors of the ganglia, which decrease acetylcholine output. Receptors are those components of responsive target cells with which hormones and drugs interact.

A purinergic or peptidergic system has been identified as part of the autonomic system, in addition to the parasympathetic and sympathetic systems. This third nervous system is the predominant inhibitory nervous pathway to airways smooth muscle. Vasoactive intestinal peptide (VIP) is a transmitter in this system (Barnes, 1984).

Although the principal function of the lung is gas exchange, that is, adding oxygen and removing carbon dioxide from the blood, the lung also synthesizes and selectively metabolizes a variety of chemicals and functions as an endocrine organ by regulating concentrations of vasoactive substances, such as bradykinin, serotonin, and angiotensin I. Vasoactive hormones that pass through the lung without change in activity include epinephrine, prostaglandins A_1 and A_2, prostacyclin (PGI_2), bradykinin-like peptins, angiotensin II, vasopressin or antidiuretic hormone (ADH), and vasointestinal peptide (VIP).

Pulmonary defense mechanisms include mechanical barriers, physical clearance of foreign particles, and detoxification within the lung. Foreign particles, including infectious agents, greater than 10 μ in diameter are cleared by mucociliary or aerodynamic transport. Particles of about 1 μ in diameter may reach the respiratory unit and are phagocytosed by alveolar macrophages whose lysosomal membranes fuse around the particles, which are then digested by hydrolytic enzymes. In addition, an abundant lymphatic network, located in the peribronchial and perivascular connective tissue sheets and in the bronchial walls and underlying the pulmonary pleura, forms a plexiform network with valves that direct the flow of lymph centripetally. Lymphoid aggregates are located along the bronchi, especially at sites of branching. Immune mechanisms, including blood-borne immunoglobulins; cell-mediated immunity; and, especially, locally secreted IgA make important contributions to the defense of the lung.

Pulmonary Mechanics. (O'Brodovich and Chernick, 1983). An understanding of static lung volumes is important in assessing the influence of disease on the mechanical properties of the lung and chest wall and in evaluating the effects of therapy.

The lung volume at which the outward recoil of the chest wall is equal to the inward recoil of the lung is called the *functional residual capacity* (FRC) and is the sum of the *residual volume* (RV) and *expiratory reserve volume* (ERV). FRC or resting lung capacity (a capacity is the sum of two or more lung volumes) is determined by the compliance of the lung and chest wall. It is reduced when lung compliance decreases or chest wall compliance increases and is increased when lung compliance increases or chest wall compliance decreases. FRC is increased with partial lower airway obstruction; this leads to an increase in diameter of intrathoracic airways, which aids in relieving the obstruction and decreasing the work of breathing. (See Chapter 38 for discussion of measurements of pulmonary functions.)

Airway Resistance. The pressure required to generate a given flow of gas through a tube is directly proportional to the length of the tube and the viscosity of the gas and is indirectly proportional to the radius of the tube raised to the fourth power ($1/r^4$). The resistance (R) to airflow is calculated as the ratio of driving pressure to airflow as follows:

$$R = \frac{\text{driving pressure (cm } H_2O)}{\text{flow (L/sec)}}$$

The driving pressure for airflow in the lower respiratory tract is the difference in pressure between the alveoli and the mouth. The measurement of alveolar pressure requires special techniques, such as body plethysmography. In practice, therefore, an estimate of airway resistance is obtained by measuring the *peak expiratory flow rate* (PEFR) or the amount of air exhaled during the first second of the forced vital capacity maneuver (FEV_1). Since these tests depend on the subject's effort in performing the test, interpretation of the results may be difficult in young children.

In young children, the small airways account for about 50 percent of the airway resistance, and any change in small airways resistance, such as that which occurs in bronchiolitis or asthma, seriously affects them. In children above the age of about 5 years and in adults, 80 percent of the airway resistance lies in airways larger than 2 mm in diameter. In older children and adults, considerable increase in small airways resistance may occur in the absence of symptoms, and the usual pulmonary function tests (PEFR, FEV_1) done in the physician's office, which indirectly reflect airways resistance, may be normal. Several approaches to measuring the contribution of small airways to airway resistance have recently been introduced.

Expiratory flow rates are greatly influenced by lung volume. At high lung volume, there is a "tethering" effect of the lung that tends to keep airways widely patent; this tethering effect diminishes or disappears at low lung volumes. Thus, flow is measured continuously during the vital capacity maneuver and related to the volume of air expired, the so-called flow-volume curve. For example, the flow at 75 percent, 50 percent, and 25 percent of the vital capacity may be reported. In small airway disease, the flow may be markedly diminished at 25 percent of the vital capacity.

Airway resistance depends to a very great extent on airway diameter. Forces that tend to narrow airways include smooth muscle contraction and an increase in peribronchial (pleural) pressure. Forces that tend to open airways are increased intraluminal pressure and the tethering action of the surrounding lung, particularly at high lung volumes. Airway closure tends to occur at low lung volumes even in the healthy individual. The lung volume at which airway closure occurs may be determined by measuring the washout of nitrogen from the lung following the inspiration of 100 percent oxygen from RV. Those airways that are open at RV receive less oxygen than those that are closed and, therefore, have higher nitrogen concentrations. During expiration, nitrogen concentration rises sharply at the point of airway closure. The volume at which this occurs is called the *closing volume*; the closing volume plus residual volume is called the *closing capacity*. Closing volume is high in young children and may exceed FRC in children under the age of 6 years. The closing volume decreases to a nadir during the late teenage years and then gradually increases with age. Above the age of about 50 years, closing volume is again above FRC.

Gas Exchange

Carbon Dioxide. The primary function of the lung is to excrete carbon dioxide and to oxygenate the pulmonary capillary blood. Carbon dioxide, produced in the tissues as a result of aerobic metabolism, is transported to the lung by the blood. Two thirds of the CO_2 in blood is in the plasma, chiefly as bicarbonate; one third is in the red cell as bicarbonate and hemoglobin carbonate. When pulmonary capillary blood is exposed to fresh alveolar air containing little CO_2, CO_2 diffuses from the blood into the alveolar air and is eliminated during expiration. In the red blood cell, carbonic anhydrase rapidly converts blood bicarbonate to CO_2 and H_2O, facilitating rapid equilibration with alveolar gas.

The concept of alveolar ventilation ($\dot{V}_A$), therefore, is an important one. The term refers to that proportion of minute ventilation that is involved with gas exchange in the lung, principally CO_2. The relationship between $\dot{V}_A$ and carbon dioxide production ($\dot{V}_{CO_2}$) and alveolar P_{CO_2} (equivalent to arterial P_{CO_2} [$Paco_2$]) is described as follows:

$$\dot{V}_{CO_2} = \dot{V}_A (Paco_2) \times k$$

$$\text{or } Paco_2 \, \alpha \, \frac{1}{V_A}$$

Thus, for a steady rate of CO_2 production, when alveolar ventilation doubles, $Paco_2$ must halve, and when $\dot{V}_A$ halves, $Paco_2$ must double. The measurement of $Paco_2$ thus is an indication of the adequacy of alveolar ventilation for a given CO_2 production.

In the blood, CO_2 is in equilibrium with bi-carbonate, and their relationship (Henderson-Hasselbach equation) is as follows:

$$pH = \log pK + \log \frac{HCO_3^-}{\alpha \, P_{CO_2}}$$

where α is the solubility coefficient for CO_2.

A clinically useful form of this equation is as follows:

$$H^+ \text{ concentration (nanomoles/1)} =$$
$$24 \times \frac{Paco_2}{HCO_3^-}$$

When HCO_3^- concentration is normal (24 mEq/L), a $Paco_2$ of 40 is equivalent to a H^+ concentration of 40 nm/l (pH = 7.40). H^+ concentration at pH of 7.00, 7.10, 7.20, 7.30, and 7.50 are 100, 80, 62.5, 50, and 32 nm/L, respectively.

The lung excretes about 300 mEq/kg per day of acid in the form of CO_2, while the kidney excretes 1 to 2 mEq/day.

Oxygen. CO_2 in the lung diffuses nearly 21 times faster than oxygen. The transfer of oxygen from alveoli to the red blood cell in the capillary is dependent on the driving pressure (alveolar PO_2 minus capillary PO_2) and the resistance of the alveolar tissue and red blood cell barriers. About half of the resistance to diffusion exists in the alveolar membrane, the other half in the red blood cell.

Clinically, a reduced arterial PO_2 rarely is the result of a diffusion barrier to oxygen. The most common cause of hypoxemia in a patient with lower respiratory tract disease is ventilation-perfusion inequality, which may be treated by increasing inspired oxygen concentration (Fio_2). Another cause is hypoventilation ($Paco_2$), which also may require an increase in alveolar ventilation, often by mechanical means, as well as an increase in Fio_2. In patients with extrapulmonary right to left shunting, neither method of therapy is successful in raising Pao_2 significantly.

When the patient breathes room air at sea level, the sum of alveolar PO_2 ($P_{A_{O_2}}$) and PCO_2 cannot exceed 150 mm Hg, since the rest of the total pressure is occupied by nitrogen and water vapor. Normally, $Paco_2$ is about 40 mm Hg, and $P_{A_{O_2}}$ is about 110 mm Hg. The alveolar PO_2 can be approximated by the following equation:

$$P_{A_{O_2}} = \text{inspiratory } PO_2 - (Paco_2 \times R^{-1}).$$

For example, if inspiratory PO_2 is 150 mm Hg and $Paco_2$ is 40 mm Hg, then $P_{A_{O_2}}$ is 110 mm Hg. This equation assumes a respiratory quotient of 1. The ratio of a/APO_2 should normally exceed 0.8, regardless of F_{IO_2}. This calculation is useful in following the progress of patients who require oxygen therapy and is the only way one can detect changes in the ability to oxygenate the blood in the presence of a changing $Paco_2$ or F_{IO_2}.

In contrast to CO_2, over 98 percent of the oxygen in the blood is carried in the red blood cell as oxyhemoglobin, the rest being dissolved oxygen. The relationship between Po_2 and hemoglobin oxygen saturation is curvilinear (oxyhemoglobin dissociation curve) and affected by blood pH, temperature, 2,3-diphosphoglycerate (2,3-DPG), and the type of hemoglobin present. 2,3-DPG binds to hemoglobin and reduces its affinity for oxygen, thus shifting the curve to the right, as does an increase in temperature or a reduction in pH.

Ventilation/Perfusion $(\dot{V}/\dot{Q})$ *Relationships.* The fact that mismatched $\dot{V}/\dot{Q}$ in the lung is a common cause of hypoxemia has been mentioned. Normally, the ratio $\dot{V}/\dot{Q}$ is about 0.8. If ventilation is disproportionately low in relation to blood flow in an area of the lung, then $Paco_2$ will be disproportionately high, and Pao_2, low. The blood leaving this area of lung will have a low Pao_2 and will mix with blood from relatively normal areas of the lung. This so-called venous admixture may be corrected by letting the patient breathe high oxygen concentrations. Thus, if hypoxemia is present when the patient is breathing room air, Pao_2 will rise to 500 mm Hg or higher when 100 percent oxygen is given, if hypoxemia is a result of mismatched $\dot{V}/\dot{Q}$. If the hypoxemia is caused by true right to left shunting of blood, such as with transposition of the great vessels, 100 percent oxygen will not reverse hypoxemia.

When there are low $\dot{V}/\dot{Q}$ areas, an increase in alveolar ventilation to the other areas of the lung will easily compensate for low CO_2 excretion in the affected area but will not result in additional oxygen uptake by the red cells, which already are virtually 100 percent saturated. $\dot{V}/\dot{Q}$ abnormality is commonly found in patients with pulmonary disease and usually requires only an inspired oxygen concentration of 25 to 30 percent to provide an arterial Pao_2 of 50 mm Hg or greater, which is adequate for tissue oxygenation. Higher concentrations of oxygen are not necessary and are known to be toxic to the lung with prolonged use.

DIAGNOSTIC PRINCIPLES

History. Common symptoms of respiratory disease are shortness of breath, cough, abnormal breath sounds, such as wheezing and stridor, sputum production, hemoptysis, chest pain, respiratory distress, and labored breathing. In infants and toddlers, nonspecific symptoms, such as refusal to suckle or eat, fussiness, and rapid breathing may herald significant respiratory tract disease. In patients of any age, it is important to establish whether symptoms are acute, recurrent, or chronic; the rate of progression of symptoms; and the effect of prior treatment on symptoms.

In order to elucidate the etiology of a patient's respiratory disease, the physician may find it useful to take a detailed history of the patient's environment. Does the patient smoke? If the patient is a child, do the parents smoke? Does the patient live in an area where air pollution is a problem? Is the patient exposed regularly to birds or other animals? Is the patient exposed to potential irritants or allergens while at work or while engaged in hobbies?

If cough is present, it is helpful to know its characteristics. Is it *paroxysmal* (a series of explosive expirations following a single inspiration), indicative of a foreign body or pertussis; *productive,* indicative of pneumonia, bronchiectasis, or cystic fibrosis; *associated with wheezing,* indicative of tracheobronchial obstruction; *barking,* indicative of involvement of glottic and subglottic areas, as in croup; *associated with aphonia or dysphonia,* indicative of laryngeal foreign body or other involvement of the larynx? Does the cough occur chiefly at night or with exercise, suggesting asthma? If asthma is mild, the cough may not be accompanied by wheezing or shortness of breath. Cough at night also may suggest congestive heart failure; cough related to food ingestion suggests tracheoesophageal fistula, or esophageal reflux; and cough associated with change in position suggests lung abscess or localized bronchiectasis. In a smoker, change in the nature of chronic cough requires prompt investigation.

Infants and young children usually do not expectorate sputum but swallow it instead; hence, it may be found in vomitus and stools. Mucus plugs may be coughed up in asthma and aspergillosis.

Hemoptysis may result from a lesion in the oropharynx; foreign body injury of the respiratory mucosa; inflammation and erosion of the respiratory mucosa, as in cystic fibrosis, tuberculosis or lung abscess; or bronchial adenoma. Gross hemoptysis is unusual in young patients. In older patients, bronchogenic carcinoma or other serious disorders such as pulmonary thromboembolism or left ventricular failure, must be considered as potential causes of hemoptysis.

Chest pain is not a common complaint in young patients. It may be associated with prolonged or frequent coughing. It also may occur in diseases of the chest wall such as costochondritis; in rib fractures; with inflammation of the diaphragmatic pleura, such as pneumonia; in disorders of the esophagus, such as ulceration or the presence of a foreign body; or in pericarditis. Severe chest pain also may be produced by myositis or intercostal neuralgia. In an adult, chest pain is more likely to suggest myocardial disease, pulmonary thromboembolism, or serious inflammatory or neoplastic disorders.

Respiratory distress associated with hoarseness suggests laryngeal involvement and distress associated with drooling and muffling of the voice suggests involvement of the epiglottis.

If labored breathing is present, its suddenness of onset and rate of progression must be noted. Provoking factors should be noted, such as choking; exercise; a "cold"; or exposure to irritants, e.g. smoke and potential allergens. Associated symptoms, such as grunting, cyanosis, stridor, and wheezing, must be ascertained.

Chronic halitosis may be noted in patients with bronchiectasis, lung abscess, sinusitis, nasal foreign body, and infectious or allergic rhinitis.

Some airway problems appear, or worsen, during sleep, so the physician should always inquire into the patient's sleeping pattern (Mark and Brooks, 1984).

In young patients, the perinatal history is important, as survivors of lung disease in infancy often have continuing disability; for example, infants with bronchopulmonary dysplasia may have recurrent wheezing, frequent lower respiratory tract infections, and heart failure in the early years of life (Smyth et al., 1981).

Presence of symptoms in other systems and presence of respiratory symptoms in other family members should be ascertained.

Physical Examination. Physical signs vary with age and, in obstructive disease, depend on air entry.

Inspection. Nonspecific signs of respiratory disease include weight loss, failure to gain weight or (in a child) stature, pallor, and lethargy. Clubbing is common in bronchiectasis, cystic fibrosis, pulmonary abscess, empyema, and various chronic pneumonias and neoplasms, as well as in cardiac, hepatic, and gastrointestinal disease.

The upper airway is examined indirectly by listening to the speech or cry of the patient, by noting whether inspiratory stridor or barking cough are present, and whether hoarseness or aphonia are present. Inspiratory retractions, particularly in the supraclavicular region, often point to upper airway obstruction. The examiner should palpate the trachea and larynx for tenderness, masses, and distortion of contour. The upper airway also should be examined directly, with care taken <u>not</u> to insert a tongue blade if epiglottitis is suspected.

Cyanosis, difficult to detect reliably, is best observed in the lips, other mucous membranes, the skin, and the nailbeds. It usually is related to the absolute amount of unoxygenated hemoglobin (deoxyhemoglobin) in the capillaries. This, in turn, may be due to alveolar hypoventilation from obstruction to air flow, suppression of the respiratory center, or weakness of the respiratory muscles; uneven distribution of blood or gas through the lungs; disturbances of alveolocapillary diffusion, as in interstitial pneumonia or pulmonary fibrosis; or anatomic shunts of blood. If cyanosis is due to an anatomic shunt, the patient's color will not improve dramatically following administration of oxygen.

The resting rate of respiration varies with age, with the normal respiratory rate at 1 year averaging 30 per minute; the normal average adult rate of 14 per minute is reached at about age 14 years. Orthopnea, or inability to breathe while recumbent, is characteristic of pulmonary edema and of obstructive disorders, such as asthma. Hyperpnea (deep breathing) may occur in the absence of respiratory disease in the child with fever, severe anemia, salicylism, metabolic acidosis, or respiratory alkalosis. Hypopnea (shallow breathing) occurs with metabolic alkalosis, as in pyloric stenosis, and with respiratory acidosis.

Dyspnea in the infant or child may be evidenced by flaring of the alae nasi, head bobbing due to contraction of the accessory muscles of inspiration (including the scalene and sternocleidomastoid muscles), and grunting. In the older patient, grunting usually is associated with chest pain.

Retractions usually indicate increased inspiratory effort. They may be localized to the lower intercostal areas in infants in whom the diaphragm is the major muscle of respiration. Intercostal bulging may be a sign of great expiratory effort.

In severe obstructive disease of the lung, the anteroposterior diameter of the thorax exceeds the transverse diameter. This sign is more useful in older children and adults than in infants, who normally may have somewhat round chests.

Palpation. Tracheal palpation in the suprasternal notch can indicate whether there has been a volume or pressure change in the thoracic cavity. For example, a foreign body in the right main stem bronchus that completely occludes the bronchus and produces atelectasis of the right lung will cause the mediastinum and the trachea to shift to the right. A pneumothorax or any space-occupying lesion on the left will cause the trachea to shift to the right.

Percussion. Indirect percussion of the chest should be performed in order to localize areas of dullness (atelectasis or consolidation) or to detect hyperinflation. In infants and young children, it is preferable to leave percussion until the end of the physical examination.

Auscultation. Auscultation over each bronchopulmonary segment should be performed using a stethoscope head of appropriate size. The relative duration of expiration to inspiration, normally 2 : 1, should be noted. The quality of breath sounds should be described, as follows: *tracheal* (high-pitched tubular sounds evident throughout both phases of respiration), *vesicular* (soft, low-pitched inspiration and soundless expiration), *bronchovesicular* (soft, low-pitched expiratory note heard in the early part of expiration), and *bronchial* (tubular note throughout all of expiration). Diminished ventilation in a given segment or through the entire lung is significant, since a patient with severe airways obstruction may have little stridor or wheezing, owing to the poor air exchange.

Wheezes are continuous high- or low-pitched musical sounds produced by air moving rapidly past a fixed obstruction in the airway. They result from the vibration of the walls of compressed bronchi, and their pitch is determined by the mass and elastic properties of the walls, the tightness of the stenosis, and the rate of gas flow through it. Thus, they can be generated only in the larger airways. Crackles are discontinuous, nonmusical, and crackling or bubbling sounds produced by explosive reopening of the airway or by air bubbling through secretions (Loudon and Murphy, 1984).

In some patients, wheezes will be heard during forced expirations but not during quiet breathing. In young children who cannot perform forced expiration maneuvers, manual compression of the chest wall during the expiratory phase (a hug by the patient's parent or a nurse) will facilitate auscultation of wheezes. Infants should be auscultated when they are prone, as well as upright or supine. In the prone position, the intensity of transmitted rhonchi caused by excessive secretions in the upper respiratory tract is diminished. Infants also should be auscultated when placed on the side with the neck flexed, in order to accentuate any inspiratory stridor present.

The cardiovascular system should be examined carefully; a loud snapping second heart sound in the second and third left interspace may be evidence of pulmonary hypertension. Tachycardia, gallop rhythm, cardiomegaly, and extracardiac signs, such as elevation of the jugular venous pressure, hepatomegaly, and peripheral edema or anasarca, are evidence of congestive heart failure.

Evidence of impending *respiratory failure* includes change in level of consciousness, such as agitation, restlessness, or inability to be aroused; extreme respiratory distress and diminished or absent air entry (a "silent chest"); or cyanosis (Pagtakhan and Chernick, 1983). Patients may complain of headache or even dimness of vision. Tachycardia or hypertension or (late) hypotension may be present. If hypoxemia is chronic, polycythemia may be present. In hypercapnia, engorgement of the fundal veins, muscular twitching, depressed tendon reflexes and extensor plantar responses, papilledema, and miosis may be present.

Differential Diagnosis. Respiratory disorders are best classified according to the predominant functional abnormality, as this forms a basis for rational approach to therapy. A useful functional classification of respiratory disorders in infancy, childhood, and adulthood is presented in Table 37–1.

In the differential diagnosis of obstructive airways disease, it is important to note the effect of the phase of respiration on increasing or decreasing the obstruction. *Extrathoracic* obstruction is primarily manifest in the *inspiratory* phase, because in forced inspiration the pressure in the main airways is negative (less than atmospheric), and the normal pressure in surrounding tissues tends to compress the airway and increase the obstruction. *Intrathoracic* obstruction is generally manifest in the *expiratory* phase, because in forced expiration all intrathoracic airways decrease in diameter, owing to a reduction in the tethering force of the lung as the lung volume decreases. Airways that are between the mouth and the equal pressure point, but still in the thorax, also tend to collapse as pleural pressure exceeds intra-airway pressure, and only the structural rigidity of the airways resists the collapse.

TABLE 37-1. Functional Classification of Lower Respiratory Tract Disorders*

Disturbance	Disorder
OBSTRUCTIVE DISEASE	
UPPER RESPIRATORY TRACT	
Anomalies	Tracheal stenosis, vocal cord paralysis, vascular ring, laryngotracheomalacia
Aspiration	Foreign body,† vomitus
Infection	Laryngitis,† laryngotracheobronchitis,† epiglottitis,† peritonsillar or retropharyngeal abscess
Tumor	Papilloma, hemangioma, lymphangioma, teratoma, gross hypertrophy of tonsils and adenoids
Other	Laryngospasm from local irritation (aspiration, intubation, drowning), tetany, hereditary angioedema, anaphylaxis
LOWER RESPIRATORY TRACT	
Anomalies	Bronchomalacia, lobar emphysema, aberrant vessels
Aspiration	Tracheoesophageal fistula, foreign body,† vomitus, pharyngeal incoordination (Riley-Day syndrome), drowning
Infection/Inflammation	Pertussis,† bronchiolitis,† tuberculosis, cystic fibrosis, pneumonia, bronchiectasis, chronic bronchitis and emphysema (COPD)
Tumor	Bronchogenic cyst, teratoma, atrial myxoma, primary and secondary malignancies
Allergic or reflex	Asthma,† bronchospasm secondary to inhalation of noxious gases
RESTRICTIVE DISEASE	
PARENCHYMAL	
Anomalies	Hypoplasia, congenital cyst, pulmonary sequestration
Atelectasis	Viscous secretions (e.g., postoperative state), foreign body
Infection	Pneumonia, cystic fibrosis, bronchiectasis, pneumatocele
Alveolar rupture	Pneumothorax (spontaneous or secondary to trauma or asthma)
Others	Allergic alveolitis, pulmonary edema, lobectomy, chemical pneumonitis, pleural effusion, near drowning
CHEST WALL	
Muscular	Amytonia congenita, poliomyelitis, diaphragmatic hernia or eventration, myasthenia gravis, muscular dystrophy, botulism
Skeletal malformations	Kyphoscoliosis, hemivertebrae, absent ribs
Others	Obesity, flail chest
INEFFICIENT GAS TRANSFER	
PULMONARY DIFFUSION DEFECT	
Increased diffusion path between alveoli and capillaries	Pulmonary edema, pulmonary fibrosis, collagen disorders, *Pneumocystis carinii* infection, sarcoidosis, pneumoconiosis, lung contusion
Decreased alveolocapillary surface area	Pulmonary embolism, sarcoidosis, pulmonary hypertension (primary or secondary), mitral stenosis, fibrosing alveolitis
Inadequate erythrocytes and hemoglobin	Anemia, hemorrhage
Other	Arteriovenous malformation
RESPIRATORY CENTER DEPRESSION	
Increased cerebrospinal fluid pressure	Cerebral trauma, intracranial tumors, central nervous system infection (meningitis, encephalitis, sepsis)
Excessive central nervous system depressant drugs	Sedation, overdosage with barbiturates, opiates, benzodiazepines, or other drugs
Excessive chemical changes in arterial blood	Severe asphyxia (hypercapnia, hypoxemia) carbon monoxide poisoning
Toxic	Tetanus

*Modified from Pagtakhan, R.D. and Chernick, V.: Intensive Care for Respiratory Disorders. *In* Kendig, E.L., Jr., Chernick, V. (eds.), Disorders of the Respiratory Tract in Children, 4th ed., Philadelphia, W.B. Saunders Co., 1983.
† *Common causes* of pulmonary disease in childhood.

The differential diagnosis of many common respiratory disorders is reviewed in the following references: Berquist et al., 1981; Blaser et al., 1980; Crystal et al., 1981; Goldstein, 1985; Latimer and Sharp, 1980; Levison et al., 1982; Mark and Brooks, 1984; Petty, 1984; Turner et al., 1981; Wohl and Chernick, 1978; and Wood et al., 1976.

Diagnostic Laboratory Procedures

Radiologic Procedures. Plain posteroanterior and lateral radiographs of the chest should be examined systematically with regard to appropriateness of the views; technical variations; the chest wall (congenital or acquired defects of ribs, sternum, or spine); diaphragm (lines intact and domes in normal position); pleura (costophrenic angle, presence or absence of pneumothorax, position of fissures); mediastinum (normal position, heart size, position of aortic arch, clarity of heart borders); clarity of cervical airways, hila, and pulmonary vessels (normal position, size, and caliber); and, finally, pulmonary parenchyma (presence of abnormal densities, nodules, air bronchogram, Kerley lines, areas of hyperaeration, atelectasis, or consolidation).

Radiographs of the neck and thoracic inlet may be helpful in investigation of masses, such as cellulitis in the retropharyngeal soft tissue and tumors or foreign bodies in the cervical esophagus or the upper airway; epiglottitis; and vascular rings, such as double aortic arch and right aortic arch with aberrant right subclavian artery. Esophagrams, performed under fluoroscopic control using colloidal barium, may be helpful in evaluation of patients with airflow obstruction; gastroesophageal reflux; tracheoesophageal fistula; and mediastinal masses, causing esophageal displacement.

Bronchography is valuable in the demonstration of bronchiectasis and certain congenital abnormalities, such as bronchomalacia and vascular rings.

Computerized tomography (CT) scanning produces images in various anatomic planes and is particularly useful for a cross-sectional display of anatomy. It is the current preferred method of evaluating a mediastinal mass demonstrated on the chest radiograph and is useful in detection and evaluation of lung and pleural nodules, aortic aneurysms, and excess fluid in the pleural space. Conventional tomography is used less frequently now, having been supplanted by newer techniques.

Nuclear magnetic resonance (NMR) is a method of gaining chemical information from the magnetic properties of atomic nuclei. This information can be used to obtain cross-sectional tomographic images with proton resonance or to measure the spectrum of phosphorus nuclear resonance and provide chemical analysis of tissue energy metabolism. NMR techniques for studying vascular flow, mass lesions, diffuse lung disease, and lung water are undergoing evaluation (Cohen, 1984).

Angiography is used for investigation of anomalies of the pulmonary vasculature and for localization of sites of hemoptysis in patients in whom bronchoscopy is not feasible.

Isotope scan may be helpful if perfusion defects are suspected, and it can be useful in identifying foreign bodies in patients in whom plain films and fluoroscopic assessments are not definitive.

Nonradiologic Tests

BLOOD COUNT. The complete blood count should be checked for evidence of anemia, polycythemia, leukocytosis, esoinophilia, and lymphopenia.

PULMONARY FUNCTION TESTS. Pulmonary function tests are useful for diagnosis and follow-up (see Chapter 38). In patients under age 6 years, techniques requiring cooperation generally cannot be used, and special tests may be required (Morgan, 1986).

BLOOD GAS VALUES. Arterial puncture of the radial vessel is a safe and simple procedure at all ages, if the ulnar collateral arterial supply is assured (by compressing the radial artery and noting that the palm does not blanch). Use of the femoral artery should be avoided. Use of arterialized capillary blood for measurement of P_{CO_2} and pH is preferable to not measuring these values at all, but serious underestimation of P_{O_2} may result, particularly if the peripheral perfusion is poor or if the extremity is not vasodilated by warmth or iontophoresis, using a histamine-containing cream. Respiratory failure, suspected on the basis of clinical findings, is confirmed if Pa_{CO_2} is greater than 60 torr or is rising rapidly (>10 torr per hour) in an exhausted patient, or if Pa_{O_2} is less than 55 or 60 torr when the patient is breathing 100 percent oxygen.

MICROBIOLOGIC STUDIES. Infants and young children seldom produce sputum for Gram stain and culture. A sample of tracheal secretions may be obtained by passing a sterile catheter by mouth, but unless a single species is isolated, results may be misleading. Documentation of specific viral infections by means of cultures for viruses, fluorescent antibody studies, and paired acute and convalescent sera is useful.

Lung puncture with a 20 to 22 gauge needle is used to obtain aspirates for histologic study or culture (for example, in severe pneumonia of unknown etiology) and requires only local anesthesia. Complications include pulmonary hemorrhage, empyema, and pneumothorax.

Open lung biopsy may be required if a specific diagnosis has not been made using less invasive techniques (Waring, 1983).

LARYNGOSCOPY. Indirect laryngoscopy is difficult or impossible to perform in most infants and young children. Direct laryngoscopy, usually under general anesthesia, must be performed to identify congenital abnormalities (e.g., laryngomalacia, webs, atresias, paralysis) and tumors and cysts of the larynx. Nasopharyngolaryngoscopy, using a fiberscope, can be helpful in children and adults.

BRONCHOSCOPY. Considerable improvements have been made in rigid bronchoscopes in recent years. The flexible bronchofiberscope, now available in a wide variety of sizes, has revolutionized pulmonary medicine (Wood, 1984). Bronchoscopy permits visualization of the larger branches of the tracheobronchial tree. It is performed to identify, localize, and remove foreign bodies and in other situations when less invasive procedures have failed, e.g., when the origin of bleeding or purulent secretions must be ascertained. Anomalies and site of compression may be identified. Specimens for culture, cytologic studies, and histologic studies can be obtained. *In inexpert hands, bronchoscopy is hazardous. Timing of the procedure and premedication may be critical. In patients with hyperirritable airways (e.g., in asthma), bronchoscopy may trigger massive vagal reflex and severe bronchospasm.*

Bronchoalveolar lavage (BAL), with enumeration and identification of respiratory cells and immunochemical analysis of lung lining fluid, provides important information in interstitial lung diseases, such as sarcoidosis, hypersensitivity pneumonitis, idiopathic pulmonary fibrosis, and eosinophilic granuloma of the lungs. At present, BAL analysis is a research tool, and its precise role in clinical practice is still being defined (Crystal et al., 1981).

SWEAT CHLORIDE TEST. Quantitation of sweat chloride by the pilocarpine iontophoresis method should be performed to rule out cystic fibrosis in any patient with a history of cystic fibrosis in a sibling or first cousin (Shwachman and Mohmoodian, 1979) or in any patient with wheezing, recurrent pneumonia, or other pulmonary disease associated with gastrointestinal symptoms or failure to thrive.

OTHER LABORATORY INVESTIGATIONS. Quantitation of immunoglobulins G, A, and M is necessary in patients with recurrent pneumonia and bronchiectasis to rule out immunodeficiency. Quantitation of the IgG subtypes is helpful in selected patients. Quantitation of total IgE may be of prognostic value in patients with bronchiolitis.

Alpha-1-antitrypsin should be measured to rule out deficiency in a patient with a clinical picture suggesting emphysema (Latimer and Sharp, 1980).

Esophageal manometrics, esophagoscopy, and the acid reflux (intraluminal pH) test are helpful in documenting gastroesophageal reflux in patients with chronic pulmonary disease (Berquist et al., 1981).

THERAPEUTIC PRINCIPLES

Goals of treatment of respiratory diseases are the following: preservation of life; facilitation of normal life style, including regular school or work attendance and participation in normal physical activity; minimization of morbidity from chronic pulmonary disorders; maintenance of normal physical and psychosocial growth and development; prevention of complications, such as thoracic deformity, bronchiectasis, and cor pulmonale; and prevention of iatrogenic disease.

Severe late sequelae of acute respiratory disease in childhood have long been known. For example, bronchiolitis may be followed by asthma, bronchiectasis, or hyperlucent lung syndrome (Wohl and Chernick, 1978). Less obvious pulmonary sequelae probably occur much more frequently than recognized. For instance, croup or bronchiolitis may result in residual pulmonary abnormalities years later, even in patients who appear to be symptom free (Fig. 37–2) (Kattan et al., 1977)

General principles of treatment of respiratory disorders are summarized next.

Environment. The environment surrounding the patient with respiratory disease should be as free as possible from air-borne irritants and allergens (Strope and Stempel, 1984).

Hydration. Removal of mucus from the airways is aided by adequate fluid intake. Patients with acute respiratory disorders may develop fluid and electrolyte deficits because of hyperpnea, tachypnea, vomiting, and fever. Fluid balance must be restored, but fluids should never be "forced" by mouth because of the high risk of aspiration, particularly in the dyspneic

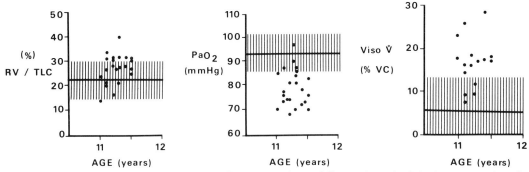

FIGURE 37–2. Evidence for residual parenchymal or airways' lesion following bronchiolitis. Asymptomatic patients with abnormal residual volume/total lung capacity ratio, PaO_2 and volume of isoflow about 11 years after uncomplicated bronchiolitis. Individual data points and mean and 2 standard deviations above and below mean are shown. (From Kattan, M., Keens, T. G., Lapierre, J.G., Levison, H., Bryan, A. C., and Reilly, B. J.: Pulmonary function abnormalities in symptom-free children after bronchiolitis. Pediatrics 591:683, 1977.)

infant or toddler. Intravenous fluid therapy should be adequate for maintenance and repair of dehydration, but *overhydration and its complication of pulmonary edema must be avoided.*

Mist treatment, delivered by ultrasonic nebulizer, jet nebulizer, or natural fog generator, may be useful for croup. In lower respiratory tract disease, such as bronchiolitis or asthma, benefits from mist treatment are not clear since particles that pass beyond the major airways tend to deposit in the least obstructed airways, and adverse effects, such as reflex bronchoconstriction, may occur from stimulation of irritant receptors.

Chest Physiotherapy. Chest physiotherapy in its simplest form consists of encouraging a patient to cough and breathe deeply. Balloons, blow bottles, and rebreathing tubes may be used. However, forced inspiration and forced expiration maneuvers may provoke further bronchospasm in a patient with irritable airways. Postural drainage, accomplished by positioning the patient so that the involved segment of lung is uppermost, is useful in removal of mucus and other foreign material from the lung. Percussion with cupped hands and vibration may be performed over the involved area. Oxygen and suction should be readily available.

These measures are more useful in bronchiectasis and cystic fibrosis (Wood, 1976) than in a nonsuppurative respiratory disorder, in which there is little evidence of benefit. The measures may be helpful in asthma only if atelectasis or excessive secretions predominate over bronchospasm. Postural drainage and suctioning are necessary in any patient who is mechanically ventilated for any reason.

Bronchoscopy. Bronchoscopy may be of fundamental importance in restoring airway patency when a foreign body has been inhaled into the tracheobronchial tree or in the rare instance when tenacious mucus plugs must be removed, as in bronchopulmonary aspergillosis. It should be used with care in patients with hyperreactive airways.

Oxygen. Oxygen deprivation leads to clouding of the sensorium, unconsciousness, cardiac arrhythmias, and decreased mental function. In patients with respiratory distress, adequate oxygenation must be ensured. Dependence on a hypoxic drive to ventilation is so rare that for practical purposes, the physician need not worry about "turning off" ventilation by increasing inspired oxygen. In any case, the patient who responds to oxygen inhalation with hypoventilation can be identified with frequent arterial blood gas determinations or continuous monitoring of oxygen and carbon dioxide tensions, using electrodes applied to the skin.

All patients in acute respiratory distress should receive oxygen that has been fully saturated with water and warmed to body temperature, initially in a concentration of 30 to 40 percent by face mask and nebulizer, with the concentration later adjusted as needed to maintain arterial oxygen tensions of 50 to 80 torr. Skin surface oxygen and carbon dioxide electrodes are convenient to use, provided appropriate correction formulae are applied (Burki and Albert, 1983). An oxygen analyzer should be used to monitor inspired oxygen concentration.

In infants and young children, administration of oxygen by head box may be necessary if a mask is not tolerated. Nasal prongs cannot be used if nasal obstruction is present. They often are poorly tolerated by children and by uncooperative patients of any age. Administration of oxygen by a mist tent is possible in concentrations up to 30 percent if the tent is opened infrequently. However, *tents interfere with observation of the patient and with nursing care and are not generally recommended.*

If a patient requires mechanical ventilation for respiratory failure over several days, attempts should be made to reduce inspired oxygen concentration by institution of positive end-expiratory pressure (PEEP) and to maintain optimal fluid and electrolyte balance, since use of concentrations of even 60 to 70 percent oxygen for 4 or 5 days may be harmful.

The biochemical basis of oxygen toxicity lies in increased production of highly reactive, partially reduced metabolites of oxygen by cells in hyperoxia. The metabolites include hydrogen peroxide and oxygen free radicals. The pathologic changes of oxygen toxicity are not specific. There may be collapsed alveoli at low lung volumes; decreased surfactant activity; intra-alveolar, interstitial, and perivascular edema; hyaline membrane formation; and destruction of type I cells. In the chronic phase, hyperplasia of type II cells, septal thickening, capillary hyperplasia, and interstitial fibroelastic proliferation occur. Symptoms of oxygen toxicity include substernal pain, paresthesias, and cerebral symptoms, resulting from vasoconstriction. There are no pathognomonic radiologic features. Physiologic manifestations include decreases in vital capacity, diffusing capacity, and lung compliance. No effective pharmacologic means exist for lessening pulmonary oxygen toxicity in humans (Jackson, 1985).

The occurrence of oxygen toxicity depends on the inspired oxygen tension and duration of treatment and does not develop in patients breathing 100 percent oxygen for 24 hours or less. Therefore, oxygen toxicity is never a consideration in transport or resuscitation procedures or in the emergency treatment of tension pneumothorax, pending insertion of a chest tube with an underwater seal.

Pharmacologic Treatment. *Bronchodilators* including beta-adrenergic agonists, methylxanthines, and inhaled anticholinergic drugs, such as ipratropium bromide, are discussed in Chapter 19. They are important in restoration and maintenance of airway patency in asthma, laryngotracheo bronchitis, and cystic fibrosis, and possibly in bronchiolitis. Mast cell–

stabilizing drugs, such as cromolyn sodium, and anti-inflammatory drugs, such as corticosteroids, are also discussed in Chapter 19.

Expectorants, such as guaifenesin (guaiacol glycerol ester), ammonium chloride, and iodide, are without demonstrable benefit. Some beta-adrenergic drugs, such as terbutaline, may increase tracheal mucous velocity, however. Cough suppressants (e.g., codeine, dextromethorphan, and noscapine) may depress spontaneous respiration and should be used with extreme caution during acute respiratory disease. The use of antihistamines in patients with asthma has been controversial, but evidence is accumulating that these agents generally do more good than harm.

Antimicrobials are of primary importance in the treatment of tonsillitis, bacterial tracheitis, epiglottitis, pertussis, bacterial and mycoplasmal pneumonias, mycoses, psittacoses, bronchiectasis, cystic fibrosis, pulmonary abscess, and tuberculosis, in which a susceptible organism is involved. There is no justification for "prophylactic antibiotics" in respiratory diseases, particularly for children who have normal immune systems (see Chapter 23 for discussion of antimicrobial therapy).

Sedatives and tranquilizers are contraindicated with rare exceptions in the conscious, spontaneously breathing patient with acute respiratory disease, no matter how anxious or irritable the patient appears. *The anxiety associated with dyspnea and labored breathing is almost always due to hypoxia and is treated by ensuring that the airways are patent and by administering supplemental oxygen.* Sedatives are necessary in patients who are mechanically ventilated for respiratory failure.

Alkali Therapy. Respiratory acidosis is treated by establishing adequate ventilation in the patient. For correction of metabolic acidosis (pH < 7.3; base deficit > 5 mEq/L), sodium bicarbonate (7.5 percent solution) is the drug of choice. It is given in a dose of 2 to 5 mEq/kg (maximum 45 mEq) and may be repeated every 10 or 15 minutes.

Intermittent Positive Pressure Breathing (IPPB). IPPB is contraindicated in spontaneously breathing patients who have normal muscles of respiration and can take deep breaths. IPPB does not enhance peripheral deposition of aerosols in the lungs and tends to deliver medication to the least obstructed areas. It also may increase airway resistance and in diseases such as asthma may induce or aggravate pneumomediastinum or pneumothorax. In laryngotracheobronchitis, delivery of epinephrine by IPPB has been superceded by the use of face masks (Levison et al., 1982).

Surgical Therapy. Management of a tension pneumothorax requires aspiration of air and placement of a chest tube in the second intercostal space in the midclavicular line; the tube is connected to an underwater seal. Suction will be required if the leak is large. Accumulation of liquid in the pleural space also necessitates tube drainage, but in this instance, the tube is placed in the dependent part of the pleural space. Thoracotomy is required for evacuation of purulent thick pleural fluid and for control of massive pulmonary hemorrhage or persistent air leak.

In summary, the young patient with respiratory symptoms requires a unique diagnostic and therapeutic approach, based on understanding of the influence of normal growth and development of anatomy and physiology of the respiratory tract. In patients of any age, the risks versus the benefits of any diagnostic or therapeutic procedure should be carefully weighed.

REFERENCES

Barnes, P.J.: The third nervous system in the lung: physiology and clinical perspectives. Thorax 39:561–567, 1984.

Berquist, W.E., Rachelefsky, G.S., Kadden, M., Siegel, S.C., Katz, R.M., Fonkalsrud, E.W., Ament, M.E.: Gastroesophageal reflux–associated recurrent pneumonia and chronic asthma in children. Pediatrics 68:29–35, 1981.

Blaser, S., Naveh, Y., Friedman, A.: Foreign body in the airway: A review of 200 cases. Am. J. Dis. Child. 134: 68–71, 1980.

Burki, N.K., Albert, R.K.: Noninvasive monitoring of arterial blood gases—a report of the ACCP section on respiratory pathophysiology. Chest 83:666–670, 1983.

Cohen, A.M.: Magnetic resonance imaging of the thorax. Radiol. Clin. North Am. 22:829–846, 1984.

Crystal, R.G., Gadek, J.E., Ferrans, V.J., Fulmer, J.D., Line, B.R., Hunninghake, G.W.: Interstitial lung disease: Current concepts of pathogenesis, staging and therapy. Am. J. Med. 70:542–568, 1981.

Gail, D.B., Lenfant, C.J.M.: Cells of the lung: biology and clinical implications. Am. Rev. Respir. Dis. 127:366–387, 1983.

Goldstein, R.A. (ed.): Advances in the diagnosis and treatment of asthma. Chest 87:1S–113S, 1985.

Inselman, L.S., Mellins, R.B.: Growth and development of the lung. J. Pediatr. 98:1–15, 1981.

Jackson, R.M.: Pulmonary oxygen toxicity. Chest 88:900–905, 1985.

Kattan, M., Keens, T.G., Lapierre, J.G., Levison, H., Bryan, A.C., Reilly, B.J.: Pulmonary function abnormalities in symptom-free children after bronchiolitis. Pediatrics 59:683–688, 1977.

Latimer, J.S., Sharp, H.L.: Alpha-1-antitrypsin deficiency in childhood. Curr. Prob. Pediatr. 11:1–36, 1980.

Levison, H., Tabachnik, E., Newth, C.J.L.: Wheezing in infancy, croup and epiglottitis. Curr. Prob. Pediatr. 12: 1–65, 1982.

Loudon, R., Murphy, R.L.H.: Lung sounds. Am. Rev. Respir. Dis. 130:663–673, 1984.

Mark, J.D., Brooks, J.G.: Sleep-associated airway problems in children. Pediatr. Clin. North Am. 31:907–918, 1984.

Morgan, W.J.: Pulmonary function testing in infants and pre-school children. *In* Estelle, F., Simons, R. (eds.), The Child with Asthma, Report of the Sixth Canadian Ross Conference in Paediatrics. Montreal, Ross Laboratories, 1986.

O'Brodovich, H.M., Chernick, V.: The Functional Basis of Respiratory Pathology. *In* Kendig, E.L., Jr., Chernick, V. (eds.), Disorders of the Respiratory Tract in Children, 4th ed., Philadelphia, W.B. Saunders Co., 1983.

Pagtakhan, R.D., Chernick, V.: Intensive Care for Respiratory Disorders. *In* Kendig, E.L., Jr., Chernick, V. (eds.) Disorders of the Respiratory Tract in Children, 4th ed., Philadelphia, W.B. Saunders Co., 1983.

Petty, T.L.: Twenty-sixth Aspen Lung Conference: Chronic Obstructive Pulmonary Disease. Chest 85:1S–89S, 1984.

Shwachman, H., Mohmoodian, A.: Quality of sweat test performance in the diagnosis of cystic fibrosis. Clin. Chem. 25:158–161, 1979.

Smyth, J.A., Tabachnik, E., Duncan. W.J., Reilly, B.J., Levison, H.: Pulmonary function and bronchial hyperreactivity in long term survivors of bronchopulmonary dysplasia. Pediatrics 68:336–340, 1981.

Strope, G.L., Stempel, D.A.: Risk factors associated with the development of chronic lung disease in children. Pediatr. Clin. North Am. 31:757–771, 1984.

Turner, J.A.P., Corkey, C.W.B., Lee, J.Y.C., Levison, H., Sturgess, J.: Clinical expressions of immotile cilia syndrome. Pediatrics 67:805–810, 1981.

Waring, W.W.: Diagnostic and therapeutic procedures. *In* Kendig, E.L., Jr., Chernick, V. (eds.), Disorders of the Respiratory Tract in Children, 4th ed., Philadelphia, W.B. Saunders Co., 57–78, 1983.

Wohl, M.E., Chernick, V.: Bronchiolitis. Am. Rev. Respir. Dis. 118:759–781, 1978.

Wood, R.E.: Spelunking in the pediatric airways: explorations with the flexible fiberoptic bronchoscope. Pediatr. Clin. North Am. 31:785–799, 1984.

Wood, R.E., Boat, T.F., Doershuk, C.F.: Cystic fibrosis. Am. Rev. Respir. Dis. 113:833–878, 1976.

38

The Assessment of Lung Function: Pulmonary Function Testing

MARK C. WILSON, M.D.
GARY L. LARSEN, M.D.

There are many ways to assess lung function in the patient with pulmonary-related complaints. After a detailed history and physical examination, with particular emphasis on the respiratory tract, it is a common procedure to obtain a chest roentgenogram and, occasionally, an arterial blood gas determination to further this assessment. Various measurements of pulmonary function are also available and important in the evaluation and management of respiratory disease, and some tests can be performed by children as young as 5 or 6 years of age. Pulmonary function tests can assist patient evaluation and serve as important and indispensable aids in the care of many acute and chronic pulmonary disorders. This fact is especially true in the diagnosis and care of patients with asthma and other obstructive airway disorders, because wheezing, often used as an index of airflow limitation, does not occur in the smaller airways. Auscultation also is a grossly imperfect way of assessing obstruction to airflow. This chapter will review common tests of lung function and particularly those that can be performed and interpreted in the physician's office or other clinical setting. Table 38–1 indicates the clinical applications and limitations of these tests that aid in the diagnosis, evaluate precipitants of the symptoms, assess the effects of therapy, and follow the course of the disease. Although many of the examples in the figures are from the assessment of pediatric patients, the general principles apply to adults as well. The emphasis of this chapter is on asthma, but the physiology of diseases that may be mistaken for asthma will be presented as well.

Tests of lung function most easily conducted and interpreted within the physician's office may be grouped into two broad categories: lung volumes (or capacities) and flow rates (volume per unit of time).

Definition of Lung Volumes and Capacities. Air within the lung is partitioned into various functional compartments called volumes. Sums of volumes are termed capacities. The proportion of these compartments is similar among healthy individuals. The absolute values of these subdivisions change with age and body size (primarily height) and may differ among races and sexes. Various lung volumes and capacities are displayed in Figure 38–1. The volume of air that is inspired and expired during normal, quiet breathing is the tidal volume (V_T) and normally equals approximately 10 percent of the maximum amount of air contained within the lung. The maximal volume of air that can be inhaled over and above the tidal volume is the inspiratory reserve volume (IRV); the maximal volume of air that can be exhaled from normal breathing is the expiratory reserve volume (ERV). The air in the lung that cannot be expelled with maximal effort is termed the residual volume (RV).

As noted, the sums of the volumes in the lung make up various functional components termed capacities. Thus, the sum of all of the volumes ($RV + ERV + V_T + IRV$) is the total lung capacity (TLC). The total amount of air that can be exhaled (from the point of maximum inspiration) is the vital capacity (VC) and is thus the sum of the inspiratory reserve volume, the tidal volume, and the expiratory reserve volume. The functional residual capacity (FRC) is composed of the ERV and the RV. Normally, the VC equals approximately 75 percent of the TLC, with the RV accounting for the remaining 25 percent. The FRC is approximately 40 percent of the TLC in healthy individuals. These relationships may be altered in obstructive airways diseases, such as asthma, in which the absolute values of the RV and FRC increase, as does the ratio of either to the TLC (see the right side of Fig. 38–1 and Fig. 38–2A).

Measurements of Lung Volumes and Capacities. Many of the volumes and the VC discussed previously can be measured with the use

TABLE 38–1. Pulmonary Function Tests: Clinical Applications and Limitations

Applications

Aid in diagnosis
Quantitate disease severity
Define precipitants of symptoms
Evaluate therapy
Follow the disease course

Limitations

Wide range of normal values
Dynamic changes with age
Variable patient cooperation
Lack of tests for infants, small children

of a simple spirometer as displayed in Figure 38–1. The maximal expiratory vital capacity maneuver is employed to measure these functions. The subject is instructed to perform a slow, full inhalation of air to maximum inflation, hold his or her breath for a brief period of time, and then perform a sudden, sustained maximal exhalation to RV that lasts a minimum of 3 seconds. From the volume-time tracing produced (spirogram) shown in Figure 38–1, the VC plus all lung volumes except the RV can be calculated. It is important to stress, however, that the RV (and thus the FRC and TLC, both of which include the residual volume) cannot be calculated from this record. Other methods

must be employed to measure these compartments. Although the techniques used in these assessments are more complicated than simple spirometry, and the equipment needed is not usually found within the physician's office or a clinic, it is important to review briefly the principles involved in the determination of these compartments that may be useful clinically.

The TLC and the RV both can be computed if the FRC is known. The FRC usually is determined by one of two techniques, i.e., gas dilution or body plethysmography. With gas dilution, the changes in concentration of a relatively insoluble gas (helium or nitrogen) are monitored as the subject breathes either single or multiple breaths in a closed (rebreathing) or an open (nonrebreathing) system. In most laboratories where this principle is applied, helium is utilized as the reference gas in a closed circuit technique. The subject breathes from a spirometer containing a mixture of helium and air until the concentration of helium is the same in both the lungs and spirometer. The volume of gas in the system is noted before the test begins, and the helium concentration is noted once equilibration occurs; a simple formula can then be used to calculate the volume of air in the lung at the initiation of inspiration (FRC) from the spirometer (Cherniack, 1977). With this method of assessing FRC, all areas of the lung must com-

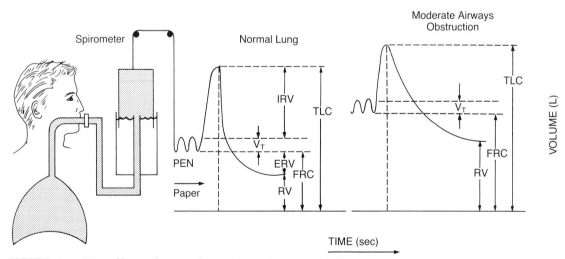

FIGURE 38–1. Normal lung volumes and capacities and an example of those found with moderate airway obstruction are displayed as a spirogram (volume versus time tracing). The volumes and capacities include tidal volume (V_T), inspiratory reserve volume (IRV), expiratory reserve volume (ERV), residual volume (RV), vital capacity (VC), functional residual capacity (FRC), and total lung capacity (TLC). The VC and all volumes except the RV can be measured with a simple spirometer, as displayed. To assess RV as well as TLC and FRC, spirometry has to be combined with either body plethysmography or a gas dilution technique (see text). With moderate airways obstruction, expiratory airflow is decreased, as represented by less volume of air exhaled per unit of time; lung volumes (RV, FRC) are increased.

municate with the airways to be measured. Thus, if some air containing units do not communicate with the central airways because of complete airways obstruction, the FRC may be underestimated.

The other method employed to assess the FRC is body plethysmography. A plethysmograph is an airtight chamber in which the subject sits and performs various respiratory maneuvers through a mouthpiece. This application takes advantage of Boyle's law, which states that the volume of a gas in a container varies inversely with the pressure to which it is subjected. For measuring lung volume in the plethysmograph, the airway is occluded at the end of a quiet expiration (at FRC). Through continued respiratory efforts against an occluded airway, the subject compresses and decompresses the gas within the chest. By measuring pressure and volume changes in the plethysmograph produced by this maneuver, the FRC may be determined, again through use of a simple formula (Cherniack, 1977). With this technique, air containing units do not need to communicate with airways to be measured; thus, lung volume assessed by this method will not be underestimated in the presence of severe or complete obstruction of airways. In general, the plethysmographic method of determining FRC is utilized more widely because it is quicker to perform, and airways resistance may be determined at the same time. The RV and TLC may be derived from the FRC, as determined by either method.

Definition and Measurement of Flow Rates. By analyzing the volume of air that can be expired from the lung in a defined period of time, various flow rates can be derived. Because maximal flow rates reflect the degree of resistance to airflow or airways obstruction, they are useful measurements of lung function that are commonly assessed in diseases such as asthma.

Flow rates vary with lung size, lung volume, and patient effort. Airway caliber increases with age and height, leading to a decrease in the resistance to airflow and the ability to produce higher flow rates. At any given age and height, the flow rate also depends on the lung volume at which it is measured; one reason for this is that the elastic recoil pressure is greater at higher lung volumes. As discussed in more detail elsewhere (Cherniack, 1977), recoil pressure is one of the major determinants of flow rates generated during maximal expiratory maneuvers.

The most common measurements of flow include the peak expiratory flow rate (PEFR), the forced expiratory volume at one second (FEV_1) and the maximum midexpiratory flow rate (MMEF). The PEFR is the maximal flow recorded during a forced expiratory maneuver from TLC and is expressed in L/sec. This test of lung function, which correlates with FEV_1, is simple to perform, easily learned, and reproducible. In addition, PEFR may be assessed by a number of hand-held devices specifically made for this one pulmonary function. These devices include a sturdy professional model (Wright peak-flow meter) as well as less durable plastic models (Mini-Wright peak-flow meter, Vitalograph Pulmonary Monitor) suited for monitoring of PEFR in the home and at work when clinically indicated. It is possible to measure this flow rate from the volume-time tracing (spirogram shown in Fig. 38–1 and Fig. 38–2B) by drawing a tangent to the steepest part of the curve. However, this method is inaccurate and is not recommended. PEFR may be derived more reliably from a flow-volume curve.

FEV_1 is the most commonly measured flow rate within a physician's office or clinic and is easily determined from a spirogram (see Fig. 38–1 and Fig. 38–2B) or from flow-volume curves. This function is obtained from a recording of a maximal forced expiratory maneuver that goes from full inspiration to full expiration. It is often compared with the forced vital capacity as a ratio (FEV_1/FVC). A value greater than 0.80 in children and young adults is consistent with normal airflow, without limitation (Polgar and Promadhat, 1971) (Fig. 38–3 and Fig. 38–4).

The maximum midexpiratory flow rate (MMEF or $FEF_{25-75\%}$) is the mean flow rate during the middle portion of an FVC maneuver. It may be calculated from the spirogram as the slope of a straight line between the points representing 25 percent and 75 percent of the VC. A steeper slope describes a higher flow rate, whereas a decline in this slope describes a lower flow rate. The decrease in volume exhaled per unit of time that is characteristic of diseases due to airways obstruction is shown diagramatically in Figure 38–1 and Figure 38–2B.

Aside from the spirogram (volume-time tracing), flow rates may also be determined from flow-volume curves (Fig. 38–2A). Instead of displaying volume and time, flow and volume are exhibited. The maneuver employed to generate the expiratory flows is the same (maximal FVC), but in many instances, the maximal expiratory maneuver is followed by a maximal in-

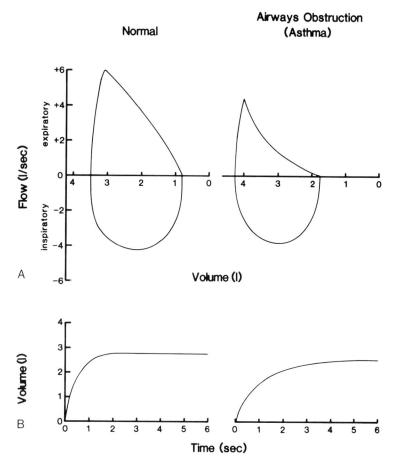

FIGURE 38-2. Flow-volume loops are compared with volume-time tracings (spirograms) in a patient with asthma at two time points. Pulmonary functions displayed on the left, when disease is well controlled (Normal), are compared with a time when the patient is unstable (Airways Obstruction). In A, flow is on the y-axis, and volume on the x-axis. Normal maximal inspiratory and expiratory curves that constitute the flow-volume loop are shown on the left. Maximal inspiration (total lung capacity) is the point of zero flow on the left side of the loop (approximately 3.5 L; maximal exhalation (residual volume) is at the point of zero flow at the right side of the loop (0.8 L in this example). With a forced vital capacity maneuver, expiratory flow reaches a maximum value soon after the onset of effort and then decreases to zero flow as a straight line or with some concavity to the volume axis. With airways obstruction (right), hyperinflation is noted (increase in residual volume), and flow rates decrease as manifest in the curve that becomes convex to the volume axis. Note that the inspiratory loop is relatively preserved with moderate lower airway obstruction (compare with Fig. 38-5). In B, volume is plotted on the y-axis against time on the x-axis. A normal expiratory curve is shown on the left. With a forced vital capacity maneuver, volume reaches a plateau within 2 seconds (approximately 2.7 L). Forced expiratory volume at 1 second (FEV_1) is read from the y-axis, where the 1-second time mark intersects the curve (approximately 2.4 L). With airways obstruction on the right, the volume-time curve is less steep. The FEV_1 is therefore decreased, and a longer period of time is required for the curve to plateau at vital capacity. Although minimally diminished in this example, forced vital capacity may be more decreased, especially with more severe obstruction.

spiratory maneuver so that both inspiratory and expiratory flows can be assessed. One consequence of this method of recording is that instantaneous flow rates at any point in the maneuver may be read directly from the curves. Thus, the highest flow generated after the onset of the expiratory maneuver is the PEFR. On some equipment, a small deflection of the expiratory limb of the flow-volume loop signifies 1 second has elapsed since expiration began, allowing computation of the FEV_1 (not shown in Fig. 38-2A).

In the physician's office setting, where FRC, RV, and TLC are usually not measured, instantaneous flow is related to a percentage of VC. For example, flow after exhalation of 50 or 75 percent of the VC is computed by finding the volume on the x-axis and reading the flow rate directly from the y-axis. Where body plethysmography or gas dilution techniques are available to measure FRC (and hence TLC), instantaneous flow may be related to an absolute lung volume (as in Fig. 38-2A) or reported as a percentage of TLC (usually flow at 60 or 50 percent of TLC) read from the y-axis. For example, at a lung volume of 2 L in the normal subject in Figure 38-2A, the flow rate is approximately 3.5 L/sec.

Spirograms Versus Flow-Volume Curves. Both methods of recording forced expiratory maneuvers can be employed alone or in combination with a complete assessment of lung volumes and capacities (via a gas dilution technique or body plethysmography) to obtain a

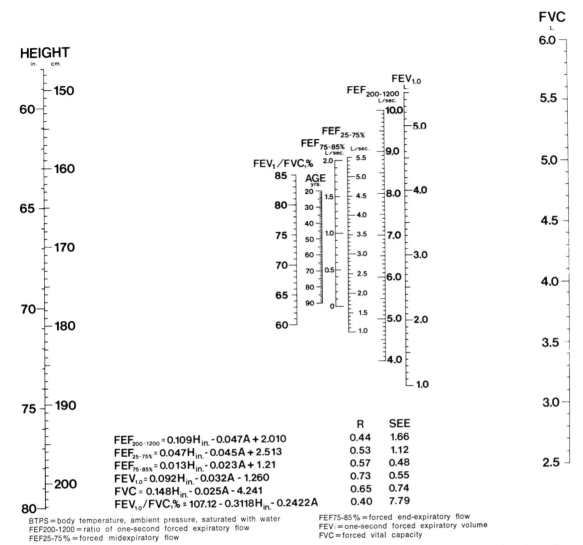

FIGURE 38–3. Spirometry in the evaluation of pulmonary function. Shown are normal predicted values for males. (From Morris, et al: West. J. Med. *125*:110–118, 1976.)

The figure includes the following equations and statistics:

Equation	R	SEE
$FEF_{200-1200} = 0.109H_{in.} - 0.047A + 2.010$	0.44	1.66
$FEF_{25-75\%} = 0.047H_{in.} - 0.045A + 2.513$	0.53	1.12
$FEF_{75-85\%} = 0.013H_{in.} - 0.023A + 1.21$	0.57	0.48
$FEV_{1.0} = 0.092H_{in.} - 0.032A - 1.260$	0.73	0.55
$FVC = 0.148H_{in.} - 0.025A - 4.241$	0.65	0.74
$FEV_{1.0}/FVC,\% = 107.12 - 0.3118H_{in.} - 0.2422A$	0.40	7.79

BTPS = body temperature, ambient pressure, saturated with water
FEF200-1200 = ratio of one-second forced expiratory flow
FEF25-75% = forced midexpiratory flow

FEF75-85% = forced end-expiratory flow
FEVₗ = one-second forced expiratory volume
FVC = forced vital capacity

more complete picture of pulmonary physiology. There are differences, however, between the two tracings that should be pointed out. As mentioned, flow rates from a spirogram reflect mean flows, whereas flows from a flow-volume curve represent instantaneous flows. Thus, it is easier by visual inspection to examine the expiratory portion of the flow-volume curve, and from the shape of the curve alone, determine if airflow limitation exists (Hyatt and Black, 1973). For example, on the normal curve depicted in Figure 38–2A, the descending limb of the expiratory portion of the flow volume loop is straight or slightly concave to the volume axis. However, when airways obstruction exists, as shown in the right hand portion of

Figure 38–2A, the descending curve becomes "scooped out" and is convex to the volume axis. Mild degrees of airways obstruction are harder to identify by inspection of the spirogram and are more obvious on the flow-volume curve. Artifacts also are easier to identify when instantaneous flow is displayed. Common artifacts include less than maximal effort in the initiation of the forced expiratory maneuver, premature termination of the test (not blowing completely to residual volume), and coughing during the expiratory maneuver. On the flow-volume curve flow does not increase to a maximum value within the first 25 percent of the VC when the initial effort is suboptimal, and flow precipitously returns to the point of zero flow when

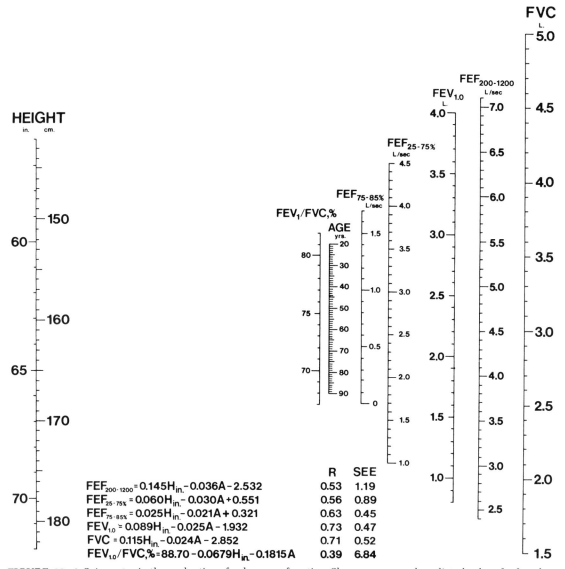

FIGURE 38–4. Spirometry in the evaluation of pulmonary function. Shown are normal predicted values for females. (From Morris, et al: West. J. Med. 125:110–118, 1976.)

effort is terminated prematurely. Coughing during the maneuver leads to very uneven flow rates.

Another advantage of a flow-volume analysis is that both inspiratory and expiratory curves can be examined. The contour of a normal inspiratory curve is shown in Figure 38–2A, and as can be seen, the inspiratory flow rate is roughly equivalent to the expiratory flow rate at 50 percent of VC. With diffuse airways obstruction, such as that observed with mild to moderate asthma (right portion of Figure 38–2A), the expiratory curve is more abnormal than the inspiratory curve. This differential effect of diffuse lower airways obstruction on the inspiratory and expiratory curves is due partly to transmural pressures generated by these maneuvers; sections of the intrathoracic airways are normally compressed during expiration, and during inspiration the opposite (dilatation) tends to occur.

Other types of pathology within the airways may result in different patterns on the flow-volume loop (Miller and Hyatt, 1973). As shown in Figure 38–5, with fixed airways obstruction within the central airways (larynx, trachea) that is either intrathoracic or extrathoracic, truncation of both the inspiratory and expiratory limbs of the flow-volume loop occurs. This type of abnormality can be seen in a patient with subglottic stenosis, in whom the pathology involves the total circumference of the airway. Tumors invading the walls of the airways may also produce such a pattern. With an extrathoracic lesion that is variable, i.e., the airway still undergoes dilatation and compression during the respiratory cycle, flow limitation is more marked on inspiration during which the normal tendency is for the extrathoracic airway to collapse. Laryngomalacia produces this type of pattern. When a lesion affects a major intrathoracic airway (trachea or main stem bronchus) and dynamic movements with respiration still occur, a variable intrathoracic pattern is seen in which flow limitation is greatest on expiration. Certain types of vascular rings as well as other masses compressing the airways can produce this pattern. The configuration of the flow-volume loop found with a diffuse disease (asthma) within the intrathoracic airways (right side of Fig. 38–2A) should be contrasted to the configuration found with a lesion within the major airways that produces variable compression during expiration (right side of Fig. 38–5). In the latter, there is more truncation of the expiratory flow at high lung volumes.

Other Tests. In addition to spirometry performed in the physician's office, an occasional patient may require more sophisticated tests that are performed only in a well-equipped pulmonary function laboratory. The techniques of assessing absolute lung volumes (TLC, FRC, RV) are but some examples and have been discussed previously. Three other tests deserve brief mention.

Measurement of the more detailed mechanical properties of the lung by obtaining a pressure-volume curve may aid in the diagnosis of a patient with a confusing clinical picture or spirometric values or both. For example, in a patient with emphysema, a marked loss of elastic recoil pressure (decreased compliance) is noted on a pressure-volume curve, whereas in a patient with a disease, such as interstitial fibrosis, an increase in elastic recoil (increased compliance) is noted. When a defect in gas diffusion is suspected, the diffusing capacity of carbon monoxide (DL_{CO}) across the alveolar-capillary membrane can be assessed. Low DL_{CO} values are found in diseases characterized by loss of surface area (emphysema) or interstitial processes within the lung (interstitial fibrosis). Another group of tests may be used to assess small airway function. These tests include the closing volume or the volume above RV at which small airways within the dependent areas of the lung begin to narrow and close. The principles behind these tests of lung function as well as the indications for their use and the methods employed in their assessment are reviewed in Cherniack (1977) and Macklem (1975).

INDICATIONS FOR USE OF PULMONARY FUNCTION TESTS

Pulmonary function tests may be used for many purposes. In the initial assessment of a patient, they aid in the evaluation of complaints, often aiding in the differential diagnosis. For those patients with asthma, tests of lung function may be especially helpful in

FIGURE 38–5. Flow-volume loops are displayed for various types of obstructing lesions of the proximal airways (trachea and larynx) that may present as wheezing. For comparison, the normal configuration of a flow-volume loop is shown on the left side of Figure 38–2A. With a lesion that is circumferential, preventing either compression or dilation of the airway with respiratory efforts, a "fixed" pattern is seen with truncation of both the inspiratory and expiratory curves. If a lesion permits compression or dilation with respiration, the pattern will depend on whether the lesion is extrathoracic or intrathoracic. With the extrathoracic lesion, the inspiratory curve is more affected. The intrathoracic lesion will have more of an effect on expiratory airflow.

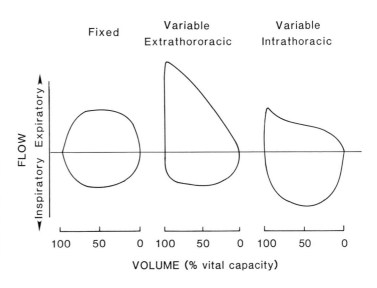

Fixed   Variable Extrathororacic   Variable Intrathoracic

FLOW

Expiratory ▲

Inspiratory ▼

VOLUME (% vital capacity)

100   50   0   100   50   0   100   50   0

identifying specific precipitants of airways obstruction. With the institution of therapy, the assessment of pulmonary function may indicate the efficacy of acute therapy and also offer an objective means for following the course of a patient's disease over time.

Aid in Diagnosis. Pulmonary function tests are used commonly to confirm the presence of airway lability in patients suspected of having asthma. This confirmation is most often accomplished by performing lung functions before and after the administration of an inhaled bronchodilator. An example of the type of response expected on a flow-volume curve in a patient with asthma is shown in Figure 38–6. Before administration of the drug, there is evidence of mild airflow limitation in that the expiratory limb of the flow-volume curve is slightly convex to the volume axis. After administration of the drug, flow rates improve markedly.

For any test of lung function, the magnitude of change (percent increase or decrease) considered significant will vary with the function examined. Some tests, such as VC and FEV_1, are more reproducible from effort to effort, whereas MMEF and flows at lower lung volumes on the expiratory flow-volume curve are variable or less reproducible (Lemen, 1983). Thus, an increase in the FEV_1 of 15 to 20 percent or an increase in the MMEF of 25 to 30 percent often is taken to represent significant reversibility to an inhaled bronchodilator, assuming that the maneuver has been performed correctly, without artifacts in the record. No matter which tests are employed, the interpretation of functions must take into account the variability of the functions employed. It also is necessary to know that the tests have been performed correctly, and for that purpose, a permanent copy of the record (spirogram or flow-volume curve

or loop) is helpful (see subsequent discussion).

Other studies are capable of demonstrating airways hyperreactivity and can be employed as diagnostic aids in patients suspected of having asthma. However, because these studies by nature are intended to assess the production of bronchoconstriction, it is of utmost importance to know the degree of impairment present before challenge is undertaken. In general, subjects who undergo such challenges should be symptom free at the time of study and have lung functions of at least 80 percent of their best previous efforts. The procedures must be conducted in a standardized fashion by personnel well versed in the performance of provocation tests as well as assessments of pulmonary function. Equipment and medications always must be on hand to reverse severe airways obstruction that can develop over a short period of time.

A common physiologic method to demonstrate airways lability is the exercise challenge. Exercise is a frequent precipitant of airways obstruction in patients with asthma. Documenting the presence of exercise-induced bronchoconstriction not only helps to establish the diagnosis of asthma but also pinpoints a precipitant in an individual patient that can be approached through therapy (see further discussion in Chapter 44).

Normal lung functions with flow rates and volumes that do not change appreciably with administration of bronchodilators do not in themselves preclude the existence or diagnosis of asthma. In addition to the quiescent phase of this disorder, this finding occurs in patients in whom chronic cough is the only manifestation of reactive airways disease (Cloutier and Loughlin, 1981). An exercise test, however, may demonstrate airways lability. A bronchial

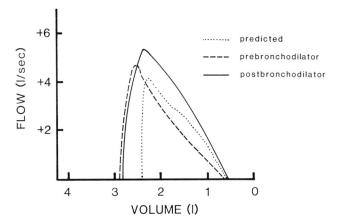

FIGURE 38–6. The expiratory flow-volume curve for a child with asthma is shown before and after administration of an inhaled adrenergic drug. For comparison, the predicted values are also shown. Lung function is only mildly abnormal before administration of the bronchodilator, with only mild convexity of the descending portion of the curve, and no significant increase in residual volume. Following treatment, lung function improves significantly; the curve is now concave to the volume axis, with flows greater than predicted values. The test results confirmed reactivity of the airways and helped define the optimal lung function for the patient.

challenge with either histamine or methacholine is a diagnostic study that may be employed to determine whether airways hyperreactivity exists. In this test, serial lung functions are performed before and successively after increasing doses of one of these bronchoconstricting drugs. The objective of the challenge is to determine whether airways obstruction will occur at concentrations of a drug that do not lead to airways obstruction in normal subjects. It is a potentially dangerous procedure; the test must be performed in a standardized fashion with a medical and technical staff well versed in procedure and interpretation of a challenge (Cropp et al., 1980). In general, a 20 percent decrease in the FEV_1, following inhalation of a drug, is considered a positive response. Normal subjects will not exhibit significant declines in lung functions in response to the maximally selected doses of either drug employed for challenges.

Exposure to air that is dry or cold or both also can induce airways obstruction in patients with asthma. Such exposure also has been used to assess airways hyperreactivity (Aitken and Marini, 1985). Because of the special equipment needed for this type of bronchoprovocation, this technique remains a research tool at this time.

It is important to bear in mind that many types of lung disease may appear with dyspnea, or other respiratory symptoms, not due to asthma. In addition, airways reactivity may be a component of other lung diseases, such as cystic fibrosis, which have different long-term consequences than asthma. Thus, a thorough assessment of lung function to help define pathophysiology and to assess bronchial hyperreactivity (see previous discussion) should be considered an important part of most evaluations of possible respiratory disease.

Assessment of pulmonary physiology can help to define diagnostic possibilities when history and physical findings are not enlightening. An important diagnostic consideration, for example, relates to whether the pulmonary problem is based on an obstructive or a restrictive process. Examples of obstructive problems include asthma, chronic bronchitis, emphysema, and cystic fibrosis; restrictive problems include chest wall deformities limiting lung expansion as well as interstitial disorders due to collagen vascular diseases, hypersensitivity pneumonitis, sarcoidosis, and intersititial fibrosis. It is important to recognize that certain diseases may produce both obstruction and restriction. Thus, the distinction between obstructive and restrictive disorders may not be as clear as the example that follows.

Physiologically, the characteristics of obstructive and restrictive disorders are compared in Figure 38–7. In an obstructive disorder, there is airflow limitation with decrease in maximal expiratory flows as demonstrated by the convex characteristics of the flow-volume curve as well as decrease in the FEV_1/FVC ratio. In addition, there commonly is evidence of hyperinflation with an increase in RV and FRC. In a restrictive disorder, on the other hand, lung volumes including TLC, VC, and RV, all tend to be low. Although the FEV_1 may be less than predicted,

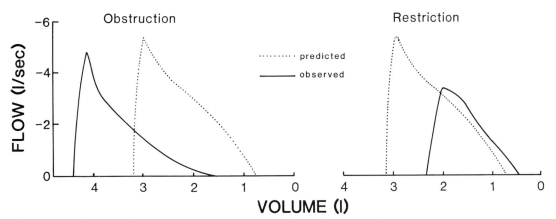

FIGURE 38–7. Expiratory flow-volume curves demonstrate the findings in an obstructive versus a restrictive pulmonary disease. The patient on the left had asthma and demonstrated gas trapping (increased RV) as well as a decrease in flow rates. On the right, the child with a restrictive disorder (idiopathic interstitial pneumonia) had low lung volumes and no evidence of obstruction to airflow, as defined by a normal FEV_1/FVC ratio and above normal flow rates when corrected for lung volumes. This patient was thought to have asthma until tests of lung function pointed to a restrictive process.

the FEV_1/FVC ratio is normal, indicating a lack of airflow limitation. Also, flow related to volume is not subnormal but higher than predicted. This fact can be appreciated by plotting flows on an absolute lung volume axis, as in Figure 38–7. An important feature of this type of pulmonary problem is that flow corrected for lung volume often is elevated, which may be due to interstitial fibrosis produced by the disease process, causing the lung to become "stiffer" with greater elastic recoil. Since this recoil is one of the determinants of maximal expiratory flow rates, flows can be supernormal.

The patient whose pulmonary functions are displayed as the example of restriction in Figure 38–7 presented with a diagnosis of "asthma" because of vague symptoms she experienced with exercise. Her evaluation included the flow-volume curve shown as well as an evaluation of the pressure-volume characteristics of her lung (Macklem, 1975). The last evaluation demonstrated noncompliant or "stiff" lungs, consistent with a restrictive and not an obstructive process. A subsequent lung biopsy specimen demonstrated an interstitial process of undefined etiology. It is stressed that patients who present or are referred for evaluation of asthma may not have evidence of reversible airways obstruction. A thorough evaluation of any pulmonary problem is dependent on acquiring information on the physiology of the underlying process.

The various patterns the flow-volume loop assumes with fixed or variable obstruction of either the intrathoracic or extrathoracic airways have already been reviewed (see Fig. 38–5). It is important to emphasize that disorders that lead to these abnormalities may appear with wheezing, which is interpreted by patients or medical personnel to be due to asthma.

The Evaluation of Precipitants. Pulmonary function tests also can facilitate the evaluation of precipitants that can lead to airways obstruction. One example mentioned is exercise as a trigger in asthma. As with some other precipitants, when exercise is recognized as a factor, therapy can be directed at preventing this problem.

Pulmonary function tests also can be used to assess other potential triggers. For example, antigens to which an asthmatic has IgE antibody may or may not be triggers for disease. Even though the probable importance of a particular antigen may be gauged by the history and the degree of the positive skin test reaction (Cavanaugh et al., 1977), these relationships often are unclear. In certain instances, it may be important clinically to determine if exposure to a particular allergen can induce respiratory symptoms in the patient. The simplest and possibly the safest approach to this problem may be to measure PEFR in the home or work environment after natural exposure of the patient to the antigen in question. This also may be a critical diagnostic tool in evaluating adults when there is concern about occupational lung disease. At other times, especially if considering an antigen that is perennial or for which the intensity of natural exposure is hard to gauge, bronchial challenge with antigen may be indicated (Fig. 38–8). It is important to stress that this is not a routine office procedure, and if contemplated should be cause for referral to a hospital or clinic where the procedure is carried out frequently. A major reason for this precaution is that severe airways obstruction to inhaled antigen may be precipitated immediately after antigen challenge (immediate asthmatic response) or hours after exposure (late asthmatic response). The time course of both the immediate and late responses is shown in Figure 38–8.

The immediate asthmatic response occurs within minutes of the exposure, peaks within

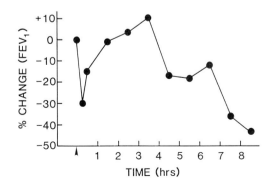

FIGURE 38–8. Changes in lung function (FEV_1) from baseline values versus time after antigen challenge (arrow) are shown for a patient with both an immediate and a late asthmatic response after antigen challenge. While the immediate response is easily reversed with inhaled or injected adrenergic agents, the late response may be more resistant to therapy and require steroids for early resolution.

15 to 30 minutes, and resolves over 1 to 2 hours. The late response has an onset 2 to 4 hours after challenge, and usually peaks within 8 to 12 hours, but may take several days to resolve. Patients who respond to antigen challenge may have an immediate reaction, an immediate and late reaction, or an isolated late reaction. The first two patterns are the most frequent. Whereas the immediate response is reversed easily with inhaled or injected adrenergic drugs, the late response may be incompletely or only temporarily reversed with adrenergic drugs and requires steroids for resolution. Thus, observation of a subject for a minimum of 12 hours after antigen challenge is recommended to document the response and to treat appropriately. Another potential sequela of bronchial challenge is that nonspecific airways reactivity may increase after a late asthmatic response, making the airways of the patient more susceptible to other triggers and possibly intensifying the problem of asthma. This is usually a short-lived problem, however. Nevertheless, it underscores the importance of performing antigen challenges only when clinically indicated and in a proper setting. The reader is referred to Bhagat et al. (1985) and Cropp et al. (1980) for more extensive discussions of antigen challenges in asthma.

Other potential triggers also can be assessed with the aid of pulmonary function tests. The responses to ingested substances, such as aspirin, tartrazine, and metabisulfite, are common concerns in patients with asthma (Mathi-son and Stevenson, 1979; Stevenson and Simon, 1981). Pulmonary function tests help quantitate any untoward response to these agents and define its time course. As with bronchial challenges, these challenges are not without risks and should be performed cautiously in a setting where deterioration in lung function can be controlled and treated appropriately.

Evaluation of Therapy. Pulmonary function tests are an important aid in evaluating both acute and chronic effects of treatment in patients with various lung diseases (Table 38–2). An example of their usefulness in the initial care of a child with severe asthma is demonstrated in Figure 38–9. On patient presentation (left side of figure), the flow-volume curve demonstrated evidence of significant obstruction with marked increase in the residual volume, descending limb of the expiratory curve that was convex to the volume axis, and flow rates that were depressed. After inhalation of a bronchodilator, no significant change in lung function was noted. Because of a history compatible with asthma that was poorly controlled over the recent past, oral corticosteroids were started. After several days of therapy, the response to repeat administration of inhaled bronchodilator is seen. Although pretreatment lung functions did not improve measurably from those performed earlier, there was a significant response to inhaled drug with a decrease in RV, an increase in the FVC, and increases in flow rates. This pattern (no initial objective response to adrenergic agents until institution of steroid

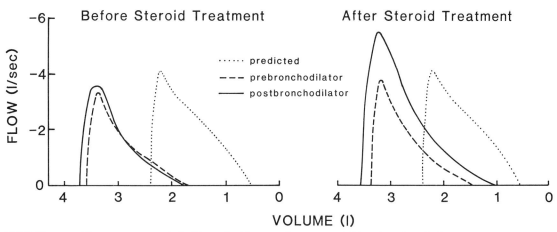

FIGURE 39–9. The response to inhaled bronchodilator is shown in a child with asthma before and after a course of oral steroids. As shown on the left, the functions reveal a marked increase in residual volume as well as significant airflow limitation. Inhaled adrenergic drugs are ineffective in reversing this obstruction. After administration of oral steroids, as shown on the right, the same inhaled bronchodilator leads to a marked increase in flow and a decrease in residual volume. Despite this beneficial response, lung function never completely normalized in the patient.

TABLE 38-2. Average (50 percent) Pulmonary Function
Values in Children*

| Height | | FVC (L) | | | FEF$_{25-75\%}$ | | PEFR | |
CM	IN	BOYS	GIRLS	FEV$_1$ (L)	L/MIN	L/SEC	L/MIN	L/SEC
100	39.4	1.00	1.00	.70	55	.91	100	1.67
102	40.2	1.03	1.00	.75	60	1.00	110	1.83
104	40.9	1.08	1.07	.82	64	1.06	120	2.00
106	41.7	1.14	1.10	.89	70	1.17	130	2.17
108	42.5	1.19	1.19	.97	75	1.25	140	2.33
110	43.3	1.27	1.24	1.01	80	1.33	150	2.50
112	44.1	1.32	1.30	1.10	86	1.43	160	2.67
114	44.9	1.40	1.36	1.17	90	1.50	174	2.90
116	45.7	1.47	1.41	1.23	96	1.60	185	3.08
118	46.5	1.52	1.49	1.30	100	1.67	195	3.25
120	47.2	1.60	1.55	1.39	105	1.75	204	3.40
122	48.0	1.69	1.62	1.45	110	1.83	215	3.58
124	48.8	1.75	1.70	1.53	118	1.97	226	3.77
126	49.6	1.82	1.77	1.59	121	2.01	236	3.93
128	50.4	1.90	1.84	1.67	127	2.12	247	4.11
130	51.2	1.99	1.90	1.72	132	2.20	256	4.27
132	52.0	2.07	2.00	1.80	139	2.32	267	4.45
134	52.8	2.15	2.06	1.89	142	2.37	278	4.63
136	53.5	2.24	2.15	1.98	149	2.48	289	4.82
138	54.3	2.35	2.24	2.06	153	2.55	299	4.98
140	55.1	2.40	2.32	2.11	159	2.65	310	5.17
142	55.9	2.50	2.40	2.20	163	2.72	320	5.33
144	56.7	2.60	2.50	2.30	170	2.83	330	5.50
146	57.5	2.70	2.59	2.39	173	2.88	340	5.67
148	58.3	2.79	2.68	2.48	180	3.00	351	5.85
150	59.1	2.88	2.78	2.57	183	3.05	362	6.03
152	59.8	2.97	2.88	2.66	190	3.17	373	6.22
154	60.6	3.09	2.98	2.75	195	3.25	384	6.40
156	61.4	3.20	3.09	2.88	200	3.33	394	6.57
158	62.2	3.30	3.18	2.98	205	3.42	404	6.73
160	63.0	3.40	3.27	3.06	210	3.50	415	6.92
162	63.8	3.52	3.40	3.18	215	3.58	425	7.08
164	64.6	3.64	3.50	3.29	220	3.67	436	7.28
166	65.4	3.78	3.60	3.40	225	3.75	446	7.43
168	66.1	3.90	3.72	3.50	230	3.83	457	7.62
170	66.9	4.00	3.83	3.65	236	3.93	467	7.78
172	67.7	4.20	3.83	3.80	241	4.01	477	7.95
174	68.5	4.20	3.83	3.80	246	4.10	488	8.13
176	69.3	4.20	3.83	3.80	251	4.18	498	8.30

* Data from Polgar, G., Promadhat, V.: *Pulmonary Function Testing in Children:
Techniques and Standards.* Philadelphia, W.B. Saunders Co., 1971.

therapy) is not uncommon in children or adults with severe asthma and persistent wheezing (Ellul-Micallef and Fenech, 1975).

The benefit of assessing lung function in the emergency treatment of asthma in children (Lulla and Newcomb, 1980) and adults (Fanta et al., 1982) has been documented. While there is little doubt that these objective measures can be of assistance in assessing the degree to which the acute airways obstruction is reversed, it is important to stress that pulmonary function tests should supplement and not replace a careful history and serial examination of the patient with acute wheezing.

An evaluation of the effectiveness of therapy also is frequently undertaken before elective surgery in patients with asthma or other chronic lung diseases. The indications for such assessments, the tests employed, and the benefits that can be derived have been reviewed recently (Tisi, 1979).

Following the Course of a Disease. Assessment of pulmonary function is helpful in charting the course of a disease. This is especially true when dealing with a process that is progressive, such as cystic fibrosis or interstitial lung disease. The assessment provides an objective means for measuring the effectiveness of therapy in delaying the progression of the disease and also allows realistic counseling of the patient and family about prognosis. Although asthma generally is thought of as a disease in which irreversible damage does not occur, it is evident that many patients with severe disease do, in fact, have irreversible damage, limiting airflow (Loren et al., 1978). Whether this represents a sequela of poorly controlled asthma or is the result of a separate insult to the airways (e.g., viral illness in childhood) often is not apparent. Close observation of alterations in physiology over time is likely to provide useful information concerning factors that predispose the patient to irreversible obstruction.

Regular home or work place peak flow measurements by the patient may be invaluable to the physician and the patient in following the course of various pulmonary disorders, including asthma. Using one of the home peak flow devices (mentioned previously) and charting the measurements can offer a guide to the judicious use of drugs on an outpatient basis, especially in the patient requiring multiple medications. Peak-flow devices also can be employed to give a patient with a poor perception of the disease an awareness of a decrease in lung function, thus allowing earlier therapeutic intervention.

CAVEATS IN PULMONARY FUNCTION TESTS

As with any laboratory tests, limitations of pulmonary function tests must be appreciated in order to utilize them appropriately. Major limitations of clinical importance are summarized next.

Wide Range of Normal Values. Ranges of normal are defined by an analysis of large groups of subjects who are free of obvious disease when tested. Normal pulmonary function values are based primarily on height, sex, and race (Polgar and Promadhat, 1971). Despite the ability to form subgroups of individuals in these categories, there is a wide range of normal values, and there are many practical applications of this point. First, the physician must have a knowledge of the magnitude of change necessary for an alteration in lung function to be of clinical significance. As noted previously, some tests are more reproducible than others. This topic is dealt with in more detail in other discussions of pulmonary function tests (Lemen, 1983). Second, values within a normal range may not be normal for the patient. For example, note the change in lung function in the case of the asthmatic patient illustrated in

Figure 38–6. Lung function varied from a normal range before therapy to an above "predicted" range, with bronchodilator treatment. Also, a single determination may not give an accurate picture of the patient's overall lung function. Serial measurements in the physician's office or at the patient's home (e.g., with a peak flow meter) over time will be more enlightening in this regard than measurements obtained only during visits to the physician's office.

Dynamic Changes with Age. In contrast to arterial blood gas tensions, which are fairly constant throughout life, major physiologic alterations take place in lung volumes and flows with growth and aging (Knudson et al., 1983). Consequently, serial determinations of lung functions tend to be much more informative than isolated tests. This is especially true for children and adults with chronic diseases that may be progressive; both the lung function at a point in time and the overall pattern of change in volumes and flows with time are critical to their care. Employing graphs that demonstrate plots of functions versus time (similar to plots of height, weight, and head circumference in the growing infant and child) should enhance our ability to detect problems at an earlier time in the course of the disease (Lemen, 1983).

Patient Cooperation. In all tests of lung function performed in a physician's office or a clinic, the cooperation of the patient is paramount. Pulmonary function tests, although not especially difficult or unpleasant to perform, do rely on a certain level of psychomotor maturation. Thus, it is possible to test lung function in children less than 5 years of age, only with special techniques. There also is a learning effect associated with repeated testing; as the subject becomes more comfortable with the equipment and individuals conducting the tests, the reproducibility of results generally improves. This effect applies to adults as well as children and must be taken into consideration in interpreting the results of the test. Some children and adults have a great deal of difficulty in performing lung function tests properly and may require an unusual amount of repeated efforts in order to obtain valid and reproducible information.

LACK OF AVAILABLE TESTS FOR INFANTS AND SMALL CHILDREN

Although various methods have been and are being developed and employed for assessment of lung function in preschool children, these remain research tools not available for routine office use. The inability to assess lung function in preschool children is a serious drawback in assessing their pulmonary status. Many respiratory illnesses (asthma, cystic fibrosis) may first manifest symptoms within children of this age group. The airways during this period of rapid growth may be subjected also to significant insults, such as viral infections, that can have lifelong consequences. Reliable tests of lung functions in this preschool group will be essential to measure more precisely the degree of impairment caused by these diseases and to assess objectively effectiveness of therapy. One hopes that specialized techniques now limited to research laboratories will become available for general clinical use in the near future.

EQUIPMENT FOR ASSESSMENT OF PULMONARY FUNCTION TESTS

A number of pieces of equipment are available for the routine assessment of lung function. Every primary care office should have a peak flow meter. In addition, inexpensive peak flow meters may be used in the home. Spirometers analyze either volume or time, with measurement of FEV_1, FVC, MMEF ($FEF_{25-75\%}$), flow and volume signals, and depiction of maximal inspiratory and expiratory maneuvers. Several spirometers have been reviewed recently and are acceptable for primary care office use (Gardner et al., 1980). In considering various pieces of equipment, aside from expense, a desirable feature is a permanent copy of the spirogram or the flow-volume curve so that this record can be reviewed to insure the maneuver is technically acceptable. Whereas a direct readout of the numerical results is convenient, the ability to inspect the test visually will decrease errors in assessment. The decision to purchase a unit that provides test results from a volume-time tracing versus a flow-volume curve or a unit that provides information from both types of analysis must be based on cost and preference for viewing the data. Although most offices will not have (and will not need) equipment to measure lung volumes by gas dilution or body plethysmography, the value of assessing lung volumes for certain clinical problems must be borne in mind. This ordinarily can be accomplished through referral to medical centers where equipment and those with expertise for such measurements are available.

Ideally, normal data should be generated for each practice setting, thereby standardizing a local healthy population with specific equipment and technicians, for comparison with patients with pulmonary complaints. Since this is impractical in a busy office or clinic, the use of either published normal values or standards furnished by the manufacturer ordinarily will suffice. When employing a new machine for testing lung functions, it is helpful to test several normal subjects and to compare their values to values obtained in older equipment that has been standardized through past use and maintenance. The need to maintain and calibrate equipment routinely before use is critical to accurate acquisition of data. Reference to standards of spirometry is recommended for all those who employ tests of lung function (see Fig. 38–3, Fig. 38–4, and Table 38–2) (Gardner et al., 1979; Taussig et al., 1980).

PERSONNEL AND ENVIRONMENT FOR CONDUCTING PULMONARY FUNCTION TESTS

The need for a motivated office nurse or assistant who is knowledgeable about pulmonary functions, who can teach and coach patients patiently through new procedures, and who can recognize technical problems that interfere with accurate assessments cannot be overstated. This person also should be responsible for assuring routine calibration of the equipment.

In testing of children, the environment should be friendly, free of distractions, and removed from areas where painful procedures take place. When the same child-oriented technician helps the patient during each visit to perform the test in an unhurried, nonthreatening setting, more consistent results are insured. Time should be allowed for the child to become comfortable with the equipment and to practice blowing through the unattached disposable mouthpiece or other similar devices (Fig. 38–10). An opportunity to see the curve simultaneously develop on the spirometer paper or screen may serve visually to reinforce better effort. Even if their trials are suboptimal, familiarity with staff and equipment will foster a willingness to correctly perform the test during subsequent visits. The same principles can

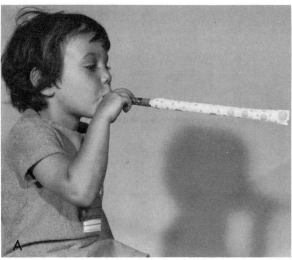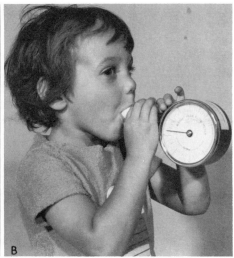

FIGURE 38–10. Use of a party favor to teach lung function maneuver to small children.

apply to older patients, who may have equal difficulties in performing these effort dependent tests.

REFERENCES

Aitken, M.L., Marini, J.J.: Effect of heat delivery and extraction on airway conductance in normal and in asthmatic subjects. Am. Rev. Respir. Dis. 131: 357–361, 1985.

Bhagat, R.J., Strunk, R.C., Larsen, G.L.: The late asthmatic response. Ann. Allergy 54: 272, 297–301, 1985.

Cavanaugh, M.J., Bronsky, E.A., Buckley, J.M.: Clinical value of bronchial provocation testing in childhood asthma. J. Allergy Clin. Immunol. 59: 41–47, 1977.

Cherniack, R.M.: Pulmonary Function Testing. Philadelphia, W.B. Saunders Co., 1977.

Cloutier, M.M., Loughlin, G.M.: Chronic cough in children: a manifestation of airway hyperreactivity. Pediatrics 67: 6–12, 1981.

Cropp, G.J.A., Berstein, I.L., Boushey, H.A., Hyde, R.W., Rosenthal, R.R., Spector, S.L., Townley, R.G.: Guidelines for bronchial inhalation challenges with pharmacologic and antigenic agents. Am. Thor. Soc. News 6: 11–19, 1980.

Ellul-Micallef, R., Fenech, F.F.: Effect of intravenous prednisolone in asthmatics with diminished adrenergic responsiveness. Lancet 2: 1269–1271, 1975.

Fanta, C.H., Rossing, T.H., McFadden, E.R.: Emergency room treatment of asthma. Relationships among therapeutic combinations, severity of obstruction and time course of response. Am. J. Med. 72: 416–422, 1982.

Gardner, R.M.: American Thoracic Society. Snowbird Workshop on Standardization of Spirometry. Am. Rev. Respir. Dis. 119: 831–838, 1979.

Gardner, R.M., Hankinson, J.L., West, B.J.: Evaluating commercially available spirometers. Am. Rev. Respir. Dis. 121: 73–82, 1980.

Hyatt, R.E., Black, L.F.: The flow-volume curve. A current perspective. Am. Rev. Respir. Dis. 107: 191–199, 1973.

Knudson, R.J., Lebowitz, M.D., Holberg, C.J., Burrows, B: Changes in the normal maximal expiratory flow-volume curve with growth and aging. Am. Rev. Respir. Dis. 127: 725–734, 1983.

Lemen, R.J.: Pulmonary function testing in the office and clinic. In Kending, E.L., Jr., Chernick, V. (eds.), Disorders of the Respiratory Tract in Children. Philadelphia, W.B. Saunders Co., 1983.

Loren, M.L., Leung, P.K., Cooley, R.L., Chai, H., Bell, T.D., Buck, V.M.: Irreversibility of obstructive changes in severe asthma in childhood. Chest 74: 126–129, 1978.

Lulla, S., Newcomb, R.W.: Emergency management of asthma in children. J. Pediatr. 97: 346–350, 1980.

Macklem, P.T.: New tests to assess lung function. N. Engl. J. Med. 293: 339–342, 1975.

Mathison, D.A., Stevenson, D.D.: Hypersensitivity to nonsteroidal anti-inflammatory drugs: indications and methods for oral challenges. J. Allergy Clin. Immunol. 64: 669–674, 1979.

Miller, R.D., Hyatt, R.E.: Evaluation of obstructive lesions of the trachea and larynx by flow-volume loops. Am. Rev. Respir. Dis. 108: 475–481. 1973.

Polgar, G., Promadhat, V. (eds.): Pulmonary Function Testing in Children. Philadelphia, W.B. Saunders Co., 1971.

Stevenson, D.D., Simon, R.A.: Sensitivity to ingested metabisulfites in asthmatic subjects. J. Allergy Clin. Immunol. 68: 26–32, 1981.

Taussig, L.M., Chernick, V., Wood, R., Farrell, P., Mellins, R.B.: Standardization of lung function testing in children. Proceedings and recommendations of the GAP Conference Committee, Cystic Fibrosis Foundation. J. Pediatr. 97: 668–676, 1980.

Tisi, G.M.: Preoperative evaluation of pulmonary function. Validity, indications and benefits. Am. Rev. Respir. Dis. 119: 293–310, 1979.

39

Obstructive Diseases of the Larynx and Trachea

PEYTON A. EGGLESTON, M.D.

Patients with obstructive lesions of the larynx and trachea frequently present with stridor and spasmodic cough; thus, the symptoms may be confused occasionally with those of asthma. This especially is true of disorders that are recurrent, such as croup, and disorders that produce chronic cough. This chapter deals with the more common obstructive conditions of the larynx and trachea with particular reference to important clinical features that can help to distinguish these conditions from asthma.

EPIGLOTTITIS

Epiglottitis is a "cellulitis" of the larynx, pharynx, and epiglottis which occurs largely in young children but can occur in adults. It is induced by a specific organism, *Haemophilus influenzae*, type b. Fortunately, children rapidly develop immunity to the causative organism, thus making this an uncommon disease (Mayosmith et al., 1986). The widespread availability of *H. influenzae*, type b immunization should reduce its frequency further. The onset of epiglottitis is abrupt (8 to 24 hours), and the child develops stridor with or without a croupy cough. Characteristically, the child is febrile, toxic, and lethargic and complains of marked pharyngeal pain, frequently so severe that the child will drool rather than swallow. There is marked leukocytosis and frequently bacteremia (80 percent) with *H. influenzae*. The combination of croup, dysphagia, and severe toxicity should alert the physician to the possibility of epiglottitis. Any attempt to confirm the diagnosis by visualization of the epiglottis should be approached with extreme caution since abrupt, fatal obstruction occurs commonly (10 to 40 percent). If epiglottitis is suspected, an anesthe-

siologist, an otolaryngologist, or a surgeon accustomed to emergency resuscitation should be present, with equipment for intubation ready, before the child is examined. Laryngoscopy is less hazardous in adults.

Other diseases usually considered in the differential diagnosis of epiglottitis are spasmodic croup and laryngotracheobronchitis. Neither of these two syndromes is associated with extreme toxicity or pharyngeal pain. In borderline situations in which fever and leukocytosis are present, a lateral neck roentgenogram to demonstrate the presence or absence of an enlarged epiglottis is appropriate. This is not the procedure of choice when epiglottitis is strongly suspected in children, since abrupt obstruction may occur while the roentgenogram is being taken, but it is thought by some clinicians to be indicated in adults.

Epiglottitis is an emergency, and the patient so affected should be hospitalized promptly. Because of the high mortality rate (30 percent) and because death usually results from abrupt airway obstruction, it generally is accepted that emergency creation of an artificial airway, either through insertion of a nasotracheal tube (Milko et al., 1974) or tracheostomy (Margolis et al., 1972), should be performed as soon as the diagnosis is made in adults and children. Intravenous antibiotic treatment with ampicillin, 150 mg/kg/day and chloramphenicol, 50 to 100 mg/kg/day, should be instituted immediately.

CROUP

Croup in children occurs in two clinical patterns, spasmodic croup and laryngotracheobronchitis. Both appear most commonly between 3 months and 3 years of age, and both are characterized by inspiratory stridor and barking cough. Spasmodic croup begins abruptly, usually in early morning hours, and ends abruptly after a few hours or less. Laryngotracheobronchitis begins more gradually, is more prolonged, and is frequently more severe.

In the majority of cases of laryngotracheobronchitis, the infecting agent is a parainfluenza virus, most often type 1, but many other viruses also have been implicated, including influenza, adenovirus, rhinovirus, and enterovirus (Glezen et al., 1971). Infection with these

528

viruses in older children and adults usually is associated with nonspecific upper respiratory symptoms, so it appears that an unusual host response as much as a specific organism is responsible for the syndrome. The importance of specific host response also is suggested by the demonstration that IgE antibodies specific for parainfluenza virus can be found in secretions from infected children who manifest the croup syndrome or wheezing but not from those who only have coryzal symptoms (Welliver et al., 1982). IgE antibodies, by activating mucosal mast cells, could trigger immediate hypersensitivity reactions that result in the edema and inflammation which have been found in the rare case that was studied at autopsy.

Typically, croup begins with an upper respiratory infection or "cold," without unusual toxicity or fever. Initial symptoms progress to a dry, hacking cough that becomes brassy as inspiratory stridor and hoarseness develop. Alternatively, the brassy cough, hoarseness, and stridor may develop abruptly. Croup usually begins at night, most often reaching a peak at about 10 to 11 p.m. Depending on the severity of obstruction, the child may be anxious, air hungry, and dyspneic with substernal and intercostal refractions. Crying and agitation may lead to frequent spasms of coughing, which increase obstruction. In severe cases, children are anxious, agitated, and cyanotic. Chest examination reveals only stridor and transmitted sounds of upper airway secretions.

There is no specific therapy, and the most important aspect of management is careful, expectant observation. Hospitalization is indicated if close observation is not possible at home, if there is any question about the severity, or if the process appears to be worsening. The usual treatment at home consists of the use of a vaporizer, increased oral intake of fluids, and bed rest. Syrup of ipecac in subemetic doses (1 drop per month of age up to 2 years) is believed to help resolve spasmodic croup syndrome. Caution should be exercised when using ipecac in any child with severe obstruction to avoid aspiration of the vomitus.

After examination in the emergency room has determined that the child does not have epiglottitis, inhalation of 2.25 percent racemic epinephrine nebulization may be tried (Adair et al., 1971). Even if the patient shows improvement after such inhalation, response may be temporary (Westley, 1978). The patient therefore should be observed in the emergency room for at least 4 hours after a satisfactory response.

In the hospital, the respiratory rate, the sternal retractions, the amount of stridor, and the development of cyanosis should be monitored carefully. The patient should be placed in a room close to a nursing station. At the same time, every effort must be made to keep the child quiet and undisturbed since agitation and apprehension may exacerbate obstruction. The use of blood gas determinations, which would otherwise be an extremely helpful method of assessing severity, therefore should be limited. Moisture and increased inspired oxygen tension can be provided in a mist tent. However, the potential benefits must be balanced against the disadvantages of increasing the child's anxiety and making observation more difficult. Effective drug treatment is limited. If symptoms respond to racemic epinephrine, treatment may be continued with doses given every 1 to 2 hours; however, the patient should be observed carefully for marked or persistent tachycardia. Leipzig and coworkers (1979) suggested that corticosteroid therapy may be helpful, but this therapy is still controversial.

The major complications of the syndrome are respiratory failure and cardiorespiratory arrest. These are uncommon, and tracheostomy is required in only 2 to 8 percent of hospitalized cases.

A small number of children develop croup repeatedly. These children usually have abnormal airways reactivity, as demonstrated by inhalation challenge tests; they may eventually have typical asthma attacks (Zach et al., 1980). Recurrent croup may represent a variant of asthma, and treatment with bronchodilators should be attempted.

DIFFERENTIAL DIAGNOSIS OF ACUTE OBSTRUCTION

In addition to epiglottitis, croup, and atypical asthma, other acute illnesses should be considered, as noted in Table 39–1 and Table 39–2. Acute pharyngeal infections, such as peritonsillar abscess, are rare but potentially fatal. They should be considered in a child thought to have epiglottitis and should be sought with careful examination of the pharynx or lateral neck roentgenogram, observing the same precautions noted earlier. Aspirated foreign bodies rarely cause upper airway obstructions in children but instead cause wheezing and pneumonia. They should be suspected when abrupt

TABLE 39–1. Acute Laryngeal Obstruction in Children

Croup
Epiglottitis
Foreign body
Pharyngeal infection (peritonsillar, retropharyngeal)
Trauma (physical, thermal, chemical)
Pertussis
Diphtheria
Anaphylaxis
Vocal cord paralysis

onset of obstruction and croup exist, and a history of aspiration should be identified. Laryngeal obstruction may occur with physical trauma, inhalation of smoke, or ingestion and aspiration of irritant chemicals (e.g., caustics, hydrocarbons).

Pertussis and diphtheria both are rare causes of respiratory obstruction in children. Pertussis and croup are characterized by a tight spasmodic cough, and both are observed in younger children. Immunization history, peripheral lymphocytosis, and duration of the illness should facilitate differentiation. Diphtheria may be confused with epiglottitis and should be considered if immunizations are not complete or if a dense pharyngeal membrane is present. Laryngeal edema and obstruction may occur during anaphylaxis but almost never occur without accompanying urticaria, angioedema, and wheezing.

In adults, the most common cause of acute obstruction is local trauma. Aspirated foreign bodies including food, lodge in the larynx much more commonly in adults than in children. Obstruction is severe and may be fatal unless the object is quickly dislodged with the Heimlich maneuver or unless the object is small. Direct laryngoscopy is diagnostic. Hereditary angioedema is rare in adults and unheard of in children. A history of recurrent angioedema, of recurrent painful gastrointestinal obstruction, or of peripheral angioedema suggests the diagnosis. Iatrogenic causes of obstruction include

TABLE 39–2. Acute Laryngeal Obstruction in Adults

Trauma
Epiglottitis
Foreign body
Angioedema
Iatrogenesis
Infection
Hysterical aphonia

thyroid surgery, producing recurrent laryngeal nerve paralysis and acute obstruction; tracheal intubation, producing delayed obstruction; and inhaled steroid therapy, producing myopathy of the vocal cords. Epiglottitis and severe pharyngitis are much less common causes of obstructions in adults than in children. Hysterical aphonia rarely causes severe obstruction and characteristically disappears.

DIFFERENTIAL DIAGNOSIS OF CHRONIC AIRWAY OBSTRUCTION

The differential diagnosis of chronic airway obstruction in children and adults is outlined in Table 39–3 and Table 39–4. It should be apparent that the most common causes are infectious and congenital in children. In adults, the etiology is more frequently degenerative, traumatic, or cancerous.

Vocal cord paralysis is a common cause of laryngeal obstruction in the neonatal period. Infants typically are aphonic with mild to severe inspiratory stridor. Approximately a third of cases are not explained by birth or surgical trauma or by structural, infectious, or functional central nervous system disease. Rarely, vocal cord paralysis may be familial (Cunningham et al., 1985).

Obstructive sleep apnea occurs in children and adults. In children it almost invariably is associated with hypertrophied tonsils and adenoids, whereas in adults it seems to occur in the absence of structural abnormalities, with the possible exception of obesity, and is thought to be caused by muscular hypotonia and incoordination. Thus, obstruction is apparent to some extent when children are examined while awake but is not apparent when adults are examined while awake.

TABLE 39–3. Chronic Upper Airway Obstruction in Children

Laryngotracheomalacia
Congenital malformations
Structural
Neurologic
Adenotonsillar hypertrophy
Obstructive sleep apnea
Iatrogenesis
Postintubation, steroids
Neoplasms
Hemangiomas
Polyps
External compression

TABLE 39–4. Chronic Upper Airway Obstruction in Adults

Neoplasm
Trauma
Physical
Smoking
Iatrogenesis
Postoperative
Postintubation
Steroid myopathy
Obstructive sleep apnea
Congenital (neurologic)
Polyp
Cricoarytenoid ankylosis
Hypothyroidism
Hysterical aphonia

Tracheomalacia and bronchomalacia are syndromes caused by excessive flexibility of the larynx, trachea, and bronchi. The syndromes are characterized by signs of obstruction, chiefly during expiration, noisy breathing, and recurrent infections. The conditions occur predominantly in infancy, usually early infancy, and spontaneous resolution occurs with age.

Expiratory obstruction is associated with tracheomalacia because intrathoracic airways are affected by pressures generated during respiration. During quiet respiration, with normal, compliant lungs, intrathoracic pressure changes are minor. Expiration occurs as the elasticity of the lungs and thorax restores expiratory volume, and little positive pressure is developed. However, during a cough with normal lungs, or during quiet respiration with obstructive lung disease, pressures of 20 cm H_2O or greater may be found.

Expiratory compression forces are not present throughout the tracheobronchial tree. In the very narrow airway at the upper trachea, airway pressure is near atmospheric level (zero); it is here that intrathoracic pressure exerts its chief effect. Progressing from the trachea toward the alveoli, pressure inside the airways approaches that in the surrounding lung. At some point, airway and lung pressures are equal, and there are no collapsing forces in the more distal airways. This equal pressure point is in the segmental bronchi of the normal lung. It is believed by some that tracheomalacia almost always is due to coincident lung disease and secondary tracheal compression, since cases studied at autopsy rarely demonstrate absent cartilage (Baxter and Dunbar, 1963) and since tracheomalacia usually is most apparent in the upper trachea (Wittenborg et al., 1967). An obvious exception is the localized deformity of the trachea or bronchi that follows removal of an extrabronchial mass.

The onset of symptoms may be abrupt, beginning with a respiratory infection in early infancy, but the syndrome may have a more insidious onset. A barking, croupy cough is prominent and resolves more slowly than does the usual croup. There may be an associated stridor, but evidence of loose, moist expiratory obstruction and wheezing is more common. Crying or exertion may promote obstruction and thus precipitate bouts of coughing. Recurrent infections are common, and with each one the pattern of respiratory distress with obstruction, brassy cough, and slow resolution repeats itself.

In the rare case of localized absence of bronchial cartilage, the chest roentgenogram may show localized hyperinflation of a lobe or lung. More commonly, one sees only peribronchial or interstitial infiltrates and generalized hyperinflation. Inspiratory and expiratory radiograms show excessive motion in the trachea, just under the glottis. This excessive motion is even more apparent with cinefluorography. In the occasional case in which bronchoscopy is performed, the tracheal and bronchial walls may be seen to flex inward during expiration. In general the prognosis is good. Mortality is low, and most children improve spontaneously by 3 to 4 years of age. Treatment is nonspecific and supportive. Humidified oxygen may be necessary, and chest percussion and postural drainage may be helpful. Bacterial infections should be treated aggressively with antibiotics. Above all, careful follow-up should be maintained in order to detect any significant increase in respiratory difficulty. Surgical therapy rarely is indicated. In general, even the localized deformity associated with extrabronchial obstruction is too extensive for successful resection. Lobar resection for localized bronchomalacia may improve oxygenation by removing hyperinflated lung that may be compressing adjacent normal lung. It is important to investigate and manage any suspected associated lung disease.

OBSTRUCTIVE LESIONS OR MASSES

Many patients with lesions in and around airways present with symptoms that mimic croup or asthma. These lesions may be categorized into extrabronchial, intrabronchial, and intramural.

Pulmonary function test results may provide important information about the site and nature of obstructive lesions, as shown in Figure 39–1 (see also Chapter 38). The flow-volume loop is much more helpful in this regard than the simple spirogram. Fixed obstructive lesions reduce both maximal inspiratory and expiratory flows; a characteristic limitation of maximal flow in both inspiration and expiration is produced. Variable (flexible) extrathoracic obstruction is reduced during inspiration, since luminal pressure is negative in the airways at that phase of respiration, and constriction is accentuated. On the other hand, variable intrathoracic lesions produce maximal obstruction during expiration when extraluminal pressures compress the airways.

Extrabronchial Lesions

Neoplasms may involve intrathoracic structures and thus impinge on airways (Whittaker and Lynn, 1973). The most common include lymphoid tissue (Hodgkin disease, lymphosarcoma, leukemia, lymph node metastases); neural crest tissue (neuroblastoma, ganglioneuroma, ganglioneuroblastoma); thymus (thymoma, lymphosarcoma, teratoma); and miscellaneous tissues (teratoma, cystic hygroma).

Lymphoid tissue may be involved in nonneoplastic inflammatory processes. The thymus is large characteristically in infants and may sometimes impinge in the airway if located high in the thoracic outlet. Similarly, lymphadenopathy associated with tuberculosis or fungal or bacterial lung disease may compromise the airway. Primary pulmonary tuberculosis almost invariably appears with hilar adenopathy; in most instances, a parenchymal lesion cannot be demonstrated, even though it necessarily exists. Sarcoidosis occasionally involves paratracheal nodes and almost always produces bilateral hilar lymphadenopathy; parenchymal lesions are present in about half the cases. Bronchogenic cysts are uncommon. They usually are single and are more common in the area of the right main stem bronchus and to the right of the trachea.

A variety of vascular anomalies can compress the airways. They most commonly produce a vascular ring syndrome (right aortic arch with persistent ligamentum of ductus arteriosus; double aortic arch), with compression of both the esophagus and trachea. In addition, a pulmonary sling may be produced by an aberrant left pulmonary artery, arising from the right and crossing the trachea and left main stem bronchus to supply the left lung, or by an innominate artery, arising to the left of the trachea. Finally, hemangiomas may compress the airways.

It should be apparent that most lesions causing extrabronchial compression are located in the mediastinum. The anterior mediastinum contains the thymus and the anterior aspect of the heart. The most common anterior medias-

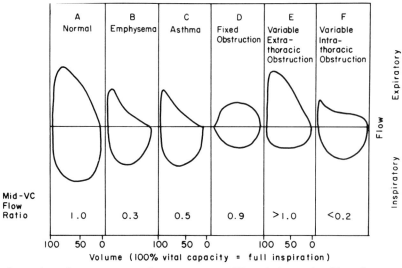

FIGURE 39–1. Flow volume loops in various obstructive states. VC = vital capacity. (From Lazarus, A.: Pulmonary function tests in upper airway obstruction. Basics of RD. 3:8, 1980.)

tinal masses are hyperplastic thymus and tera-tomas; when enlarged, they frequently cause respiratory symptoms. The posterior mediastinum contains principally neural tissue and the esophagus. The most common posterior mediastinal masses are neurogenic tumors; respiratory symptoms are encountered only late in the course. The middle mediastinum contains the heart, airways, great vessels, and lymph nodes. The most common middle mediastinal masses are hyperplastic or neoplastic lymph nodes and bronchogenic cysts; they induce respiratory symptoms early.

Certain lesions tend to be related to age. Bronchogenic cysts, cystic hygromas, and tera-tomas are most common before 2 years of age. Lymphomas, leukemic adenitis, and fungal adenitis appear more frequently in school-age children and adolescents.

Symptoms are produced either by direct compression of the airway or by secondary complications. Compression may lead to a persistent wheeze, atelectasis, or air trapping and hyperinflation. Stridor is unusual unless the lesion is high in the superior mediastinum. Vagal reflexes may lead to more widespread wheezing. Secondary problems may arise when secretions cannot be cleared and become infected or when a vessel eroded by the mass bleeds into the airway or mediastinum. Symptoms begin insidiously unless bleeding or infection occurs or unless a cyst ruptures into the airway. Usually an irritative cough, stridorous respiration, and wheezing or dysphagia constitute the earliest symptoms. Chest discomfort, pain, fever, and weight loss usually appear later.

Routine posteroanterior and lateral chest roentgenograms usually will localize the lesion to a particular mediastinal section. Examination of the tracheobronchial air columns may demonstrate local compression. A barium esophagram may further help define the extent and location of the mass. Tomograms are useful but have been replaced by computerized axial tomography, which depicts structural detail more clearly. Laboratory studies furnish supporting evidence. A hemogram may demonstrate anemia or leukocytosis; the sedimentation rate may be elevated. Skin tests for tuberculosis and serology for fungal infections should be performed in all cases. Sputum or tracheal aspirates may be examined for cytologic and fungal cultures. Urinary vanillylmandelic acid and homovanillic acid levels will be elevated with neuroblastomas.

Bronchoscopy may be extremely helpful, especially with the availability of the flexible bronchoscope. The site of the lesion can be identified, and culture, cytology, and biopsy obtained as appropriate. Although major technical problems still exist with bronchoscopy in young children, rapid progress is being made so that bronchoscopy may be a reasonable diagnostic procedure even in young children in the near future.

The treatment of most lesions is surgical, and prognosis depends on the specific lesion.

Intrabronchial lesions, which will be discussed subsequently, and asthma constitute the major conditions in the differential diagnosis. It is well to recognize that a more common disease, such as asthma, may coexist with one of these lesions and may further complicate diagnosis and treatment. For this reason, every child with *severe asthma* should have a chest roentgenogram.

Intrabronchial Lesions

Intrabronchial obstructive lesions usually are due to foreign bodies or neoplasms. Foreign bodies consist most often of particles of food, which usually lodge in the trachea or main stem bronchi. However, anything may be aspirated and may lodge anywhere. Intrabronchial neoplasms most often reported in children are bronchial adenomas and papillomas. Papillomas may be multiple, recurrent, and sometimes are associated with laryngeal papillomas.

Obstruction from intrabronchial lesions may be partial, leading to localized wheezing and distal hyperinflation, or may be complete, leading to absorptive atelectasis. Infection frequently develops, usually localized to the involved bronchus or to the lobe served by that bronchus. Generalized wheezing may occur, presumably mediated by vagal reflexes, and can confuse the clinical picture of localized obstruction.

Patients with intrabronchial obstruction usually present with cough, which may be irritative at first and then productive, with dyspnea and wheezing. Foreign bodies should be suspected when symptoms begin abruptly, especially when associated with gagging and apneic episodes, particularly in children 6 months to 6 years of age. The usual radiographic finding is localized hyperinflation or atelectasis. This is associated with a visible foreign object, if the foreign body is radiopaque. Localized air trapping may be suggested in expiratory films or fluoroscopy by marked deviation away from the involved lobe on expiration. Alternatively, decubitus films may demonstrate that mediastinal structures shift toward the normal lung when it is dependent but not toward the hyperinflated lung.

If an intrabronchial lesion is suspected, bronchoscopy should be performed as soon as possible but only by an experienced bronchoscopist and anesthesiologist. This procedure in infants requires special equipment and expertise and should be performed in a hospital that is equipped for the study of infants. Occasionally, pneumonia or severe respiratory distress must be treated prior to bronchoscopy. The foreign body usually can be removed at bronchoscopy. Excisional biopsy specimens of tumors may be obtained in this way as well. Only bronchial adenomas require lobectomy.

Intrabronchial lesions should be suspected in any child with sudden onset of wheezing who resists the usual therapy for asthma, especially if there is any suggestion in the history, physical examination, or laboratory evaluation of a bronchial lesion. It is well to remember that wheezing may be generalized and may respond briefly or partially to bronchodilator therapy.

Intramural Lesions

Intramural lesions include neoplasms and postinflammatory mural thickenings. Purely intramural neoplasms are rare and include hamartomas, bronchial adenomas, fibromas, leiomyosarcomas, and angiomas. In general, most lesions expand into the airway to produce intraluminal obstruction, rather than infiltrate into the bronchial wall. Postinflammatory intramural obstruction occurs most often after prolonged intubation or after removal of a foreign body or tumor. An acute obstruction may be related to a reversible process (edema and inflammation), which may become both irreversible and more severe as a cicatrix forms.

Depending on the level of obstruction, illness may begin with stridor or wheezing observed chiefly during expiration. In general, cough is not prominent and when present is productive. With upper respiratory infections or other conditions that increase tracheal secretions and inflammation, respiratory distress becomes more severe and may lead to acute respiratory failure.

Chest roentgenogram may show a localized constriction in the air bronchogram. Neoplasms almost invariably are associated with masses apparent in nodes around the airways or in lung parenchyma. Barium esophagrams, tomograms, and computerized axial tomography can be helpful in defining the nature and extent of the lesion. Bronchoscopy may be helpful but should be employed with particular caution when significant obstruction is present. The major lesions to be differentiated are other mass obstructive lesions. For this reason, bronchoscopy, careful radiologic examination, and exploratory thoracotomy should be considered when the diagnosis is in question.

Treatment is nonspecific in the case of inflammatory lesions, but humidification may be helpful. It is appropriate to use bronchodilators to relieve any bronchospastic components and to reduce local vasodilation; epinephrine or phenylephrine aerosols may accomplish both. Steroids may be helpful in preventing or treating postintubation obstruction. Surgical dilatation, resection, or tracheostomy has been the only recourse in chronic cases.

REFERENCES

Adair, J.C., Ring, W.H., Jordan, W.S., et al.: Ten-year experience with IPPB in the treatment of acute laryngotracheobronchitis. Anesth. Analg. 50:649, 1971.

Baxter, J.D., Dunbar, J.S.: Tracheomalacia. Ann. Otol. Rhinol. Laryngol. 72:1013, 1963.

Cunningham, M.J., Eavey, R.D., Shannon, D.C.: Familial vocal cord dysfunction. Pediatrics 76:750–753, 1985.

Glezen, W.P., Loda, F.A., Clyde, W.A., Jr., et al.: Epidemiologic patterns of acute lower respiratory disease of children in a pediatric group practice. J. Pediatr. 78:397, 1971.

Holinger, L.D., Holinger, P.C., Hollinger P.H.: Etiology of bilateral abductor vocal cord paralysis: A review of 389 cases. Ann. Rhinol. Laryngol. Otol. 85:428–435, 1976.

Lazarus, A.: Pulmonary function tests in upper airway obstruction. Basics RD. 3:8, 1980.

Leipzig, B., Oski, F.A., Cummings, C.W., et al.: A prospective randomized study to determine the efficacy of steroids in treatment of croup. J. Pediatr. 94:194, 1979.

Margolis, C.Z., Ingram, D.L., Meyer, J.H: Routine tracheostomy in *Hemophilus influenzae* type b epiglottitis. J. Pediatr. 81:1150, 1972.

Mayosmith, M.F., Hirsch, P.J., Wodzinski, S.F., Schiffman, F.J.: Acute epiglottitis in adults: An eight-year experience in the state of Rhode Island. New Engl. J. Med. 314:1133–1139, 1986.

Milko, D.A., Marshall, G., Striker, T.W.: Nasotracheal intubation in the treatment of acute epiglottitis. Pediatrics 53:674, 1974.

Miller, R.D., Hyatt, R.E.: Obstructing lesions of the larynx and trachea: Clinical and physiologic characteristics. Mayo Clin. Proc. 44:145–161, 1969.

Welliver, R.C., Wong, D.T., Middleton, F., Jr., et al.: Role of parainfluenza virus specific IgE in pathogenesis of croup or wheezing subsequent to infection. J. Pediatr. 101:889–896, 1982.

Westley, C.R., Cotton, E.K., Brooks, J.B.: Nebulized racemic epinephrine by IPPB for the treatment of croup: A double-blind study. Am. J. Dis. Child. 132:484, 1978.

Whittaker, L.D., Jr., Lynn, H.B.: Mediastinal tumors and cysts in the pediatric patient. Surg. Clin. North Am. 53:893, 1973.

Wittenborg, M.H., Gyepes, M.T., Crocker, D.: Tracheal dynamics in infants with respiratory distress, stridor and collapsing trachea. Radiology 88:563, 1967.

Zach, M.S., Schnall, R.P., Landau, L.I.: Upper and lower airway hyperreactivity in recurrent croup. Am. Rev. Respir. Dis. 11:979–983, 1980.

40

Acute Bronchopulmonary Infections

ELLIOT F. ELLIS, M.D.

ACUTE BRONCHITIS

Acute bronchitis is a frequently diagnosed but poorly characterized condition in both children and adults. It is scarcely mentioned in four of the five major American pediatric and internal medicine textbooks (Hoekelman et al., 1978; Rudolph, 1982; Petersdorf et al., 1983; Wyngaarden and Smith, 1985) and is, in a sense, an obsolete diagnostic term which reflects a concept that various inflammation-causing agents affect anatomically distinct divisions of the respiratory tract. Although signs and symptoms referable to one part of the airway may predominate, the entire respiratory tract usually is involved when inflammation is induced by infectious agents (especially viral) or toxins (e.g., chemical fumes, smoke). Adult patients who are diagnosed as having a "cold" have evidence of peripheral airway dysfunction (Cate et al., 1973; Picken et al., 1972). Children with viral croup have evidence of lower respiratory tract involvement (Newth et al., 1972). Since the term "bronchitis" is so firmly implanted in medical practice, however, it will be employed, recognizing its limitations, as noted.

Acute bronchitis is a common manifestation of a viral respiratory tract infection. All the major viral agents, including respiratory syncytial virus, parainfluenza virus, adenovirus, rhinovirus, and influenza virus, may act as etiologic agents. There is little evidence that bacterial agents, other than *Bordetella pertussis* and *Mycobacterium tuberculosis,* have primary roles in acute bronchitis, either in children or adults.

Cough is the principal symptom of bronchitis and is due to stimulation of afferent vagal receptors in the airway. During the early stage of the illness, the cough is dry and irritative in

character, and adventitious sounds in the chest characteristically are absent. After 3 to 4 days, the cough becomes moist and looser, and at this time rhonchi and rattling sounds may be heard on auscultation. Sputum generally is not produced in significant quantities. Typically, the chest roentgenogram is normal. There is no specific treatment. Suppression of cough with a codeine-containing expectorant is indicated during the acute phase of the illness. Proven secondary bacterial infection is rare, and antimicrobials are not indicated. Use of a humidifier may make the patient more comfortable but does not influence the course of the illness. Individuals subjected to recurrent attacks of acute "bronchitis" should be carefully examined for evidence of underlying illness, particularly asthma.

Asthmatic bronchitis, "wheezy bronchitis," or capillary bronchitis are diagnostic terms applied to children, particularly those under 5 years of age, who wheeze with each respiratory infection but who are essentially free of respiratory symptoms in between. Williams and McNicol (1969), in a careful, long-term epidemiologic study, were unable to separate "wheezy bronchitis" as a distinctive entity from asthma during early life. There were no discernible differences in clinical features nor in outcomes of children diagnosed as having wheezy bronchitis from those with asthma. When applied to infants and children, the terms asthmatic bronchitis, capillary bronchitis, and wheezy bronchitis are euphemisms used by physicians who do not fully comprehend the spectrum of asthma in childhood (see Chapter 41). The young child who has recurrent episodes of wheezing with viral respiratory infections should be considered as having asthma until proved otherwise. The term "asthmatic bronchitis" often is used by internists and pulmonologists to describe adults who have chronic bronchitis and periodic episodes of acute airway obstruction with wheezing. The distinction between asthma and asthmatic bronchitis is fuzzy, and for this reason the term should be abandoned. In most major internal medicine textbooks, "asthmatic bronchitis" is scarcely mentioned, and if so, only in the aforementioned context.

Pertussis, which represents the most severe and best example of bacterial bronchitis, occurs principally in children and is due to a gram-negative rod, *B. pertussis.* Other agents, such as *B. parapertussis* and adenovirus, also have been reported to cause a similar clinical picture (Connor, 1970; Krugman and Ward, 1977). The illness begins with a highly infectious catarrhal stage that lasts 1 to 2 weeks, followed by several weeks of severe paroxysmal coughing. Coughing episodes may be severe enough to cause cyanosis and apnea. The greatest morbidity and mortality are recorded in infants less than 1 year of age, and particularly less than 6 months of age (Brooks and Buchanan, 1970). In young infants, *Chlamydia trachomatis* infections may be confused with pertussis.

When pertussis was prevalent in the past, the disease was noted to be the provocateur of the initial attack of asthma in some children. This observation is of particular interest because of the ability of *B. pertussis* to produce beta-adrenergic blockade that persists for many weeks in animals. Furthermore, airway irritability in individuals recovering from pertussis appears to persist for many months. Children who have had pertussis recently may respond to subsequent viral illnesses with paroxysms of coughing similar to those observed during the pertussis illness. The frequency of asthma does not appear to be higher in pertussis-immunized children compared with those who have not been immunized, and thus there is little to suggest that pertussis vaccination may predispose children to asthma. Pertussis in adults usually occurs in a modified form, reflecting the partial immune status of previously vaccine-inoculated individuals. The cough may be nonparoxysmal and of brief duration. Lymphocytosis may not be present. This form of pertussis, because of its atypical clinical manifestations, may not be considered in the differential diagnosis of severe, persistent, and particularly bothersome nocturnal cough. Hospital employees so affected may represent sources of infection to infants and children (Editorial, 1968; Kurt et al., 1972).

The characteristic whooping cough during the paroxysmal or spasmodic stage of the illness suggests a diagnosis of pertussis. An additional aid includes the peripheral white blood cell count, which usually demonstrates an absolute lymphocytosis (counts as high as 150,000 to 200,000/mm³ have been reported); but this finding may be absent in infants or partially immune patients. The lymphocytosis, consisting of mostly small mature T and B cells, is due to a disturbance in the normal pattern of lymphocyte recirculation, in which the rate of entry

of lymphocytes from the blood into the lymphoid tissue is substantially decreased (Morse, 1976). Although culture of the posterior nasopharynx is an excellent method to establish the diagnosis, most clinical bacteriology laboratories do not maintain the special media (Bordet-Gengou agar) needed to isolate the organism. Fluorescent antibody staining of nasopharyngeal secretions is a rapid and reasonably reliable diagnostic technique. Although antimicrobial therapy does not influence the course of the disease in its paroxysmal stage, erythromycin should be given for 14 days to render the patient noninfectious (Bass et al., 1969; Altemeier et al., 1977). In several European studies, albuterol (salbutamol) reduced the frequency of paroxysms of coughing and severity of illness. Corticosteroids alter the severity and duration of pertussis, and their use should be considered in patients with severe disease (Zoomboulakis et al., 1973). Pertussis is a preventable disease, and while current vaccines do not confer complete or lifelong immunity, immunization of all susceptible infants and children is clearly indicated. From a public health perspective, the risks of serious adverse reactions (encephalopathy, 1/300,000 immunizations) to pertussis vaccine pale in significance to the dangers of the disease (see also Chapter 8).

Primary tuberculosis with endobronchial involvement may produce true bronchitis with signs and symptoms of large airway involvement. Fungal involvement of the bronchi rarely is encountered in children or adults on a primary basis; it is encountered principally in immunocompromised patients. Bronchopulmonary aspergillosis occasionally is diagnosed in children in the United States; in adults with asthma, its prevalence is substantially higher. (This disorder is discussed in Chapter 47.) The increasing use of potent surface-active corticosteroids in patients with asthma has not, despite concerns, led to monilial bronchitis secondary to local depression of cell-mediated immunity.

Chemical causes of acute bronchitis in children and adults include aspiration of gastric contents due to gastroesophageal reflux, smoke inhalation from burning buildings, air pollution in heavily polluted areas, and either active or passive exposure to cigarette smoke. Of great concern is the adverse effect of cigarette smoke on children reared in homes where the parents, particularly the mother, smoke cigarettes. Children so exposed have a significantly increased incidence of symptoms referable to the respiratory tract (Ferris et al., 1985). Furthermore, passive exposure to cigarette smoke has a deleterious effect on the natural history of asthma in childhood (Weiss, 1980). In adults, the combination of a history of childhood respiratory problems, particularly of the "bronchial" type, and cigarette smoking is a malignant combination, leading to more rapid deterioration in pulmonary function as compared with nonsmoking subjects. Therapy of noninfectious acute bronchitis initially is symptomatic and subsequently is directed toward treatment or avoidance of the causative factor.

PNEUMONIA

Pneumonia both in children and in adults is secondary to failure of pulmonary defense mechanisms, to infection with a particularly virulent microorganism, or to exposure to an overwhelming inoculum. Particularly in adults, factors that interfere with normal host defenses are known to predispose them to infections of the lower respiratory tract. These include (1) alteration in the state of consciousness (alcoholism, stroke, seizures, drug intoxication, anesthesia), leading to aspiration of oropharyngeal flora; (2) exposure to cigarette smoke, leading to inhibition of mucociliary clearance and macrophage function; (3) serious underlying disease states (congestive heart failure, diabetes, chronic obstructive pulmonary disease, immune deficiency that includes acquired immune deficiency syndrome); (4) preceding viral upper respiratory infection; (5) malnutrition; and (6) use of immunosuppressive agents. In one large series of adults with pneumonia, 82 percent were found to have an underlying disease as a predisposing cause (Dorff et al., 1973). In infants and children, impairment of host defense mechanisms as a cause predisposing them to pneumonia is less evident. Susceptibility to

infection on the basis of lack of prior exposure to the infectious agent, overwhelming inoculum, and impairment of immune mechanism by preceding viral infection appear to be responsible for most instances of pneumonia.

Pneumonia is one of the most frequent and serious infections of children and adults. Infants less than 1 year of age and the elderly are prone to develop the most severe illness. Almost every class of microorganism has been shown to produce pneumonia, e.g., bacteria, viruses, bacteria-like agents (mycoplasma, chlamydia), fungi, mycobacteria, parasites, and rickettsia.

In neonates, in the elderly (especially nursing home residents), and in alcoholics, bacterial infections predominate. Viruses account for most respiratory illness in childhood and in adulthood, whereas *Mycoplasma* causes a significant proportion of disease in school-age children, adolescents, and young adults.

Identification of the infectious agents that cause pneumonia frequently is difficult. There are, however, certain features of bacterial pneumonias that help to differentiate them from viral or mycoplasma disease (Table 40–1). The onset of bacterial illness usually is sudden, and the patient appears toxic. In the infant, examination of the chest may be normal, but in the older child and adult evidence of consolidation is present. Radiographs of the chest often demonstrate lobar or segmental consolidation, and pleural effusions frequently are present. The white blood cell count usually is in excess of $15,000/mm.^3$

There is no simple method to identify the specific bacteria that may be etiologic in children. Sputum generally is unavailable, and throat cultures are of little value in establishing the diagnosis since pathogenetic bacteria, such as *Streptococcus pneumoniae*, inhabit the nasopharynx of healthy children (Loda et al., 1975).

TABLE 40–1. Characteristic Findings in Bacterial and Viral Pneumonia

Findings	Bacterial	Viral
Onset	Sudden	Gradual
Progression	Rapid	Slow
Toxicity	Severe	Mild to moderate
Cough	Productive	Nonproductive
Fever	High	Low
Physical findings	Unilateral evidence of consolidation	Bilateral rales
Radiographic findings	Lobar or segmental infiltrate; pleural effusions common	Diffuse, patchy bronchopneumonia; pleural effusions uncommon
White blood cell count	$>15,000/mm^3$	$\leq 15,000/mm^3$
Response to antibiotics	Good	None

Blood cultures yield the causative agent in only about 25 percent of cases. Lung aspiration represents the most direct method to establish the diagnosis, but it usually is reserved for the seriously ill child or for the child who fails to respond to therapy.

In adults the value of examination and culture of expectorated sputum have received substantially more emphasis than in children. Gram stains of sputum are routinely made, and the number of neutrophils, eosinophils, and epithelial cells per high power field are counted. (Many epithelial cells indicate significant contamination of the specimen with oropharyngeal contents and diminish the value of the specimen.) The morphology and staining characteristics of the bacteria are noted. Low carrier rates of pneumococci and *Haemophilus influenzae* in normal adults make the presence of these organisms in sputum samples in disease states easier to interpret. However, some investigators question the value of Gram stain and culture as a means of etiologic diagnosis of pneumonia in adults. Transtracheal aspiration and percutaneous lung aspiration are carried out when the clinical circumstances indicate that a specific microbiologic diagnosis is essential for the patient's well being.

Streptococcus pneumoniae remains the most common bacterial cause of pneumonia in children and in adults. In particular, 50 to 90 percent of cases of community acquired suppurative pneumonias are due to *S. pneumoniae* (McFarlane et al., 1982). The clinical picture of pneumococcal pneumonia is similar in children and adults; however, abdominal pain often is present in children and may lead to the mistaken diagnosis of appendicitis. Patients with pneumococcal pneumonia respond rapidly to penicillin therapy. Small pleural effusions when present often resolve without drainage.

Staphylococcus aureus causes a severe, rapidly progressive pneumonia in the young infant. Empyema and pneumatoceles are common. The diagnosis often is established when the empyema fluid is drained and yields the organism. Unlike pneumococcal pneumonia, staphylococcal pneumonia is slow to resolve despite effective treatment with penicillinase-resistant penicillins. Ultimately, pneumatoceles and pleural changes disappear, leaving no sequelae (Ceruti et al., 1971). In adults, *S. aureus* accounts for up to 10 percent of community acquired pneumonias. In adults, the disease often strikes within a few days after the onset of influenza. Mortality may be high (30 to 50 percent). The

diagnosis is suggested by poor response to antipneumococcal therapy, appearance of multiple areas of pulmonary consolidation, rapid cavitation of bronchopneumonic infiltrate, or development of pleural empyema.

Haemophilus influenzae type b is being recognized more often as a cause of pneumonia in both children and adults. Unfortunately, there are no distinctive signs or symptoms that suggest *H. influenzae* as the etiologic agent. However, it should be suspected in the patient who fails to respond to penicillin therapy. Unlike pneumococcal disease, *Haemophilus* has a more insidious onset and tends to produce a subacute process with segmental, lobar, bronchopneumonic, or interstitial infiltrates. The illness is slow to respond to appropriate therapy. Effusions occur in 50 percent of cases (Honig et al., 1973). The diagnosis may be established through blood culture results or demonstration of the organism in pleural fluid. Countercurrent immunoelectrophoresis may prove helpful in establishing the diagnosis. Since the appearance of ampicillin-resistant *H. influenzae*, chloramphenicol has become the drug of choice in the seriously ill child. The true incidence of this disease remains to be established, but reports suggest that few childhood pneumonias are due to *H. influenzae* (Ginsburg et al., 1979). In adults, 2 to 18 percent of acute community acquired pneumonias are thought to be due to *H. influenzae* (Dorff et al., 1973; Hirschmann and Everett, 1979).

The elderly and nursing home residents have substantially different microbiologic etiologies of acute community acquired pneumonia. Gram-negative organisms, especially *Klebsiella pneumoniae*, *Enterobacter aerogenes*, *H. influenzae*, and *S. aureus*, are commonly the causes of bacterial pneumonia in older individuals. Aspiration pneumonia often yields multiple bacterial pathogens, including organisms' residing in the mouth, such as aerobic and nonaerobic streptococci, *Bacteroides spp.*, staphylococci, and gram-negative enteric bacteria. The lobes of the lung most often involved in aspiration pneumonia are the posterior segments of the upper lobes and the basilar segments of the lower lobes. Initially, treatment is begun empirically with clindamycin and gentamicin. Cefataxime, a third generation cephalosporin, may be added later.

Mycobacterium tuberculosis is an infrequent cause of pneumonia in children today (Kendig, 1977). The diagnosis often is considered only after the child fails to respond to routine antibiotic therapy. The presence of hilar adenopathy on the chest roentgenogram suggests the diagnosis, and a positive skin test reaction with PPD provides supportive evidence. Isolation of the organism from sputum, gastric washings, or urine confirms the diagnosis. In adults, tuberculosis continues to be an important communicable disease problem with approximately 25,000 new cases each year. Treatment with a combination of isoniazid and rifampin daily for 9 months currently is the best therapeutic regimen (Cynamon, 1986).

Mycoplasma pneumoniae accounts for 10 to 20 percent of all cases of pneumonia in children and is the primary cause of pneumonia among teenagers and young adults. It characteristically produces headache, low-grade fever, pharyngitis, and dry cough. Young infants may acquire the infection, but they manifest little or no disease (Fernald et al., 1975). Physical examination of the chest demonstrates rales. A chest radiograph shows an interstitial peribronchial infiltrate, which often is more impressive in extent than the physical examination suggests. Pleural effusion may be seen in 20 percent of cases. The diagnosis is suggested by the presence of serum cold agglutinins, which are found in 70 to 90 percent of patients with mycoplasma pneumonia (Chanock, 1965). Other infectious agents also have been shown to induce cold agglutinins (Sussman et al., 1966). Culture, which requires 2 to 3 weeks, and a specific complement fixation test remain the best methods to definitely establish the diagnosis. Numerous antibiotics have been used, but only erythromycin and tetracycline seem effective. Despite treatment, patients continue to excrete the organism (Foy et al., 1966). Immunity to *Mycoplasma* is not long lived, and repeated infections occur (Foy et al., 1977).

Chlamydia trachomatis, an organism known to be a cause of urethritis in adults, has been identified as a significant cause of respiratory tract disease in children. Estimates of incidence range as high as 30 percent of all pneumonias in infants hospitalized during the first 6 months of life. Respiratory symptoms appear at 2 to 3 weeks of age, with the diagnosis made typically at 6 weeks. Conjunctivitis is determined by history in 50 percent of the affected infants. Systemic signs are minimal, and the affected infants are not febrile. Nasal obstruction and mucoid discharge are common. Tachypnea in the range of 50 to 60 breaths per minute is the most prominent finding. A staccato-like cough is present, similar to that of pertussis but without a whoop. On examination of the chest, hyperinflation is evident, breath sounds are not diminished, and crepitant rales are heard throughout. Expiratory wheezing is absent or minimal. Chest roentgenogram shows hyperinflation and diffuse interstitial and patchy alveolar infiltrates. Blood gas values show a decreased PaO_2, with a normal or low $PaCO_2$. IgG and IgM are increased, and there is a mild absolute eosinophilia. The course of the illness is protracted. Cough and tachypnea may last for several weeks, and rales and abnormal X-ray findings for a month or more (Harrison et al., 1978; Hammarschlag, 1984). The organism requires tissue culture for diagnosis. Most recently, an enzyme linked immunosorbent assay (ELISA) has been developed. The illness is of particular interest because of its many similar features to bronchiolitis and asthma in early infancy.

At the present time, viruses are believed to be the most common cause of pneumonia in children and in adults as well. The clinical picture of viral pneumonia helps to distinguish it from bacterial disease (see Table 40–1). Most often, viral pneumonia is found concurrently with upper respiratory illness. The illness progresses gradually over several days. Although the majority of patients are not very ill, severe disease may occur, especially in the very young and the chronically ill. Tachypnea is a common finding as are other signs of pneumonia, such as crepitant rales.

There is little radiographic distinction between the various viral pneumonias. Roentgenograms show diffuse and localized involvement with both interstitial and alveolar patterns. Pleural effusions are uncommon. The total white blood cell count may be normal or minimally elevated.

Respiratory syncytial virus (RSV) is the single most important agent that causes lower respiratory tract disease in children. RSV rarely causes pneumonia in adults. It may be responsible for as much as 25 percent of all pneumonias in hospitalized children (Kim et al., 1973). It tends to occur in outbreaks in midwinter and early spring. Very young children are likely to develop severe disease, but the reasons are not well understood. Although maternal antibody was thought to play a direct role in the pathogenesis of the disease (Chanock et al., 1970), currently it is believed that cell-mediated immune reaction mounted by the infant or child is associated in some way with the evolution of the disease (Scott et al., 1978).

Parainfluenza virus is the second most frequent cause of viral pneumonia in children and, similar to RSV, is not a cause of pneumonia in adults. It cannot be distinguished clinically from other viral pneumonias.

Adenoviruses 1 and 5 commonly cause disease in children, and types 7 and 21 have been reported to cause severe disease with necrotizing bronchiolitis (Lang et al., 1969; Brown et al., 1973). Children less than 2 years of age are the most susceptible. Hospital outbreaks of adenovirus have resulted in mortality rates approaching 25 percent (Brown et al., 1973). Among survivors, significant sequelae, including pulmonary fibrosis, bronchiectasis, and obliterative bronchiolitis, have been observed (Lang et al., 1969). Adenoviral infections in civilian populations are infrequent. Military recruits, however, develop acute respiratory disease (ARD) and atypical pneumonia due to types 2, 4, and 7.

Influenza virus has the potential to produce croup and bronchiolitis as well as pneumonia in children. Fever may be the only clinical sign in very young infants. In a single report, temperatures greater than 39°C occurred in more than 50 percent of infected children (Wright et al., 1977). Pneumonitis may be severe and lead to death. Secondary bacterial pneumonia is not uncommon. Chronic pulmonary changes have been reported in children developing disease in the first 4 years of live. These changes include radiographic evidence of fibrosis, bronchiectasis, and obliterative bronchiolitis. Obstructive and restrictive pulmonary function defects also have been observed during long-term follow-ups (Laraya-Cuasay et al., 1977; Winterbauer et al., 1977). In contrast to the major causes of viral pneumonia in children, RSV and parainfluenza virus, influenza virus is a major cause of lower respiratory tract disease in adults. Influenza is primarily a tracheobronchitis which, despite causing significant morbidity, most often does not progress to pneumonia unless a secondary bacterial complication is present due to *S. aureus, S. pneumoniae,* or *H. influenzae.* Primary influenza pneumonia occurs principally in the elderly or those with underlying chronic pulmonary, cardiac, renal, or metabolic disease. In these populations, progression of disease with a hemorrhagic pneumonitis is rapid despite treatment, and mortality is high (Louria et al., 1959; Schwarzmann et al., 1971).

Although no specific treatment for influenza exists, amantadine has been effective in the chemoprophylaxis of type A but not type B.

Influenza vaccine prevents infection or reduces the severity of disease when the vaccine is matched with the prevailing strain of virus. Although indicated primarily for those at risk of serious complications of influenza infection (the elderly, those with chronic debilitating illness), many allergists and pulmonologists also recommend its use in adults with asthma. In asthmatic children, influenza is generally a milder illness and flu vaccine may or may not be indicated depending upon the clinical circumstances. In young asthmatic children in particular, influenza does not appear to be an asthmogenic virus. Whole virus vaccines are used in adults. The split virus (subvirion) vaccine should be given to children under 12 years to reduce the frequency of febrile responses (Gross et al., 1977).

Pneumonia may occur as part of the clinical picture in such common childhood viral diseases as rubeola, varicella-zoster, and rubella. Rubeola produces a giant cell pneumonia that is seen during large outbreaks of disease, especially in malnourished populations. As with influenza, secondary bacterial pneumonia may complicate the clinical picture. Varicella pneumonia is uncommon in normal children but is observed especially in immunosuppressed patients, such as those with leukemia. Normal adults who acquire varicella also are susceptible to primary varicella pneumonia. Pneumonia due to rubella is unusual; however, congenitally infected infants may develop a chronic form of pneumonia due to the virus. Pneumonia due to cytomegalovirus and pneumocystis is most often seen in immunocompromised hosts.

Occasionally, parasites are responsible for pneumonia in children and rarely in adults. In the United States, *Ascaris lumbricoides* and *Toxocara canis* both produce a symptom complex of wheezing, pulmonary infiltrates, and eosinophilia.

BRONCHIOLITIS

Bronchiolitis is an acute inflammatory disease of airways that range in caliber from 75μ to approximately $300\ \mu$. The principal pathologic features of acute bronchiolitis are necrosis of bronchiolar epithelium, which sloughs into the lumen; increase in mucous secretions; and inflammatory exudate; all of which combine to form dense plugs. A peribronchial infiltrate composed principally of lymphocytes occurs with some involvement of plasma cells and macrophages as well. There is edema of the submucosa and adventitial tissues but no damage to smooth muscle or elastic fibers. The degree and extent of bronchiolar obstruction determines whether acute obstructive emphysema (hyperinflation) or atelectasis occurs. Collateral ventilation is less well developed in the immature lung, small airways are disproportionately narrow, and elastic recoil properties of the lung are diminished. These factors make the infant particularly vulnerable to bronchiolar inflammatory disease.

Infants affected with bronchiolitis show clinical findings that have been correlated physiologically in adults with small airways disease, namely tachypnea, hypoxemia (often profound), and hyperinflation. Limited studies of mechanics of breathing in infants with bronchiolitis have shown a functional residual capacity (FRC) of about twice normal, decreased dynamic compliance, and increased total respiratory resistance. The abnormal physiologic findings generally revert to normal within 2 weeks after the acute illness. Bronchiolitis is principally a disease of the winter and spring months and affects males predominantly. Its peak incidence is during the first 6 months of life, at which time morbidity and mortality are higher. Epidemic bronchiolitis most often is due to RSV and, to a lesser extent, parainfluenza virus. *M. pneumoniae* can cause the bronchiolitis syndrome in older children.

Signs, Symptoms, and Laboratory Findings. Patients with the illness commonly present with signs and symptoms of a cold, which usually has been transmitted from another member of the family. Low-grade fever, with temperatures generally not in excess of 39°C, is present in the majority of patients. Tachypnea with respiratory rates of 50 to 60 breaths per minute, but sometimes as high as 80 breaths per minute, develops rapidly and is accompanied by cough, wheezing, and retractions. The infant appears dyspneic. Hyperinflation of the chest, which sometimes is extreme, is evident upon inspection, and hyperresonance is noted upon percussion. Crepitant rales may be heard in addition to diffuse wheezing. The liver often is palpable as a result of diaphragmatic depression by the overinflated lungs. Radiographic examination of the chest shows hyperlucency with increase in the anteroposterior diameter of the chest, retrosternal air, and flattening of the diaphragm. Small areas of increased density may be seen, representing atelectasis, and lung markings commonly are

increased. Blood gas analysis almost always shows arterial hypoxemia as a result of $\dot{V}/\dot{Q}$ abnormality. The $PaCO_2$ is variably altered as is the pH, depending upon the severity and stage of the illness. When acidosis (due to accumulation of organic acids) is present, a metabolic component may cause a substantial base deficit. The white blood cell count usually is moderately elevated.

Differential Diagnosis. The great majority of infants with bronchiolitis do not require hospitalization. In infants with more severe disease, various causes of airway obstruction in addition to congestive heart failure must be considered. Asthma is the disorder with which bronchiolitis most often is confused. If RSV is prevalent in the community and the infant is less than 6 months of age, the diagnosis of bronchiolitis is most likely. However, in the older infant, there is no way to distinguish with certainty between the two conditions. Actually, there are more similarities than differences between the two entities, and physicians spend too much time for little purpose at the bedside trying to distinguish between the two disorders. Symptoms and physical, radiographic, physiologic, and blood gas findings are virtually identical. On the one hand, the response to epinephrine, which often is used by clinicians as a differential point, is by definition poor in status asthmaticus. On the other hand, an infant with bronchiolitis due to RSV can have a good response to epinephrine; thus, the test is of little diagnostic value. It appears that the response to adrenergic agents is determined more by the severity of the airway obstruction than by some fundamental difference between asthma and bronchiolitis.

The argument that airway obstruction in bronchiolitis is due to an infection whereas in asthma it is due to an allergic reaction is not tenable. Asthma during infancy, like bronchiolitis, is most often due to viral infection. Measurement of total IgE (a marker of the atopic constitution) may be of some value in older infants in distinguishing between those who probably have infectious bronchiolitis without asthma and those who probably have asthma. In a single study of this nature, it was observed that only 6 percent of infants with epidemic bronchiolitis had serum IgE concentrations increased over the 95th percentile, whereas 35 percent of infants with nonepidemic (sporadic) bronchiolitis had such serum IgE concentrations (Polmar et al., 1972). Welliver and associates (1981) in an interesting study of infants and children with various forms of respiratory disease (upper respiratory infection, pneumonia without wheezing, pneumonia with wheezing, bronchiolitis) due to RSV, showed the association of wheezing illness with the presence of RSV-specific IgE in nasopharyngeal secretions. Histamine was detected significantly more often and in higher concentrations in the subjects who wheezed.

The association of bronchiolitis with the subsequent development of asthma is generally accepted on the basis of published studies and clinical experience. The unresolved question is whether the bronchiolitis episode itself in some way alters airway reactivity and predisposes to subsequent wheezing or whether RSV simply identifies those infants genetically destined to wheeze. Eisen and Bacal (1963) and Wittig and Glaser (1959) showed that 25 and 32 percent of infants with bronchiolitis developed asthma, but these are retrospective reports. Thus, one is unable to determine how many of the infants diagnosed as having bronchiolitis actually were suffering from their first episode of asthma.

Similarly, the question whether RSV-positive bronchiolitis is more or less likely to result in the subsequent development of asthma cannot be resolved on the basis of published data. Simon and Jordan (1967) in a study of children with RSV-positive and RSV-negative bronchiolitis, concluded (with little follow-up data) that those with RSV-induced bronchiolitis were not at risk of subsequent asthma. To the contrary, Rooney and Williams (1971), in a follow-up of infants with RSV-positive bronchiolitis, found a significant incidence of subsequent wheezing and a positive personal and family history of atopic disease. Other follow-up studies of children with histories of bronchiolitis in infancy, both with and without data on RSV infection, show a high frequency of abnormal bronchial lability, utilizing methacholine or histamine responsiveness or exercise challenge when studied 10 years later (Kattan et al., 1977; Pullan and Hey, 1982). McConnochie and Roghmann (1984), in a carefully conducted historical cohort–design retrospective study, found a strong association between bronchiolitis in infancy and wheezing almost 8 years later. This association persisted even after adjusting for a genetic predisposition to wheezing illness or atopy.

Treatment. The treatment of acute bronchiolitis is directed toward maintaining adequate gas exchange (Ellis, 1977; Outwater and Crone, 1984). Oxygen sufficient to maintain the PaO_2 between 70 and 90 mm Hg must be adminis-

tered, since hypoxemia almost invariably is present. Hydration (with great care not to overhydrate) also is indicated. Despite the fact that adrenergic aerosols were not shown in one study to be helpful in relieving the airway obstruction of bronchiolitis (Phelan and Stocks, 1974), it is clear that some patients respond favorably to inhalation of bronchodilator aerosol (isoetharine, metaproterenol, or albuterol). Since the adverse effects of this treatment are virtually nonexistent, a therapeutic trial always is indicated. Similarly, intravenous aminophylline often is useful. Even in the face of minimal bronchodilator response to aminophylline, the extrapulmonary effect of theophylline in increasing diaphragmatic contractility and delaying onset of fatigue (Aubier et al., 1981) may make the drug particularly useful in the infant with respiratory distress and greatly increased work of breathing. Corticosteroid usage is more controversial because of older studies that showed no benefit in bronchiolitis (Leer et al., 1969). However, in the extremely ill infant, the short-term use of high-dose steroid does no harm and would seem prudent. Since there is little to suggest significant bacterial superinfection in infants with viral bronchiolitis, the routine administration of antimicrobial agents is not indicated (Aherne et al., 1970). Most recently, the efficacy of aerosolized ribavirin (a synthetic triazole nucleoside) in treatment of RSV bronchiolitis has been established in well-controlled studies (Editorial, 1986). Administration of ribavirin for 20 hours per day by aerosol lessened cough, rales, retractions, lethargy, and overall severity of illness scores and improved arterial oxygen saturation by the second to fourth day. Adverse effects were not observed. The treatment is expensive and thus should be reserved for appropriately selected patients.

REFERENCES

Aherne, W., Bird, T., Court, S.D.M., Gardner, P.F., McQuillin, J.: Pathological changes in virus infections of the lower respiratory tract in children. J. Clin. Pathol. 23:7, 1970.

Altemeier, W.A., Jr., Ayoub, E.M.: Erythromycin prophylaxis for pertussis. Pediatrics 59:623, 1977.

Aubier, M., DeTroyer, A., Sampson, M., et al.: Aminophylline improves diaphragmatic contractility. N. Engl. J. Med. 305:249, 1981.

Bass, J.W., Klenk, E.L., Kotheimer, J.B., Linneman, C.C., Smith, M.H.D.: Antimicrobial treatment of pertussis. J. Pediatr. 75:768, 1969.

Brooks, G.F., Buchanan, T.M.: Pertussis in the United States. J. Infect. Dis. 122:123, 1970.

Brown, R.S., Nogrady, M.B., Spence, L., Wigglesworth, F.W.: An outbreak of adenovirus type 7 infection in children in Montreal. Can. Med. Assoc. J. 108:434, 1973.

Cate, T.R., Roberts, J.S., Russ, M.A., Pierce, J.A.: Effects of common colds on pulmonary function. Am. Rev. Respir. Dis. 108:858, 1973.

Ceruti, E., Contreras, J., Neira, M.: Staphylococcal pneumonia in childhood. Am. J. Dis. Child. 122:386, 1971.

Chanock, R.M.: Mycoplasma infections in man. N. Engl. J. Med. 273:1199, 1257, 1965.

Chanock, R.M., Kapikian, A.Z., Mills, J., Kim, H.W., Parrott, R.H.: Influence of immunological factors in respiratory syncytial virus disease of the lower respiratory tract. Arch. Environ. Health 21:347, 1970.

Connor, J.D.: Evidence for an etiologic role of adenoviral infection in pertussis syndrome. N. Engl. J. Med. 283:390, 1970.

Cynamon, M.H.: Tuberculosis and other mycobacterial diseases. In Rakel, R.E. (ed.), Conn's Current Therapy. Philadelphia, W.B. Saunders Co., 1986.

Dorff, G.J., Rytel, M.W., Farmer, S.G., et al.: Etiologies and characteristics of pneumonias in a muncipal hospital. Am. J. Med. Sci. 266:349, 1973.

Editorial: Pertussis in adults. Ann. Int. Med. 68:953, 1968.

Editorial: Ribavirin and respiratory syncytial virus. Lancet 1:362, 1986.

Eisen, A.H., Bacal, H.L.: The relationship of acute bronchiolitis to bronchial asthma. A 4- to 14-year followup. Pediatrics 31:859, 1963.

Ellis, E.F.: Therapy of acute bronchiolitis. Pediatr. Res. 11:263, 1977.

Fernald, G.W., Collier, A.M., Clyde, W.A.: Respiratory infections due to *Mycoplasma pneumoniae* in infants and children. Pediatrics 55:327, 1975.

Ferris, B.G., Jr., Ware, J.H., Berkey, C.S., et al.: Effects of passive cigarette smoking on the health of children. Environ. Health Perspect. 62:289, 1985.

Foy, H.M., Grayston, J.T., Kenny, G.E., Alexander, E.R., McMahon, R.: Epidemiology of *Mycoplasma pneumoniae* in families. J.A.M.A. 197:859, 1966.

Foy, H.M., Kenny, G.E., Sefi, R., Ochs, H.D., Allan, I.D.: Second attacks of pneumonia due to *Mycoplasma pneumoniae*. J. Infect. Dis. 135:673, 1977.

Ginsburg, C.M., Howard, J.B., Nelson, J.D.: Report of 65 cases of *Haemophilus influenzae* penumonia. Pediatrics 64:283, 1979.

Gross, P.A., Ennis, F.A., Gaerlan, P.F., Denson, L.J., Denning, C.R., Schiffman, D.: A controlled double-blind comparison of reactogenicity, immunogenicity, and protective efficacy of whole-virus and split-product influenza vaccines in children. J. Infect. Dis. 136:623, 1977.

Hammarschlag, M.R.: Infections due to chlamydia trachomatis. Pediatr. Ann. 13:673, 1984.

Harrison, H.R., English, M.G., Lee, C.K., Alexander, E.R.: *Chlamydia trachomatis* infant pneumonitis. Comparison with matched controls and other infant pneumonitis. N. Engl. J. Med. 298:702, 1978.

Hirschmann, J.V., Everett, E.O.: *Haemophilus influenzae* infections in adults: Report of nine cases and a review of the literature. Medicine 58:80, 1979.

Hoekelman, R.A., Blatman, S., Brunell, P.A., Friedman, S.B., Seidel, H.M.: Principles of Pediatrics. New York, McGraw-Hill Book Co., 1978.

Honig, P.J., Pasquariello, P.S., Stool, S.: Influenzae pneumonia in infants and children. J. Pediatr. 83:215, 1973.

Kattan, M., Keens, T., LaPierre, J.G., Levison, H., Reilly, B.J.: Pulmonary function abnormalities in symptom-free children ten years after bronchiolitis. Pediatrics 59:683, 1977.

Kendig, E.L., Jr.: Tuberculosis. In Kendig, E.L., Jr. (ed.), Disorders of the Respiratory Tract in Children, 3rd ed. Philadelphia, W.B. Saunders Co., 1977.

Kim, H.W., Arrobio, J.O., Brandt, C.D., Jeffries, B.C., Pyles, G., Reid, J.L., Chanock, R.M., Parrott, R.H.: Epidemiology of respiratory syncytial virus infection in Washington, D.C. I. Importance of the virus in different respiratory tract disease syndromes and temporal distributions of infection. Am. J. Epidem. 98:216, 1973.

Krugman, S., Ward, R.: Pertussis (whooping cough). In Krugman, S., Ward, R. (eds.), Infectious Diseases of Children and Adults, 6th ed. St. Louis, C.V. Mosby Co., 1977.

Kurt, T.L., Yeager, A.S., Guenette, S., et al.: Spread of pertussis by hospital staff. J.A.M.A. 221:264, 1972.

Lang, W.R., Howden, C.W., Laws, J., Burton, J.F.: Bronchopneumonia with serious sequelae in children with evidence of adenovirus type 21 infection. Br. Med. J. 1:73, 1969.

Laraya-Cuasay, L.R., DeForest, A., Huff, D., Lischner, H., Huang, N.N.: Chronic pulmonary complications of early influenza virus infections in children. Am. Rev. Respir. Dis. 116:617, 1977.

Leer, J.A., Green, J.L., Heimlich, E.M., Hyde, J.S., Moffet, H.L., Yung, G.A., Barron, B.A.: Corticosteroid treatment in bronchiolitis. A controlled, collaborative study in 297 infants and children. Am. J. Dis. Child. 117:495, 1969.

Loda, F.A., Collier, A.M., Glezan, W.P., Strangert, K., Clyde, W.A., Jr., Denny, F.W.: Occurrence of *Diplococcus pneumoniae* in the upper respiratory tract of children. J. Pediatr. 87:1087, 1975.

Louria, D.B., Blumenfeld, H.L., Ellis, J.T., et al.: Studies on influenza in the pandemic of 1957–1958. II. Pulmonary complications of influenza. J. Clin. Invest. 38:213, 1959.

McConnochie, K.M., Roghmann, K.J.: Bronchiolitis as a possible cause of wheezing in childhood: new evidence. Pediatrics 74:1, 1984.

McFarlane, J.T., Finch, R.G., Ward, M.J., et al.: Hospital study of adult community acquired pneumonia. Lancet 2:255, 1982.

Morse, S.I.: Biological activities of *Bordetella pertussis*. Adv. Appl. Microbiol. 20:9, 1976.

Newth, C.J.L., Levison, H., Bryan, A.C.: The respiratory status of children with croup. J. Pediatr. 81:1068, 1972.

Outwater, K.M., Crone, R.K.: Management of respiratory failure in infants with acute viral bronchiolitis. Am. J. Dis. Child. 138:1071, 1984.

Petersdorf, R.G., Adams, R.G., Braunwald, E., Isselbacher, K.J., Martin, J.B., Wilson, J.D.: Harrison's Principles of Internal Medicine, 10th ed. New York, McGraw-Hill Book Co., 1983.

Phelan, P.D., Stocks, J.G.: Management of severe viral bronchiolitis and severe acute asthma. Arch. Dis. Child. 49:143, 1974.

Picken, J.J., Niewoehner, D.E., Chester, E.H.: Prolonged effects of viral infections of the upper respiratory tract upon small airways. Am. J. Med. 52:738, 1972.

Polmar, S.H., Robinson, L.D., Minnefor, A.B.: Immunoglobulin E in bronchiolitis. Pediatrics 50:279, 1972.

Pullan, C.R., Hey, E.N.: Wheezing, asthma and pulmonary dysfunction 10 years after infection with respiratory syncytial virus in infancy. Br. Med. J. 284:1665, 1982.

Rooney, J.C., Williams, H.E.: The relationship between

proven viral bronchiolitis and subsequent wheezing. J. Pediatr. 79:744, 1971.

Rudolph, A.M. (ed.): Pediatrics, 17th ed. New York, Appleton-Century-Crofts, 1982.

Schwarzmann, S.W., Adler, J.L., Sullivan, R.J., et al.: Bacterial pneumonia during the Hong Kong influenza epidemic of 1968–1969. Arch. Int. Med. 127:1037, 1971.

Scott, R., Kaul, A., Scott, M., Chiba, Y., Ogra, P.: Development of in vitro correlates of cell-mediated immunity to respiratory syncytial virus infection in humans. J. Infect. Dis. 137:810, 1978.

Simon, G., Jordan, W.S.: Infectious and allergic aspects of bronchiolitis. J. Pediatr. 70:553–558, 1967.

Sussman, S.J., Magoffin, R.L., Lennette, E.H., Schieble, J.: Cold agglutinins, Eaton agent, and respiratory infections of children. Pediatrics 38:571, 1966.

Weiss, S.T., Tager, I.B., Speizer, F.E., Rosner, B.: Persistent wheeze: Its relationship to respiratory illness, cigarette smoking and level of pulmonary functions in a population sample of children. Am. Rev. Resp. Dis. 122:697–707, 1980.

Welliver, R.C., Wong, D.T., Sun, M., et al.: The development of respiratory syncytial virus–specific IgE and the release of histamine in nasopharyngeal secretions after infection. N. Engl. J. Med. 305:841, 1981.

Williams, H., McNicol, K.N.: Prevalence, natural history and relationship of wheezy bronchitis and asthma in children. An epidemiological study. Br. Med. J. 4:321, 1969.

Winterbauer, R.H., Ludwig, R.W., Hammar, S.P.: Clinical course, management, and long-term sequelae of respiratory failure due to influenza viral pneumonia. Johns Hopkins Med. J. 141:148, 1977.

Wittig, H.J., Glaser, J.: The relationship between bronchiolitis and childhood asthma. J. Allergy 30:19, 1959.

Wright, P.F., Ross, K.B., Thompson, J., Karson, D.T.: Influenza A infections in young children. Primary natural infection and protective efficacy of live vaccine–induced or naturally acquired immunity. N. Engl. J. Med. 296:829, 1977.

Wyngaarden, J.B., Smith, L.H., Jr.: Cecil's Textbook of Medicine, 17th ed. W.B. Saunders Co., Philadelphia, 1985.

Zoomboulakis, D., Anagnostakis, D., Albanis, V., et al.: Steroids in the treatment of pertussis. A controlled clinical trial. Arch. Dis. Childh. 48:51, 1973.

41

Asthma (Bronchial Asthma)

DAVID S. PEARLMAN, M.D.
C. WARREN BIERMAN, M.D.

Asthma is a chronic obstructive disorder of the tracheobronchial tree characterized by paroxysmal episodes of respiratory distress generally interspersed with prolonged periods of apparent complete well-being. Typically, there are wide variations in the degree of obstruction over relatively short periods of time; the obstruction may subside spontaneously or only as a result of therapy. The hallmark of the disease is *wheezing*, a squeaky sound made by air rushing through the larger but narrowed airways. Cough also is a characteristic part of the disorder and may constitute the major symptom with which an asthmatic presents. A patient with asthma may even present with "croup," other subtle symptoms of bronchopulmonary obstruction *without wheezing*, or both, a fact not fully appreciated until the 1970's (McFadden, 1975a and 1975b; Corrao et al., 1979). The more subtle symptoms and signs of asthma often are unappreciated, and asthma is a commonly underdiagnosed disorder. Because of this underdiagnosis and the prevalence of erroneous concepts of the etiology, course, and prognosis, asthma also tends to be a greatly undertreated disorder in childhood and adulthood (Speight et al., 1983; Pearlman, 1984).

PATHOLOGY (Reid, 1977; Hogg, 1985)

Examination of postmortem lung specimens of patients' dying of asthma shows marked hyperinflation with smooth muscle hyperplasia of bronchial and bronchiolar walls, thick tenacious mucus plugs often completely occluding airways, markedly thickened basement membrane, and variable degrees of mucosal edema and denudation of bronchial and bronchiolar epithelium. Eosinophilia of the submucosa and secretions is prominent whether or not allergic (IgE-mediated) mechanisms are present. Plasma cells that contain IgG, IgM, and IgA may be seen, and in some patients plasma cells that contain IgE also are seen. Occasionally, the inflammatory response is indicative of infection, a finding more common in adults, especially those with concurrent chronic bronchitis. Mucus plugs contain layers of shed epithelial cells, which may form Creola bodies (sloughed epithelial clumps) and eosinophils, and may contain polymorphonuclear neutrophils, lymphocytes, and plasma cells. Charcot-Leyden crystals from eosinophils and mucus casts of the airways with epithelial cell clumps (Curschmann spirals) also are observed. Toxic products from eosinophils, in particular, may play an important role in the destructive changes observed (Frigas and Gleich, 1986). The mucosal edema with separated columnar cells and stratified nonciliated epithelium, which replace ciliated epithelium, results in abnormal mucociliary clearance. Mast cells often are absent, possibly reflecting degranulation and discharge of the chemical mediators. Submucous gland hypertrophy and increased goblet cell size are not constant features of asthma, being more characteristic of chronic bronchitis. The long recognized inflammatory nature of the bronchial response with desquamation of the bronchial epithelium has only recently been emphasized in the contexts of both pathophysiology and important clinical therapeutic implications (see subsequent discussion). The development of bronchial hyperresponsiveness, considered to be an important pathogenetic feature in patients with current symptomatic asthma, has been attributed to "late" cellular inflammatory responses initiated by allergic and other nonimmune mechanisms (Cockroft, 1985; Larsen, 1985; Hargreave et al., 1986).

The thickened basement membrane is a striking feature of asthma and has been reported even in "mild" asthmatics, sometimes associated with deposition of various immunoglobulins. Part of the apparent thickening is due actually to submembrane deposition of collagen and various other materials. Basement membrane thickening is thought to occur early in the disease, but its pathogenetic significance remains to be determined. All of these findings have been observed in symptom-free asthmatic individuals following accidental deaths. On the one hand, although an occasional patient may show localized bronchiectasis and small focal areas of alveolar destruction, these are not characteristic of asthma, and there is little evidence that asthma leads to destructive emphysema. On the other hand, "distensive emphysema," clinically significant diminution in pulmonary elasticity, may be a concomitant of long-standing alveolar hyperinflation. Bronchiectasis is rare in asthma but may occur in association with allergic bronchopulmonary aspergillosis where it involves the proximal branches (see Chapter 47) and in a small number of patients with similar disorders. Incomplete reversibility of airflow limitation seen in some asthmatics suggests that some of the pathologic changes noted may, in fact, have long-term clinical implications.

EPIDEMIOLOGY

Asthma commonly begins in childhood and has been considered mistakenly to be a disorder confined largely to early life. Much childhood asthma persists through adulthood: almost half of all asthma in adulthood begins in childhood. The vast majority of childhood asthma begins before the age of 8 years, most begins before the age of 6 years, and about half begins before the age of 3 years. Until puberty, males are affected twice as frequently as are females. In the teens and in early adulthood, there is a reversal of this trend, so that by mid to late adult life, females are affected more frequently than are males.

Asthma is a deceptively common disorder; the exact figures on incidence and prevalence vary from study to study, related at least in part to different criteria for diagnosis and different methodologies used in the studies (see Chapter 9). In addition, there is some reason to believe that the incidence and prevalence may be increasing. At any given time, approximately 3 percent of a population is considered to have asthma, but this undoubtedly is a gross underestimate (Speight et al., 1983; Pearlman, 1984). It is probable that the true prevalence is at least three to five times this figure in the United States and other Western nations. The mortality rate among asthmatics is less than 0.1 percent/year, a relatively low yet significant rate, and appears to be increasing in many Western countries (Asthma Deaths, 1986). However, the morbidity in asthma is extraordinarily high. It is a source of chronic fatigue and may interfere with sleep, with school and work performance, and with normal exercise and physical development. Asthma may affect a child's psychologic growth and development. At all ages it may affect interactions with family and peers, disturb family life, and cause economic hardship —because of medical costs as well as time lost from work by the patient or by the parent who cares for the child with asthma.

NATURAL COURSE

It is a common belief that childhood asthma generally is "outgrown" by adulthood. Indeed, in various studies, 30 to 50 percent of asthmatic children have been reported to be symptom free at puberty. Remissions occur somewhat earlier in girls than in boys, as do pubertal changes. However, many children who have "outgrown" asthma in puberty develop recurrent asthmatic symptoms in later adult life, as is clearly shown in a series of studies by Flensborg (1945) and Ryssing (1959).

Asthmatic children and adults examined during "symptom-free" periods frequently have clinically significant evidence of obstruction by objective testing. In addition, pharmacologic hyperactivity of the airways in asthmatic individuals generally persists for many years even in the absence of overt asthmatic attacks (Townley et al., 1975), and pathologic evidence of pulmonary obstructions can be found in patients many years after the apparent cessation of asthmatic symptoms. Though many asthmatic children improve significantly by puberty, a small subpopulation may actually develop more severe asthma. It is clear also that in only a relatively small proportion does asthma completely disappear. More often ". . . it is the pediatrician rather than the disease that is outgrown" (Levison et al., 1974). The natural history of asthma in adults is unclear, but it appears to take the same form as does asthma in children, becoming chronically or frequently symptomatic in some and episodic and occasional in others. In some cases, it may be lost altogether. Whether or not airway hyperreactivity is the basis for asthma, it does play an important role in most patients with asthma, and an understanding and appreciation of this phenomenon is important to an understanding of the pathogenesis and treatment of asthma (Pearlman, 1984; Hargreave et al., 1986).

ETIOLOGY

An extraordinary tracheobronchial hyperreactivity to acetylcholine and to other neurotransmitters and mediators of inflammation, such as prostaglandin F_{2a}, leukotriene C_4, D_4, and E_4, platelet activating factor (PAF), and kinins, is a characteristic of symptomatic asthma and occurs at some time or other in most patients with asthma irrespective of the presence or absence of demonstrable allergic mechanisms. Though some workers consider that this "nonspecific" hyperreactivity is a basic characteristic of asthma and may employ the term *reactive airways disorder* as a synonym for asthma, currently it is not clear that it is present in all asthma. This pharmacologic hypersensitivity is the basis of a diagnostic test for asthma (methacholine or histamine bronchial challenge). Responsiveness to these agents correlates well with responsiveness to other more natural stimuli, such as exercise and hyperventilation in cold air. Bronchial hyperresponsiveness in asthma, however, is not entirely "nonspecific," and bronchial reactivity to different stimuli can be more selective than implied by the terminology used, reflecting different pathways through which bronchial reactivity occurs. Szentivanyi (1968) proposed that hypersensitivity to pharmacologic mediators in asthma is due to an imbalance in the autonomic nervous system concerned with counterbalancing the effects of various chemical mediators.

The fact that chemical mediators to which the tracheobronchial tree is hypersensitive can be liberated by various mechanisms, both immune and nonimmune, may explain the observation that in most asthmatic individuals numerous factors, such as inhalant irritants, allergens, exercise, infections, and psychologic factors, act as triggers of bronchoconstriction. Moreoever, the degree of reactivity can vary from time to time, creating an inconsistency in the susceptibility or tolerance of the lung to various potential asthmogenic stimuli (Cockroft, 1983), as diagrammed in Figure 41–1.

Heightened tracheobronchial sensitivity can be demonstrated also in chronic bronchitis, following some viral respiratory tract infections, and in family members of asthmatic patients, without asthmatic symptoms but generally not to the degree observed in asthmatic patients. Bronchial hyperresponsiveness can be initiated by allergens; by industrial chemicals (allergic and nonallergic mechanisms); by atmospheric irritants, such as ozone; and by infectious

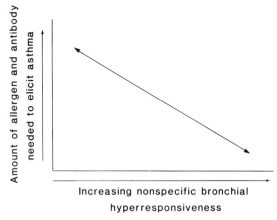

FIGURE 41–1. Relationship between bronchial hyperreactivity and amount of allergen exposure required to induce bronchial obstruction. As the degree of nonspecific bronchial responsiveness increases, the amount of antigen-antibody reacting required to induce obstruction diminishes. Thus, casual encounter with allergen in a highly sensitive individual with marked nonspecific bronchial hyperresponsiveness may induce asthma, but intense antigen exposure may be required to do so in the asthmatic with relatively little IgE antibody or relatively little nonspecific bronchial hyperresponsiveness. (Modified from Cockroft, D.W., et al.: Determination of allergen-induced asthma: dose of allergen, circulating IgE antibody concentration, and bronchial responsiveness to inhaled histamine. *Am. Rev. Resp. Dis.*, *120*:1053, 1979.)

agents (Hargreave et al., 1986). It also is of interest that in some individuals, airway hyperresponsiveness induced by industrial chemicals, for example, disappears when contact with the chemicals ceases, whereas, in others, it persists.

The basis for the pharmacologic hypersensitivity in asthma may be genetic. There is a familial association of the clinical asthmatic state and tracheobronchial hypersensitivity and, separately, a familial association of the heightened IgE antibody responses. The coexistence of asthma, airway hyperreactivity, and increased IgE antibody production is far greater than in the population at large (Cockroft et al., 1984), but each is separable and seems to be genetically independent. Within a given family constellation, some members may have asthma and also manufacture large amounts of IgE; others may manufacture IgE antibody extraordinarily well but have no evidence of tracheobronchial hypersensitivity (Townley et al., 1976; Sibbald et al., 1980). The exact mode of inheritance of asthma is still not clear. Although in twin studies, concordance for asthma generally has been greater for identical twins compared with nonidentical twins or other nontwin siblings; concordance nevertheless is lower than 50 percent (Bias, 1973).

Though most children and young adults with asthma have specific skin-sensitizing (IgE) antibodies, the proportion of older asthmatic adults with demonstrable IgE antibodies is much lower. The presumption that all asthma was "allergic" or had an immune basis led to the concept of "extrinsic" asthma, due to exogenous allergens, and "intrinsic" asthma, due to "normal" bacterial allergens from the respiratory tract (Rackemann, 1940). However, in many individuals with asthma, no evidence can be found that allergic mechanisms are operative in the disease. Moreover, even when allergy is present, it rarely is the only important factor, and sometimes the IgE antibody present may be irrelevant to the asthma (Aas, 1970). However, in the presence of even small amounts of IgE antibody, acute asthma can be provoked by inhalation of allergen with clinical reactivity a factor of the combined variables of the amount of antibody present, the amount of allergen exposure, and the degree of bronchial irritability (Cockroft et al., 1979) (see Fig. 41–1). Moreover, allergic sensitization, particularly that which results in induction of "late" responses, may be the critical initiating process of asthma in many patients. There is a strong association between allergic sensitization and the increasing prevalence of asthma in some underdeveloped countries (Dowse et al, 1985).

Environmental factors play critical roles in the expression of asthma in "susceptible" individuals. In childhood and in adulthood, the onset of asthma frequently is associated with a respiratory tract infection (viral). Certain viruses (respiratory syncytial virus, adenovirus, parainfluenza virus, possibly corona virus, influenza virus) and *Mycoplasma* are particularly important in causing asthmatic episodes (Ellis, 1977) (see Chapter 14). In addition to initiating asthma, inhalation of allergens and irritants can increase tracheobronchial reactivity further in asthmatic patients. Maternal smoking appears to be a risk factor for the occurrence of childhood asthma (McConnochie and Roghmann, 1986).

PRECIPITATING AND AGGRAVATING FACTORS IN ASTHMA

Allergens. In some individuals with asthma, it is possible to induce an asthmatic reaction to substances to which IgE and possibly other skin-sensitizing antibody can be demonstrated. In others, allergens may play only an ancillary or a negligible role. Allergic reactions may induce bronchoconstriction directly, may increase tracheobronchial sensitivity in general, or may be obvious or subtle precipitating factors. In addition, the role played by an allergen may appear to be inconsistent and therefore historically confusing or unclear as an asthma precipitant, related not only to intensity of exposure but the degree of airway hyperreactivity, which may change from time to time. Although "immediate" responses to allergens via IgE antibody–induced mediator release are striking, it may be that "late" reactions (which occur 4 to 12 hours after antigen contact and which appear to be mediated also by IgE antibody–related mechanisms) are more important in the disease. Allergens that can induce asthma include foods (mainly in early life), animal allergens, mold spores, pollens, insects (mainly by inhalation but also by sting), infectious agents (especially fungi but perhaps viruses, as discussed subsequently), and, occasionally, drugs.

Irritants. Numerous upper and lower respiratory irritants have been implicated as precipitants of asthma. These include paint odors, hairsprays, perfumes, chemicals, air pollutants, cigarette smoke (also cigar and pipe smoke), cold air, cold water, cough, and positive ions. Some allergens may act as irritants. As indicated previously, some irritants such as ozone and industrial chemicals also may initiate bronchial hyperresponsiveness by inducing inflammation. Active and passive exposure to cigarette and cigar smoke, in addition to acting as precipitants and aggravators of asthma, also can be associated with an accelerated irreversible loss of pulmonary function (Barter and Campbell, 1976).

Weather Changes. Atmospheric changes commonly are associated with an increase in asthmatic activity. The mechanism of this effect has not been defined (see Chapter 13).

Infections. By far, the most common infectious agents responsible for precipitating or aggravating asthma are viral respiratory pathogens. In some instances, however, fungal infections (e.g., bronchopulmonary aspergillosis), bacterial infections (e.g., pertussis), and parasitic infestations (e.g., toxocariasis and ascariasis) can be important triggers. The importance of viral infections as precipitants and possible initiators of asthma and bronchial hyperreactivity cannot be overemphasized. Various mechanisms have been implicated to explain the role of viruses in asthma and other allergic diseases, including IgE-mediated mechanisms (Welliver, 1986) (see Chapter 14).

Exercise. Strenuous exercise ordinarily associated with breathlessness, such as running, bicycle riding, and cross-country skiing (downhill skiing generally is not associated with this problem), may induce bronchial obstruction in the vast majority (at least 70 to 80 percent) of individuals with asthma. In some instances, exercise is a major asthmatic precipitant, whereas in others it is a minor or an insignificant one altogether (see Chapter 44). Exercise can be a subtle though significant problem associated with only cough or excessive breathlessness. Exercise can induce late asthmatic responses, but it is unclear whether these responses are associated with bronchial hyperreactivity.

Emotional Factors. The influence of the psyche on asthma is unquestioned, and in some instances suggestion has been shown to alter airway resistance significantly. Emotional upsets clearly aggravate asthma in some individuals. However, there is no evidence indicating that psychologic factors are the basis for asthma. The elegant studies of Kinsman and associates (1977) strongly indicate that coping styles of patients, their families, and their physicians can intensify or lead to more rapid amelioration of asthma. Conversely, denial of asthma by patients, parents, or physicians may delay therapy to the point that reversibility of obstruction is more difficult. Psychologic factors have been implicated in deaths from asthma in children (Strunk et al., 1985). The influence of psychosocial factors on compliance and the effect of hostility or fear on the ability or propensity to comply are yet other important facets of treatment failure or success.

Just as psychologic factors may influence the course of asthma in a given patient, it is important to recognize that asthma itself can strongly influence the emotional state of the patient, of the family, and of other individuals associated with the patient. Indeed, asthma probably is more frequently "somatopsychic" than it is "psychosomatic" (see Chapter 22).

Gastroesophageal Reflux. Reflux of gastric contents into the tracheobronchial tree can aggrevate asthma in children as well as in adults (see Chapter 24) and is one of the causes of nocturnal asthma. There also is suggestive information that gastroesophageal reflux (GER) may increase airway reactivity.

Allergic Rhinitis, Sinusitis, and Upper Respiratory Tract Inflammation. Acute or chronic sinusitis can be associated with aggravation of asthma and can be a cause of recalcitrant asthma (Slavin, 1986). Evidence from experimental animal studies also suggests that sinusitis may be capable of increasing bronchial responsiveness. It is probable that allergic rhinitis also can aggravate asthma through irritant or "reflex" mechanisms. Irritation of the upper respiratory tract by any of a variety of mechanisms appears capable of triggering asthmatic symptoms.

Nonallergic Hypersensitivity to Drugs and Chemicals. Though allergic sensitivity to aspirin has been reported on occasion with manifestations that include asthma, aspirin and nonsteroidal anti-inflammatory drugs (NSAIDs), such as indomethacin and ibuprofen, are more likely to exacerbate asthma on a nonallergic basis. Aspirin ingestion may diminish pulmonary functions in up to one third of children and adolescents with severe asthma (Rachelefsky et al., 1975). In many instances, this effect may be subtle. Consequently, as a general rule, it is wise to restrict aspirin and aspirin-containing products for all individuals who have asthma. Patients who react to aspirin are likely to react to other NSAIDs that should be avoided, but most are able to tolerate acetaminophen. The importance of sensitivity to tartrazine (FD & C Yellow No. 5), a common dye found in many foods and drugs, in aspirin-sensitive or other asthmatics is unclear, but early reports that it can induce asthma have not been confirmed. Metabisulfite can be an important precipitant or aggravator of asthma, both by allergic and nonallergic mechanisms (Bush et al., 1986) (see Chapter 53). A small proportion of severe asthmatics appear to be extremely sensitive, but it is probable that all asthmatics are sensitive to some degree to sulfur dioxide that is released from metabisulfite.

Endocrine Factors. Aggravation of asthma occurs in some patients in relation to the menstrual cycle, beginning shortly before menstruation. Whether this reflects changes in water and salt balance, irritability of bronchial smooth muscle, or other factors is unknown. The use of birth control pills occasionally also aggravates asthma. Hyperthyroidism has been reported to worsen or precipitate asthma severely in an occasional patient. Treatment of hyperthyroidism usually ameliorates the asthma. Relationships between endocrine disorders, pregnancy, and asthma are discussed in Chapter 15.

TABLE 41–1. Bronchial Asthma Patterns

Precipitants	Examples* A	Examples* B	Examples* C	Estimated Involvement (percent of cases)
Viral infections	+	(+)	+	90
Irritants	+	(+)	(+)	100
Exercise	+	(+)	(+)	70
Allergens	+	+	−	40 (Adults), 80 (Children)
Emotions	+	(+)	−	?

* + = major importance; (+) = minor importance; − = no importance.

Sleep or Nocturnal Asthma. Sleep or nocturnal asthma is a risk factor for asthma severity and even death in some asthmatics. Although nocturnal asthma may result from late phase reactions to earlier allergen exposure, GER, or sinusitis in some patients, these conditions are not present in most patients with severe nocturnal asthma. Nocturnal asthma does not appear to be related to recumbency or to sleep per se. One possible explanation is an exaggeration of a normal circadian variation in bronchomotor tone (Barnes 1986). Abnormalities in central nervous system control of respiratory drive, in particular with defective hypoxic drive, also may be present in some patients and can pose serious risks to those with asthma (Martin, 1984; Lancet Commentary, 1983).

Interaction of Various Precipitating Factors. Not infrequently, concurrent exposure to various precipitating or aggravating factors may induce additive effects in asthma. For example, some individuals experience exercise-induced asthma only when exercising in cold air or during a pollen allergy season. Others recognize increased symptoms from specific allergen exposure after respiratory infections. As indicated previously, this may be due to increased bronchial responsiveness caused by inflammation (allergic or infectious).

ASTHMATIC PATTERNS

In some asthmatics, most of the factors listed previously appear to play important roles in asthma, whereas in other asthmatics only some appear to be important. Table 41–1 provides examples of various reaction patterns in patients with asthma. For example, patient A's asthma may be precipitated by each of the factors listed, whereas for patient B, allergic triggers are of predominant influence in the disease, and other factors are of minor influence. Patient C is one with "nonallergic" asthma. The estimated importance of each of the precipitating factors in the asthmatic population is noted in the table. Table 41–2 relates the importance of various asthmatic precipitants to age. For example, viral infections are of great importance in precipitating asthma early in the child's life, become relatively less important as the child grows older, and assume a major role again in the adult.

Since the development of allergy is dependent on duration and intensity of exposure to allergens, allergy to foods in infancy generally precedes allergy to inhaled substances. Thereafter, inhaled allergens become progressively more important, as prolonged exposure to such perennial factors as salivary proteins and

TABLE 41–2. Precipitants of Asthmatic Symptoms in Various Age Groups

	Infancy	Early Childhood	Later Childhood	Adulthood
Viral infections	++++*	+++	+(+)	+++
Exercise	+	++	+++	+++
Irritants	+	++	+++	+++
Foods	++	+	(+)	(+)
Indoor inhalants	+(+)	+++	+++	+++
Pollens		++	+++	++(+)
Emotions†	(+)	+	+	+

* Relative importance denoted, in order, by ++++, +++, ++, ++(+), and (+).
† See text.

danders from domestic animals, house dust–mite antigens, and air-borne mold spores results in allergic sensitization. As the child grows older, repeated pollen exposure results in "pollen" asthma. In later childhood and in adulthood, exercise becomes an important factor, as the patient participates in more strenuous activities and in competitive sports. In later adulthood, allergens tend to assume much less or no importance, possibly because of age-related waning of immune responsiveness.

THE PRESENTATION OF ASTHMA

A patient with asthma may present with any or all of a variety of symptoms, which can include wheezing, cough, shortness of breath, and complaints of "chest congestion," "tight chest," exercise intolerance, and recurrent "bronchitis" or recurrent "pneumonia." Often asthma appears subtly as coughing without overt wheezing, especially in conjunction with colds or during pollen seasons. On the one hand, the adage attributed to Chevalier Jackson that ". . . not all the wheezes is asthma" has been well publicized, and indeed causes for wheezing other than asthma are numerous (Table 41 – 3). On the other hand, it has become apparent also that ". . . not all asthma wheezes" (at least not overtly), a presentation in fact that is not uncommon. In many instances, cursory physical examination fails to reveal evidence of obvious pulmonary obstruction (although careful examination might do so), and obstructive disease of the lower respiratory tract may be overlooked unless pulmonary function is tested. Thus, the physician should consider the diagnosis of asthma not only when the patient has recurrent wheezing but when there are repeated complaints referable to the lower respiratory tract even in the absence of wheezing.

"Wheezing" may be a late sign in asthma. It is caused by air rushing past a narrowed portion of the airway in sufficient force to generate air vibrations perceived as sound, and *it occurs only in the larger airways where airflow is turbulent. The small airways are "silent,"* since the air flow there is laminar rather than turbulent. Consequently, marked small airway obstruction can be present that may not be recognized on physical examination. In most instances, airway narrowing in asthma is sufficiently generalized that large and small airways obstruction coexist, so that wheezing is audible either overtly or by auscultation. Before wheezing is perceptible to the patient or the patient's parent, however, there generally are more subtle symptoms of obstruction, such as cough or a feeling of chest

TABLE 41 – 3. Differential Diagnosis of Asthma

Condition	Relative Frequency of Occurrence			
	INFANCY	CHILDHOOD	ADOLESCENCE	ADULTHOOD
Laryngomalacia-tracheomalacia-bronchomalacia	++	±	−	−
Cystic fibrosis	+++*	+*	±	±†
Chronic viral infection	+++	++		
Foreign body	++	+++	±	±
Croup	++	+	−	−
Epiglottitis	+++	+	−	−
Pertussis	+++	+	−	−
Congenital anomalies	+++	+	−	−
Hyperventilation syndrome	−	+	++	++
Bronchiectasis	+	+	+	+
Mitral valve prolapse	−	−	+	+
Laryngeal (physical or psychologic)	−	−	±	±
Tumors (extra- or intraluminal)	−	−	−	+
COPD (includes emphysema, chronic bronchitis)	−	−	−	++*
Cardiac	−	−	−	+
Pulmonary embolism	−	−	−	±
Collagen-vascular	−	−	±	±
Aspiration syndromes	+	±	±	+

* Often coexists with an element of "asthma." Information obtained from various sources. See, in particular, MacDonnell and Chawla, 1985.
† Many patients with cystic fibrosis are now living into adulthood. The minus sign denotes never or extremely rare.

discomfort. *Moreover, in many patients, there may not be signs or symptoms until airflow limitation, easily measured by spirometry, is moderately severe (forced expiratory volume in 1 second or FEV₁ below 50 percent of normal). It cannot be overemphasized that auscultation is a useful but highly imperfect device for determining whether or not there is any airflow limitation and, if so, the degree that exists.*

This phenomenon may be more readily appreciated using as an analogy the concept of an iceberg (Fig. 41 – 2). By this analogy, the ocean floor represents completely normal pulmonary function, and the ocean surface the point at which pulmonary obstruction is obvious clinically. Wheezing, in other words, is the tip of the iceberg. Just as most of the iceberg is not evident, pulmonary obstruction begins well before wheezing is heard. In some instances, the slope to the tip of the iceberg is slight, and obstruction progresses slowly (days); in others, it is steep, and pulmonary obstruction advances rapidly to overt symptoms in minutes to hours. Auscultation may detect wheezing or prolonged expiration before wheezing is overt, and sensitive pulmonary function measurements may detect obstruction before wheezing can be heard by auscultation.

Figure 41 – 2 contains various examples of asthma patterns selected for illustrative purposes. In some instances, as illustrated in example I, the obstructive phenomenon is short lived, beginning and ending over a period of hours to days. In other instances, obstruction may be constant, surfacing periodically as wheezing and apparent paroxysms of asthma interspersed with minor or no obvious symptoms (example II) or associated with virtually constant wheezing of varying intensity (example III). Example IV is an illustration of the patient who never wheezes despite significant pulmonary obstruction; the obstruction may not be recognized unless the examiner is alert enough to perform pulmonary function tests. Figure 41 – 2 also illustrates the point that there are two sides to the asthma iceberg. Although overt asthmatic symptoms may cease after a relatively short period of time, there is a prolonged phase of diminishing but significant pulmonary obstruction. This phase has been well documented by various investigators, including McFadden (1973) who studied adults and Levison and coworkers (1974) who studied children and showed that days to weeks after an asthma attack, at a time when patients claim to be completely asymptomatic, abnormal flow rates, hyperinflation, or both remain. The "pattern" can vary substantially from time to time, influenced by treatment, natural exposure to allergens or irritants or both.

This concept of asthma may be developed into a classification of disease severity that considers frequency of asthmatic attacks, severity of attacks, functional impairment between attacks, and overall functional disability. Such a classification is useful in defining therapy as well as in following the course of the disease (Table 41 – 4).

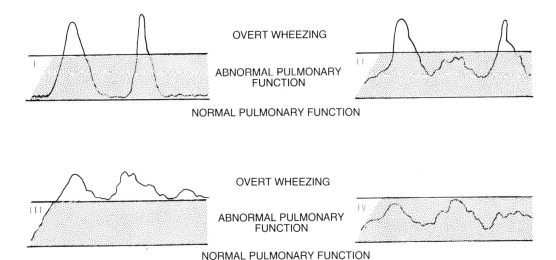

FIGURE 41 – 2. Iceberg concept of asthma. The "ocean floor" represents pulmonary normality; the surface of the ocean, the point at which asthmatic symptoms (e.g., wheezing) are obvious.

TABLE 41–4. Classification of Severity of Asthma

Classification*	Definition
Mild (Example I)	Less than six mild attacks per year *and* asymptomatic between attacks *and* no functional impairment between attacks *and* no medication used between attacks.
Moderate to moderately severe (Examples II, IV)	Up to eight severe attacks per year *and* mild to moderate symptoms between attacks *and* mild to moderate functional impairment between attacks *and* on continuous medication.
Severe (Example III)	More than eight severe attacks per year while on continuous medication *and* moderate to severe functional impairment between attacks, steroid dependent, *or* at least two episodes of status asthmaticus per year.

Continuous medication is defined as medication used on more than 25 percent of the days in the past year.

Functional impairment is defined as:

Normal functional activity — on par with peers

Minimal functional impairment — 1 or 2 disability days/quarter

Moderate functional impairment — 1 or 2 disability days/month

Severe functional impairment — 1 or more disability days/week

A *disability day* is defined as a day on which a person stays in bed most of the day because of asthma or a work or school day loss.

* Examples in Figure 41–2.

Recognition of the various patterns has important therapeutic implications. First, early treatment of asthma is more successful than is late treatment, and even subtle signs of pulmonary obstruction should be signals to institute therapy. In the patient who wheezes with upper respiratory tract infection, the characteristic cough that precedes overt wheezing should be a signal to initiate therapy. In addition, pharmacologic therapy should be continued even when overt symptoms of asthma have cleared and until pulmonary obstruction has reversed or pulmonary functions have become stable at an acceptable functional level.

In asthmatics who have chronic pulmonary obstruction, pharmacologic treatment must be continuous or round-the-clock. *It is emphasized that asthma is a chronic disorder that may surface periodically but in which chronic obstruction may be more severe than frequently is appreciated.*

PROGNOSIS

In children and adolescents, asthma frequently is a completely "reversible" obstructive airways disease, and indeed no abnormalities in pulmonary functions can be detected in many asthmatic patients when they become symptom free. However, there is a significant subpopulation of asthmatic children and adults who, even in the absence of symptoms for prolonged periods of time, have persistent abnormalities in pulmonary functions, with chronic hyperinflation, decreased pulmonary flow rates, or both, with or without mild hypoxemia. The potential reversibility of abnormal pulmonary functions —even in severely asthmatic children— towards or to normal by intensive therapy was demonstrated by Tooley and colleagues (1965). However, it is clear that in many children and adults with severe asthma, normal pulmonary functions cannot be maintained without continuous intensive therapy, including corticosteroids. Reversibility of pulmonary function abnormalities with therapy is transient in that withdrawal of constant therapy usually leads to the return of pulmonary functions to initial abnormal baselines (Cade and Pain, 1973).

As noted previously, even severe asthma generally does not progress to emphysema. However, asthma appears to progress to chronic nonreversible obstructive disease in some individuals with the disorder. Chronic mucus plugging, tracheobronchial ciliary dysfunction, smooth muscle hyperplasia, and persistent hyperinflation possibly may lead to pulmonary abnormalities in adult life. Recent findings of residual pulmonary function abnormalities following respiratory viral infections early in life (Kattan et al., 1977) and the fact that viral respiratory tract infections occur more commonly in asthmatic children than in their nonasthmatic siblings (Minor et al., 1974) further confuse the issue. Similar arguments may be made with regard to irreversible pulmonary changes in asthmatic adults. In addition, passive or active smoking in asthmatic children as well as adults has been shown to be related to more rapid decline in small airways function in comparison with nonasthmatics (Barter and Campbell, 1976). Thus, it is not clear that asthma per se leads to irreversible pulmonary changes. Evidence suggests, however, that asthma significantly predisposes patients to irreversible damage from various noxious environmental agents (Pearlman, 1984).

Since the natural course of continued bronchial obstruction is not known, a therapeutic dilemma arises about the extent to which asthma should be treated. Should the patient be treated until pulmonary function is totally normal or until he or she can function reasonably and normally even though pulmonary functions are abnormal? Whether intensive therapy early in the course of asthma or persistent therapy to achieve constant pulmonary normality can prevent any irreversible changes later, in childhood or adulthood, needs to be determined.

Information on the relationship between age of onset, severity of asthma, and ultimate prognosis is conflicting. It appears, however, that a patient with asthma that begins before 6 months of age may have a worse prognosis in terms of severity and longevity than one with asthma that begins later in childhood. Those with *severe* asthma earlier in life also appear to have less favorable prognoses than those with mild asthma. The onset of asthma after the age of 6 months, but before the age of 2 or 3 years, does not imply a worse prognosis than onset of asthma that begins later in childhood. Asthma in childhood tends to be more severe, and the patient is less likely to become symptom free, if allergic mechanisms are involved in the disease. The disease also tends to be more severe if associated with atopic dermatitis. Conversely, there is some suggestion that patients with nonallergic asthma precipitated mainly by viral respiratory tract infections ("wheezy bronchitis" or "asthmatic bronchitis") more likely will become symptom free in later childhood. Nonallergic asthma in adulthood, however, has a significantly worse prognosis than does allergic asthma. Asthma tends to be more severe in general and occurs earlier if there is a family history of atopic disease in close relatives or if there is a personal history of other atopic disorders (atopic dermatitis or allergic rhinitis). Patients who are not symptom free during puberty are unlikely to outgrow their symptoms as young adults (Blair, 1977). There is little data on the outcome of adult asthma; from clinical experience, the prognosis would appear to be highly variable, with a few patients becoming essentially free of asthma as a significant problem.

Although morbidity from asthma is high, mortality from asthma fortunately occurs at a low rate. Nevertheless, deaths from asthma do occur, attributable to a variety of causes and occurring mainly in patients with severe asthma. Foremost amongst these causes are the failure by patient, physician, or both to appreciate the severity of asthma and to treat it appropriately. Although deaths have been attributed to overuse of isoproterenol and similar inhaled bronchodilators, as well as inappropriate administration of sedatives and misuse of aminophylline and theophylline, by far the greatest contributor to death from the disease is undertreatment. The underdiagnosis of the severity of asthma by physicians, hospital personnel, and attendants undoubtedly contributes to the fact that an emergency room constitutes a risk factor for death in asthmatics! The lability of asthma, regardless of severity, also is a risk factor, as are respiratory infections, nocturnal asthma, history of respiratory failure, and marked diurnal variation in airflow limitation with low pulmonary functions in the morning ("morning dippers"). It is important to recognize that some patients cannot perceive severe airflow obstruction, especially when it occurs gradually. Such patients must be taught to recognize warning signs of airflow obstruction. A simple device for measuring airflow, such as a portable peak flow meter, will help the patient to recognize the development of severe asthma. Finally, psychologic factors have been implicated in deaths from asthma, particularly in sudden deaths in asthmatic adolescents (Strunk et al., 1985; Benatar, 1986; Asthma Deaths, 1986).

DIAGNOSIS

Clinical Diagnosis

History. The history in the patient with suspected asthma should be designed to accomplish several things as follows: (1) to elucidate the disease process from its onset to the present and to learn what type of medication has been employed to this point in terms of management; (2) to learn about other members of the family with asthma, which may provide insight not only into the diagnosis but also into the type of understanding that the patient or family has about the disease; and (3) to identify factors that are etiologically important in inducing acute exacerbations of the disease or in prolonging or intensifying the process.

Though patients with asthma may present in a variety of ways, most share certain common historic features, and asthma often can be diagnosed by history alone. The wheezing associated with asthma characteristically is expiratory; in severe obstruction, it may be heard both in inspiration and expiration. Wheezing only in inspiration suggests obstruction high in the airway (e.g., laryngeal area) and is uncharacteristic of asthma. (As the asthmatic attack becomes more severe, patients may feel it is harder "to get air in" than to get air out, however!) During the history taking, it is essential that the patient's parent or patient understands the meaning of the term "wheezing." Wheezing usually is accompanied by cough; occasionally, cough may be the only symptom. Asthmatic attacks are episodic at first, with intervals of symptom-free periods, but as the disease becomes more chronic, the number of symptom-free periods tends to diminish progressively.

Symptoms often are more severe at night or in the early morning and improve through the day. A history of symptoms with improvement after an injection of epinephrine, inhaled or oral adrenergic drugs, or oral theophylline, suggests the diagnosis. A typical "attack" usually lasts 5 to 7 days and may clear spontaneously (though lung function abnormalities generally last much longer and often persist between attacks).

Symptoms vary with age. The infant and young child may have histories of recurrent bronchitis, bronchiolitis or pneumonia, persistent coughing with colds, recurrent "croup," or just a chronic "chest rattle." Older children and adults often develop "tight" chests with colds, recurrent "chest congestion," "bronchitis," or persistent coughing or wheezing. Respiratory symptoms may be precipitated or exacerbated also by exposure to animals, moldy or dusty areas, tobacco smoke, or cold air or by exercise. In the review of the systems, one needs to inquire about such allergic manifestations as gastrointestinal problems, including vomiting or diarrhea; skin conditions, such as atopic dermatitis or hives; and the presence or absence of factors such as recurrent colds, perennial nasal obstruction, hay fever, ear infections, sinus infections, bronchitis, asthma, pneumonia, and

exercise intolerance. One needs to ask specifically about factors that may aggravate symptoms, such as exposure to house dust, animals, grass cuttings, and irritants such as hairsprays, aerosol sprays, and cigarette smoke, or reactions to outdoor air pollutants. Drug reactions are particularly important, especially idiosyncratic or allergic reactions to antibiotics, bronchodilators, or antihistamines. One should also inquire about unusual reactions to insect stings, hospitalizations, and past illnesses. Details about whether the patient has previously had an allergy related work-up, with studies for specific IgE level and immunotherapy (hyposensitization), and lung functions, should be recorded.

The environmental history is a unique and important element in the patient with suspected asthma or other respiratory allergies, since many of the symptoms may be exacerbated by factors found in the surroundings, whether at home, school, work, or play (see Chapters 16 and 18). The environmental history is of importance primarily because it provides information on potential allergens to which the patient is exposed, and it is the cornerstone of therapy in terms of avoidance of specific factors that may be identified by allergy testing. The patient's environment includes the home, neighborhood, and work or school. Materials used in hobbies or at work may prove to be of significance in inducing symptoms.

Physical Examination. The physical examination should focus on overall growth and development in children and on respiratory mechanics: a careful examination of the chest and an examination for the associated signs of allergic disease are included. In children, weight and height should be recorded and plotted on a growth grid. Asthma itself as well as therapy with steroids can affect growth. Growth retardation may be caused by chronic hypoxemia, and under such a circumstance, control of asthma may be associated with a growth spurt. The blood pressure should be recorded, since steroids, adrenergic agents, and possibly theophylline prescribed for asthma may elevate blood pressure. Cardiac rate and rhythm also should be noted since, in addition to asthma itself in some patients, these and possibly other therapeutic drugs may exert effects on the cardiovascular system. The physician should observe respiratory rates, color of lips and nail beds, evidence of clubbing of the fingers (*not* a concomitant of asthma), dyspnea or prolongation of expirations, retractions, and use of accessory muscles by which the patient lifts the shoulders in breathing. A round-shouldered posture with an increase in anterior-posterior diameter results from hyperinflation. In children who develop asthma early, there may be a "pseudorachitic" chest deformity from long-standing airway obstruction in a growing chest. In small children, the lungs are best examined first when they are cooperative, before they are frightened by a flashlight or otoscope.

Examination of the lungs frequently reveals rhonchi, which may clear on changing position or coughing, or unequal breath sounds. On the one hand, compression of the chest during expiration may produce latent wheezes, a maneuver especially useful in children. On the other hand, older children and adults can generate lower pitched wheezing sounds on greatly forced expiration normally, without abnormal airflow limitation. Also, with sufficient effort, an expiratory wheezing sound can be made on forced expiration from the laryngotracheal area in normal individuals. Though wheezing can be elicited frequently with a forced expiratory maneuver, occasionally there is only prolongation of expiration, without wheezing. Frequently, it is difficult to persuade the older child or adult to exhale forcefully to induce latent wheezes, because the patient has discovered intuitively that such a maneuver may induce coughing that can increase bronchospasm. It is important to note air exchange because some patients with severe asthma do not wheeze — too little air is exchanged to generate a wheezing sound. With marked hyperinflation, the heart and liver both may be displaced downward as the diaphragm is depressed, shifting the point of cardiac maximal impact, decreasing precardiac dullness, and making the liver palpable. Though examination of the heart may be difficult when heart sounds are obscured by wheezing, it is important, since both asthma and its therapy may alter cardiac rate and rhythm.

The recognition of signs of upper respiratory allergy that coexist frequently with asthma (aggravating factors, e.g., sinusitis, or coexistent physical disability, e.g., serous otitis with conductive deafness) may aid in achieving better control of asthma. If nasal polyps are present, they should suggest cystic fibrosis in the young child or paranasal sinusitis possibly with aspirin sensitivity in the adolescent or adult. Eardrums should be examined with a pneumatic otoscope for serous otitis. The conjunctivae should be examined for edema, inflammation, and tearing. A slit lamp examination for cataracts also is

indicated in the patient who is receiving long-term corticosteroid treatment. Note also the texture of the skin and subcutaneous tissue, as it relates to nutrition and fluid balance, and examine flexor creases and other areas of skin for active or healed atopic dermatitis.

DIFFERENTIAL DIAGNOSIS

Table 41–3 notes the more common conditions to be differentiated from asthma at various ages. Almost all can coexist with asthma. A comprehensive list of conditions associated with wheezing is found elsewhere (Siegel et al., 1978).

Laryngotracheobronchomalacia. A congenital disorder of cartilage, laryngotracheobronchomalacia can coexist with asthma. Symptoms increase with respiratory infections. The condition usually subsides spontaneously by age 2 years (see Chapter 39).

Cystic Fibrosis. Cystic fibrosis should be suspected in any infant who has recurrent bronchial infection with poor growth. A diagnosis of cystic fibrosis does not rule out asthma, since the two may coexist (Chapter 48).

Chronic Disease due to Respiratory Viral Infections. Both adenovirus and respiratory syncytial virus infections may cause chronic pulmonary disease in infants. The ultimate prognoses for such patients are not known at present, though several prospective studies are in progress (Chapter 40).

Foreign Body. The presence of a foreign body must be distinguished from asthma at any age. *The sudden onset for the first time of persistent nonremitting wheezing is due to a foreign body until proved otherwise.* Some foreign bodies may not induce immediate symptoms, however, depending on their composition and the regions in which they lodge. For instance, an aspirated peanut may cause progressive symptoms not only because it induces progressive inflammation per se but also because it may induce allergic sensitization that may lead to progressive allergic reaction to peanut antigens. Inflammation caused by a foreign body may further cause localized bronchiectasis. If foreign body is suspected chest x-rays in inspiration and expiration should be obtained, followed if necessary by fluoroscopy, bronchoscopy, or both (Chapter 39).

Croup and Acute Epiglottitis. Croup is a

common condition due to a respiratory virus; acute epiglottitis is a fulminating infection due to *Haemophilus influenzae* infection (Chapter 39). In both, "wheezing" is mainly inspiratory. Often, children have asthma have histories of recurrent croup.

Hyperventilation Syndrome. This condition is more likely to occur in adolescence and adulthood than in childhood; it may be mistaken for asthma or may coexist with it. Typically, the patient is anxious, complains of marked dyspnea and difficulty getting her or his breath in the presence of excellent air exchange on auscultation and in the absence of wheezing. Often, there are associated complaints of headache and tingling of fingers and toes. Pulmonary function tests are helpful in differentiating hyperventilation syndrome from asthma, if the patient's cooperation can be obtained. (The patient sometimes will refuse to perform them because of fear of "smothering.") Immediate therapy consists of reassurance and possibly rebreathing into a paper bag to elevate $Paco_2$ levels. Long-term therapy involves evaluation of the cause of anxiety and psychotherapy as appropriate.

Mitral Valve Prolapse. Mitral valve prolapse occurs in asthenic (slender) adolescents and adults and is more frequent in females than males. Patients with this condition may have symptoms of chest pain during or following strenuous exercise; it is this symptom that could be confused with asthma induced by exercise. On physical examination, diagnosis may be suspected by hearing systolic "clicks" in the mitral area and can be confirmed by echocardiography (Devereux et al., 1978). An exercise test would rule out exercise-induced asthma but should be performed only with a cardiac monitor.

Other Conditions. Conditions occurring almost exclusively in the adolescent, adult, or both age groups include laryngeal wheezing due to either physical or psychologic factors; tumors, either extraluminal or intraluminal; and chronic obstructive pulmonary disease (COPD), either emphysema or chronic bronchitis. Patients with COPD often have reversible components to their obstructive diseases, altered either with bronchodilators or corticosteroids. Other conditions include cardiac failure with wheezing, pulmonary embolism, collagen vascular disease, and aspiration syndromes, such as GER which may be associated with hiatal hernias in adults.

LABORATORY TESTS

Table 41–5 lists laboratory tests useful in asthma.

Complete Blood Count. The complete blood count often is normal. Eosinophilia, if present, does not indicate an allergic etiology, since eosinophil counts may vary with adrenal function and severity of asthma. Leukocytosis greater than $15,000/mm^3$ does not necessarily indicate infection, since both epinephrine administration and the "stress" of acute asthma can induce leukocytosis.

Sputum and Nasal Mucus. Examinations of sputum and nasal mucus are simple, noninvasive tests. Asthma in older children and adults is characterized by abundant, thick tenacious sputum. In young children, sputum rarely is observed since they ordinarily swallow it. When obtained, it usually is white or "clear"; it may be interspersed with small yellow plugs (often containing eosinophils), even when infection is not present. On microscopic examination, eosinophils usually are present, along with other findings listed in Table 41–5. Sputum eosinophilia is present in both nonallergic and allergic asthma.

Nasal secretions are obtained readily in patients of all ages. When eosinophils predominate, they suggest accompanying nasal allergy in children, though adolescents and adults can have nasal eosinophilia in the absence of proven allergy. A predominance of polymorphonuclear neutrophils and lymphocytes occurs with viral respiratory infections; PMNs and ingested bacteria are seen frequently in patients with sinusitis.

Serum Tests. Quantitative immunoglobulin levels of IgG, IgM, and IgA are useful only to rule out immunodeficiency syndromes in children with recurrent or chronic infections. In patients with asthma, IgG levels usually are normal, IgA levels occasionally are low, and IgM levels may be elevated. Determination of IgE levels rarely are needed; an exception is suspected bronchopulmonary aspergillosis. *Normal IgE levels do not rule out allergy; elevated ones only suggest it.* They may be useful occasionally in infants with recurrent bronchitis or in patients with questionable "allergy." In the patient with shifting pulmonary infiltrates, tests for precipitating antibody to *Aspergillus* species and agents causing hypersensitivity pneumonitis are indicated (see Chapter 47).

Sweat Test. A sweat test should be consid-

TABLE 41–5. Laboratory Tests in Asthma

Tests	Possible Abnormalities in Asthma	Comments
Complete blood count	Leukocytosis (occasionally)	Induced by infection, epinephrine administration, "stress" (?)
	Eosinophilia (frequently)	Varies with medication, time of day, adrenal function; not necessarily related to "allergy." (Often higher in "intrinsic" than "extrinsic" asthma.)
Sputum examination	Eosinophils	In both "intrinsic" and "extrinsic" asthma.
White or "clear" and small yellow plugs	Charcot-Leyden crystals	Derived from eosinophils.
	Creola bodies	Clusters of epithelial cells.
	Curschmann spirals	Threads of glycoprotein.
Nasal smear	Eosinophils	Suggests concomitant nasal allergy.
	Lymphocytes, PMNs, macrophages	Sometimes replace eosinophils in upper respiratory infections.
	PMNs with ingested bacteria	Bacterial rhinitis or sinusitis.
Serum tests	IgG, IgA, IgM	Often normal. May be abnormal— various patterns seen.
	IgE	Sometimes elevated in "allergic" asthma; markedly elevated in active bronchopulmonary aspergillosis. Often normal.
	Aspergillus-precipitating antibody	Suggestive, not diagnostic of bronchopulmonary aspergillosis.
Sweat test	Normal in asthma	
	Perform to rule out cystic fibrosis	Cystic fibrosis and asthma can coexist.
Chest x-ray	Hyperinflation, infiltrates, pneumomediastinum, pneumothorax	Indicated once in all patients with asthma; should be considered on hospitalization for asthma.
Lung function tests	$\downarrow FEV_1$, $\downarrow FVC$, $\downarrow FEF_{25-75\%}$, $\downarrow PEFR$; $FEV_1/FVC \downarrow$	Useful for following course of disease, response to treatment.
Response to bronchodilators	> 15 percent improvement FEV_1; PEFR	Safest diagnostic test for asthma.
Exercise tests	Decreased lung function after 6 minutes of exercise PEFR and $FEV_1 > 15$ percent $\downarrow$ $FEF_{25-75\%} > 25$ percent $\downarrow$	Useful to diagnose asthma. Often abnormal when resting lung function is normal.
Methacholine inhalation test (mecholyl test); histamine inhalation test	20 percent fall in lung function with dose tolerated by "normal" subjects	Should be performed by specialists only.
Antigen inhalation test	20 percent fall in lung function immediately after challenge; may cause delayed response 6 to 8 h later	Potentially dangerous; should be performed by specialist only.
Allergy skin tests	Identifies allergic factors that *might* be causative factors	Test likely factors only — select by history.
Serologic tests for IgE antibody (e.g., RAST)	Same significance as skin tests	More expensive than skin tests.

ered in infants and children with chronic respiratory symptoms to rule out cystic fibrosis. However, cystic fibrosis and asthma (or at least a large reactive airways component) may coexist (see Chapter 48).

Chest X-rays. All patients with asthma should have chest x-rays at some time to rule out parenchymal disease, congenital anomaly, and foreign body. A chest x-ray should be considered for every patient admitted to a hospital with asthma, depending on the presentation and severity of asthma and any suspicion of complications, such as pneumonia and pneumothorax (Fig. 41–3). Chest x-ray findings in asthma may range from normal to hyperinflation with peribronchial interstitial infiltrates and atelectasis. In a 3-year study of children hospitalized for asthma, the following abnormalities were seen: 76 percent had hyperinflation with increased bronchial markings; 20 per-

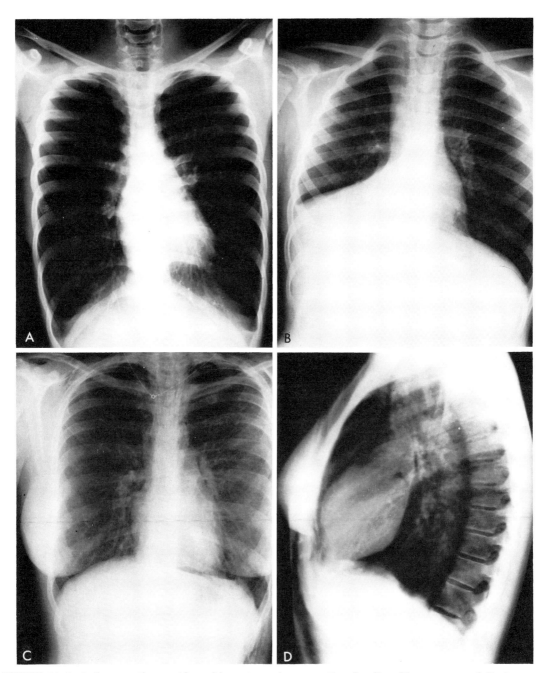

FIGURE 41–3. *A*, Severe asthma evidenced by extreme hyperaeration, "scalloped" appearance of diaphragm as insertions are visualized, and mediastinal air seen along right heart border.

B, There is almost complete collapse of right middle and right lower lobes with considerable shift of the mediastinum and elevation of the right hemidiaphragm.

C, Extensive mediastinal and subcutaneous emphysema is present without pneumothorax. The lungs are hyperexpanded and the diaphragm is flattened, consistent with the clinical diagnosis of asthma.

D, Lateral view of C showing extensive mediastinal air. (Continued on following page.)

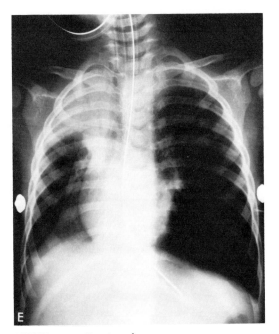

FIGURE 41–3. Continued.
E, Marked right pneumothorax with shift of pneumo-mediastinum to the right and hyperaeration of left lung.

cent had infiltrates, atelectasis, pneumonia, or a combination of the three; and 5.4 percent had pneumomediastinum often with infiltrates (Eggleston et al., 1974). Pneumothorax occurs rarely. Paranasal sinus x-rays also should be considered in patients, especially children, with persistent nocturnal coughing and headaches (see Chapter 35).

Lung Function Tests. Lung function tests are objective, noninvasive, and cost effective in diagnosing and following the patient with asthma (see Chapter 38). A simple mechanical spirometer, from which an FEV_1 and forced vital capacity (FVC) can be calculated, or a Wright Peak Flow Meter (pediatric meters are available for younger children) is useful in office practice. Children as young as 2 years can be taught to perform pulmonary function maneuvers with birthday party favors (Fig. 41–4). Results can be compared with normal standards (Chapter 38).

Response to Bronchodilators. The safest diagnostic test for asthma is to look for an improvement in lung function before and after administration of bronchodilators, such as epinephrine (epinephrine hydrochloride (1 : 1000) 0.01 ml/kg up to a maximum dosage 0.3 ml subcutaneously) and beta-2 agonists (inhalation of albuterol or equivalent by pressurized metered dose inhaler or 5- to 10-minute aerosolized solution). A greater than 15 percent improvement is virtually diagnostic of asthma.

Exercise Tolerance Tests. In older children and adolescents, a free-running exercise tolerance test is simple to perform and requires little equipment (see Chapter 44). A fall of greater than 15 percent in FEV_1 and in peak expiratory flow rate (PEFR) or 25 percent in forced expiratory flow of 25 to 75 percent ($FEF_{25-75\%}$) is diagnostic of asthma.

Bronchial Challenge Tests. Extreme airway sensitivity characterizes the patient with

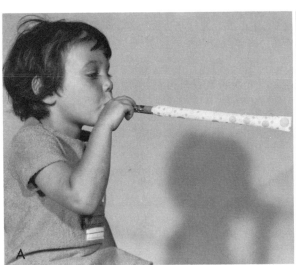
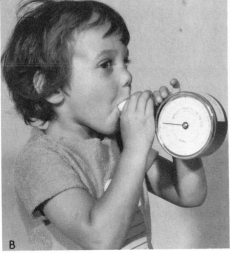

FIGURE 41–4. Illustration of the use of a party favor to teach young children the technique applicable to the use of equipment for measuring pulmonary functions.

asthma, whose airways are 50 to 1000 times more sensitive to methacholine than are those of the normal person. This has been developed as a diagnostic test for asthma (Chai et al., 1975). Histamine is used as an alternative. Inhalation of nebulized water or cold dry air also has been used.

Another challenge test involves the inhalation of allergens in various concentrations to determine the patient's bronchial sensitivity to them (bronchial provocation test). Often this test induces a biphasic reaction, an initial fall in lung function with recovery followed in 6 to 8 hours by more severe protracted bronchospasm. *All bronchial challenge tests (both methacholine-type and allergen challenge) are potentially dangerous; they should be performed only by specialists who have special training in their use.*

Allergy Testing. Allergy testing (skin testing or serologic testing, such as radioallergosorbent testing or RAST) is indicated in patients in whom specific allergic factors are believed to be important. Testing is done through selective allergens based on history and known or potential allergen exposure (see Chapter 17).

THERAPEUTIC CONSIDERATION

Philosophy of Management

A comprehensive approach to treatment of asthma requires an understanding of the disease, the manner in which patients present, and how the disease may affect physical and psychologic growth and development in children and interfere with work and normal interpersonal relationships in adolescents and adults. *The ultimate goals are to prevent disability and to minimize physical and psychologic morbidity.* These include facilitating social adjustment of the patient with the family, school, work, and community, including normal participation in recreational activities and sports. This adjustment is achieved in steps and should begin with early diagnosis and appropriate management of acute episodes. Irritant and allergic factors should be identified and eliminated from the patient's environment. *Education of the patient's parents, the patient, or both to the long-term course of asthma and to the management of exacerbations is an essential part of asthma therapy.* Unnecessary and illogical restrictions of the patient's and family's life styles should be avoided. Associated conditions that exacerbate asthma and predispose the patient to school or

work absenteeism or interfere with school or work performance must be recognized and treated. The ultimate goal should be "functional" normality—in which maximal benefit is achieved from total therapy, with the fewest detrimental effects.

Achieving these goals requires time, knowledge, and experience. The demands on the physician will vary depending on the severity of the disease, the age of the patient, and the resources of the patient or family. The family physician, internist, or pediatrician *who is willing to devote the time* can care adequately for the patient with mild or moderate asthma. However, the patient with severe asthma and chronic obstructive pulmonary changes will benefit by referral to an allergist who has the knowledge, experience, and time to initiate appropriate therapy, to follow the patient's progress, and to act as an advisor to the primary care physician. Such a referral should help ensure prompt and effective treatment of acute attacks to minimize the need for hospitalization (or, when hospitalization is necessary, to reduce length of hospital stay). A team approach that includes regular communication between the primary care physician and the specialist is essential for consistent and comprehensive long-term care.

Compliance by patient, family, or both is the keystone of any therapy. Compliance is influenced by many factors—the physician's attitude; the family's and the patient's understanding of the disease; and peer pressure. It is in *compliance* that psychologic factors are of overwhelming importance. The attitude of the patient towards the disease is paramount in his or her willingness to follow the physician's recommendations. The child's attitude towards asthma and the willingness to comply with recommendations reflect the parents' attitudes towards the disease. The physician's guidance can prevent overprotection or neglect by helping the family of a younger child to cope with such aspects of asthma as the inconvenience of a round-the-clock medication schedule and environmental control. As the child grows, the physician and family should give the patient the responsibility for his or her own medication, though the physician should help by providing the most convenient medication schedule possible—ideally one that avoids the need to take medication in school. When medication is needed at school, the patient should be permitted to take it privately without embarrassment. The physician should aid patient and family in making decisions on such activities as sports, overnight visits, and camping trips, taking care to avoid overprotection while ensuring appropriate control of asthma. The physician also can help to change attitudes of teachers, principals, and coaches (and, in some cases, school nurses) by educating them to the needs of the individual child and by showing them how the school program can be adjusted to the child's physical capacity, so that the child is not penalized or ridiculed.

Finally, when a patient fails to comply, the physician should try to find out the reasons and should work out a reasonable solution, acceptable to the patient and the family. Noncompliance in the face of severe disease, particularly in an adolescent, places the patient at great risk with regard to both morbidity from the disease and death.

Management of Asthma through the Physician's Office

The means available for management of asthma through the physician's office include pharmacologic therapy; identification and elimination of exacerbating or aggravating factors; immunotherapy (hyposensitization), when appropriate, for major allergens that cannot be eliminated or avoided; provision of optimal physical exercise; and *education of the patient and family about the disease.*

Avoidance. Allergic and irritant factors that exacerbate asthma should be identified and removed from the patient's environment. Major allergic or irritant factors in the home, school, or work place suggested by a detailed history and confirmed when applicable by skin test reactions should be eliminated or avoided to the extent possible within the framework of normal physical and psychologic growth and development (Chapter 22). Of major importance is evidence that antigen avoidance not only reduces frequency of attacks but may diminish severity of asthma itself by reducing bronchial hyperreactivity both in children (Murray et al., 1983) and adults (Platts-Mills et al., 1982). Though the removal of important allergic and irritant factors from the home is essential, the physician also must be flexible and reasonable. Often, effective environmental control may involve a compromise between what is desirable medically and what is acceptable emotionally to the family and patient.

Maximum Exercise Function. Participation in normal family, school, work, and community functions requires reasonably normal exercise tolerance. Regular exercise should be encouraged. The patient with asthma does particularly well in such sports as swimming, downhill skiing, gymnastics, and soccer (selected positions), in which acceptance as a normal team member strengthens ego and builds self respect. Pretreatment with appropriate medication and a "warm-up," consisting of a short period of mild exercise before more active exercise, are especially helpful (see Chapter 44).

Allergy Injection Therapy. Hyposensitization (immunotherapy) is indicated for major environmental allergens that cannot be avoided, such as pollen antigens. Many children and adults have allergic rhinitis, for which hyposensitization has proved efficacious. Immunotherapy may reduce the incidence of late phase reactions and thereby could reduce bronchial hyperreactivity, although this possibility remains to be firmly established (see Chapter 20). Hyposensitization also can ameliorate asthma in allergic children (Warner et al., 1978).

Management of the Acute Attack. Acute asthma can develop as a mild illness that responds promptly to bronchodilators, or it can develop into a medical emergency over a matter of a few hours, especially in the young child who is unable to retain oral medications and fluids or in the older adult who has underlying chronic pulmonary disease. In such patients, decreasing wheezing may be ominous, signaling an increasing obstruction of airways with concomitant decreases in air exchange. If the asthma fails to respond to treatment at home, the patient should be seen on an emergency basis in the physician's office or in a hospital emergency room.

Drugs of choice for treating acute asthma are epinephrine by injection or aerosolized adrenergic agents (Table 41–6). Epinephrine or terbutaline may be repeated by subcutaneous injection up to three times. This initial therapy can be followed by an injection of epinephrine suspension (Sus-Phrine), which may provide bronchodilation up to 6 hours duration (Josephson et al., 1979).

Increasingly, aerosolized bronchodilators have become the treatment of choice. Studies comparing aerosolized isoproterenol with injected epinephrine showed equivalent bronchodilation but fewer side effects by inhalation (Rossing et al., 1980). More selective adrenergic agents have been studied. Shapiro and colleagues (1987) studied three different dosages

TABLE 41–6. Adrenergic Drugs for Treatment of Acute Attack

Drug	Administration*	Dosage		Frequency	Notes
		CHILD	ADULT		
Terbutaline	Subcutaneous	0.01 mg/kg	0.25 ml	20 mins(×2)	
Epinephrine aqueous 1:1000 sol (1 mg/ml)	Subcutaneous	0.01 mg/kg	0.3 ml	20 mins(×3)	
Suspension epinephrine 1:200 (Sus-Phrine) (5 mg/ml)	Subcutaneous	0.005 ml/kg	0.2 ml	Single dose	To follow treatment, if appropriate (see text).
Isoetharine 1:100 (10 mg/ml)	Nebulized aerosol	0.25 to 0.60 ml in 2.0 ml saline†	0.25 to 1.0 ml in 2.0 ml saline	30 mins(×3)	
Metaproterenol 1:20 (50 mg/ml)	Nebulized aerosol	0.1 to 0.2 ml in 2.5 ml saline†	0.2 to 0.3 ml in 2.5 ml saline	30 mins(×3)	‡
Albuterol 1:200 (5 mg/ml)	Nebulized aerosol	0.02 ml/kg up to 0.5 ml† (100 μg/kg)	0.5 to 1.0 ml in 2.0 ml saline	30 mins(×3)	‡
Terbutaline 1:1000 (1 mg/ml)	Nebulized aerosol	1 ml in 1 ml saline†	2.0 ml in 1.0 ml saline	30 mins(×3)	‡

* In moderately severe or severe attack, it is best to administer drug via or concomitant with oxygen.
† Authors' recommendation.
‡ Safety and effectiveness of the inhaled solution in patients younger than 12 years have not been established.

of metaproterenol in 100 children with acute asthma. In this study 5 mg and 10 mg in aerosolized saline provided maximal bronchodilation with minimal side effects. Becker and coworkers (1983) compared inhaled albuterol (0.02 ml/kg of a 0.5-percent solution, maximum dosage 1 ml) with injected epinephrine in 40 children with acute asthma. The two drugs provided similar clinical improvement although 50 percent of those treated with epinephrine had such adverse effects as nausea, vomiting, palpitations, excitability, and pallor. These symptoms did not occur in the albuterol-treated group. Ahrens and associates (1980) studied terbutaline in acute asthma and found that 1 mg of terbutaline for children or 2 mg for adults diluted in saline provided longer bronchodilation than did metaproterenol.

Patients responding incompletely to adrenergic agents may benefit from short bursts (5 to 7 days) of prednisone or methylprednisolone. These will provide more rapid returns to normal pulmonary functions without significant adverse effects (Shapiro et al., 1983).

Intermittent positive pressure breathing (IPPB) should not be used because it might induce or worsen pneumomediastinum or pneumothorax (Lancet, 1978). If the patient can and will cooperate, pulmonary function testing employing measurement of peak expiratory flow or spirometry before and after therapy is quite helpful, since apparent improvement conveyed by stethoscope may be misleading in the presence of severe bronchial obstruction.

If an adequate trial of injected or aerosolized adrenergic drug fails to produce a significant response, the patient should be admitted to the hospital and treated for status asthmaticus.

Management of Mild Asthma. Mild asthma, in which the patient has only intermittent episodes of asthma but is completely symptom free between episodes, can often be managed by aerosolized adrenergic solutions. In the small child, an adrenergic bronchodilator (Table 41–7 and Table 41–8) can be administered by an electric compressor–driven nebulizer. In the older child and adult, metered dose inhalers can be used alone or with a spacer device, minimizing the need to coordinate inspiration with activation of the pressurized canister. Often, even an adult patient who has difficulty with coordination of inspiration will benefit from the use of a spacer.

TABLE 41–7. Pharmacotherapy of Mild Asthma (Intermittent, Acute Episodes and Asymptomatic Between)*

Inhalant beta-2 adrenergic drugs: metaproterenol, isoetharine, albuterol, terbutaline, bitolterol
  Delivery: metered dose inhaler (spacer if necessary); electric or oxygen driven compressor (solution)
Oral beta-2 adrenergic drugs: albuterol or metaproterenol
Oral theophylline: solution, immediate release, sustained release
Cromolyn sodium: solution, turboinhaler, metered dose inhaler

* See Table 41–8 for dosages of drugs.

TABLE 41–8. Pharmacotherapy of Moderate Asthma

Drug	Formulation	Dosage	Frequency	Comments
Theophylline	Timed-release spansule/ tablet	16–24 mg/kg/day	98–12 h	Follow theophylline levels.
Cromolyn sodium	Turboinhaler Aerosol solution MDI*	20 mg 20 mg 2 mg (2 inhalations)	Begin qid; reduce to tid or bid	Can be used as preventative (prn).
Adrenergic Agents				
Albuterol	MDI	2 inhalations	q4–6 h	‡
	Nebulizer solution	0.2 ml/kg up to 1 ml	q4–6 h	‡
	Oral solution/ tablets	0.1 mg/kg maximum of 4 mg	q6–8 h	Little data on children under 6.†
Metaproterenol	MDI	2 inhalations	q4–6 h	‡
	Nebulizer solution	0.1–0.2 ml in 2 ml saline	q4–6 h	‡
	Oral solution tablets	1.3–2.6 mg/kg/ day; maximum of 20 mg tid	q6–8 h	Little data on children under 6.
Terbutaline	MDI	2 inhalations	q4–6 h	‡
	Tablets	2.5–5 mg	q4–6 h	Little data on children under 12.
	Ampules	0.25 mg IM or SC	Repeat in 20 mins × 1	
Bitolteral mesylate	MDI	2 inhalations	q4–6 h	‡
Isoetharine	1 percent	0.30–0.75 ml	q4–6 h	
	MDI	2 inhalations	q4–6 h	
Ipratropium bromide	MDI	2 inhalations	qid	‡
				Marketed for those with chronic bronchitis but effective in some with asthma.
Steroids	See Table 41–9.			Short bursts used occasionally when not adequately responsive to nonsteroidal bronchodilators.

* MDI = metered dose inhaler.
† Drug used round-the-clock or prn as appropriate (see text).
‡ Safety and effectiveness in patients below 12 years of age have not been established, according to manufacturer.

Oral administration of adrenergic agents, theophylline, or both represents an alternative form of therapy for acute attacks, although oral adrenergic agents and theophylline are associated with increased systemic adverse effects compared with inhaled adrenergic drugs.

Aminophylline suppositories should be avoided because of erratic and slow absorption and potential overdosage. Rectal theophylline preparations, in the marketed solution form, however, are well absorbed and can be used for short periods in place of oral theophylline. Cromolyn sodium may be effective if used prior to anticipated exposure to known allergens (e.g., cats) or prior to exercise.

Management of Moderately Severe Asthma. Asthma that interferes with activity, sleep, or exercise and is characterized by per- sistently abnormal lung functions requires a regular maintenance medication for control. Either aerosolized cromolyn or sustained-release theophylline can be employed as a first-line, maintenance drug (Table 41–8). Both appear to be equivalent in asthma control in children with moderate asthma (Furukawa et al., 1984). Cromolyn does not have the side effects of theophylline (see Chapter 19), including adverse effects on school performance (Rachelefsky et al., 1986), and does not require regular monitoring of serum concentrations that are obligatory for theophylline. Cromolyn, however, is not a bronchodilator and is not effective in acute asthma. Cromolyn may be administered as a metered dose aerosol, as a powder by a turboinhaler, or as a solution by motor driven nebulizer. The initial dosage of four times daily may be reduced to thrice or even twice daily, once the medication's effect has been achieved (usually in a 4-week period).

When theophylline is prescribed as a primary drug, a timed-release formulation is administered every 8 to 12 hours in a dose that provides a peak concentration of less than 20 μg/ml (we prefer to keep peak levels less than 15 μg/ml). A back-up adrenergic agent is appropriate for exacerbation of acute asthma, or one can be added to the long-term therapeutic regimen. Theophylline dosages and formulations are discussed fully in Chapter 19. Exacerbations of acute asthma are treated as previously described, adding short bursts of short-acting steroids as necessary.

Management of Severe Asthma. In severe asthma, the patient continues to have incapacitating dyspnea, cough, and obstructed airways in spite of treatment as described for moderate asthma. Long-term corticosteroid therapy is essential to the treatment of such patients as an adjunct to other therapy (Table 41–9). After controlling the asthma with a burst of short-acting steroids (prednisone, prednisolone, methylprednisolone), the patient may be placed on every-other-day steroids, beginning with 2.5 times the minimal daily steroid dosage that controlled the asthma, or on inhaled steroids (beclomethasone dipropionate, triamcinolone acetonide, or flunisolide). Inhaled steroids are usually initiated with a dosage of three inhalations four times daily. The dosage of oral

TABLE 41–9. Pharmacotherapy of Severe Asthma

Theophylline, adrenergic drugs, cromolyn: as outlined in Table 41–8 for moderately severe asthma.
Steroids including prednisone, prednisolone, methylprednisolone: Begin at 30 to 40 mg/day (once daily in a.m. or split into 2 to 3 doses/day). Taper to lowest daily (early a.m.) dose that controls asthma and maintains adequate lung functions. Short bursts (3 to 10 days) used occasionally may suffice without long-term therapy. Long-term therapy involves shifting to every second day (qod), using 2.5 times the lowest daily dosage that controlled asthma. (Give before 8 a.m.) Dosage reductions should be attempted at 2-week intervals. Reassess dosage requirements periodically.
Aerosolized steroids including beclomethasone dipropionate, triamcinolone acetonide, flunisolide: Begin with 2 to 3 inhalations, four times daily (qid), and reduce to lowest dosage that controls asthma. Dosage reductions should be attempted at 2-week intervals. Reassess dosage requirements periodically. Larger doses may be required in patients with resistant diseases.

or inhaled steroids is slowly reduced to the smallest one that will control the asthma. Often, the frequency of inhaled steroids can be reduced to thrice daily and occasionally to twice daily. Oral candidiasis, the major complication of aerosolized steroid therapy, can be minimized by rinsing the mouth with water after each treatment.

When a patient has received oral steroids for a prolonged period, prednisone should be tapered slowly when attempting to replace them with aerosolized steroids, since the hypothalamic-pituitary-adrenal axis may take up to a year to recover normal responsiveness. If the patient is on alternate-day or aerosolized steroid therapy, short courses of daily steroid therapy should be considered for acute exacerbations of asthma, major surgery (see Chapter 58), and acute, severe illness in general.

When systemic steroids cannot be changed to every-other-day dosage or to aerosolized steroids, troleandomycin (TAO) has been found to have a unique steroid-sparing effect. This effect is exclusively associated with methylprednisolone therapy (Spector et al., 1974). TAO and methylprednisolone have been found useful in treating steroid-dependent children between 7 and 13 years of age (Eiches et al., 1985). In 11 steroid-dependent children, TAO therapy resulted in improved clinical and pulmonary function within 7 days of initial treatment. Side effects of treatment were increased cushingoid features, abdominal pain, and increased liver enzyme concentrations. After a methylprednisolone reduction to the lowest effective dosage, TAO was begun at 14 mg/kg/day with a weekly reduction over 4 weeks to 3.5 mg/kg/day and a concomitant reduction of methylprednisolone. Patients on daily steroids were shifted to every-other-day, if possible, and those on oral steroids were shifted to aerosolized steroids. *TAO affects the metabolism of theophylline, so that the theophylline dosage should be reduced 30 to 50 percent to avoid toxicity.* Weekly liver tests, spirometry, and theophylline serum levels should be performed on patients who are taking TAO.

Further studies in adults recommend a starting dosage of 250 mg once daily and shifted, if possible, to every other day with the methylprednisolone every other day. Those patients whose asthma cannot be controlled on every-other-day steroids should be considered TAO failures, and TAO should be discontinued (Wald et al., 1986).

The mechanism of action of TAO is not clear;

it does not act as an antibiotic. Although it appears to have a steroid-sparing action, responsive patients become cushingoid at lower steroid dosages. TAO has a direct adverse effect on the liver and induces abnormal liver chemistry findings in some patients. However, neither its steroid-sparing or hepatic action explains its effectiveness.

Other Drugs. Other agents sometimes prescribed for asthma include expectorants, sedatives, tranquilizers, and antihistamines. All expectorants depend upon adequate hydration for effective action. Iodides, the traditional expectorants of the past, should be avoided in children because of many side effects that make their use unacceptable (A.A.P. Committee on Drugs, 1976). Other expectorants, such as glycerol guaiacolate, add little at best to adequate hydration. Antibiotics are indicated only when there is substantial evidence of bacterial or mycoplasma infection (see Chapter 23). Sedatives are contraindicated in asthma therapy. Mild tranquilization may be appropriate for treatment of concomitant conditions but not for treatment of asthma per se. Drugs with H1 antihistamine action appear to have prophylactic antiasthma action, as reported in some studies. These drugs include azatadine, azelastine, ketotifen, and perhaps astemizole and terfenadine. Further studies will be needed to define the role of these agents in asthma therapy.

Psychologic Problems. In chronic asthma, various psychologic problems may require referral to specialists. The types of problems requiring consultation include the patient or family whose denial of asthma leads to treatment delays or noncompliance and repeated hospitalizations; estranged parents whose child's asthma is a focal point in their quarrels; parents who overprotect the child into adult life, unable to allow him or her to grow up; parents who are overcontrolled by the child who has asthma; and patients who use their asthma consistently to avoid responsibility or uncomfortable situations (Chapter 22).

SPECIAL PROBLEMS IN ASTHMA THERAPY

Nocturnal Asthma. Asthma that greatly intensifies at night is one of the risk factors for death from the disease (Hetzel et al., 1977). In addition to patients with this specific complaint, nocturnal asthma should be suspected in patients who awaken in the morning with se-

vere asthma and in those who have marked diurnal variations in peak flow rates. Causes of increased asthma at night are numerous and include late reactions to allergen exposure or other asthmogenic factors, such as exercise, GER and secretions from the sinuses or nasopharynx. These can be further intensified simply by poor control of asthma, with persistent gross abnormalities in pulmonary functions. Normalization of lung functions and identification with elimination or treatment of factors responsible for nocturnal exacerbations are the obvious optimal therapeutic approaches to this problem. The intensification of asthma during sleep appears unrelated to recumbency or to sleep per se but may be related to an exacerbation of a normal circadian variation in bronchomotor tone (Barnes, 1986). Abnormalities in central nervous system control of respiratory drive also may be operative in some patients and can pose serious risks to patients with asthma (Martin, 1984). Suggested therapy includes the use of long-acting bronchodilators, particularly long-acting theophylline preparations, in addition to other round-the-clock medications, including steroids, with intensification of the regimen at bedtime and provision of a warm humidified atmosphere through the night (Barnes, 1986). Sedatives or hypnotics are contraindicated in such patients. In rare circumstances, therapeutic nocturnal awakening may be necessary to avoid dangerous drops of airflow. Suspicion of possible abnormal respiratory patterns requires investigation in a "sleep laboratory," available in many major medical centers. In a patient with severe asthma and abnormal hypoxic drive, the use of oxygen during sleep may be life saving.

Asthma in Infancy and Early Childhood. Asthma in infancy and early childhood presents a special problem because of unique anatomic, pathophysiologic, and pharmacologic characteristics (Siegel and Rachelefsky, 1985; Rachelefsky and Siegel, 1985). Anatomically, peripheral airways are disproportionately narrow, which results in increased peripheral resistance to airflow when compared with that of children over age 6 years. There is poorly developed collateral ventilation, with fewer and smaller interalveolar communications (pores of Kohn), fewer communications of bronchi to alveoli (Lambert canals), and fewer openings between alveolar ducts of different acini. Further, there are increased numbers of mucus glands in major bronchi, as compared with older children or adults, and there is a relative paucity of smooth muscle in the walls of peripheral airways. Accordingly, airways obstruction in acute asthma is due to edema and copious secretions rather than to broncho-spasm. Thus, bronchodilators are less effective in general in this age group than in older individuals (see Chapter 37).

In the infant and small child, viral infections are the major precipitants of asthma (see Table 41–1), and there is evidence of an IgE antibody response to respiratory syncytial virus and perhaps other respiratory viruses (Welliver et al., 1981), which could lead to prolonged periods of active asthma.

Few therapeutic studies have been carried out in this age group. Theophylline therapy is associated with many side effects in patients under 1 year of age (irritability, insomnia, vomiting, and seizures from overdosage), and many workers believe that it should be avoided entirely in patients under 6 months of age because of erratic absorption of sustained release granules and rapidly changing metabolic half-life of drug inactivation.

Newth and colleagues (1982) studied 24 children between 1 and 6 years of age and compared aerosolized cromolyn, oral theophylline, and their combination in a three-way crossover design. The children had significantly fewer symptomatic days on cromolyn or the combination than on theophylline. Gastrointestinal and central nervous system symptoms occurred frequently during the early days of theophylline therapy; ten had vomiting while on theophylline and two, on cromolyn. The combined drug phase was associated with statistically less need for supplementary albuterol.

In this age group, we use topical (aerosolized) medications over oral whenever feasible for treating mild to moderate asthma. (It should be recognized, however, that the majority of studies on the effectiveness of adrenergic agents in this age group have not indicated great therapeutic benefit.) Cromolyn nebulization at home by motor driven nebulizer can be supplemented with 0.1 ml (5 mg) metaproterenol nebulizer solution (Shapiro et al., 1987) or 0.02 ml/kg of 0.5 percent albuterol nebulizer solution for exacerbations of asthma (Becker et al., 1983). Either can be added to the cromolyn nebulizer solution or administered in 2.5 ml of saline or water. Alternatively, metaproterenol syrup or albuterol syrup can be administered in a dose ranging from 1 to 2 ml every 4 to 6 hours as needed.

For more severe asthma, theophylline sus-tained-release granules can be added for children over 6 months with a starting dosage of 2 to 4 mg/kg every 8 hours. This dosage is increased gradually to provide a peak serum concentration of 5 to 15 μg/ml.

In the child with severe chronic asthma, a burst of prednisone can be followed by a dosage of 5 to 10 mg or less, every other day. It is essential that the child's growth be plotted on a growth grid and the steroid dosage be reduced, if the rate of growth decreases.

In this age group, particularly, it is essential that airway irritants such as tobacco smoke or wood smoke be eliminated from the home and that environmental control for allergens be enforced in order to reduce to a minimum the need for pharmacologic therapy.

REFERENCES

Aas, K.: Bronchial provocation tests in asthma. Arch. Dis. Child. 45:221, 1970.

Ahrens, R.C., Hendles, L., Weinberger, M.: Clinical Pharmacology of Drugs Used in Treatment of Asthma. In Yaffe, S.J. (ed.), Pediatric Pharmacology. New York, Grune and Stratton, 1980.

American Academy or Pediatrics Committee on Drugs: Adverse reactions to iodide therapy of asthma and other pulmonary diseases. Pediatrics 57:272, 1976.

Asthma Deaths. N.E.R. Allergy Proc. 7:421–470, 1986.

Barnes, P.J.: Nocturnal asthma: Underlying mechanisms and implications for therapy. Immunol. Allergy Pract. 3:9–15, 1986.

Barter, C.E., Campbell, A.H.: Relationship of constitutional factors and cigarette smoking to decrease in 1-second forced expiratory volume. Am. Rev. Resp. Dis. 113:305–314, 1976.

Becker, A.B., Nelson, N.A., Simons, F.E.R.: Inhaled salbutamol (albuterol) vs. injected epinephrine in the treatment of acute asthma in children. J. Pediatr. 102:465–469, 1983.

Benatar, S.R.: Fatal asthma. N. Engl. J. Med. 314:423–488, 1986.

Bias, W.B.: The Genetic Basis of Asthma. In Austen, K.F., Lichtenstein, L.M. (eds.), Asthma. New York, Academic Press Inc., 1973.

Blair, H: Natural history of childhood asthma. Arch. Dis. Child. 52:613–619, 1977.

Bronchial Asthma: See Weiss, E.B., Segal, M.S., Stein, M.

Bush, R.K., Taylor, S.L., Busse, W.: A critical evaluation of clinical trials in reactions to sulfites. J. Allergy Clin. Immunol. 78:191–201, 1986.

Cade, J.F., Pain, M.C.F.: Pulmonary function during clinical remission of asthma. How reversible is asthma? Aust. N.Z.J. Med. 3:545–551, 1973.

Chai, H., Farr, R.S., Froehlich, L.A., Mathison, D.A., McLean, J.A., Rosenthal, R.R., Sheffer, A.L., Spector, S.L., Townley, R.G.: Standardization of bronchial inhalation challenge procedures. J. Allergy Clin. Immunol. 56:323–327, 1975.

Clark, T.J.H., Godfrey, A.: Asthma. London, Chapman and Hall, 2nd ed. 1983.

Cockroft, D.W.: Mechanism of perennial allergic asthma. Lancet 2:253–255, 1983.

Cockroft, D.W.: The bronchial late response in the pathogenesis of asthma and its modulation by therapy. Ann. Allergy 55:857–862, 1985.

Cockroft, D.W., Murdock, K.Y., Berscheid, B.A.: Relationship between atopy and bronchial responsiveness to histamine in a random population. Ann. Allergy 53:26–29, 1984.

Cockroft, D.W., Ruffin, R.E., Frith, P.A, Cartier, A., Juniper, E.F., Dolovich, J., Hargreave, F.E.: Determinants of allergen-induced asthma: Dose of allergen circulating IgE antibody concentration and bronchial responsiveness to inhaled histamine. Am. Rev. Resp. Dis. 120:1053–1058, 1979.

Corrao, W.M., Braman, S.S., Irwin, R.S.: Chronic cough as the sole presenting manifestation of bronchial asthma. N. Engl. J. Med. 300:633–637, 1979.

Dawson, A., Simon, R.A.: The Practical Management of Asthma. New York, Grune and Stratton, 1984.

Devereux, R.B., Perloff, J.K., Reichele, N., Josephson, M.F.: Mitral valve prolapse. Circulation 54:3, 1978.

Dowse, G.K., Turner, K.J., Stewart, G.A., Alpers, M.P., Woolcook, A.J.: The association between *Dermatophagoides* mites and the increasing prevalence of asthma in village communities within the Papua New Guinea highlands. J. Allergy Clin. Immunol. 75:75–83, 1985.

Editorial: Alveolar rupture. Lancet 2:137, 1978.

Eggleston, P.A., Ward, B.H., Pierson, W.E., Bierman, C.W.: Radiographic abnormalities in acute asthma in children. Pediatrics 54:442–449, 1974.

Eitches, R.W., Rachelefsky, G.S., Katz, R.E., Mendoza, G.R., Siegel, S.C.: Methylprednisolone and troleandomycin in treatment of steroid-dependent asthmatic children. Am. J. Dis. Child. 139:264–268, 1985.

Ellis, E.F.: Role of infection in asthma. Adv. Asth. Allergy Pulmon. Dis. 4:28, 1977.

Flensborg, E.W.: The prognosis for bronchial asthma arisen in infancy after the nonspecific treatment hitherto applied. Acta Paediatr. 33:4–23, 1945.

Frigas, E., Gleich, G.J.: The eosinophil and the pathophysiology of asthma. J. Allergy Clin. Immunol. 77:527–537, 1986.

Furukawa, C.T., Shapiro, G.G., Bierman, C.W., Kraemer, M.J., Ward, D.J., Pierson, W.E.: A double blind study comparing the effectiveness of cromolyn sodium and sustained-release theophylline in childhood asthma. Pediatrics 74:453–459, 1984.

Gershwin, M.E.: Bronchial Asthma, Principles of Diagnosis and Treatment. New York, Grune and Stratton, 1981.

Hargreave, F.E., Dolovich, J., O'Byrne, P.A., Ramsdale, E.H., Daniel, E.E.: The origin of airway hyperresponsiveness. J. Allergy Clin. Immunol. 5:825–832, 1986.

Hetzel, M.R., Clark, T.J.H., Branthwaite, M.A.: Asthma: Analysis of sudden deaths in ventilatory arrests in hospital. Br. Med. J. 1:808–811, 1977.

Hogg, J.C.: The Pathology of Asthma. In Weiss, E.B., Siegel, M.S., Stein, M. (eds.), Bronchial Asthma. Mechanisms and Therapeutics, 2nd ed. Boston, Little, Brown and Co., 1985.

Josephson, G.W., MacKenzie, E.J., Lietman, P.S., Gibson, G.: Emergency treatment of asthma. J.A.M.A. 242:639–643, 1979.

Kattan, C.M., Keens, T.G., Lapierre, J.G., Levison, H., Bryan, C., Reilly, B.J.: Pulmonary function abnormalities in symptom-free children after bronchiolitis. Pediatrics 59:683–688, 1977.

Kinsman, R.A., Dahlein, N.W., Spector, S., Studenmayer, H.: Observations on subjective symptomatology, coping behavior, and medical decision in asthma. Psychosomat. Med. 39:102–119, 1977.

Lancet Commentary: Asthma at Night. Lancet 1:220–222, 1983.

Lancet Editorial. Alveolar Rupture. Lancet 2:137, 1978.

Larsen, G.L.: Late phase reactions: Observations on pathogenesis and prevention. J. Allergy Clin. Immunol. 76:665–669, 1985.

Levison, H.S., Collins-Williams, C., Bryan, A.C., Reilly, B J., Orange, R.P.: Asthma. Curr. Con. Pediatr. Clin. N. Am. 21:951–965, 1974.

MacDonnell, K.F., Chawla, S.S.: Differential Diagnosis of Asthma. In Weiss, E.B., Segal, M.S., Stein, M. (eds.), Bronchial Asthma. Mechanisms and Therapeutics 2nd ed. Boston, Little Brown and Co., 1985.

Martin, R.J.: Cardiorespiratory Disorders During Sleep. Futura Publishing Co., Inc., Mount Kisco, New York, 1984.

McConnochie, K.M., Roghmann, K.J.: Breast feeding and maternal smoking as predictors of wheezing in children age 6 to 10 years. Pediatr. Pulm. 2:260–268, 1986.

McFadden, E.R., Jr.: Exertional dyspnea and cough as preludes to acute attacks of bronchial asthma. N. Engl. J. Med. 292:555–559, 1975a.

McFadden, E.R., Jr.: The chronicity of acute attacks of asthma—mechanical and therapeutic implications. J. Allergy Clin. Immunol. 56:18–26, 1975b.

McFadden, E.R., Jr., Kisser, R., DeGroot, W.J.: Acute bronchial asthma: Relations between clinical and physiological manifestations. N. Engl. J. Med. 288:221–228, 1973.

Minor, T.E., Baker, J.W., Dick, E.C., DeMeo, A.N., Oulette, J.J., Cohen, M., Reed, C.E.: Greater frequency of viral respiratory infections in asthmatic children as compared with their nonasthmatic siblings. J. Pediatr. 85:472–477, 1974.

Murray, A.B., Ferguson, A.C.: Dust-free bedrooms in the treatment of asthmatic children with house dust or house dust mite allergy: a controlled trial. Pediatrics 71:418–423, 1983.

Newth, C.J.L., Newth, C.V., Turner, J.A.P.: Comparison of nebulized sodium cromoglycate and oral theophylline in controlling symptoms of chronic asthma in preschool children: A double blind study. Aust. N.Z.J. Med. 12:232–238, 1982.

Pearlman, D.S.: Bronchial Asthma. A perspective from childhood to adulthood. Am. J. Dis. Child. 138:459–466, 1984.

Platts-Mills, T.A.E., Michel, E.B., Nock, P., Tovey, E.R., Moszoro, H., Wilkins, S.R.: Reduction of bronchial hypersensitivity during prolonged allergen avoidance. Lancet 2:675–678, 1982.

Rachelefsky, G.S., Coulson, A., Siegel, S.C., Stiehm, E.R.: Aspirin intolerance in chronic childhood asthma: detected by oral challenge. Pediatrics 56:443–448, 1975.

Rachelefsky, G.S., Siegel, S.C.: Asthma in infants and children—Treatment of childhood asthma: Part II. J. Allergy Clin. Immunol. 76:409–425, 1985.

Rachelefsky, G.S., Wo, J., Adelson, M.A., Mickey, M.R., Spector, S.L., Katz, R.M., Siegel, S.C., Rohr, A.S.: Behavior abnormalities and poor school performance due to oral theophylline use. Pediatrics 78:1133–1138, 1986.

Rackemann, F.M.: Intrinsic asthma. J. Allergy 11:147, 1940.

Reid, L.: Pathological Changes in Asthma. In Clark, T.J.H.,

Godfrey, S. (eds.), Asthma. Philadelphia, W.B. Saunders Co., 1977.

Rossing, T.H., Fanta, C.H., Goldstein, D.H., Snapper, J.R., McFadden, E.R., Jr.: Emergency treatment of asthma: Comparison of the acute effects of parenteral and inhaled sympathomimetics and infused aminophylline. Am. Rev. Respir. Dis. 122:365–374, 1980.

Ryssing, E.: Continued follow-up investigation concerning the fate of 298 asthmatic children. Acta Pediatr. 48:255–260, 1959.

Shapiro, G.G., Furukawa, C.T., Pierson, W.E., Chapko, M.K., Sharp, M., Bierman, C.W.: Double-blind, dose-response study of metaproterenol inhalant solution in children with acute asthma: J. Allergy Clin. Immunol. 79:378–386, 1987.

Shapiro, G.G., Furukawa, C.T., Pierson, W.E., Gardinier, R., Bierman, C.W.: Double-blind evaluation of methylprednisolone versus placebo for acute asthma episodes. Pediatrics 71:510–514, 1983.

Sibbald, B., Horn, M.E.C., Brain, E.A., Gregg, L.: Genetic factors in childhood asthma. Thorax 35:671–674, 1980.

Siegel, S.C., Katz, R.M., Rachelefsky, G.S.: Asthma in infancy and childhood. In Middleton, E., Reed, C.E., Ellis, E.F. (eds.), Allergy: Principles and Practice. St. Louis, C.V. Mosby Co., 1978.

Siegel, S.C., Rachelefsky, G.S.: Asthma in infants and children. Part I. J. Allergy Clin. Immunol. 76:1–15, 1985.

Slavin, R.G.: Recalcitrant asthma: Have you looked for sinusitis? J. Resp. Dis. 7:61–68, 1986.

Speight, A.N.P., Lee, D.A., Hey, E.N.: Underdiagnosis and undertreatment of asthma in childhood. Brit. Med. J. 286:1253–1256, 1983.

Strunk, R.D., Mrazek, D.A., Fuhrmann, G.S., LaBreoque, J.F.: Physiologic and psychological characteristics associated with deaths due to asthma in childhood. J.A.M.A. 254:1193–1198, 1985.

Spector, S.L., Katz, F.H., Farr, R.S.: Troleandomycin: effectiveness in steroid-dependent asthma and bronchitis. J. Allergy Clin. Immunol. 54:367–379, 1974.

Szentivanyi, A.: The beta adrenergic theory of the atopic abnormality in bronchial asthma. J. Allergy 42:203–232, 1968.

Tinkelman, D.G., Falliers, C.J., Naspitz, C.K.: Childhood Asthma. Pathophysiology and Treatment. New York, Marcel Dekker Inc., 1987.

Tooley, W.H., DeMuth, C., Nadel, J.A.: The reversibility of obstructive changes in severe childhood asthma. J. Pediatr. 66:517–524, 1965.

Townley, R.G., Guirgis, H., Bewtra, A., Watt, G., Burke, K., Carney, K.: IgE levels and methacholine inhalation responses in monozygous and dizygous twins. (Abstract). J. Allergy Clin. Immunol. 57:227, 1976.

Townley, R.G., Ryo, U.Y., Kolokin, B.M., Kang, B.: Bronchial sensitivity to methacholine in current and former asthmatic and allergic rhinitis patients and control subjects. J. Allergy Clin. Immunol. 56:429–432, 1975.

Wald, J.A., Friedman, B.F., Farr, R.S.: An improved protocol for the use of troleandomycin (TAO) in the treatment of steroid dependent asthma. J. Allergy Clin. Immunol. 78:36–43, 1986.

Warner, J.O., Price, J.F., Soothill, J.F., Hey, E.N.: Controlled trial of hyposensitization to *dermatophagoides pteronyssinus* in children with asthma. Lancet 2:912–915, 1978.

Weiss, E.B., Segal, M.S., Stein, M. (eds.): Bronchial Asthma: Mechanisms and Therapeutics, 2nd ed. Boston, Little, Brown and Co., 1985.

Welliver, R.C.: Allergy and the syndrome of chronic Epstein-Barr virus infection. (Editorial.) J. Allergy Clin. Immunol. 78:278–281, 1986.

Young, S.H., Shulman, S.A., Shulman, M.D.: The Asthma Handbook: A Complete Guidebook for Patients and their Families. New York, Bantam Books, 1985. (Recommended for patients and their parents.)

42

Treatment of Acute Asthma in Children

HERBERT C. MANSMANN, JR., M.D.
C. WARREN BIERMAN, M.D.
DAVID S. PEARLMAN, M.D.

The management of the patient with acute asthma requires prompt assessment of severity to determine appropriate therapeutic requirements and to provide them in a logical systematic fashion. The goals of treatment should provide for maximal pulmonary gas exchange, decrease of pulmonary inflammation, relaxation of bronchospasm, and clearing of tracheobronchial secretions. These goals are reached in a stepwise approach to management, which must be adapted in regard to both the age of the patient and the severity of the disease. With improved understanding of asthma and its therapy, status asthmaticus has been treated in at least four major children's hospitals without a death for over 10 years (Mansmann, 1987).

Classification of patients according to asthma severity facilitates a logical approach to therapy. This classification is based upon reviews by Mansmann (1980, 1983, and 1987). Therapeutic considerations are reviewed also by Heurich et al. (1978), Kurland and Leong (1985), Sybert and Weiss (1985), and Bierman et al. (1985). Classification of disease severity based on initial signs and symptoms and their progression is noted in Table 42–1. Patients seeking medical care for acute asthma can be classified into five distinct categories; *mild episodic asthma, acute severe asthma, early status asthmaticus, advanced status asthmaticus,* and *acute respiratory failure.* Status asthmaticus is defined as severe asthma poorly responsive or unresponsive to therapy. It is a "relative" term, since almost all asthma is responsive eventually to appropriate treatment. As the disease progresses, the patient moves through each stage in a continuum though the rate of progression and length of time in each stage varies from patient to patient.

Successful management of acute illness is based upon three cornerstones as follows: (1) *education*—parents, and ultimately the patient, must be educated about the multiple facets of asthma and the appropriate selection and use of medications to modify them; (2) *medical supervision*—patients with asthma require regular, careful medical supervision; and (3) *prompt recognition and treatment*—the physician, parents, and patient must recognize and treat increasingly severe asthma promptly, since *the best treatment of respiratory failure is prevention by effective early treatment of acute asthma.*

PATHOPHYSIOLOGY

Acute bronchial asthma is a disease of the airways, which results in progressive, but reversible, airflow limitation with hyperinflation throughout the lungs. Obstruction to airflow is due to bronchial smooth muscle constriction, with edema and infiltration by inflammatory cells, and to desquamation of cells lining the airway mucosa coupled with bronchial and bronchiolar plugging by intraluminal secretions. Acute asthmatic attacks frequently are superimposed upon a chronic asthmatic process, with underlying prolonged pathophysiologic changes that include all of the aforementioned ones as well as smooth muscle hypertrophy, basement membrane thickening, and hyperplasia of the mucous glands. The acute obstructive process is unevenly distributed in the lungs, resulting in ventilation-perfusion imbalance and predisposing the patient to hypoxemia. In the infant and young child, mucosal edema and mucous plugging are prominent (Field, 1968); in the older patient, bronchospasm predominates more often. Even without acute provocation, the child with chronic asthma can develop hypoxemia during sleep and, with progressive hypoxemia, can develop a decreased ventilatory response (Smith and Hudgel, 1980).

In the acute attack, minute ventilation initially is increased and $PaCO_2$ falls, producing respiratory alkalosis. Pulmonary flow rates fall while lung volumes increase from air trapping.

571

TABLE 42–1. Stages of Acute Asthma

Stage	1a	1b	2	3	4
Designation	Mild Episodic	Acute Severe	Early	Advanced	Respiratory Failure
	Asthma		Status Asthmaticus		
Characteristics by Stage					
Initial Clinical Features	Sudden mild cough, wheeze No dyspnea	Mild dyspnea Tachypnea Hypocarbia	Moderate dyspnea Tachypnea Unresponsive to epinephrine Normocarbia	Severe dyspnea Tachypnea Hypercarbia Central cyanosis	Respiratory failure
Frequency of Initial Presentation (1b thru 4)	Unknown	69 percent	20 percent	10 percent	1 percent (patient may arrive in coma)
Progression	None	11 percent	40 percent	Rarely	None
Physical Signs					
Pulsus paradoxus (mm Hg)	0–10	0–13	10–20	>20	20–50
Supraclavicular indrawing	None	Rare	Often	Usual	All
Sternocleido-mastoid contraction	None	Rare	Usual	All	All
Blood Gas Values					
$PaCO_2$ (torr)	35–42	<35	35–45	>45	55–100+
pHa	7.40	>7.40	7.40	<7.35	<7.2
PaO_2 (torr)	80–65	65–55	55–45	<45	<45
Pulmonary Function					
FEV_1	>75 percent of predicted	>50 percent of predicted (2.0 L)*	>25 percent of predicted (2.0–1.0 L)*	<25 percent of predicted (1.0–0.5 L)*	Unable to perform
PEFR	>75 percent of predicted (300 L/min)*	>50 percent of predicted (200 L/min)*	>20 percent of predicted (200–100 L/min)*	<20 percent of predicted (100 L/min)*	Unable to perform

* Values in older children and adults.

With continuing distention of the lungs, the development of respiratory muscle inefficiency due to fatigue, and the worsening of airflow obstruction, CO_2 begins to accumulate. The patient develops hypocarbia, then normocarbia, and then hypercarbia. Thus, normocarbia in the presence of airflow limitation in asthma indicates early respiratory failure. In addition to the development of respiratory acidosis associated with CO_2 retention, a child often has a metabolic component to the acidosis (Weng et al., 1970). Poor oral intake, vomiting, extra work of breathing, apprehension, fever, and infection can contribute to ketosis and lactic acidosis. The lack of aggressive treatment or unresponsiveness to therapy as all of the aforementioned occurs, can lead to cardiovascular collapse and death.

AGE-DEPENDENT FACTORS

Young children are particularly susceptible to status asthmaticus. Over a 3-year period, 512 children were hospitalized for status asthmaticus in a major children's hospital (Eggleston et al., 1974). Half were 3 years of age or less and two thirds were less than 6 years of age. The reasons for this predilection are primarily anatomic and appear to be related to respiratory surface area, airway diameter, quantity of bronchial smooth muscle, and concentration of mucous glands in the airway.

Bronchial smooth muscle is relatively poorly developed in infants and children under 3 years of age; edema rather than bronchospasm is the predominant obstructive feature of asthma in this age group. The density of mucous glands is increased in the infant, and the ratio of mucous glands to bronchial wall (Reid Index) also is higher (Field, 1968). Moreover, a low proportion of fatigue-resistant diaphragmatic muscle fibers, an increased peripheral pulmonary resistance, and a small alveolar surface contribute to the increased incidence of respiratory failure in infants during severe asthma (Tabachnik and Levison, 1981). These factors account for the greater severity of asthma, the more frequent need for hospitalization, and the relatively poorer response to bronchodilator drugs in children less than 6 years of age and, in particular, children less than 3 years.

CLINICAL ASSESSMENT OF SEVERITY

A brief history and physical examination of the chest when therapy is begun must be followed by a comprehensive evaluation while awaiting the initial response to treatment. This evaluation should include assessment in the patient of known risk factors for status asthmaticus (Table 42–2). It is necessary to ascertain the duration of each symptom and specific sign; the medications used including name, dose, and time of administration during the past 24 to 48 hours; the estimation of oral fluids retained; the dates of previous episodes with forms of treatment needed and the patient's response; the presence of other diseases or the use of other medications; and a review of suspected

TABLE 42–2. Risk Factors for Status Asthmaticus

Asthma since infancy
Males with severe chronic asthma
Barrel-chest deformity
Short stature
Underweight
Steroid dependency
Poor coping style
Sudden changes in asthma pattern
Previous episodes of status asthmaticus
Previous failure usually to respond to appropriate therapy
Short-term relief of symptoms by adrenergic agents

precipitating factors. It is important to learn and follow the rate of progression of such symptoms as restlessness, altered consciousness, increasing fatigue, inability to speak, degree of air exchange as assessed by auscultation, tachypnea, degree of chest hyperexpansion, and heart rate.

It also is generally considered optimal, in pediatric practice, to record at least hourly, the presence or absence of subjective dyspnea, subjective wheeze, auscultatory wheeze with and without end-expiratory chest compression, prolonged expiration, flaring of ala nasi, supraclavicular retraction, and scalene and sternocleidomastoid muscle contraction. Of these, only sternocleidomastoid contraction and supraclavicular retractions actually have been found to correlate clearly with the severity of airflow obstruction in children. When the forced expiratory volume in one second (FEV_1) and the peak expiratory flow rate (PEFR) were below 50 percent of predicted, most patients had supraclavicular retractions, and all had sternocleidomastoid contractions (Commey and Levison, 1976). Pulsus paradoxus is another prognostic sign; a mean value of 22.2 mm Hg was observed in children when the $PaCO_2$ was above 40 mm Hg (Galant et al., 1978). With practice, the pulsus paradoxus can be measured, in spite of marked tachypnea, by obtaining the highest initial point when the irregular fading pulse sound begins and by subtracting from it the point when the pulse sound becomes uniform in intensity. Predictive index scoring systems are poor substitutes for frequent (every 30 to 60 minutes) observations by a concerned, experienced physician (Mansmann, 1983 and 1987), although some workers disagree on this point (Kurland and Leong, 1985).

PEFR or FEV_1 should be obtained in all patients initially and at 30 to 60 minute intervals. Baseline arterial or arterialized blood gas values should be obtained on admission to the hospital. These should be repeated as often as every 15 to 30 minutes if the patient does not appear to respond adequately to therapy. A rise of 10 torr in the $PaCO_2$ per hour is a poor prognostic sign.

Since viral infections frequently cause acute asthma, fever is not uncommon in children. An evaluation for bacterial infection should be made, nevertheless. The finding of leukocytosis may be of little value, since it follows injection of epinephrine. Also, yellow discoloration of sputum can be caused by eosinophil accumulation, which in turn is more likely to be a reflec-

TABLE 42–3. Indications for Hospitalization for Treatment of Acute Severe Asthma

Historical Reasons

Recurrent status asthmaticus
Previous respiratory failure
Previous use of intravenous isoproterenol
Previous use of controlled ventilation

Clinical Findings

Disturbance of consciousness
Exhaustion
Sternocleidomastoid contraction
Supraclavicular retractions
Pulsus paradoxus > 15 mm Hg
PEFR < 35 percent
FEV_1 < 35 percent
$Paco_2$ > 40 mm Hg
Pao_2 < 60 mm Hg
Electrocardiography abnormalities
Diaphoresis
Unresponsiveness to initial therapy in the first hour
Emergency treatment 2 successive days

tion of the asthma's severity than of etiology (e.g., "infection").

An understanding of the various components of management is essential to optimal outcome. The physician should be knowledgeable about the pharmacology of all medications used for treatment of acute asthma. Table 42–3 lists indications for hospitalization. Specific points relevant to acute asthma are discussed under each medication below. A protocol and an algorithm for treatment of asthma are provided in the following outlined section and in Figure 42–1.

MANAGEMENT PROTOCOL FOR ACUTE BRONCHIAL ASTHMA

I. Patients with Acute Severe Asthma
   A. Adrenergic Therapy
      1. *Epinephrine 1-1000,* 0.01 ml/kg (maximum of 0.3 ml), subcutaneously, every 15 to 20 minutes, for up to three doses. Maximum dose of 0.6 ml the first hour, and q. 4 h. Last dose should be Sus-Phrine (epinephrine suspension 1 : 200) (Shake Well), 0.005 ml/kg, subcutaneously, then q. 6 to 12 h OR
      2. Sus-Phrine (Shake Well), 0.005 ml/kg, subcutaneously, q. 6 to 12 h (20 percent is immediately released). Maximum single dose 0.2 ml OR
      3. *Terbutaline,* 0.01 mg/kg (maximum of 0.25 mg), subcutaneously, repeat in 20 minutes (maximum of 0.5 mg/4 h) OR

      4. *Aerosolized adrenergic agents,* see Table 42–4, may be used if PEFR or FEV_1 is greater than 40 percent of predicted.
   B. Oxygen, humidified, to maintain PaO_2 between 80 and 100 mm Hg.
   C. Response to treatment: if unresponsive in 1 hour, consider admitting to hospital and proceed as follows.
   D. Corticosteroids, if patient not immediately responsive, start steroids.
II. Patients with Early Status Asthmaticus
   A. Draw blood sample for STAT studies, serum theophylline level, arterial blood gas values, pHa, serum electrolyte levels, complete blood count, and differential.
   B. Aminophylline
      1. Obtain STAT theophylline level on all patients. For patients with 0 level, use loading dose of 7.0 mg/kg over 15 minutes. If level is under 10 μg/ml, give a sufficient dose to reach a therapeutic level. The maintenance infusion should be initiated at a rate of 0.85 mg/kg/hr for those 1 to 6 years old, 0.65 mg/kg/hr for those 7 to 16 years old, and 0.45 mg/kg/hr for those older than 16 years for a level between 10 and 15 μg/ml. Repeat levels at 1, 6, 12, and 24 hours of intravenous therapy.
      2. In the patient who has not received theophylline-containing medication, a loading dose is usually given followed by maintenance therapy. The loading dose in a patient not taking oral theophylline ranges from 5 to 7 mg/kg diluted in 25 to 50 ml of saline and given over 20 minutes. *An initial loading dose should not be administered to a patient who is receiving an oral theophylline preparation if the initial serum theophylline concentration is unknown.*
   C. Intravenous fluids: these are administered as 5-percent glucose in normal saline for hydration with fluids as appropriate for maintenance and depletion repair.
      1. Initial hydration—12 ml/kg or 360 ml/m² for the first hour (5 percent glucose in normal saline).
      2. Maintenance—50 ml/kg/24 h depending on age or 1500 ml/m²/24 h (5 percent glucose in water).
      3. Depletion repair—normal saline, 10

ALGORITHM FOR THE TREATMENT OF ACUTE ASTHMA

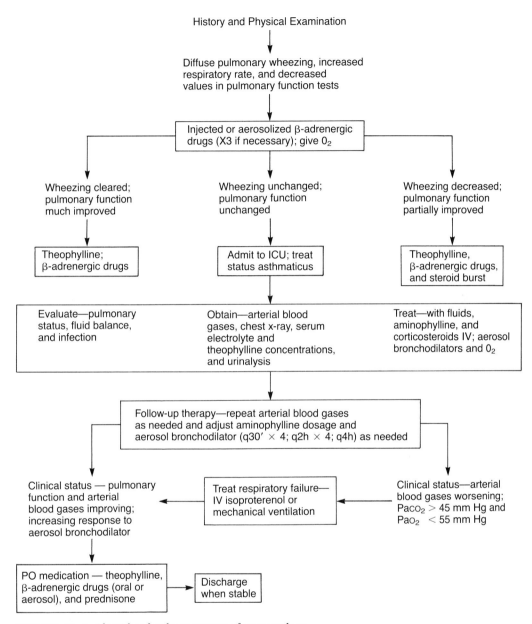

FIGURE 42–1. Algorithm for the treatment of acute asthma.

to 15 ml/kg/24 h or 300 to 500 ml/m² and water (5 percent glucose in water), 10 to 15 ml/kg/24 h or 300 to 500 ml/m²/24 h.

4. Maintenance of normal pH and electrolyte concentrations—the following is recommended for maintenance of normal potassium and sodium concentrations:

   a. Potassium—2 mEq/100 ml of maintenance intravenous fluids (after urination established).

   b. Sodium—3 mEq/100 ml of maintenance intravenous fluids.

   c. Buffers—if pH is below 7.30 and base deficit is greater than 5 mEq/L, correct to normal range with intravenous sodium bicarbonate as follows:

     (1) mEq bicarbonate = negative

base excess $\times$ 0.3 $\times$ kg (body weight)

    (2) Administer half the calculated dose initially and the other half after repeating blood gas determinations.

D. Corticosteroids

  1. Hydrocortisone hemisuccinate, 7 mg/kg stat and 7 mg/kg/24 h.

  2. Solu-Medrol (paraben-free methylprednisolone sodium succinate) or equivalent, 2 mg/kg STAT, I.V., slowly over 10 minutes and 4 mg/kg/24 h.

  3. Dexamethasone phosphate, 0.3 mg/kg stat and 0.3 mg/kg/24 h.

  4. Betamethasone, 0.3 mg/kg stat and 0.3 mg/kg/24 h by constant infusion or divided into four 6-hour doses.

E. Diagnostic Studies

  1. Posteroanterior and lateral x-ray of chest

  2. Urinalysis

  3. Nose, throat, and sputum cultures

III. Patients with Advanced Status Asthmaticus

A. Admit to Intensive Care Unit

B. Corticosteroids, as noted.

C. Vital Signs

  1. Record and evaluate blood pressure, pulse, respiratory rates, and pulsus paradoxus.

  2. Observe for sternocleidomastoid contraction and supraclavicular indrawing every 15 minutes.

  3. Repeat blood gas analysis, pHa every 30 to 60 minutes, and Na, K, and Cl every hour as appropriate.

D. Antibiotics, as indicated for obvious bacterial infection.

E. Medical Staff Coordination

  1. The same physician should evaluate the patient *at least* hourly for several hours.

  2. Document review of vital observations and that administration of medications and fluids are given on schedule.

  3. Associated staff physicians should be kept current on patient's condition.

  4. Alert controlled ventilation team (pediatrician, allergist, critical care physician, and pediatric pulmonologist or anesthesiologist) in the event

of impending respiratory failure, if the $Paco_2$ is increasing by 5 mm Hg/h.

IV. Patients with Acute Respiratory Failure

A. Follow protocol noted in II and III.

B. If the patient is stuporous or unconscious or if the patient's condition is rapidly deteriorating (e.g., an increase in $Paco_2$ of 5 mm Hg or more per hour), proceed as follows:

  1. Assemble controlled ventilation team.

  2. Examine bag and mask and ensure readiness to resuscitate patient.

  3. Have endotracheal tubes, tracheostomy set, cut-down set, and good suction equipment at the bedside.

C. Intravenous isoproterenol, via a calibrated constant infusion pump, beginning with 0.1 μ/kg/min, increasing the dosage 0.1 μ/kg/min every 15 to 20 minutes until clinical improvement or tachycardia (200/min) develops, as observed by electrocardiography (ECG) monitoring (Downs et al., 1973). *This step is not for children who are past their early teens.*

D. *Mechanical ventilation* may be necessary if the patient is unresponsive to isoproterenol, unable to receive it, or comatose.

  1. Endotracheal intubation, neuromuscular paralysis, sedation, and mechanical ventilation with a volume ventilator, with constant monitoring of ECG and frequent blood gas determinations are necessary.

  2. Once asthma is controlled with the aforementioned medications, the patient can be provided assisted ventilation and usually extubated in 24 to 48 h (Simons et al., 1977).

E. Additional Options: the following options are available if controlled ventilation is unsuccessful, prolonged, or complicated:

  1. The use of halothane anesthesia (O'Rourke and Crane, 1982)

  2. Bronchopulmonary lavage (Rogers et al., 1972)

  3. Extracorporeal membrane oxygenation (Zapol et al., 1977)

  4. Ether anesthesia (Robertson et al., 1985) should be seriously considered (Mansmann, 1983 and 1987).

  5. Because of its lesser myocardial de-

pression and arrhythmogenic potential than halothane, the administration of isoflurane should be entertained (Bierman et al., 1986).

V. Follow-up Therapy
   A. Monitor pulmonary function and blood gas values.
   B. Change patient's therapy to oral theophylline and corticosteroids (prednisone, 1 to 2 mg/kg is initiated as a single morning dose for at least 5 days or tapered gradually over 7 to 10 days).
   C. Continue aerosolized adrenergic agents.
   D. Taper steroid therapy as rapidly as patient's condition permits.
   E. Discharge patient as soon as stable and on oral medication.
   F. Follow-up within 1 week of hospital discharge.

GENERAL TREATMENT

The child in status asthmaticus should be managed in an intensive care unit or other facility where vital signs and overall condition can be monitored closely in a setting in which the physician, nurse, respiratory therapist, and any other medical person, such as a consulting anesthesiologist, can function as a team. Although the management of the child with status asthmaticus must be individualized, certain general principles apply to all patients.

Oxygenation

Humidified oxygen delivered by nasal cannula, face mask, or mechanical ventilator at a final concentration (FiO_2) to maintain PaO_2 of 80 to 100 torr (at sea level, with proportionally lower values at higher altitudes) is an important adjunct in managing status asthmaticus. *All patients who require hospitalization because of refractory asthma have hypoxemia.* Certain drugs (e.g., epinephrine) that are employed frequently in treatment may increase the myocardial oxygen need when the arterial oxygen is low. In addition, the potential toxicity of such medications is increased under conditions of hypoxemia and acidosis. Leukotriene mediators, which appear to be so important in severe asthma, also may reduce coronary artery blood flow and induce myocardial depression (Lewis and Austen, 1981). The appropriate use of oxy-gen supports the myocardium and helps prevent arrhythmias.

Hydration

Administration of intravenous fluids is essential for treatment of status asthmaticus, since a child so affected often is dehydrated on admission to the hospital because of vomiting, inadequate fluid intake, and greater insensible water loss from the increased work of breathing. Fluid therapy should be designed to replace deficits as well as to provide normal maintenance requirements. Excessive fluid administration should be avoided, however, since pulmonary edema and hypovolemia with water intoxication may result (Segar and Chesney, 1981).

Overhydration may increase microvascular hydrostatic pressure and reduce plasma colloid osmotic pressure. These changes can lead to formation of pulmonary edema in the child who has asthma with substantial negative pleural pressure (Stalcup and Mellins, 1977). Specific recommendations for fluid and electolyte therapy are given in the section Management Protocol for Acute Bronchial Asthma.

Aminophylline (Theophylline Ethylenediamine) Therapy

Aminophylline or theophylline is an effective bronchodilator for children with status asthmaticus (Pierson et al., 1971) and has become the most frequently administered intravenous drug for severe asthma. If the patient has not been receiving theophylline and has a zero theophylline level, a loading dose is usually administered followed by a maintenance dosage.

If the patient has an adequate serum theophylline level, obviously an initial loading dose should not be administered, and only a maintenance dosage given. Intravenous aminophylline treatment, consisting of a fourth of the calculated dose administered intravenously every 6 hours, may be preferred when consistent infusion is not practical (Maselli et al., 1970).

During intravenous aminophylline therapy, serum theophylline concentrations should be monitored for safety and effectiveness. Levels should be maintained above 10 μg/ml and below 20 μg/ml. Such levels should be obtained after the loading dose has equilibrated (approximately 1 hour after administration) and again after 6, 12, and 24 hours of intravenous therapy. Additional determinations of levels should be obtained if the patient has persistent heartburn, nausea, vomiting, seizures, nervousness, anxiety, insomnia, headache, diarrhea, irritability, or cardiac arrhythmia, to rule out theophylline intoxication (Weinberger et al., 1976). Also, theophylline can drive the respiratory center and increase the pulse rate.

Use of Adrenergic Agonists

For acute asthma these agents are the mainstay in treatment, often used also as "add ons" for those on maintenance theophylline. Whereas subcutaneously injected epinephrine is commonly employed in treating acute asthma, its short duration of action and side effects (stimulation of beta 1- as well as beta 2-receptors) make it less desirable than drugs that can be administered by aerosol (Becker et al., 1983). Inhalation of this class of drugs is preferred generally, in fact, to injection. However, a patient with severe obstruction (PEFR < 25 percent of predicted) is likely to have a more rapid recovery after subcutaneous medication because of greater dilatation of both larger and more peripheral small airways (Tashkin et al., 1980; Pliss and Gallagher, 1981). Multiple injections of epinephrine, although not cumulative in their action, have a sustaining therapeutic effect (Ownby and Anderson, 1986). Ben-Zvi and colleagues (1983) found that a single injection of epinephrine resulted in two to three times more failures than multiple injections. However, a single injection of Sus-Phrine (1:200 epinephrine suspension) had the same beneficial results at 1 hour as did multiple injections, but with fewer side effects, and has been recommended for initial therapy. Though the child may respond poorly to beta-adrenergic agents on hospital admission, he or she will become progressively more responsive as other therapy is administered.

Aerosolized metaproterenol solution (Shapiro et al., 1987), terbutaline, or albuterol (salbutamol) in 3 ml saline (Beck et al., 1985) should be given every half hour for the first 2 hours and at longer intervals as the patient improves. Dosages are noted in Table 42–4. These drugs are administered by low-pressure ultrasonic or wall-mounted nebulizer for 5 to 10 minutes every half hour ($\times 4$), then as indicated by the patient's condition. The pulse should be monitored, and treatment should be stopped when the pulse is ≥ 190 beats/min. Continuous administration of aerosolized beta-adrenergic drugs (e.g., terbutaline, 1 to 2 mg/hr) has been employed successfully in the treatment of acute asthma in children and adults.

Positive pressure ventilation (IPPB) is contraindicated in children because of the danger of inducing greater bronchoconstriction, pneumomediastium, and pneumothorax. Hypokalemia is a potential complication of beta-adrenergic therapy even with inhalation (Haalboon et al., 1985); hence, serum electrolyte levels should be monitored.

Corticosteroid Therapy

Patients requiring hospitalization, those already on steroids or previously on long-term oral steroids, and those on aerosolized steroids in the previous 6 weeks, should receive cortico-

TABLE 42–4. Aerosolized Adrenergic Agents

Drugs (Solution)	Dose
Metaproterenol (5 percent)	0.1 to 0.3 ml in 3 ml saline or water
Isoetharine (1 percent)	0.25 to 0.5 ml in 3 ml saline or water
Isoproterenol (1–200)	0.1 to 0.3 ml in 3 ml saline or water
Terbutaline (1 mg/ml)*	0.1 mg/kg q. 4–6 h (maximum of 6 mg/dose)
Albuterol (salbutamol)	2.5 mg in 2 ml saline or water

Administration
Low-pressure ultrasonic or wall nebulizer for 5 to 10 min, q. ½ h ($\times 4$), then as indicated by patient's conditions. Monitor pulse and discontinue if > 190/min.

* Some clinicians use injectable solutions for nebulization, since only this form is available in the United States.

steroids immediately. Short-term intravenous administration of steroids in high doses rarely, if ever, causes adverse effects. Recommendations of steroid dosages are given in the section Management Protocol for Acute Bronchial Asthma.

Corticosteroids accelerate the recovery from status asthmaticus with a maximal effect occurring 2 to 3 days after the beginning of treatment. Pierson and coworkers (1971) documented better arterial oxygen tensions in children who were treated with glucocorticosteroids compared with children who received placebo. In a recent study of children with acute asthma, steroid therapy improved small airways obstruction 24 hours after it was instituted but had minimal effectiveness on large airways obstruction, as compared with placebo-treated children (Shapiro et al., 1983). This finding may explain why several published studies have failed to show any beneficial effects of steroid therapy on lung function, since these studies employed measurements of airflow only in large airways (Luksza, 1982).

Another important effect of steroids appears to be the increase in effectiveness of beta-adrenergic drugs, an effect that may occur earlier than previously appreciated (Arnaud et al., 1979). Even in hospitalized infants with "bronchiolitis," there is evidence that steroids potentiate the effectiveness of beta-adrenergic drugs (Tal et al., 1983). The beneficial effect of steroids in the treatment of acute severe asthma also has been well documented in adults (Littenberg and Gluck, 1986).

Antibiotic Therapy

Antibiotics are indicated only in children in whom bacterial diseases are suspected (Shapiro et al., 1974). Viral respiratory infections induce acute severe asthma far more frequently than do bacterial infections, and current antibiotics are not effective in treating viral infections. There are no special indications for the use of antibiotics in asthma or other allergic disorders.

It is well to remember that asthma is frequently accompanied by patchy atelectasis that is often misinterpreted on a radiograph as bronchopneumonia (Eggleston et al., 1974). Leukocytosis of 15,000/mm³ or more may occur in severe asthma in the absence of a demonstrable infection, particularly after administration of epinephrine.

Use of Sedatives

Patients with severe asthma have good reason to experience extreme anxiety, and their anxiety is the result of respiratory distress and hypoxemia rather than the cause of them. *Sedatives are contraindicated in patients with status asthmaticus.*

Anticholinergic Drug Therapy

Anticholinergic agents, atropine sulfate, atropine methylnitrate, and ipratropium bromide, have been used in treatment of acute and chronic asthma with some success, although results have been variable. There is relatively little data on the use of these agents in acute severe asthma in children, but data in adults would suggest that they probably add little to the therapy of acute severe asthma and may disproportionately increase undesirable effects (Karpel et al., 1986). However, Beck and colleagues (1985) did find a small but significant beneficial effect from combining ipratropium bromide with albuterol in children.

Use of Cromolyn Sodium in Status Asthmaticus

Patients on the powdered form of cromolyn should discontinue this drug when acutely ill because the powder is irritating and may increase coughing. It is not contraindicated if employed in the aerosolized or nebulized form, but there is no evidence that it aids in therapy of acute severe asthma. When the previous schedule has been two or three times daily, it should be increased to four times daily until the patient has returned to preattack or baseline condition completely. Following status asthmaticus, therapy may be initiated with cromolyn solution by a nebulizer combined with a beta agonist solution, such as metaproterenol or albuterol.

Special Considerations Regarding Therapy of Infantile Asthma

For reasons previously stated, infants and toddlers often require aggressive therapy in the hospital. Although the ability of wheezing infants to respond to bronchodilators has been questioned, Tal and associates (1983) found that combined treatment with dexamethasone and aerosolized salbutamol (albuterol) resulted in more than twice the rate of improvement of other treatments for "bronchiolitis" or asthma. These investigators believe that theophylline should not be employed or should be used with extreme caution in those infants under 8 months of age. The risk of toxicity is very great; when theophylline is employed, it must be monitored frequently. For infants less than 1 year of age, the maintenance dosage can be derived from the following formula (Kurland and Leong, 1985):

Theophylline Dose in
  mg/kg/hr = [age in weeks $\times$ 0.008] + 0.21

MONITORING OF THERAPY

Clinical. Regular and systematic clinical, physiologic, and laboratory observation helps to ascertain the effectiveness of treatment and aids in the early recognition of complications. Frequent assessment of the patient's clinical course often is overlooked, but it is an important aspect of medical management of the patient with severe asthma.

Radiography. A "routine" chest x-ray is not considered to be necessary in every patient with status asthmaticus. However, a chest x-ray should be obtained for any patient who is doing poorly or who suddenly develops increased respiratory distress. Atelectasis and pulmonary infiltrates occur commonly (1 in 3 patients) and sometimes may involve an entire lobe; pneumomediastinum, the next most common complication, occurs in 1 of 20 children with status asthmaticus (Eggleston et al., 1974); and pneumothorax occurs in approximately 1 of 1000 patients admitted with acute severe asthma.

Pulmonary Function Tests. Pulmonary function tests provide valuable data that cannot be obtained by physical examination. *Clinical impressions of airflow by patient or physician are highly imperfect in children, as they are in adults. Frequently, lung functions are overestimated in children who are severely compromised.* Baseline objective measurements should be followed during the therapy of acute asthma. As pulmonary obstruction is relieved by therapy, the lung function should improve. A sudden worsening of lung function may be the first evidence of disease progression or pulmonary complication, such as pneumomediastinum or atelectasis. In children as young as 3 years of age, the

PEFR can be followed. Older children can usually use spirometers, which provide information concerning the forced vital capacity (FVC) (air trapping or atelectasis), FEV_1 (larger airway function), and forced expiratory flow during midexpiration ($FEF_{25-75\%}$) (smaller airway function). Ideally, lung function tests should be repeated every 4 to 6 hours during the first day of hospitalization and twice daily thereafter, until the patient's asthma is controlled.

Cardiovascular Monitoring. An early physiologic consequence of acute asthma is hypoxemia (McFadden and Lyons, 1968). This condition by itself can produce adverse cardiovascular effects; the use of beta-adrenergic drugs and aminophylline stimulates the heart and increases its need for oxygen when the patient is relatively hypoxemic. Certain inflammatory mediators including the leukotrienes may induce coronary artery constriction that further decreases the blood flow to the cardiac muscle. Arrhythmias may occur unexpectedly, owing to these factors during the course of status asthmaticus, even in children. Continuous monitoring of heart rate and rhythm should be carried out during treatment until the patient's asthma has improved sufficiently to reinstitute oral therapy.

Monitoring of Blood Gas and Serum Electrolyte Levels. The measurements of arterial blood gas tensions are extremely important in the child with severe asthma in that they provide objective measurements of the adequacy of alveolar ventilation and blood oxygenation. Arterial blood gas analysis is most accurate, but for baseline or follow-up values, "arterialized" blood (warming the patient's hand for 10 minutes prior to drawing the capillary blood) can be a useful substitute in small children (Stamm, 1967). As an alternative, oximetry can be used to monitor the degree of oxygenation. In the very sick patient, the insertion of an intra-arterial line facilitates repeated sampling without further discomfort. If the initial $PaCO_2$ is 40 mm Hg or higher, the patient must be considered to be in respiratory failure. A $PaCO_2$ value greater than 50 mm Hg indicates gross respiratory failure. Immediate provision should be made to treat respiratory failure (see subsequent section, Respiratory Failure).

Serum electrolyte values should be obtained on hospital admission as a guide to intravenous fluid therapy. They are especially important in a child who is vomiting or febrile. Inappropriate antidiuretic hormone (ADH) response can occur in patients with severe asthma (Baker, 1976; Segar and Chesney, 1981), which is manifested by low urine output and reduced serum sodium concentration in association with excessive urinary sodium output (see subsequent section, Complications of Severe Asthma).

Monitoring of Theophylline Levels. Therapeutic monitoring of serum theophylline levels is essential for patients with severe asthma, both to assure adequate therapy and to avoid theophylline toxicity. A number of factors may influence theophylline serum levels, even in a patient whose preadmission theophylline levels have been in a steady state for weeks to months. Theophylline metabolism can be decreased by high fever, liver disease, and macrolide antibiotics, including erythromycin (Ellis, 1985). Influenza B infections may reduce theophylline metabolism for weeks to months, and even influenza immunizations may alter theophylline serum half-life (Kraemer et al., 1982). Periodic monitoring of theophylline levels is also important in the child who is vomiting, who has cardiac arrhythmias, or who is not improving.

COMPLICATIONS OF SEVERE ASTHMA

Complications of asthma may be pulmonary or extrapulmonary. Pulmonary complications include (1) acute respiratory failure, (2) atelectasis, (3) pneumomediastinum and pneumothorax, and (4) superimposed infections (pneumonia, empyema). Extrapulmonary complications include (1) excessive vasopressin, (2) flaccid paralysis of an arm or leg, (3) sudden alteration in theophylline metabolism, (4) cardiac arrhythmia, and (5) hypoxemic brain damage. Pulmonary and extrapulmonary factors may combine to cause acute respiratory failure, resulting in brain damage or death.

Pulmonary Complications

Respiratory Failure. Respiratory failure occurs in a small but significant number of children admitted to the hospital with status asthmaticus (Simons et al., 1977). It often is the result of failure by the physician, patient, or family to recognize the severity of the child's asthma. Signs of overt respiratory failure can include decreased or absent pulmonary breath sounds, severe intercostal retraction, pulsus paradoxus, use of accessory muscles of respiration, cyanosis with treatment by FiO_2 of 40 percent, reduced response to pain, poor skeletal muscle tone, and profuse diaphoresis. The use of accessory muscles of respiration, as previously noted, is one of the early signs of respiratory failure.

These signs indicate an extreme emergency and mandate immediate treatment for acute respiratory failure with intravenous isoproterenol or mechanical ventilation for the child who is already on isoproterenol treatment. Other methods, such as continuous aerosolized beta-adrenergic agents and intranenous salbutamol or terbutaline, are employed in other countries or experimentally in the United States.

Arterial blood gas tensions and pH must be monitored frequently in a distressed child. Impending respiratory failure cannot be diagnosed from clinical signs alone. For example, a rise of $PaCO_2$ from 39 to 44 mm Hg in 1 hour in an exhausted child who is receiving maximal therapy should be considered progressive respiratory failure and treated as discussed subsequently.

Although several groups have reported extensive experience in management of respiratory failure with intravenous isoproterenol, there have been many treatment failures by this method that have necessitated mechanical ventilation (Parry et al., 1976). In general, the use of intravenous isoproterenol has been useful in children with borderline respiratory failure. We consider it to be contraindicated in adolescents and adults because of a greater likelihood of serious cardiovascular side effects from intravenously administered isoproterenol in these age groups.

Therapy with Intravenous Isoproterenol. Therapy with intravenous isoproterenol must be carried out in a properly equipped intensive care unit with continuous cardiac monitoring and a calibrated constant-infusion pump. *Intravenous isoproterenol therapy should never be initiated without all facilities and personnel for intubation and mechanical ventilation on hand.* A staff thoroughly familiar with this form of treatment is essential. An intra-arterial catheter must be in place for monitoring blood gas tension. Before administration of the drug, an anesthesiologist or a physician similarly skilled in intubation of children should be consulted so that all facilities for mechanical ventilation are immediately available. This arrangement is especially important for the child who has received excessive quantities of B-adrenergic agents before admission, since isoproterenol may precipitate worsening of respiratory failure (Parry et al., 1976). After an initial starting dosage of 0.1 μg/kg/min delivered with a constant-infusion pump, dosage is increased at the rate of 0.1 μg/kg/min every 15 to 20 minutes until there is clinical improvement, tachycardia of 200 beats/min, or development of arrhythmia. Hazards of intravenous isoproterenol include cardiac arrhythmia, myocarditis, subendocardial necrosis, and induction of massive mucorrhea.

A proposed alternative to intravenous isoproterenol is administration of terbutaline in saline as a continuous aerosol with an oxygen driven nebulizer in a dosage of 2 mg/hour. Again, cardiac monitoring should be continuous, and arterial blood gas tensions should be monitored frequently.

Use of Mechanical Ventilation in Respiratory Failure. Mechanical ventilation requires endotracheal intubation, neuromuscular blockade, and sedation (Simons et al., 1977). A *volume-controlled ventilator* with constant cardiac monitoring and an intra-arterial line for fre-

quent blood gas determinations must be employed to ensure adequate alveolar ventilation. Once stabilized, the patient can be given intermittent mandatory ventilation and generally can be weaned in 24 to 48 hours. Pneumomediastinum, pneumothorax, cardiac arrhythmia, and unintentional extubation make mechanical ventilation a complicated procedure that should be performed only in adequately equipped and staffed tertiary care centers.

Atelectasis. Up to one third of all hospitalized asthmatic children have had pulmonary complications, such as pneumonia and atelectasis, and 20 percent have had pulmonary infiltrates involving multiple lobes (Eggleston et al., 1974). Perihilar interstitial infiltrates will vary in severity from increased bronchovascular markings to shaggy, diffuse peribronchial viral pneumonia. Atelectasis of all or part of a lobe, the next most common complication, will occur in 10 percent of admissions. The right middle lobe is most frequently involved because of anatomic factors, e.g., the right main stem bronchus tends to twist with hyperinflation, resulting in its partial occlusion. Why right-middle

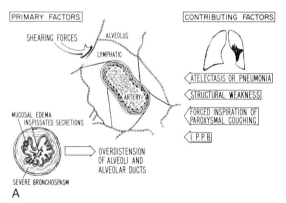

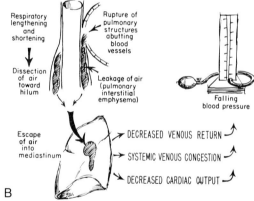

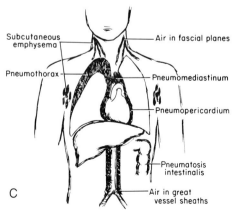

FIGURE 42–2. Mechanism of pneumomediastinum in acute asthma.

lobe atelectasis develops more frequently in girls than in boys is not clear (Dees and Spock, 1966).

The treatment of atelectasis should be conservative. In most cases it will resolve when the asthma is controlled. Respiratory therapy consisting of postural drainage and clapping as tolerated clinically is helpful. Intermittent positive pressure breathing (IPPB) therapy should be avoided, since it is likely to induce pneumomediastinum or pneumothorax (Bierman, 1967). If atelectasis persists, the presence of a foreign body, an anatomic defect, or an obstructing peribronchial lymph node should be considered. Fiberoptic bronchoscopy may be useful if a foreign body is suspected.

Pneumomediastinum and Pneumothorax. In status asthmaticus, 5 percent of patients may develop extrapulmonary air (Eggleston et al., 1974). Shearing forces, from coughing and bronchospasm superimposed on hyperinflation also related to atelectasis or pneumonia and possible structural weakness, cause air to rupture alveolar bases and to dissect along blood vessel sheaths (Bierman, 1967) (Fig. 42–2). These effects result in pulmonary interstitial emphysema. It manifests as a worsening clinical course associated with reduced venous return, cardiac output, and blood pressure. Air dissects along the great vessel sheaths to the mediastinum and pericardium and along the aorta to the intestinal wall or along the fascial planes into the neck (Fig. 42–3). While this air

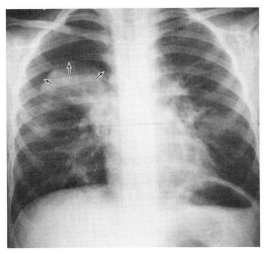

FIGURE 42–4. Pneumothorax secondary to paroxysmal coughing in asthma.

remains under high pressure, asthma symptoms worsen and precardiac dullness disappears. Air may escape into the relatively low pressure subcutaneous tissue of the neck and axilla, resulting in crepitant subcutaneous emphysema.

Rarely, pneumothorax complicates childhood asthma. It may be self limited if small, or tension pneumothorax can occur that may severely compromise breathing. Bilateral pneumothorax can be the cause of sudden death in asthma (Jorgensen et al., 1963). Tension pneumothorax that results from the rupture of a pleural bleb needs decompression with a chest tube and underwater suction (Fig. 42–4). A pneumothorax secondary to air rupturing through parietal pleura into the pleural space from a pneumomediastinum is less serious and may be treated conservatively. Often it will clear with treatment of the asthma.

Extrapulmonary Complications

Vasopressin Excess (Inappropriate ADH Secretion). The release of ADH is regulated through mechanisms such as (1) pain, fear, and drugs acting on higher central nervous system centers; (2) drops in arterial pressure; (3) increases in plasma concentration ($\geq$280 mOsm/L) of nondiffusible solute perfusing the hypothalamus, and (4) decreases in stimulation of stretch receptors in the left atrium. When filling of the left atrium is reduced, the vagus nerve stimulates the hypothalamus to secrete vaso-

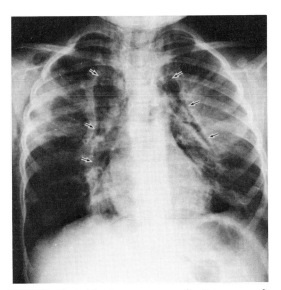

FIGURE 42–3. Massive pneumomediastinum complicating asthma.

pressin. In severe asthma, vasopressin levels are elevated regardless of the serum sodium concentrations, apparently because of the effect of severe asthma on the pulmonary circulation. Vasopressin levels fall as the patient improves (Benfield et al., 1982; Segar and Chesney, 1981).

Criteria for the diagnosis of vasopressin excess are as follows:

1. Hyponatremia that is associated with plasma hypo-osmolality.

2. Continuing renal excretion of sodium in presence of hyponatremia.

3. Absence of any evidence of dehydration.

4. Urinary osmolality value that is greater than plasma osmolality value.

5. Normal kidney and adrenal function.

The treatment of excessive vasopressin involves three general principles. First, severe asthma must be corrected with appropriate therapy. Second, water intake and body weight, plasma electrolyte concentration and osmolarity, and urine volume and osmolality must be monitored closely; fluid intake should be restricted to the minimal amount compatible with control of asthma. Third, complications such as water intoxication with seizures should be treated with hypertonic saline and furosemide. Hypertonic saline and furosemide are rarely needed if the underlying asthma is treated successfully.

Sudden Alteration in Theophylline Metabolism. Theophylline clearance may be decreased by a number of factors (see Monitoring of Theophylline Levels). Aminophylline should be used cautiously in febrile patients, and dosage should be regulated by serial monitoring of serum theophylline concentrations in order to avoid theophylline toxicity. The theophylline requirement may increase because of third compartment filling secondary to edema and inappropriate ADH secretion. This condition could lead to sudden theophylline toxicity when the patient's pulmonary function improves.

Flaccid Paralysis. In 1974, Hopkins reported ten children with flaccid paralysis after acute asthma severe enough to require hospitalization. The paralysis developed during the recovery phase from asthma. In all patients, paralysis was permanent and involved one arm or one leg. To date, 19 children with this syndrome from Australia, England, Sweden, and the United States have been reported in the medical literature (Shapiro et al., 1979); we have knowl-

edge of at least four other unreported cases in North America.

Patients had similar characteristics as follows: (1) all were between 1 and 11 years of age; (2) all had asthma that was severe enough to require hospitalization; (3) all developed paralysis 4 to 11 days after onset of asthma (average = 5 days); (4) all had only one affected limb; more frequently it was the arm rather than the leg; (5) all had flaccid paralysis that affected only the motor nerves with no sensory involvement; and (6) all had progressive paralysis that was permanent (Commentary, 1980). All reported patients had been immunized for poliomyelitis and no polio virus was obtained on culture. Although this paralysis is presumed to be a disease of viral etiology, no pathogenetic virus has yet been identified in these patients. There also is no explanation why these phenomena occurred only in children who had severe asthma.

Transient phrenic nerve paralysis also has been reported in status asthmaticus, possibly as a complication of assisted ventilation (Rohatigi et al., 1980).

Cardiorespiratory Arrest with Brain Damage. Permanent hypoxic brain damage due to cardiorespiratory arrest can be a complication of severe asthma and is particularly unfortunate because it is preventable with appropriate

TABLE 42–5. Causes of Death from Asthma

Failure of physician or patient to appreciate severity
  Lack of objective measurements
  Lack of intensified therapy
Inappropriate therapy given
  Too late due to delay by patient or physician
  Too little (e.g., low steroid dose or recent discontinuation)
  Too much (e.g., beta agonists, theophylline, sedative abuse)
Progressive unresponsive asthma
Prolonged attack
Pulmonary complications
  Infection (often undiagnosed)
  Pneumothorax
  Barotrauma
  Aspirations of gastric contents
  Malfunction of ventilator
Cardiac complications
  Arrhythmias
  Hypotension
  Myocardial toxicity
  Sudden cardiac arrest
Underlying cardiopulmonary disease
Hemodynamic
  Hypovolemia, shock
  Pulmonary edema

---

therapy. In virtually all cases, it has been the result of the parent's or the physician's failure to recognize the severity of asthma and to institute appropriate therapy (Bierman et al., 1975).

Death. Table 42–5 lists the causes of death associated with asthma in children. Virtually all are potentially preventable and can be avoided with appropriate education and treatment (Strunk and Mrazek, 1986).

REFERENCES

Arnaud, A., Vervoet, D., Dogue, P.: Treatment of acute asthma: effect of intravenous corticosteroids and beta-2 agonists. Lung 156: 43–48, 1979.

Baker, J.W., Yeager, S., Segar, W.E.: Elevated plasma antidiuretic hormone levels in status asthmaticus. Mayo Clin. Proc. 51:31–34, 1976.

Beck, R., Robertson, C., Galdes-Sebaldt, M., Levinson, H.: Combined salbutamol and ipratropium bromide by inhalation in the treatment of severe asthma. J. Pediatr. 107:605–608, 1985.

Becker, A.B., Nelson, N.A., Simons, F.E.R.: Inhaled salbutamol (albuterol) vs. injected epinephrine in the treatment of acute asthma in children. J. Pediatr. 102:465–469, 1983.

Benfield, Q.F., Odoherty, K., Davies, B.H.: Status asthmaticus and the syndrome of inappropriate secretion of antidiuretic hormone. Thorax 37:147–148, 1982.

Ben-Zvi, Z., Lam, C., Spohm, W.A., Gribetz, I., Mulvihill, M.N., Kattan, M.: An evaluation of repeated injections of epinephrine for the initial treatment of acute asthma. Am. Rev. Respir. Dis. 127:101–105, 1983.

Bierman, C.W.: Pneumomediastinum and pneumothorax complicating asthma in children. Am. J. Dis. Child. 114:42, 1967.

Bierman, M.I., Brown, M., Muren, O., Keenan, R.L., Glauser, F.L.: Prolonged isoflurane anesthesia in status asthmaticus. Crit. Care Med. 14:832–833, 1986.

Bierman, C.W., Pierson, W.E., Shapiro, G.G., Simons, F.E.R.: Brain damage from asthma in children. J. Allergy Clin. Immunol. 55:126, 1975.

Bierman, C.W., Shapiro, G.G., Furukawa, C.T., Pierson, W.E.: Status Asthmaticus. In Dickerman, J.D., Lucey, J.F. (eds.), Smith's The Critically Ill Child. W.B. Saunders Co., Philadelphia, 1985.

Commentary: Post-asthmatic pseudopolio in children. Lancet 1:860, 1980.

Commey, J.O.O., Levison, H.: Physical signs in childhood asthma. Pediatrics 58:537–541, 1976.

Dees, S.C., Spock, A.: Right middle lobe syndrome in children. J.A.M.A. 197:8, 1966.

Downs, J.J., Wood, D.W., Harwood, I., Scheinhopf, H.N., Raphaelz, R.C.: Intravenous isoproterenol infusion in children with severe hypercapnia due to status asthmaticus. Crit. Care Med. 1:63–68, 1973.

Eggleston, P.A., Ward, B.H., Pierson, W.E., Bierman, C.W.: Radiographic abnormalities in acute asthma in children. Pediatrics 54:442–449, 1974.

Ellis, E.E.: Theophylline toxicity. J. Allergy Clin. Immunol. 76:297–301, 1985.

Field, W.E.: Mucous gland hypertrophy in babies and children aged 15 years or less. Brit. J. Dis. Chest. 62:11, 1968.

Galant, S.P., Groncy, C.E., Shaw, K.C.: The value of pulsus paradoxus in assessing the child with status asthmaticus. Pediatrics 61:46–51, 1978.

Garra, B., Shapiro, G.G., Dorsett, C.S., et al.: A double-blind evaluation of the use of nebulized metaproterenol and isoproterenol in hospitalized asthmatic children and adolescents. J. Allergy Clin. Immunol. 60:63–68, 1977.

Glauser, F.L.: Signs and Symptoms in Pulmonary Medicine. Philadelphia, J.B. Lippincott Co., 1983.

Haalboon, J.R.E., Deenstra, M., Struyvenberg, A.: Hypokalaemia induced by inhalation of fenoterol. Lancet 1:1125–1127, 1985.

Harfi, H., Hanissian, A.S., Crawford, L.V. Treatment of status asthmaticus in children with high doses and conventional doses of methyloprednisolone. Pediatrics 61:829–831, 1978.

Heurich, A.E., Huang, C.T., Lyons, H.A.: Status asthmaticus — Definition, criteria for diagnosis and clinical causes. In Weiss E.B. (ed.), Status Asthamticus. Baltimore, University Park Press, 1978.

Hopkins, I.J.: A new syndrome: poliomyelitis-like illness associated with acute asthma in childhood. Aust. Paediatr. J. 10:273–273, 1974.

Jorgensen, J.R., Fallure, C.J., Bukantz, S.C.: Pneumothorax and mediastinal and subcutaneous emphysema in children with bronchial asthma. Pediatrics 3:824, 1963.

Karpel, J.P., Appel, D., Breidbart, D., Fusco, M.J.: A comparison of atropine sulfate and metaproterenol sulfate in the emergency treatment of asthma. Am. Rev. Resp. Dis. 133:727–729, 1986.

Kattan, M., Gurwitz, D., Levision, H.: Corticosteroids in status asthmaticus. J. Pediatr. 96:596–599, 1980.

Kraemer, M.J., Furukawa, C.T., Kaup, J.R., et al.: Altered theophylline clearance during an influenza B outbreak. Pediatrics 69:476–480, 1982.

Kurland, G., Leong, A.B.: The management of status asthmaticus in infants and children. Clin. Rev. Allergy 3:37–67, 1985.

Lewis, R.A., Austen, K.E.: Mediation of local homeostasis and inflammation by leukotrienes and other mast cell–dependent compounds. Nature 293:103–108, 1981.

Littenberg, B., Gluck, E.H.: A controlled trial of methylprednisolone in the emergency treatment of acute asthma. N. Engl. J. Med. 314:150–152, 1986.

Luksza, A.R.P.: Acute severe asthma treated without steroids. Brit. J. Dis. Chest. 76:15–19, 1982.

Mansmann, Jr., H.C.: The evaluation, control, and modification of continuing asthma. Clin. Chest Med. 1:339–360, 1980.

Mansmann, Jr., H.C.: A 25-year perspective of status asthmaticus. Clin. Rev. Allerg. 1:147–162, 1983.

Mansmann, Jr., H.C.: A 29-year perspective of status asthmaticus in children. In An International Symposium on Status Asthmaticus and Asthma Deaths. N.E.R. Allergy Proc., 1987.

Maselli, R., Casal, G.L., Ellis, E.F.: Pharmacologic effects of intravenously administered aminophylline in asthmatic children. J. Pediatr. 76:777–782, 1970.

McFadden, Jr., E.R., Lyons, H.A.: Airway resistance and uneven ventilation in bronchial asthma. J. Appl. Physiol. 25:365, 1968.

O'Rourke, P.P., Crane, R.K.: Halothane in status asthmaticus. Crit. Care Med. 10:341–343, 1982.

Ownby, D.R., Anderson, J.: Response to epinephrine in children receiving oral B-agonists. Am. J. Dis. Child. 140:122–123, 1986.

Parry, W.H., Martorano, F., Cotton, E.I.C.: Management of life threatening asthma with intravenous isoproterenol infusions. Am. J. Dis. Child. 130:39–46, 1976.

Pierson, W.E., Bierman, C.W., et al.: Double-blind trial of aminophylline in status asthmaticus. Pediatrics 46:642, 1971.

Pierson, W.E., Bierman, C.W., Kelly, V.C.: A double-blind trail of corticosteroid therapy in status asthmaticus. Pediatrics 54:282–288, 1974.

Pliss, L.B., Gallagher, E.J.: Aerosol vs. injected epinephrine in acute asthma. Ann. Emerg. Med. 10:353–355, 1981.

Robertson, C.E., Sinclair, C.J., Steedman, D., Brown, D., Malcom-Smith, N.: Use of ether in life-threatening acute severe asthma. Lancet 1:182–187, 1985.

Rogers, R.M., Braunstein, M.S., Shuman, J.F.: Role of bronchopulmonary lavage in the treatment of respiratory failure: A review. Chest 62S;95S–106S, 1972.

Rohatigi, N., Fields, A., Sly, R.M.: Status asthmaticus complicated by phrenic nerve paralysis. Ann. Allery 45:177–178, 1980.

Segar, W.E., Chesney, R.W.: Disorders of electrolyte metabolism. Pediatr. Ann. 10:288, 1981.

Shapiro, G.G., Bierman, C.W., Furukawa, C.T., Pierson, W.E.: Double-blind dose-respone study of metaproterenol inhalant solution in children with acute asthma. J. Allergy Clin. Immunol. 79:378–386, 1987.

Shapiro, G.G., Chapman, J.I., Pierson, W.E., Bierman, C.W. Poliomyelitis-like illness after acute asthma. J. Pediatr. 94:767–768, 1979.

Shapiro, G.G., Eggleston, P.A., Pierson, W.E., et al.: Double-blind study of the effectiveness of a broad spectrum antibiotic in status asthmaticus. Pediatrics 53:867–873, 1974.

Shapiro, G.G., Furukawa, C.T., Pierson, W.E., et al.: Double-blind evaluation of methylprednisolone versus placebo for acute asthma episodes. Pediatrics 71:510–514, 1983.

Siegel, D., Sheppard, D., Gelb, A., Weinberg, P.F.: Aminophylline increases the toxicity but not the efficacy of an inhaled beta-adrenergic agonist in the treatment of acute exacerbations of asthma. Am. Rev. Respir. Dis. 132:283–286, 1985.

Simons, F.E.R., Pierson, W.E., Bierman, C.W.: Respiratory failure in childhood status asthmaticus. Am. J. Dis. Child. 131:1097, 1977.

Smith, T.F., Hudgel, D.W.: Decreased ventilation response to hypoxia in children with asthma. J. Pediatri. 97:736–741, 1980.

Stalcup, S.A., Mellins, R.B.: Mechanical forces producing pulmonary edema in acute asthma. N. Engl. J. Med. 297:592–596, 1977.

Stamm, S.J.: Reliability of capillary blood for measurement of paO_2, PaO_2 and O_2 saturation. Dis. Chest 52:191–194, 1967.

Strunk, R.C., Mrazek, D.A.: Deaths from asthma in childhood. Can they be predicated? N. Engl. Reg. Allergy Proc. 7:454–461, 1986.

Sybert, A., Weiss, E.B.: Status Asthmaticus. In Weiss, E.B., Segal, M.S., Stein, M.S. (eds.), Bronchial Asthma, Mechanisms and Therapeutics. Boston, Little, Brown and Co., 1985.

Tabachnik, E., Levison, H.: Infantile bronchial asthma. J. Allergy Clin. Immunol. 67:339, 1981.

Tal, A., Bavilsk, C., Yohai, D., Bearman, J.E., Gorodischer, R., Moses, S.W.: Dexamethasone and salbutamol in the treatment of acute wheezing in infants. Pediatrics 71:13–18, 1983.

Tashkin, D.P., Trevor, E., Chopra, S.K., Taplin, G.V.: Sites of airway dilatation terbutaline. Comparison of physiologic tests with radionuclide lung images. Am. J. Med. 68:14–26, 1980.

Weinberger, M.W., Matthay, R.A., Ginihansky, E.J., et al.: Intravenous aminophylline dosage: use of serum theophylline measurement for guidance. J.A.M.A. 235:2110–2113, 1976.

Weng, T.R., Langer, H.M., Featherby, E.A., Levison, H.: Arterial blood gas tensions and acid-base balance in symptomatic and asymptomatic asthma in childhood. Am. Rev. Respir. Dis. 101:274, 1970.

Zapol, W.M., Snider, M.T., Schneider, R.C.: Extracorporeal membrane oxygenation for acute respiratory failure. Anesthesiology 46:272–285, 1977.

43

Treatment of Asthma in Adults*

ROBERT K. BUSH, M.D.
WILLIAM W. BUSSE, M.D.

Bronchial hyperreactivity is a feature of asthma shared by children and adults (McFadden, 1984). Furthermore, the same precipitants trigger asthma in patients of all ages. Nevertheless, certain features of asthmatic disease are unique to adults and must be appreciated in diagnosis and treatment.

PRECIPITATING FACTORS OF ASTHMA

Allergens

In allergic adult asthmatic patients, allergen exposures can induce asthma, as it does in children. Pollens, molds, animal danders and proteins, and house dust mites are common allergens. Although the majority of adult asthmatics have positive immediate skin test responses to these aeroallergens (Barbee et al., 1985), the correlation of such responses to asthma provocation is less well defined in adults than in children. Moreover, with an ever-growing list of work-place materials, special attention must be paid to occupational exposures in adults.

Infections

Viral, not bacterial, upper respiratory infections provoke asthma in patients of all ages. In infants and children, respiratory syncytial virus infections are the most common precipitants, whereas in adolescents and adults, rhinovirus, influenza virus, and parainfluenza virus as-

sume greatest importance. The mechanisms of virus-induced asthma remain unknown but include virus cytotropic effects on airway epithelium with inflammation and sensitization of vagal sensory fibers, IgE antibody sensitization to the respiratory virus, nonimmune enhancement of mediator release, and diminished beta-adrenergic responsiveness (Busse, 1985). An important factor is that most severe attacks of asthma in adults are preceded by respiratory infections. Antibiotic therapy is not necessary unless sinusitis, pneumonia, or other evidence of bacterial infection is present.

Exercise

Almost all asthmatics develop airways obstructions with strenuous exercise (Anderson, 1983). The intensity of symptoms relates to the severity of underlying airways obstructions and the particular kind of exercise, with running being the most asthmogenic. With the current focus of society on regular aerobic exercise, this and other forms of exercise have become major triggers for many asthmatic adults. The physician's responsibility is further increased when it involves the care of athletes with asthma, since small changes in airway function can translate into compromised performance, and treatment must consist of bronchodilators that are approved for sporting events (Fitch, 1984; see also Chapter 44).

Aspirin and Nonsteroidal Anti-Inflammatory Drugs (NSAIDs)

Aspirin and NSAIDs can provoke attacks of asthma in susceptible individuals. The intensity of these reactions is variable and may be associated with naso-ocular symptoms (Stevenson, 1984). The incidence of aspirin sensitivity in adults with asthma is difficult to determine, but best estimates place the prevalence between 8 and 20 percent. In certain subsets of asthma patients, particularly those with chronic rhino-sinusitis, nasal polyps, and steroid dependency, the prevalence may approach 30 to 40 percent. Aspirin commonly cross-reacts with the NSAIDs, particularly those that inhibit prostaglandin synthetase. In contrast, the nonpros-

* This work was supported in part by the Veterans Administration. We wish to express our sincere appreciation to Carol Steinhart for editorial assistance in the preparation of this manuscript.

taglandin-synthesis inhibitor acetaminophen rarely cross-reacts with aspirin. Asthmatic children with aspirin sensitivity have been identified, but the prevalence appears less than in asthmatic adults (Rachelefsky et al., 1975).

The pathogenic mechanism of aspirin sensitivity is not known, although several hypotheses have been proposed. To date, no evidence for an IgE antibody mechanism has been identified. The role of tartrazine (F.D.A. Yellow Dye No. 5) in provoking asthma in the aspirin-sensitive patient is unclear. Earlier reports suggested that up to 20 percent of aspirin-sensitive patients may experience asthma upon ingestion of this dye, but recent, more carefully conducted studies fail to substantiate these claims (Simon, 1984).

Sulfite Sensitivity

Sulfiting agents, such as the bisulfites and metabisulfites of sodium and potassium, are antimicrobial agents and antioxidants used to prevent discoloration of and to preserve various foods and medications. Some asthmatics experience profound bronchospasm upon ingestion of sulfited foods (Stevenson and Simon, 1981). The exact prevalence and mechanism of sulfiting agent sensitivity is not known, but we find sensitivity to be confined primarily to the steroid-dependent asthma patient (Bush et al., 1986). Sources of sulfite exposure include lettuce from salad bars, where solutions of sulfiting agents are sprayed on vegetables to prevent discoloration; dried fruits; wines; and certain beers. Adverse responses to sulfited aerosol bronchodilators, such as isoetharine, also have been reported (Koepke et al., 1984). Because of these reactions, the use of sulfite is being restricted by the U.S. Food and Drug Administration.

Allergic Bronchopulmonary Aspergillosis (ABPA)

ABPA is an uncommon but not rare complication of asthma, more likely to affect adults than children. Its presence should be considered in asthma patients with recurrent pulmonary infiltrates, proximal bronchiectasis, striking peripheral blood eosinophilia, and IgE sensitivities to *Aspergillus* and other inhalants (Greenberger, 1984). Because untreated ABPA can lead to irreversible pulmonary fibrosis, its identification is of utmost importance (see Chapter 47).

Coexistent Illnesses

Coexistent diseases in adults can influence the severity of bronchospasm and complicate the diagnosis and treatment of asthma. These effects are true particularly in patients with underlying obstructive lung diseases, such as chronic bronchitis or emphysema, which can mask the presence of asthma and limit responses to treatment. Moreover, patients with reactive airway disease can develop "cardiac asthma." In these cases, the differentiation between nocturnal asthma and shortness of breath of cardiac origin frequently is difficult, unless careful attention is given to the detection of signs of congestive heart failure. A patient with preexisting cardiac disease should have an electrocardiogram prior to administration of theophylline or beta-adrenergic drugs. The physician also should be aware that systemically administered beta-agonists can cause nonspecific S-T wave changes and arrhythmias in some patients. Furthermore, coexisting cardiac decompensation should be treated with diuretics and digitalis. The physician prescribing these agents should realize, however, that methylxanthines may potentiate the action of diuretics, and these agents along with corticosteroids can increase calcium loss significantly. In the asthmatic with cardiac decompensation, salt-retaining corticosteroids must be administered cautiously, with attention to minimizing weight gain and scrutinizing serum potassium levels especially with concomitant diuretics. Many antiarrhythmic and antihypertensive agents have sedative properties and can depress respiratory drive. Gastroesophageal reflux, especially when it occurs at night, can provoke asthma; this can be further complicated by methylxanthine therapy, which diminishes cardioesophageal sphincter tone.

Pregnancy

The effect of pregnancy on asthma is variable and largely dictated by the severity of preexisting disease (Greenberger and Patterson, 1985). If exacerbations of asthma occur during pregnancy, they are more likely after the fourth month. Unless existing airway disease is severe, there is little evidence to indicate undue risk to the fetus. Oral beta-agonists must be stopped at term, since they inhibit uterine contraction. Of special concern is the effect of maternal medication on the fetus. Theophylline, corticosteroids, and most beta-adrenergic drugs are safe during pregnancy (Greenberg, 1985). Theophylline metabolism often slows during the third trimester of pregnancy, and the physician must guard against theophylline toxicity at this time.

Vocal Cord Dysfunction

Some adult asthmatics appear unresponsive to all treatment efforts. Occasionally, this lack of response is due to upper airway obstruction secondary to vocal cord dysfunction rather than to asthma (Christopher et al., 1983). Such patients exhibit what appears to be severe airway obstruction by effort-dependent spirometric testing, yet arterial blood gas values are normal. This finding should lead the clinician to suspect this condition. Inspiratory and expiratory flow volume loops are helpful in diagnosis, and direct vocal cord visualization will verify the suspected defect. These patients tend to benefit from psychiatric treatment and retraining of vocalization. Surgery is not indicated since the obstruction is functional rather than anatomic.

BRONCHODILATOR THERAPY IN THE ADULT ASTHMA PATIENT

Bronchial smooth muscle spasm is a major factor in the airway obstruction of asthma. Beta-adrenergic agonists, theophylline, and now anticholinergic preparations relax airway smooth muscle. Since each of these drugs acts by a different mechanism, their combined use may afford added benefit.

Specific Adrenergic Bronchodilators

EPINEPHRINE

Epinephrine (Adrenalin) is a potent, rapidly acting parenteral and aerosol bronchodilator. Therapeutic use is limited by its short duration of action (unless it is combined with alum, as in injectable Sus-Phrine) and its possession of both alpha-adrenergic and beta-adrenergic agonist properties. Subcutaneous doses of epinephrine, 0.01 mg/kg (maximum doses of 0.3 to 0.5 mg), produce acute bronchodilation, but

the coexistence of potent alpha-adrenergic activity may limit its safe use in adult patients with underlying cardiac disease or hypertension (Sly et al., 1985). There are no absolute contraindications to parenteral epinephrine use in acute asthma on an age basis alone. However, in patients known to have hypertension, coronary artery disease, and angina or arrhythmias, we suggest that aerosolized beta-adrenergics be given as the initial treatment. Nonetheless, the physician must be aware that a small portion of the inhaled beta-agonist is absorbed and can stimulate the myocardium to increase heart rate.

EPHEDRINE

Ephedrine is a weak bronchodilator often found combined with a fixed dose of theophylline and a sedative in oral bronchodilators (Tedral, Marax). Its use is limited to mild cases of asthma.

ISOPROTERENOL

Isoproterenol administered by metered-dose aerosolization or nebulization gives rapid bronchodilation, with a peak response occurring within 5 minutes. Because of its short duration of action (less than 2 hours) and the availability of new selective beta-2 adrenergic bronchodilators, its use is limited. Some clinicians have advocated intravenous isoproterenol in severe, intractable asthma. In our opinion, this is potentially a risky approach in adults, as major cardiac side effects can follow intravenous isoproterenol.

METAPROTERENOL

Metaproterenol has a structural shift in the hydroxyl group to the meta position on the benzene ring, which diminishes its susceptibility to catechol-*O*-methyl transferase degradation and gives longer bronchodilation (3 to 4 hours). This compound does not have exclusive selectivity for the beta-2 receptor but is relatively beta-2 selective, when used by inhalation because of its slow absorption from the lung.

NONCATECHOL BETA-2 ADRENERGIC SELECTIVE BRONCHODILATORS

Noncatechol, beta-2 adrenergic bronchodilators (terbutaline, albuterol, and bitolterol) offer adrenergic selectivity and prolonged bronchodilation. Each of these compounds has a unique structure, but all give equivalent bronchodilation. Principal side effects include tremor and tachycardia; their intensity is patient variable. Side effects occur more frequently with systemic administration but diminish with continued use.

Use of Beta-Adrenergic Drugs in Adult Asthma Treatment

Beta-adrenergic agonists provide first-line treatment of adult asthma. Aerosol delivery provides prompt and effective bronchodilation in mild asthma. Moreover, premedication with aerosolized beta-agonists successfully prevents exercise-induced asthma in most patients. With more severe asthma, scheduled dosing with beta-adrenergic drugs, through either metered-dose or oral administration, gives sustained bronchodilation.

ORAL, AEROSOL, OR PARENTERAL ADMINISTRATION

Advantages can be cited for oral, parenteral, and aerosol delivery. Metered-dose delivery has many advantages, including prompt action, minimal side effects, and prolonged bronchodilation. Systemic administration with oral beta-agonists is convenient and dilates both large and small airways, but with stable asthma or with the use of spacer devices, metered-dose aerosols may be equally effective in this regard. During asthma attacks, aerosol distribution to the airways is more unpredictable but can be improved by the use of spacer devices or nebulizers. When distribution and delivery are critical, e.g., in status asthmaticus, parenteral administration may be combined with nebulized beta-agonist treatment to insure optimal bronchodilation.

BETA-ADRENERGIC RECEPTOR DESENSITIZATION

Tolerance to beta-adrenergic drugs can develop during continual administration, as membrane receptors are either lost or uncoupled. The consequence of desensitization can be noted by a diminished maximal bronchodilation, a shorter duration of bronchodilation, or both. The development of beta-adrenergic "down-regulation" in asthma is not a consistent finding, nor should it mitigate against scheduled daily dosing (Jenne, 1982).

CONCOMITANT ADMINISTRATION WITH THEOPHYLLINE

Treatment with beta-agonists or theophylline alone is not sufficient to control airway obstruction in most symptomatic asthmatics. The concomitant administration of beta-agonists (preferably by metered dose) and theophylline may give additional bronchodilation. Moreover, in patients unable to tolerate therapeutic doses of either beta-agonists or methylxanthines, submaximal doses of each will increase bronchodilation and minimize side effects (Wolfe et al., 1978). Concern has recently been raised about the possibility of augmented cardiac toxicity with combination regimens of methylxanthines and beta-adrenergics (Nicklas et al., 1984). Such findings have yet to be substantiated in humans, but caution should be extended to patients with underlying heart disease (Kemp et al., 1984).

BETA-ADRENERGIC ANTAGONISTS AND ASTHMA

Beta-adrenergic antagonists are effective antihypertensive agents, but they constitute a major risk for almost all asthmatics. Sensitivity can be striking; some patients develop asthma from a beta-antagonist, timolol, used in eye drops for glaucoma treatment. The risk may be reduced, but not always eliminated, with lower doses of "selective" beta-adrenergic antagonists (e.g., atenolol and metoprolol). Mild hypertension in asthma, especially if precipitated by systemic corticosteroid use, is treated with a thiazide diuretic. More substantial hypertension can be safely treated with a vasodilator (e.g., prazosin, methyldopa, and clonidine). For more severe hypertension, drugs such as captopril can be considered. The newer calcium channel antagonists also have been safely used as antihypertensives and do not exacerbate asthma.

Theophylline

Theophylline, another first-line drug in asthma therapy, is available in a variety of formulations. For acute asthma, plain tablets act rapidly but are not useful for maintenance therapy, owing to their short duration of action. Sustained-release products are now most frequently selected for long-term therapy and provide a slow onset of action but prolonged (12 to 24 hours) bronchodilation. The convenience of once or twice daily dosing increases patient compliance and decreases fluctuation in peak-to-trough plasma theophylline concentrations.

For adults, initial therapy with 400 mg/day given either as a single dose or as two doses (200 mg each) daily is a reasonable starting level. If this initial dose is tolerated, a 25 percent increase is given at 3-day intervals to the maximum premeasured dose, which in the adult is 13 mg/kg/day (based on the ideal body weight) or 900 mg/day, whichever is less. After the patient has been on this regimen for at least 48 hours, a plasma theophylline level is obtained 4 hours after the administration of a sustained release preparation (peak level). At that point, if the medication is tolerated and the disease controlled, the patient is maintained on this dose until such time as the disease may be in remission. If the medication is tolerated but the disease is not controlled and the theophylline level is not in the therapeutic range, slow, cautious increases may be made until the plasma concentration is at a therapeutic level and the disease is managed. If the disease is not controlled in spite of an adequate theophylline level, additional therapeutic measures are necessary. If the patient does not tolerate the dose of theophylline, whether or not the patient's theophylline level is within the therapeutic range, the dose should be decreased until the patient can tolerate the medication, or it is discontinued and another medication is substituted. Since many patients will experience transient side effects, such as nausea and irritability, when large initial doses are employed, it is best to proceed with slow initial titration procedure as outlined. Further, once daily theophylline may provide better control of asthma with fewer side effects, especially when given in the evening as opposed to in the morning (Busse and Bush, 1985).

Optimal therapeutic concentrations of plasma theophylline have been considered by some workers to fall between 10 and 20 μg/ml. Because many adults with mild asthma experience significant bronchodilation at plasma theophylline levels of less than 10 μg/ml, the window of efficacy for these patients should be expanded to 5 to 20 μg/ml, with the knowledge that some patients will have excellent control of their asthma even at plasma levels of less than 5 μg/ml. The clinical response to theophylline always must be considered along with the plasma theophylline concentration in asthma therapy. Moreover, some patients experience gastrointestinal side effects, headaches, and irritability at levels in the so-called therapeutic range.

It no longer appears that the mechanism of action of theophylline is entirely related to an inhibition of the phosphodiesterase degradation of cAMP; in vitro concentrations of theophylline needed to produce this effect are toxic in vivo. Theophylline may antagonize adenosine-induced bronchoconstriction (Cushley et al., 1984), stimulate endogenous catecholamine release (Bukowskyj et al., 1984), affect intracellular calcium flux, increase binding of cAMP to cAMP binding proteins, and reduce fatigue of diaphragmatic muscles.

Elderly patients metabolize theophylline at much slower rates than do children and young adults, and underlying illnesses, such as congestive heart failure, liver disease, and viral upper respiratory infections, also prolong plasma half-life. Interactions with erythromycin, propranolol, allopurinol, and cimetidine, but not ranitidine (Powell et al., 1984), also prolong the half-life of theophylline. Specific recommendations are available for appropriate reduction in doses (Bukowskyj et al., 1984).

Theophylline freely crosses the placenta, and the infant's blood level at the time of birth parallels that of the mother's (Labovitz and Spector, 1982). Theophylline therapy in pregnant women has not been associated with any significant birth defects, but it can lead to transient theophylline toxicity in the newborn.

Anticholinergic Drugs

Atropine, the anticholinergic prototype, has limited use in asthma treatment due to side effects from mucosal absorption (Gross and Skorodin, 1984). Modification of atropine into quaternary ammonium congeners decreases systemic absorption yet maintains potent local anticholinergic activity. Among the synthetic quaternary derivatives being evaluated for the treatment of obstructive lung disease are ipratropium bromide (Atrovent), atropine methylnitrate, and glycopyrrolate (Robinul), all of which are nearly twice as effective as atropine in bronchodilation with a significantly greater duration of action.

Anticholinergic agents induce prompt bronchodilation but require 60 to 90 minutes to reach peak activity and continue bronchodilation up to 12 hours (Gal et al., 1984). Some reports indicate that anticholinergic agents are more effective than albuterol in asthma patients over 40 years of age, who have long-standing disease and profound bronchoconstriction due to emotional stimuli. Moreover, atropine derivatives show greater efficacy in patients with chronic bronchitis and emphysema than with asthma. Anticholinergic therapy has been particularly safe, with little evidence to suggest detrimental effects on mucus clearance.

Increased efficacy in bronchodilation occurs with the combined use of anticholinergic and beta-adrenergic drugs (Rebuck et al., 1983). This combination gives rapid onset (from the beta-agonist) and long duration (from the anticholinergic agent) of action. Such a combination metered-dose aerosol is available in Europe (Duo-Vent: fenoterol and ipratropium). Because the aerosolized anticholinergics have yet to be licensed for sale in the United States, their role in asthma therapy is not fully established. Nonetheless, the use of anticholinergic drugs for asthma treatment promises effective bronchodilation for many asthma patients.

Corticosteroids

Corticosteroids may be used for several purposes in the treatment of asthma. A patient suspected of having asthma who has not responded to bronchodilator therapy should be given a trial of oral prednisone (10 to 15 mg, 4 times a day for 1 week, followed by 10 to 20 mg as a single morning dose for an additional week) to determine whether the obstruction is fixed (chronic obstructive pulmonary disease) or substantially reversible (asthma). Patients exhibiting improvement in pulmonary functions in such circumstances may benefit from long-term maintenance steroid therapy. The morbidity of acute, severe exacerbations of asthma can be reduced by administration of a 5- to 7-day course of oral prednisone (0.5 to 1.0 mg/kg/day in 4 divided doses) in addition to regular bronchodilators. Courses of oral corticosteroids given in pharmacologic doses for up to 2 weeks do not require a tapering schedule.

Inhaled corticosteroids (Table 43–1) are preferred for long-term maintenance, since they avoid the adrenal suppression and complications of corticosteroids administered systemically. Aerosolized steroids should be initiated after the patient achieves maximal improvement of pulmonary function (usually following a short course of oral steroids) in order to ensure maximal delivery of medication to the airways. Side effects of aerosolized steroids include intermittent hoarseness or sore throat and oral candidiasis, which is preventable by rinsing the mouth immediately after steroid administration.

A few patients require long-term maintenance therapy with corticosteroids because of continued pulmonary function abnormalities or persistent asthma symptoms in spite of intensive bronchodilator therapy. Ultimately, the oral dose should be reduced to the minimum amount required for control of asthma. The dose should be taken upon arising. Every attempt should be made to achieve an alternate-day dosing schedule if possible, with short-acting steroid preparations, such as prednisone or methylprednisolone, rather than long-acting corticosteroid preparations, such as dexamethasone.

Even though complications of long-term steroid administration are well known, these should not prevent the use of steroids in the treatment of asthma when necessary. Most of the short-term complications of corticosteroid therapy are readily reversible or easily controlled if proper precautions are taken. The most common short-term complications are central nervous system effects, such as insomnia, agitation, or depression, when steroids are administered on an acute basis. Peptic ulceration may occur, but can be prevented by administration of antacids. Disturbances in fluid

TABLE 43–1. Aerosolized Corticosteroid Preparations

Drug		Dose/Activation (μg)*	Usual Adult Dose	Recommended Maximum Adult Dosage (μg/day)†
Beclomethasone dipropionate	(Beclovent, Vanceril)	42	2 puffs, 3 to 4 times daily	840
Flunisolide	(AeroBid)	250	2 puffs, 2 times daily	2000
Triamcinolone acetonide	(Azmacort)	100	2 puffs, 3 to 4 times daily	1600

* Dose reported as delivered to the patient.
† Selected patients may require higher doses.

and electrolyte balance, such as sodium retention and edema, can be managed with diuretics; hypokalemia can be treated with potassium replacement. Hyperglycemia may require institution of insulin therapy temporarily during treatment with high-dose corticosteroids. Patients should be advised that they will experience an increase in appetite and that restricted caloric intake may be necessary to prevent rapid weight gain. For long-term maintenance therapy, aerosolized steroids or alternate-day schedules of steroids should be used to prevent the serious complications of corticosteroid administration. These complications include posterior subcapsular cataracts; osteoporosis; aseptic necrosis of bone; and endocrinologic disturbances, such as hyperglycemia, hypertension, and sodium retention. For the pregnant asthmatic patient, corticosteroids, when indicated for the treatment of severe asthma, do not appear to increase the risk of maternal or fetal complication aside from that of premature birth (Schatz et al., 1975).

Cromolyn

Cromolyn has several important clinical effects. It prevents both the immediate and the late phase asthmatic response after bronchial challenge with allergens. In this way, cromolyn is protective in a patient naturally exposed to allergens during the course of a pollen season and prevents reflex bronchoconstriction induced by inhalation of sulfur dioxide. Finally, cromolyn protects against exercise-induced asthma. The effectiveness of cromolyn is greater in children than in adults.

Cromolyn is not effective for reversal of acute asthma. It is useful on only a prophylactic basis for which the usual dose is one 20-mg powdered capsule; 2-ml solution by nebulization, inhaled three to four times daily or approximately 15 minutes before exposure; or two inhalations (1.6 mg total) of a metered-dose inhaler. In adults, cromolyn may prevent asthma associated with exposure to specific allergens, such as animal danders or those found in an occupational situation. Inhalation of cromolyn immediately before exercise can prevent bronchospasm. Often this effect is enhanced if it is preceded by one to two inhalations of a metered-dose, beta-agonist bronchodilator.

Cromolyn is an exceptionally safe drug, and adverse reactions are usually not life-threatening and are reversible. Two percent of 375 patients experienced adverse reactions, consisting of dermatitis, myositis, or gastroenteritis (Settipane et al., 1979). In addition, a few isolated cases of pulmonary infiltrates with eosinophilia have been reported. The safety of cromolyn use in pregnancy has not been established.

IMMUNOTHERAPY

Immunotherapy is used as adjunctive therapy in a patient who has IgE-mediated component to asthma. Unfortunately, the data supporting the effectiveness of immunotherapy in adult asthmatics are limited as is the knowledge of its mechanisms of action (Zeiger and Schatz, 1981). Preliminary data suggest that immunotherapy may be more effective in preventing the late phase bronchial reaction to antigen than the immediate reaction (Metzger et al., 1983; Warner et al., 1978).

Maintenance doses of immunotherapy appear to be safe in the pregnant asthmatic patient (Turner et al., 1980); however, it probably is best to reserve institution of immunotherapy until after the patient has delivered. Treatment with unconventional techniques, such as the Rinkel method, has not been shown to be effective (Van Metre et al., 1979) (see Chapter 57).

TREATMENT OF ACUTE ASTHMA

An acute attack of asthma poses a medical emergency. The intensity of the acute episode will be dictated by the severity of the underlying illness, the duration of the current episode, the history of the previous hospitalizations with respiratory failure, and the age of the patient, with the very young and the very old being at particular risk.

Physical examination confirms the diagnosis of acute asthma but does not reliably indicate its severity. Wheezing is present unless the obstruction to airflow is diminished markedly, and then few sounds are heard. More objective signs of a severe attack include the use of accessory muscles of ventilation, increased heart rate and blood pressure, exaggerated pulsus paradoxus (difficult to measure in acute asthma), intercostal retractions, and cyanosis. None of these findings can substitute for measurements of pulmonary functions, which should be obtained to assess precisely the severity of airway obstruction and to serve as guides for treatment. Peak expiratory flow rates (PEFR) below

20 percent predicted (< 100 L/min) or forced expiratory volumes in one second (FEV_1) below 25 percent of predicted (< 1L) represent severe obstruction and are likely to be associated with severe hypoxemia and carbon dioxide retention.

Table 43–2 suggests an initial treatment approach for the adult patient with acute asthma. Sympathomimetics are given immediately by either parenteral administration (epinephrine or terbutaline) or nebulized solution. Less severe episodes of asthma should respond to nebulized sympathomimetics with fewer side effects than are found with parenteral administration. Intravenous aminophylline can increase bronchodilation primarily when given

TABLE 43–2. General Treatment Program for Use in the Emergency Room

Time (min)	Treatment	Assessment
0	Injectable epinephrine or terbutaline OR Nebulized aerosol* Metaproterenol, 0.3 ml (5 percent) + 2.2 ml saline OR Terbutaline, 1 mg/ml + 2 ml saline Aminophylline IV (with severe asthma) Oxygen by nasal prongs (flow rates of 2 to 6 L/min)	FEV_1, FVC Arterial blood gas determinations, if cyanosis or severe airway obstruction
20	Epinephrine	
30	Nebulized aerosol OR Injectable terbutaline Aminophylline IV	FEV_1, FVC If improved, watch for additional 30 minutes and discharge with bronchodilator therapy
40	Epinephrine	
60	Repeat evaluation, determine need for further treatment	FEV_1, FVC If improved, discharge with bronchodilator therapy†; if not improved, admit to hospital for further treatment

* Would use nebulized aerosol in adults with underlying cardiac disease, hypertension, coronary artery disease, or arrhythmias.

† If the patient has been on aerosolized corticosteroids or systemic corticosteroids, it is suggested that a short course of prednisone (e.g., 10 mg t.i.d. or q.i.d. for 7 days) be considered at discharge. Further, if the patient has not shown complete reversibility of airway obstruction, a short "burst" of prednisone (10 mg t.i.d. or q.i.d. for 7 days) may be appropriate (see text).

with beta-adrenergic drugs to patients with low plasma theophylline values. Treatment in the emergency room or physician's office of the patient with an acute attack should not continue for longer than 1 hour before a decision is made whether or not to admit the patient to a hospital, since little additional improvement in airway obstruction is likely after the first hour of intensive treatment (Fanta et al., 1982). Patients showing improvement but not complete recovery may benefit from short bursts of prednisone, following initial bronchodilator therapy (Fiel et al., 1983). Patients with severe airway obstructions (FEV_1 of < 1.0 L), those with histories of previous episodes of respiratory failure, and those who are elderly should be admitted to intensive care units for close monitoring. The need to use intensive care facilities for all other patients in status asthmaticus is less well substantiated but probably wise (Hetzel et al., 1977).

TREATMENT OF THE HOSPITALIZED ADULT PATIENT WITH STATUS ASTHMATICUS

Failure to achieve significant improvement (as measured by spirometry) with bronchodilator therapy during an acute attack of asthma is defined as status asthmaticus and requires hospitalization for further care. Resistance to bronchodilator treatment occurs because of bronchial obstruction caused by bronchospasm, airway inflammation, and mucus plugs. On hospital admission, spirometry (FEV_1 and FVC) should be performed, and an arterial blood sample obtained to monitor the impact of airway obstruction on pulmonary gas exchange. Special caution must be given to the patient with moderately severe obstruction when the arterial blood gas determinations indicate hypoxemia with "normal" $Paco_2$ and pH values. In this circumstance, the arterial $Paco_2$ and pH values in fact are not "normal" (since $Paco_2$ should be decreased from the increased ventilatory effect) but rather are indications that the patient's condition is quickly deteriorating, with eventual hypercarbia, acidosis, and respiratory failure the possible outcomes. With respiratory failure, the patient will usually require endotracheal intubation and assisted ventilation. Early aggressive therapy is needed to prevent respiratory failure.

Bronchodilator therapy must be continued. The physician has the choice between nebulized or parenteral (subcutaneous) administration. Nebulized therapy appears to be as effective as parenteral treatment in severe asthma. Nebulized terbutaline or metaproterenol or albuterol can be given every 2 to 3 hours. The choice for parenteral therapy is epinephrine suspension (Sees-Phrine) or terbutaline every 6 to 8 hours. In some cases, the nebulized and parenteral forms may be given concomitantly. By alternating the administration of nebulized and parenteral sympathomimetics every 3 hours, maximum bronchodilation can be achieved. With severe attacks of asthma, these beta-adrenergic drugs appear well tolerated and safe.

Beta-agonists, either by injection or by nebulization, are far superior to intravenous aminophylline in acute asthma. For the hospitalized patient, intravenous aminophylline remains an appropriate treatment. For patients who have not previously received theophylline, an intravenous loading dose of 5.6 mg/kg is followed by an infusion appropriate for the age of the patient (Hendeles and Weinberger, 1983). Patients should have plasma theophylline levels monitored, with subsequent adjustment of dosages to achieve levels of 10 to 20 µg/ml. For patients who have received theophylline prior to hospital admission, the plasma theophylline concentrations should be determined; if there are no signs of clinical toxicity, patients should be given 2.5 mg/kg loading doses over 30 minutes, followed by constant intravenous infusions. As for the loading dose in the patient who has not previously received theophylline, the plasma concentration 30 minutes after the loading dose administration should be measured to ascertain if additional theophylline is required. Intravenous theophylline is usually continued for at least 24 hours after parenteral corticosteroid preparations are discontinued. At that time, the patient may be started on oral sustained-release theophylline therapy, which may be calculated from the total theophylline requirement in a 24-hour period that produced a therapeutic plasma theophylline concentration.

Early institution of corticosteroid treatment reduces the morbidity of status asthmaticus (Fanta et al., 1983) and possibly also the associated mortality. Therapy should be initiated with intravenous hydrocortisone, 3 to 4 mg/kg every 2 to 3 hours, or an equivalent dose of methylprednisolone. These doses are designed to achieve plasma cortisol levels in excess of 100 µg/ml (Seigel, 1985). The intravenous route is

continued until the patient shows improvement in pulmonary function, usually after 24 to 48 hours. At that time, an oral steroid preparation, such as prednisone 10 to 15 mg q.i.d. is substituted, until pulmonary functions reach maximum bronchodilation (7 to 10 days). At this point, steroids are discontinued or tapered as necessary.

Supplemental oxygen also should be given. Although it is commonly recommended that fluids be "pushed," there is little evidence to support this recommendation and in fact overhydration may predispose the patient to pulmonary edema. Unless an infectious complication, such as pneumonia, sinusitis or purulent bronchitis, is found, antibiotics are not needed.

Morbidity in asthma is increased in the elderly and in those with previous episodes of respiratory failure. Morbidity also is greater in those who have received sedatives or in those who have had corticosteroid therapy withheld. Status asthmaticus is a medical emergency that should have a favorable outcome with proper treatment. To accomplish this goal, the physician must heed the warning of severe disease, use bronchodilators and corticosteroids, and monitor pulmonary functions and arterial blood gas determinations carefully.

REFERENCES

Anderson, S.D.: Recent advances in the understanding of exercise-induced asthma. Eur. J. Respir. Dis. 64:225, 1983.

Barbee, R.A., Dodge, R., Lebowitz, M.L., Burrows, B.: The epidemiology of asthma. Chest 87:215, 1985.

Bernstein, I.L.: Cromolyn sodium in the treatment of asthma: coming of age in the United States. J. Allergy Clin. Immunol. 76:381, 1985.

Bukowskyj, M., Nakatsu, K., Munt, P.W.: Theophylline reassessed. Ann. Intern. Med. 101:63, 1984.

Bush, R.K., Taylor, S.L., Holden, K., Nordlee, J.A., Busse, W.W.: Prevalence of sensitivity to sulfiting agents in asthmatic patients. Am. J. Med. 81:816, 1986.

Busse, W.W.: The precipitation of asthma by upper respiratory infections. Chest 87:445, 1985.

Busse, W.W., Bush, R.K.: A comparison of AM and PM dosing with a 24-hour sustained release theophylline, rhiniphyl, for nocturnal asthma. Am. J. Med. 79(6A):62, 1985.

Christopher, K.L., Wood, R.P., Eckert, R.C., Blager, F.B., Raney, R.A., Souhrada, J.F.: Vocal-cord dysfunction presenting as asthma. N. Engl. J. Med. 308:1566, 1983.

Cushley, M.J., Tattersfield, A.E., Holgate, S.T.: Adenosine-induced bronchoconstriction in asthma. Antagonism by inhaled theophylline. Am. Rev. Respir. Dis. 129:380, 1984.

Fanta, C.H., Rossing, T.H., McFadden, E.R., Jr.: Emergency room treatment of asthma. Am. J. Med. 72:416, 1982.

Fanta, C.H., Rossing, T.H., McFadden, E.R., Jr.: Glucocorticoids in acute asthma: a critical controlled trial. Am. J. Med. 74:485, 1983.

Fiel, S.B., Swartz, M.A., Glanz, K., Francis, M.E.: Efficacy of short-term corticosteroid therapy in outpatient treatment of acute bronchial asthma. Am. J. Med. 75:259, 1983.

Fitch, K.D.: Management of allergic Olympic athletes. J. Allergy Clin. Immunol. 73:722, 1984.

Gal, T.J., Suratt, P.M., Lu, J.-Y.: Glycopyrrolate and atropine inhalation: comparative effects on normal airway function. Am. Rev. Respir. Dis. 129:871, 1984.

Grammer, L.C., Shaughnessy, M.A., Patterson, R.: Modified forms of allergen immunotherapy. J. Allergy Clin. Immunol. 76:397, 1985.

Greenberg, F.: The potential teratogenicity of allergy and asthma treatment in pregnancy. Immunol. Allergy Prac. 7:15, 1985.

Greenberger, P.A.: Allergic bronchopulmonary aspergillosis. J. Allergy Clin. Immunol. 74:645, 1984.

Greenberger, P.A., Patterson, R.: Management of asthma during pregnancy. N. Engl. J. Med. 3:897, 1985.

Gross, N.J., Skorodin, M.S.: Anticholinergic, antimuscarinic bronchodilators. Am. Rev. Respir. Dis. 129:856, 1984.

Hendeles, L., Weinberger, M.: Theophylline. A "state of the art" review. Pharmacotherapy 3:2, 1983.

Hetzel, M.R., Clark, I.J.H., Branthwaite, M.A.: Asthma: Analysis of sudden deaths and ventilatory arrests in hospital. Brit. Med. J. 1:808–811, 1977.

Jenne, J.W.: Whither beta-adrenergic tachyphylaxis? J. Allergy Clin. Immunol. 70:413, 1982.

Kaliner, M.: Mechanisms of glucocorticosteroid action in bronchial asthma. J. Allergy Clin. Immunol. 76:321, 1985.

Kemp, J.P., Chervinsky, P., Orgel, H.A., Meltzer, E.O., Noyes, J.H., Mingo, T.S.: Concomitant bitolterol mesylate aerosol and theophylline for asthma therapy, with 24 hour electrocardiographic monitoring. J. Allergy Clin. Immunol. 73:32, 1984.

Koepke, J.W., Christopher, K.L., Chai, H., et al.: Dose-dependent bronchospasm for sulfites in isoetharine. J.A.M.A. 251:2982, 1984.

Labovitz, E., Spector, S.: Placental theophylline transfer in pregnant asthmatics. J.A.M.A. 247:786, 1982.

Levinson, A.I., Summers, R.J., Lawley, T.J., et al.: Evaluation of the adverse effects of long-term hyposensitization. J. Allergy Clin. Immunol. 62:109, 1978.

McFadden, E.R., Jr.: Pathogenesis of asthma. J. Allergy Clin. Immunol. 73:413, 1984.

Metzger, W.J., Donnelly, B.A., Richerson, H.B.: Modification of the late asthmatic responses (LAR) during immunotherapy for *Alternaria*-induced asthma. (Abstract) J. Allergy Clin. Immunol. 71:119, 1983.

Morris, H.G.: Mechanisms of action and therapeutic role of corticosteroids in asthma. J. Allergy Clin. Immunol. 75:1, 1985.

Nicklas, R.A., Whitehurst, V.E., Donohue, R.F., Balazs, T.: Concomitant use of beta-adrenergic agonists and methylxanthines. J. Allergy Clin. Immunol. 73:20, 1984.

Powell, J.R., Rogers, J.F., Wargin, W.A., et al.: Inhibition of theophylline clearance by cimetidine but not ranitidine. Arch. Intern. Med. 144:484, 1984.

Rachelefsky, G.S., Coulsen, A., Siegel, S.C., Strehm, E.R.: Aspirin intolerance in chronic childhood asthma detected by oral challenge. Pediatrics 56:443, 1975.

Rebuck, A.S., Geut, M., Chapman, K.R.: Anticholinergic and sympathomimetic combination therapy of asthma. J. Allergy Clin. Immunol. 71:317, 1983.

Rocklin, R.E.: Clinical and immunologic aspects of allergen-specific immunotherapy in patients with seasonal allergic rhinitis and/or allergic asthma. J. Allergy Clin. Immunol. 72:323, 1983.

Schatz, M., Patterson, R., Zeitz, S., et al.: Corticosteroid therapy for the pregnant asthmatic patient. J.A.M.A. 233:804, 1975.

Seigel, S.C.: Overview of corticosteroid therapy. J. Allergy Clin. Immunol. 76:312, 1985.

Settipane, G.A., Klein, D.E., Boyd, G.K., et al.: Adverse reactions to cromolyn. J.A.M.A. 241:811, 1979.

Simon, R.A.: Adverse reactions to drug additives. J. Allergy Clin. Immunol. 74:623, 1984.

Sly, R.M., Anderson, J.A., Bresman, C.W., et al.: Adverse effects and complications of treatment with beta-adrenergic agonist drugs. J. Allergy Clin. Immunol. 75:433, 1985.

Stevenson, D.D.: Diagnosis, prevention, and treatment of adverse reactions to aspirin and non-steroidal anti-inflammatory drugs. J. Allergy Clin. Immunol. 74:617, 1984.

Stevenson, D.D., Simon, R.A.: Sensitivity to ingested metabisulfite in asthmatic subjects. J. Allergy Clin. Immunol. 68:26, 1981.

Stiles, G.L., Caron, M.G., Lefkowitz, R.J.: Beta-adrenergic receptors: biochemical mechanisms of physiological regulation. Physiol. Rev. 64:661, 1984.

Turner, E.S., Greenberger, P.A., Patterson, R.: Management of the pregnant asthmatic patient. Ann. Intern. Med. 93:905, 1980.

Van Metre, T.E., Jr., Adkinson, N.F., Jr., Amodio, F.J., et al.: A comparative study of the effectiveness of the Rinkel method and the current standard method of immunotherapy for ragweed pollen hay fever. J. Allergy Clin. Immunol. 66:500, 1979.

Warner, J.O., Soothill, J.F., Price, J.F., et al.: Controlled trial of hyposensitization to *Dermatophagoides pteronyssinus* in children with asthma. Lancet 2:912, 1978.

Wasserman, S.I.: Mediators of immediate hypersensitivity. J. Allergy Clin. Immunol. 72:101, 1983.

Wolfe, J.D., Tashkin, D.P., Calvarese, B., Simmons, M.: Bronchodilator effects of terbutaline and aminophylline alone and in combination in asthmatic patients. N. Engl. J. Med. 298:363, 1978.

Zeiger, R.S., Schatz, M.: Immunotherapy of atopic disorders. Med. Clin. North Am. 6:987, 1981.

44

Exercise-Induced Asthma

SIMON GODFREY, M.D., PH.D.

Towards the end of the seventeenth century, Sir John Floyer, a physician who suffered from asthma, made detailed observations on his condition which he reported in his *Treatise on the Asthma*. Among other factors that could provoke asthmatic attacks he noted that "all violent Exercise makes the Asthmatic to breathe short" and related how different types of exercise had different potentials for provoking asthmatic attacks. Little interest was taken in the subject of exercise-induced asthma (EIA) until recent times, even though the phenomenon was clearly recognized by clinicians. In some asthmatic individuals, EIA was the most prominent feature of their disease. Consequently, EIA was sometimes considered a disease in its own right. Careful clinical and physiologic observations have shown clearly that significant EIA occurs only in asthmatics and is not an independent disorder. It is emphasized that EIA is but another manifestation of the bronchial hyperreactivity which is characteristic of asthma. Not all asthmatic patients develop EIA. Even in a given patient, the ability to provoke bronchoconstriction from exercise may vary widely from time to time. EIA tends to be more common in a younger patient, in whom it may be a very troublesome symptom. In our clinic, exercise was reported as a significant provoking factor by 97 percent of 63 asthmatic children and was the single most common provoking factor noticed by these children (Table 44–1). Older patients report this as less of a problem. However, they also tend to exercise less.

Because of its easy provocation under controlled conditions in the laboratory, EIA has been of considerable interest to investigators seeking a model of clinical asthma. Scientific investigation of this subject began with the remarkable pioneering observations by R.S. Jones and his colleagues in Liverpool (1962). These investigators showed EIA to be a normal feature of childhood (and young adult) asthma, related the pattern of EIA to clinical severity, and noted persistence of EIA in young adults who had "grown out" of childhood asthma. Other early studies described the diminution of response to further exercise after an attack of EIA, i.e., a refractory period. There also was considerable interest in the use of EIA as a model for studying the effects of drug therapy in asthma. In the past few years, the interest in EIA has been reawakened by some remarkable new observations on the effect of climate in which exercise is undertaken. Advances in biochemical techniques also have led to better data on the role of mast cell–derived mediators in the pathogenesis of EIA. Thus, some 300 years after Sir John first brought attention to this topic, we are still actively investigating why "all violent Exercise makes the Asthmatic to breathe short."

PULMONARY FUNCTION CHANGES IN EXERCISE-INDUCED ASTHMA

The response of the asthmatic child or adult to exercise is remarkably consistent and is illustrated in Figure 44–1. There is an initial mild bronchodilatation that often is maintained throughout the exercise period, although in more responsive subjects bronchoconstriction not uncommonly begins towards the end of the exercise period. After stopping exercise, bronchospasm takes over, and pulmonary functions reach their lowest levels after 3 to 5 minutes in children and 5 to 7 minutes in adults. All pulmonary function tests reflecting airway obstruction are similarly affected. We now prefer the forced expiratory volume in 1 second (FEV_1) because it is simple and more reproducible than the peak expiratory flow rate (PEFR). Correct timing of measurements is important since too long a delay after exercise in measuring the response can result in an underestimation of the severity of EIA. If measurements are made at 5 and 10 minutes after exercise, it is unlikely that important changes in pulmonary function will be missed. Also, if pulmonary function at 15 minutes differs little from that at 10 minutes, it is unlikely that further meaningful change will occur, and the test can be stopped.

During all or most of the exercise period that

TABLE 44–1. Incidence of Symptoms in 63 Asthmatic Children

Asthma Provoked By	Percent
Exercise	97
Allergy	73
Night time	71
Emotions	60
Weather change	59
Infection	56

precedes bronchoconstriction, there is generalized bronchodilatation. After exercise, when overt asthma develops, evidence is present of generalized airways obstruction with hyperinflation. Various attempts have been made to partition airways obstruction of EIA between large and small airways using helium and oxygen mixtures. These studies have shown considerable variation among individuals, with some apparently having larger airways obstruction and others having smaller airways obstruction (McFadden et al., 1977). Other studies have implied that there is widespread airway closure and, in addition, that some subjects increase their total lung capacity because of reduced elastic recoil pressure. Loss of elastic recoil would also contribute to the reduction of maximal expiratory flow at low lung volumes.

The usual pattern of lung function change in EIA closely resembles an immediate type of bronchial response to the inhalation of allergen. However, after antigen challenge there is often a secondary decrease of lung function after 4 to 6 hours. This late asthmatic reaction is probably of an inflammatory nature and more closely resembles persistent and clinically troublesome asthma than acute reactions provoked either by exercise or allergen. Evidence has begun to accumulate, as a result of work by Lee and coworkers (1983) and by Bierman and coworkers (1984) that suggests exercise, similar to allergens, might induce inflammatory changes in the airways. These investigators found that some asthmatics developed late bronchial responses to exercise and that these were accompanied by second (late) rises in the levels of circulating neutrophil chemotactic factor (NCF), similar to antigen-induced late phase responses. From lung function studies of the effect of breathing helium, they suggested that early responses to exercise were predominantly in the large airways (flow rates improved with helium), whereas late responses were predominantly in the small airways (no change with helium). Late responses to exercise are not seen in the majority of asthmatics, and the importance of this phenomenon has yet to be assessed.

The effect of exercise on arterial blood gas determinations in EIA is much as would be predicted from the changes in pulmonary function. During exercise, Pa_{O_2} and Pa_{CO_2} remain essentially normal, whereas pH falls owing to the accumulation of lactic acid. During an attack of EIA, there is moderate arterial hypoxemia and occasional hypercapnia. Despite early enthusiasm for their causation of EIA, changes in blood gas values or acid-base balance have not been shown to serve as the triggering factors of EIA.

QUANTITATION OF THE RESPONSE IN EXERCISE-INDUCED ASTHMA

Various indices have been proposed for quantitation of EIA, but for the sake of simplicity, those illustrated in Figure 44–2 are most widely accepted. EIA itself is measured by the percent fall in FEV_1 or ΔFEV_1, which is the percent decrease, postexercise, from the baseline, pre-exercise. Bronchodilatation during exercise can similarly be measured by the percent rise in FEV_1; total exercise-induced bronchial lability is the sum of these two indices. For practical purposes, the ΔFEV_1 is the only index needed to quantitate EIA. This type of index does pose some problems in comparisons of the relative severities of EIA, if pre-exercise baseline lung functions vary much between experi-

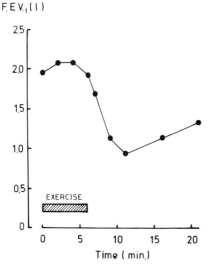

FIGURE 44–1. Typical pattern of lung function changes in response to 6 minutes of running by an asthmatic child.

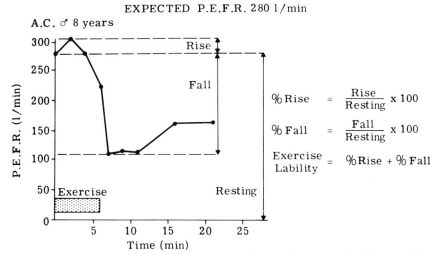

FIGURE 44–2. Method of calculation of indices commonly used to quantitate exercise-induced asthma. The percent fall (% Fall) is equivalent to the ΔFEV_1. (From Godfrey, S., et al.: J. Allerg. Clin. Immunol. *52*:199, 1973.)

ments. For this reason, it is important that baseline FEV_1 values be as close to each other as possible whenever comparative studies are made.

To date, little attention has been paid to the duration of the attack when quantitating EIA. In children, lung functions have usually returned to baseline levels by about 30 minutes after a standard of 6 minutes of exercise. In adults, normalization of lung functions generally takes somewhat longer. A problem, as yet unresolved in analyzing the severity of EIA, concerns whether a given absolute fall in lung function that takes a short time to recover indicates the same severity as the same absolute fall that takes a longer time to recover.

The response to exercise also has been assessed by performing short periods of progressively intense exercise separated by brief pauses for the measurement of lung function. From this type of test it is possible to construct a dose-response curve for EIA similar to that used to quantitate the response to methacholine or histamine inhalation. Unfortunately, this approach ignores the fact that EIA results in a refractory period, which is dependent upon the severity of the exercise, when the subject is less responsive to repeated exercise (Edmunds et al., 1978). This can profoundly affect the severity of EIA as illustrated in Figure 44–3, which shows the results we found when patients undertook a progressive type of test and also one

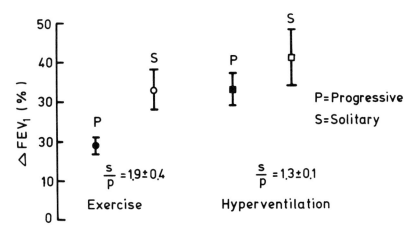

FIGURE 44–3. Severity of exercise-induced and hyperventilation-induced asthma, comparing the results from a steady state test with a corresponding single level test taken from a progressively increasing workload test. The severity of asthma was reduced in the progressive test when the challenge was exercise. There was little difference when the challenge was hyperventilation.

single level test of the same duration at an equivalent work level. Interestingly, this phenomenon was far less marked with isocapnic hyperventilation-induced asthma (HIA) undertaken by the same patients. Thus, results of progressive tests cannot be compared with results of steady state tests for EIA.

RANGE OF EXERCISE-INDUCED BRONCHIAL LABILITY

In normal subjects, exercise has little effect on lung functions. Using a simple test involving 6 minutes of running at about two thirds of maximum working capacity under ordinary room conditions, we found that the average rise in PEFR during exercise was about 3 to 4 percent, and the maximum fall after exercise was about 9 to 10 percent (Anderson et al., 1975). Burr and colleagues (1974) studied a group of 812 children aged 12 years who were not only healthy themselves but had no close relatives who were asthmatics. These workers found that 92 percent of the youngsters had postexercise falls in peak flow rates of less than 10 percent, and 98 percent had falls of less than 15 percent. This type of study has not been performed in an adult population, and results would be difficult to interpret because of such complicating factors as age, fitness, smoking habits, and other coincidental diseases.

The reported incidence of EIA in individuals and the reproducibility of tests of EIA are greatly influenced by the nature of the exercise tests and the conditions under which they are performed. These factors were unappreciated when studies of incidence and reproducibility originally were undertaken. In various studies, the incidence of EIA among unselected asthmatic children and adults has been reported to vary from 71 to 89 percent. It seems likely that all asthmatics will develop EIA if they exercise hard enough under appropriate conditions. However, many asthmatics, especially adults, never experience EIA because of little exercise participation. Also, it has become apparent that the severity of EIA varies from time to time in an individual patient. Consequently, the formulation of a standardized exercise test protocol has become more and more problematic.

In some patients with other pulmonary disorders, most notably cystic fibrosis, bronchial lability can be demonstrated in association with exercise due to marked bronchodilatation. Bronchoconstriction after exercise does not occur except in those with concomitant asthma. A similar pattern of moderately increased total bronchial lability with an improvement of lung function during exercise is sometimes found in the healthy relatives of asthmatic children or in those who had bronchiolitis in infancy. These patients or healthy subjects do not develop significant postexertional bronchospasms except when asthma coexists, and this type of bronchial lability should not be confused with EIA. Some patients with allergic rhinitis have been found to develop exercise-induced bronchospasm. However, careful inquiry of such an individual, concerning symptomatology, reveals the presence of at least mild asthma.

FACTORS THAT INFLUENCE THE SEVERITY OF EXERCISE-INDUCED ASTHMA

Since the time of Sir John Floyer it has been known to both asthmatics and their physicians that some kinds of exercise are more troublesome than others. For example, running causes more asthma than swimming, and free-range running causes more asthma than treadmill running, which in turn causes more than cycling. For a given type of asthmogenic exercise, such as running or cycling, the severity of the EIA depends upon the severity and duration of the exercise. Silverman and Anderson (1972) showed that the severity of EIA was greater with increasing work rate and with increasing duration of exercise up to certain plateau values, as illustrated in Figure 44–4 and Figure 44–5. Children exercised in random order for various times at constant treadmill settings and with various treadmill slopes for constant periods. The overall conclusion was that the maximum response was seen after 6 to 8 minutes of treadmill running at slopes of 10 to 15 percent. It was noted that patients who developed severe EIA after 6 to 8 minutes often had less severe EIA after more prolonged exercise— and patients often reported that they could "run through" their asthma. The severity of the exercise usually raised the heart rate to 170 to 180 beats/min in children (rather lower in adults), a level of work that corresponded to approximately 70 percent of the maximum oxygen uptake of all subjects. The treadmill test is particularly useful, since the work performed depends on body weight; hence, at a given setting, such as 3 mph (5 kmph), and a 10-percent slope, all subjects work at a similar relative

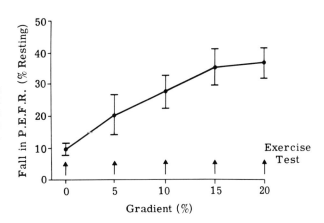

FIGURE 44–4. Effect of gradient (work rate) on asthma induced by treadmill running at a constant speed for 6 minutes. Each point represents the mean of tests in nine children who performed each gradient on a different occasion. (From Godfrey, S., et al.: J. Allerg. Clin. Immunol. *52*:199, 1973.)

level. Another study by Eggleston and Guerrant (1976) essentially confirmed these findings, and they recommended a test consisting of 5 minutes continuous treadmill exercise, adjusting slope and speed to produce a heart rate of 90 percent of the predicted maximal heart rate for the age and sex of the subject. In view of the plateau effects seen in Figure 44–4 and Figure 44–5, it probably is unnecessary to be overly exact about work rates and times provided they are near values producing the plateau effects.

Recommendations, previously mentioned, for exercise challenges apply to young healthy subjects. It is unwise to undertake such a test in anyone over 40 years of age or with any suspected ischemic heart disease, without appropriate precautions. Minimal requirements should include a full pre-exercise electrocardiogram (ECG) and continuous ECG monitoring during exercise. On the one hand, we have never encountered a dangerous asthmatic response to exercise for which the patient has required resuscitation. On the other hand, a patient can develop severe EIA and, in such a case, the test should be terminated immediately by the administration of a selective beta-2 stimulant via a nebulizer, preferably oxygen driven. This equipment should be available and ready for use whenever exercise tests are performed.

The asthmatic patient often is unable to participate in continuous exercise lasting a few minutes yet is capable of playing games such as tennis or football. In most games, the exercise actually is brief and intermittent. These short bursts of exercise may not activate the mechanism that results in bronchospasm. In addition, it has been shown that brief warming-up sprints can markedly diminish EIA, resulting from a subsequent and more prolonged period of exercise. This inactivation of the asthma-provoking mechanism also may be responsible for the lack of EIA while participating in some sports and may account for the well-recognized phenomenon of the refractory period that follows EIA. The response to a second exercise challenge is diminished following an attack of EIA and may be almost completely abolished by repeating the exercise (Fig. 44–6). This refractoriness wears off quite quickly, however, with a half-life of refractoriness of about 1 hour.

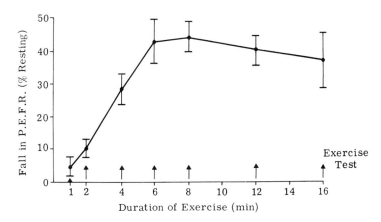

FIGURE 44–5. Effect of duration rate on asthma induced by treadmill running at a constant speed and gradient. Each point represents the mean of tests in ten children who performed each exercise test on a different occasion. (From Godfrey, S., et al.: J. Allerg. Clin. Immunol. *52*:199, 1973.)

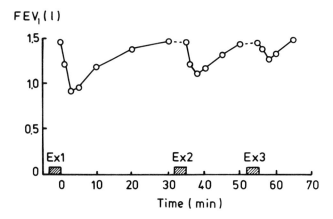

FEV₁ (l)

FIGURE 44–6. Refractoriness to exercise-induced asthma demonstrated by a decreasing amount of asthma following each of a series of equally severe exercise tests. (From Godfrey, S. *In* Asthma, Clark, T.J.H., Godfrey, S., (eds.), London, Chapman and Hall Medical, 1983.)

Although easy to perform, running up and down stairs or up and down a hill is a form of intermittent exercise and is not recommended as a test for EIA.

Environmental conditions under which exercise is performed also have profound influence on the induction of EIA. Contrary to the previously held opinion that a dry climate was good for asthma patients, a number of investigators showed that EIA was markedly diminished if the climate and, therefore, the air breathed was warm and humid. This finding led Deal and colleagues (1979) to develop what has been termed the "respiratory heat loss hypothesis" for EIA. These investigators conceived the idea that the effect of humidity was in reality due to the prevention of cooling of the airways; they showed that breathing cold or dry air enhanced EIA and that hyperventilation with chilled, dry air could evoke asthma even without exercise (hyperventilation-induced asthma or HIA). The considerable influence of ambient temperature and, even more so, humidity could account for some of the variations in asthmogenic properties found in earlier studies of EIA, e.g., swimming in comparison with running, as well as the variations among different studies using similar types of exercise. This influence makes it imperative that environmental factors be standardized in all studies of EIA.

As indicated previously, the severity of EIA varies widely in the same patient at different times, and it is likely that this is due to variations in basic airway hyperreactivity. Reactivity to histamine is considerably increased following antigen challenge, and air pollution and exercise may interact to potentiate asthma. Recently, we found a considerable increase in the severity of EIA during the week following an antigen challenge (Mussaffi et al., 1986). Thus, the response of a patient to exercise may depend in part upon the prevailing levels of antigenic stimulation or other respiratory irritant that can vary markedly from time to time.

VALUE OF EXERCISE CHALLENGE IN ASTHMA

A 6-minute run in a child or young adult is simple to perform, requires minimal equipment, and confirms the diagnosis of asthma if EIA is produced. However, this is an inconsistent and highly imperfect method for detecting asthma, reasons for which have been discussed, and a lack of response does not rule out the existence of asthma. Also, the severity of EIA does not appear to accurately reflect the overall severity of asthma, and, therefore, the response to exercise is not a useful guide to the need for treatment. For practical purposes, a bronchial provocation test with methacholine or histamine is more likely to provide a method for establishing the diagnosis and possibly the severity of asthma (see Chapter 17). Exercise testing is worthwhile when EIA appears to be the major clinical problem and it is important that this be documented, for example, in athletes or in military recruits in whom it is essential to ascertain that exercise associated with their activities is not likely to put them at undue risk. Provocation of asthma by exercise also provides a natural stimulus and response and is a valuable tool for research studies aimed at investigating the basic mechanisms of the disease. As previously noted, exercise testing is not recommended for anyone with cardiac or other health problems. When performed, precautions including ECG monitoring if appropriate should be taken for any untoward cardiopulmonary problems that may result.

EFFECT OF DRUGS ON EXERCISE-INDUCED ASTHMA

Various antiasthmatic medications can partially or completely prevent or reverse EIA. Because initiation of EIA performed with appropriate safeguards is a safe and simple diagnostic and investigative tool, it frequently has been used as a model for testing the effectiveness of various drugs used in the treatment of asthma. Controlled studies have shown that EIA can be inhibited by the prior administration of sympathomimetic agents but generally not by steroids. The effectiveness of theophylline derivatives and atropine is less impressive than that of sympathomimetic agents. Antihistamines have little or no value in EIA. An important theoretic advance was made when it was shown that cromolyn sodium also could prevent EIA, since this drug is believed to act primarily by preventing the release of mediators from mast cells and lacks a bronchodilator effect. Silverman and Andrea (1972) showed that cromolyn sodium prevented EIA only if given before exercise and not if given at the end of exercise but prior to the development of bronchospasm. This finding implied that EIA is due, at least in part, to the liberation of meditors during exercise.

The response of EIA to common antiasthmatic medications is shown in Figure 44–7, which was derived from a study in which each agent was administered to a group of asthmatic children. Because several of the agents used were bronchodilators, results are expressed on an absolute scale of PEFR to show the postdrug bronchodilatation, further exercise-induced bronchodilatation, and exercise-induced bronchoconstriction. It can be seen that the interpretation of the relative efficacy of the various agents becomes a problem if postdrug, pre-exercise bronchodilatation occurs. Absolute postexercise PEFR after atropine and theophylline was better than after placebo and near predrug, pre-exercise values. Nevertheless, exercise caused a deterioration in lung function from the postdrug, pre-exercise values. The problem of judging a response when the baseline lung function is altered is probably responsible for much of the lack of agreement concerning the efficacy of atropine and theophylline and their derivatives in EIA. Cromolyn sodium does not change baseline lung function and inhibits EIA to a considerable degree, whereas salbutamol (albuterol), although a bronchodilator, so completely abolishes any postexercise change that there is no doubt as to its efficacy.

The question of the effect of steroids on EIA has been asked again recently after it was long believed that steroids did not influence acute responses, following either exercise or antigen stimulation. Regular treatment of asthma with an inhaled steroid has been shown to diminish or abolish EIA, but interpretation of this effect is complicated by the coincident improvement in baseline lung function. It is not clear, therefore, that steroids can influence the immediate response to exercise in the absence of change in basal airway caliber. The only other agent that has been shown consistently to prevent EIA is a calcium channel blocker, nifedipine; it is believed to act in a manner similar to that of cro-

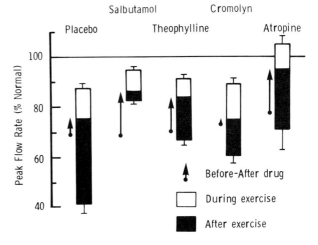

FIGURE 44–7. The effect of various drugs on exercise-induced asthma. The results are expressed as percentage of the expected normal peak expiratory flow rate for each subject. The arrows indicate the response to the drug at rest before the start of exercise. The bars indicates ±SEM. (From Anderson, S.D., et al.: Br. J. Dis. Chest 61:1, 1975.)

molyn by preventing the calcium-dependent liberation of mediators from mast cells.

In practice, the simplest way to protect a patient against EIA is to give either an inhaled selective beta-2 sympathomimetic agent or cromolyn sodium. Both drugs work if given immediately before exercise by inhalation. Sympathomimetic agents are more potent with longer durations of effectiveness, but proper inhalation technique is important for this effect. The powder inhaler type of device through which cromolyn sodium can be given is rather easier to master. The time until protection falls to about 50 percent of initial protection is about 4 to 5 hours for albuterol and 1 to 2 hours for cromolyn sodium. Oral sympathomimetic agents are less effective. In my opinion, there is little reason to use theophylline for the sole purpose of inhibiting EIA for it appears to be relatively inefficient in doing so, and superior EIA blocking drugs are available. Before testing for EIA it is necessary to omit all medications, except perhaps steroids, for 8 hours. Long-acting theophylline preparations should be discontinued at least 24 hours prior to testing. This factor means that exercise testing simply may not be possible in many chronic perennial asthmatics who cannot omit ongoing therapy without serious risks.

PATHOGENESIS OF EXERCISE-INDUCED ASTHMA

Understanding of the pathways underlying exercise- and hyperventilation-induced asthma has increased greatly in recent years. Nevertheless, a great deal of controversy over the mechanisms of EIA remains (Godfrey, 1975). Although it was generally accepted for a long time that exercise itself triggered EIA in some undefined manner, the influence of the type of exercise and the lack of asthma after swimming appeared to contradict this notion. The recognition of the importance of temperature and humidity of inspired air to the occurrence of EIA led to the respiratory heat loss (RHL) hypothesis, which proposed that cooling of the airways served as the trigger for EIA and HIA. This hypothesis provides an attractive unifying concept that could explain differences in EIA and HIA under varying environmental conditions. However, a number of observations cast some doubt on its validity. According to the RHL hypothesis, asthma should not occur following exercise in which there is no respiratory heat loss, i.e., exercise during which the subject breathes air warmed and humidified to body conditions. Whereas EIA generally is abolished or markedly diminished under such conditions, a small number of individuals develop marked EIA and a large number develop some degree of EIA when breathing warmed and humidified air. Experiments by Anderson and her colleagues (1983) showed that inhalations of hypotonic or hypertonic saline solutions could provoke asthma similar to EIA or HIA. This finding led to the suggestion that the trigger of EIA and HIA, rather than respiratory heat loss, is airway water loss with consequent osmotic change. In fact, it is difficult to separate completely the effects of temperature from those of humidity; in any case, the water loss hypothesis suffers from deficiencies similar to those of the heat loss hypothesis, since asthma can be induced in some subjects breathing warm humid air when neither heat nor water loss occurs. Thus, a study by Eschenbacher and Sheppard (1985) concluded that neither the RHC nor the RWC hypotheses could account entirely for the triggering of EIA.

There also is doubt whether the mechanism for EIA and HIA is the same. Bar-Yishay and colleagues, (1983), studying the refractory period after HIA, found that hyperventilation when breathing warm humid air neither induced asthma nor refractoriness to a subsequent hyperventilation challenge when breathing cold dry air. In a previous study of EIA, Ben-Dov and associates. (1982) had shown that the majority of subjects became refractory to a subsequent exercise challenge in cold dry air after an initial exercise test in warm humidified air, which did not itself provoke EIA. These results suggest that exercise per se and not respiratory heat (or water) loss is important in the development of refractoriness to EIA, but in the case of HIA climatic conditions assume critical importance. This led us to suggest that the trigger site for HIA might lie in the larger, more central airways in which temperature changed markedly during hyperventilation or exercise and that the trigger site for EIA lies more deeply in the lung tissue where temperature changes are less (McFadden et al., 1985). Support for different trigger sites came from a study in which it was shown that cromolyn sodium was more effective in preventing EIA, if baseline lung function was good, but more effective in preventing HIA, if baseline lung function was poor (Ben-Dov et al., 1984).

Neutrophil chemotactic activity (NCA) studies also provide evidence that EIA and HIA are different, since NCA is released by EIA (Lee et al., 1982) but not by HIA (Deal et al., 1980).

The manner by which the stimulus of EIA or HIA is transferred to the effector site is still being investigated. One obvious possibility is that EIA is simply the result of a neural reflex mediated via the vagus nerve, and the stimulus is cooling or drying of the airways leading to cholinergic-mediated bronchospasm. Evidence for vagal involvement in EIA based on the inhibition of EIA by atropine or other anticholinergic agents is conflicting. A strong argument against the idea that EIA is due to a neural reflex is to be deduced from the time course of changes in lung function and airway cooling in response to exercise. The temperature falls soon after the exercise starts and returns to baseline soon after the exercise ends, whereas lung function falls only when exercise ends and returns to baseline after about 30 minutes. The lag between temperature change and asthma is far too long to be explained by simple neural reflex action.

Alternatively, exercise may stimulate release of chemical mediators, which in turn act directly or through neural reflex on bronchial smooth muscle to provoke asthma. This hypothesis was based originally on circumstantial evidence related to the existence of a refractory period after EIA and to the effect of cromolyn sodium in prevention of EIA. Some subjects also become refractory to antigen challenges after repeated exercise, which has made them refractory to EIA (Weiler-Ravell and Godfrey, 1981). More recently, direct support for the mediator hypothesis has come from the work of Lee and colleagues (1982). They showed that the mast cell mediator, neutrophil chemotactic factor, is liberated into the circulation of patients who develop EIA. This mediator release correlates with the fall in pulmonary function, and both phenomena can be prevented by pretreatment with cromolyn. Because of the nonuniform response of patients to various challenges, it is possible that there may be some diversity in intermediary pathways, which can be involved in EIA. Specifically, not all patients can be made refractory to EIA or HIA; exercise while breathing warm humidified air does not render all patients refractory to subsequent challenges while breathing cold dry air. Only half of the subjects tested could be made refractory to antigen challenge after repeated exercise.

These observations suggest a model of EIA in which a combination of exercise intensity, duration, and environmental conditions acts as the trigger that releases mediators from mast cells. The increased sympathetic drive during exercise largely prevents bronchospasm so long as exercise continues. If exercise is sufficiently prolonged, the continued sympathetic discharge may allow time for the liberated mediator to be metabolized so that EIA does not occur. The process of mediator release may be somewhat analogous to that induced by allergen with mast cell mediators acting on bronchial smooth muscle to produce the immediate episode of EIA and, in some instances, also invoking a late asthmatic response. The severity of EIA may depend on the amount of mediator remaining from the balance between the quantity liberated and that destroyed by metabolism. However, the actual severity of asthma induced also undoubtedly depends upon the intrinsic reactivity of the airways, which in turn is influenced by antigenic stimulation and other environmental factors. It is apparent, therefore, that the interaction of several factors important in the response to exercise makes it impossible to predict the severity of EIA in an individual test. We have learned a great deal about EIA since the time of Sir John Floyer, and clearly there is still much more to learn.

REFERENCES

Anderson, S.D., Schoeffel, R.E., Finney, M.: Evaluation of ultrasonically nebulised solutions for provocation testing in patients with asthma. Thorax 38:284–291, 1983.
Anderson, S.D., Silverman, M., Konig, P., Godfrey, S.: Exercise-induced asthma. Brit. J. Dis. Chest 69:1–39, 1975.
Bar-Yishay, E., Ben-Dov, I., Godfrey, S.: Refractory period following hyperventilation-induced asthma. Am. Rev. Resp. Dis. 127:572–574, 1983.
Ben-Dov, I., Bar-Yishay, E., Godfrey, S.: Refractory period following exercise-induced asthma unexplained by respiratory heat loss. Am. Rev. Resp. Dis. 125:530–534, 1982.
Ben-Dov, I., Bar-Yishay, E., Godfrey, S.: Relation between efficacy of sodium cromoglycate and baseline lung function in exercise and hyperventilation-induced asthma. Isr. J. Med. Sci. 20:130–135, 1984.
Bierman, C.W., Spiro, S.G., Petheram, I.: Characteristics of the late response in exercise-induced asthma. J. Allergy Clin. Immunol. 74:701–706, 1984.
Burr, M.L., Eldridge, B.A., Borysiewicz, L.K.: Peak expiratory flow rates before and after exercise in school children. Arch. Dis. Child. 49:923–926, 1974.
Deal, E.C., McFadden, E.R., Ingram, R.H., Strauss, R.H., Jaeger, J.J.: Role of respiratory heat exchange in production of exercise-induced asthma. J. Appl. Physiol. 46:467–475, 1979.
Deal, E.C., Wasserman, S.I., Sother, N.A., Ingram, R.A.,

McFadden, E.R.: Evaluation of the role played by mediators of immediate sensitivity in exercise-induced asthma. J. Clin. Invest. 65:659–665, 1980.

Edmunds, A.T., Tooley, M., Godfrey, S.: The refractory period after exercise-induced asthma, its duration and relation to severity of exercise. Am. Rev. Resp. Dis. 117:247–254, 1978.

Eggleston, P.A., Guerrant, J.L.: A standardised method of evaluating exercise-induced asthma. J. Allergy Clin. Immunol. 58:414–425, 1976.

Eschenbacher, W.L., Sheppard, D.: Respiratory heat loss is not the sole stimulus for bronchoconstriction induced by isocapnic hyperpnea with dry air. Am. Rev. Resp. Dis. 131:894–901, 1985.

Godfrey, S.: Controversies in the pathogenesis of exercise-induced asthma. Eur. J. Resp. Dis. 68:81–88, 1986

Jones, R.S., Buston, M.H., Wharton, M.J.: The effect of exercise on ventilatory function in the child with asthma. Brit. J. Dis. Chest 56:78–86, 1962.

Lee, T.H., Nagy, L., Nakagura, T., Walport, M.J., Kay A.B.: Identification and partial characterisation of an exercise-induced neutrophil chemotactic factor in bronchial asthma. J. Clin. Invest. 69:889–899, 1982.

Lee, T.H., Toshikazu, N., Papageorgiov, N., Ikura, Y., Kay, A.B.: Exercise-induced late asthmatic reactions with neutrophil chemotactic activity. N. Engl. J. Med. 308:1502–1505, 1983.

McFadden, E.R., Ingram, R.H., Haynes, R.L., Wellman, J.J.: Predominant site of flow limitation and mechanisms of postexertional asthma. J. Appl. Physiol. 42:746–752, 1977.

McFadden, E.R., Pichurko, B.M., Bowman, H.F., Ingenito, E., Burns, S., Dowling, N., Solway, J.: Thermal mapping of the airways in humans. J. Appl. Physiol. 58:564–570, 1985.

Mussaffi, H., Springer, C., Godfrey, S.: Increased bronchial responsiveness to exercise and histamine after allergen challenge in asthmatic children. J. Allergy Clin. Immunol. 77:48–52, 1986.

Silverman, M, Anderson, S.D.: Standardisation of exercise tests in asthmatic children. Arch. Dis. Childh. 47:882–889, 1972.

Silverman, M., Andrea, T.: Time course of effect of disodium cromoglycate on exercise-induced asthma. Arch. Dis. Childh. 47:419–422, 1972.

Weiler-Ravell, D., Godfrey, S.: Do exercise and antigen-induced asthma utilize the same pathways? Antigen provocation in patients rendered refractory to exercise induced asthma. J. Allergy Clin. Immunol. 67:391–397, 1981.

45

Asthma and Institutional Care

HYMAN CHAI, M.D.

It is estimated that between 5 and 10 percent of the population of the United States have asthma. Whatever the exact prevalence, it is clear that there are millions of children and adults who suffer from asthma. Units specializing in asthma and other allergic diseases deal with a selected population of asthmatics. Patients treated in these specialized institutions constitute a subpopulation of patients whose asthma, or problems associated with asthma, has gone beyond the ability of their physicians to cope with the problem. Well-trained allergists are capable of treating most asthmatics equally as well as specialized institutions devoted to care of asthmatics. Nevertheless, some patients in whom the severity of the disease and multiplicity of contributing clinical factors involved, as well as the very serious and debilitating accompanying psychosocial problems, dictate the need for both medical and psychologic care on a more or less round-the-clock daily basis. It is this group of individuals for whom admission to an institution that deals specifically with asthma is most appropriate.

WHAT DO SPECIAL ASTHMA CENTERS HAVE TO OFFER?

Although specialized investigations of severely asthmatic children and adults can be achieved on an outpatient basis, some require highly specialized tests that must be repeated at a high frequency and can be managed only with extreme difficulty over time in a physician's office. Some examples of these include the use of frequent pulmonary function tests (such as spirometry); for instance, such tests three times a day, 7 days a week, for prolonged periods in order to determine a pattern of the patient's asthma and evaluate the success of a therapeutic program may be needed. In addition, the availability in "one house" of special facilities and staff with expertise to analyze the pulmonary aspects of asthma thoroughly and to perform numerous other pertinent analytic tests is an important advantage, since some patients are found to have other medical or even psychologic disorders rather than asthma. Inhalation challenge, exercise testing, and radiographic, immunologic, pharmacologic, and psychiatric expertise for diagnosing and treating asthma or problems associated with it are included. This multidisciplinary expertise is of potential critical value in analyzing a patient's problem and in constructing a maximal therapeutic program. It often is possible to make observations on precipitating or aggravating factors, compliance, psychosocial behavior, and therapeutic effects of programs outlined on an inpatient, close, round-the-clock setting crucial for successful treatment of asthma, which cannot be made even in a closely supervised outpatient setting. Psychologic, social, and educational services, important to a rehabilitative program, also are available, permitting the kind of coordinated effort necessary for successful therapy; these services are often impossible to bring together through an office-based approach. The ability to have all personnel and facilities on hand to cope with severe asthma while diagnostic investigations and therapeutic programs are undertaken also is an important if not crucial advantage.

Some Comments on Psychologic Aspects of Asthma and its Therapy as They Relate to Special Asthma Centers

Chronic disease that interferes with breathing is a frightening experience for asthmatic adults and children and for their families. Psychologic consequences of chronic severe asthma can be totally disabling for a patient and for an entire family, especially with regard to the implications from the fear of death from the disease. Moreover, the socioeconomic impact of uncontrolled asthma on the individual, family, and sometimes community can be enormous. The availability of psychologists, psychiatrists, social workers, physical therapists, and others who understand the disease as well as nursing staff equally able to care for those patients with the problem is a phenomenon virtually unique to asthma institutions. This ability is an essential ingredient for restoring normality following the immense psychologic harm that affects asthmatic patients and their families, which can be just as disabling as the disease itself. For successful long-term outcome of any asthma therapy, it cannot be overemphasized that the patient and everyone involved with the patient must be educated. All should understand what problems the asthmatic patient may face and how the disease can be handled once the patient returns home. Above all else, the patient and family need to be given realistic hope that the disease can be controlled and managed. For many patients with severe asthma and for their families, intense and prolonged psychosocial support and education on how to cope with the disease and its manifestations may be necessary.

INDICATIONS FOR ADMISSION TO A SPECIAL ASTHMA CARE FACILITY

Frequency and Severity of Asthmatic Episodes

If the asthma is perennial, the attacks are severe, the emergency visits to a physician's office or hospital emergency room are frequent despite the use of the best available outpatient management, institutionalization for intensive investigation of causes and for management of the disease should be considered. Although a lack of control of asthma may be due to a lack of compliance with an otherwise adequate program of therapy, this in itself may be an indication for admission to a special facility (see subsequent discussions).

Psychosocial Problems

Psychosocial problems related to asthma are not easily managed by office-based practitioners or by psychiatrists and psychologists who are inexperienced in dealing with the disease itself. These problems may have many causes as follows: (1) the severity of the asthma itself; (2) family breakdown (often because of the stress of dealing with a family member with severe asthma); (3) strained family financial resources; (4) single parent families, with the attendant problems of coping with an asthmatic

family member's management while attempting to work; and (5) a home environment that is not suited to management of a family member with such a chronic disease. The need for psychologic intervention is essential and may require a high degree of continuing psychologic intervention and social involvement with their peers over time.

Compliance

The asthmatic patient has to be taught repeatedly to comply with directions for prescribed therapy as scheduled for control of his or her disease. Often this is a long-term commitment, which requires endless repetition. In severely asthmatic patients, in whom lack of compliance is a major factor interfering with control of the disease, reasons for noncompliance must be determined in order to address them. Education to improve compliance may be achieved in such institutions when it cannot be achieved on an outpatient basis.

The High Risk Asthmatic Patient

Certain clinical and psychologic aspects of asthma place some patients at risk of death. Recognition of these factors is crucial both to identify such patients and to manage them appropriately. Such factors identified in asthmatic children are noted in Table 45–1. Identification of pertinent factors and education of patients and their families to understand and manage the disease themselves are of primary importance. These include recognition and management of important "warning factors" of disease severity that need to be handled expeditiously not only to reduce morbidity from the disease, but also to minimize the risk of death.

Education and Rest for the Family

A family unit can be destroyed by the emotional and financial strain of a patient with chronic asthma, particularly a patient who has repeated severe attacks. An inpatient unit provides temporary alleviation of the extreme psychologic tensions associated with the daily concern and care for a patient with severe asthma. It allows some restoration of physical and socioeconomic stability for the family and can be invaluable to the rehabilitation of the patient.

TABLE 45–1. High Risk Factors of Asthmatic Children Hospitalized at The National Jewish Center for Immunology and Respiratory Medicine*

Seizures with asthma
Poor self care
Denial of wheezing
Depression
Parent and staff conflict
Prednisone reduction of greater than 50 percent of the initial dose
Increased wheezing the week prior to discharge

Associated Factors

Emotional disturbance
History of emotional, behavioral, and physical reactions to separation or loss
Manipulative use of asthma within the family
Family dysfunction
Patient and staff conflict
Patient and parent conflict
Use of inhaled beclomethasone at hospital discharge

* Adapted from Strunk, R. C. et al.: Physiologic and psychological characteristics associated with deaths due to asthma in childhood. A case controlled study. J.A.M.A. 254:1193–1198, 1985. Copyright 1985. American Medical Association.

The first goal of hospitalization (in some patients) may be to create a family environment that is conducive to education and compliance with recommended therapy.

SPECIAL CONSIDERATIONS CONCERNING "LONG-TERM" HOSPITALIZATION

In the mid-1950's and the early 1960's, long-term asthma care facilities assumed the role of removing the asthmatic child from the home surroundings that were considered by some allergists at the time to be major problems contributing to the continuation of chronic asthma. This concept was called "parentectomy." The degree of devotion to this aspect of therapy in those days can be well demonstrated by the numerous pages of notes devoted to the psychologic work-ups and interviews compared with the few notes devoted to the medical aspects of the diseases. It is highly probable, in my view, that at least one aspect of parentectomy achieved the goals for which children were referred at the time for long-term institutionalization but for other reasons. Children stayed away from the home for at least 2 years. Therefore, they were under a round-the-clock medical and nursing umbrella for 7 days a week, and asthma could be handled quickly;

moreover, daily treatment tended to be more structured and consistent than at home. (Indeed, in many children from disadvantaged homes, simply having medicine to take regularly was a change, as was being in a new environment in which the distractions of a poor psychosocial setting no longer interfered with therapy.) In addition, the family had 2 years of peace and rest from the management of the child, without having to face the problems of constant asthma and repeated emergency room visits. In all, the continuous availability of immediate help for 2 years, while the child attended school, was associated with a decrease of asthma either because of the different physical environment or because of the provision of maximum psychologic and medical care. Time to mature in a setting of maximized psychologic and medical care and highly structured education in regard to the disease and its medical management led to significant immediate and long-term benefit for many of these children.

Long-term institutionalization tends to be much shorter now (weeks to months) because of the availability of therapeutic equipment for home care, effective drugs for home care, and better education of physicians for care of asthma. In addition, economic constraints, in large part from third party payers, have diminished the length of hospitalization financially feasible for many patients. Nevertheless, the goals of therapy for many asthmatics are similar to those of this previous era. Whether these goals can be achieved without more prolonged institutionalization than currently is available remains to be seen.

REFERENCES

Creer, T.L.: Asthma Therapy: A Behavioral Health Care System for Respiratory Disorders. New York, Springer Publishing Co., 1979.

Creer, T.L., Chritin, W.P.: Chronically Ill and Handicapped Children. Champaign, Illinois, Research Press Co., 1976.

Creer, T.L., Kotses, H.: Long Term Management and Prevention of Asthma: Assessment of Ability and Goal Setting. In Allergy: Principles and Practice, vol. II. Ellis, E.F., Middleton, E., Reed, C. (eds.), St. Louis, C.V. Mosby Co., 1983.

Dirks, J.F., Kinsman, R.A., Horton, D.J., Fross, K.H., Jones, N.F.: Panic-fear in asthma: Rehospitalization following intensive long-term treatment. Psychosom. Med. 40:5, 1978.

Dirks, J.H., Schraa, J., Brown, E.L., Kinsman, R.A.: Psychomaintenance in asthma: Hospitalization rates and financial impact. Brit. J. Med. Psychol. 53:349, 1980.

Ellis, E.F., Middleton, E.: Asthma in Children. In Current

Therapy in Allergy and Immunology, 1983–1984. Lichtenstein, L.M., Fancl, A., (eds.), St. Louis, C.V. Mosby Co., 1984

Godfrey, S.: Childhood Asthma. In Asthma, 2nd ed., Clark, T.J.H., Godfrey, S. (eds.), London, Chapman and Hall, 1983.

Holroyd, K.A., Creer, T.L.: Self Management of Chronic Disease. Orlando, Florida, Academic Press, Inc., 1986.

Klieger, J.H., Kirks, J.F.: Medication compliance in chronic asthmatic patients. J. Asthma Res. 16:93, 1979.

Staudenmayer, H., Kinsman, R.A., Jones, N.F.: Attitudes toward respiratory symptomatology and treatment response. J. Ner. Ment. Dis. 41:109, 1979.

46

Occupational Asthma

H. WILLIAM BARKMAN JR., M.D.
JOHN E. SALVAGGIO, M.D.

Occupational asthma is one of the oldest of the environmentally induced lung diseases. In 1700, Bernardino Ramazzini, who has been called the father of occupational medicine, enumerated the diseases of tradesmen in his treatise, *De Morbis Artificum*. His characterization of the respiratory health effects of exposure to grain dust is one of the earliest descriptions of occupational asthma. Since then over 200 compounds, both natural and synthetic, have been implicated in causing occupational asthma. Currently, some of these compounds are not restricted to occupational settings, and individuals may develop effects of exposure to these compounds while involved with hobbies. This chapter is intended to be an overview of the diagnosis and management of occupational asthma.

DEFINITION OF OCCUPATIONAL ASTHMA

The commonly accepted definition of asthma is a disease manifested by recurrent reversible airflow obstruction. Unfortunately, the definition of occupational asthma is much less precise. Some investigators would suggest that the definition be restricted to airflow obstruction induced by only those compounds that can clearly be shown to be sensitizers, while others would expand the definition to include all causes of reversible airflow obstruction found in a working environment. For the purpose of discussion, an individual can be diagnosed as having occupational asthma if the following criteria are met: (1) respiratory symptoms and recurrent reversible airflow obstruction can be documented objectively; (2) a temporal relationship exists between the occupational exposure and the occurrence of respiratory symptoms, and a reversible reduction of lung function can be measured objectively across the working shift or in a laboratory setting; and (3) no other plausible explanation exists for the reversible airflow obstruction.

Currently, there are no accurate statistics on the overall prevalence or incidence of occupational asthma. Due to the great variability of the compounds, of the industrial processes, and of the working conditions, there are wide ranges of prevalence rates ascribed to working with different compounds. For instance, the prevalence of asthma among workers exposed to proteolytic enzymes may vary from 10 to 45 percent (Murphy, 1976; Brooks, 1977), whereas workers exposed to volatile isocyanates or western red cedar dust appear to have a prevalence rate of approximately 5 percent (Chan-Yeung et al., 1978; Diem et al., 1982). "Occupational asthma" also may occur occasionally in adults and children who live close to an industrial source of an inhalant allergen or irritant. This has been demonstrated, for instance, in castor bean processing, pharmaceutic manufacturing, and grain loading.

PATHOPHYSIOLOGY

Occupational asthma is manifested in three different patterns of reaction as follows: immediate, late, and dual. Immediate reactions appear within an hour and generally improve within 2 hours. The onset of late reactions is between 2 and 12 hours after exposure. Many investigators have suggested that the late reaction is more common in occupational asthma; however, the significance of that observation remains to be determined (Chan-Yeung et al., 1982; Cockcroft, 1983; Maestrelli et al., 1983).

Pathogenetic mechanisms proposed to induce bronchoconstriction include those that are reflex-irritant mediated, pharmacologic, and allergic. Table 46–1 lists the most well-recognized families of agents causing occupational asthma by proposed mechanism. Detailed lists of agents are published elsewhere (Chan-Yeung et al., 1986; Brooks, 1983; Bernstein, 1981).

Cold air is a good example of a physical stimulant that can lead to bronchoconstriction in an occupational as well as an environmental setting. The reflex bronchoconstriction resulting

TABLE 46–1. Causes of Occupational Asthma by Mechanism

Mechanisms	Industries or Workers
Reflex-irritant	
Cold air	Meat processing
	Laboratory workers
Talc	Pharmaceutical
Irritant gases	
Ammonia	Chemical
Chlorine	Chemical
Sulfur dioxide	Chemical
Pharmacologic	
Cotton dust	Textile
Isocyanates	Polyurethane foam
Organophosphates	Pesticide workers
Allergic	
Animal proteins	Farmers
	Animal handlers
Plant proteins	
Flour	Millers, bakers
Coffee	Food
Wood	Lumber
Enzymes	
Papain	Food
Subtilisn	Detergent
Trypsin	Pharmaceutical
Metals	
Nickel	Metal plating
Platinum	Metal refining
Drugs	
Cephalosporins	Pharmaceutical
Phenylglycine acid chloride	Pharmaceutical
Ampicillin	Pharmaceutical
Tetracycline	Pharmaceutical
Anhydrides	
Trimellitic anhydride	Plastics
Isocyanates	
Toluene diisocyanate	Polyurethane foam
Methylene-diphenyl diisocyanate	Polyurethane foam
Hexylmethylene diisocyanate	Paint

from cold air exposure is thought to be secondary to a direct effect on irritant receptors in the submucosa of the bronchial wall (Horton and Chen, 1979; Frank et al., 1972; Brooks et al., 1972; Widdicombe et al., 1962).

Inflammatory bronchoconstriction also is usually a result of exposure to respiratory irritants. Respiratory irritants represent a diverse group of exogenous gases and vapors, which produce a nonspecific inflammatory reaction of the bronchial membranes. The extent and severity of the injury largely depend on the material's physical classification, concentration, and water solubility, and the individual's susceptibility. The concentration of the irritant largely determines the severity of the acute injury. Water solubility in conjunction with the dose of irritant inhaled determines the site of injury. Extremely water soluble gases (e.g., ammonia) tend to cause more upper airway injury in contrast to insoluble gases (e.g., nitrogen oxide), which tend to cause alveolar injury. Brooks and Lockey (1981) have suggested a new term, reactive airways disease syndrome (RADS), to describe the asthma-like syndrome that develops in patients secondary to irritant exposure. The pathogenesis of RADS is unknown, and its significance is undetermined. Overall, the inflammatory mechanism probably represents one of the most common forms of airway injury. However, it is unclear how often these injuries lead to development of asthma or its long-term outcome.

Pharmacologic bronchoconstriction refers to asthma caused by modulation of mediators. In the case of isocyanates, the cyclic adenosine monophosphate response is impaired and may play a pathogenetic role in some cases (Butcher and Salvaggio, 1986). Organophosphates inhibit acetylcholine, which potentially can result in bronchoconstriction (Weiner, 1961).

As seen in Table 46–1, a great number of occupational agents are suspected of having allergenic properties. In the case of high molecular weight organic compounds (e.g., animal danders, wood dusts, coffee and castor bean products, insect materials, and enzymes, such as papain), an IgE-mediated mechanism usually is implicated, as based on positive skin test reactions and elevated specific IgE levels. In addition, atopic individuals appear to be more susceptible to this form of asthma. Asthma secondary to an exposure to a proteolytic enzyme, from *Bacillus subtilis*, is an example of IgE-mediated occupational asthma. Newhouse and colleagues (1969) showed a clear relationship between sensitization and level of exposure to the allergen; all who developed asthma had immediate positive skin test reactions and the presence of specific IgE antibodies to the enzyme.

Low molecular weight compounds are the fastest growing group of compounds associated with occupational asthma; isocyanate, western red cedar (plicatic acid), and trimellitic anhydride are all excellent examples. In many cases, the pathogenesis is not clearly established or may be multifactorial; however, there is evidence (usually elevated specific IgE antibody levels) that suggests an allergic mechanism. In the case of late asthmatic reactions, observations are available to support involvement of IgE and IgG antibody and participation of chronic inflammatory cells, particularly eosinophils, attracted to the airways and lungs by chemotactic mediators released during the immediate (early) reaction.

The most commonly used isocyanates include toluene diisocyanate (TDI), methylenediphenyl diisocyanate (MDI), and hexylmethylene diisocyanate (HDI) (Henschler et al., 1962; Brugsen and Elkins, 1963; Butcher et al., 1970; Butcher, 1979; Taylor, 1970; O'Brien, et al., 1970). These are highly reactive low molecular weight chemicals used in the polyurethane foam and painting industries. Although the pathogenesis is not fully understood, approximately 15 to 20 percent of exposed workers develop a tolyl-specific positive radioallergosorbent test result, suggesting an immune mechanism in some cases. Approximately 5 percent of the workers exposed will develop asthma. Again, late or dual reactions appear to be more common than immediate reactions.

Trimellitic anhydride (TMA) has been associated with four clinical syndromes as follows: asthma and rhinitis, late respiratory systemic syndrome, pulmonary disease – anemia syndrome, and irritant syndrome. TMA is a highly reactive chemical used as a bonder in the plastics industry. Patterson and colleagues (1978 and 1979) and Zeiss and colleagues (1977) have demonstrated that the immunopathology from exposure to TMA is a likely result of TMA-protein complexes that induce the formation of new antigenic determinants or "neoantigens." The same phenomenon has been noted in the case of isocyanates.

A number of metals have been associated with induction of asthma. The complex salts of platinum have been the most extensively studied. Platinum salts have been implicated in the induction of asthma, rhinitis, and urticaria. Asthmatic reactions may be immediate, late, or dual and may be reproduced in challenge tests. Specific IgE has been found in affected workers (Cromwell et al., 1979).

DIAGNOSIS

In assessing individuals for suspected occupational asthma, one must first document the diagnosis of asthma and a temporal relationship with an occupational exposure. In the typical case, the individual presents with a history of episodic attacks of cough, wheezing, and shortness of breath at work. In the case of the late type asthmatic reaction, the symptom of nocturnal dyspnea may be overlooked or misinterpreted. A thorough search for a family history of asthma, atopy, and pre-existing asthma is important. Other plausible explanations, such as nonoccupational allergic exposures and viral respiratory tract infections, must be excluded. A smoking history also is important.

A complete occupational history is essential when attempting to establish a temporal relationship with suspected occupational exposure. Several important questions to ask include the following: What is your job? How long have you been employed? What happens to the symptoms during the work shift? Do the symptoms improve while on vacation or during the weekend away from the work place? What are the exposures? Often the patient's exposure information is sketchy, and one may be forced to obtain data from the employer's safety officer or industrial hygienist. Was there an overexposure (i.e., spill)? Has there been a change in the industrial process? Are any other workers ill?

The physical examination may be unrewarding, since the findings may be normal between attacks. Signs of allergic disease, such as nasal polyps, rhinitis, and skin rash, should be sought.

Once the provisional diagnosis of occupational asthma has been established, several of the following laboratory tests usually are performed in an effort to establish the diagnosis objectively. These tests usually include the following: (1) pulmonary function, (2) methacholine challenge, (3) immunologic studies (when appropriate antigens are available), and (4) inhalation challenge.

Pulmonary function tests include baseline spirometry, prebronchodilator and postbronchodilator spirometry, lung volumes, and diffusion capacity. If there is no evidence of airflow obstruction or of reversibility of obstruction that does exist, one should proceed to a methacholine challenge to assess the underlying degree of nonspecific bronchial hyperreactivity, a phenomenon generally associated with active asthma. The methodology of testing has been standardized and is published elsewhere (Chai et al., 1975). The presence of nonspecific bronchial hyperreactivity does not in itself establish a diagnosis of occupational asthma, nor does the absence of nonspecific bronchial hyperreactivity rule out occupational asthma, but it does make the diagnosis much less probable. Nonspecific bronchial hyperreactivity has been suggested as being useful potentially as a predictor of individuals who may develop occupational asthma or decreased lung function or both. However, there is no good prospective, large scale epidemiologic information to determine whether this concept, in fact, is correct.

Immunologic studies can be useful in the diagnosis of occupational asthma. In particular, the presence of IgE antibody to the suspected allergen should be assessed, but it is often of limited value in establishing the diagnosis of occupational asthma. Table 46–2 shows the number of compounds in which skin testing has been used to determine probable etiology in occupational asthma. One should be extremely cautious in establishing the diagnosis of occupational asthma on the basis of skin testing alone.

Currently, the standard for establishing the diagnosis of occupational asthma resides with inhalation challenge testing. Indications and contraindications are summarized in Table 46–3. There are two types of challenges that are performed, natural and laboratory based. The natural challenge involves testing the individual in the work place. In general, the methodology requires the individual to be removed from the work place for several days, taken off medication, and on the day prior to returning to the work place, baseline pulmonary function is assessed either by peak flow measurements or by repetitive FEV_1 measurements. The individual

TABLE 46–2. Types of Occupational Asthma in Which Skin Tests Have Been Used to Determine Probable Etiology

Agents	Industries or Workers
METALS	
Platinum	Metal refining
Nickel	Metal refining
BIOLOGIC SOURCES	
Animal danders	Laboratory workers, animal handlers
Castor beans	Food industry
Soybeans	Food industry
Green coffee beans	Food industry
Flour	Millers, bakers
Grain	Grain elevator workers
Wood dust	Lumber
Vegetable gums	Printers
Pancreatic extracts	Pharmaceutical
Bacillus subtilis	Detergent industry
CHEMICALS	
Cephalosporins	Pharmaceutical
Phenylglycine acid chloride	Pharmaceutical

TABLE 46–3. Bronchoprovocation Testing

Indications

To quantitate the degree of bronchial reactivity to compounds encountered in the occupational environment

To allow the physician to objectively correlate signs and symptoms with exposure to the compounds

To longitudinally assess an individual's degree of specific bronchial reactivity

Contraindications

An FEV_1 of less than 50 percent of predicted

Inability to complete the test because of any underlying medical or psychologic problem

Inability to discontinue bronchodilator therapy

then returns to the work environment, and the lung function is tested repetitively through the work shift and overnight. A 20-percent decline in the FEV_1 is considered a positive result. The advantages of a work place challenge include less expense and testing in the suspected environment. The disadvantages of the work place challenge are a less stringent quality control of lung function testing, a potential for multiple confounding exposures, and an inability to obtain a dose response curve to the suspected inhalant. In contrast, the laboratory based inhalation challenge test is more expensive but allows assessment in a very controlled environment at subirritant levels of exposure to potentially sensitizing compounds. Thus, once a dose response curve has been established, the individual can be retested and a direct comparison of the degree of bronchial reactivity obtained. As in the work place challenge, the individual's medications are stopped and, a day after the baseline lung function and methacholine test have been performed, a mock challenge is performed to establish baseline FEV_1. All challenges are carried out in a chamber where very stable exposures can be established. Generally, the first day the individual is challenged to the suspected compound, extremely low doses (i.e., 5 ppb of TDI) for a short period of time (i.e., 15 minutes) are given. If no response occurs within 24 hours, the exposure is repeated at a higher dose for a longer period of time. Figure 46–1 is an example of a patient's positive late response to an isocyanate challenge.

TREATMENT

If the diagnosis of occupational asthma can be established, the treatment of choice is re-

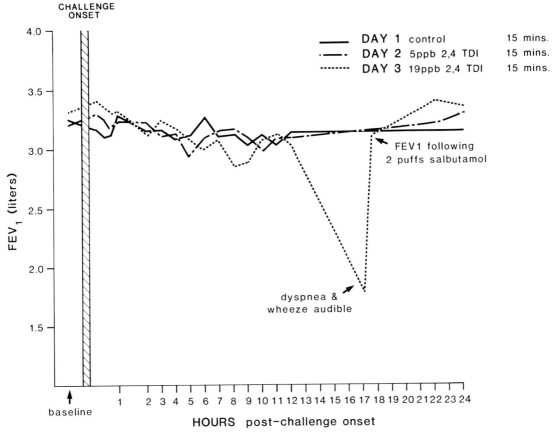

FIGURE 46-1. The graph depicts the results of specific challenge testing in a worker who developed sensitivity to toluene diisocyanate following viral pneumonia.

moval of the individual from exposure. Depending on the circumstances, this recommendation may be met with resistance from patient, management, or both. In that particular case, every effort should be made to improve environmental controls. The treatment of occupational asthma beyond removal from exposure is similar to that of nonoccupational asthma.

Though the lung functions of individuals with occupational asthma usually improve when they are no longer exposed, Chan-Yeung and Lam (1986) indicated that these patients may retain increased bronchial reactivity to such compounds for years. These investigators also reported that individuals with persistent asthma, lower levels of lung function, and more severe bronchial reactivity have poorer prognoses. There also is a suggestion that those with late or dual reactions in response to occupational exposures have poorer prognoses than those with immediate reactions. It is unclear, however, whether longstanding exposure to

compounds that cause occupational asthma will lead to permanent respiratory injury.

The pharmacologic treatment of occupational asthma is similar to that of nonoccupational asthma. Oral theophylline compounds and inhaled beta-2 selective sympathomimetics alone or in combination have been the mainstay of therapy. If the pattern of reactions can be established, prophylactic therapy with sodium cromolyn for immediate reactions and inhaled or oral corticosteroids for late reactions may be beneficial in the allergic-mediated forms of occupational asthma.

In summary, patients with occupational asthma are an important subgroup of patients with asthma. From a clinical standpoint, it is one of the most difficult respiratory diagnoses to establish. It is extremely important to have well-outlined criteria and verifiable objective data, as these cases often enter the arena of forensic medicine. Current and future research directed toward mechanisms as well as epidemiology should lead to better understanding of the disease and ultimately to better management. Until then, the most appropriate treatment for individuals with occupational asthma is removal from exposure.

REFERENCES

Bernstein, I.L.: Occupational asthma. Clin. Chest Med. 2:255–272, 1981.

Brooks, S.M.: Bronchial asthma of occupational origin. Scand. J. Work Environ. Health 3:53, 1977.

Brooks, S.M.: Bronchial asthma of occupational origin. In Environmental and Occupational Medicine. Rom, W.N. (ed.), Boston, Little, Brown and Company, 1983.

Brooks, S.M., Lockey, J.: Reactive airways dysfunction syndrome (RADS). A newly defined occupational disease. (Abstract.) Am. Rev. Respir. Dis. 123:133, 1981.

Brooks, S.M., Mintz, S., Weiss, E.: Changes occurring after freon inhalation. Am. Rev. Respir. Dis. 105:640–643, 1972.

Brugsch, H.G., Elkins, H.D.: Toluene diisocyanate (TDI) toxicity. N. Engl. J. Med. 268:353–357, 1963.

Butcher, B.T.: Inhalation challenge testing with toluene diisocyanate. J. Allergy Clin. Immunol. 64:655–657, 1979.

Butcher, B.T., Salvaggio, J.E.: Occupational Asthma. J. Allergy Clin. Immunol. 78:547–556, 1986.

Butcher, B.T., Salvaggio, J.E., Weill, H., Ziskind, M.M.: Toluene diisocyanate (TDI) pulmonary disease: immunologic and inhalation challenge studies. J. Allergy Clin. Immunol. 58:89–100, 1970.

Chai, H., Farr, R., Froehlich, L.A., et al.: Standardization of bronchial inhalation procedures. J. Allergy Clin. Immunol. 56:323–327, 1975.

Chan-Yeung, M., Ashley, M.J., Corey, P., Willson, G., Dorken, E., Grzybowski, S.: A respiratory survey of cedar mill workers. I. Prevalence of symptoms and lung function abnormalities. J. Occup. Med. 20:323, 1978.

Chan-Yeung, M., Lam, S.: State of art: Occupational asthma. Am. Rev. Respir. Dis. 133:686–703, 1986.

Chan-Yeung, M., Lam, S., Koener, S.: Clinical features and natural history of occupational asthma due to western red cedar *(Thuja plicata)*. Am. J. Med. 72:411, 1982.

Cockcroft, D.W.: Mechanisms of perennial allergic asthma. Lancet 2: 253, 1983.

Cromwell, O., Pepys, J., Parish, W.E., Hughes, E.G.: Specific IgE antibodies to platinum salts in sensitized workers. Clin. Allergy 9:109–117, 1979.

Diem, J.E., Jones, R.N., Hendrick, D.J., Glindmeyer, H.W., et al.: Five-year longitudinal study of workers employed in a new toluene diisocyanate manufacturing plant. Am. Rev. Respir. Dis. 126:420–428, 1982.

Frank, N.R., Amdur, M.O., Worcester, J., Whittenberger, J.L.: Effects of acute controlled exposure to SO_2 on respiratory mechanics in healthy male adults. J. Appl. Physiol. 17:252–258, 1962.

Henschler, D., Assman, W., Meyer, K.O.: The toxicology of the toluene diisocyanates. Arch. Toxicol. 19:364–387, 1962.

Horton, D.J., Chen, W.Y.: Effects of breathing warm humidified air on bronchoconstriction induced by body cooling and by inhalation of methacholine. Chest 75:24–28, 1979.

Maestrelli, P., Alessandri, M.V., Polato, R., Rossi, A.: Occupational asthma in workers exposed to flux-cored solder-containing colophony. Folia Allergol. Immunol. Clin. 30/45:118, 1983.

Murphy, R.L.H., Jr.: Industrial disease with asthma. In Bronchial Asthma: Mechanisms and Therapeutics. Weiss, E.B., Segal, M.S. (eds.), Boston, Little, Brown and Company, 1976.

Newhouse, M.L., Tagg, B., Pocock, S.L.: An epidemiological study of workers producing enzyme washing powders. Lancet 1:1181, 1969.

O'Brien, I.M., Harries, M.G., Burge, P.S., Pepys, J.: Toluene diisocyanate–induced asthma. Reactions to TDI, MDI, HDI and histamine. Clin. Allergy 9:1–6, 1979.

Patterson, R., Addington, W., Banner, A., et al.: Anti-hapten antibodies in workers exposed to trimellitic anhydride fumes: a potential immunopathogenetic mechanism for the trimellitic anhydride pulmonary disease-anemia syndrome. Am. Rev. Respir. Dis. 120:1259–1267, 1979.

Patterson, R., Zeiss, C.R., Roberts, M., et al.: Human anti-hapten antibodies in trimellitic anhydride inhalation reactions: immunoglobulin classes of antitrimellitic anhydride antibodies and hapten inhibition studies. J. Clin. Invest. 62:971–978, 1978.

Ramazzini, B.: Diseases of workers. Translated by W.C. Wright from De Morbis Artificum. New York, Hafner Publishing Company, 1964.

Taylor, G.: Immune response to tolulene diisocyanate (TDI) exposure in man. Proc. Royal Soc. Med. 63:379–380, 1970.

Weiner, A.: Bronchial asthma due to organic phosphate insecticide. Ann. Allergy 19:397–401, 1961.

Widdicombe, J.T., Kent, D.C., Nadel, J.A.: Mechanisms of bronchoconstriction during inhalation of dust. J. Appl. Physiol. 17:613–616, 1962.

Zeiss, C.R., Patterson, R., Pruzansky, J.J., Miller, M., et al.: Trimellitic anhydride–induced airway syndromes: clinical and immunologic studies. J. Allergy Clin. Immunol. 60:96–103, 1977.

47

Hypersensitivity Pneumonitis and Allergic Bronchopulmonary Aspergillosis

F. STANFORD MASSIE, M.D.

HYPERSENSITIVITY PNEUMONITIS

A patient with hypersensitivity pneumonitis (HP) typically presents with fever, cough, malaise, and severe nonwheezing dyspnea several hours after inhalation of organic dust that contains any of a wide variety of antigenic materials from thermophilic organisms; bird, fungi, and animal proteins; chemicals; or drugs (Table 47–1). HP occurs primarily in nonatopic individuals. Pulmonary reactions resembling asthma or diffuse pulmonary disease also may be induced by drugs and chemicals and occur in atopic and nonatopic individuals with equal frequency. Because there is a delay in onset of symptoms following exposure to the causative agent, the patient and physician may fail to notice a relationship. Early diagnosis and prompt therapy are essential in order to prevent irreversible lung damage, with fibrosis and progressive pulmonary disability (Bierman et al., 1983).

HP, also called extrinsic allergic alveolitis, involves the distal airways and pulmonary parenchyma. It can occur as an acute intermittent systemic and respiratory illness or as an insidious, chronically progressive pulmonary disease. HP is found in 5 to 20 percent of persons regularly exposed to etiologic agents.

The Acute Form

Chills, fever, malaise, cough and dyspnea, basilar rales, leukocytosis, pulmonary infil-trates, and restrictive type pulmonary function test defects usually begin 4 to 6 hours after exposure to the causative organic dust. Symptoms and signs are frequently mistaken for those of infectious pneumonitis. Temperature may be as high as 40° C (104° F). Rapid respirations and moist crepitant rales may be heard predominantly at the lung bases, and there usually is no wheezing and minimal hyperinflation. These abnormalities ordinarily resolve within 12 to 18 hours but occasionally may persist for several days, unless terminated by corticosteroid therapy.

The Insidious Form

With prolonged and continuous exposure to the offending dust, cough and dyspnea may be progressive without acute episodes. Dyspnea on exertion, anorexia, weight loss, and fatigue may occur without fever, and positive findings may be limited to fine basilar rales and, rarely, clubbing of the fingers.

Laboratory Features

In the acute form, leukocytosis may be as high as 25,000 white blood cells/mm^3, with a predominance of segmented polymorphonuclear leukocytes and up to 10 percent eosinophils, in association with chills and fever. These findings return to normal as symptoms subside, usually 12 to 18 hours after onset. Serum immunoglobulin levels may be elevated. IgE is usually normal, except in atopic individuals with bird fancier's lung or allergic bronchopulmonary aspergillosis (ABA). Nonspecific serologic findings, such as the presence of rheumatoid factor and positive mononucleosis spot test results may be seen in those with the acute illness. The erythrocyte sedimentation rate occasionally is elevated. Smears and cultures of the throat, sputum, and blood are negative for pathogenic organisms. Leukocytosis and other nonspecific abnormal findings are usually absent in the chronic intermittent exposure form of the disease (Fink, 1984; Levy and Fink, 1985).

TABLE 47-1. Classification of Hypersensitivity Pneumonitis*

Type of Exposure	Disease	Source	Antigen
Environment	Humidifier lung	Home or work humidifiers	Thermophilic actinomycetes,
	Ventilation system disease	and air conditioning systems	ameba, various fungi
Hobbies and pets	Pigeon breeder's disease	Pigeon, parakeet, or parrot	Avian protein antigen
	Bird fancier's lung	droppings	
Occupation	Bagassosis	Moldy sugar cane	*Thermoactinomyces sacchari*
	Cheese worker's disease	Cheese mold spores	*Penicillium casei*
	Enzyme worker's lung	Bacterial products (inhalation)	*B. subtilis* enzymes
	Farmer's lung	Moldy hay, oats, corn	*Micropolyspora faeni*
	Mushroom worker's disease	Compost	*Thermoactinomyces vulgaris*
	Malt worker's lung	Germinating barley	*Aspergillus clavatus, A. fumigatus*
	Maple bark disease	Moldy maple bark	*Cryptostroma corticale*
	Mill worker's disease	Mill dust, wheat flour	*Sitophilus granarius* (weevil)
	Poultry worker's disease	Poultry sheds	Chicken dander
	Sequoiosis	Moldy redwood sawdust	*Graphium pullularia*
	Wood worker's lung	Moldy wood chips	*Alternaria* species
	Suberosis	Moldy cork dust	*Penicillium frequentans*
Chemicals	Isocyanate hypersensitivity pneumonitis	Isocyanates	Toluene diisocyanate
	Porcelain refinisher's lung	Paint catalyst	Diphenyl methane diisocyanate
	Epoxy resin worker's lung	Epoxy resin	Phthalic anhydride
	Plastic worker's lung	Trimellitic anhydride	Trimellitic anhydride
Animals	Laboratory worker's lung	Rodent urine	Rodent proteins
	Furrier's lung	Hair dust	Dander proteins
Medications	Pancreatic extract lung	Pancreatic enzymes (inhalation)	Pig pancreatic protein
	Pituitary snuff-taker's lung	Pituitary powder (inhalation)	Ox or pig protein

* Modified from Bierman, C. W., et al.: Nonasthmatic Allergic Pulmonary Disease. In *Disorders of the Respiratory Tract in Children.* Kendig, E. L., Jr., Chernick, V. (eds.), Philadelphia, W. B. Saunders, Co., 1983.

Roentgenographic Features

In the acute form, the chest x-ray film shows a diffuse interstitial infiltrate with fine reticular densities, multiple small nodules, and patchy infiltration at the lung bases. In the chronic phase, diffuse interstitial fibrosis, with coarsening of the bronchovascular markings and contraction of lung tissue, is seen. Hyperinflation is uncommon but can occur (Fig. 47-1).

Pulmonary Function Tests

Restrictive impairment of pulmonary function, with reduced forced vital capacity (FVC), is the primary abnormality of HP. This may return to normal between acute episodes; but in the chronic phase of the disease, FVC is reduced irreversibly because of pulmonary fibrosis. Increased stiffness of the lung, with decreased compliance, may be accompanied by an alveolar-capillary blockade with reduced gas transfer and diminished carbon monoxide diffusion.

Functional residual capacity and total lung capacity are low. Arterial blood gas values reveal diminished Po_2, decreased oxygen saturation, and diminished Pco_2. The pH is slightly elevated, with a mild respiratory alkalosis during acute episodes. Airways resistance as measured by plethysmography, forced expiratory volume at one second (FEV_1), and other flow rates are usually normal unless the patient has significant bronchiolitis or superimposed asthma (as in bird fancier's lung). In the insidious form of the disease, increased residual volume and decreased flow rates may be seen, indicating loss of pulmonary elasticity, as is found in emphysema.

Immune Responses

Antigens that induce HP appear to be of appropriate size ($< 10 \mu$) for reaching the bronchial tree, where they are processed by pulmonary macrophages. The antigens are nondigestible by lysosomal enzymes, are particulate in

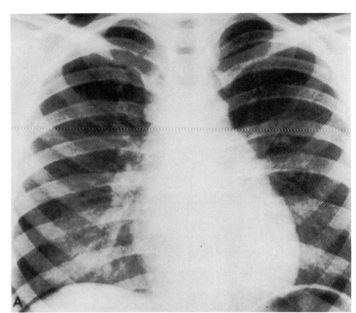

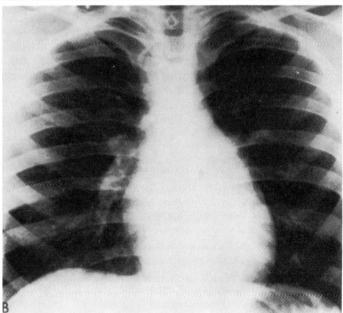

FIGURE 47-1. Acute (A) and convalescent (B) chest films of a child with hypersensitivity pneumonitis due to exposure to doves in the home. (From Cunningham, A. S., Fink, J. N., and Schleuter, D. P.: Pediatrics 58:436, 1976)

nature, are capable of directly activating complement, and have an adjuvant effect on pulmonary immune responses (Fink, 1984). In the serum of patients with HP, precipitating IgG antibodies characteristically are found to suspect, organic dust–containing fungal antigens; thermophilic actinomycetes; or avian proteins. These antibodies may be detected in up to 50 percent of asymptomatic, similarly exposed individuals, and therefore their presence per se is not indicative of disease. Epidemiologic studies have suggested that they simply reflect predominant antigen exposure. Early studies postulated that they were responsible for a type III or local Arthus hypersensitivity reaction in the lung. Although type III reactions appear to occur in these diseases, recent experimental and human studies have implicated monocytes and lymphocytes (and presumably type IV reactions) in the pathogenesis of the pulmonary reaction. Precipitating antibodies may play a protective role in antigen-clearing mechanisms. Antibody titers generally are higher in symptomatic individuals. Cross reactions have been noted between various organic dust antigens and are believed to indicate a wide degree of exposure to the antigens capable of inducing HP in patients with the disease. Patients with farmer's lung disease have been found to have broad immune responses with elevated specific antibodies to a panel of respiratory viruses and *Mycoplasma* compared with normal individuals, perhaps indicating wide antigenic exposure or unknown peculiarities in host responsiveness.

Serum complement level has been reported to be decreased in asymptomatic, but not in symptomatic, pigeon breeders upon inhalation challenge with pigeon antigens; however, in other studies, alveolar-fluid levels of complement from patients with hypersensitivity lung disease did not differ from levels from patients with idiopathic pulmonary fibrosis or normal controls. Furthermore, extracts of *Micropolyspora faeni,* important in farmer's lung disease, have been found to consume complement *in vitro* in the absence of detectable antibodies. The immunopathogenic role of complement activation directly by causative antigens (alternative pathway?) or through antigen-antibody interaction (classic pathway) requires further elucidation.

Cellular Immune Studies

Peripheral blood lymphocytes and bronchoalveolar lavage (BAL) T cells from patients with HP undergo blast transformation and release lymphokines when cultured *in vitro* with appropriate fungal or avian antigens. In contrast, lymphocytes from asymptomatic individuals do not react in this manner even though there may be serum-precipitating antibodies present to the antigens. In pigeon breeder's disease, BAL T cells are increased with normal T and B cell ratios and helper and suppressor cell ratios. Abnormalities in T cell immunoregulation with decreased suppressor cell function exist and may be important in the pathogenesis of HP. In animal models of HP, lymphocytes appear to be of prime importance. Animal transfer experiments with infusion of sensitized lymphocytes were followed by pulmonary lesions on antigen challenge by inhalation. In most studies, serum transfer was less likely to induce typical HP lesions after inhalation challenge.

Genetic control of the pulmonary response is suggested by studies in animals and humans.

Human leukocyte antigen (HLA) linkage has not been confirmed, however. Pulmonary damage appears to develop after an immune response that combines both antigen-specific humoral antibodies and cellular hypersensitivity, with mononuclear cells releasing lymphokines. Complement activation in the lung and irritant effects of the thermophilic agents also may be important. Cellular hypersensitivity to organic dusts may lead to HP, after being triggered by a nonspecific inflammatory process, such as a respiratory infection.

Skin Tests

Scratch, prick, or intradermal tests are useful with bird-derived antigens in pigeon breeder's disease or bird fancier's lung disease. Extracts of thermophilic actinomycetes are irritating and cannot be used for testing in farmer's lung and other related HP. The usual skin response is erythema and edema at 4 to 8 hours. A biopsy specimen of the skin reveals a perivascular infiltrate consistent with an immune complex or Arthus reaction.

Inhalation Challenge Studies

All the signs and symptoms of HP can be reproduced when appropriate extracts of causative agents are used for inhalation challenge. Care must be taken in performing these tests, since reactions may be severe. Re-exposure to suspect environmental areas, such as pigeon coops, may be necessary.

Histologic Studies

Lung biopsy specimens from patients with acute HP reveal interstitial pneumonitis with involvement of alveolar walls, spaces, and bronchioles. Infiltrations with lymphocytes, plasma cells, foamy histiocytes, and increased numbers of alveolar macrophages are seen with an alveolar proteinaceous exudate. Focal granulomas and minimal vasculitis may be present. In the chronic phase, fibrosis with destruction of lung parenchyma is seen. A "honeycomb" pattern of cystic changes and obliteration of bronchioles by deposition of collagen and granulation tissue are associated with severe interstitial fibrosis.

Experimental Studies

Many different animal models of HP have been reported in which all features of the human disease have been reproduced. Detailed information on immunopathogenesis has been reviewed (Richerson, 1983; Fink, 1983).

Diagnosis

A high index of suspicion and a detailed history of the patient's home environment, hobbies, and work environment are necessary for diagnosis of HP. Infectious pneumonia is frequently misdiagnosed in the acute form, but attention should be paid to recurrence of symptoms on returning to the previous environment. Symptoms may occur 5 nights of the week after work. Cultures of the environment for airborne fungi and serologic tests for precipitins should be considered. Lung biopsy and inhalation challenge with pulmonary function tests may be necessary, particularly in the patient with the insidious form. Differentiation from allergic bronchopulmonary aspergillosis is discussed subsequently.

Therapy

Careful avoidance of re-exposure to causative agents and corticosteroid therapy will achieve remission of the acute form. Steroid therapy should begin with a single early morning dose of 40 mg of prednisone, with a gradual daily dose reduction. Chest x-ray films and lung function tests should be carefully monitored. If long-term steroid therapy is necessary, an alternate day regimen should be tried. Avoiding reexposure may be difficult, since occupation or lifestyle may need to be changed. Lack of compliance may be followed by recurrence or progression of pulmonary disease.

SPECIFIC SYNDROMES

Disease Related to Home Environment

Interstitial Lung Disease Due to Contamination of Forced Air Systems. Home and office air conditioning systems present specific hazards of HP. It has been reported after exposure to office air conditioners, home furnace humidifiers, room humidifiers, home air conditioners, car air conditioners, and cool mist vaporizers. Etiologic agents have been identified as *Thermoactinomyces candidus, T. vulgaris,* and *T. sacchari.* The thermophilic agents contaminated the air conditioning or humidifying equipment and led to sensitization. Thermotolerant bacteria and amebae also may be involved in some cases. In one report, the source of such agents was a contaminated water supply delivered to the humidifier. In children with persistent respiratory problems, such as cystic fibrosis, long-term use of humidifiers, vaporizers, or tents should be suspected as possible causes of further lung disease.

Disease Due to Hobbies

Pigeon Breeder's Disease (PBD). PBD is the most common and best studied pediatric hypersensitivity pneumonitis (Fink, 1983). It has been reported after long-standing exposure to avian antigens from pigeons, parrots, doves, parakeets (budgerigars), and chickens. HP has been reported after exposure to mice, rats, gerbils, and guinea pigs. There usually is an insidious onset with a prolonged course. Weight loss is a common sign. Clinical features include cough, dyspnea, basilar rales, absence of wheezing, abnormal chest x-ray films with infiltrates, and restrictive lung disease with reduced FVC and diffusing capacity. There is a history of exposure to avian antigens, with a variable duration from 6 weeks to 7 years. Skin testing with pigeon serum or extracts of feathers and droppings may reveal both an immediate and a late onset skin reaction. Precipitating antibodies to avian proteins are present in the serum. Careful inhalation challenge with bird-derived extracts in a hospitalized patient will be followed by an acute syndrome with cough, dyspnea, and rales 4 to 8 hours after exposure and abnormal pulmonary function studies. Lung biopsy specimen reveals a chronic interstitial mononuclear infiltration. Therapy consists of elimination of birds and a course of corticosteroids. These produce clearing of the abnormal signs and normal chest x-ray film findings, providing exposure has not been sufficient to produce pulmonary fibrosis.

Occupational Lung Disease

As outlined in Table 47–1, HP may be seen in workers exposed to organic dust, containing thermophilic actinomycetes or other fungi from sugar cane (bagassosis), cheese, laundry detergent enzymes (Bacillus subtilis), moldy hay (farmer's lung disease), mushroom compost, or wood dust; in chemical workers exposed to isocyanates and phthalic and trimellitic anhydrides; in animal workers exposed to laboratory rodents; in furriers; and in individuals exposed to medications containing pig or cow proteins. Clinical features of HP have been reported in parents caring for children with cystic fibrosis (pancreatic enzymes) and in patients with diabetes insipidus (pituitary snuff). Synthetic vasopressin (Pitressin) has significantly reduced the incidence of this latter problem.

A high index of suspicion and a careful environmental history are essential in diagnosis of any individual with chronic cough and interstitial pneumonitis. Failure to recognize a relationship between environmental exposure to causative agents and preventable chronic lung disease may lead to insidious pulmonary deterioration, with fibrosis as the end result.

Drug- and Chemical-Induced Pulmonary Disease

Numerous industrial materials and drugs are known to produce pulmonary disease. The types of reactions are obstructive, with asthma-like syndromes (e.g., aspirin, industrial chemicals); restrictive, with diffuse pulmonary disease suggesting pneumonitis (e.g., nitrofurantoin); and combined obstructive and restrictive (e.g., metal fumes). Mediastinal and hilar changes have been reported from phenytoin and corticosteroids. An asthma-like syndrome, a late-onset asthma with chills and fever, and a restrictive lung disease or HP have been reported with trimellitic anhydride, isocyanate, and sodium diazobenzene sulfate exposure (Schatz et al., 1983; Zeiss et al., 1977).

ALLERGIC BRONCHOPULMONARY ASPERGILLOSIS (ABA)

Definition

ABA is an immune bronchial disease occurring in asthmatics. Pulmonary infiltrates and eosinophilia in blood and sputum are characteristic. It was first described in adults in England in 1952 and in children in 1970. It may be distinguished from other forms of lung disease due to Aspergillus fumigatus (Af), such as invasive or septicemic aspergillosis, aspergilloma, IgE-mediated asthma from Af sensitivity, and HP due to A. clavus, growing in barley, in "malt worker's lung."

Aspergillus is found year-round in air; soil; decaying vegetation, such as cut grass, potting soil, and mulches; basements; bedding; house dust; and swimming pool water. Individuals with episodic bronchial obstructive disease, such as patients with asthma and, occasionally, patients with cystic fibrosis, are susceptible to colonization of the bronchial tree with Af. Presumably because of thick tenacious mucus and possibly other host factors, ABA may develop. There have been occasional reports of at least

TABLE 47–2. Criteria for Diagnosis of Allergic Bronchopulmonary Aspergillosis

Primary

Obstructive airway disease
Eosinophilia $> 1000/mm^3$
Immediate skin test positive reaction to Aspergillus fumigatus (Af)
Serum precipitating antibodies against Af
Elevated serum IgE level
History of transient or fixed pulmonary infiltrates
Central bronchiectasis in upper lobes
Elevated serum IgE/IgG antibodies to Af

Secondary

Positive sputum culture for Af
History of golden brown sputum plugs
Late skin test reactivity to Af (4 to 8 hours)
Fall in total IgE level after prednisone therapy

two family members having the disease. HLA studies have revealed no genetic predisposition.

Clinical symptoms include anorexia, malaise, fever, attacks of wheezing, and productive cough with solid sputum plugs. Rales over areas of pulmonary infiltrates and wheezing may be heard on auscultation of the chest. Laboratory studies reveal a profound eosinophilia frequently greater than $1000/mm^3$ and elevated IgE level as high as 80,000 ng/ml. Most reported patients have been adults, but the diagnosis should be suspected in wheezing children even under 2 years of age who exhibit recurrent infiltrates, eosinophilia, and Af in the sputum.

Diagnosis

Diagnostic aids for ABA are outlined in Table 47–2. All asthmatic patients with pulmonary infiltrates should have skin testing with Af antigen. A dual reaction with an immediate (10 to 15 minutes) and a late (4 to 8 hours) reaction occurs in a third of patients with ABA. The immediate response is IgE mediated; the late response also may be largely IgE mediated, since biopsy specimens of the late reaction fail to show vasculitis, as in a true Arthus reaction, despite the presence of IgG, IgM, IgA, and C3. Similarly, immediate and late immune reactions are believed to be pathogenetic for the bronchial disease that occurs. When levels of IgE-Af or IgG-Af antibodies, or both, are compared between ABA patients and asthmatics who are Af skin test positive but have no evidence of ABA, ABA patients are found to have at least twice the levels of antibody as asthmatics without ABA. This Af antibody "index" is helpful in diagnosis and follow-up of the ABA patient. Antibodies are measured by radioimmunoassay (RIA) and enzyme-linked immunosorbent assay (ELISA) techniques. Total IgE concentration is elevated at least two-fold

over baseline measurements in all patients with acute infiltrates and is a useful aid in following disease activity.

Roentgenographic Features

Roentgenographic findings in ABA are outlined in Table 47–3 and vary according to disease activity and stage. There is an upper lobe predilection to the abnormalities with bronchial wall edema, inflammation, obstruction, and damage presenting as "tramlines," "ring and toothpaste shadows," and infiltrates. In advanced ABA, damaged proximal bronchi with central bronchiectasis appear as hilar shadows best delineated by tomography. This is in contrast to postinfectious bronchiectasis in which large bronchi are normal, but there is distal bronchial damage. Late stage findings may include cavitation, honeycomb-like fibrosis, and contracted upper lobes.

Differential Diagnosis

The differential diagnosis of ABA includes abnormalities listed in Table 47–4. Steroid-dependent asthmatics should be investigated carefully for the presence of ABA. Other causes for the pulmonary infiltrate with eosinophilia (PIE) syndrome should be considered. ABA appears to be increased in patients with cystic fibrosis (CF), with increased IgE, with atopy, and with positive skin test reactions to Af. Positive sputum cultures for Af may be seen in this disease with a frequency of 20 to 50 percent. Ten percent of 100 CF patients aged 2 to 34 years had features indicating ABA (Laufer et al., 1984). Differentiating features of ABA and HP are listed in Table 47–5.

During the acute stage of ABA, pulmonary function tests reveal an obstructive airway pattern with reductions in FVC, FEV_1, total lung

TABLE 47–3. Roentgenographic Abnormalities in Allergic Bronchopulmonary Aspergillosis

Perihilar or parenchymal infiltrates
Air fluid levels in central bronchi
Homogeneous consolidation
"Toothpaste" shadows in impacted bronchi
"Gloved-finger" shadows in distal bronchi
Tramline shadows (two parallel hair lines) and ring shadows in the hila
Proximal upper lobe bronchiectasis (hilar tomography)
Cavitation, contracted upper lobes, and honeycomb-like fibrosis

TABLE 47–4. Differential Diagnosis of Allergic
Bronchopulmonary Aspergillosis

Poorly controlled asthma with mucoid impaction/atelectasis
Pneumonitis, viral or bacterial
Tuberculosis with eosinophilia
Sarcoidosis
Pulmonary infiltrates with eosinophilia syndrome
Parasitism
Churg-Strauss vasculitis
Pulmonary neoplasm
Hypersensitivity pneumonitis
Cystic fibrosis (with or without ABA)
Immotile cilia syndrome

capacity, and the ratio of diffusion capacity to total lung capacity. These abnormalities return to baseline measurements with clinical remission. Restrictive lung disease may be seen in advanced disease, however. Staging of the disease process is useful in following ABA. The five following stages are identified: acute, remission, recurrent exacerbation, corticosteroid-dependent asthma, and fibrosis. The goals of management are early recognition and prevention of exacerbation and end-stage chronic lung disease. Exacerbations have occurred after 7 years in remission, thus making long-term follow-up essential.

Pathologic Features

Bronchiectasis' involving segmental bronchi with sparing of distal branches, particularly in the upper lobes, is characteristic. Inspissated mucus contains Curschmann spirals, Charcot-Leyden crystals, eosinophils, fibrin, and mononuclear cells. Fungal hyphae may be seen, Af may be cultured, but there is no invasion of bronchial walls. A granulomatous bronchiolitis sometimes is seen. Microabscesses containing Af, eosinophilic pneumonia, lipid pneumonia, lymphocytic interstitial pneumonia, desquamative interstitial pneumonia, fibrosis, bron-

TABLE 47–5. Differential Diagnosis of Hypersensitivity Pneumonitis (HP) and Allergic
Bronchopulmonary Aspergillosis (ABA)*

Diagnostic Feature	HP	ABA
Nature of patient	Nonatopic (nonallergic)	Atopic (allergic)
Symptoms and physical findings	Cough, dyspnea, fever, no wheezing, weight loss, rales at lung bases	Asthma, fever, ± hemoptysis, chest pain
Skin tests	± (positive immediate and late reactions in some cases of pigeon breeder's lung)	+ (immediate and late responses)
Blood count	Normal or lymphopenia	Eosinophilia
Immunoglobulins	Elevated IgG and IgA, IgG precipitating antibodies	Elevated IgE, IgG precipitating antibodies
Sputum	Normal	Eosinophilia, mycelia
Chest x-ray film	Pulmonary interstitial infiltrates	Pulmonary lobar infiltrates
Complications	Pulmonary fibrosis	Atelectasis, proximal bronchiectasis, fibrosis (late)
Pulmonary function tests	Restrictive	Obstruction (restrictive late)
Inhalation challenge tests	Late restriction (±immediate/late obstruction) (positive immediate and late reactions in some cases of pigeon breeder's lung)	Immediate and late obstruction
Immune mechanism	Immune complexes and delayed hypersensitivity	Immediate hypersensitivity and immune complexes (± delayed hypersensitivity)
Treatment	Avoidance, corticosteroids	Bronchodilators, corticosteroids

* Modified with permission from Slavin, R. G.: Allergic bronchopulmonary aspergillosis. In Middleton, E., Jr., Reed, C. E., Ellis, E. F. (eds.), Allergy: Principles and Practice. St. Louis, C. V. Mosby Co., 1983.

TABLE 47-6. Treatment and Follow-up of Allergic Bronchopulmonary Aspergillosis

Prednisone 0.5 mg/kg, at 8 a.m., q.d. for 2 weeks (40 to 60 mg/d in adults); check for improvement in pulmonary infiltrates.
Prednisone 0.5 mg/kg, at 8 a.m., q.o.d. for 3 months after clearing of infiltrates.
Taper q.o.d. dose (5 mg/month) over 3 months with continued improvement.
Obtain total serum IgE levels monthly for 2 years, then every 2 months.
Obtain chest x-ray films every 4 months for 2 years, every 6 months for 2 years, and yearly thereafter.
Reinstitute daily prednisone with two-fold rise in serum IgE level and new pulmonary infiltrates.

chiolitis obliterans, or bronchocentric granulomatosis may be reported from pathology specimens of patients with ABA. Bronchoprovocation tests with Af and bronchography have attendant risks and are not generally necessary for diagnosis. Lung biopsy is best reserved for questionable cases, when other diseases must be excluded.

Treatment

Once the diagnosis of an acute or exacerbated stage is determined, corticosteroid therapy is begun (see Table 47-6). The acute stage is characterized by asthma, pulmonary infiltrates, or proximal bronchiectasis on chest x-ray, with positive immediate skin test reaction to Af, precipitating antibodies to Af, elevated total IgE level, eosinophilia, and twice the value for IgE-Af or IgG-Af antibodies or both, when compared with Af asthmatics prick positive reactions. Many episodes may be asymptomatic. Following initiation of prednisone therapy, pulmonary infiltrates should disappear. A decline in total serum IgE level of up to 35 percent may be seen within 6 weeks. A decrease in peripheral eosinophilia and asthma symptoms accompanies improvement. Prednisone decreases the inflammatory response and aids in removal of the fungus by relieving airway obstruction. Antifungal agents, cromolyn sodium, and topical inhalant steroids have been used but are not effective. Corticosteroid-dependent asthma and ABA in fibrotic stages are less responsive to prednisone because of the damage to the bronchial tree already present. In order to prevent these stages, follow-up with frequent total serum IgE levels and chest x-rays as outlined in Table 47-6 is essential. A declined and stabilized serum IgE level and a clearing of pulmonary infiltrates for at least 6 months are seen in the remission stage. Prednisone can then be tapered and stopped. A sharp rise in serum IgE level and a new pulmonary infiltrate herald an exacerbation. Prednisone should be instituted and given as in the acute stage. Bronchodilator therapy should be continued through all stages. Heavy mold spore exposure and allergen immunotherapy with *Aspergillus* should be avoided. The prognosis of patients with ABA is good if detected early and treated with prednisone; however, a long-term study of patients with untreated ABA revealed progressive declines in lung functions. The clinician should maintain a high index of suspicion for ABA in asthmatic patients.

REFERENCES

Bierman, C.W., Pierson, W.E., Massie, F.S.: Non-asthmatic allergic pulmonary disease. In Disorders of the Respiratory Tract in Children. Kendig, E.L., Jr., Chernick, V., (eds.), Philadelphia, W. B. Saunders Co., 1983.

Cunningham, A.S., Fink, J.N., Schleuter, D.P.: Childhood hypersensitivity pneumonitis due to dove antigens. Pediatrics 58:436, 1976.

Fink, J.N.: Pigeon breeder's disease. Clin. Rev. Allergy 1:497–508, 1983.

Fink, J.N.: Hypersensitivity pneumonitis. J. Allergy Clin. Immunol. 74:1–9, 1984.

Greenberger, P.A.: Allergic bronchopulmonary aspergillosis. J. Allergy Clin. Immunol. 74:645–653, 1984.

Laufer, P., Fink, J.N., Bruns, W.T., Zinger, G.F., Kalbfleisch, J.H., Greenberger, P.A., Patterson, R.: Allergic bronchopulmonary aspergillosis and cystic fibrosis. J. Allergy Clin. Immunol. 73:44–48, 1984.

Levy, M.B., Fink, J.N.: Hypersensitivity pneumonitis. Ann. Allergy 54:167–171, 1985.

Richerson, H.B.: Hypersensitivity pneumonitis—pathology and pathogenesis. Clin. Rev. Allergy 1:469–486, 1983.

Ricketti, A.J., Greenberger, P.A., Mintzer, R.A., Patterson, R.: Allergic bronchopulmonary aspergillosis. Chest 86:773–778, 1984.

Schatz, M., Patterson, R.: Hypersensitivity pneumonitis—general considerations. Clin. Rev. Allergy 1:451–467, 1983.

Slavin, R.G.: Allergic bronchopulmonary aspergillosis. Clin. Rev. Allergy 3:167–182, 1985.

Zeiss, C.R., Patterson, R., Pruzansky, J.J., Miller, M.M., Rosenberg, M., Levitz, D.: Trimellitic anhydride–induced airway syndromes: Clinical and immunologic studies. J. Allergy Clin. Immunol. 60:96, 1977.

48

Nonallergic Chronic Pulmonary Diseases

ROBERT H. SCHWARTZ, M.D.

Acute illnesses usually subside spontaneously or with therapy within 3 weeks. Illnesses that last from 3 weeks to 3 months can be considered subacute. Chronicity is implied when abnormal signs and symptoms last 3 or more months. When episodes of illness are separated by periods of health, a respiratory condition is considered recurrent, and a chronic underlying disorder should be considered.

Though bronchial asthma has remained the most common chronic pulmonary disease of childhood and adolescence, there have been changes in the etiologies of other chronic pulmonary diseases over the past several decades. Prior to the institution of public health sanitation measures, immunizations for respiratory pathogens, and antibiotics, recognized childhood chronic lung diseases consisted of tuberculosis and complications of pertussis, rubeola, and bacterial pneumonias. These have been replaced by other chronic pulmonary diseases whose etiologies and natural histories may not be known. For example, hereditary risk factors, such as alpha-1-antitrypsin deficiency, in combination with environmental irritants (air pollution, smoking) or respiratory viral infections (respiratory syncytial virus, influenza, adenovirus HTLV-III) or both may predispose individuals of all ages to chronic lung disease (Hall et al., 1984). As newer techniques are developed in the fields of immunology and recombinant DNA molecular biology, greater understanding of pathogenesis and therapy will emerge. The isolation of the human gene for alpha-1-antitrypsin, the synthesis of antiprotease for therapy, or the introduction of normal alpha-1-antitrypsin genes into the chromosomes of cells may provide a means of treatment or even a cure (Schroeder et al., 1985). Perhaps an understanding of the molecular genetic basis for cystic fibrosis, the most common lethal inherited

chronic pulmonary disease, may soon be achieved.

This chapter discusses the more important nonallergic chronic pulmonary diseases of infancy, childhood, and adolescence, many of which also apply to adults, that either share some signs and symptoms of allergic pulmonary disease or must be considered in its differential diagnosis (Table 48–1).

CONDITIONS ASSOCIATED WITH PULMONARY DISEASES

Cough, labored breathing (tachypnea, dyspnea), wheezing, and sputum production are the usual cardinal signs and symptoms of pulmonary disease. These signs often are associated with clubbing and hemoptysis, abnormal pulmonary functions, and abnormal chest x-ray findings.

Clubbing of Fingers and Toes

The association of clubbing of the fingers and toes with lung disease has been recognized since the time of Hippocrates. Finger clubbing is common in cystic fibrosis (CF) but unusual in asthma. Clubbing in asthmatics should always prompt a search for the other conditions more commonly associated with it (Table 48–2).

Accurate clinical assessment of finger clubbing is helpful both in detecting serious lung disease and in following its course. Clubbing occurs in the following order:

1. *Development of a floating nail.* This sign can be demonstrated by pressing the mantle (nail root) with the examining finger and finding it soft and mushy.

2. *A diminution in the angle the nail makes with the extrapolated axis of the digit.* This change is often accompanied by an increased longitudinal curvature of the nail.

3. *An increase in the DPD/IPD (see following discussion).* This change is accompanied by broadening of the terminal phalanx as viewed from the palmar surface, leading to a "drumstick" finger.

A metric micrometer or caliper is used to measure the finger depth at the nail base. This is

626

TABLE 48–1. Chronic Pulmonary Diseases in Children and Adolescents*

Allergic

Bronchial asthma
Hypersensitivity pneumonitis
Allergic bronchopulmonary aspergillosis
Hypersensitivity reactions to drugs and chemicals

Infectious

Chronic tuberculosis and atypical mycobacterial infection
Histoplasmosis
Other mycoses
Cytomegalic inclusion disease
Chlamydia, including psittacosis and ornithosis
Pneumocystis carinii infection
Visceral larva migrans

Postinfectious

Bronchiectasis*
Bronchiolitis obliterans
Unilateral hyperlucent lung syndrome
Interstitial fibrosis

Congenital and Hereditary

Anomalies of the lung (cysts and sequestration)
Congenital lobar emphysema
Cystic fibrosis*
Immune deficiency disorders*
Alpha-1-antitrypsin deficiency*
Dysmotile cilia syndrome and Kartagener syndrome*
Ectodermal dysplasia*
Williams-Campbell syndrome*
Familial dysautonomia

Associated with Underlying Systemic Disease

Sarcoidosis
Collagen diseases
Malignancy
Reticuloendothelioses
　Liporeticuloses
　　Gaucher disease
　　Niemann-Pick disease
　Histiocytosis-X
　　Letterer-Siwe disease
　　Hand-Schüller-Christian disease
　　Eosinophilic granuloma
Wegener granulomatosis

Complicating Management of Pre-existing Disease

Bronchopulmonary dysplasia
Radiation pneumonitis
Musculoskeletal disorders
Central nervous system disorders

Idiopathic

Pulmonary hemosiderosis*
Pulmonary fibrosis*
Fibrosing alveolitis (usual intersititial pneumonia, UIP)
Desquamative intersitial pneumonia (DIP)*
Lymphoid interstitial pneumonia (LIP)*
Giant cell interstitial pneumonia (GIP)
Bronchiolitis obliterans with interstitial pneumonia (BIP)
Pulmonary alveolar microlithiasis

---

* Familial or hereditary implications discussed in this chapter.

TABLE 48–2. Conditions Associated with Clubbing

Pulmonary

Cystic fibrosis
Bronchiectasis of other etiologies
Pulmonary abscess
Empyema
Chronic interstitial pneumonitis
Alpha-1-antitrypsin deficiency with lung disease
Primary and metastatic pulmonary neoplasms
Cavitary tuberculosis

Cardiac

Congenital cyanotic heart disease
Subacute bacterial endocarditis

Hepatic

Hepatic cirrhosis
　Postinfectious
　Associated with alpha-1-antitrypsin deficiency
Intrahepatic biliary atresia
Thalassemia

Gastrointestinal

Chronic ulcerative colitis
Regional enteritis
Multiple intestinal polyposis
Chronic dysentery (amebic or bacillary)

Other

Thyrotoxicosis

---

called the distal phalangeal depth (DPD). The depth of the finger is also measured at the interphalangeal fold. This measurement is the interphalangeal depth (IPD). A ratio of the DPD/IPD greater than 1.0 is considered indicative of clubbing. The left index finger should be used, as the normal ratio may be different for other fingers.

Progressive fingertip deformity is accompanied by increased blood flow to the digits, overgrowth of vascular elements, hyperplasia of fibrous tissue, and edema. The pathophysiologic mechanisms that induce these changes are not well understood. A variety of factors implicated include hypoxemia, vasoactive substances (prostaglandin E, serotonin, and bradykinin), and autonomic reflexes. Clubbing also has been observed in association with vascular abnormalities, leading to differences in blood flow to the extremities (arteriovenous fistulas of the subclavian artery and aortic aneurysms).

Clubbing usually is painless. However, it may be accompanied by hypertrophic pulmonary osteoarthropathy (HPO), which is manifested by stiffness, swelling, and arthralgia of the fingers, wrists, ankles, and knees. Formation of new subperiosteal bone most frequently occurs along the distal portions of the tibia, fibula, radius, and ulna. Less commonly, the humerus, femur, metacarpal, and metatarsal bones may be involved. Pain and tenderness are exacerbated by cold and relieved by warmth and rest.

Hemoptysis

Hemoptysis is defined as the spitting or coughing of blood, ranging from streaks of blood admixed with sputum to massive, exsanguination originating from a lesion anywhere in the respiratory tract. Although hemoptysis is uncommon in children, when it occurs it is a frightening experience for the patient and parent and should be considered with alarm by the physician because it usually implies either significant trauma or serious pulmonary disease. Bleeding of esophageal or gastric origin (hematemesis) may be mistaken for hemoptysis. In some infants, blood from the bronchopulmonary tree is swallowed without coughing and then vomited; therefore, when one encounters unexplained hematemesis in an infant with abnormal chest film findings, a pulmonary source of bleeding should be considered. History and careful physical examination of the nose, mouth, and throat will usually provide clues to bleeding from the gums or other oral lesions. Blood originating from the trachea and distal bronchopulmonary areas may occur under a variety of circumstances (Table 48–3).

Bronchiectasis is one of the most frequent causes of hemoptysis. Hemoptysis hardly ever occurs in primary tuberculosis, but can occur occasionally, usually in secondary tuberculosis (adult form) when a pulmonary abscess ruptures into a bronchus with subsequent bleeding of the granulation tissue lining the walls. Blood streaking of mucus is frequent in CF in which widespread bronchiectasis is the rule. Fifty percent of adult patients with CF have such minor bleeding. Massive hemoptysis, defined as acute bleeding of at least 300 ml, is life threatening. Five percent of older CF patients have acute arterial bleeding that originates from the erosion of destroyed lung parenchyma, which erodes into enlarged, tortuous blood vessels and bronchopulmonary arterial anastomoses adjacent to bronchiectatic airways. In CF, *Pseudomonas aeruginosa* may also cause hemorrhagic pneumonitis. Hemoptysis may also complicate systemic vasculitis syndromes.

TABLE 48–3. Conditions Associated with Hemoptysis

Infections

Bronchitis/bronchiectasis
Tuberculosis (adult)
Lung abscess
Intracavitary fungus balls (aspergillomas)
Certain bacterial pneumonias *(Pseudomonas, Staphylococcus, Klebsiella)*
Fungal diseases (the mycoses)
Parasitic infections (e.g., paragonimiasis)

Neoplasms

Tracheal tumors
Bronchial adenomas
Bronchogenic cancer
Endobronchial metastases

Vascular Disorders

Arteriovenous malformations
Pulmonary embolism and infarction
Mitral stenosis
Cardiac failure with pulmonary edema

Vasculitic Disorders

Churg-Strauss syndrome
Systemic lupus erythematosus
Wegener granulomatosis

Coagulation and Bleeding Disorders

Primary (inherited)
Secondary (acquired)

Trauma

Lung contusion
Rib fracture
Foreign bodies

Other

Cystic fibrosis
Neonatal pulmonary hemorrhage
Pulmonary sequestration
Idiopathic and primary pulmonary hemosiderosis
Goodpasture syndrome
Myocarditis
Cow's milk sensitivity

Patients may be able to identify the area of lung that is bleeding by describing a feeling of warmth or a gurgling sensation in their chests. The best diagnostic method to localize the site of bleeding is bronchoscopy or arteriography during or immediately after an acute episode. Conservative medical management (antibiotics, rest, blood replacement, oxygen, correction of bleeding diathesis) usually is adequate to treat blood streaking and small acute bleeds. Bronchial artery embolization with gelatin sponge (Gelfoam) has been successful about 90 percent of the time in patients with life-threatening hemoptysis. Transverse myelitis may complicate this procedure if the spinal arteries are inadvertently embolized. Pulmonary infarction and embolization of the mesenteric arteries also may occur.

CYSTIC FIBROSIS

CF is the most common genetic disease of white children, adolescents, and young adults. CF is an autosomal, recessively inherited, chronic multisystem disease. It is lethal because of its progressive pulmonary destruction. It shares many signs and symptoms with respiratory and nonrespiratory diseases of allergic origin. Allergy and CF can coexist or allergy can exist as a complication of CF. CF should be considered in the differential diagnosis of respiratory conditions in which the signs and symptoms given in Table 48–4 are present.

Incidence and Heredity

The incidence of CF is estimated at between 1 : 1600 and 1 : 2500 white live births. It is less

TABLE 48–4. Respiratory Signs and Symptoms of Cystic Fibrosis

Chronic cough with or without sputum production
Chronic wheezing
Chronic rhinitis
Hemoptysis
Recurrent infections (bronchitis, bronchiolitis, pneumonia)
Chest findings
  Barrel chest
  Tachypnea
  Retractions
  Rales
Digital clubbing
Head and upper airways abnormalities
  Nasal polyposis
  Pansinusitis
  Mucocele of paranasal sinuses
Sputum culture
  Staphylococcus aureus
  Pseudomonas aeruginosa (both mucoid and nonmucoid)
  Pseudomonas cepacia
  Haemophilus influenzae
  Aspergillus fumigatus
Chest x-ray abnormalities
  Overaeration
  Peribronchial thickening, cuffing, or both
  Bronchial plugging
  Atelectasis (especially right upper lobe)
  Bronchiectasis
  Pneumothorax
  Consolidation

common in non-European whites, and has been reported only sporadically in other races. Its incidence is higher among central and western European populations than among northern (Sweden) and southern (Italy) populations. Although several different modes of inheritance have been proposed, including autosomal dominant and dominant alleles at two interacting polymorphic loci, the autosomal recessive mode of inheritance is strongly supported by most family and population studies. The variable expression of CF, from a mild disease with slow progression to severe disease with more rapid progression, suggests genetic heterogeneity arising from multiple mutant alleles at a single locus. Heterozygote detection and prenatal diagnosis offer the best methods for control of the disease until the CF gene is isolated, inheritance is completely understood, and specific therapy is developed.

Genetic Counseling

Specialists who provide genetic counseling practice at most university medical centers. With the increasing potential for specific genetic testing, the involvement of such specialists in the activities of the CF patient's care, teaching, and resource centers and clinics has become a necessity. However, counseling is best initiated and performed with the guidance of the health professional who understands the patient and the family most thoroughly. This process begins at the time of diagnosis, when parents learn that CF is an inherited disease and that mother and father each are carriers of a single autosomal recessive gene. Various issues, including misplaced guilt and blame, must be dealt with from the beginning. The risks and odds of the parents, siblings, and other relatives having a CF child in the future need to be addressed (Table 48–5).

Each sibling's chance of being a carrier is 2 : 3 or 66 percent, and the chance of the same parents producing a carrier with each subsequent pregnancy is 2 : 4 or 50 percent. Although the sweat test cannot reliably identify the heterozygote (carrier), all siblings should be tested. They may have CF and may have been overlooked because the extent of the disease was clinically mild, in the CF spectrum.

Males of reproductive age contemplating marriage should consider sperm analysis. Most (98 percent) are sterile due to obliteration of the vas deferens system. The difference between

TABLE 48–5. Risks of Producing a Child with Cystic Fibrosis

One Parent	Other Parent	Risk in Each Pregnancy
No CF history	No CF history	1 : 1600
No CF history	First cousin with CF	1 : 320
No CF history	Aunt or uncle with CF	1 : 240
No CF history	Sibling with CF	1 : 120
No CF history	CF child by previous marriage	1 : 80
No CF history	Parent with CF	1 : 80
No CF history	CF	1 : 40
Sibling with CF	Sibling with CF	1 : 9
CF child	CF child	1 : 4

sterility and virility (not impaired) should be made clear. Many females with CF have had children of their own, although their fertility is frequently impaired owing to thick cervical mucus or anovulation accompanying chronic illness. At least two CF children have been borne of CF mothers. All non-CF children of a mother with CF will be carriers.

Pathophysiology and Diagnosis

Cystic fibrosis is considered to be a disease of exocrine gland epithelial cells as follows: the cells that line the airways, the cells that are associated with submucosal glands bordering the airways, and the cells that line the ducts of the sweat glands (Quinton and Bijman, 1983). The defect may be a primary abnormality of the chloride channel or an abnormality in its regulation. Reabsorption of chloride ions across epithelial membranes is sterically or electrochemically inhibited. This results in electronegativity of surface membranes (nasal and bronchial epithelium) and increased chloride excretion by sweat glands. Indirectly, this defect results in abnormal passive transport of sodium and water, affecting the hydration of mucus, which becomes thickened and viscous and obstructs ducts and tubes of various organs. This obstruction leads to inflammation in some organs (pancreas, liver) and stagnation and infection in other organs (bronchopulmonary tree, sinuses).

Recent advances in molecular technologies have enabled scientists to make rapid progress in cystic fibrosis research. It is now established that the gene for CF, both in outbred and in inbred families, is located on the long arm of chromosome 7 (Watkins et al., 1986). Although the CF gene has not been isolated, several DNA linkage markers have been discovered that are sufficiently close to the CF gene to permit tracking of the CF gene in those families who have had children with CF. Prenatal diagnosis and carrier detection are now available for at-risk families.

The pathophysiologic and diagnostic hallmarks of CF are (1) pancreatic enzyme deficiency; (2) progressive chronic bronchial and bronchiolar obstruction; (3) infection (usually *Staphylococcus* and eventually *Pseudomonas*); (4) destructive inflammatory pulmonary disease; and (5) elevated sweat chloride, sodium, and potassium concentrations. CF is a clinical diagnosis that is confirmed by the presence of a positive sweat test result. The sweat test performed by the method of Gibson and Cooke — pilocarpine iontophoresis followed by quantitative analysis of chloride in sweat collected on and eluted from filter paper or gauze pads — has excellent discriminative power for CF in both children and adults. Ninety-six percent of normal people have sweat chloride concentrations below 30 mmol/L and the remainder, below 60 mmol/L. Persons with CF have sweat chloride concentrations between 60 and 160 mmol/L.

CF should be suspected and a sweat test performed on pediatric patients with one or more of the following clinical features: failure to thrive, steatorrhea or maldigestion, meconium ileus, recurrent rectal prolapse, hypoprothrombinemia with purpura (beyond the newborn period), hyponatremia and hypochloremia (in infants), metabolic alkalosis (in older children), heat prostration, and cirrhosis (in children). Sweat tests should also be considered in children with unexplained chronic cough, recurrent or chronic pneumonia, *Staphylococcus* or

Pseudomonas (especially mucoid form) cultured from sputum, and nasal polyps.

Pulmonary Complications

Lung function usually is normal at birth. The first sign of pulmonary involvement is hyperexpansion or increased radiolucency of lung fields on chest x-ray films. This sign is due to the earliest lesion of CF—bronchiolar obstruction with mucus. This obstruction predisposes the individual to infection and inflammation, progressing with time to the larger airways and destruction of airway walls. Mucociliary clearance is impaired. Bronchiolitis, bronchitis, bronchiectasis, peribronchial fibrosis, and large cystic bronchial dilatation occur that may involve all subsegmental bronchi. Alveolar destruction ensues, with infection of atelectatic areas or with episodes of patchy pneumonia and hemorrhagic pneumonia. There is progressive loss of pulmonary function, which may be complicated by massive hemoptysis, recurrent pneumothorax, hypercapnia, hypoxia, and cor pulmonale, all of which are poor prognostic signs. The presence of mucoid strains of *Pseudomonas* in CF sputum also seems to separate the more severe from the milder cases. Mucoid *Pseudomonas* organisms are almost unique to CF. *Pseudomonas cepacia* colonization may also occur during the course of hospitalization of those with severe disease and is increasingly associated with an adverse clinical outcome.

Allergic and Asthmatic Complications

Immediate wheal and flare skin test reactions can be demonstrated in 25 to 50 percent of patients with CF. However, the parallel development of these immune phenomena does not prove cause and effect. Although atopic asthma and CF can coexist, the frequently observed airways hyperreactivity in CF is probably based upon nonimmune mechanisms. Airways hyperreactivity has been demonstrated by histamine and methacholine inhalation challenges and by exercise testing. Increased bronchomotor tone has been demonstrated by its reversibility with isoproterenol, theophylline, and atropine. If either airways hyperreactivity or rhinitis occurs in CF on a specific immune basis, this relationship has yet to be proved by inhalation challenge or provocative nasal challenge with specific allergens.

Pharmacotherapy should be individualized and used in those patients who demonstrate significant improvements in airways obstruction with oral or inhaled bronchodilators. Immunotherapy is not warranted unless there are symptoms present that are associated with clear-cut allergen exposure, as with seasonal allergic asthma or allergic rhinitis.

Nasal polyps can appear either on an allergic or on a chronic inflammatory basis (Oppenheimer and Rosenstein, 1979). In children, nasal polyps most commonly are associated with CF (Schramm and Effron, 1980). Since CF can be present in extremely mild forms, children with nasal polyps should have sweat tests. Pansinusitis occurs in over 90 percent of cases. The overall incidence of nasal polyposis in CF patients is 10 to 15 percent and has been reported to approach 50 percent in the adult population. Ninety percent have pansinusitis, but there is no association between these findings and aspirin idiosyncrasy (Noritake et al., 1981).

Allergic Bronchopulmonary Aspergillosis (ABA) Complication

An association between CF and ABA has been known since 1965 (Mearns et al.). Thirty percent of CF patient groups in the United States (Schwartz et al., 1970) and in London, England (Mearns et al., 1967) have been reported to have serum precipitins to *Aspergillus* antigens. This high prevalence, verified in other studies, indicates a ubiquitous exposure to *Aspergillus* and suggests that ABA might be anticipated as a frequent complication of CF. As can occur in asthma, *Aspergillus* mold spores are easily trapped by mucus in the proximal bronchi, thus providing a milieu for germination, hyphal growth, and antigen stimulation of local and systemic immune responses. One study reported that 57 percent of 46 CF patients were colonized with *Aspergillus fumigatus*; 37 percent had serum precipitins to antigenic extracts of this fungus; 39 percent had positive immediate skin test reactions; and 22 percent had elevated total serum IgE concentrations (Nelson et al., 1979). Seven of the 46 (15 percent) patients developed ABA (Schwartz and Hollick, 1981), according to the accepted diagnostic criteria (Rosenberg et al., 1977). A similar incidence has been reported in a second study (Laufer et al., 1984). The true incidence of ABA in CF is difficult to determine because of variations in mold exposure in different locales (urban vs. rural) and sporadic case-finding efforts among clinics. However, ABA should be anticipated as a complication of CF, and in the milder cases treated with steroids. In the more severe cases, concomitant bacterial antibiotic therapy also may be necessary.

Complications Resembling Other Immune Diseases

In early infancy, CF has been mistaken for gastrointestinal allergy to cow's milk. In these instances, the substitution of soybean formulas has delayed diagnosis and treatment of maldigestion and malabsorption and has contributed to the development of a syndrome of severe failure to thrive, edema, anemia, and hypoproteinemia. This syndrome, amyloidosis (Ristow et al., 1977), and other conditions for which immune complex phenomena have been implicated are listed in Table 48–6 (Berdischewsky et al., 1980; Moss and Lewiston, 1980; Church et al., 1981; Moss, 1983).

Altered Immune Processes

Alterations in immunity may contribute to the pathogenesis of CF (Matthews et al., 1980; Wheeler et al., 1984), and these have been the subject of an extensive review (Shapira and Wilson, 1984). A working hypothesis, outlining these interrelationships and their possible sequence, is presented in Table 48–7.

Approach to Management and Prognostic Considerations

The natural history of CF has changed in the past 50 years. A disease formerly lethal in the first years of life is now one in which the median age of survival has surpassed 18 years. There are many patients in their twenties and

TABLE 48–6. Complications of Cystic Fibrosis that Resemble Other Immune Diseases

Gastrointestinal allergy to cow's milk
Systemic amyloidosis with renal involvement
Vascular purpura and cutaneous vasculitis
Erythema nodosum
Arthritis of pulmonary osteoarthropathy
Transient episodic polyarticular or monarticular arthritis

TABLE 48–7. Hypothesis of Impairment of Immune Function and Hyperimmune Processes that Contribute to the Pathophysiology of Cystic Fibrosis

Basic Defect

1. Basic genetic defect leads to the production of a thickened mucus that coats mucosal surfaces.
2. Thickened mucus
   a. acts as a barrier to antigen penetration.
   b. slows mucociliary clearance.
   c. traps bacteria or fungi, which then proliferate.

Benign Hypogammaglobulinemia

3. Early in the course before (c) occurs, hypogammaglobulinemia is present because gammaglobulin synthesis is not driven by antigenic stimulation due to (a).

Chronic Infection

4. In some patients at early stages and in all at varying stages, (a) is broken down because of (b) and (c) and other intercurrent factors (irritants, pollutants, viral infection).

Hypersensitivity

5. The immune sytem is then chronically stimulated, eventually by antigen excess.
6. Large amounts of specific antibodies are synthesized and hypergammaglobulinemia ensues.
7. Serum IgE and specific IgE antibody production is stimulated in genetically primed subjects, leading to clinical or laboratory findings, or both, similar to atopy.

Immune Complex Formation

8. In antigen excess, soluble complexes occur in local sites (lungs).

Chronic Inflammation

9. The complement system is activated locally with release of vasoactive and chemotactic factors, encouraging neutrophilic inflammation and subsequent tissue injury due to release of proteolytic enzymes by inflammatory cells and by the formation of toxic oxygen radicals.
10. Immune complexes spill over into the circulation, sometimes localizing at distant sites. Immune complexes may form within the bronchial lumen, the bronchial wall, or the alveoli.

Autoimmune Phenomena

11. Chronic antigenic stimulation may also occur from autogenous antigens due to tissue destruction secondary to mucus obstruction of tubes (pancreatic ducts, bile canaliculi).

Secondary Immune Impairment

12. Chronic stimulation of the immune system results in the production of homeostatic regulatory substances that in turn inhibit normal immune function (inhibitory substances for phagocytic and bactericidal function of neutrophils and alveolar macrophages). T-helper/suppressor cells may also be inhibited.

Adapted from Talamo and Schwartz, 1984.

TABLE 48–8. Services Provided by Cystic Fibrosis Centers

Sweat testing and confirmation of diagnosis
Evaluation and outline of therapeutic and prophylactic programs
Education of the patient and the entire family
Instruction in pulmonary physiotherapy and inhalation therapy
Instruction in nutrition, diet, and enzyme replacement
Genetic counseling
Vocational counseling
Financial counseling
Teenage, adult, and parent discussion and support groups
Other consultative services (surgery, allergy, psychiatry)
Hospitalization and treatment for complications
Voluntary research by patients and relatives

thirties who are leading productive lives despite their disabilities. Proper management of patients requires a broad understanding of the pathology of CF; a knowledge of its variable patterns of onset, expression, and complications; and an appreciation of the imposed psychologic, social, and financial stresses. The most capable physician can no longer be the sole provider of the multiple services needed. Pediatricians and internists with specialized training direct CF centers that provide the services summarized in Table 48–8. Personnel at CF centers are trained to coordinate care of patients within the context of family, community, and religious life styles. An informed case manager, whether the primary physician, CF specialist, nurse practitioner, family counselor, or other health professional, is a necessity. Despite progress, the prognosis remains poor. The goal of therapy is not only to increase the span of life but to improve the quality of life. Patients, their families, their caregivers, scientists, and the Cystic Fibrosis Foundation (6931 Arlington Road, Bethesda, Maryland 20814) are working in concert to find an ultimate answer to and cure for this disease.

THE KARTAGENER SYNDROME AND IMMOTILE (DYSKINETIC) CILIA SYNDROME

The Kartagener syndrome consists of a triad of dextrocardia with situs inversus totalis, chronic sinusitis or agenesis of the frontal sinuses, and bronchiectasis. The incidence of the Kartagener syndrome has been estimated at 1 per 50,000 population, whereas the incidence of situs inversus is 1 per 8000 (Adams and Churchill, 1937). Bronchiectasis, which occurs in less than 0.5 percent of the general population, is found in up to 25 percent of patients with situs inversus (Olsen, 1943). Dextrocardia with or without situs inversus may be associated with other anomalies, such as single ventricle, arterial transposition, pulmonary stenosis, ventricular and atrial septal defects, and asplenia. Other associated conditions include nasal polyps, transient deficiency of immunoglobulin A, and mesangiocapillary glomerulonephritis with hypocomplementemia (Egbert et al., 1977).

Kartagener syndrome has been reported among family members; in these cases, the mode of inheritance is thought to be autosomal recessive. Penetrance is variable, as siblings may have bronchiectasis without situs inversus (see subsequent discussion). Transmission from an affected parent to a child has not been reported. An important component of this syndrome is male infertility. Women with Kartagener syndrome have borne children, however.

Pathogenesis

Mucociliary transport is maintained by the rhythmic beating of cilia. Cilia and sperm tails both contain nine microtubular doublet filaments that are arranged symmetrically and radially around a central doublet and are connected to each other by nexin links and to the central sheath by radial spokes. Energy for the shortening of the outer microtubular filaments is provided by the hydrolysis of ATP by ATPase contained in dynein arms, which are attached to one of each doublet. The bending motion and the direction of ciliary beating occurs because of the orientation of the outer microtubules to the central tubules. Absence of dynein arms, radial spokes, or shortening of central tubules have been detected by electron microscopy in patients with immotile cilia, dysmotile cilia, and Kartagener syndrome. Similar structural and functional abnormalities also may be found in bronchitis and other bronchial inflammatory conditions. However, in these cases, the abnormalities are transient, reverting to normal when inflammation subsides. Ciliated epithelia are present in the respiratory tract, paranasal sinuses, eustachian tubes, oviducts, and vas efferentia. Inborn errors of ciliary function explain upper and lower respiratory tract pathology in these syndromes. Additionally, immotile cilia may account for situs inversus

(Afzelius, 1976). Unidirectional embryonic ciliary beating determines organ spiral orientation. There is an even chance of rotation to either side in the absence of ciliary movement. Thus, situs inversus occurs by chance. Immotile cilia and sperm may be found in patients without situs inversus, and 50 percent of those with this defect will have normal organ orientation.

Respiratory Manifestations

Impaired removal of secretions results in sinusitis, otitis media, and recurrent bronchitis. Symptoms of cough, rhinitis, wheezing, and other respiratory difficulties may begin in the first year of life. *Haemophilus influenzae* and *Streptococcus pneumoniae* cause recurrent pneumonia in contrast to *Staphylococcus* and *Pseudomonas* organisms, which are the common pathogens of CF. Chronic pulmonary changes resemble postinfectious interstitial pneumonitis and cylindric, follicular, and saccular bronchiectasis. Persistent cough, sputum production, and recurrent fevers ensue when bronchiectasis becomes severe. Patients with situs inversus may develop left middle lobe pneumonia, atelectasis, and bronchiectasis.

Management and Prognosis

Situs inversus should be diagnosed in the newborn period. As many as 25 percent of these infants will develop bronchiectasis. Anticipatory and preventive measures should be started at the time of diagnosis. These should include immunization against respiratory pathogens — rubeola, pertussis, influenza, pneumococci, and *Haemophilus influenzae* type B — according to age and dosage recommendation; early detection of bacterial infection by culture and treatment with antibiotics; and postural drainage to prevent pooling of secretions. Reproductive and genetic issues must be addressed. However, with proper treatment, these disorders are compatible with normal life expectancies (Rott, 1979).

THE YOUNG SYNDROME

Despite different mechanisms of pathogenesis, both CF and the dysmotile cilia syndromes are associated with male infertility and chronic bronchial inflammation. Men with obstructive azoospermia and chronic sinopulmonary infections have been described (Young, 1970; Hendry et al., 1978; Handelsman et al., 1984). This condition has some features similar to both CF and the dysmotilia syndromes, and it is impossible to exclude the chance that this syndrome is a variant of either CF or the dysmotile syndromes.

THE ECTODERMAL DYSPLASIAS

The ectodermal dysplasias (ED) are a heterogeneous group of disorders (at least 117 separate clinical entities) related to disorganization of tissues derived from primitive ectoderm. The spectrum of disease is great; patients with the mildest forms probably never seek medical attention or remain undiagnosed. Two main forms, the anhidrotic type and the hypohidrotic type, have certain similarities to CF, which include heritability, abnormalities of sweating, abnormalities of respiratory mucus production, increased susceptibility to upper and lower respiratory infections, and high frequency of wheezing. The hypohidrotic type has an increased incidence of atopic sensitization as defined by multiple positive immediate skin tests to common inhalant allergens (Vanselow et al., 1970; Beahrs et al., 1971).

Anhidrotic Type

This disease is inherited as an X-linked recessive disorder. Males inherit the complete form, whereas females usually inherit a partial form. Anhidrosis (no sweating) or severe hypohidrosis, anodontia (no teeth) or severe hypodontia, and hypotrichosis (sparse hair) are the cardinal features that should lead directly to the diagnosis. Other physical findings include prominant frontal bossing, saddle-shaped nose, protruding or deformed ears, thin wrinkled eyelids with prominant supraorbital ridge, thick and protruding lips, and delayed or absent dentition. When present, the incisors are widely spaced and the canines are conically shaped. Anodontia and hypodontia affect both the deciduous and permanent teeth. Other abnormalities found in most patients include sparse, fine, blond hair and absent eyebrow, eyelash, body, axillary, and pubic hair. The skin is smooth and dry; fingernails are dystrophic. Flexural eczema typical of atopic dermatitis has been reported in several cases (Reed et al., 1970; Vanselow et al., 1970).

External manifestations are the result of absent or reduced numbers of skin appendages — hair follicles and sweat, sebaceous, and apocrine glands. Mammary, salivary, and lacrimal glands may be absent in some cases. The cutaneous pathology produces the inability to regulate body temperature in warm weather, resulting in high fevers. Involvement of entodermal elements accounts for both chronic upper and lower respiratory tract disease. Mucous glands of the respiratory tract often are atrophied and in some cases, absent (DeJager, 1965; Capitanio et al., 1969). Deficiency of seromucus interferes with mucociliary clearance in the respiratory tract and leads to dryness, bronchitis, and infection, especially with staphylococci. Allergen sensitization via the respiratory tract may be due to increased permeability of mucosal surfaces. Allergic rhinitis and asthma (both seasonal and perennial) have been described.

Hypohidrotic Type

A positive sweat test result (elevated sodium and chloride concentrations) may occur in the hypohidrotic form, presumably because shortened sweat ducts are unable to reabsorb sodium and chloride maximally from the fluid secreted by sweat coils as an isotonic solution. This type may be associated with sensorineural deafness. Although this condition has only rarely been reported, confusion with CF can occur, and it seems likely that some patients having the hypohidrotic form of ectodermal dysplasia have been misdiagnosed as having CF.

In contrast to the anhidrotic type of ectodermal dysplasia, the hypohidrotic type is inherited as an autosomal dominant trait with complete penetrance. Males and females are equally affected. Female carriers of the X-linked form may have similar clinical findings. These include sparse, thin, fragile hair on the head, eyebrows, and body and dystrophic, thick nails with subungual infections. The skin of the palms and soles is thick, with brownish pigmentation. There may be generalized hypopigmentation, with hyperpigmentation present on the extensor surfaces of the elbow, areolar areas of the breasts, umbilicus, and interphalangeal joints. Fingernails may be dystrophic, occasionally absent, thin, or thickened with striations. Generally, there is no aplasia or hypoplasia of the sweat, sebaceous, and mucous glands. Ci-

liary dyskinesia or dysgenesis in the bronchial epithelium contributes to severe recurrent chest infections (Pabst, 1983).

Management

Anhidrotic patients with respiratory abnormalities require proper environmental humidification and temperature regulation. Patients eventually learn to place damp cloths on their bodies to provide cooling by evaporation. They should be advised to limit exercise in hot weather. Since mucociliary clearance is impaired, those with cough may also benefit from regular postural drainage. Patients should be treated promptly with appropriate antibiotics when upper and lower respiratory infections occur and they should be immunized against respiratory viral and bacterial pathogens. Dentures should be made for those with anodontia and hypodontia.

THE WILLIAMS-CAMPBELL SYNDROME

The Williams-Campbell syndrome (Williams and Campbell, 1960; Mitchell and Bury, 1975; Wayne and Taussig, 1976) is a distinct entity due to a congenital defect in cartilage development in which cartilage is absent, diminished, or soft. The subsequent abnormalities are distributed symmetrically throughout the proximal bronchi and can be demonstrated by bronchography, which shows collapse of proximal bronchi during expiration. Symptoms begin in early infancy, suggesting a congenital origin. Autosomal recessive inheritance, in some cases, has been proposed because of familial occurrence. The prognosis depends upon the extent of the cartilage defect and intercurrent complications and may range from death in infancy to survival to adulthood.

BRONCHIECTASIS

Cylindric, tubular, and pseudobronchiectasis (absence of normal bronchial tapering) frequently follows acute lower respiratory infections and is reversible. Saccular bronchiectasis (irregular bronchial dilitations and narrowings) is irreversible. Large dilitations are referred to as cystic bronchiectasis. Proximal or central bronchiectasis is a late complication of allergic bronchopulmonary aspergillosis. Bronchiectasis usually is acquired, occurring commonly in disorders such as CF, immune deficiency disorders, Kartagener syndrome, alpha-1-antitrypsin deficiency, and rarely severe chronic asthma. Postinfectious bronchiectasis is seen less frequently than in former years. The decreased incidence is due to the decline in measles and pertussis infections, former common precursors of bronchiectasis; the effective use of antibiotics in lingering lower respiratory infections; the control of influenza by current vaccines; the decrease of primary tuberculosis in infancy and early childhood; and the better management of atelectasis and chronic bronchial inflammation (Nemir, 1977). Most acquired postinfectious bronchiectasis now may be a sequela of viral infection, such as influenza (Laraya-Cuasay et al., 1977) and adenovirus, particularly types 3, 7, and 21 (Becroft, 1971). For instance, acute adenoviral infections induce a necrotizing bronchiolitis, which may proceed to bronchiolar obliteration (bronchiolitis obliterans). The consequences of this include atelectasis and inflammation in areas of stagnant secretions, both thought to be the main causes of bronchiectasis. Chronic airways obstruction, due to mucus plugging, foreign body aspiration, and compression or erosion of bronchi by tuberculous lymph nodes, also can lead to bronchiectasis.

Clinical Features and Diagnosis

The cardinal clinical feature of bronchiectasis is chronic cough productive of mucopurulent sputum, which on culture usually yields *Haemophilus influenzae* or *Streptococcus pneumoniae*. Gram-negative organisms, such as *Escherichia coli*, *Proteus*, and *Klebsiella*, also may be cultured after multiple courses of antibiotics. *Staphylococcus* and *Psuedomonas* are the predominant organisms in CF. Bronchiectasis should be anticipated when acute lower respiratory illnesses are slow to resolve, when there is a history of recurrent pulmonary infections, or when there is persistent atelectasis. Lesions may be localized or diffuse. Localized lesions most commonly involve the left lower lobe except with foreign body aspiration, which most commonly involves the right lower lobe. For unknown reasons, the right upper lobe commonly is the first and most severely involved in CF. Physical examination usually reveals rales and crackles in the affected areas. Digital club-

bing occurs usually with diffuse disease but may occur with localized lesions and has been noted to disappear when these are resected.

Bronchiectasis frequently is associated with chronic maxillary sinusitis and each may contribute to the chronicity of the other. *Staphylococcus*, *Streptococcus*, and anaerobic *Bacteroides* organisms may infect the sinuses. The spectrum of bronchiectasis may range from almost asymptomatic localized disease to full-blown chronic diffuse disease. Malnutrition, clubbing, hypoxemia, pulmonary hypertension, and cor pulmonale are late complications. Pneumonia and atelectasis are frequent complications. Bronchopleural fistula and metastatic brain abscess are less common complications since the advent of antibiotics.

Chest roentgenograms may appear normal or may exhibit increased linear markings ("tramline" tracks and ring shadows) due to peribronchial thickening and inflammation. If disease is allowed to progress, small cystic and nodular lesions show a honeycomb-like pattern. Large cysts and bullae occur with most advanced disease. These may be filled with air or with air/fluid and predispose patients to aspergillomas (mycetomas). Today, bronchography is no longer used to diagnose but is reserved to evaluate the extent of involvement when surgery is contemplated.

Management

Nemir (1977) has discussed the medical and surgical treatment of childhood bronchiectasis. Medical management is preferred for patients with minimal disease who are asymptomatic, patients with early disease that may be reversible, and patients with advanced diffuse disease who are unable to tolerate surgery because of greatly impaired pulmonary function. Medical management should include chest physiotherapy, bronchodilators, and appropriate antibiotics. Respiratory bacterial and viral vaccination should be kept current. Medical management should be given for 2 to 4 weeks prior to bronchography to eliminate obstructing bronchial secretions, to minimize infection, and to allow time for resolution of reversible lesions. Surgical treatment is reserved for those symptomatic patients whose disease is localized to one segment or lobe with either a persistent or recurrent obstruction, an infection uncontrolled by antibiotic therapy, a recurrent hemoptysis from a localized source, or a foreign body that cannot be removed by bronchoscopy. In CF, prognosis may be improved by resection when one segment or lobe has far-advanced bronchiectasis and the remaining lung involvement is mild. This situation is unusual, however. Resection should be an elective procedure, if possible.

PULMONARY HEMOSIDEROSIS

Pulmonary hemosiderosis is the result of intra-alveolar hemorrhage (hemorrhagic alveolitis) and deposition of iron as hemosiderin in the interstitium of the lung. Though patients with this condition may exsanguinate, they more frequently develop iron deficiency anemia because of recurrent hemoptysis, sequestration of iron in the lung, or both. After repeated bleeding, pulmonary hemosiderosis and fibrosis ensue with impairment of lung function, including decreased diffusion, decreased compliance, and airways obstruction. Clubbing, pulmonary hypertension, and cor pulmonale may occur in chronic cases. In children, cor pulmonale secondary to adenoidal upper airway obstruction, alveolar hypoventilation especially during sleep, and pulmonary hypertension has been described in association with pulmonary hemosiderosis (Boat et al., 1975). Initially, roentgenograms show diffuse perihilar infiltrates and patchy alveolar densities. Later, diffuse reticular markings and septal thickening are seen with pulmonary fibrosis.

Pathogenesis and Diagnostic Considerations

Pulmonary hemosiderosis may be a primary pulmonary problem or associated with other conditions, such as mitral stenosis with increased pulmonary venous pressure, collagen vascular disease with vasculitis, and other chronic bleeding diatheses. Most cases occur in infants and children except for Goodpasture syndrome (Proskey et al., 1970), which usually afflicts young male adults. In Goodpasture syndrome, the initial acute respiratory episode is soon followed by glomerulonephritis, progressing to renal failure. This arises from the deposition of antibodies, which are formed against glomerular basement membrane, along lung and kidney basement membrane. In infants and children, milk sensitization, milk aspiration, or both are thought to play roles in the

genesis of idiopathic pulmonary hemosiderosis (see subsequent discussion). Heredity may be an additional risk factor because several cases have been described in families (Thaell et al., 1978; Breckenridge and Ross, 1979; Beckerman et al., 1979). There is epidemiologic data to suggest that common environmental factors (insecticides) superimposed on genetically predisposed persons may precipitate recurrent episodes of pulmonary hemorrhage (Cassimos et al., 1983). A history of possible exposure to inhaled toxins (organic phosphate insecticides, chlorobenzene derivatives, and indan derivatives) should be included in the evaluation of all patients with known or suspected idiopathic pulmonary hemosiderosis.

Pulmonary Hemosiderosis in Children Associated with Immune Phenomena

Heiner and Sears (1960) reported the association of chronic respiratory disease in children with multiple circulating precipitins to cow's milk proteins. Heiner et al. (1962) implicated sensitivity to milk proteins as the basis of the chronic disease and added pulmonary hemosiderosis to a syndrome consisting of poor growth, pulmonary and gastrointestinal symptoms, and iron deficiency anemia. Episodic pulmonary bleeding is accompanied by fever, tachycardia, tachypnea, leukocytosis, and elevated erythrocyte sedimentation rate. Hepatosplenomegaly is found in 20 percent of cases. In many cases, symptoms resolve with complete removal of cow's milk from the diet (Levy et al., 1985).

A unique pathogenetic immune mechanism has not been demonstrated for idiopathic pulmonary hemosiderosis with milk precipitins. However, the immune phenomena associated with this syndrome suggest that immune mechanisms are operative. These are peripheral eosinophilia, elevated IgE serum level, LE or tart cells on peripheral blood smear, positive direct Coombs test, circulating cold agglutinins, and increased lymphocyte incorporation of tritiated thymidine on stimulation with milk protein (Stafford et al., 1977).

Some investigators believe that milk sensitization occurs via the gastrointestinal tract. Others have postulated that aspiration accounts both for sensitization and for development of the pulmonary lesions. Milk precipitins have been found in children with defects in swallowing (Peterson and Good, 1962). These precipitins have also been found in association with other pathologic conditions in which there is likelihood of aspiration, e.g., in children with esophageal atresia or stenosis (Handleman and Nelson, 1964) and with Down syndrome (Nelson, 1964; McCrea et al., 1968). Animal experiments further support this aspiration hypothesis (Richerson, 1974; Hensley et al., 1978; Scherzer and Ward, 1978). Acute hemorrhagic alveolitis with inflammation of capillaries can be induced in actively or passively immunized animals by respiratory insufflation of animal proteins or by endotracheal instillation of preformed immune complexes. The reaction has characteristics both of the immune complex disease and of the Arthus reaction.

Diagnosis

The disease should be suspected in any young child with chronic pulmonary symptoms, especially with hemoptysis associated with iron deficiency anemia and typical roentgenographic findings. Many children have chronic rhinitis, recurrent otitis media, failure to thrive, persistent cough, wheezing, tachypnea, pallor, and cyanosis. Others have been described with cor pulmonale secondary to adenoidal upper airway obstruction, alveolar hypoventilation especially during sleep, and pulmonary hypertension (Boat et al., 1975). The diagnosis of intra-alveolar bleeding is confirmed by the finding of hemosiderin-laden alveolar macrophages in sputum, tracheobronchial washings, or gastric aspirates. Since needle biopsies have resulted in massive pulmonary hemorrhage, open lung biopsies should be done only after repeated efforts have been made to find these macrophages in other fluids.

Treatment

In view of the aforementioned considerations, milk should be eliminated completely from the diet in children with chronic or recurrent lower respiratory disease in whom multiple milk precipitins are found. The physician should ask about possible aspiration and should observe the infant's feeding. Dynamic radiologic studies of swallowing (deglutition) may need to be pursued for evidence of subtle aspiration and for evidence of gastroesopha-

geal reflux. If such evidence is found, the elimination of milk, the use of smaller but more frequent feedings, the use of thickened feedings, and the proper positioning of the child after feeding may prevent aspiration and sensitization. Potential environmental toxins should be searched for and eliminated if present. Blood transfusions may be necessary for acute hemoptysis or for severe chronic anemia. Steroids and other immunosuppressive drugs (azathioprine, cyclophosphamide, chlorambucil) have been used empirically. There are no controlled studies to assure their effectiveness in idiopathic pulmonary hemosiderosis. Effective immunosuppressive therapy protocols have been developed for treatment of rapidly progressive glomerulonephritis with pulmonary hemorrhage, including Goodpasture syndrome (Bolton, 1985).

BRONCHOPULMONARY DYSPLASIA

Bronchopulmonary dysplasia (BPD) is a common form of chronic pulmonary disease occurring in neonates and infants who have been treated with high oxygen concentrations and prolonged mechanical positive pressure ventilation for respiratory distress syndrome (RDS). The reported incidence varies from 7 to 36 percent of survivors of neonatal lung disease and its therapy. It may occur also in infants who survive meconium aspiration, persistent fetal circulation, or certain surgically correctable conditions, including diaphragmatic hernia and tracheoesophageal fistula. The condition includes a wide clinical spectrum as the process producing BPD depends upon the necessity for and intensity of prolonged respiratory support therapy of the underlying condition. There is a 30 to 50 percent mortality for severe BPD in the first year of life.

Pathogenesis, Progression, and Prevention

High oxygen tensions produce interstitial edema and epithelial necrosis. Mechanical ventilation produces airway damage that creates edema, increased secretions, and disruption of elastic tissue. The progression of BPD can be classified radiographically through four stages (granular pattern, opacification, fine sponge, coarse sponge) (Northway et al., 1967), which have pathologic correlations (Edwards et al., 1979). Tracheobronchial aspirate cytopathology analysis gives a more dynamic picture of the inflammatory nature of the process (Merritt et al., 1981). After 1 to 4 days, specimens show organized sheets and single cells of bronchial epithelium. After 4 to 10 days of ventilation, bronchial cells appear damaged with cytoplasmic deterioration and smudged and pyknotic nuclei. Polymorphonuclear leukocytes predominate, followed by monocytes and macrophages which then predominate. These cells are vacuolated and contain abundant mitochondria, suggesting activation. After 10 days of ventilation, bronchial epithelial cells with increased nuclear/cytoplasmic ratios, multiple nucleoli, and large chromocenters appear and suggest regeneration. Multinucleated histiocytes appear late and are associated with pulmonary "air leaks," especially pulmonary interstitial emphysema. It is thought that lung injury is initiated by toxic oxygen radicals and proteolytic enzymes released from polymorphonuclear leukocytes attracted to the site by chemotactic substances released from alveolar macrophages that have been activated by high oxygen tensions. Alveolar macrophages also release toxic, oxygen-free radicals and proteases (e.g., elastase). Anti-inflammatory therapy and anti-oxidant therapy (vitamin E) are potential avenues to modify the progressive events occurring in BPD. The more recent successful use of insufflated surfactant to prevent RDS may very well prevent the induction of its iatrogenic sequela, BPD (Shapiro et al., 1985). (Nebulized cromolyn sodium has appeared to be useful in a pilot clinical trial.)

Long-Term Management and Prognosis

Infants who survive the initial airways obstruction, air trapping, bleb formation, decreased compliance, and maldistribution in gas exchange frequently exhibit long-term abnormal roentgenographic findings. These include hyperaeration, coarse interstitial markings, atelectasis, and bilateral cystic changes, which may persist for months. Chronic or recurrent tachypnea and retractions and wheezing are not unusual; periodic respiratory exacerbations with wheezing, especially with viral respiratory infections, are common especially in infancy. Children with BPD require close follow-up. Mild chronic symptoms can be managed with

chest physiotherapy and bronchodilators to create an optimal pulmonary toilet and minimize atelectasis. Those with severe BPD may require permanent tracheostomy and assisted ventilation. Because of the pulmonary growth potential early in life, sufficient recovery from BPD to minimize development of chronic obstructive lung disease is possible. Long-term survivors of BPD may have evidence of airway obstruction, hyperinflation, and airway hyperreactivity (Bader et al., 1987).

SARCOIDOSIS

Sarcoidosis is a multisystem, noncaseating granulomatous, inflammatory disorder that primarily affects the lung. Its etiology is unknown. Genetic factors may be important because it occurs most commonly among northern European and American blacks. The diagnosis is most frequently made between the ages of 20 and 40 years. Although fewer than 200 cases of sarcoidosis have been reported in children, it may be underdiagnosed in this age group (Kendig, 1977). Sarcoidosis has been seen as early as 2 months of age, but the diagnosis usually is made later, at 9 to 15 years of age. The disease most commonly resolves spontaneously and completely, but in 20 percent of cases proceeds to fibrosis. Reactivation of quiescent disease is known.

Clinical Manifestations

Symptoms at first may be protean, the most common being lassitude, apathy, and malaise. Symptoms referrable to the respiratory tract often consist of dry, hacking cough, and mild to moderate shortness of breath. Patients present with other complaints, such as fever, weight loss, adenopathy, and vision loss. Other diseases that produce granulomatous lesions, which should be considered in the differential diagnosis, include tuberculosis, histoplasmosis, cocciodioidomycosis, chronic granulomatous disease, berylliosis, farmer's lung (hypersensitivity pneumonitis), and aspergillosis. The chest roentgenogram of advanced sarcoidosis may be indistinguishable from that of advanced CF, but bilateral hilar adenopathy is of particular importance as a diagnostic point.

Sarcoidosis may affect any organ or part of the body. The following also are seen in sarcoidosis: enlarged lymph nodes (54 percent of cases); eye involvement with uveitis and iritis (42 percent of cases); skin lesions (45 percent of cases), consisting of small discrete nodules, large conglomerate masses, or large flat plaques varying in color from waxy yellow to reddish blue; uveoparotid fever (12 percent of cases) with uveitis, parotid gland swelling, and fever frequently associated with facial nerve palsy; and hepatic (18 percent of cases) and splenic (23 percent of cases) involvement, leading to portal hypertension, hypersplenism, and in some cases massive sarcoid splenomegaly. In addition, bone lesions (24 percent of cases) are found in patients with chronic skin lesions and consist of either single or multiple punched out areas in metacarpals or metatarsals. Hypercalcemia and hypercalciuria, caused by increased absorption of dietary calcium as a result of increased sensitivity to vitamin D, result in nephrocalcinosis, nephrolithiasis, and chronic renal disease. Sarcoid granulomas may involve the myocardium, central nervous system, and endocrine glands. Cardiac arrhythmias, seizures, hypopituitarism, diabetes insipidus, adrenal insufficiency, and thyroiditis have been reported in both adults and children.

Etiology and Immunology

The etiology of sarcoidosis is unknown. The pulmonary lesion begins as alveolitis, with helper T cells and alveolar macrophages the predominant cell types. Their presence indicates active inflammation that may be reversible. Neutrophil infiltration is the forerunner of fibrotic end-stage pulmonary disease, which occurs in a minority of patients. Concomitant with active alveolitis, there is depressed cell-mediated immunity as manifested by delayed skin test anergy. This anergy is thought to be due to the paucity of peripheral circulating helper T cells. Hypergammaglobulinemia is common.

The Kveim Test

This test has been used to confirm the diagnosis of sarcoidosis and is positive in 80 percent of cases. The antigen, however, has not been standardized and its safety has not been established. It is prepared and used by those individuals who are engaged in research on sarcoidosis. Skin test antigen is prepared from extracts of spleens from patients with active sarcoidosis.

The material is injected intradermally as in the tuberculin test, and the site is observed for 6 weeks. If a nodule forms, this is biopsied; the specimen is considered positive if a granuloma typical of sarcoid is seen.

Management and Prognosis

Staging of disease involvement and activity provides a rational approach to therapy (Albelda and Daniele, 1985). This is done by history, physical examination, chest roentgenograms, and pulmonary function tests. Active inflammation can be distinguished from end-stage pulmonary fibrosis by open lung biopsy. Noninvasive techniques provide safer additional approaches to serial evaluations. Bronchoalveolar lavage, gallium-67 scanning, and serum angiotensin converting–enzyme (SACE) measurement are helpful methods, which are becoming available in specialized medical centers. Activated T lymphocytes in lavage fluid reflect active alveolitis. Chronic stages have increased numbers of polymorphonuclear leukocytes. Increased pulmonary uptake of gallium-67 by alveolar macrophages suggests active alveolitis. Gallium-67 scanning also localizes nonpulmonary areas of activity. SACE is found in pulmonary endothelial cells. Increased levels are from granulomatous tissue. Elevated SACE levels are found in 50 to 75 percent of sarcoid patients. However, SACE levels may be elevated in patients with cirrhosis, hyperthyroidism, and diabetes mellitus. When SACE levels are elevated in sarcoidosis, their measurement may be useful in following disease activity and response to therapy.

Systemic steroid therapy is indicated when there is progressive or severe systemic involvement without pulmonary disease (Stage 0). Topical steroids are effective in the treatment of anterior uveitis and skin lesions. In some cases, chloroquine is helpful in therapy of skin disease. Colchicine and other nonsteroidal anti-inflammatory agents have been used to treat systemic symptoms (fevers, arthralgias, erythema nodosum). Patients with hilar adenopathy and normal pulmonary function test results (Stage I) are treated only if there is deterioration of pulmonary function or roentgenographic abnormalities on serial determinations. Patients with pulmonary parenchymal disease with or without hilar or mediastinal adenopathy (Stages II and III) are treated if and when they develop pulmonary function abnormalities. Since so few cases of sarcoidosis have been described in children, the long-term prognosis is difficult to determine as is the efficacy of steroid therapy. Prognosis appears to be better in children than in adults. Most cases resolve spontaneously. When steroids are used, prompt resolution of clinical manifestations occurs (Kendig and Brummer, 1976).

PULMONARY FIBROSIS

Pulmonary fibrosis is the end stage of several different inflammatory processes of the alveolar wall (interstitial pneumonitis) initiated by known and unknown etiologic events. Some cases may be genetically determined (Bonnani et al., 1965). Familial associations of both desquamative interstitial pneumonia (Tal et al., 1984) and lymphoid interstitial pneumonia (O'Brodovich et al., 1980) have been reported in children. Pulmonary fibrosis and interstitial fibrosis occur with connective tissue diseases (systemic lupus erythematosus, dermatomyositis, scleroderma, rheumatoid arthritis), other diseases with immune features (Sjögren syndrome, Hashimoto thyroiditis, chronic active hepatitis, hypergammaglobulinemic renal tubular acidosis, ulcerative colitis, sarcoidosis, chronic hypersensitivity pneumonitis), the use of cytotoxic drugs (bleomycin, busulfan, cytoxan, hexamethonium, hydantoin, hydralazine, mecamylamine, melphalan), drug sensitivity (nitrofurantoin) (Rosenow, 1972), and viral infections (Laraya-Cuasay, 1978). When its etiology is unknown, pulmonary fibrosis has been called idiopathic or referred to in other clinical nonetiologic terms (e.g., Hamman-Rich syndrome, interstitial fibrosis, cryptogenic fibrosing alveolitis, honeycomb lung).

Histopathologic Classification of Interstitial Pneumonias

Liebow (1975) has classified the interstitial pneumonias on the basis of the type and location of the inflammatory process as follows: usual interstitial pneumonia (UIP), desquamative interstitial pneumonia (DIP), lymphoid interstitial pneumonia (LIP), giant cell interstitial pneumonia (GIP), and bronchiolitis obliterans with interstitial pneumonia (BIP). These descriptions give little etiologic information but provide prognostic and therapeutic information that justify open lung biopsy for initial de-

finitive diagnosis. When viral cultures are positive, an etiologic diagnosis can be established. A histologically confirmed diagnosis of chronic LIP in a child (under 13 years of age) is considered indicative of acquired immune deficiency syndrome (AIDS) unless test results for HTLV-III (HIV) are negative. An inflammatory alveolitis precedes pulmonary fibrosis of varying degrees, frequently progressive and ultimately fatal. Less invasive techniques can be used to assess the alveolitis longitudinally and its response to treatment. Gallium-67 scanning of the lung detects the extent and location of alveolitis. Gallium-67 is taken up by neutrophils and activated macrophages, which constitute most of the inflammatory cells in idiopathic pulmonary fibrosis. Bronchoalveolar lavage and analysis of cellular components can detect lymphocytes, neutrophils, and eosinophils. High intensity alveolitis, the precursor of fibrosis, is characterized by neutrophilia or eosinophilia (Applebaum and Hunninghake, 1985).

Clinical Course, Treatment, and Prognosis

Alveoli, their lining cells, basement membranes, capillaries, and connective tissues become involved in the inflammatory reaction. Macrophages, lymphocytes, neutrophils, and eosinophils destroy and derange pulmonary components through the action of mediators, enzymes, and toxic oxygen radicals. The chronic alveolitis results in the fibrotic process affecting not only alveoli but also alveolar ducts, bronchioles, and supporting structures. Early in the process, the chest roentgenogram shows a diffuse ground glass appearance, accentuated perihilar markings, and patchy infiltrates. Late in the disease process, the characteristic honeycomb-like lung is seen. Alveolar wall fibrosis in both children and adults implies a poor prognosis (Patchefesky et al., 1973). Infants, children, and adults with desquamative interstitial pneumonias respond to steroid therapy. A patient may present with a variable clinical picture (including cough, tachypnea, cyanosis, and failure to thrive). A careful history may detect that this has occurred 1 day to several weeks after a viral respiratory infection. The course can be rapid as in the Hamman-Rich syndrome, with dry cough and severe progressive dyspnea ending in respiratory failure and cor pulmonale within months of the onset of symptoms. The course also can be slower, incomplete, or nonprogressive. Pulmonary fibrosis is a restrictive lung disease; pulmonary function studies demonstrate reductions in lung volumes, carbon monoxide diffusing capacity, and compliance. Hypoxemia that becomes more severe with exercise also is a common feature and reflects disruption of the alveolar-capillary unit. The mainstay of therapy is to retard or to abort the inflammatory reaction if this is not spontaneous. Conventional therapy is with glucocorticosteroids. If this fails, cytotoxic agents (cyclophosphamide) are added. Since these conditions are uncommon in children, the initiation and type of therapy must be based upon experience with adults.

REFERENCES

Adams, R., Churchill, E.D.: Situs inversus, sinusitis, bronchiectasis: Report of five cases including frequency statistics. J. Thorac. Surg. 7:206, 1937.

Afzelius, B.A.: A human syndrome caused by immotile cilia. Science 193:317, 1976.

Albelda, S.M., Daniele, R.P.: Sarcoidosis. In Current Therapy in Allergy, Immunology and Rheumatology. Lichtenstein, L.M., Fauci, A.S. (eds.), 1985–1986. Philadelphia, B.C. Decker Inc.

Applebaum, M.L., Hunninghake, G.W.: Idiopathic Pulmonary Fibrosis. In Current Therapy in Allergy, Immunology and Rheumatology, 1985–1986. Lichenstein, L.M., Fauci, A.S. (eds.), Philadelphia, B.C. Decker Inc., 1985–1986.

Bader, D., Ramos, A.D., Lew, C.D., Platzker, A.C.G., Stabile, M.W., Keens, T.G.: Childhood sequelae of infant lung disease: Exercise and pulmonary function abnormalities after bronchopulmonary dysplasia. J. Pediatr. 110:693–699, 1987.

Beahrs, J.O., Lillington, G.A., Rosa, R.C., Russin, L., Lindgren, J.A., Rowley, P.T.: Anhidrotic ectodermal dysplasia: Predisposition to bronchial disease. Ann. Int. Med. 74:92, 1971.

Beckerman, R.C., Taussig, L.M., Pinnas, J.L.: Familial idiopathic pulmonary hemosiderosis. Am. J. Dis. Child. 133:609, 1979.

Becroft, D.M.O.: Bronchiolitis obliterans, bronchiectasis and other sequelae of adenovirus type 21 infection in young children. J. Clin. Pathol. 24:72, 1971.

Berdischewsky, M., Pollack, M., Young, L.S., et al.: Circulating immune complexes in cystic fibrosis. Pediatr. Res. 14:830–833, 1980.

Boat, T.F., Polmar, S.H., Whitman, V., Kleinerman, J.I., Stern, R.C., Doershuk, C.F.: Hyperreactivity to cow milk in young children with pulmonary hemosiderosis and cor pulmonale secondary to nasopharyngeal obstruction. J. Pediatrics, 87:23, 1975.

Bois, E., Feingold, J., Demanais, F., Runavot, Y., Jehanne, M., Toudic, L.: Cluster of cystic fibrosis cases in a limited area of Brittany (France). Clin. Genet. 14:73, 1978.

Bolton, W. K.: Goodpasture's syndrome and rapidly progressive glomerulonephritis. In Current Therapy in Allergy, Immunology and Rheumatology. Lichtenstein, L.M., Fauci, A.S. (eds.), Philadelphia, B.C. Decker, Inc., 1985.

Bonnani, P.P., Frymoyer, J.W., Jacox, R.F.: A family study of idiopathic pulmonary fibrosis: A possible dysproteinemic and genetically determined disease. Am. J. Med. 39:411, 1965.

Breckenridge, R.L., Ross, J.S.: Familial pulmonary hemosiderosis. A report of familial occurrence. Chest 75:5, 1979.

Brock, D.J.H.: Amniotic fluid alkaline phosphatase isoenzymes in early prenatal diagnosis of cystic fibrosis. Lancet 2:941, 1983.

Bryan, M.H., Hardie, M.J., Reilly, B.J., Swyer, P.R.: Pulmonary function studies during the first year of life in infants recovering from respiratory distress syndrome. Pediatrics 52:169, 1973.

Capitanio, M.A., Chen, J.T.T., Arey, J.B., Kirkpatrick, J.A.: Congenital anhidrotic ectodermal dysplasia. Am. J. Roentgen. 103:168, 1968.

Carswell, F., Oliver, J., Silverman, M.: Allergy in cystic fibrosis. Clin. Exp. Immunol. 35:141–146, 1979.

Cassimos, C.D., Chryssanthopoulos, C., Panagiotidou, C.: Epidemiologic observations in idiopathic pulmonary hemosiderosis. J. Pediatr. 102:698, 1983.

Church, J.A., Jordan, S.C., Keens, T.G., Wang, C-I.: Circulating immune complexes in patients with cystic fibrosis. Chest 80:405–411, 1981.

Coury, A.J., Fogt, E.J., Norenberg, M.S., Untereker, D.F.: Development of a screening system for cystic fibrosis. Clin. Chem. 29/9:1593–1597, 1983.

Davis, P.B., Hubbard, V.S., McCoy, K., Taussig, L.M.: Familial bronchiectasis, J. Pediatr. 102:177, 1983.

De Jager, H.: Congenital anhidrotic ectodermal dysplasia: Case report. J. Path. Bacteriol. 90:321, 1965.

Denning, C.R., Huang, N.N., Cuassay, L.R., Shwachman, H., Tocci, P., Warwick, W.J., Gibson, L.E.: Cooperative study comparing three methods of performing sweat tests to diagnose cystic fibrosis. Pediatrics 66:752, 1980.

di Sant'Agnese, P.A., Davis, P.B.: Cystic fibrosis in adults. 75 cases and a review of 232 cases in the literature. Am. J. Med. 66:121, 1979.

Edwards, D.K., Colby, T.V., Northway, W.H.: Radiographic-pathologic correlations in bronchopulmonary dysplasia. J. Pediatr. 95:835, 1979.

Egbert, B.M., Schwartz, E., Kempson, R.L.: Kartagener's syndrome: Report of a case with mesangiocapillary glomerulonephritis. Arch. Pathol. Lab. Med. 101:95, 1977.

Gell, P.G.H., Coombs, R.R.A.: Clinical Aspects of Immunology. Philadelphia, F.A. Davis Co., 1964.

Gorvoy, J.D.: Allergic bronchopulmonary aspergillosis in a patient with cystic fibrosis and prolonged use of marihuana. Cystic Fibrosis Club Abstracts, 25th Annual Meeting. San Jose, Cal., April 27–30, 25:79, 1984.

Gusella, J.F., Wexler, N.S., Conneally, P.M., Naylor, S.L., Anderson, M.A., Tanzi, R.E., Watkins, P.C., Ottina, K., Wallace, M.R., Sakaguchi, A.Y., Young, A.B., Shoulson, I., Bonilla, E., Martin, J.B.: A polymorphic DNA marker genetically linked to Huntington's disease. Nature, 306:234, 1983.

Hall, C.B., Hall, W.J., Gala, C.L., et al.: Long-term prospective study in children after respiratory syncytial virus infection. J. Pediatr. 105:358, 1984.

Handleman, N.I., Nelson, T.L.: Association of milk precipitins with esophageal lesions causing aspiration. Pediatrics 34:699, 1964.

Handelsman, D.J., Conway, A.J., Boylan, L.M., Turtle, J.R.: Young's syndrome: Obstructive azoospermia and chronic sinopulmonary infections. N. Engl. J. Med. 310:3, 1984.

Heiner, D.C., Sears, J.W.: Chronic respiratory disease associated with multiple circulating precipitins to cow's milk. Am. J. Dis. Child. 100:500, 1960.

Heiner, D.C., Sears, J.W., Kniker, W.T.: Multiple precipitins to cow's milk in chronic respiratory disease. Am. J. Dis. Child. 103:40, 1962.

Hendry, W.F., Knight, R.K., Whitfield, H.N., Stansfield, A.G., Pryse-Davies, J., Ryder, T.A., Pavia, D., Bateman, J.R.M., Clarke, S.W.: Obstructive azoospermia: Respiratory function tests, electron microscopy, and results of surgery. Brit. J. Urol. 50:598, 1978.

Hensley, G.T., Fink, J.N., Barboriak, J.J.: Hypersensitivity pneumonitis in the monkey. Arch. Pathol. 97:33, 1974.

Hinson, K.F.W., Moon, A.J., Plummer, W.S.: Bronchopulmonary aspergillosis. Thorax 7:317–333, 1952.

Jaffe, B.F., Strome, M., Khaw, K.T., Shwachman, H.: Nasal polypectomy and sinus surgery for cystic fibrosis—a 10 year review. Otolaryngol. Clin. N. Am. 10:81–90, 1977.

Kendig, E.L.: Chronic lung disease in children. Hosp. Pract. 87–98, 1977.

Kendig, E.L., Brummer, D.L.: Prognosis of sarcoidosis in children. Chest 70:351, 1976.

Klinger, K.W.: Cystic fibrosis in the Ohio Amish: Gene frequency and founder effect. Hum. Genet. 65:94, 1983.

Laraya-Cuasay, L.R.: Pulmonary sequelae of acute viral infections. Pediatr. Ann. 7:21, 1978.

Laraya-Cuasay, L.R., DeForest, A., Huff, D., Lischner, H., Huang, N.N.: Chronic pulmonary complications of early influenza virus infection in children. Am. Rev. Respir. Dis. 116:617, 1977.

Larsen, G.L., Barron, R.J., Cotton, E.K., Brooks, J.G.: A comparative study of atropine sulfate and isoproterenol hydrochloride in cystic fibrosis. Am. Rev. Respir. Dis. 117:298, 1978.

Laufer, P., Fink, J.N., Bruns, T., Unger, G.F., Kalbfleisch, J.H., Greenberger, P.A., Patterson, R.: Allergic bronchopulmonary aspergillosis in cystic fibrosis. J. Allergy Clin. Immunol. 73:44–48, 1984.

Levy, J., Kolski, G.B., Scanlin, T.F.: Hemoptysis and anemia in a 3-year-old boy. Ann. Allergy 55:441, 1985.

Liebow, A.A.: Definition and classification of interstitial pneumonias in human pathology. Hum. Pathol. Prog. Respir. Res. 8:1, 1975.

Matthews, W.J., Williams, M., Oliphint, B., Geha, R., Colten, H.R.: Hypogammaglobulinemia in patients with cystic fibrosis. N. Engl. J. Med. 302:245–249, 1980.

McCrea, M.G., Heston, J.F., Wood, H.F., Sullivan, J.E.: Milk precipitins: A serologic survey of 932 individuals. J.A.M.A. 203:557, 1968.

Mearns, M., Longbottom, J., Batten, J.C.: Precipitating antibodies to *Aspergillus fumigatus* in cystic fibrosis. Lancet 1:538–539, 1967.

Mearns, M., Young, W., Batten, J.: Transient pulmonary infiltrations in cystic fibrosis due to allergic aspergillosis. Thorax 20:385–392, 1965.

Mellis, C.M., Levison, H.: Bronchial reactivity in cystic fibrosis. Pediatrics 61:446–450, 1978.

Merritt, T.A., Stuard, I.D., Puccia, J., Wood, B., Edwards, D.K., Finkelstein, J., Shapiro, D.L.: Newborn tracheal aspirate cytology: Classification during respiratory distress syndrome and bronchopulmonary dysplasia. J. Pediatr. 98:949, 1981.

Middleton, E., Reed, C.E., Ellis, E.F. (eds.): Allergy: Principles and Practice, 2nd ed. St. Louis, C.V. Mosby Co., 1983.

Mitchell, R.E., Bury, R.G.: Congenital bronchiectasis due to deficiency of bronchial cartilage. J. Pediatr. 87:230, 1975.

Moss, R.B.: Immunology of cystic fibrosis: immunity, immunodeficiency and hypersensitivity. In Textbook of Cystic Fibrosis. Lloyd-Still, J.D. (ed.), Boston, John Wright PSG, 1983.

Moss, R.B., Lewiston, N.J.: Immune complexes and humoral responses to *Pseudomonas aeruginosa* in cystic fibrosis. Am. Rev. Respir. Dis. 121:23–29, 1980.

Nadler, H.L., Ben-Yoseph, Y.: Genetics. In Cystic Fibrosis. Taussig, L.M. (ed.), New York, Thieme-Stratton Inc., 1984.

Nelson, L.A., Callerame, M.L., Schwartz, R.H.: Aspergillosis and atopy in cystic fibrosis. Am. Rev. Respir. Dis. 120:863–873, 1979.

Nelson, T.L.: Spontaneously occurring milk antibodies in mongoloids. Am. J. Dis. Child. 108:494, 1964.

Nemir, R.L.: Bronchiectasis. In Disorders of the Respiratory Tract in Children. Kendig, E.L., Chernick, V. (eds.), Philadelphia, W.B. Saunders Co., 1977.

Noritake, D., Hen, J., Dolan, T.F.: Effects of aspirin on pulmonary function in patients with cystic fibrosis. Cystic Fibrosis Club Abstracts, 22nd Annual Meeting. San Francisco, Cal., May 1, 22:144, 1981.

Northway, W.H., Rosan, R.C., Porter, D.Y.: Pulmonary disease following respiratory therapy of hyaline membrane disease. N. Engl. J. Med. 276:357, 1967.

O'Brodovich, H.M., Moser, M.M., Lu, L.: Familial lymphoid interstitial pneumonia: A long-term follow-up, Pediatrics 65:523, 1980.

Olsen, A.M.: Bronchiectasis and dextrocardia: Observations on aetiology of bronchiectasis. Am. Rev. Tuberc. 47:435, 1943.

Oppenheimer, E.H., Rosenstein, B.J.: Differential pathology of nasal polyps in cystic fibrosis and atopy. Lab. Invest. 40:445–449, 1979.

Pabst, H.F., Groth, O., McCoy, E.E.: Hypohidrotic Ectodermal Dysplasia with Hypothyroidism. In Mendelian Inheritance In Man, 6th ed. McKusick, V.A., (ed.), Baltimore, The Johns Hopkins University Press, 1983.

Patchefesky, A.S., Fraimow, W., Hoch, W.S.: Desquamative interstitial pneumonia: Pathologic findings and follow-up in thirteen patients. Arch. Int. Med. 132:222, 1973.

Peterson, R.D.A., Good, R.A.: Antibodies to cow's milk proteins—their presence and significance. Pediatrics 31:209, 1962.

Proskey, A.J., Weatherbee, L., Easterling, R.E., et al.: Goodpasture's syndrome: A report of five cases and review of the literature. Am. J. Med. 48:162, 1970.

Quinton, P.M., Bijman, J.: Higher bioelectric potentials due to decreased chloride absorption in the sweat glands of patients with cystic fibrosis, N. Engl. J. Med. 308:1185–1189, 1983.

Rachelefsky, G.S., Coulson, A., Siegel, S.C., Stiehm, E.R.: Aspirin intolerance in chronic childhood asthma detected by oral challenge. Pediatrics 56:443, 1975.

Rachelefsky, G.S., Osher, A., Dooley, R.E., Ank, B., Stiehm, E.R.: Coexistent respiratory allergy and cystic fibrosis. Am. J. Dis. Child. 128:355–359, 1974.

Reed, W.B., Lopez, D.A., Landing, B.: Clinical spectrum of anhidrotic ectodermal dysplasia. Arch. Dermatol. 102:134, 1970.

Richerson, H.B.: Varieties of acute immunologic damage to the rabbit lung. Ann. N.Y. Acad. Sci. 221:340, 1974.

Ricketti, A.J., Greenberger, P.A., Patterson, R.: Serum IgE as an important aid in management of allergic bronchopulmonary aspergillosis. J. Allergy Clin. Immunol. 74:68–71, 1984.

Ristow, S.C., Condemi, J.J., Stuard, I.D., Schwartz, R.H.,

Bryson, M.F.: Systemic amyloidosis in cystic fibrosis. Am. J. Dis. Child. 131:886, 1977.

Rosenberg, M., Patterson, R., Mintzer, R., et al.: Clinical and immunologic criteria for the diagnosis of allergic bronchopulmonary aspergillosis. Ann. Intern. Med. 86:405–414, 1977.

Rosenow, E.C.: The spectrum of drug-induced pulmonary disease. Ann. Int. Med. 77:977, 1972.

Rott, H.D.: Kartagener's syndrome and the syndrome of immotile cilia. Hum. Genet. 46:541, 1979.

Scherzer, H., Ward, P.A.: Lung and dermal vascular injury produced by preformed immune complexes. Am. Rev. Respir. Dis. 117:551, 1978.

Schiotz, P.O., Hoiby, N., Juhl, F., et al.: Immune complexes in cystic fibrosis. Acta Microbiol. Scand. 85:67–74, 1977.

Schramm, V.L., Effron, M.Z.: Nasal polyps in children. Laryngoscope 90:1488–1495, 1980.

Schroeder, W.T., Miller, M.F., Woo, S.L.C., Saunders, G.F.: Chromosomal localization of the human alpha-1-antitrypsin gene(PI) to 14q31–32. Am. J. Hum. Genet. 37:868, 1985.

Schwartz, R.H., Doherty, R.A.: Thirty-one cases of cystic fibrosis in an Amish-Mennonite kindred. Cystic Fibrosis Club Abstracts. Rockville, Maryland, Cystic Fibrosis Foundation, 25:213, 1984.

Schwartz, R.H., Hollick, G.E.: Allergic bronchopulmonary aspergillosis with low serum immunoglobulin E. J. Allergy Clin. Immunol. 68:290–294, 1981.

Schwartz, R.H., Johnstone, D.E., Holsclaw, D.S., Dooley, R.R.: Serum precipitins to *Aspergillus fumigatus* in cystic fibrosis. Am. J. Dis. Child. 120:432–433, 1970.

Shapira, E., Wilson, G.B.: Immunological Aspects of Cystic Fibrosis: CRC Series in Immunology and Lymphoid Cell Biology. Boca Raton, Florida, CRC Press, Inc., 1984.

Shapiro, D.L., Notter, R.H., Morin, F.C., Deluga, K.S., Golub, L.M., Sinkin, R.A., Weiss, K.I., Cox, C.: Double-blind, randomized trial of a calf lung surfactant extract administered at birth to very premature infants for prevention of respiratory distress syndrome. Pediatrics 76:593, 1985.

Shen, J., Brackett, R., Fischer, T., Holder, A., Kellog, F., Michael, J.G.: Specific *Pseudomonas* immunoglobulin E antibodies in sera of patients with cystic fibrosis. Infect. Immunol. 32:967–968, 1981.

Silverman, M., Hobbs, F.D.R., Gordon, I.R.S., Carswell, F.: Cystic fibrosis, atopy, and airways lability. Arch. Dis. Child. 53:873–877, 1978.

Sorensen, R.U.: Immune responses to *Pseudomonas* and other bacteria in cystic fibrosis patients. In Immunolog-

ical Aspects of Cystic Fibrosis. Shapira, E., Wilson, G.B., (eds.), Boca Raton, Florida, CRC Press, 1984.

Soter, N.A., Mihm, M.C., Colten, H.R.: Cutaneous necrotizing venulitis in patients with cystic fibrosis. J. Pediatr. 95:197–201, 1979.

Stafford, H.A., Polmar, S.H., Boat, T.F.: Immunologic studies in cow's milk–induced pulmonary hemosiderosis. Pediatr. Res. 11:898, 1977.

Tal, A., Maor, E., Bar-Ziv, J., Gorodischer, R.: Fatal desquamative interstitial pneumonia in three infant siblings. J. Pediatr. 104:873, 1984.

Talamo, R.C., Schwartz, R.H.: Immunologic and Allergic Manifestations. In Cystic Fibrosis. Taussig, L.M. (ed.), New York, Thieme-Stratton Inc., 1984.

Thaell, J.F., Greipp, P.R., Stubbs, S.E., et al.: Idiopathic pulmonary hemosiderosis: Two cases in a family. Mayo Clin. Proc. 53:113, 1978.

Tobin, M.J., Maguire, O., Reen, D., Tempany, E., Fitzgerald, M.X.: Atopy and bronchial reactivity in older patients with cystic fibrosis. Thorax 35:807–813, 1980.

Vanselow, N.A., Yamate, M., Adams, M.S., Callies, Q.: The increased prevalence of allergic disease in anhidrotic congenital ectodermal dysplasia. J. Allergy 45:302, 1970.

Warner, J.O., Norman, A.P., Soothill, J.F.: Cystic fibrosis heterozygosity in the pathogenesis of allergy. Lancet 1:990–991, 1976.

Warner, J.O., Taylor, B.W., Norman, A.P., Soothill, J.F.: Association of cystic fibrosis with allergy. Arch. Dis. Child. 51:507–511, 1976.

Watkins, P.C., Schwartz, R.H., Hoffman, N., Stanislovitis, P., Doherty, R., Klinger, K.: A linkage study of cystic fibrosis in extended multigenerational pedigrees. Am. J. Hum. Genet. 39:735–743, 1986.

Wayne, K.S., Taussig, L.M.: Probable familial congenital bronchiectasis due to cartilage deficiency (Williams-Campbell syndrome). Am. Rev. Respir. Dis. 114:15, 1976.

Wheeler, W.B., Williams, M., Matthews, W.J., Colten, H.R.: Progression of cystic fibrosis lung disease as a function of serum immunoglobulin G levels: a 5-year longitudinal study. J. Pediatr. 104:695–699, 1984.

Williams, H., Campbell, P.: Generalized bronchiectasis associated with deficiency of cartilage in the bronchial tree. Arch. Dis. Child. 35:182, 1960.

Young, D.: Surgical treatment of male infertility. J. Reprod. Fertil. 23:541, 1970.

Zambie, M.F., Gupta, S., Lemen, R.J., Hilman, B., Waring, W.W., Sly, R.M.: Relationship between response to exercise and allergy in patients with cystic fibrosis. Ann. Allergy 42:290–294, 1979.

49

Chronic Obstructive Pulmonary Diseases in Adults

E. FERNANDEZ, M.D.
R. MASON, M.D.

Difficulty on expiration is the hallmark of certain diseases of the lung. Etiologies of "obstructive disease of the airways" are diverse, but degrees of impediment to expiration can be assessed quantitatively with similar types of function tests. Consequently, nonspecific designations commonly are used to refer to various disease entities, such as chronic obstructive pulmonary disease (COPD), chronic obstructive lung disease (COLD), and chronic airway obstruction (CAO).

MAGNITUDE OF THE PROBLEM

In the last 35 years, COPD has grown to become a major health problem. Morbidity, disability, and death due to chronic bronchitis and emphysema have become increasingly common. This trend was preceded by a substantial increase in cigarette smoking. The National Health Survey, from information collected through questionnaires to 42,000 households representative of the population of the United States, estimated the 1970 prevalence of emphysema to have been 9.8 per 1000 and of bronchitis, 29.5 per 1000. Limitation of activity from these conditions was reported in 5 percent of persons with bronchitis and 37.3 percent of those with emphysema (Wilson, 1973). In 1973, 41,042 deaths in the United States were attributed to bronchitis, emphysema, asthma, and COPD. At least 60,000 deaths were recorded in which these diseases were thought to be contributory causes. For the last 15 years, approximately 35,000 Americans have become totally disabled from these diseases each year. Emphysema has been second to only coronary heart disease as a social security–compensated

disability. The economic cost has been great; direct costs for hospital and nursing care, physician's services, and drugs amounts to nearly 1 billion dollars, and indirect cost from lost productivity due to morbidity and mortality amounts to more than 1 billion dollars.

DEFINITION AND MORPHOLOGIC CHARACTERISTICS

In 1962, a committee of the American Thoracic Society defined chronic bronchitis as a clinical condition characterized by excessive tracheal-bronchial mucus secretions and chronic recurrent productive cough, with symptoms present on most days for a minimum of 3 months for not less than 2 successive years. It was recognized that many other lung diseases, such as tuberculosis, lung abscess, bronchiectasis, tumors, and even congestive heart failure, also might cause similar clinical states. Pathologically, bronchitis is a disease in which there is hypertrophy of bronchial mucous glands and peribronchial inflammation with damage to the bronchial lumen. The morphometric counterpart of excess clinical mucus production is enlargement of the mucous secretory glands. Quantification of mucous gland enlargement is provided as follows by the Reid Index (RI) (Reid, 1960):

$$RI = \frac{\text{mucous gland thickness}}{\text{bronchial wall thickness}}$$

In bronchitis the volume of the mucous glands increases and the RI increases. In normal subjects, the RI is 0.26 with a range of 0.14 to 0.36; in those with chronic bronchitis, the RI is 0.59 with a range of 0.41 to 0.79 (Reid, 1960; Thurlbeck and Angus, 1964). Inflammatory and obliterative changes in the small airways of the lung (less than 2 mm in diameter) have been observed in a large number of people who smoke (Macklem, 1972). When the changes are mild, they may have relatively little effect on the overall lung function. For this reason, the small airways have been called the "quiet zone" of the lung. Abnormalities in the small airways of people who smoke often can be detected by sensitive pulmonary function tests. When abnormalities of the small airways are quite extensive, changes in more standard spir-

645

ometric tests, such as the forced expiratory volume in 1 second (FEV_1), are detectable. As this disease produces a decrease in clinically significant forced expiration results, it is called "chronic obstructive bronchitis."

By contrast, emphysema is defined anatomically as an alteration of lung architecture, characterized by an irreversible enlargement of the airspaces distal to the terminal bronchiole accompanied by destruction of alveolar walls. By its focus on airspaces, emphysema is considered a parenchymal disease. The increase in airspaces must be abnormal in order to distinguish emphysema from the normal increase in airspaces that occurs with aging. Destruction must be present in order to differentiate emphysema from the compensatory dilatation of airspaces in a lung remaining after pneumonectomy. Emphysema is defined as destruction of the airspaces in the acinar region or that portion of the lung distal to the terminal bronchiole. According to the portion of the acinus that is involved, emphysema is classified as follows: (1) paraacinar or panlobular, i.e., uniform involvement of the acinus; (2) centrilobular, i.e., involvement of the proximal portion of the acinus with predominant enlargement of the respiratory bronchioles; and (3) paraseptal, i.e., involvement of the distal portion of the acinus with predominant enlargement of the alveolar sacs.

EPIDEMIOLOGIC AND ETIOLOGIC CONSIDERATIONS

Smoking. The 1979 Surgeon General report concluded that "Epidemiologic, autopsy, and experimental data presented in previous editions of this report indicate that cigarette smoking is the primary cause of chronic bronchitis and emphysema." Evidence reviewed demonstrates a strong association between prevalance of COPD and resulting mortality in both men and women. Mortality from bronchitis in smokers was 3.6 to 21.2 greater than that of nonsmokers, and mortality from emphysema was 6.9 to 25.3 times greater. Among both male and female cigarette smokers, there were higher incidences of symptoms and pulmonary function impairments characteristic of COPD than among nonsmokers. These parameters improved with cessation of smoking. Pipe smokers and cigar smokers were at greater risk than nonsmokers but less than cigarette smokers. Former smokers had a declining mortality rate as the years passed, and after fifteen

years had no greater mortality rate than lifelong nonsmokers (Friedman et al., 1981). Based on current data, tobacco smoke impairs ciliary activity and macrophage function and induces infection, inflammation, edema, increased mucus, scarring, and obstruction in small bronchioles. Similar changes occur in large airways, and result in productive cough. Finally, emphysema is thought to be caused by proteases released from macrophages and neutrophils, which are increased in number because of tracheobronchial inflammation. Cigarette smoke also may impair the antiprotease defenses by inactivating alpha$_1$-antiprotease.

Air Pollution. There appears to be a relationship between air pollution and prevalence of respiratory symptoms, airways reactivity, pulmonary function, and mortality and morbidity of disease in different populations and in different segments of populations. The levels of the various pollutants that produce untoward respiratory effects and the durations of exposure that induce these effects are not yet known. Current primary ambient air quality standards do not consider the type or size distribution of particulate matter that also may affect lung function adversely. The interaction between different types of pollutants also may be an important variable. Recent studies by the Environmental Protection Agency have suggested that the concentration of acid sulfates in the air may be more hazardous to health than either total suspended particulates or SO_2 content.

Hereditary Factors. Eriksson (1964), in Sweden, discovered that there was an association of obstructive lung disease with hereditary deficiency of alpha$_1$-globulin. A glycoprotein, referred to as alpha$_1$-antitrypsin, was specifically deficient in the individuals studied. This substance is responsible for much of the antiprotease activity of human serum. Ninety percent of the antitryptic activity of serum was shown to be localized in the alpha$_1$-globulin zone (Jacobsson, 1955). Alpha$_1$-antitrypsin has been found to be a polymorphic protein with more than 30 phenotypes that can be distinguished by specialized electrophoretic techniques. Inheritance is hypothesized as being controlled by a single autosomal locus with multiple codominant alleles. The various proteinase inhibitor (Pi) alleles and phenotypes that result are presented by letters. The normal allele is Pi^M, and the normal Pi type is homozygous MM. Allelic frequencies have been determined; Pi^M is the most common, and Pi^Z and Pi^S are the next most common. The homozygous ZZPi type is associated with extremely low levels of alpha$_1$-antitrypsin (less than 20 mg/100 ml). The normal range of alpha$_1$-antitrypsin (geometric mean ± 2 standard deviations) is 90 to 178 mg/100 ml (Alpha$_1$-Antitrypsin Laboratory Manual).

It is estimated that 70 to 80 percent of patients with homozygous ZZ type deficiency will develop emphysema (Eriksson, 1964; Jacobsson, 1955; Alpha-Antitrypsin Laboratory Manual; Lieberman, 1973). Less than 5 percent of the general population have this phenotype. There are conflicting data on the prevalence of emphysema in patients with the heterozygous MZ type. Some studies suggest an increased prevalence (Mittman et al., 1971), whereas others do not (Eriksson, 1965; Talamo et al., 1968). MZ patients who smoke may have a higher incidence of COPD than nonsmoking heterozygotes or those with the MMPi type who smoke (Mittman et al., 1971).

It has been hypothesized that alpha$_1$-antitrypsin is essential in protection of the lung against the destructive action of naturally occurring proteases. The sources of such proteases include bacteria, leukocytes, macrophages, and serum. Thus, persons with normal serum trypsin inhibitory activity may have intrinsic protection against these factors, whereas those with deficient activity develop progressive pulmonary disease. Alveolar macrophage and neutrophil elastases appear to be the proteolytic enzymes that are most important in inducing lung damage and emphysema (Kimbel, 1980; Guenter et al., 1981).

Diagnosis of homozygous deficiency is relatively simple, since alpha$_1$-globulin is so severely reduced it appears nearly absent on routine serum protein electrophoresis. Quantitative assessment should be carried out by radial immunodiffusion (Talamo et al., 1968) or by assay of trypsin inhibitory capacity of serum for confirmation (Eriksson, 1965). Since there is overlapping of values of normal subjects and certain unusual Pi types in identification of heterozygous (MZ) deficiency, phenotyping requires special electrophoretic techniques.

Occupational Exposure. Exposure to a wide variety of dusts contributes to the development of chronic bronchitis and emphysema. Coal, gold, and fluorspar miners and foundry, furnace, cotton, and flax workers have been found, therefore, to have a higher prevalence of respiratory symptoms of chronic bronchitis and a lower average ventilatory function than persons of the same age living in the same area who are not exposed to such occupational dusts.

Exposure to vegetable dusts appears more likely to cause chronic bronchitis than exposure to most mineral dusts. Thus, apart from byssinosis, a specific occupational disease of cotton workers, workers exposed to flax and hemp dust also experience an increased prevalence of bronchitis. A high prevalance of respiratory symptoms also has been reported among grain handlers. Exposure to fumes and gases at work has received much less study than exposure to dusts. Oxides of nitrogen have been incriminated as causes of obliterative bronchitis in silofillers and in miners, following blasts in enclosed underground spaces.

Infection. The possible role of infection in early life as a predisposing cause of chronic bronchitis and emphysema has received little objective evaluation. Tager and Speizer (1975) have reviewed studies that suggest that adults who develop bronchitis have had more frequent childhood or early adult respiratory illnesses compared with normal controls. Bronchiolitis may be an especially frequent precursor of chronic respiratory disease. Patients with chronic bronchitis often develop acute exacerbations, with purulent sputum from which *Haemophilus Influenzae* or *Streptococcus pneumoniae* may be cultured (May, 1953). Whether these organisms lead to progression of bronchitis is not known, since many subjects from whom the organisms are cultured fail to produce antibodies to them. These organisms are also present in the upper respiratory tracts of many normal subjects and the lower respiratory tracts of bronchitics between acute exacerbations. The roles of viral and mycoplasmal agents in exacerbations of chronic bronchitis need particular study, since acute exacerbations of chronic bronchitis appear to hasten progression of COPD. Available data suggest that the progressive decline in pulmonary functions in patients with COPD is not greatly affected by mild exacerbations of symptoms or mild respiratory tract infections.

CLINICAL PRESENTATION

The typical patient with COLD presents with a mixed form of chronic bronchitis and emphysema, with wheezing similar to that in asthma, often complicated by manifestations of right-sided heart failure. As a result, it is a common tendency to place patients with various kinds of obstructive lung disease in a single diagnostic category and to treat them all in the same manner. However, this tendency results in overmedication for those with severe emphysema and little reversible disease and in inadequate therapy for those with predominant chronic bronchitis.

Chronic Bronchitis

PATHOPHYSIOLOGY

Eighty percent of airways resistance occurs in central airways. Narrowing and inflammation of such airways in bronchitis increase resistance, the immediate functional consequences of which include inspiratory and expiratory airflow obstruction, hyperinflation, and maldistribution of ventilation.

Flow Obstruction. The determinants of maximal expiratory flow ($\dot{V}_{max}$) are muscular pressure (P_{mus}), airway resistance (RAW), and elastic recoil pressure (P_{el}). In bronchitis, expiratory flow is decreased as a function of increased RAW. The combination of decreased $\dot{V}_{max}$ and increased RAW identifies central airways disease.

Overinflation. There is an increase in total lung capacity (TLC) and an increase in the volume of air remaining after maximal expiration or increased residual volume (RV) and RV/TLC.

Maldistribution of Ventilation. The increased RAW in regional lung units causes abnormal time constants, with resultant inhomogeneous ventilation. In bronchitis, there is increased blood flow to units of lungs with low ventilation/perfusion ($\dot{V}/Q$) ratios, which causes a significant right-to-left shunting of blood (Wagner et al., 1977). Because of these abnormalities, arterial blood gas determinations in chronic bronchitis show the following characteristic changes: moderate to severe arterial hypoxemia, arterial hypercapnia, and a degree of right-to-left shunting of blood (PaO_2 between 400 and 500 mm Hg, breathing 100 percent O_2).

Signs and symptoms of chronic bronchitis are variable, depending on when in the natural history of the disease the patient seeks medical attention or which complications the patient develops. Six major groups of patients can be identified as follows: (1) patients with cough and sputum production, without expiratory flow obstruction; (2) patients with cough and sputum production, with expiratory flow ob-

struction; (3) patients with cough and sputum production and progressive airway disease and with mild derangements in $\dot{V}/Q$ and arterial blood gas values; (4) patients with severe airway disease and severe abnormalities in $\dot{V}/Q$ and arterial blood gas values; (5) patients with pulmonary hypertension; and (6) patients with right-sided heart failure (cor pulmonale).

Emphysema

PATHOPHYSIOLOGY

Elastin rather than collagen is the chief connective tissue element responsible for the lung's elasticity. Destruction of this connective tissue within alveolar walls reduces the lung's elasticity. The amount of elastin in the emphysematous lung is normal (Pierce et al., 1961); reduced elasticity has been attributed to disruption in the normal arrangement of the elastic fibers (Kuhn et al., 1976). The functional expression of reduced elasticity is increased pulmonary compliance. Three diagnostic criteria for increased pulmonary compliance are as follows: (1) an upward and leftward shift of the volume pressure curve, (2) a transpulmonary pressure (PTP) at total lung capacity (TLC) of less than 19 cm H_2O, irrespective of a patient's age, and (3) a coefficient of retraction of less than 2.5 cm H_2O/L.

Air Trapping. A patient with emphysema can deliver a larger vital capacity during a slow expiration than during a maximally forced expiration. During a slow expiration the highest positive pleural pressures of a maximal expiration are avoided, and airway compression and closure are minimized. During a maximally forced expiration the airways are compressed and air trapping occurs.

Flow Obstruction. In emphysema, expiratory flow is reduced but P_{mus} and RAW are normal. Since RAW reflects primarily the caliber of central airways, the site of narrowing responsible for the decreased flow must be the in the peripheral airways, the so-called silent zone of the lungs. The pattern of peripheral airway disease is defined as decreased $\dot{V}_{max}$ with a normal P_{mus} and RAW. The mechanism responsible for peripheral airway disease can be determined by measuring P_{el}. The combination of decreased $\dot{V}_{max}$, normal P_{mus} and RAW, and decreased P_{el} characterizes the peripheral airway disease as emphysema.

Overinflation. A second result of airway narrowing and closure in emphysema is overinflation (increased RV, RV/TLC, and TLC). Since the thoracic cage increases its anteroposterior diameter as emphysema progresses, the vital capacity (VC) is protected or preserved until late in the course of disease. This is a contrasting feature to the pattern of overinflation seen in bronchitis in which there is less increase in TLC.

Maldistribution of Ventilation. The loss of elasticity in a regional lung unit results in an abnormal time constant for that unit and, as a result, underventilation of the lung unit. The $\dot{V}/Q$ patterns in patients with emphysema have been studied by Wagner and associates (1977); they demonstrated that there is very little blood flow to units of lung with the low $\dot{V}/Q$ ratio of emphysema. There is very little right-to-left shunting, and there is increased ventilation to units of lung with high $\dot{V}/Q$ ratios (wasted ventilation). These findings are to be contrasted with the pattern of chronic bronchitis, in which there is increased right-to-left shunting. The ventilation-perfusion scans in patients with emphysema show that the distribution of ventilation appears to be uniform in all lung zones and closely matches perfusion so that there are not large areas of low ventilation and high perfusion, as seen in chronic bronchitis. The probable explanation for this relative matching of ventilation and perfusion in emphysema is that units of lung that are underventilated owing to loss of elasticity also are underperfused because of loss of capillary bed. The $\dot{V}/Q$ pattern in emphysema is the explanation for the arterial blood gas patterns of these patients with arterial normoxemia or mild hypoxemia, normocapnia, and no right-to-left shunting (PaO_2 greater than 500 mm Hg, breathing 100 percent O_2).

Since alveolar destruction occurs over decades, the development of symptoms in patients with emphysema is insidious. The principal clinical components of emphysema are progressive expiratory flow obstruction and overinflation, along with progressive dyspnea and exercise limitation. The severity of symptoms is related to the severity of anatomic destruction. The clinical presentation of patients who have homozygous deficiency in alpha$_1$-antitrypsin (ZZ phenotype) is characteristic in that the emphysema is panlobular, occurs at an earlier age (45 compared with 60 years), and occurs predominately at the lung bases.

One of the early attempts to categorize the distinctive clinical syndromes in the heterogeneous population of patients with chronic obstructive pulmonary disease was done by Dornhorst in 1955. He coined the term *blue bloaters* for bronchitis patients, and *pink buffers* for emphysematous patients. Burrows and associates (1964) referred to patients with bronchitis as *Type B,* and patients with emphysema as *Type A.* Robin and O'Neill (1963) labeled the emphysematous patient as a *fighter* and the bronchitic patient as a *quitter.* This former description focused on the fact that the emphysematous patient "fights and mounts" a large minute ventilation to maintain normal arterial blood gas concentrations. The latter or bronchitic patient "quits," maintains a lower minute ventilation, and develops arterial hypoxemia and hypercapnia.

PRECLINICAL COURSES AND EARLY DETECTION OF THE DISEASE

The preclinical courses of bronchitis and emphysema are not well known. Fletcher and associates (1976) found a good relationship between the rate of decline in FEV$_1$ over an eight-year period and the mean FEV$_1$ over the same period of time. This finding implies a sensitivity of lung functions in susceptible individuals to the effects of smoking and excessive rates of decline in lung functions over the entire period that such individuals smoke. Also, by about 60 years of age, smoking will have been associated with a significant level of dysfunction in such patients. These investigators also have found that the presence of productive cough does not influence the rate of decline in lung function. It also seems likely that intercurrent infections are not related to functional loss. However, other investigators found that smokers with chronic productive coughs have proportionately lower lung functions and those with previous chest illnesses show more severe disease. In the susceptible smoker who will develop disabling obstruction by age 60, a reduced FEV$_1$ can be found early in the course of the disease; screening for such a patient should be done in order to have the patient stop smoking. This should slow down the rate of loss of function before clinically significant symptoms occur. Screening with standard spirometric tests raises some questions, however. Although low FEV$_1$ correlates with rapid declines in lung function, there is no proof that a single FEV$_1$ measurement will predict subsequent fall in function. Also, there is little relationship between the level of FEV$_1$ and its rate of fall when the FEV$_1$ is more than 70 percent of predicted. Furthermore, patients have been observed in whom the FEV_1 measurements have been normal and stable throughout middle age, only to decline rapidly to the point of severe disability. Other subjects show considerable fluctuations in lung functions before the development of irreversible obstruction. Nevertheless, FEV_1, which has been criticized as an insensitive prognosticator is always abnormal before the age of 30 years in any individual who is likely to die of obstructive disease by age 70 years (Burrows, 1974). Similarly, as Bates (1974) has suggested, seldom is the maximum mid-flow rate (MMFR) normal at age 40 (and probably at age 30) in a subject who will be severely disabled from obstructive lung disease at age 50. Fletcher's calculations have determined that cessation of smoking corrects the rapid pulmonary function decline of the COPD patient to a normal rate of decline (Fletcher, 1976). Thus, by not smoking, the patient at risk of COPD might avert premature death.

Since the FEV_1 is a reproducible though a relatively insensitive indicator of airway dysfunction, new tests have assumed increasing popularity as probable indicators of small airways disease. Some of the test results purported to measure small airways disease include abnormalities in $\dot{V}_{max}$ 75%, closing volume, phase III of nitrogen washout, response of the maximal expiratory flow volume (MEFV) curve to inhalation of helium, and comparison of compliance measurements at increasing respiratory rates with static compliance determination (Cdyn/Cst). However, the relevance of these abnormal test results to clinical problems in patients with COPD remains unknown. For example, although these tests detect subtle airway dysfunction common in smokers, there is no evidence that they can identify those smokers who will later develop disabling irreversible airway obstruction. Currently, an abnormal FEV_1 or a downward change in FEV_1 from a previously measured FEV_1 is the accepted means of identifying middle-aged smokers who are likely to progress to respiratory insufficiency.

COURSE AND PROGNOSIS OF ESTABLISHED DISEASE

The course of severe COPD appears to be progressive regardless of conventional therapeutic measures (Renzetti et al., 1965; Burrows et al., 1969; Petty et al., 1969). Symptoms of COPD tend to worsen slowly with time. A major exception is cough, which often improves if smoking is discontinued. Most investigators believe that the course of the disease is more rapid if the patient continues to smoke.

Normally, there is a minor decrease in FEV_1 (L) of approximately 28 ml/year between the ages of 20 and 60. Although the variability in FEV_1 makes the true rates of decline difficult to measure in individual patients until there are many years of follow-up, studies of COPD patients indicate a linear fall in FEV_1 of approximately 80 ml/year, i.e., approximately $2\frac{1}{2}$ times greater than the normal decrease of 28 ml/year (Renzetti et al., 1965; Burrows et al., 1969; Petty et al., 1969).

Burrows and associates (1969) have analyzed prognosis in COPD in terms of the degree of flow obstruction and the presence or absence of other variables, such as hypercapnia, diffusion capacity less than 50 percent of predicted, resting pulse greater than 100/min, and clinical evidence of cor pulmonale. Survival has been shown to be closely related to the initial severity of disease and the percent predicted FEV_1 obtained following administration of a bronchodilator.

TREATMENT

There are four basic goals of treatment as follows: (1) attempt to prevent progression of the disease, (2) attempt to prevent those complications leading to acute deterioration (exacerbation), (3) treat the potentially reversible components of the disease, (4) and teach the patient how to participate in his or her management. Cigarette smoking has been shown to be the major cause of COPD; it is highly probable that cessation will abort the progression of pulmonary dysfunction. The more advanced the functional loss, the less the impact will be. *Early detection of the disease and cessation of smoking seem to be the strongest management measure to "prevent" the progression of illness.*

The most common complications in chronic obstructive pulmonary disease are pulmonary infection secondary to virus or bacteria. Prophylactic use of influenza and pneumococcal vaccinations is especially important. The prompt use of antibiotics (ampicillin, tetracycline) during exacerbation of cough and sputum production or the use of broad-spectrum antibiotics for 1 week of every month during the peak months of respiratory infections decreases the severity and duration of these episodes but does not appear to decrease the number of episodes of infection. Elimination or reduction of exposure to environmental or occupational air pollution is another preventive approach. Postnasal discharge, often associated with nocturnal bouts of cough and wheeze, and gastroesophageal reflux (GER), which also can aggravate respiratory symptoms, need to be treated aggressively. The chronic postnasal drip can be associated with chronic sinusitis, and the GER, with hiatus hernia. These need to be treated if present.

Complete pulmonary function testing is mandatory in the patient with COPD in order to assess the severity of disease, to aid in decisions about therapy, and to recognize potentially reversible components of the disease. The therapeutic goal is reduction of airflow resistance. Measures used may vary in different patients but are directed towards reducing production of secretions, increasing elimination of secretions, and reversing bronchospasm.

There are several approaches to reducing excessive airways secretions. These include adequate oral hydration (2½ to 3 quarts of fluid/day), mobilization of secretions by chest physiotherapy, postural drainage by devices producing chest vibration (3000 cycles/min), or hand clapping of the chest. Bronchial hygiene maneuvers always should be tried in patients with increased secretions. Because of the risk of hypoxemia with postural drainage and chest percussion, the procedure should be accompanied by supplemental oxygen in those patients who are hypoxemic. If secretions are not a problem, these procedures are not necessary, but adequate hydration nevertheless still is important. Relief of bronchospasm with methylxanthine, beta-adrenergic drugs, or both is an important mainstay in the treatment of a patient with chronic airflow obstruction. A trial of bronchodilators is warranted in virtually every patient in order not to miss an opportunity to treat a potentially reversible element of the disease. It should be remembered that the absence of an acute response to bronchodilators does not preclude benefit from their long-term use; it is not unusual for a patient who fails to show reversibility to benefit subsequently. Inhaled or systemic steroids, anticholinergic agents, and inhaled cromolyn sodium are other treatment options directed to reduce bronchospasm. Since airway hyperreactivity is common among patients with COPD, the long-term use of bronchodilators also may serve to prevent airway constriction due to inhaled irritants.

Mild to severe hypoxemia can occur in acute episodes. Hypoxemia is due primarily to ventilation-perfusion mismatching. Hypoxemia causes reactive pulmonary hypertension and subsequent cor pulmonale, which clearly worsens the prognosis (Mitchell et al., 1964). The Nocturnal Oxygen Therapy Trial Group (NOTT, 1980) established that continuous oxygen therapy (COT) affords a better clinical outcome than does nocturnal oxygen therapy (NOT). The Medical Research Council Working Party (1981) of Britain also compared 15 hours/day oxygen with no oxygen and found a significantly greater survival in patients who received oxygen 15 hours/day compared with patients who did not receive oxygen. Patients who are candidates for oxygen therapy include those with chronic persistent hypoxemia with a PaO_2 of 55 mm Hg or less after optimal control of any reversible component, those with documented pulmonary hypertension or congestive heart failure, and those with significant hypoxemia during exercise or sleep. Patients with right-sided heart failure often respond to gentle diuresis and initiation of long-term oxygen therapy. The use of digitalis is controversial. It is unclear if the positive inotropic effect of digitalis on the right ventricle is clinically beneficial, and its use can be associated with significant toxicity.

Exercise tolerance is significantly greater after a program of gradually increasing exercise loads for 3 to 6 weeks. Although mechanical lung function is not improved, the maximum oxygen uptake and the ability to perform work improves. Ventilatory muscles also can respond to training, although not every patient improves clinically. Greater respiratory muscle strength and endurance after respiratory muscle training improve exercise tolerance (Grassino et al., 1979) and can modify the clinical course of respiratory failure.

Comprehensive care of a patient with chronic airflow limitation is based upon well-established data, experience, and clinical judgment. Benefits are numerous and include reduction of symptoms (cough, sputum, dyspnea), reduction of anxiety and depression, improvement of ego strength, decrease of hospitalization, improvement of exercise tolerance, maintenance of or return to gainful employment, and enhancement of ability to carry out daily activity. Comprehensive pulmonary rehabilitation programs can improve significantly the quality of life, although therapy per se does not improve lung function.

BRONCHIOLITIS OBLITERANS

Bronchiolitis obliterans is a rapidly progressive, usually irreversible disorder of the small airways (Seggev et al., 1983). The list of factors that leads to the development of bronchiolitis obliterans is extensive. These factors include exposure to irritating or toxic chemicals and vapors and viral infections, particularly influenza, adenoviruses 7 and 21, and measles. Bronchiolitis obliterans also is associated with collagen diseases, particularly rheumatoid arthritis; with interstitial pneumonitis; and with miscellaneous disorders, such as myasthenia gravis, lymphomas, and pulmonary alveolar proteinosis. In many cases, however, the cause is unknown. Bronchiolitis obliterans is primarily a pathologic diagnosis characterized by a widespread obliterative process of the bronchioles. There is extensive damage to the bronchial walls, and the lumina are partially or totally occluded by organizing bronchial exudate.

Symptoms of bronchiolitis obliterans are relatively nonspecific. All patients so affected have severe shortness of breath, cough, and sputum production. Chest roentgenograms are variable, ranging from hyperinflation alone to nodular or alveolar opacities which may be segmental or diffuse. Pulmonary function tests reveal airflow limitation in all such patients; most have hyperinflation.

Bronchiolitis obliterans often is irreversible. A trial of corticosteroids may be appropriate, but unless there is definitive objective improvement, they should be tapered or stopped. Steroids have dramatic effects in cases of NO_2 exposure, of postviral disease, and of eosinophilic pneumonia with bronchiolitis obliterans. A role for immunosuppressive agents is not clear, but these may be used as a therapeutic last resort.

REFERENCES

Alpha$_1$-Antitrypsin Laboratory Manual. U.S. Department of Health, Education and Welfare. Publication No. (NIH)78-1420 Public Health Service. National Institute of Health, Bethesda, Maryland.

Bates, D.V.: The prevention of emphysema. Chest 65:437, 1974.

Burrows, B.: Early detection of airway obstruction. Chest 65:239, 1974.

Burrows, B., Earle, R.H.: Course and prognosis of chronic obstructive lung disease. N. Engl. J. Med. 280:397, 1969.

Burrows, B., Neden, A.J., Fletcher, C.M., Jones, J.L.: Clinical types of chronic obstructive lung disease in London and Chicago. Am. Rev. Respir. Dis. 90:14, 1964.

Definitions and Classification of Chronic Bronchitis, Asthma, and Pulmonary Emphysema. Am. Rev. Respir. Dis. 85:762, 1962.

Dornhorst, A.C.: Respiratory insufficiency. Lancet 1:1185, 1955.

Eriksson, S.: Pulmonary emphysema and alpha$_1$-antitrypsin deficiency. Acta Med. Scand. 175:197, 1964.

Eriksson, S.: Studies in alpha$_1$-antitrypsin deficiency. Acta Med. Scand. 177(Suppl 432):1, 1965.

Fletcher, C.M., Jones, J.L., Burrows, B., Neden, A.J.: American emphysema and British bronchitis: A standardized comparative study. Am. Rev. Respir. Dis. 90:1, 1964.

Fletcher, C.M., Peto, R., Tinker, C.M., et al.: The Natural History of Chronic Bronchitis and Emphysema. Oxford, England, Oxford University Press, 1976.

Friedman, G.D., Petitti, D.B., Bawol, R.D., Siegelaub, A.B.: Mortality in cigarette smokers and quitters. N. Engl. J. Med. 304:1407, 1981.

Grassino, A., Gross, D., Macklem, P.T., et al.: Inspiratory muscle fatigue as a factor limiting exercise. Bull. Eur. Physiopathol. Respir. 15:105, 1979.

Guenter, C.A., Coalson, J.J., Jacques, J.: Emphysema associated with intravascular leukocyte sequestration: Comparison with papain induced emphysema. Am. Rev. Respir. Dis. 123:79, 1981.

Jacobsson, K.: Studies on the trypsin and plasmin inhibitors in human blood serum. Scand. J. Clin. Lab. Invest. 7(Suppl 14):55, 1955.

Kimbel, P.: Proteolytic lung damage. Chest 77:274, 1980.

Kuhn, C., III, Yu, W., Chraphyvy, M., Linder, H.E., Senior, R.M.: The induction of emphysema with elastase II. Changes in connective tissue. Lab. Invest. 34:372, 1976

Lieberman, J: Alpha$_1$-antitrypsin deficiency. Med. Clin. N. Am. 57:691, 1973.

Macklem, P.T.: Obstruction in small airways — A challenge to medicine. Am. J. Med. 52:721, 1972.

May, J.R.: The bacteriology of chronic bronchitis. Lancet 2:534, 1953.

Medical Research Council Working Party. Long-term domicilliary oxygen therapy in chronic hypoxic cor pulmonale complicating chronic bronchitis and emphysema. Lancet 1:681, 1981.

Mitchell, R.S., Wess, N.C., Filley, G.F.: Chronic obstructive bronchopulmonary disease III. Factors influencing prognosis. Am. Rev. Respir. Dis. 89:878, 1964.

Mittman, C., Lieberman, J., Macasso, F., Miranda, A.: Smoking and chronic obstructive lung disease in alpha$_1$-antitrypsin deficiency. Chest 60:214, 1971.

Nocturnal Oxygen Therapy Trial Group: Continuous or Nocturnal Oxygen Therapy in Hypoxemic Chronic Obstructive Lung Disease. A Clinical Trial. Ann. Intern. Med. 92:391, 1980.

Petty, T.L., Nett, L.M., Finigan, M.M., Brink, G.A., Corsello, P.R.: A comprehensive care program for chronic airway obstruction. Ann. Intern. Med. 70:1109, 1969.

Pierce, J.A., Hocott, M.S., Bert, R.V.: The collagen and elastin content of the lung in emphysema. Ann. Intern. Med. 55:210, 1961.

Reid, L.: Measurement of bronchial mucous gland layer: a diagnostic yardstick in chronic bronchitis. Thorax 15:132, 1960.

Renzetti, A.D., Jr., McClement, J.H., Litt, R.D.: Veterans administration cooperative study of pulmonary function. 3. Mortality in relation to respiratory function in chronic obstructive pulmonary disease. Am. J. Med. 39:941, 1965.

Robin, E.D., O'Neill, R.P.: The fighter versus the non-fighter. Arch. Environ. Health 7:125, 1963.

Seggev, J.S., Mason, U.G., Worthen, S., et al.: Bronchiolitis obliterans. Report of three cases with detailed physiologic studies. Chest 83:169, 1983.

Tager, I., Speizer, F.E.: Role of infection in chronic bronchitis. N. Engl. J. Med. 292:563, 1975.

Talamo, R.C., Allen, J.D., Kahan, M.G., Austen, K.F.: Hereditary alpha$_1$-antitrypsin deficiency. N. Engl. J. Med. 278:345, 1968.

Thurlbeck, W.M., Angus, G.E.: A distribution curve of chronic bronchitis. Thorax 19:436, 1964.

US Public Health Service: Smoking and Health: A report of the Surgeon General. Part I. The health consequences of smoking. US Department of Health and Welfare. Publication No. 75-50066, 1979.

Wagner, P.D., Dantzker, D.R., Duek, R., Clausen, J.L., West, J.B.: Ventilation-perfusion in equality in chronic pulmonary disease. J. Clin. Invest. 59:203, 1977.

Wilson, R.W.: Cigarette smoking, disability days and respiratory conditions. J. Occup. Med. 15:23, 1973.

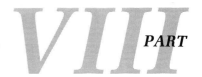
MANAGEMENT OF OTHER ALLERGIC DISEASES

50

Diseases of the Eye
S. LANCE FORSTOT, M.D.

The eye and ocular adnexae are the sites of allergic reactions from infancy to adulthood. Eye function can be critically affected by reactions that cause even minor alterations in ocular structure. The eye, therefore, is exquisitely sensitive to allergic inflammation. The visibility of the ocular structures also makes the signs of allergic disease easily observable. Because of certain anatomic and physiologic peculiarities, the eye may respond in a slightly different manner in allergic reactions than do many other tissues.

ANATOMIC AND PHYSIOLOGIC CONSIDERATIONS

In contrast to most other tissues in which allergic reactions take place, the cornea, lens, and vitreous are normally avascular structures. The cornea is nourished by contents of the tear film, aqueous humor, and limbal circulation. The lens possesses a capsule that further isolates it from the aqueous humor and vitreous. The globe (corneoscleral shell) and its contents do not have lymphatic drainage. In addition, there is a blood-aqueous barrier which is selective, in that the contents of the aqueous humor are not proportional to the contents of the blood.

The conjunctiva, as an exposed epithelial surface, comes in contact with a variety of microorganisms and noninfective allergens. The ability of the conjunctiva to mount an inflammatory response is relatively limited. The inflamed "red" eye reflects dilatation of conjunctival blood vessels; chemosis (edema) of the conjunctiva occurs with transudation of fluid through vessel walls; and cellular elements may exude with transudation, and together with glandular mucous secretions and tears, may produce an ocular "discharge."

With acute inflammation, the palpebral conjunctiva can develop follicles and papillae. Follicles are collections of lymphoid cells (lymphocytes, macrophages, and plasma cells) in the conjunctiva (Fig. 50–1). Conjunctival lymphoid tissue develops in the first month of life. The intensity (size and number) of the follicular response is determined by the stimulus. As follicles form, they displace vessels and appear to have a vascular coat. Follicles occur most often in the inferior palpebral conjunctiva and lower fornix. The papilla is a vascular structure more often seen on the upper palpebral conjunctiva (Fig. 50–2 A). A papilla has a vessel in the central core and is composed of various "acute" inflammatory cells (polymorphonuclear leukocytes, basophils, and eosinophils). As discussed subsequently, examination of the type of conjunctival response (follicular or papillary) as well as examination of the cellular makeup (conjunctival cytologic smear) of the discharge (exudate) can aid in the diagnosis of the disease.

The cornea is normally clear and transparent. Corneal inflammation is characterized by stromal infiltrates that produce granular opacities. If these opacities originate in avascular corneas, they often are of limbal vessel origin and are marginal in location. In vascularized (inflamed) corneas, stromal infiltrates originate near the new vessels and can occur more centrally.

Another important physiologic consideration in ocular allergy is the "lymph node" phenomenon. Since the eye itself has no lymphatic drainage, it is believed that antigen is processed at a distant site and that sensitized lymphocytes return to the site of origin. The uveal tract (iris, ciliary body, and choroid) is the vascular coat of the eye and is the principal site of the lymphoid cell supply of the eye. The vascular watershed area of the cornea, the limbus, also may be a site of sensitized cells in which the antigen is of corneal origin. Repeated exposures to antigen,

655

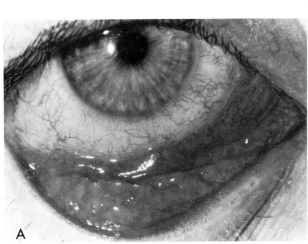
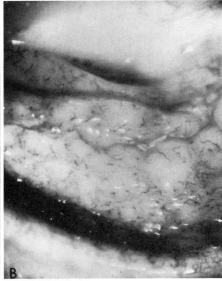

FIGURE 50-1. *A*, Chlamydial inclusion conjunctivitis with follicles in the conjunctiva. *B*, Close-up of follicles.

either at the eye or a more remote area of the body, could trigger local antibody formation and local "lymph node" activity with the production of recurrent uveitis or keratitis (Silverstein, 1968).

GENERAL DIAGNOSTIC AND THERAPEUTIC CONSIDERATIONS

Diagnostic Considerations. In dealing with conjunctival disease, cytologic smears, microbial smears (Gram stain for bacteria, Giemsa stain for various organisms), and microbial cultures for bacteria and fungi are of paramount diagnostic importance. In atopic conjunctivitis and vernal conjunctivitis, eosinophils are abundant in epithelial scrapings. In viral (herpes simplex or adenovirus) conjunctivitis, lymphocytes are predominant, whereas in bacterial conjunctivitis and *Chlamydial* infections, polymorphonuclear leukocytes are predominant. In addition, conjunctivitis of viral or chlamydial origin is characterized by a predominantly follicular conjunctival reaction. In vernal and atopic conjunctivitis, the reaction is mainly papillary.

In uveal tract disease, serologic tests may be helpful. Systemic-onset juvenile rheumatoid arthritis (JRA) and polyarticular JRA are not usually associated with iridocyclitis. However, one type of pauciarticular JRA may be associated with the presence of antinuclear antibody (ANA) in as many as 50 percent of cases and has severe morbidity from chronic anterior uveitis, whereas another type of pauciarticular JRA is ANA negative and is associated with acute iritis and HLA-B27 histocompatibility antigen (Wedgwood and Schaller, 1977). Posterior uveitis due to toxoplasmosis can be diagnosed with both morphologic findings and positive serologic test results for antibody to the organism.

Therapeutic Considerations. Care of both lid inflammation and exudative conjunctivitis requires good lid hygiene. The lid may become encrusted with exudate or inflammatory scaling that can hinder antibiotic effectiveness. Removal of this encrustation is important in therapy. A mild soap, such as baby shampoo, diluted from full strength, is an effective lid cleanser, applied either with a washcloth or cotton-tipped applicator to the lid margin and eyelash base.

Both acute and chronic allergic conjunctivitis respond symptomatically to oral antihistamines. Topical decongestants/vasoconstrictors (Table 50–1) and topical antihistamines (Table 50–2) are of value as adjunctive therapy. Topical steroids also may be required to relieve more severe symptoms, especially of vernal conjunctivitis. However, the long-term use of topical steroids can lead to the development of cataracts. In susceptible patients, intraocular pressure may rise, causing secondary glaucoma. Topical steroids also can potentiate herpes simplex keratitis and secondary bacterial infection. Because of these side effects, *long-term use of*

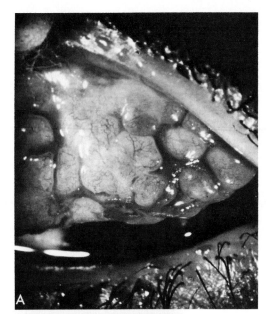

FIGURE 50-2. Vernal conjunctivitis. *A*, Tarsal (palpebral) form. Everted upper lid with giant "cobblestone" papillae. *B*, Limbal form. Gelatinous conjunctival hypertrophy.

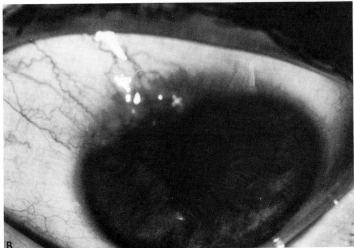

topical steroids is best managed in conjunction with an ophthalmologist. The choice of a topical steroid preparation involves a decision regarding the type of steroid compound (solution versus suspension) (Table 50–3). If profuse epiphora is prominent, the efficacy of drops may be diminished through dilution by tears. An ointment may be required in vernal conjunctivitis with severe tearing.

Prednisolone acetate is a particularly effective steroid preparation (Leibowitz and Kupferman, 1975). However, this suspension can be irritating because of its particulate nature; the importance of shaking such preparations before administration should be emphasized for full effectiveness.

Cromolyn sodium is available topically as a 4-percent ophthalmic solution. It inhibits release of histamine and other mediators by blocking mast cell degranulation and is useful in ameliorating mild to moderate allergic conjunctivitis.

In patients with uveitis, intraocular inflammation can cause cataracts and glaucoma. These may be difficult to distinguish from drug-induced and disease-induced problems. Chronic topical steroids can induce local problems, as indicated. Systemic steroids for ocular conditions, such as uveitis, can cause severe systemic side effects, especially in children. Periocular injections may circumvent these side effects, but systemic absorption of drugs may

TABLE 50-1. Decongestants/Vasoconstrictors

Preparation	Vasoconstrictor (percent)	Preservative
Ak-Con	NZ 0.1	BAC, EDTA
Ak-Nefrin	PE 0.12	BAC, EDTA
Albalon	NZ 0.1	BAC, EDTA
Collyrium 2*	THZ 0.05	BAC, EDTA
Clear Eyes	NZ 0.012	BAC, EDTA
Degest 2	NZ 0.012	BAC, EDTA
Murine Plus	THZ 0.05	BAC, EDTA
Muro's Opcon	NZ 0.1	BAC, EDTA
Naphcon	NZ 0.012	BAC, EDTA
Naphcon Forte	NZ 0.1	BAC, EDTA
Prefrin Liquifilm	PE 0.12	BAC, EDTA
VasoClear	NZ 0.02	BAC, EDTA
VasoClear A*	NZ 0.02	BAC, EDTA
Vasocon Regular	NZ 0.1	BAC, EDTA
Visine	THZ 0.05	BAC, EDTA
Visine A.C.*	THZ 0.05	BAC, EDTA
Zincfrin*	PE 0.12	BAC

* Contains astringent (zinc sulfate 0.25 percent). (NZ = naphazoline; PE = phenylephrine; THZ = tetrahydrazoline; BAC = benzalkonium chloride; and EDTA = disodium edetate.)

occur and can be associated with systemic steroid side effects.

Antibiotic therapy is indicated in diagnosed bacterial disease. Although bacterial conjunctivitis often is self limited, topical antibiotic therapy will shorten its course as well as decrease the opportunity for patient-to-patient spread. Since most cases of bacterial conjunctivitis are due to gram-positive cocci, the use of sulfacetamide or erythromycin (drops or ointment) is of value. Topical drops combining gramicidin, neomycin, and polymyxin B (or ointments combining bacitracin, neomycin, and polymyxin B) provide broad-spectrum coverage in acute conjunctival disease. These drugs treat both gram-positive and gram-negative organisms. Initially, a drop every 1 to 4 hours may be required, depending on the severity; after a therapeutic response, this may be tapered to 4 times a day. Therapy should be continued 24 to 48 hours beyond cessation of signs and symp-

TABLE 50-2. Antihistamines

Preparation	Antihistamine (percent)	Vasoconstrictor (percent)	Preservative
Ak-Con-A	PhM 0.3	NZ 0.025	BAC, EDTA
Albalon-A	AZ 0.5	NZ 0.05	BAC, EDTA
Muro's Opcon-A	PhM 0.3	NZ 0.025	BAC, EDTA
Naphcon-A	PhM 0.3	NZ 0.025	BAC, EDTA
Prefrin-A	PyM 0.1	PE 0.12	BAC, EDTA
Vasocon-A	AZ 0.05	NZ 0.05	BAC, EDTA

(AZ = antazoline; PhM = pheniramine maleate; PyM = pyrilamine maleate; NZ = naphazoline; PE = phenylephrine; BAC = benzalkonium chloride; and EDTA = disodium edetate.)

TABLE 50-3. Relative Anti-inflammatory Activity*

Compound†	Strength (percent)	Preparation
Prednisolone acetate	1.0	Suspension
Dexamethasone	1.0	Suspension
Fluorometholone	0.1	Suspension
Prednisolone sodium phosphate	1.0	Solution
Prednisolone acetate	0.125	Suspension
Prednisolone sodium phosphate	0.125	Solution
Dexamethasone phosphate	0.1	Solution
Dexamethasone phosphate	0.05	Ointment

* Data compiled from Leibowitz, H.M., Kupferman, A.: Bioavailability and therapeutic effectiveness of topically administered corticosteroids. Trans. Am. Acad. Ophthalmol. Otolaryngol. 79:OP-78, 1975.
† Decreasing order—cornea with intact epithelium.

toms or after a negative response on culture. Because neomycin has a high rate of sensitization, preparations containing this drug can be used on a short-term basis but not on a long-term basis.

Antiviral therapy is required for herpes simplex keratitis. Frequent and intensive treatment is needed. Idoxuridine (0.1-percent solution or 0.5-percent ointment), vidarabine (3-percent ointment), and trifluridine (1-percent solution) currently are available.

DISEASES OF THE EYELIDS

The lids may be involved in a generalized acute allergic reaction, with urticaria or angioedema. Foods, drugs, insect bites, and contact allergens can initiate the reaction (see Chapter 31).

Contact dermatitis and blepharoconjunctivitis may occur with ocular drug therapy. These can be due to the active drug, the preservative, or the ointment base. Over-the-counter preparations cannot be excluded as offending agents. Compositions of artificial tear preparations and ocular lubricants, including their preservatives, are listed in Table 50-4 and Table 50-5. Preservatives found in topical decongestants/vasoconstrictors and antihistaminic preparations are included in Table 50-1 and Table 50-2. Preservatives in contact lens solutions may cause allergic contact blepharoconjunctivitis. These preservatives include thimerosal, benzalkonium chloride, sorbic acid, chlorobutanol, phenylmercuric nitrate, chlorhexidine gluconate, and parabens, and the enzyme cleanser, papain (Fisher, 1985). Cosmetics also may cause contact dermatitis (see Chapter 30). Therapy consists of withdrawal of the contact allergen and treatment of the symptoms. Topical steroid ointments can be used as well as oral antihistamines. Chronic steroid ointments applied to the lids have the same risks (cataract

formation, induced glaucoma, and suprainfection) as topical steroids in the eye.

Blepharitis is either microbial or seborrheic in origin. *Staphylococcal blepharoconjunctitvitis* is the most common form of bacterial blepharitis. The lid margin often is red, with ulceration and crusting around the lashes. A concomitant, superficial punctate keratitis may exist. Therapy consists of good lid hygiene, employing lid scrubs with mild soap. Antibiotic therapy, such as sulfacetamide or erythromycin ointment on the lids, is indicated. In severe inflammation, application of a mild topical steroid for a short period also can be helpful. Acute recurrent hordeola (styes) are of staphylococcal origin and also require good lid hygiene and antibiotic therapy. In recalcitrant cases, systemic antibiotics may be beneficial. In adults, oral tetracycline is used. Because of growth and developing dentition, other antibiotics, such as erythromycin, are preferred in children.

Seborrheic blepharitis occurs in patients with

TABLE 50-4. Artificial Tear Solutions

Preparation	Polymer*	Preservative*
AKWA Tears	PVA	CB, EDTA, MP
Adsorbotear	Povidone, HEC	TM, EDTA
Comfort Tears	HEC	BAC, EDTA
Hypotears	Lipiden, PVA	BAC, EDTA
Lacril	HPMC	CB
Liquifilm Forte	PVA (3 percent)	TM
Liquifilm Tears	PVA (1.4 percent)	CB
Lyteers	HEC	BAC, EDTA
Muro Tears	HPMC	BAC, EDTA
Murocel	MC (1 percent)	MP, PP
Neo-Tears	PVA, HEC	TM, EDTA
Tearisol	PVA, HEC	TM, EDTA
Tears Naturale	Duasorb (HPMC)	BAC, EDTA
Tears Plus	PVA, Povidone	CB

* (HEC = hydroxyethyl cellulose; HPMC = hydroxypropyl methylcellulose; MC = methylcellulose; PVA = polyvinyl alcohol; PVP = polyvinylpyrrolidone; BAC = benzalkonium chloride; CB = chlorobutanol; EDTA = disodium edetate; MP = methylparaben; PP = propylparaben; and TM = thimerosal.)

TABLE 50-5. Lubricating Ointments

Preparation	Ingredients	Preservative
AKWA Tears	White petrolatum, mineral oil, lanolin	None
Duolube	Sterile ointment, white petrolatum, mineral oil	None
Duratears	Sterile ointment, white petrolatum, mineral oil, anhydrous liquid lanolin	Methylparaben Propylparaben
Lacri-Lube S.O.P.	Sterile ointment, white petrolatum, mineral oil, nonionic lanolin derivatives	Chlorobutanol

seborrhea of the scalp and eyebrows. The lids characteristically have dandruff-like deposits known as "scurf." Treatment consists of lid hygiene and control of seborrhea on the scalp and brows with appropriate shampoo (see Chapter 32).

DISEASES OF THE CONJUNCTIVA

Ophthalmia Neonatorum. Ophthalmia neonatorum is any conjunctivitis within the first month of life. "Chemical conjunctivitis," due to silver nitrate instillation for gonococcal prophylaxis, is the condition with earliest onset. This mild conjunctivitis begins in 24 hours after drug instillation, with hyperemia and watery discharge. It usually is self-limited and requires no specific treatment. Gonococcal conjunctivitis is a purulent inflammatory condition, beginning between the third and fifth day of life. It is associated with chemosis and lid edema. The cornea may be involved. Because corneal ulceration can be devastating, both systemic and topical penicillin are used in treatment. Diagnosis is made through cultures and smears, showing gram-negative intracellular diplococci. Chlamydiae are the most common cause of microbial ophthalmia neonatorum. "Inclusion conjunctivitis" (blennorrhea) usually has its onset 5 days or more after birth. Follicles are not present, as the neonate has no conjunctival lymphoid tissue. Late untreated disease may progress to follicular conjunctivitis after 6 weeks. Basophilic cytoplasmic inclusions are found in high percentage of Giemsa-stained conjunctival scrapings. Inclusions also may be identified rapidly and accurately with immunofluorescent antibody techniques. Topical therapy consists of erythromycin or tetracycline. Systemic therapy is necessary, since there is a high association with systemic chlamydial disease acquired at birth, e.g., pneumonitis, rhinitis, and otitis. Systemic erythromycin is the drug of choice. Other causes of bacterial ophthalmia neonatorum include staphylococci, streptococci, *Escherichia coli,* and *Haemophilus spp.* Each requires specific topical antibiotic therapy. *Pseudomonas* conjunctivitis may occur in premature newborn infants.

Atopic Conjunctivitis. Atopic conjunctivitis may be acute, subacute, chronic, or seasonal in nature. The conjunctivitis of hay fever is characterized by conjunctival injection and edema. The discharge is watery, occasionally with a mucoid component. The most prominent symptom is itching. Cytology of conjunctival scrapings often reveals eosinophils. Treatment consists of topical decongestants/vasoconstrictors and oral antihistamines to relieve itching. Topical steroids occasionally are necessary for symptomatic relief, and topical cromolyn may be helpful. Recurrent bouts of atopic conjunctivitis can lead to chronic conjunctival changes that predispose the patient to keratitis (atopic keratoconjunctivitis) (Hogan, 1953). Corneal vascularization and opacification can occur. When corneal changes cause abnormal tear patterns with rapid tear film breakup, wetting agents such as artificial tears may be helpful in preventing further scarring.

Vernal Conjunctivitis. Vernal conjunctivitis, bilateral recurrent inflammation of the conjunctiva, derives its name from the fact that it occurs in the spring and the summer months. The tarsal (palpebral) form is characterized by "cobblestone-like" (flat-topped) papillae (Fig. 50–2 A), and the limbal form (Fig. 50–2 B), by limbal papillary hypertrophy often associated with white spots (Trantas dots). Both forms can coexist. Symptoms include itching, tearing, and photophobia. Excess mucus production is common. Patients also may complain of foreign body sensation. The diagnosis can be made clinically on the appearance of the giant cobblestone-like papillae or Trantas dots. Cytologic smears reveal numerous eosinophils. The disease is most common between the ages of 5 and 10 years and is more common among males. More than 50 percent of children with vernal conjunctivitis have atopic disorders (asthma, eczema, allergic rhinitis) and high concentrations of IgE in tears have been found by some investigators. However, an immune basis for this disorder has not been established.

The mainstay of therapy in vernal conjunctivitis is topical steroids; systemic steroids are almost never necessary. Soluble steroids are recommended over suspensions because suspensions contain particles that may become trapped between papillae and cause irritation. When tearing is profuse, ointments should be considered, since steroid drops may be diluted to the point of ineffectiveness. Because of the side effects of topical steroids, the dose should be titrated to the minimum required to control the disease.

The thick lardaceous mucus produced in vernal conjunctivitis often contributes to irritation. Mucolytic agents, such as acetylcysteine in a 10 or 20-percent solution, may be helpful in decreasing symptoms (Rice et al., 1971). This drug is not currently available in the United States for ophthalmic use. Antibiotic therapy usually is not needed. If vernal corneal ulcers develop, prophylactic antibiotics to prevent secondary infections are indicated. Topical cromolyn sodium has been evaluated and found to be effective in decreasing symptoms and topical steroid requirements (Easty et al., 1971). Cromolyn sodium 4-percent solution is available.

The cornea may become involved with superficial punctate keratitis. Occasionally, a large shallow oval ulcer occurs in the upper third of the cornea; the ulcer tends to be indolent but eventually heals, often leaving a corneal opacity at the level of the Bowman membrane and anterior stroma. Therapeutic soft contact lenses may help in protecting the eroded cornea from the trauma of the papillae.

Giant Papillary Conjunctivitis in Contact Lens Wearers. Allansmith and coworkers (1977) described a syndrome of conjunctival inflammation characterized by giant papillae on the upper tarsal conjunctiva, with increased mucus production, mild itching, and decreased tolerance to contact lenses (hard or soft). The clinical picture resembles that of vernal conjunctivitis. However, all patients so affected were wearers of contact lenses, had no seasonal variation in symptoms, had no tendency towards atopic disease, and had resolution of symptoms with discontinuation of lens wear. All lenses contained deposits. Conjunctival scrapings revealed eosinophils; histology of the conjunctiva revealed basophils, eosinophils, and mast cells in the epithelium. In the stroma, lymphocytes and plasma cells were seen in large numbers; eosinophils and basophils also were seen in the stroma. An immune etiology has been postulated, with material in the lens' deposits suspected as constituting the antigenic stimulus. Because of the character of the cellular infiltrate, delayed hypersensitivity of the cutaneous basophilic type is suspected. Therapy, as noted, consists of removal of the old contact lens: almost immediate cessation of symptoms is expected within 5 days. Topical cromolyn has been found a helpful adjunct to comfortable lens wear when lens wear is resumed.

Phlyctenular Keratoconjunctivitis. Formation of nodules (phlyctenules), 1 to 2 mm in size, of the conjunctiva, cornea, or limbus characterizes phlyctenular keratoconjunctivitis. The nodules evolve as microabscesses with ulceration but leave no scarring. It has been suspected as being an allergic reaction to tuberculoprotein, but sensitivity to staphylococci also

has been implicated. Symptoms include irritation and itching when the phlyctenules are conjunctival. Corneal phlyctenules produce pain, tearing, and photophobia. Treatment for corneal disease consists of the use of topical steroids. A cycloplegic may be necessary if the keratitis is severe. If there is also a staphylococcal conjunctival infection with purulent discharge, antibiotics should be employed. Conjunctival phlyctenules may not need treatment if the symptoms are minimal, as they resolve spontaneously. Children should also be evaluated for tuberculosis with skin tests and chest x-rays.

Erythema Multiforme. Erythema multiforme, an acute bullous inflammation of the skin and mucous membranes, in its mild form may involve only the skin. In the more severe form, extensive skin and mucous membrane involvement can occur. This severe form, in patients who are toxic and febrile and who have severe ocular involvement, is known as Stevens-Johnson syndrome (Baum, 1973). The etiology is unknown, but inciting factors implicated include systemic bacterial and viral infections as well as drugs (see Chapter 53). Ocular involvement occurs with mucopurulent conjunctivitis and mucosal blistering occurs. As the disease progresses, pseudomembranous or membranous conjunctivitis is common. It may become purulent if a secondary infection develops. The conjunctiva heals with progressive cicatrization and symblepharon formation. Conjunctival scarring causes a secondary aqueous tear deficiency. Corneal drying and scarring may occur with eventual corneal vascularization. Conjunctival scarring also may lead to lid deformity and trichiasis with secondary corneal scarring. Conjunctival smears examined early in the disease show polymorphonuclear leukocytic response with some eosinophils. Ocular therapy is supportive and involves the use of systemic steroids. *Topical steroids may be helpful in relieving ocular symptoms but usually do not change the cicatrizing course and may predispose the patient to secondary infection.* Mechanical lysis of adhesions of the conjunctiva may be necessary. Topical antibiotics are used if secondary infections are present. Artificial tears will be required if deficiency of tears ensues. "Bandage," soft contact lenses may aid in protecting and moistening the cornea.

Viral Conjunctivitis. Viral conjunctivitis usually caused by adenovirus, is characterized by an acute follicular inflammation with serous discharge. It generally is bilateral and is associated with preauricular node enlargement. Symptoms include itching, a feeling of grittiness, and a foreign body sensation in the eye. Signs include redness, chemosis, and marked follicular conjunctival response. A syndrome in children may consist of fever and pharyngitis (i.e., pharyngeal-conjunctival fever or PCF). Conjunctival smears show predominantly mononuclear cells. The disease itself is self limited and benign, unless more severe keratitis ensues (typically with adenoviris type 8 or type 19). Initially, it is punctate epithelial keratitis, which any progress to subepithelial opacities. The epithelial lesions often cause severe photophobia; occasionally, the late subepithelial opacities may decrease vision. Steroids can be of symptomatic benefit in the patients so affected. Antibiotics do not alter the course. If the late subepithelial opacities impair vision, topical steroids can be used to dissolve the infiltrates, although 50 percent of patients will have infiltrates return with discontinuation of topical steroids. These lesions spontaneously resolve without therapy over months.

A mild, self-limited viral conjunctivitis can be associated with both measles and chickenpox infections. The conjunctivitis is catarrhal with serous discharge. Symptoms are minor and usually require no treatment.

Chlamydia. Chlamydiae are the most common causes of oculogenital disease in the neonate, child, adolescent, and adult (Ostler, 1976a). The disease in children is somewhat different from ophthalmia neonatorum. It manifests itself as a mucopurulent follicular conjunctivitis, most prominent in the lower fornix and tarsal conjunctiva (see Fig. 50–1). Neonates have no conjunctival lymphoid tissue to manifest this follicular reaction, however. In addition, older children have less of a tendency to form pseudomembranes from the exudate. Preauricular adenopathy is present. A superficial epithelial keratitis may develop, with small peripheral subepithelial infiltrates. Conjunctival smears show a polymorphonuclear leucocytic response and inclusion bodies may be seen with Giemsa stain or with immunofluorescent antibody stain. The conjunctivitis often is self limited in older children and adults but responds well to topical tetracycline, erythromycin, or sulfa drugs. Systemic therapy should be employed as well because of the oculogenital transmission of the conjunctival disease.

Though not common in the United States, *trachoma* is an extremely prevalent chlamydial conjunctivitis in children and adults throughout the world and is a leading cause of blindness. It is characterized by chronic follicular conjunctivitis, with follicular hypertrophy more prominent in the upper tarsus. Some papillary reaction of the conjunctiva is present. With progression of the disease, conjunctival scarring occurs. Late sequelae include tear deficiency and lid deformity with trichiasis, leading to progressive scarring. Direct corneal involvement may develop in epithelial keratitis, with subsequent corneal vascularization and pannus formation. The diagnosis is made on the basis of the clinical picture ard smears containing inclusion bodies. Treatment is with topical tetracycline, erythromycin, or sulfonamides.

Parinaud Oculoglandular Conjunctivitis. This syndrome consists of unilateral focal granulomatous lesion and follicular conjunctival reaction associated with prominently enlarged preauricular, cervical, and submandibular lymph nodes. The etiologic agent in most cases is unknown, although there is often a history of an association with cats. This entity, in fact, may be related to cat scratch fever, since fever and malaise may accompany the other features of the syndrome. There is no specific therapy.

Ocular Cicatricial Pemphigoid. Cicatricial pemphigoid (also known as benign mucous membrane pemphigoid and essential shrinkage of the conjunctiva) is a severe, bilateral blinding disease. It often occurs in the seventh decade, and women are affected more often than men. It is a chronic bullous disease of the mucous membranes; conjunctivae, oral mucosae, pharynx, esophagus, anus, and urethra may be involved. Ulceration and scarring may follow the bullous changes. The chronic nonspecific conjunctivitis progresses to symblepharon formation, with obliteration of the conjunctival fornices. There may be total adhesion of the lid to the globe. In the late stages, the eye becomes dry because of tear deficiency and loss of goblet cells. The cornea often develops keratitis with subsequent neovascularization and opacification. The scarred conjunctivae may cause entropion of the lid and trichiasis, giving rise to further corneal scarring.

The basic pathology is that of an immune process at the level of the epithelium and basement membrane. Antibodies have been demonstrated to be bound at the basement membrane; rarely, circulating autoantibodies are found.

Systemic steroids appear to ameliorate the inexorable course. Cytotoxic agents, such as cyclophosphamide and azathioprine, have been useful adjuncts in therapy. Topical therapy is directed towards the dry eye. Occasionally, mild topical steroids are helpful.

DISEASES OF THE CORNEA

Thygeson Superficial Punctate Keratitis. This disease is characterized by multiple, discrete, epithelial corneal opacities, occurring bilaterally. These small lesions usually require utilization of a slit lamp for accurate diagnosis. This allows good visualization of the pathognomonic epithelial lesions. The conjunctiva is not affected. The disease has a chronic course, usually 6 months to years, with waxing and waning symptomatic periods of photophobia, tearing, and foreign body sensation. These symptoms are caused by microerosions of the corneal epithelium overlying the opacities. The etiology of this disease is unknown. Attempts at viral isolation or identification with electron microscopy have been fruitless. Topical steroids usually induce remission of symptoms. Therapeutic soft contact lenses also have been used to alleviate symptoms from the microerosions.

Keratoconjunctivitis Medicamentosus. This condition is characterized by superficial punctate erosions. The desquamated epithelial cells give rise to symptoms of foreign body irritation and photophobia. This reaction can be caused by almost any ocular drug or preservative when the preparation is used frequently. Therapy consists of discontinuation of the drug. Patching the eye and cycloplegia may provide symptomatic relief until the epithelium heals.

Catarrhal Marginal Ulcers. These ulcers are peripheral corneal infiltrates often associated with chronic staphylococcal blepharoconjunctivitis. Coagulase-positive staphylococci are often but not always isolated from the conjunctiva. The lesions begin as small infiltrates close to the limbus. The infiltrates break down and may coalesce to form crescentic ulcers. The etiology of the marginal ulcers is believed to be hypersensitivity to staphylococcal toxins. Therapy with topical steroids usually is effective. Antibiotic therapy is indicated if bacteria are isolated in culture.

Herpes Simplex Keratitis. Herpes simplex virus (HSV) infections can cause a self-limited follicular conjunctivitis with preauricular adenopathy. However, primary infection with HSV usually is asymptomatic, involving vesicular lesions of the lip and buccal mucosa. This infection occurs in infancy when protection from maternal antibodies has declined. Most children have antibodies to HSV by the age of 10 years (Ostler, 1976b). Recurrent ocular herpetic infection may be in the form of blepharitis or blepharoconjunctivitis but is most common as dendritic keratitis. This dendritic keratitis is a linear branching epithelial ulcer, which can be demonstrated with rose bengal vital stain. The adjacent epithelial tissue is abnormal and usually is infected with the virus. Corneal sensation often is decreased or lost. Most dendritic ulcers heal spontaneously in 7 to 10 days. Occasionally, the ulcer will progress to a large broad area of ulceration, with borders resembling a map (geographic) or an ameba (ameboid). These ulcers have a longer clinical course and often follow prior inadvertent use of topical steroids in dendritic disease. *Topical steroids are contraindicated in ocular herpetic disease.*

HSV also can invade the corneal stroma. These lesions may or may not be associated with epithelial keratitis. They can become progressively necrotic, with ultimate corneal thinning and perforation.

Another form of keratitis is the indolent ulcer or metaherpetic disease. In this entity, the ulcer has a protracted course unresponsive to antiviral therapy. There usually is marked corneal anesthesia. On cultures, these ulcers do not produce virus and are believed to be related to recurrent epithelial erosions that fail to heal because the epithelium poorly attaches to the Bowman membrane.

An additional form of stromal keratitis is a disciform lesion characterized by a central round stromal opacity with corneal thickening and edema. The opacity is a fine granular infiltrate. The Descemet membrane may have striae. Uveitis usually is a concomitant finding, with keratic precipitates on the endothelium behind the disc of edema. Rarely, an immune ring is seen surrounding the central lesion. The vision generally is blurred, with some tearing and photophobia.

Therapy of lesions with active viral epithelial disease (dendritic and geographic ulcers) requires antiviral therapy of idoxuridine, vidarabine, trifluridine. Débridement of the epithelium also is of benefit. Antiviral therapy is indicted in active stromal disease. Disciform stromal disease and uveitis are thought to be due to an immune response to viral antigen without active viral replication. Judicious use of topical steroids in conjunction with antiviral therapy is employed.

A similar disciform stromal keratitis with edema, after chickenpox (varicella) conjunctivitis with keratitis or herpes zoster keratitis, also is thought to represent an immune response to viral antigen. As in HSV disciform keratitis, topical steroid therapy is indicated, but antviral therapy is not required.

Keratoconus. This is a corneal degeneration of unknown etiology, which usually is bilateral. It manifests with apical corneal thinning, scarring, and conical ectasia of the central cornea. It is noninflammatory and results in a painless, progressive visual loss due to slowly developing and irregular myopic corneal astigmatism. It becomes apparent most often during puberty. Patients with previous histories of atopic or vernal conjunctivitis have more of a tendency to develop keratoconus, and there is a high incidence of prior atopic disease in patients with keratoconus. The irregular corneal astigmatism can be corrected in its initial form with rigid contact lenses to provide good vision. If the disease progresses, a corneal transplant may be necessary. Because the cornea is avascular, success rates for corneal transplants in this condition are greater than 90 percent.

Mooren Ulcer. This is a chronic, progressive, marginal corneal ulceration not associated with any systemic disease. It occurs in older patients and is very painful. The ulcer begins as a stromal infiltrate that destroys the overlying epithelium, then spreads both circumferentially and centripetally. It has a prolonged course that may be unresponsive to any form of therapy. The overhanging edge of the ulcer contains mainly polymorphonuclear leukocytes, the base contains numerous plasma cells and leukocytes, and giant cells may be found. The adjacent conjunctiva contains mostly plasma cells. Proteolytic enzymes are present in the conjunctiva, and this has been the basis for therapeutic conjunctival resection. Keratectomy to remove corneal tissue that is believed to contain the antigenic reservoir has been tried. Cryotherapy has been applied to conjunctiva and cornea. Cytotoxic drugs (cyclophosphamide and methotrexate) have been used to systemically ameliorate the disease.

DISEASES OF THE LENS

Atopic Cataract. Cataract formation usually is related to congenital development problems, changes due to senility, or trauma. It may be drug (steroid) induced or secondary to intraocular inflammation. However, patients with atopic dermatitis have an increased incidence (8 to 10 percent) of cataracts in early adult life. Typically, the cataract develops as an irregular plaque located in the posterior cortex, although changes may occur in the anterior cortex. Another form of cataract is located in the posterior subcapsular epithelial region. The exact link between atopic disease and cataract formation is not known, but steroid use in an atopic patient is not the cause of the characteristic type of "atopic" cataract.

Lens-induced or Phacogenic Uveitis. Following traumatic or surgical rupture of the lens capsule, a sterile inflammation of the iris and ciliary body can occur due to release of lens material into the aqueous humor. This uveitis develops 1 to 14 days after insult to the lens. The anterior chamber is clouded with inflammatory debris. The inflammation is an immune response to the liberated lens protein that is "foreign" to the immune system, since the lens has been both structurally and anatomically isolated. Keratic precipitates (KP) are seen on the endothelium; these are accumulations of inflammatory cells on the corneal endothelium. The "mutton-fat" KP, as seen in phacogenic uveitis, are large precipitates consisting of macrophages, monocytes, and histiocytes. (The KP in more acute inflammations with polymorphonuclear leukocytes are granular and punctate in shape.) Posterior synechiae from iris to lens and even a cyclitic membrane may develop. The histologic picture reveals the cells of a polymorphonuclear leukocytic infiltration of the disrupted remnant lens material; these cells are surrounded by a zone of mononuclear cells, with some epithelioid and multinucleate giant cells. The iris and ciliary body are primarily involved (with the choroid secondarily affected) and are infiltrated with mononuclear cells, lymphocytes, and plasma cells.

Rarely, the opposite uninjured eye may develop uveal inflammation at a later time. This uveitis also is characterized by a cellular exudation in the anterior chamber, KP, and often a hazy cornea. The phenomenon usually occurs if the second lens is traumatized or developes a cataract. The mechanism is thought to be related to restimulation of the previously primed lymphoid tissue, similar to sympathetic ophthalmia, discussed subsequently.

DISEASES OF THE UVEAL TRACT

Inflammation of the uveal tract (iris, ciliary body, or choroid) accurs mainly in adults. It is relatively uncommon in children and adolescents and almost nonexistent in infants (Giles, 1975). In infants, the two following entities may mimic anterior uveitis: juvenile xanthogranuloma of the iris, with recurrent hyphema, and retinoblastoma, with free-floating cells from the tumor that form a pseudohypopyon in the anterior chamber.

Uveitis Associated with Juvenile Arthritis. The most common type of uveal inflammation in children and adolescents is associated with arthritis. (Arthritic entities are discussed elsewhere in this text.) Associated with pauciarticular or monoarticular arthritis is chronic iridocyclitis. The patient may present with a red eye with decreased vision or with quiet uveitis with few symptoms. If unilateral, the episode may pass unnoticed because vision is only unilaterally affected. Examination often will reveal a dense flare in the anterior chamber and a few KP. Posterior synechiae can occur with the iris adherent to the lens. Long-term changes include posterior subcapsular cataract and band keratopathy. Retinal edema, cystoid macular edema, and hypotony can also occur. Three fourths of the cases are bilateral. Females are affected five times more often than males. Serologically, patients' tests results are negative for rheumatoid factor (RF), but about 50 percent are positive for antinuclear antibody (ANA).

A second type of pauciarticular juvenile arthritis is associated with more acute symptomatic iridocyclitis. Males greatly outnumber females in those affected. Serologically, these patients do not have RF or ANA. Characteristically, they have HLA-B27 haplotypes. The spine usually is affected, and a pattern of early ankylosing spondylitis is present. The acute iridocyclitis is marked by a red eye with ciliary injection, and the anterior chamber has marked flare. The aqueous humor may look thickly proteinaceous, and synechiae may form. The acute iridocyclitis of pauciarticular (ankylosing spondylitis–like) arthritis often will resolve with topical steroid therapy. In the therapy of juvenile uveitis, the use of systemic steroids should be avoided as much as possible. Occasionally, a short course of oral steroids is necessary. Chronic iridocyclitis poses a more difficult therapeutic problem. It may not be controlled totally with topical steroids. Long-term systemic steroids administered in children cause severe side effects, including growth and hormonal problems. Periocular injections can be used, but they are less well tolerated by children than adults.

Uveitis Associated with Infection. Uveitis may occur on an infectious or an immune basis. Even in uveitis associated with known infection, it is not clear whether the uveitis is due to active infection or to the immune response to the infective organism and antigens present. An anterior iridocyclitis may be seen with viral corneal disease or as a sequela of it. This is true for herpes simplex and varicella-zoster virus. A posterior uveitis is associated with toxoplasmosis and usually is congenitally acquired when the parasites reach the fetus via the placenta. The initial inflammation may leave residual organisms encysted in the retina. Periodically, these cysts may rupture and give rise to clinically recurrent attacks of retinochoroiditis. This inflammation usually is suppressed with systemic steroids. Antiparasitic therapy consists of sulfadiazine in conjunction with pyrimethamine, with folic acid supplement to circumvent the folic acid block in humans. (*Toxoplasma* organisms cannot utilize folic acid.) The clinical picture is that of characteristic retinochoroiditis. The classic Sabin-Feldman dye test is less frequently used, since it requires live parasites. Diagnosis can be confirmed by a positive serologic test result. Most commonly, an indirect fluorescent antibody test is used in which IgA and IgM antibodies can be detected. Indirect hemagglutination and complement fixation tests also detect antibodies to the organism. The serologic test is considered significant at any titer, if associated with a retinal lesion morphologically compatible with toxoplasmosis.

Chronic Cyclitis or Pars Planitis. This entity is a bilateral uveitis of children and young adults. It has a subtle onset, and patients are asymptomatic or develop floaters or blurred vision. The eye appears uninflamed externally, but the anterior chamber may have a mild cellular reaction. The anterior vitreous may have cells, and exudates may form on the inferior pars plana ("snowbanks"). Round white opacities ("snowballs") may occur in the vitreous. Diffuse edema of the retina or macula may occur. The course may be benign, or vision-limiting complications may occur. If required, treatment is steroid therapy, usually by injection, although systemic steroids can be used.

Fuchs Heterochromic Iridocyclitis. This ocular condition is an anterior uveitis associated with loss of iris pigment and heterochromia. The etiology is unknown, but there is some evidence for an immune process. Immune complexes have been found in the serum and aqueous humor of patients. The disease usually is unilateral, but bilateral disease is possible. The first sign may be the discolored iris. A mild anterior chamber reaction is present. KP are typically small. Steroids do not usually alter the course, but a brief trial may be employed. Careful follow-up to check for secondary glaucoma and cataract formation is necessary.

Sympathetic Ophthalmia. Sympathetic ophthalmia is a rare granulomatous uveitis that follows an ocular perforating injury involving the uveal tract. The onset of the uveitis is at least 2 weeks and usually 4 to 8 weeks after the injury. The anterior chamber develops a leukocytic reaction and serous exudation. Inflammation spreads throughout the entire uveal tract, including the iris, ciliary body, and choroid. The "sympathizing eye" develops a similar inflammation simultaneously or after the "exciting eye." It is postulated that the inflammation arises owing to an autoimmune phenomenon, with the uveal pigment acting as the antigenic stimulus. Treatment in the past required enucleation of the potentially exciting eye within 2 weeks following the injury to prevent sympathetic uveitis. With the advent of steroids to suppress inflammation, enucleation of the exciting eye probably is not indicated except in those traumatized beyond repair.

REFERENCES

Allansmith, M.R., Korb, D.R., Greiner, J.V., Henriquez, A.S., Simon, M.A., Finnemore, V.M.: Giant papillary conjunctivitis in contact lens wearers. Am. J. Ophthalmol. 83:697, 1977.

Baum, J.L.: Systemic disease associated with tear deficiencies. Int. Ophthalmol. Clin. 13:154, 1973.

Bron, A.J., Tripathi, R.C.: Corneal Disorders. In Goldberg, M.G. (ed.); Genetic and Metabolic Eye Diseases. Boston, Little, Brown and Co., 1974.

Dawson, C.R., Togni, B.: Herpes simplex eye infections: Clinical manifestations, pathogenesis and management. Surv. Ophthalmol. 21:121, 1976.

Duane, T.D. (ed.): External Diseases and the Uvea. Clinical Ophthalmology, Vol. 4. Hagerstown, Maryland, Harper and Row, 1976.

Easty, D., Rice, N.S.C., Jones, B.R.: Disodium chromoglycate (Intal) in the treatment of vernal conjunctivitis. Trans. Ophthalmol. Soc. (U.K.). SCI:491, 1971.

Fisher, A.A.: Allergic reactions to contact lens solutions. Cutis Sept.:209, 1985.

Giles, C.L.: Uveitis in Childhood. In Duane, T.D. (ed.); Clinical Ophthalmology, Vol. 4. Hagerstown, Maryland, Harper and Row, 1975.

Hogan, M.J.: Atopic keratoconjunctivitis. Am. J. Ophthalmol. 36:937, 1953.

Leibowitz, H.M., Kupferman, A.: Bioavailability and therapeutic effectiveness of topically administered corticosteroids. Trans. Am. Acad. Ophthalmol. Otolaryngol. 79:OP–78, 1975.

Ostler, H.B.: Oculogenital disease. Surv. Ophthalmol. 20:233, 1976a.

Ostler, H.B.: Herpes simplex: The primary infection. Surv. Ophthalmol. 21:91, 1976b.

Rahi, A.H.S., Garner, A.: Immunopathology of the Eye. Oxford, Blackwell Scientific Publications, 1976.

Rice, N.S.C., Easty, D., Garner, A., Jones, B.R., Tripahti, R.: Vernal conjunctivitis and its management. Trans. Ophthalmol. Soc. (U.K.). XCI:483, 1971.

Silverstein, A.M.: Allergic Reactions of the Eye. In Gell, P.G.H., Coombs, R.R.A. (eds.); Clinical Aspects of Immunology. London, Blackwell Scientific Publications, 1968.

Theodore, F.H., Schlossman, A.: Ocular Allergy. Baltimore, William and Wilkins Co., 1958.

Wedgwood, R.J., Schaller, J.G.: The pediatric arthritides. Hosp. Practice 83, 1977.

51

Anaphylaxis in Children and Adults

WILLIAM T. KNIKER, M.D.

Systemic anaphylaxis is an acute allergic reaction occurring within a few minutes to a few hours following exposure to a triggering agent. It is potentially life threatening and, as such, constitutes a medical emergency that requires prompt recognition and therapy. Anaphylaxis is initiated by the generalized release of mediators from mast cells, basophils, or both, triggered by a variety of immune or nonimmune mechanisms.

This chapter addresses the common pathogenetic pathway, nature of triggering substances, clinical manifestations, and specific approaches to management of anaphylaxis. Additional details about the pathogenetic and clinical aspects of anaphylaxis can be found in numerous recent reviews (Bartolomei and McCarthy, 1984; Sheffer, 1985a; Beall et al., 1986; Kniker, 1978; Perkin and Anas, 1985; Lichtenstein, 1986; Wasserman, 1983).

COMMON PATHWAY FOR ANAPHYLACTIC REACTIONS

Although the precise pathogenetic mechanism for most anaphylactic reactions is not known, a variety of animal and human studies suggests a common pathway (Table 51–1). The first step is an alteration of mast cell and basophil cell membranes either by an immune event (e.g., binding of an allergen to IgE antibody, attachment of an antigen-antibody complex, or activated complement component) or by a nonimmune stimulus (e.g., codeine), which can induce secretion directly. This is followed by the activation of cell membrane enzymes, such as phospholipases, that initiates the breakdown of arachidonic acid into pathogenetic products and the production of internal second signals, which lead to a drop in the cAMP/cGMP ratio. There is a consequent, immediate explosive release of cell granules (modified lysosomes) and an extracellular solubilization of their stored contents.

Of those initially released mediators (see Table 51–1), histamine is the most important. It probably accounts for most of the early manifestations of anaphylaxis, such as increased vascular permeability, constriction of smooth muscle (as in bronchioles and pulmonary vessels), systemic vasodilation, and cardiac effects, such as dysrhythmia, altered myocardial contractility, and diminished coronary flow. Serotonin appears to play a negligible role in human anaphylaxis.

Following the immediate reaction, mediators that require metabolic degradation and activation become involved and contribute to the reaction. These include the arachidonic acid metabolites (prostaglandins, leukotrienes, and thromboxanes), kallikrein-generated kinins, platelet activating factor (PAF) or acetylglycerylether phosphorylcholine, and products of the Hageman factor cascade, such as complement components, plasmin, and fibrin.

The generation of these substances leads to three basic responses. The first is increased permeability of blood vessels, particularly capillaries and venules, leading to local tissue edema, hypovolemia, and hypotension or even shock. The second response is alteration in smooth muscle tone. Increased contraction is seen in circular muscles around hollow viscuses, such as the bronchioles (asthma) or the gut (hyperperistalsis, vomiting, or diarrhea). Relaxation of smooth muscles occurs in many vessels with vasodilation that leads to more edema, more hypotension, poor tissue perfusion, and augmentation of shock. (Pulmonary vessels are a notable exception, responding instead with marked vasoconstriction). If the reaction proceeds long enough, increased secretion of thickened mucus may be sufficient to contribute to laryngeal or bronchiolar obstruction. In some individuals with anaphylaxis, these pathologic reactions are short lived and relatively mild, e.g., resulting in only transient urticaria. However, even a localized reaction (e.g., laryngeal edema) can be fatal within minutes, as can be a generalized reaction in which there is vascular collapse and shock or severe respiratory obstruction with consequent hypoxia and acidosis.

TABLE 51–1. General Pathogenetic Pathway for
Anaphylactic Reactions

Steps	Events
1. Triggering of mast cell and basophil cell membranes	Triggering signals by IgE antibody–antigen or other immune aggregates or by chemical, physical, or neurogenic factors directly.
2. Activation of membrane enzymes and cytoplasmic second signals	Metabolic breakdown of arachidonic acid into active subunits and drop in cAMP/cGMP ratio internally.
3. Release of mediators of inflammation	Stored—histamine, serotonin, and neutrophil and eosinophil chemotactic factors. Activated—arachidonic acid products, such as LTB_4, LTC_4, LTD_4, thromboxanes, and PGD_2, plus kinins, platelet activating factor (PAF), and Hageman factor cascade.*
4. Functional pathologic responses	Increased vascular permeability with edema and diminished blood volume. Change in smooth muscle tone. Increased secretion of thickened mucus. Altered cardiac excitability and contractility.
5. Inflammation and involvement of secondary mediators (delayed) *(not always seen)*	Infiltration by a variety of leucocytes in response to chemoattractants with release of products that perpetuate the reaction, such as platelet aggregation, complement activation, and proteolytic digestion.

* LTB_4 = leukotriene B_4; LTC_4 = leukotriene C_4; LTD_4 = leukotriene D_4.

When a moderately severe anaphylactic reaction persists for hours, involvement of further secondary mediators occurs (see Table 51–1). Chemoattractants, including neutrophil chemotactic factor, eosinophil chemotactic factor, C3a, C5a, and leukotriene B_4 released at original sites of reaction, bring about the infiltration of neutrophils, eosinophils, basophils, monocytes, and other cells. Mediators and proteolytic enzymes released by these cells may perpetuate the reaction for hours or days. Such inflammatory processes are associated with late or delayed anaphylactic reactions; evidence of such reactions includes cellular infiltration, congestion, marked edema, and hemorrhage commonly present in the tissues of individuals who eventually died of anaphylaxis, but who survived for at least several hours.

TRIGGERS OF ANAPHYLACTIC REACTIONS

The aforementioned sequence of events cannot get underway unless an agent to which the victim is unusually susceptible triggers the process. The list of such agents continues to grow, and the incidence of anaphylactic reactions to an expanding array of triggers appears to be increasing (Lichtenstein, 1986). Most of the important causes of anaphylaxis are listed subsequently in a convenient classification scheme. However, it should be acknowledged that a particular agent may trigger anaphylaxis by more than one mechanism, and that, in a given case, the mechanism may not be precisely determined.

Anaphylactic Reactions often Associated with IgE Antibody

In this circumstance, the triggering substance serves as a complete antigen (protein or polysaccharide) or as a haptene that requires conjugation with some host substance. Upon prior exposure to allergen, the individual makes relatively large amounts of IgE antibody specific for that antigen, which fixes to the surface of mast cells and basophils in various parts of the body. Subsequent exposure to even relatively small amounts of antigen has the potential to trigger a massive release of mediators. Although injection or ingestion is the usual route of allergen entry, some reactions may follow casual contact (Munoz et al., 1985), introduction through skin abrasions (Spitalny et al., 1984), or inhalation of airborne food molecules. Many, but by no means all, individuals who develop anaphylaxis are atopic.

Typical examples of IgE antibody–mediated anaphylactic reactions are listed in Table 51–2. Chymopapain is used as a chemonucleolytic agent in the treatment of lumbar intervertebral joint disease (Shields and Arpin, 1985), and streptokinase is used as a thrombolytic agent (McGrath and Patterson, 1984). Venoms from a

TABLE 51–2. Anaphylactic Reactions that have been Associated with IgE Antibody*

Serum proteins	Heterologous antisera-antitoxins, antileukocyte globulins Monoclonal antibodies, e.g., anticancer Human IgA (in IgA deficiency)
Venoms and insects	Hymenoptera (bees, wasps, hornets, fire ants), jellyfish, snakes, spiders, kissing bugs, mosquitoes
Enzymes	Trypsin, chymotrypsin, chymopapain, penicillinase, L-asparaginase, streptokinase
Immunogens, allergens	DPT, vaccines (or their contaminants), pollen or food allergen extracts
Hormones	Insulin, ACTH, progesterone, relaxin
Seminal plasma	(In the case of a sensitized sex partner.)
Foods and micronutrients	Milk, egg, grains, nuts, seafood, chocolate, citrus, and legumes in particular, but other foods too numerous to list. Thiamine, folic acid, other vitamins.
Polysaccharides	*Acacia*, Dextran, iron-containing Dextran
Drugs and haptenes	*Antimicrobials*—penicillin, cephalosporins, tetracyclines, streptomycin, polymyxin B, nitrofurantoin, aminoglycosides (e.g., vancomycin), amphotericin B *Chemotherapeutic agents*—Adriamycin (doxorubicin), bleomycin, Cisplatin, alkylating agents, cyclophosphamide, mephalan, methotrexate, thiotepa *Miscellaneous*—heparin, protamine, muscle relaxants (tubocurarine, Suxamethonium), ethylene diamine, Azulfidine, cromolyn, psyllium

* At times the triggering mechanism may be nonimmune or involve other immune pathways.

wide array of animals and insects are common causes. Single mosquito bites and ant bites have caused numerous bouts of severe anaphylaxis in a female patient (personal communication, Reagan Hicks). Food or inhalant allergen extracts are not uncommon causes of anaphylaxis, either during an intradermal skin test or after an injection of inhalant allergen in the course of immunotherapy. A contaminant to an immunogen may cause a reaction, as is the case for beta propriolactone (a viricidal agent) added to rabies vaccine (Levenbook et al., 1986). As expected, reactions to hormones, such as insulins and ACTH, derived from other species are not rare; reactions to human-derived biologic products, such as insulin and semen, also occur. Indeed, life-threatening anaphylactic sensitivity to external and endogenous progesterone has been reported (Meggs et al., 1984). Dextran (polyanhydroglucose) is a common plasma expander added to heparin to prevent platelet adhesions in coronary angioplasty (Brown et al., 1985). It has induced anaphylactic or anaphylactic-like (anaphylactoid) reactions in which IgE antibody may not be involved.

Penicillin is by far the most common antimicrobial that causes anaphylaxis, although many others have been implicated as well. Most chemotherapeutic agents used in the treatment of cancer may induce anaphylaxis. Protamine, used in cardiopulmonary bypass surgery, also may induce complement consumption during its administration (Westaby et al., 1985). Two agents administered in the treatment of allergic disorders, ethylenediamine (in aminophylline) and cromolyn, have been implicated. Psyllium is a common ingredient of laxative preparations that may cause anaphylaxis.

Anaphylactic Reactions that have been Associated with Non-IgE Immune Mechanisms

Examples of this triggering mechanism appear in Table 51–3. Injections of immunizing materials, drugs, or other antigens into persons with relatively high levels of IgG, and perhaps IgM, may lead to anaphylactic reactions. The immune complexes activate the classic complement pathway; C3a and C5 (termed anaphylatoxins) are capable of triggering the mast cells and basophils, inducing mediator release. Other mechanisms, poorly understood, doubtless operate.

Some persons with IgA deficiency react to trace amounts of IgA in therapeutic blood prod-

ucts; this reaction may be IgG mediated, or at times, IgE mediated (Burks et al., 1986). Heterologous immunoglobulins (e.g., horse antisera) and human immune globulins given intramuscularly are decreasing in importance, the former being replaced by human products and the latter by intravenous human gamma globulin. Ethylene oxide and cuprophan (cuprammonium) both are components of dialysis membranes; reactions may involve not only complement activation (alternative pathway) but IgE-haptene albumin mediation as well (Grammer et al., 1985; Daugirdas et al., 1985). In L-asparaginase–induced anaphylaxis, IgG and IgM-containing immune complexes appear to be more common than those with IgE (Fabry et al., 1985). Monoclonal antibody therapy of cancer and other diseases will surely become a more common cause of anaphylaxis, either by IgG immune complex mechanisms or by IgE mediated mechanisms (Dillman et al., 1986).

Anaphylactic Reactions that are Presumably not Triggered Immunologically

A large number of chemical agents, usually of low molecular weight, have been found to trigger anaphylactic-like reactions. Because these agents appear to act on mast cell and basophil membranes directly without immune sensitization, these reactions formerly were termed "anaphylactoid." Common examples are found in Table 51–4. The diagnostic agent category has grown rapidly, chiefly caused by the widening use of radiocontrast media (RCM). The overall incidence of anaphylactoid reactions to RCM is about 5 percent (Erffmeyer et al., 1985). Aspirin and various nonsteroidal anti-inflammatory drugs (NSAIDs) are common causes of "allergic" reactions, including anaphylaxis, related possibly to their ability to inhibit prostaglandin synthetase. Local and systemic anesthetics are not uncommon causes; sensitivity usually is limited to members of the ester group or the amide class, although cross-reactivity between the two occurs (Bartolomei and McCarty, 1984). Cremophor EL is a castor oil–based solubilizing agent found in cyclosporine and micronazole compounds (Howrie et al., 1985). Cases of sulfite-induced reactions should diminish now that restaurants are prohibited from using sulfites. Two antiallergic medications deserve mention, antihistamine and hydrocortisone (Peller and Bardana, 1985), since both are used in the treatment of anaphylaxis.

TABLE 51–3. Anaphylactic Reactions that have been Associated with Non-IgE Immune Mechanisms*

Human blood products	IgA (in IgA deficiency), albumin, immunoglobulins, complement (C4), cryoprecipitates
Ethylene oxide and cuprophan	Hemodialysis membranes
Protamine	Cardiopulmonary bypass
L-Asparaginase	Treatment in leukemia
Murine monoclonal antibody	Treatment in cancer
Penicillin and streptokinase	Late or delayed "anaphylactic" reactions

* Commonly, these reactions involve IgG or IgM complexes with antigen and the activation of complement, including C3a and C5a. At times, the triggering mechanism may instead be IgE-mediated or nonimmune.

Physical causes of anaphylaxis are increasingly recognized. Exercise, particularly running, can induce anaphylaxis, partly through neurogenic mechanisms involving hyperventilation of cold dry air (Sheffer et al., 1985). There has been one report of anaphylaxis associated with the exertion of obstetric delivery (Smith et al., 1985). In some persons, running or food alone causes no trouble; however, anaphylaxis occurs if the running takes place within 2 hours of eating certain foods (Sheffer et al., 1985b; Beall et al., 1986). Cholinergic urticaria and anaphylaxis sometimes are associated with heating or exercise (Baadsgaard and Lindskov, 1984; Casale et al., 1986). Exposure to cold and to sunlight are other physical causes.

In some cases of anaphylaxis, no etiologic agent can be found. With repeated bouts of life-threatening disease, systematic and intensive diagnostic studies must be pursued. Stricker and coworkers (1986) reported 7 of 102 patients with "idiopathic" anaphylaxis had atopic sensitivity to a variety of foods (often unusual ones) demonstrated by history, skin test reaction, and positive reaction to challenge.

CLINICAL FEATURES AND MANIFESTATIONS

Diagnosis of acute anaphylaxis is made clinically. Often, there is a history of recent exposure to an agent to which the patient is allergic. However, many individuals can react nonim-

TABLE 51–4. "Anaphylactic" Reactions Generally not Considered to be Immunologically Triggered*

Diagnostic agents	Iodinated radiologic contrast media (RCM), dehydrocholic acid (Decheolin), Bromsulphathalein (BSP), isosulfan blue, fluorescein, indocyanine green
Analgesics	Salicylates and NSAIDs related to arachidonic acid metabolism, aminopyrine
Antimicrobials	Aminoglycosides (e.g., vancomycin) and any of the agents appearing in Table 51–2
Alkaloids	Codeine, morphine
Anesthetics	Esters (e.g., procaine, cocaine) and amides (e.g., lidocaine, bupivacaine)
Drugs and medications	Antihistamines, amphetamines, diuretics, histamine, hydrocortisone, Cremophor EL (solubilizing agent), anti-convulsants, vitamins
Food additives	Sulfites, food dyes (e.g., tartrazine), preservatives (e.g., sodium benzoate)
Physical factors	Exercise induced, sometimes food related
	Cholinergic, heat related
	Sun exposure
	Cold exposure, sometimes with exercise
Idiopathic factors	No relevant trigger found

* In some instances, the triggering mechanism may include an immune feature or a cofactor.

munologically to low molecular weight materials and may have life-threatening reactions to the first known exposure to those substances.

One should attempt to establish accurately the time that has elapsed from exposure to reaction; a reaction that begins minutes after exposure to the trigger tends to be more severe than a reaction that begins an hour or so later. It is important not only to note which medications already may have been used to treat the symptoms, but to determine which long-term medications the patient takes. Certain of these agents may potentiate anaphylaxis, hinder its treatment, or both; beta-adrenergic blockers (Lundin and Delano, 1984), NSAIDs (Bernard and Kersley, 1986), and beta-adrenergic agents themselves (Frossard et al., 1985) are notable examples.

Mild Reactions

Mild reactions tend to have delayed onsets and are manifested predominantly by urticaria, with or without edema, limited to the local area if antigen had been injected. Systemic manifestations, such as nasal stuffiness and rhinorrhea, may be absent or mild.

Serious Reactions

Serious reactions can be defined as any that are diffuse, generalized, or systemic, or that demonstrate hypotension or obstruction to respiration. The patient who has local reactions that spread proximally to involve an entire limb should be observed for several hours for possible systemic involvement. Any generalized anaphylactic reaction should be taken seriously since sudden life-threatening symptoms may not appear until several hours have elapsed.

Prodromal symptoms may include a sense of warmth, tingling, and pruritus, which spread from the head and trunk centripetally, lightheadedness, dizziness, and headache. Thereafter symptoms worsen and are found in one or more of four organ systems, as discussed.

Skin and Soft Tissues. The skin is the most common organ manifesting anaphylaxis and usually is the earliest. Initial pallor may become diffuse flushing (erythema). Deep red or purplish discoloration suggests impending shock. With severe respiratory obstruction, cyanosis is evident. Urticaria and itching most commonly involve the lips, nose, periorbital areas, ears,

hands, and feet. Angioedema is commonest in the lips and periorbital regions.

Gastrointestinal System. Reactions involving the gut are least common and never occur alone. When present, they may be disabling but not life threatening. Symptoms include nausea and vomiting, abdominal cramps or colic, uterine cramps, and diarrhea that becomes bloody or progresses to fecal incontinence.

Respiratory System. Involvement of the respiratory system accounts for the majority of deaths in anaphylaxis. Laryngospasm, laryngeal edema, bronchospasm, bronchial obstruction, or status asthmaticus all can lead to hypoxemia, hypercapnia, acidosis, and death. Partial *upper* airway obstruction is suggested by choking, hoarseness, stridor, and the sensation of a lump in the throat. Partial *lower* respiratory obstruction is suggested by chest tightness or pain, repeated coughing, dyspnea, and wheezing.

Cardiovascular System. Involvement of this system is the second most common cause of death related to anaphylaxis. A patient becomes uneasy and anxious and may have a sense of impending doom or even collapse. An extremely reliable sign is tachycardia above 140 beats/min, sometimes accompanied with dysrythmias. (Bradycardia occurs if the patient is taking beta blockers.) Hypovolemic shock with diminished left-sided heart filling, stroke volume, and cardiac output may be associated with severe hypotension unresponsive to usual vasopressors. Acidemia and hypoxemia frequently appear at this point, potentiating the physiologic abnormalities already present. Patients with severe anaphylaxis may present with severe dyspnea secondary to fulminant noncardiac pulmonary edema caused by dramatic alterations in the pulmonary vascular bed, but this is unusual (Solomon, 1986).

Differential Diagnosis

Although anaphylaxis generally causes no diagnostic problem, there are other conditions with which it can be confused. Syncopal or vasovagal reactions do show hypotension, collapse, and sometimes nausea; however, a patient so affected exhibits pallid skin, cool extremities, bradycardia and absence of respiratory obstruction, urticaria, or itching. Hyperventilation episodes and anxiety attacks associated with an inciting agent or event should cause no serious problems with the differential diagnosis. The adult respiratory distress syndrome (ARDS) may share with anaphylaxis such features as massive noncardiac pulmonary edema, dyspnea, hypotension, and hypokalemia; however, the absence of pruritus, urticaria, and an incitant history can be helpful in distinguishing ARDS from anaphylaxis (Solomon, 1986).

MANAGEMENT

Although most fatal anaphylactic reactions occur within minutes after triggering events, severe reactions may develop hours later. Because one cannot predict the outcome on early clinical grounds, patients should be observed closely (with vital signs and blood pressure measurements) in the first hours and treated aggressively if they worsen. Those patients with apparently mild reactions who are released from the physician's office or emergency department must be given strict instructions to return immediately if new symptoms appear. Patients with severe anaphylaxis should be hospitalized and monitored closely for at least a day to detect such recurrences. The elderly patient, the patient with cardiovascular disesae, and the patient with prolonged hypoxia must be observed for myocardial ischemia and cerebrovascular complications.

Mild Reactions

1. *Aqueous epinephrine* (1 : 1000) remains the drug of choice for initial treatment of anaphylactic reactions; it inhibits the release of mast cell – mediators, possibly by increasing mast cell cAMP. It also produces alpha-adrenergic mediated vasoconstriction and beta-adrenergic mediated bronchodilation. For children, the intramuscular dose is 0.01 mg/kg up to 0.3 ml and for adults it is 0.2 to 0.5 ml. The dose can be repeated every 15 minutes for several doses if necessary.

2. If the offending antigen has been introduced by insect sting or by injection, a *tourniquet* can be applied loosely proximal to the site to retard systemic absorption. Aqueous epinephrine (1 : 1000) in a dose of 0.2 to 0.3 ml also may be injected into the antigen site.

3. For a delayed effect, an *antihistamine,* such as diphenhydramine or hydroxyzine 1 mg/kg up to a total of 75 mg, can be given parentally or orally. *Aminophylline or theophyl-*

line should be considered with the occurrence of bronchospasm, using 250 mg orally (5 to 6 mg/kg for children) q6h for a few doses, if the patient is not on long-term theophylline therapy.

4. After 2 or more hours of observation, the patient whose symptoms have cleared or whose symptoms are mild can be released with strict instructions to return if symptoms worsen. However, protracted or delayed recurrence of anaphylaxis can occur and does not appear preventable by steroids administered at the onset of the immediate reaction (Stark and Sullivan, 1986). Consequently, it is important that the patient be observed for hours in a setting in which medical treatment is ready and immediately available should symptoms reappear.

Severe Reactions

The physician should move quickly and decisively because the patient may worsen in minutes. After initial outpatient treatment, transfer to an intensive care unit for further management and observation for at least 24 hours is recommended.

1. General Measures
   a. *Aqueous epinephrine* (1 : 1000) 0.01 mg/kg (up to 0.5 ml total), is given intramuscularly every 5 to 15 minutes for several repeated doses. If response is too slow or inadequate, intravenous or even endotracheal tube routes may be tried (see subsequent section 3.c.). Slow administration favors beta-adrenergic bronchodilator effects; fast administration favors alpha-adrenergic vasoconstrictive, blood pressure – raising effects. In a pregnant woman, the substitution of intravenous *ephedrine* at 25 to 50 mg in a "push dose" seems to be safer for the fetus (Entman and Moise, 1984).

   Patients on beta-adrenergic blocking drugs may not respond to epinephrine. They may, in fact, get worse because of unopposed alpha-adrenergic stimulation by epinephrine (Barach et al., 1984). In some of these patients, any drug with both alpha- and beta-adrenergic effects may be contraindicated. Alternative drugs should be considered, as follows: (1) nebulized beta selective adrenergic agents (Lundin et al., 1984); (2) intravenous glucagon, 1 to 5 mg (Sheffer, 1985); (3) nebulized atropine, 0.05 to 0.075

mg/kg every 4 hours, to elevate the heart rate; (4) intravenous aminophylline, and (5) corticosteroids.

b. For local treatment of antigen introduced by sting or injection, carry out the same measures as indicated for mild reactions.

c. *Antihistamines* are indicated, preferably the combination of H1 and H2 antagonists, since they are synergistic in their effects, particularly on blood vessels. The H1 antagonists, diphenhydramine and hydroxyzine, 1 mg/kg up to 50 to 75 mg total dose, can be given intramuscular or intravenously repeating every 6 to 8 hours as indicated. Large doses may depress respiration. For H2 blocking, oral cimetidine and ranitidine are available. Adult intravenous doses are 300 mg for cimetidine and 50 mg for ranitidine, given every 6 to 8 hours. Cimetidine is not compatible with intravenous aminophylline (Randall, 1985).

d. *Corticosteroids* probably should be given to anyone with a serious reaction, not for an immediate effect but to exert multiple antiallergic and beta-adrenergic augmenting effects in the hours that follow. Prednisone orally in relatively large doses is acceptable, if the patient is alert and ambulatory. Otherwise, consider hydrocortisone sodium succinate (Solu-Cortef), 5 to 10 mg/kg (100 to 250 mg in adults) or one fourth or one half that dose of intravenous methylprednisolone sodium succinate (Solu-Medrol) every 4 to 6 hours.

e. *Intravenous fluids* usually are indicated to replete fluids lost into the third space, to maintain fluid balance, to facilitate administration of medications, and to treat shock or acidosis if they develop.

f. *Emotional support* is an often neglected but extremely important aspect of therapy. The patient obviously is worried, sometimes agitated, and benefits greatly from calm and compassionate attention by the health care team.

2. Prevention and Management of Respiratory Problems

Respiratory obstruction and complications of hypoxemia account for the majority of deaths associated with anaphylaxis. The physician should be familiar with the evidences of hypoxia and respiratory acidosis so that appropriate care can be promptly given (Table 51–5).

a. *Maintenance of an adequate airway* is an initial and continuing, overriding concern. If the airway closes, one has up to 3 minutes to act. With laryngeal edema, cricothyrotomy or tracheostomy may be needed. For severe respiratory obstruction endotracheal intubation is necessary.

b. *Oyxgen* is an extremely important supportive measure, both for pulmonary and cardiovascular involvement. It is given 100 percent, at 4 to 6 L/min, often by nasal cannula and by assisted ventilation, if necessary.

c. *Bronchodilators* are indicated when lower ventilatory obstruction occurs; the obstruction may progress to an unresponsive form of status asthmaticus. *Aminophylline*, intravenously, often is helpful; a bolus of 5 to 7 mg/kg (250 to 500 mg for adults) in 100 to 250 ml of saline is given over 15 to 20 minutes. With the help provided through determination of theophylline levels, an appropriate dose may be repeated q6h or, in severe cases, a continuous drip of 0.5 to 1.0 mg/kg/h is preferable.

Beta-adrenergic agents should be employed aggressively, since in many cases responsiveness is reduced by the metabolic alterations associated with severe anaphylaxis. The preferred route is topi-

TABLE 51–5. Signs and Symptoms of Hypoxia and Respiratory Acidosis

Hypoxia	Hypercapnia (or Decreased pH)
Changes in judgment; euphoria	Confusion, somnolence, coma
Agitation, confusion, anxiety	Headache, papilledema, miosis
Obtundent or coma	Muscle twitching, asterixis
Tachycardia, dysrythmias	Hypertension, later hypotension
Central cyanosis, diaphoresis	Diaphoresis
Hypertension or hypotension	Cardiac failure
Cardiac or renal failure	

cal (e.g., nebulizer); beta-2 selective drugs, such as metaproterenol, albuterol, and terbutaline, appear to be more efficacious with fewer side effects by topical delivery (Lundin et al., 1984). With unremittent asthmatic obstruction, epinephrine instilled via endotracheal tube may be indicated (see 3.c.). An asthmatic patient on long-term beta-adrenergic drug therapy may have relative beta receptor desensitization, and larger than expected doses of epinephrine or beta-adrenergic drug may be required.

3. Prevention and Management of Cardiovascular Shock

In any victim of severe anaphylaxis, the possibility of developing hypovolemic shock or hypotensive shock, or both, exists. The onset may be sudden or insidious, not appearing until many hours into the reaction. Once shock begins to develop or is present, continuous monitoring with electrocardiography is desirable.

a. *Maintain adequate airway* and give *100 percent oxygen,* by assisted ventilation, if necessary.

b. Insert a *line (e.g., central venous pressure or CVP)* for rapid intravenous administration, so that extravasation of irritating or vasoactive medications into local tissues is prevented. Use the line to give adequate amounts of *colloidal plasma expanders* (e.g., albumin, and Dextran) to restore blood volume and *electrolytes* to treat acidosis. Metabolic acidosis secondary to inadequate tissue perfusion should be vigorously treated, possibly with sodium bicarbonate. Periodic measurements of CVP help protect against fluid overload.

c. If the blood pressure cannot be maintained after volume replacement, a *vasopressor or adrenergic agent* may need to be given by intravenous drip. Consider starting with *dopamine,* 200 mg in 250 ml saline, or glucose, 5 μg/kg/min, titrated to a maintenance rate of 5 to 50 μg/kg/min. Dopamine preserves renal blood flow unlike many of the other pressors. *Isoproterenol* is another possibility, administering 1 to 2 mg in 250 or 500 ml saline, titration guided by blood pressure and pulse measurements, as in severe asthma.

In the presence of profound shock or collapse, some workers recommend starting with *epinephrine* and switching to dopamine hours later, if hypotension persists. The American Heart Association currently recommends endotracheal administration of epinephrine, if vascular access is not yet available (Powers and Donorwitz, 1984). The adult dose is 1 mg or 10 ml of a 1:10,000 solution, introduced with a long needle or catheter into the endotracheal tube, followed by hyperventilation to insure rapid distribution. In children, the dose is 0.1 mg/kg of a 1:10,000 solution of epinephrine, diluted in saline to a volume of 5 ml.

Once an intravenous line is established, an initial epinephrine dose of 0.1 mg (0.1 ml) of a 1:1000 dilution mixed in 10 ml normal saline is infused over 5 to 10 minutes (Barach et al., 1984). If there is little or no improvement, a continuous infusion is begun. To prepare, add 0.5 mg (0.5 ml) of 1:1000 dilution to 100 ml D5/W; this achieves a concentration of 5 μg/ml. In children, start with 0.1 μg/kg/min, with increments of 0.1 μg/kg/min up to a maximum of 1.5 μg/kg/min. For adults, start with 1.0 μg/min, increasing to a maximum of 4 to 10 μg/min, if no effect is observed.

External counter pressure provided by Military Anti-Shock Trousers (MAST) is reported to be helpful in combating shock (Bickell et al., 1984). The trousers appear to cause increases in blood pressure and hemodynamic stability, perhaps by counteracting the effects of vasodilation and capillary leak, by increasing vascular resistance, and by promoting venous return.

Follow-up Care and Prevention of Future Anaphylactic Reactions

Once the patient has recovered sufficiently to be released from the emergency room (if the reaction was mild) or to be discharged from the hospital (if the reaction was serious), every effort should be made to prevent future reactions. If later contact with a triggering agent is possible, the patient should be provided with a kit for emergency self treatment. At the least, it should contain a form of premeasured injectable epinephrine and chewable antihistamine tablets. Additionally, a metered dose inhaler containing epinephrine, isoproterenol, or a selective beta-2 adrenergic agent seems advisable. The individual also should tell all responsible health care personnel about his or her sensitivity and wear a Medic-Alert tag.*

A careful and detailed history usually will uncover the agent or antigen that initiated the acute allergic reaction. Precise identification, at times, may be difficult, however. If an insect sting is the culprit, it often is impossible to determine which insect was responsible. If a number of drugs were concomitantly administered, identification of the individual offender may be difficult. Identification of a particular food may be possible only after repeated reactions or exhaustive tests. Skin tests (and in some cases radioallergosorbent tests) have proved to be of considerable value in identifying individuals at risk for chymopapain (Cogen et al., 1985), *Triatoma* bug bites (Rohr et al., 1984), streptokinase (McGrath and Patterson, 1984), insect venom (Reisman et al., 1985), and penicillin (O'Leary and Smith, 1986). In the case of penicillin, skin testing is particularly useful. An individual with a negative reaction to appropriate reagents can safely receive penicillin 99 percent of the time (Lichtenstein, 1986).

Once the substance that triggers anaphylaxis is identified, a number of options to reduce the likelihood of future reactions are presented. The first is to avoid contact with the offending drug, food, or substance. If one is sensitive to a drug, cross-reacting drugs need to be recognized, and safe alternative drugs need to be selected for treatment purposes (Sheffer, 1984). It may be advisable for individuals predisposed to anaphylaxis to minimize the use of beta blockers, NSAIDs, and beta-adrenergic agents. A second option in preventing subsequent anaphylactic reactions to unavoidable agents is to reduce sensitivity by immunotherapy. This is extremely successful in protecting individuals sensitive to insect venom, in particular, (Lichtenstein, 1986; Reismann et al., 1985) and *Triatoma* antigen (Rohr et al., 1984). In addition, rapid desensitization with a critically needed drug (e.g., penicillin) can be accomplished by rapidly advancing from tiny amounts to large amounts of the drug in antigen excess (Sullivan et al., 1982). Finally, in those patients who face reexposure to a substance (e.g., RCM or chymopapain) known to cause anaphylaxis, pretreatment with antianaphylactic medications can reduce the severity, if not the likelihood, of another anaphylactic episode. Often included are a combination of H1 and H2 antagonists (superior to either alone), a sympathomimetic drug, and a corticosteroid (Sage, 1985). Calcium channel blockers also offer promise.

REFERENCES

Baadsgaard, O., Lindskov, R.: Cholinergic urticaria with anaphylaxis induced by exercise or heating. Acta Derm. Venereol. (Stockh) 64:344–346, 1984.

Barach, E.M., Nowak, R.M., Lee, T.G., et al.: Epinephrine for treatment of anaphylactic shock. J.A.M.A. 251:2118–2122, 1984.

Bartolomei, F.J., McCarthy, D.J.: Anaphylaxis: mechanisms, manifestations, and management. J. Foot Surg. 23:485–488, 1984.

Beall, G.N., Casaburi, R., Singer, A.: Anaphylaxis—everyone's problem. West J. Med. 144:329–337, 1986.

Bernard, A.A., Kersley, J.B.: Sensitivity to insect stings in patients taking anti-inflammatory drugs. Brit. Med. J. [Clin. Res.] 292:378–379, 1986.

Bickell, W.H., Dice, W.H.: Military Anti-Shock Trousers in a patient with adrenergic-resistant anaphylaxis. Ann. Emerg. Med. 13:189–190, 1984.

Brown, R.I., Aldridge, H.E., Schwartz, L. et al.: The use of Dextran–40 during percutaneous transluminal coronary angioplasty: A report of three cases of anaphylactoid reactions—one near fatal. Cathet. Cardiovasc. Diag. 11:591–595, 1985.

Burks, A.W., Sampson, H.A., Buckley, R.H.: Anaphylactic reactions after gamma globulin administration in patients with hypogammaglobulinemia. N. Engl. J. Med. 314:560–564, 1986.

Casale, T.B., Keahey, T.M., Kaliner, M.: Exercise-induced anaphylactic syndromes: Insight into diagnostic and pathophysiologic features. J.A.M.A. 255:2049–2053, 1986.

Cogen, F.C., Goldstein, M., Zweiman, B.: Skin testing in chymopapain anaphylaxis. J. Allergy Clin. Immunol. 75:728–730, 1985.

Daugirdas, J.T., Ing, T.S., Roxe, D.M., et al.: Severe anaphylactoid reactions to cuprammonium cellulose hemodialyzers. Arch. Intern. Med. 145:489–494, 1985.

Dillman, R.O., Beauregard, J.C., Halpern, S.E., et al.: Toxicities and side effects associated with intravenous infusions of murine monoclonal antibodies. J. Biol. Resp. Mod. 5:73–84, 1986.

Entman, S.S., Moise, K.J.: Anaphylaxis in pregnancy. South. Med. J. 77:402, 1984.

Erffmeyer, J.E., Siegle, R.L., Lieberman, P.: Allergy grand rounds: Anaphylactoid reactions to radiocontrast material. J. Allergy Clin. Immunol. 75:401–410, 1985.

Fabry, U., Korholz, D., Jurgens, H., et al.: Anaphylaxis to L-asparaginase during treatment for acute lymphoblastic leukemia in children—evidence of a complement-mediated mechanism. Pediatr. Res. 19:400–408, 1985.

Frossard, N., Frankhuyzen-Sierevogel, J.C., Binck, M., et al.: Potential anti-anaphylactic activity of clenbuterol, a beta-agonist with calcium antagonist properties. Agent. Act. 16:166–169, 1985.

Grammer, L.C., Paterson, B.F., Roxe, D., et al.: IgE against ethylene oxide—altered human serum albumin in pa-

---

* Medic-Alert Foundation, PO Box 1009, Turlock, CA 95380.

tients with anaphylactic reactions to dialysis. J. Allergy Clin. Immunol. 76:511–514, 1985.

Howrie, D.L., Ptachcinski, R.J., Griffith, B.P., et al.: Anaphylactoid reactions associated with parenteral cyclosporine use: Possible role of Cremophor EL. Drug Intell. Clin. Pharm. 19:425–472, 1985.

Kniker, W.T.: Anaphylaxis and Anaphylactoid Reactions. In Tintalli, J. (ed.). A Study Guide in Emergency Medicine. American College of Emergency Physicians, Dallas, vol. 1:61–66, 1978.

Levenbook, I.S., Merritt, B.A., Fitzgerald, E.A., et al.: Sensitization induced in guinea pigs with beta-propriolactone–treated serum albumin: Experimental evidence for the cause of allergic reactions in humans receiving human diploid cell rabies vaccines. Int. Arch. Allergy Appl. Immunol. 80:110–111, 1986.

Lichtenstein, L.M.: Human anaphylaxis. [Editorial]. West. J. Med. 144:355–357, 1986.

Lundin, A.P., Delano, B.G.: Response to inhaled beta-agonist in a patient receiving beta-adrenergic blockers. Arch. Intern. Med. 144:1882–1883, 1984.

McGrath, K.G., Patterson, R.: Anaphylactic reactivity to streptokinase. J.A.M.A. 252:1314–1317, 1984.

Meggs, W.J., Pescovitz, O.H., Metcalfe, D., et al.: Progesterone sensitivity as a cause of recurrent anaphylaxis. N. Engl. J. Med. 311:1236–1238, 1984.

Munoz, D., Leanizbarrutia, I., Lobera, T., et al.: Anaphylaxis from contact with carrot. Cont. Derm. 13:345–346, 1985.

O'Leary, M.R., Smith, M.S.: Penicillin anaphylaxis. Am. J. Em. Med. 4:241–247, 1986.

Peller, J.S., Bardana, E.J., Jr.: Anaphylactoid reaction to corticosteroid: Case report and review of the literature. Ann. Allergy 54:302–305, 1985.

Perkin, R.M., Anas, N.G.: Mechanisms and management of anaphylactic shock not responding to traditional therapy. Ann. Allergy 54:202–208, 1985.

Powers, R.D., Donowitz, L.G.: Endotracheal administration of emergency medications. South. Med. J. 77:340–341, 346, 1984.

Randall, B.J.: Reacting to anaphylaxis. Nursing 16:34–40, 1985.

Reismann, R.E., Dvorin, D.J., Randolph, C.C., et al.: Stinging insect allergy: Natural history and modification with venom immunotherapy. J. Allergy Clin. Immunol. 75:735–740, 1985.

Rohr, A.S., Marshall, N.A., Saxon, A.: Successful immunotherapy for *Triatoma protracta*–induced anaphylaxis. J. Allergy Clin. Immunol. 73:369–375, 1984.

Sage, D.J.: Management of acute anaphylactoid reactions. Int. Anesthesiol. Clin. 23:175–186, 1985.

Sheffer, A.L.: Continuing medical education: Anaphylaxis. J. Allergy Clin. Immunol. 75:227–235, 1985.

Sheffer, A.L., Pennoyer, D.S.: Management of adverse drug reactions. J. Allergy Clin. Immunol. 74:580–588, 1984.

Sheffer, A.L., Tong, A.K.F., Murphy, G.F., et al.: Exercise-induced anaphylaxis: A serious form of physical allergy associated with mast cell degranulation. J. Allergy Clin. Immunol. 75:479–484, 1985.

Shields, C.B., Arpin, E.J.: Update on chymopapain. Neurol. Clin. 3:393–403, 1985.

Smith, H.S., Hare, M.J., Hoggarth, C.E., et al.: Delivery as a cause of exercise-induced anaphylactoid reaction: Case report. Brit. J. Obstet. Gynaecol. 92:1196–1198, 1985.

Solomon, D.R.: Anaphylactoid reaction and non-cardiac pulmonary edema following intravenous contrast injection. Am. J. Em. Med. 4:146–149, 1986.

Spitalny, K.C., Farnham, J.E., Witherell, L.E., et al.: Alpine slide anaphylaxis. N. Engl. J. Med. 310:1034–1037, 1984.

Stark, B.J., Sullivan, T.J.: Biphasic and protracted anaphylaxis. J. Allergy. Clin. Immunol. 78:76–83, 1986.

Stricker, W.E., Anorve-Lopez, E., Reed, C.E.: Food skin testing in patients with idiopathic anaphylaxis. J. Allergy Clin. Immunol. 77:516–519, 1986.

Sullivan, T.J., Yecies, L.D., Shatz, G.S., et al.: Desensitization of patients allergic to penicillin using orally administered beta-lactam antibiotics. J. Allergy Clin. Immunol. 69:275–282, 1982.

Wasserman, S.I.: Anaphylaxis. In Middleton, R.J., Reed, C.E., Ellis, E.F. (eds.), Allergy Principles and Practice. St. Louis, C.V. Mosby Co., 1983.

Westaby S., Turner, M.W., Stark, J.: Complement activation and anaphylactoid response to protamine in a child after cardiopulmonary bypass. Brit. Heart J. 53:574–576, 1985.

52

Insect Allergy (Adults and Children)*

JOHN W. YUNGINGER, M.D.

The accurate diagnosis and proper therapy of a patient with insect allergy depend on identification of the culprit insect, classification of the patient's reaction, and knowledge of the natural history of allergic reactions to insects (Levine and Lockey, 1981).

THE INSECTS

The insects commonly incriminated in producing allergic reactions are listed in Table 52–1. By far the most important are the stinging insects of the order Hymenoptera. Only about one third of victims can identify reliably the insect responsible for their stings. The culprit insect can usually be identified by determining the circumstances surrounding the sting and knowing some rudimentary entomology. Insects are often referred to by local names, such as "sweat bee" or "guinea wasp"; submission of a specimen insect to an entomologist may be required for a more scientific identification. Alternatively, a reference text may be useful (Smith, 1973).

Honeybees are mild-mannered insects that usually will not sting unless stepped or sat upon. The honeybee stinger is barbed and usually remains embedded in the sting victim. Honeybee venom is bacteriostatic, so it is unusual for honeybee stings to become secondarily infected. Bumblebees are large, slow-flying, yellow and black insects that rarely cause generalized sting reactions. Their venom crossreacts with that of honeybees, so that patients experiencing generalized reactions to bumblebees should be managed as honeybee-sensitive patients.

Wasps, yellow jackets, and hornets are col-lectively referred to as vespids. Paper wasps are widely distributed throughout the United States, building aerial nests under the overhangs of homes or of outbuildings. The coloration of paper wasps varies widely, ranging from gray to yellow to reddish orange. Yellow jackets are ill-tempered, ground-nesting insects that often sting without provocation. They frequently nest in cracks in sidewalks, in the foundations of buildings, or in abandoned animal burrows. Yellow jackets are scavengers, often feeding in garbage cans or on fallen rotten fruit or vegetables. Consequently, cellulitis is occasionally seen following yellow jacket stings. Hornets build aerial nests that resemble Japanese lanterns, usually located in trees or shrubs or on the overhangs of buildings.

Fire ants are widespread along the southern Atlantic coast and the Gulf of Mexico, building dirt mounds 1 or 2 feet in height. They anchor themselves by their mandibles when stinging, often leaving a semicircular row of vesicles at the sting site.

Biting insects, such as flies and mosquitos, frequently produce impressive large local immediate reactions, particularly in toddlers and preschool age children. A more delayed, hyperpigmented, pruritic reaction called papular urticaria can be seen at bite sites. This has been attributed to a delayed hypersensitivity reaction to the insect salivary proteins. However, the possible immune nature of these reactions has been inadequately determined; IgE-dependent mechanisms have rarely been demonstrated by rigorous techniques (Wilbur and Evans, 1975). Reactions to flies and mosquito bites are rarely systemic in nature; skin tests and immunotherapy are rarely warranted. Topical glucocorticoid creams and oral antihistamines may provide relief of itching.

Chiggers are the larval forms of several species of mites; they can produce an intensely pruritic dermatitis in humans. Chigger bites can be prevented by use of mite repellents on clothing. The dermatitis is treated with topical shake lotions, glucocorticoid creams, and oral antihistamines.

Biting insects that have been documented to cause IgE-mediated systemic reactions are the *Triatoma* or kissing bugs. These relatively large insects are stealthy nocturnal blood feeders whose saliva has been shown to contain allergens capable of inducing human anaphylaxis

*Supported in part by a U.S.P.H.S grant (AI-21398) and by Mayo Foundation.

TABLE 52–1. Common Stinging and Biting Insects

Stinging Insects (Hymenoptera)
  Bees — honeybee, bumblebee
  Vespids — wasps, yellow jackets, hornets
  Fire ants

Biting Insects
  Flies, mosquitos (Diptera)
  Chiggers (Acari)
  Kissing bugs (Hemiptera)

(Rohr et al., 1984). Management of *Triatoma*-sensitive patients should be identical to that described subsequently for stinging insects, but unfortunately diagnostic and therapeutic *Triatoma* extracts are not yet available.

CLASSIFICATION OF INSECT REACTIONS

A suggested classification of insect reactions is shown in Table 52–2 (Yunginger, 1981). Reactions are conveniently divided into immediate (up to 2 or 4 hours) or delayed (after 4 hours), depending on the time elapsed between the bite or sting and the development of signs or symptoms.

Immediate reactions are in turn divided into local, large local, systemic, and toxic. Local reactions are normal and consist of transient pain, erythema, and swelling at the sting or bite site. Large local reactions are more extensive, often involving swelling and erythema of most of an extremity; however, by definition, all signs and symptoms are contiguous with the sting or bite site. Systemic reactions are generalized and involve signs or symptoms at a site remote from the sting or bite site. For example, a sting on the forehead resulting in angioedema of the eyelids would be classified as a local or large local reaction, whereas a sting on the foot resulting in angioedema of the eyelids would be considered a systemic reaction. Systemic reactions may involve generalized urticaria and pruritus, cutaneous or laryngeal edema, bronchospasm, or

TABLE 52–2. Classification of Insect Reactions

Immediate (up to 2 to 4 hours after sting or bite)
  Local
  Large local
  Systemic
  Toxic
Delayed (4 hours or more after sting or bite)

vascular collapse. These are IgE-mediated reactions that may be life threatening, if pulmonary or cardiovascular symptoms predominate. Toxic reactions may occur after a person receives multiple stings within a short period of time. The signs and symptoms are identical to those of systemic reactions, but in this case the symptoms are produced by exogenous vasoactive amines delivered in the insect venom, rather than endogenous vasoactive materials released as a consequence of venom allergen-IgE antibody interaction on mast cell surfaces.

Delayed reactions may take several clinical forms (Light et al., 1977), including serum sickness–like reactions, transverse myelitis, or myocarditis. Many large local reactions attain maximal size 12 to 24 hours after the sting. Honeybee stings are occasionally followed by an influenza-like syndrome involving fever, myalgia, and shaking chills 8 to 24 hours after the sting. The pathophysiology of most delayed reactions is unclear; immunologic mechanisms may not be involved. Delayed reactions are rarely life threatening.

TREATMENT OF ACUTE REACTIONS

Local reactions require no therapy. Large local reactions frequently are treated with antihistamines or short courses of oral glucocorticoids. Although such therapy poses little risk to most patients, the efficacy of these medications has not been documented by formal scientific study.

The acute management of systemic reactions is in essence the treatment of anaphylaxis. For severe reactions, maintenance of the airway and administration of oxygen become the primary goals. Epinephrine is the drug of choice in most instances, unless the patient has a history of moderate to severe cardiovascular disease.

There is a deplorable tendency for emergency room personnel to withhold administration of epinephrine unless the patient is experiencing bronchospasm or cardiovascular collapse. Epinephrine is a much more efficient drug for rapid relief of generalized urticaria and pruritus than is an antihistamine; the latter medication can be used in conjunction with epinephrine, however. A short course of systemic corticosteroids is often administered during and after anaphylactic episodes. Experimental data from individual organ studies show inhibition of late-phase reactions by administration of glucocorticoids prior to antigen challenge. However, in clinical studies, glucocorticoid therapy introduced during the initial phase of anaphylaxis does not prevent the appearance of recurrent or protracted anaphylaxis (Stark and Sullivan, 1986). For long-term management, patients who sustain generalized sting reactions should be provided with epinephrine-containing emergency kits and instructed in their use. The commercially available kits include the Ana-Kit (Hollister-Stier Laboratories) and the EpiPen and EpiPen Jr. (Center Laboratories). The Ana-Kit includes a syringe containing two 0.5 ml doses of aqueous epinephrine (1:1000), along with chewable antihistamine tablets, alcohol wipes, and a string tourniquet; the patient is required to self inject the epinephrine. The EpiPen kits each contain a single 0.3 ml dose of aqueous epinephrine (1:1000 for the EpiPen; 1:2000 for the EpiPen Jr.). Each EpiPen unit contains a pressure-sensitive, spring-loaded device that automatically makes the needle puncture and injects the medication. The Ana-Kit is less expensive, but the EpiPen may be attractive to the patient who does not feel comfortable with the self-injection technique. Epinephrine-containing kits should be carried by sting-sensitive persons during the local insect "season." Patients should be reassured that exposure of the kits to ambient temperatures will not destroy the effectiveness of the epinephrine. Exposure to sunlight is more deleterious to the drug than is exposure to warm ambient temperatures. The epinephrine kits should be inspected frequently and replaced at the end of the expiration date shown on the label or if they acquire a pinkish-tan discoloration.

DIAGNOSIS OF INSECT ALLERGY

History

A carefully taken clinical history will usually permit identification of the culprit insect and accurate classification of the sting reaction, using the system shown in Table 52–2. Only persons who sustain generalized reactions need referral to an allergist for further evaluations. A search for IgE antibodies to insect allergens is not indicated for a person experiencing a local or large local reaction.

Laboratory Tests

In a person who has experienced a generalized insect sting reaction, skin testing with insect venoms is the fastest, most sensitive, and most economic method to demonstrate venom-specific IgE antibodies. Honeybee, wasp, yellow jacket, yellow hornet, and white-faced hornet venoms are marketed commercially for this purpose. These venoms are carefully standardized based on their hyaluronidase content; because they are packaged in microgram quantities, a special albumin-containing diluent is provided to prevent adsorption of venom proteins to the wall of the glass vial. Test venoms are initially placed by the scratch or puncture method to screen for extreme sensitivity; intradermal test venoms are placed subsequently if the scratch test reactions are negative. Insects deliver from 5 μg (yellow jackets) to 50 μg (honeybees) per sting; consequently, the venom skin tests, when performed as recommended, deliver less than 1/10,000 of a sting. Irritant (false positive) reactions may be produced in nonsensitive persons if venom test concentrations exceed 1 μg/ml. Positive and negative control tests with histamine phosphate and diluent, respectively, should be placed at the same time to aid in the interpretation of the skin test results.

Skin tests must always be interpreted in the context of the clinical history. The presence of a positive skin test reaction does not always imply the presence of generalized allergy. For example, many persons with histories of large local reactions following insect stings will show positive venom skin test reactions. Approximately 20 percent of persons stung recently who had only normal or local reactions will show transient positive venom skin test reactions. Furthermore, there is no correlation between the clinical severity of the previous sting reaction and the positiveness of the venom skin test reaction nor is a markedly positive venom skin test reaction an indicator of future serious reactions. Finally, sting-sensitive persons may exhibit positive skin test reactions to multiple venoms, either because of multiple previous sensitizations or, more commonly, because of shared allergens, particularly among the vespid venoms. Cross-allergenicity between bee and vespid venoms does not occur frequently.

Radioimmunoassays and enzyme immunoassays are available commercially for *in vitro* measurement of venom-specific IgE antibodies. However, elevated IgE antibody levels are seen in only 80 percent of persons who have significant positive venom skin test reactions (Sobotka et al., 1978). Moreover, there is no correlation between the magnitude of the IgE antibody level and the degree of sensitivity of the patient, as assessed by deliberate insect sting challenges (Parker et al., 1982). Because of the increased cost and the delay in obtaining test results by the *in vitro* assays, venom skin testing is the diagnostic procedure of choice.

Medical Indications for Venom Immunotherapy

The medical indications for venom immunotherapy are listed in Table 52–3. Venom immunotherapy is indicated only for adults who have clinical histories of systemic reactions following stings and who have positive venom skin test reactions. It was formerly believed that such individuals were at 100 percent risk of systemic reactions with future stings; some are still mistakenly advised that future stings will be fatal unless venom immunotherapy is received. In fact, in the absence of venom immunotherapy, such adults are at approximately 60 percent risk of repeat systemic reactions with subsequent stings (Hunt et al., 1978); venom immunotherapy will reduce this risk to approximately 2 percent. The situation is somewhat different in the case of children, in whom a subgroup experiencing milder generalized reactions (urticaria, cutaneous angioedema or both) have been shown to be at only 10 percent risk of systemic reactions with future stings (Schuberth et al., 1983). Venom immunotherapy is not routinely warranted in such children.

Nonmedical considerations often are important in an individual's decision to accept or decline immunotherapy. The cost of venom immunotherapy should be discussed with the patient or parents, along with the time commitment required. In addition, patients residing at

some distance from medical centers must frequently depend on primary care physicians for administration of immunotherapy. Occasionally, physicians refuse to administer venom injections, and patients are caught in the middle of disagreements between physicians. Although it is not possible to quantitate the "mental wear and tear" experienced by sting-sensitive persons and their family members (e.g., fear of repeat stings; maintaining an awareness of insects; alterations in occupational or leisure pursuits), the physician should attempt to assess the degree of such factors in each individual situation. *Finally, it is still appropriate to discuss venom immunotherapy as a control measure and not as a cure.*

TECHNIQUE OF VENOM IMMUNOTHERAPY

The same five insect venom preparations available for skin testing are also used for venom immunotherapy. Patients usually are treated with all venoms to which they exhibit positive skin test reactions. It is recognized that most of these multiple positive skin test reactions are due to allergens common to several vespid venoms (Hoffman, 1985), in which case immunotherapy with only one vespid venom would theoretically provide clinical protection to all vespid stings. However, the time and expense necessary to document this for each patient by immunoassay is prohibitive. A mixed vespid venom containing equal quantities of yellow jacket, yellow hornet, and white-faced hornet venoms is available for treatment of vespid-sensitive patients with skin test reactivity to all three of these venoms.

Several venom injection regimens have been compared (Golden et al., 1980), including a "rush" injection schedule involving multiple injections per patient visit and a traditional schedule involving once-weekly injection. The former is associated with fewer adverse reactions per treatment course and a shorter elapsed time required to reach maintenance dose. However, many patients are not able to spend up to 90 minutes per treatment session and prefer the single injection schedule. Both regimens provide equal clinical efficacy.

Venom injections are given subcutaneously with disposable tuberculin-type syringes in the outer midportion of the upper arm, beginning with doses of 0.01 or 0.1 μg. A patient should be observed in the office for 30 minutes after the injection; most serious reactions to injections

TABLE 52–3. Medical Indications for Venom Skin Testing and Immunotherapy

Classification of Sting Reaction by History	Venom Skin Test	Venom Immunotherapy
Local	Not indicated	No
Large local	Not indicated	No
Systemic	Positive reaction	Yes*
	Negative reaction	No
Toxic	Not indicated	No
Delayed	Not indicated	No

* Children (age 16 years or younger) who have experienced only cutaneous manifestations with their systemic reactions (generalized urticaria, cutaneous angioedema, or both without respiratory or cardiovascular signs or symptoms) are at approximately 10 percent risk of systemic reactions with future stings (Schuberth et al., 1983) and do not warrant routine venom immunotherapy.

occur during this time interval. If a patient is receiving more than one venom, it is often helpful to administer each venom as a separate injection in a different site. A patient receiving the mixed vespid venom receives one injection, however. If a patient shows a large local or systemic reaction to venom therapy, the venom responsible for the reaction can be identified more easily if the injections are separated. Subsequently, the dosage of each venom can be adjusted independently. When the patient reaches maintenance dose (100 μg for single venom; 300 μg for mixed vespid venom), the interval between injections is lengthened to 4 weeks, and separate injections may then be combined into a single injection. After 6 months of maintenance immunotherapy, the interval between injections may be lengthened to 6 weeks.

Transient local reactions at the venom injection site can be expected. These involve erythema, itching, and swelling, which appear during the first 30 minutes and may last several hours. Occasionally, these local reactions may be several centimeters in diameter and involve most of the upper arm. These reactions occur most frequently at delivered venom doses between 10 and 30 μg, and they tend to disappear when the venom doses exceed 60 μg. The local reactions may be treated with oral antihistamines, glucocorticoids, or both, but it is usually best to continue advancing the dosage administered. Conversely, the dosage should be reduced if systemic reactions (scattered urticaria or wheezing) occur after venom injections. The signs and symptoms experienced during a systemic reaction tend to be the same for a given individual; this occurrence is frequently helpful in assessing reactions to immunotherapy. Patients should be discouraged from premedicating themselves with antihistamines (or glucocorticoids) on the day that they receive venom injections; such therapy may obscure useful signs and symptoms of venom overdose. Those who administer venom injections should inquire routinely about the medication intake of patients. If large local or systemic reactions occur repeatedly, various strategies can be tried, as follows: (1) increasing the frequency of injections from once weekly to twice weekly; (2) splitting the desired dose into two or three portions and administering each portion at 30 minute-intervals; and (3) increasing the total volume in which the desired dose is delivered by adding extra diluent to the syringe.

Specific IgE antibody levels usually rise for the first 4 to 6 weeks after the initiation of venom immunotherapy, then gradually decline though they rarely disappear. IgG antibody levels usually rise following venom immunotherapy, plateau after the patient reaches maintenance dose, and decline slightly with time thereafter. Although there may be merit to measuring venom-specific antibody levels for research purposes, the clinical relevance of such measurements for individual patients is unclear. If IgE and IgG specific antibody levels are monitored, the physician should realize that what is being measured is the immune response to venom immunotherapy, rather than a parameter that will predict with certainty the clinical outcome of the patient's next hymenopteran sting. In addition to immune factors there are probably biochemical, physiologic, and psychologic factors that also are important in determining the patient's clinical response to insect stings.

Deliberate insect sting challenges under carefully controlled conditions represent the most unambiguous tests of the clinical efficacy of venom immunotherapy (Parker et al., 1982). However, besides the possible patient resistance to the procedure, such challenges pose risks and are available at only a few medical research centers.

DISCONTINUATION OF VENOM IMMUNOTHERAPY

Although some individuals have been able to discontinue venom immunotherapy after a few years of treatment without a return of sensitivity, the frequency and the underlying mechanisms are not known at present. Patients who have received the usual 100-μg maintenance dose for more than 3 years should undergo skin testing with venom again. Consideration should be given to discontinuing immunotherapy in those patients whose skin test reactions revert to negative. In our experience, however, these situations occur in only 20 to 25 percent of venom immunotherapy recipients. It has been our practice to rely on venom skin testing rather than on in vitro measurement of venom-specific IgE antibody for this assessment, because of the greater sensitivity and lower cost of venom skin testing.

INSECT AVOIDANCE

Persons who are sensitive to honeybee stings should avoid wearing brightly colored clothing or scented toiletries which may serve to attract insects, and they should avoid walking bare-footed outdoors, since honeybees often are found in the clover in lawns. Gardeners may be stung by honeybees foraging on hidden blossoms of vine crops, such as melons and cucumbers. Yellow jackets and hornets often attack after being disturbed by unwitting utility meter readers, lawn mower operators, or house painters. Vespid sting–sensitive persons should exercise caution around trash receptacles, picnic areas, and orchards, where these insects scavenge for nourishment on discarded food or rotten fruit.

UNANSWERED QUESTIONS

Although venom immunotherapy is remarkably effective in providing clinical immunity to hymenopteran stings, there are several unanswered questions concerning insect sting allergy. There is controversy whether pregnant women who are sting-sensitive should receive venom immunotherapy. Because most reactions to venom immunotherapy occur during the build-up stage of treatment, it may be prudent to defer initiation of venom immunotherapy until the pregnancy is completed. However, other risk factors, such as the likelihood of exposure to stinging insects, also must be taken into account in the decision process. Maintenance injections that are being tolerated well usually can be continued without problems in women who become pregnant after beginning immunotherapy programs.

As mentioned previously, considerable work is required to determine whether there is a minimal or optimal length of time that venom immunotherapy should be given. Finally, development of new treatment regimens, utilizing modified venom extracts, may permit clinical immunity to be achieved with fewer side effects

and fewer total injections (Patterson et al., 1985).

REFERENCES

Golden, D.B.K., Valentine, M.D., Kagey-Sobotka, A., Lichtenstein, L.M.: Regimens of Hymenoptera venom immunotherapy. Ann. Int. Med. 92:620, 1980.

Hoffman, D.R.: Allergens in Hymenoptera venom XV: The immunologic basis of vespid venom cross-reactivity. J. Allergy Clin. Immunol. 75:611, 1985.

Hunt, K.J., Valentine, M.D., Sobotka, A.K., Benton, A.W., Amodio, F.J., Lichtenstein, L.M.: A controlled trial of immunotherapy in insect hypersensitivity. N. Engl. J. Med. 299:157, 1978.

Levine, M.I., Lockey, R.F. (eds.): Monograph on Insect Allergy, 2nd ed. Pittsburgh, American Academy of Allergy, 1986.

Light, W.C., Reisman, R.E., Shimizu, M., Arbesman, C.A.: Unusual reactions following insect stings. Clinical features and immunologic analysis. J. Allergy Clin. Immunol. 59:391, 1977.

Parker, J.L., Santrach, P.J., Dahlberg, M.J.E., Yunginger, J.W.: Evaluation of Hymenoptera-sting sensitivity with deliberate sting challenges: inadequacy of present diagnostic methods. J. Allergy Clin. Immunol. 69:200, 1982.

Patterson, R., Suszko, I.M., Grammer, L.C.: Polymerized soluble venom—Human serum albumin. J. Allergy Clin. Immunol. 75:382, 1985.

Rohr, A.S., Marshall, N.A., Saxon, A.: Successful immunotherapy for *Triatoma protracta*–induced anaphylaxis. J. Allergy Clin. Immunol. 73:369, 1984.

Schuberth, K.C., Lichtenstein, L.M., Kagey-Sobotka, A., Szklo, M., Kwiterovich, K.A., Valentine, M.D.: Epidemiologic study of insect allergy in children. II. Effect of accidental stings in allergic children. J. Pediatr. 102:361, 1983.

Smith, K.G.V. (ed.): Insects and Other Arthropods of Medical Importance. London, British Museum (Natural History), 1973.

Sobotka, A.K., Adkinson, N.F., Jr., Valentine, M.D., Lichtenstein, L.M.: Allergy to insect stings. IV. Diagnosis by radioallergosorbent test (RAST). J. Immunol. 121:2477, 1978.

Stark, B.J., Sullivan, T.J.: Biphasic and protracted anaphylaxis. J. Allergy Clin. Immunol. 78:76–83, 1986.

Wilbur, R.D., Evans, R.: An immunologic evaluation of deerfly hypersensitivity. J. Allergy Clin. Immunol. (Abstract.) 55:72, 1975.

Yunginger, J.W.: Advances in the diagnosis and treatment of stinging insect allergy. Pediatrics 67:325, 1981.

53

Drug Hypersensitivity

PAUL P. VANARSDEL, JR., M.D.

Few drugs of proven effectiveness are without risk of adverse reactions. In fact, it may be a truism that the more effective the drug, the more side effects it may have. Most of society have accepted the concept that, in any therapeutic modality, a great potential benefit can make even a 100 percent risk of some adverse reaction acceptable. It should not be surprising, therefore, that as more and more potent drugs are introduced for the cure or control of life-threatening diseases, the incidence of morbidity and mortality from adverse reactions will continue to be a source of alarm to many concerned authorities.

CLASSIFICATION OF ADVERSE REACTIONS

Hypersensitivity reactions to drugs can be understood and diagnosed most reliably if one considers them within the context of all adverse drug reactions. These are classified in Table 53–1. Most adverse reactions, including those that are life threatening, are toxic; they occur because of overdosage, impaired metabolism (or excretion), or drug interaction. Toxic reactions that mimic allergic reactions are of particular importance to this discussion and are reviewed subsequently. Some disease-associated reactions also may be triggered by drugs, particularly by antimicrobials. The classic reaction of this group was first described at the turn of the century by Jarisch and Herxheimer, who observed it during the treatment of syphilis with mercury (Bryceson, 1976). When penicillin was introduced, treatment was associated with more severe reactions. Symptoms and signs included chills, fever, localized edema, skin rash, adenopathy, headache, and, most typically, a flare-up of the syphilitic skin lesions. When such a reaction develops, the knowledgeable physician will continue necessary antimicrobial

treatment while the reaction subsides. Other drugs may produce similar reactions during treatment of spirochetal, enteric, parasitic, and fungal infections (VanArsdel, 1983).

Ampicillin is associated with a high frequency of skin rashes when given to patients with infectious mononucleosis or lymphocytic leukemia and patients with gout treated also with allopurinol. The mechanisms involved remain speculative. In children particularly, the occurrence of skin eruptions during treatment with any antimicrobial drug may be entirely coincidental. Most eruptions, including urticaria, are manifestations of the illnesses being treated.

Psychophysiologic reactions can take many forms. Anxiety, lassitude, drowsiness, nausea, and headache are fairly obvious. Most physicians and other medical professionals are less aware of the possibility that allergy-like symptoms also can be psychogenic. Perhaps this is best known to those who conduct placebo-controlled clinical drug trials. Subjects not infrequently complain of nasal congestion, urticaria, angioedema, and even anaphylactoid reactions while receiving only placebos.

Definitions. The last section of Table 53–1 lists three categories which are defined here along with a few other terms:

- *Intolerance:* That condition in which a drug produces its expected toxic side effects at an unusually low dose.
- *Idiosyncrasy:* That condition in which the adverse reaction is strange and pharmacologically unexpected (i.e., different from the usual toxic reactions). Reactions of intolerance and idiosyncrasy may be related to the presence of enzyme defects in some patients.
- *Allergy:* An acquired potential for developing an adverse reaction that is immunologically mediated. *Allergy* and *hypersensitivity* will be used interchangeably in this chapter. In practice, of course, many reactions that are generally considered to be allergic, could in fact be idiosyncratic, since no immune mechanism has been identified.
- *Anaphylactoid:* An adverse reaction that mimics an allergic reaction but is produced by toxic rather than immune release of po-

TABLE 53–1. Classification of Adverse
Drug Reactions

Predictable risks

Toxic: overdose or side-effect, delayed expression (e.g.,
teratogenicity, malignancy)
Allergy-like side-effects
Superinfection
Drug interactions

Disease associated risks

Impaired degradation, excretion of drugs, or both due to
organ system failure (increased toxicity)
Conditions mimicking allergic reactions
Jarisch-Herxheimer reaction
Ampicillin reactions with infectious mononucleosis
and other diseases

Coincidental risks

Exanthematous infectious diseases
Controversial: Stevens-Johnson syndrome and other
disorders with many suspected causes
Psychogenic

Risks to a susceptible subpopulation

Intolerance
Idiosyncrasy
Allergy

---

tent vasoactive and smooth muscle reactive mediators.

- *Carrier:* A substance with immunogenic potential that, when coupled with a low molecular weight drug or metabolite, renders that chemical (the *haptene*) immunogenic.

- *Cross-reaction:* The reaction of an antibody or antigen-specific lymphocyte with an antigen other than one that induced its formation.

- *Haptene:* A substance that can react with specific antibody but is of a molecular weight too low for it to be immunogenic by itself.

GENERAL ASPECTS OF HYPERSENSITIVITY REACTIONS

By strict definition, hypersensitivity reactions should be associated with specific and reproducible abnormal immune findings. In fact, such proof is not often available. Furthermore, there is good evidence that some allergy-like reactions are not immunologically mediated. These so-called *pseudoallergic reactions* are discussed separately from allergic reactions in the sections to follow.

Allergic Drug Reactions

Background. Human hypersensitivity reactions to therapeutic agents were first recognized after the introduction of horse serum antitoxins near the turn of the century. Serum sickness was the most common major manifestation of iatrogenic allergic reactions until the 1930's. Little is known about reactions to the few specific drugs that were in general use before 1900 other than the obvious toxicity of these natural poisons. New synthetic drugs then began to appear. By 1930, adverse reactions that were presumably allergic were beginning to be reported, for example, 3 percent of patients given phenobarbital developed reactions that were probably allergic in nature. Ironically, aspirin, one of the first synthetic drugs reported after the turn of the century, to produce angioedema and asthma probably does so on a nonimmune basis (vide infra) (VanArsdel, 1984). Allergy to synthetic small molecular weight drugs did not become a prominent problem until the first sulfonamides were introduced in the late 1930's.

Characteristics. The features that characterize an allergic drug reaction are listed in Table 53–2. Perhaps the most reliable clinical feature is the latent period between the start of treatment and the onset of the adverse reaction. Even this is not absolute, because the patient may have forgotten about previous treatment or may have had some nontherapeutic exposure (e.g., penicillin in cow's milk). Ideally, hypersensitivity testing should prove or exclude the diagnosis of drug allergy. In practice, however, objective sensitivity tests are reliable for only a few categories of drugs. These are as follows:

TABLE 53–2. Features of an Allergic
Drug Reaction

Previous treatment without adverse effects.
Reaction usually appears only after several days of treatment, especially if no previous exposure to the drug.
Risk of reaction exists at doses far below therapeutic range.
Clinical manifestations do not resemble the general pharmacologic effects of the drug and cannot be predicted from animal testing.
Reaction occurs in a small proportion of the population.
Reaction usually is restricted to a limited number of syndromes generally accepted as allergic in nature.
Antibodies or T lymphocytes have been identified that react specifically with the drug or a metabolite, in a few instances.
A similar reaction can be reproduced on administration of a small amount of the suspected drug or drugs of similar chemical structure.

- Proteins and large polypeptides (xenogenic sera, hormones, enzymes).
- Drugs responsible for hematologic reactions.
- Small molecular weight drugs in which immunologically reactive intermediates have been identified (penicillin is the best example).
- Drugs responsible for allergic contact dermatitis.

The provocative challenge test is the most reliable test to confirm or exclude the diagnosis of allergy to most drugs. The suspected drug is readministered and the patient observed for a reaction similar to the previous one. Usually the risk of such a challenge is greater than any benefit one can hope to gain by such proof. One general exception is the patch test for determining the cause of allergic contact dermatitis. This test, when properly done, will provide the necessary proof safely and reliably.

Incidence and Predisposing Demographic Factors. Although adverse allergic reactions to xenogenic sera and the first sulfonamides were very common (10 percent or more of those treated reacted), recent data, based primarily on hospital populations, indicate that the incidence is relatively low. For most drugs, it is less than 2 percent. In a well-known study of hospitalized patients reported by the Boston Collaborative Drug Surveillance Program, the overall incidence of skin eruptions associated with all drugs, per course of drug therapy, was only 0.2 percent. Among the commonly used drugs, only the semisynthetic penicillins, trimethoprim-sulfamethoxazole, cephalosporins, and transfusions were associated with reactions rates over 2 percent: trimethoprim-sulfamethoxazole headed the list at 56/1000 patients treated (Bigby et al., 1986).

In *children* the incidence of all adverse drug reactions has been reported for both outpatients and inpatients by several groups. In one study, drug reactions were responsible for 2 percent of hospital admissions (McKenzie et al., 1976). Very few of these (11 of 3556) were classified as allergic. Allergic reactions are thought to be less common in children than adults, and this appears to be so at least for penicillin (Bierman and VanArsdel, 1969) and drug fever (Whyte and Greenan, 1977). However, in the Bigby study cited previously, there was no significant age association in the occurrence of skin rashes in hospitalized patients, although the reactions did occur more often in female than in male patients, independent of age.

Other Predisposing Factors. A history of a previous allergic reaction to the same drug (or one that is chemically similar) is by far the most reliable evidence that giving the drug would be risky. Perhaps multiple drug exposure (so common in hospitalized patients!) increases the risk of a reaction to a newly introduced medication, but the evidence for this is circumstantial. At one time, a history of atopic disease was generally considered to be an important risk factor. However, this assumption may not be correct. For example, the prevalence of penicillin allergy among patients with ragweed hayfever does not differ significantly from that among normal control subjects, nor is there reliable evidence for an association of atopy with allergy to any other drug (Horowitz and Parker, 1975).

The only convincing genetic influence on drug hypersensitivity is found with drug-induced systemic lupus erythematosus. Patients who are slow acetylators of certain drugs are more likely to develop this reaction than those who are fast acetylators (Woosley et al., 1978). *Immunosuppression,* surprisingly, may enhance the sensitizing potential of a few drugs. Although examples are rare, the principle is interesting. An immunosuppressed patient may become deficient in those suppressor T cells that regulate IgE antibody synthesis. A bone marrow tranplant recipient developed an allergic reaction to polymyxin B (an extremely unusual occurrence) and was found to have an IgE anti-polymyxin B antibody (Lakin et al., 1975). Finally, the risk of becoming hypersensitive to a drug is influenced by the route by which it is given. Topical medication to the skin (apparently not to the mucous membranes) is the most likely to sensitize, and oral administration the least likely. Intravenous administration of a drug is less likely to sensitize than are other parenteral approaches.

Pseudoallergic Reactions

Allergy-like side-effects can be produced directly by certain drugs in the absence of any evidence of hypersensitivity. In contrast to true allergic reactions, these occur promptly the first time the drug is given, if the dose is sufficiently high, appear only when the dose is increased, or, with an intravenous drug, when the rate of administration is increased. Table 53–3 is a

TABLE 53–3. Pseudoallergic Reactions

Histamine-releasing drugs

Deferoxamine
Metubine and tubocurarine
Opiates
Pentamidine
Phytonadione
Polymyxins
Radiographic contrast media

Autonomic drugs

Beta-adrenergic blocking agents
Reserpine and other antihypertensive agents
Parasympathetic agonists and anticholinesterases

Enzyme inhibitors

Captopril
Nonsteroidal anti-inflammatory drugs

classification of these reactions. The *histamine releasers* produce reactions that are similar to anaphylaxis. Since they are not immunologically mediated, they are referred to as *anaphylactoid* reactions. The mechanism of the anaphylactoid reaction is similar to the antigen-induced one; the drug induces a calcium-dependent and energy-dependent reaction in mast cells and basophils that results in granule exocytosis and release or activation of potent vasoactive and smooth muscle–reactive mediators. The reaction occurs most frequently when the offending substance is given rapidly and intravenously, producing a diffuse flush, pruritus, urticaria, and transient hypotension followed by headache. Phytonadione (colloidal vitamin K) also can produce such a reaction if given intravenously, and a few fatalities have been reported. The reaction may be caused by a dispersing or emulsifying agent rather than by the vitamin itself (Mandel and Cohn, 1985).

The only example of an enzyme inhibitor in common use is captopril. This antihypertensive agent acts by blocking the angiotensin-converting enzyme. This enzyme also is a kininase, and the dose-related pruritic, maculopapular skin eruptions that occur with the drug are probably caused in part by the inhibition of kinin degradation (Wilkin et al., 1980).

Antihypertensive drugs may produce or aggravate respiratory symptoms. The best known is reserpine, which produces predictable dose-related nasal stuffiness, discharge, or both. Others are hydralazine and alpha-adrenergic blockers. Anticholinesterase and histamine-releasing drugs also may produce nasal symptoms. Asthma can be made worse by beta-adrenergic blocking agents and by anticholinesterases. Rhinitis and asthma in some patients are aggravated by aspirin and other nonsteroidal anti-inflammatory drugs, possibly via their enzyme-inhibitory actions.

IMMUNE PATHOGENESIS

Immunochemical Principles

Only a few therapeutic agents are complete antigens. Foreign proteins, such as horse serum antitoxins and antithymocyte globulins, are antigenic and induce IgG antibody formation in all individuals who are capable of normal immune respones. If the titer of such antibodies is high enough, immune complexes may activate a sufficient amount of complement-derived mediators (anaphylatoxins, chemotactic factors) to produce allergic symptoms. Some individuals (not necessarily those with atopic diatheses) will produce specific IgE antibodies and develop typical anaphylactic manifestations. Larger polypeptide hormones are similarly immunogenic. Immunogenicity is weak when the molecular weight is less than 5000 daltons, and molecules containing fewer than seven amino acids are not immunogenic.

Most drugs in common use are simple organic chemicals with molecular weights under 1000 daltons. For such chemicals to produce specific immune responses, they must be conjugated to some macromolecule, usually a protein or large polypeptide, termed a *carrier*. This phenomenon was first established by Landsteiner's pioneering work over a half-century ago (Landsteiner and Jacobs, 1935). Such conjugation must be firm; the usual serum binding of drugs is not sufficient. Conjugation of virtually any drug to a carrier can be achieved artificially in the laboratory by use of such activating chemicals as the carbodiimides and diisocyanates. The drug is proved to be immunogenic by injecting the conjugate into appropriate experimental animals and demonstrating the appearance of antibodies that bind specifically to the drug (the *haptene*) rather than to the carrier protein. The role of the carrier in producing immunogenicity is not clear; it may stimulate the activation of helper T cells. Highly selective monoclonal antidrug antibodies that are induced by these conjugates are now used widely for the immunoassay of drug concentrations in biologic fluids.

Beginning with Landsteiner's findings, practically all effective conjugates prepared in the laboratory have covalent haptene-carrier bonds. Such conjugation does not occur readily *in vivo*. A few organic compounds can form covalent bonds with carriers without synthetic manipulation. These compounds are as follows: acid anhydrides, acid chlorides, aromatic halides, isocyanates, isothiocyanates, mercaptans, quinones, and diazonium salts (Levine, 1966). Few of these are known to play a role in the pathogenesis of drug hypersensitivity. Only one has been established as an important reactant in humans, i.e., the oxazolone (a type of anhydride) of penicillanic acid, a metabolite of penicillin. It forms stable covalent amide bonds with protein amino groups. This reaction was identified over 20 years ago and is used to prepare the skin-testing conjugate, benzylpenicilloyl polylysine. Other penicillin metabolites have free-SH groups and have the potential to form stable mixed disulfides with cysteine in carrier proteins. However, the immunogenicity of such conjugates has not been established in human allergy.

The experience derived from research on penicillin hypersensitivity over 20 years ago led to considerable optimism that allergic reactions to most other drugs were likely to be caused by metabolites rather than by the drugs themselves. Unfortunately, nothing has emerged from studies on other drug allergies comparable to the consistent and reproducible findings in patients with penicillin sensitivity. Acetaminophen-induced immune thrombocytopenia was shown to be a sulfate metabolite in one patient (Eisner and Shahidi, 1972), but such reports of sensitivity to other drug metabolites are rare indeed.

Mechanisms

The four Coombs and Gell types of human hypersensitivity, as originally described, are useful in classifying drug reactions and are reviewed briefly.

Conditions Associated with IgE Antibodies. A diverse number of macromolecules (allergens) are responsible for the production of anaphylaxis and urticaria and for the production or aggravation of asthma, rhinitis, and some adverse reactions to foods. In a sensitive person, an allergen reacts with specific IgE antibody on the surface of mast cells and basophils, resulting in the release or activation of histamine, leukotrienes, and other potent mediators (see Chapter 5). Macromolecular therapeutic agents can produce similar types of sensitivity. Allergenic extracts used in immunotherapy fall into this category, as do xenogenic sera, large polypeptide hormones, and macromolecular contaminants in various biologic products. Small molecular weight drugs also can produce such reactions, but, as discussed previously, the actual immunogenic haptene has been identified for the penicillin group of drugs only. Otherwise, only circumstantial immunologic evidence exists. For example, the total IgE level sometimes increases significantly during anaphylactic, urticarial, or serum sickness reactions.

Cytotoxic Antibody Reactions. Essentially all cytotoxic antibody-mediated reactions to therapeutic agents involve injury to formed elements of the blood. The most obvious ones occur when mismatched erythrocytes, leukocytes, or platelets are administered. These are injured by IgG and IgM antibodies in the presence of complement and subsequently destroyed. Drug-induced reactions fall into the three following general categories:

The Haptene-Cell Reaction. The offending drug reacts with cell surfaces to form a stable immunogenic complex, which stimulates antibody that is drug specific. The main example is penicillin-induced hemolytic anemia, confirmed by demonstrating that the patient's serum agglutinates erythrocytes that have been preincubated with penicillin. The agglutinin is an IgG antibody that does not fix complement; presumably the red blood cell destruction occurs entirely in the reticuloendothelial system.

The Immune Complex Reaction. Although this reaction belongs in the next category, it is included here for contrast. It is thought to be responsible for most allergic drug reactions involving blood cells. A drug or metabolite reacts with antibody in the circulation. The soluble immune complex that is formed, along with complement, affixes to the cell surface, and injury is produced by the membrane attack complex of complement. The drug-antibody complex may remain on the cell only transiently after activating complement, which remains behind.

Drug-Induced Autoimmune Reaction. This is a hemolytic anemia thought to be caused when the offending drug induces autoantibody production against apparently normal red blood cell determinants by an unknown mechanism. In the case of methyldopa, at least, the IgG antibody that develops reacts against Rh determinants.

Other Immune Complex Reactions. Nonhematologic reactions thought to be caused by drug-IgG antibody complexes can be systemic or local in their manifestations. The classic systemic reaction is the one produced by xenogenic serum and is called serum sickness. Much of the information about immune complex disease has been generated by the production of experimental serum sickness in animals; this is a standard model for studying immune complex nephritis. Human serum sickness differs in that renal manifestations are minor in most patients, and it almost always coexists with IgE-mediated phenomena. Serum sickness–like reactions are produced by several drugs, including penicillin. In the case of penicillin sensitivity, in which specific serum antibodies can be measured, IgG antibody is found usually in fairly high titer. However, there is no evidence that this antibody is responsible for any allergic manifestations. It does not fix complement and appears to cause no harm to the fetus after crossing the placenta. Infiltrative lung disease associated with inhaled drug allergens also is associated with the presence of IgG antibody. In the past, it developed occasionally from the inhalation of a biologic product, such as posterior pituitary powder, but rarely is seen nowadays. In any event, a T cell–mediated mechanism may play a more important role than the humoral one.

Cell-Mediated Conditions. These are mediated by specifically sensitized T lymphocytes. The great majority of the reactions occur after cutaneous contact and are characterized by infiltration of lymphocytes and other mononuclear cells. There is little reason to doubt that various lymphocyte mediators (lymphokines) are responsible for tissue injury, but little proof of this has come from *in vitro* studies on lymphocyte reactivity. Studies that measure responses, such as mitogenic transformation, tritiated thymidine uptake, and migration inhibition factor (MIF) generation from cells cultured in the presence of the suspected drug, have not led to any consistently reliable laboratory indicator for allergic contact dermatitis, let alone other drug reactions (mostly cutaneous) of uncertain pathogenesis. Although some evidence exists that cell-mediated mechanisms do

play some role in special circumstances (Rocklin, 1974; Knutsen et al., 1984), the tests are not sufficiently reliable for general use in the diagnosis of drug allergy.

The best confirmed of the systemic cell–mediated reactions are not those suspected from *in vitro* tests, but those that occur in a person with preexisting contact allergy who is given the offending agent parenterally. Such reactions from theophylline-ethylenediamine (aminophylline) given to patients with contact allergies to ethylenediamine have been reported so often in recent years that the phenomena have become model examples of systemic T cell–mediated reactions.

TYPES OF CLINICAL REACTIONS

Clinical reactions that are generally accepted as allergic or possibly allergic are outlined in Table 53–4. This outline is used in the following discussion. The listing of drugs that are pos-

TABLE 53–4. Classification of Allergic Drug Reactions

Mast cell–mediated

Systemic anaphylaxis
Urticaria and angioedema
Some pruritic maculopapular eruptions
Serum sickness (in part)
Anaphylactoid (nonimmune)

T lymphocyte–mediated

Allergic eczematous contact dermatitis

Photodermatitis

Other cutaneous reactions (mechanism uncertain)

Maculopapular or exanthematous
Fixed eruptions
Toxic epidermal necrolysis

Drug fever

Systemic lupus erythematous and other autoimmune reactions

Organ systems

Blood
    Eosinophilia, hemolytic anemia, thrombocytopenia, granulocytopenia
Lung
Liver
Kidney

Reactions with inconsistent drug associations

Erythema multiforme
Exfoliative dermatitis
Vasculitis

sible causes of the various kinds of reactions is derived from several sources. The most comprehensive are standard textbooks of pharmacology (Gilman et al., 1985), AMA Drug Evaluations (1986), and Meyler's Side Effects of Drugs (Dukes, 1984). These were supplemented by textbooks on adverse drug reactions (Cluff et al., 1975; Davies, 1985), the reports of the Boston Collaborative Drug Surveillance Program (Bigby et al., 1986), selected reviews and reports in various journals, and personal experience (VanArsdel, 1983).

Mast Cell – Mediated Reactions

Systemic Anaphylaxis. The patient who suffers this reaction develops one or more of the following symptoms, usually within a few minutes after the drug is given: generalized flush, palpitations, weakness, dizziness, tingling of the extremities or tongue, urticaria, angioedema, and apprehension. Angioedema may obstruct the upper airway. If the reaction is not treated, it may progress to difficulty breathing, shock, seizures, incontinence, coma, and death. Fortunately, anaphylaxis is rare. The most reliable information on incidence comes from the experience with penicillin treatment in venereal disease clinics. Anaphylaxis occurred in 1 of every 1820 patients treated (Rudolph and Price, 1973). One fatality from penicillin occurred in approximately 50,000. The incidence of fatal reactions to macromolecular drugs or agents is undoubtedly higher, and an important recent example is the antitumor agent, asparaginase.

Some drugs produce mast cell – mediated reactions that are not immune. As mentioned previously, mast cell release of mediators is a predictable toxic side effect of such drugs. Because their mechanism is different from the immunologically mediated one, these are called anaphylactoid reactions. Drugs that are known to produce anaphylactic or anaphylactoid reactions are listed in Table 53 – 5. The most common offenders are foreign sera, allergenic extracts, dextrans, injected enzymes, polypeptide hormones, penicillins, and radiographic contrast media. Gold sodium thiomalate, but not aurothioglucose, can produce an anaphylactoid reaction with nitritoid features; the vehicle rather than the gold is thought to be responsible. Aspirin in not included in the table because its reactions, which may be anaphylactoid when severe, are complex and are discussed in a separate section. Other drugs not listed in the

TABLE 53 – 5. Drugs Responsible for Anaphylactic or Anaphylactoid Reactions

Macromolecules	Ethambutol
Allergic extracts*	Kanamycin
Dextrans (including iron	Lincomycin
dextran)*	Penicillins*
Enzymes	Polymyxin B†
Asparaginase*	Streptomycin
Chymotrypsin	Sulfonamides
Trypsin	Tetracyclines
Chymopapain*	Vancomycin
Penicillinase*	
Heparin	**Other drugs**
Hormones (e.g., ACTH,*	Aminopyrine
insulin)	Aspirin†
Human gamma globulin	Bleomycin†
Organ extracts	Cisplatin
Protamine	Colchicine
Vaccines	Cytarabine
Xenogenic sera*	Dimethylsulfoxide†
	Gold sodium thiomalate
Diagnostic agents	Indomethacin†
Dyes	Meprobamate
Iodinated contrast media†	Mercurial diuretics
	Opiates†
Antimicrobials	Probenecid
Aminosalicylic acid	Suramin
Amphotericin B	Tolmetin
Bacitracin	Triamterene
Cephalosporins*	Tubocurarine†
Clindamycin	

* These agents either are frequent causes of anaphylaxis because of extensive use or are responsible for a relatively high incidence of reactions. They also are the most commonly implicated in urticaria and angioedema.

† These agents produce anaphylactoid (nonimmune) reactions in most instances.

table are those in which reactions are reported in the medical literature because of their rarity and not because of significant risk of anaphylaxis. Examples are glucocorticoids and tetracyclines.

Cutaneous Reactions. Most reactions are urticarial; occasionally, they can be morbilliform. Often they are accompanied by angioedema of extremities, mucous membranes, or genitalia. A reaction may appear explosively (e.g., in a previously sensitized patient) after the first dose of the drug (alone or as part of systemic anaphylaxis) or may not appear for several days. The clinical characteristics of urticaria and angioedema are described in Chapter 31. There is nothing distinctive about the appearance of drug-induced reactions. Drugs responsible for these reactions include those listed in Table 53 – 5 as well as additional drugs listed in Table 53 – 6. Most cases of urticaria clear up in a few days after treatment with the suspected drug is stopped. One should look for an alternative ex-

TABLE 53–6. Urticaria-Producing Drugs

Antimicrobials	
Aminoglycosides	Clonidine
Isoniazid	Cyclophosphamide
Metronidazole	Dantrolene
Micronazole	Digitalis*
Nalidixic acid	Doxorubicin
Quinine	Ergotamine
Rifampin	Ethchlorvynol
Spectinomycin	Ethosuximide
Suramin	Ethylenediamine
Tetracyclines*	Meprobamate
	Mercurial diuretics
Other drugs	Methaqualone
Acetaminophen/phenacetin*	Metoclopramide
Allopurinol*	Penicillamine
Anticoagulants (oral)*	Pentazocine*
Aspirin	Phenothiazines
Calcitonin	Procainamide
Chloral hydrate	Quinidine
	Tragacanth

* Reactions of urticaria and angioedema are rarely associated with these agents.

planation if the reaction lasts more than a week and should realize that many cases of chronic urticaria of unknown cause have started during some drug-treated illness.

Serum Sickness. Patients with reactions to foreign sera develop urticaria, angioedema, arthralgias with adjacent edema, and low grade fever from a few hours (the accelerated form) to 3 weeks after receiving the sera. The more severe reactions may include temporomandibular arthritis, adenopathy, and mononeuritis multiplex. A few reactions have been associated with glomerulitis. The reactions seen with small molecule–drugs usually are limited to urticaria and arthralgias. The most common causes of serum sickness today are hydralazine, penicillins, phenylbutazone, sulfonamides, thiazide diuretics, and thiouracils. Reactions to animal sera products are now rare, even with the increasing use in recent years of antithymocyte globulin (ATG) for treatment of patients with organ transplants and those with bone marrow failure. An interesting pattern has been observed in the latter group (Bielory et al., 1985); a majority of the cutaneous reactions were morbilliform rather than urticarial, and more than half the patients developed distinctive serpiginous bands of erythema on their hands and feet at the margin of palmar or plantar skin. The lesions were frequently purpuric, as might be anticipated in thrombocytopenic patients. The treatment program in this group of patients included methylprednisolone as well as ATG; this

probably is the reason for the low incidence of urticaria.

A few other drugs produce reactions that are not really similar to serum sickness but do not fit easily in any other classification. Aminosalicylic acid, for example, causes a syndrome similar to infectious mononucleosis, and phenytoin not uncommonly produces adenopathy without other stigmata of serum sickness.

One should not forget that a serum-sickness syndrome thought to be caused by a drug may actually be caused by the illness that the drug is being used to treat. Infectious diseases, in particular, may have serum sickness–like features. These diseases include hepatitis B, rubella, and infectious mononucleosis. The symptoms are likely to be mediated by immune complexes, but there is no evidence for such complexes playing any role in the production of reactions produced by small molecular size drugs. For the same reason, laboratory tests are of little value in the diagnosis of this class of drug allergy.

T Lymphocyte–Mediated Reactions

Most of these reactions result from the use of topical medications on the skin. The offending drug produces a pruritic, erythematous, papulovesicular, and even bullous eruption that is called *allergic eczematous contact dermatitis.* The general clinical, pathologic, and immune features of this condition are presented in Chapter 30. Most commonly, the reaction develops during topical therapy of a preexisting dermatosis.

Allergic contact dermatitis in general is uncommon in children; the prevalence of sensitivity increases with age. This would be true for drug sensitivity as well except that topical medications are used so frequently in treating skin rashes in young children that the development of contact sensitivity is a common event. In one study, 24 percent of 2000 patients with eczema had developed contact allergy to one or more drugs (Cronin et al., 1970).

Some drugs, notably antihistamines, penicillin, and sulfonamines, were such common sensitizers that they are now rarely used on the skin. However, these drugs and others still can sensitize the medical or manufacturing personnel who handle them. Table 53–7 lists these drugs separately from the therapeutic (topical) agents. Drugs that are fairly common sensitizers are bacitracin, benzocaine, idoxuridine, and neomycin. Other potential sensitizers are added to numerous medications as stabilizers

TABLE 53–7. Drugs that can Produce Allergic Eczematous Contact Dermatitis

Occupational	Bacitracin
Ampicillin	Benzocaine
Benzalkonium chloride	Ethylenediamine
Chlorpromazine	Fluorouracil
Formaldehyde	Formaldehyde
Glutaraldehyde	Glucocorticoids
Hexachlorophene	Idoxuridine
Local anesthetics	Iodochlorhydroxyquin
Opiates	Lanolin
Penicillin	Neomycin
Phenothiazines	Parabens
Streptomycin	Para-aminobenzoic acid
Thimerosal	Propylene glycol
	Sulfonamides
Therapeutic	Therapeutic dyes
Antihistamine (H₁)	Thimerosal
Ammoniated mercury	

and preservatives and include ethylenediamine, thimerosal, and parabens. The patient who develops contact allergy to one of these agents runs some risk of developing a generalized reaction if treated with a systemic drug containing that agent. To date, however, such reactions have been reported for ethylenediamine only (Petrozzi and Shore, 1976). Local or systemic symptoms from prosthetic implants could, theoretically, develop on the basis of T cell sensitization to metals (especially nickel) in stainless steel devices. Such sensitization is exceedingly rare, however. Recently, certain practitioners have claimed that hypersensitivity to mercury amalgam in tooth fillings could be responsible for ailments such as acne, depression, fatigue, and multiple sclerosis. In fact, such sensitivity occurs very rarely, and the resulting reaction is a local one; *there is no evidence that it is ever responsible for other symptoms* (Mackert and Fisher, 1985).

Other Cutaneous Reactions

Photodermatitis. Photosensitivity reactions occur when skin is exposed to ultraviolet light during a time when a patient is taking the offending drug, either topically or internally. There are two types, *toxic* and *allergic*. The two are differentiated as are other toxic and allergic reactions. Toxic reactions develop immediately after drug treatment is started, assuming a sufficient amount of ultraviolet light exposure occurs. The reaction is provoked by "sunburn" wavelengths (285 to 310 nm). Photoallergic reactions are activated by longer wavelengths

(320 to 450 nm) and appear only after the drug has been taken for a period of time sufficient for sensitization to develop (5 to 21 days). Whereas the toxic reaction has the characteristics of a typical sunburn, the allergic reaction may be erythematous, urticarial, edematous, eczematous, or exudative. Phototoxic drugs absorb and concentrate ultraviolet energy in the skin. Those drugs or metabolites responsible for allergic reactions may conjugate to dermal proteins and serve as haptenes to a significant degree only in the presence of ultraviolet energy.

Table 53–8 lists some systemic drugs that are responsible for photodermatitis. The most common phototoxic drugs are chlorpromazine, demeclocycline, and doxycycline. The most common systemic drugs responsible for photoallergy are griseofulvin, nalidixic acid, psoralens, and sulfonamides. With the exception of coal-tar derivatives and psoralens, the reactions to topically applied agents are photoallergic. Most topical sensitizers have been removed from the market in the United States. The halogenated salicylanilides, used as antiseptics in soaps and cosmetics, are the best known sensitizers still in common use. Others are hexachlorophene and para-aminobenzoic acid (PABA) esters.

The diagnosis of photodermatitis usually is obvious because of eruption during drug therapy and its appearance on exposed skin only. If further proof is needed, the photopatch test can be used. This is done by applying the suspected agents to skin sites in duplicate for at least 24 hours, then exposing one of the sites to natural sunlight or an artificial source of ultraviolet light for 20 minutes. The next day the sites are inspected and interpreted in the same manner

TABLE 53–8. Systemic Photosensitizing Drugs

Amiodarone
Carbamazepine
Demeclocycline*
Doxycycline*
Gold salts
Griseofulvin*
Imipramine
Lincomycin
Nalidixic acid
Phenothiazines
Psoralens*
Quinethazone
Sulfonamides*
Sulfonylureas
Thiazide diuretics
Triamterine

* Reactions to these drugs are relatively common.

as in conventional patch tests (see subsequent section on testing).

There is no way to predict who is at risk of a reaction, but it is prudent to warn the patient to avoid sunlight exposure during treatment with a known offender, such as doxycycline. Sunscreen agents may protect from unavoidable exposure, but some of them may be photoallergenic because they contain PABA esters.

Fixed Drug Eruptions. Fixed drug eruptions consist of one or more macular, erythematous, edematous, round, or oval plaques that are sharply demarcated. The more severe reactions may be eczematous or even bullous. The lesions heal with scaling after treatment with the offending drug is stopped, leaving a sharply demarcated area of dark red, violet, or brown-pink pigmentation. Lesions may occur anywhere, including mucous membranes. Occasionally, they are pruritic, but there are no systemic symptoms. Evidence for an allergic etiology is historically convincing. First, the drug may be given several times, even over the course of years, before the reaction develops. Second, the fixed eruption can be reproduced without significant risk by readministering the drug. Despite the convincing clinical evidence, the immune mechanism remains in doubt. The most likely is a localized T cell sensitivity, but numerous experimental studies using patch testing and skin grafting have produced conflicting or inconsistent results (Ackroyd, 1985). Over 50 drugs and food additives have been reported to cause fixed drug eruptions (Derbes, 1964), but most of these are rare. Drugs most commonly implicated are analgesics, barbiturates, gold salts, iodides, metronidazole, penicillins, phenolphthalein, sulfonamides, and tetracyclines.

Generalized Skin Rashes. Other drug-induced skin rashes that are thought to be allergic are characterized generally by pruritus, erythema, and maculopapular eruptions. Some are described as scarlatiniform or exanthematous. To emphasize the connection, the otherwise unenlightening term *dermatitis medicamentosa* may be used. These are the most common allergic drug reactions, amounting to 46 percent of the total in one study from a dermatology service (Kuokkanen, 1972). The onset of these eruptions usually is late in treatment, and there is nothing unique to differentiate them from infectious disease exanthemata. The reactions are thought to be allergic, possibly on a T cell–mediated basis, but definitive proof is lacking. Sometimes, as in the case of most ampicillin-induced rashes, the evidence is to the contrary; usually, the eruption is not reproduced when the patient is rechallenged with the drug. There are no helpful laboratory features to support or exclude the possibility of drug allergy.

Most drugs have produced skin eruptions at one time or another; at least 16 groups of structurally similar drugs and 52 other individual drugs are cited in Gilman et al. (1985). The most common offenders are ampicillin, aminoglycoside antibiotics, barbiturates, benzodiazepines, gold salts, and sulfonamides. Listing all drugs that have been implicated would serve no useful purpose. Instead, Table 53–9 is a list of commonly used drugs that rarely are responsible for skin eruptions.

If a maculopapular eruption develops, and for some reason treatment with the responsible drug is continued, the outcome is unpredictable. Sometimes the rash will resolve, suggesting either that it was not drug induced or that continuing the treatment has produced tolerance. The risk, of course, is that the eruption will evolve into something more severe and potentially fatal. The possibilities are *exfoliative dermatitis* and severe bullous reactions. The former is thought to be the more likely, but the evidence is scanty. Furthermore, the causal relationship is often uncertain because exfoliative dermatitis and bullous reactions are not necessarily caused by drugs. For this reason, exfoliative dermatitis is discussed in a subsequent section. However, a severe form of bullous reaction, *toxic epidermal necrolysis (TEN)* will be considered next because of an increasing con-

TABLE 53–9. Commonly used Drugs that Rarely or Never Cause Skin Eruptions

Acetaminophen	Lithium
Adrenergic agents	Local anesthetics
Androgens	Meperidine
Antacids	Morphine
Antihistamines	Nystatin
Aspirin	Paraldehyde
Atropine	Pentazocine
Bromocriptine	Prednisone
Cascara	Progesterone
Clomiphene	Spironolactone
Codeine	Tetracycline
Digoxin-digitoxin	Theophylline
Emollient laxatives	Thyroid hormones
Estrogens	Tubocurarine
Ganglionic-blocking agents	Vitamins
Glucocorticoids	Warfarin
Hydrochlorothiazide	
Levodopa	

sensus in recent years that this type of reaction more often than not is drug induced.

Toxic Epidermal Necrolysis (TEN). This reaction, also called Lyell syndrome, begins with the development of an erythematous rash, which soon is followed by the appearance of large, confluent bullae. Occasionally, the reaction may be difficult to distinguish from severe *erythema multiforme* (Stevens-Johnson syndrome, discussed in a subsequent section). TEN may be associated with, or preceded by, malaise and fever. Rarely, the reaction may be associated with eosinophilia, renal failure, or both. In the more severe reactions, bullae become widespread and confluent, and the epidermis sloughs off in large sheets, leaving large areas of raw dermis. The reaction is similar to a severe thermal injury with attendant fluid, electrolyte, and infection problems. Drugs that have been implicated as causes of TEN include allopurinol, chloramphenicol, ethambutol, ibuprofen, penicillin, phenolphthalein, phenylbutazone, phenytoin, sulfonamides, and sulindac. In rare instances, the offending drug has been given again inadvertently, and the ensuing maculopapular eruption (fortunately, self limited) has confirmed the relationship (Pegram et al., 1981).

The staphylococcal scalded skin syndrome (SSSS), usually seen in children, was classified with TEN until recently. Since it is not drug induced, the general impression developed that TEN also was not often drug induced. Skin biopsy findings, however, have proved that the two conditions are not the same. In TEN, the whole epidermis separates; in the more benign SSSS, the tissue that separates is intraepidermal.

Fever

Body temperature is regulated in the preoptic region of the anterior hypothalamus. This thermoregulatory center maintains body temperature under normal circumstances within a narrow range by controlling heat production and conservation via both autonomic and skeletal motor neural pathways. Fever can occur when macrophages are stimulated to produce endogenous pyrogen (a polypeptide now known as interleukin-1). Interleukin-1 acts by increasing the generation of E prostaglandins from arachidonic acid. This increase has an important temperature-raising influence on the hypothalamic center. Several factors are known to stimulate interleukin-1 generation. These include bacteria or bacterial products (gram-negative endotoxins and exotoxins), viruses, fungi, and antigen-antibody complexes. Since body temperature can be raised also by other mechanisms, such as inadequate heat dissipation, excessive heat production, and direct hypothalamic effect, it should not be surprising that different therapeutic agents might produce fever in different ways. Some well-recognized febrile reactions to drugs are not immunologically mediated. These are listed in Table 53–10. The first four categories in this table are self explanatory. Increased tissue metabolism often is associated with autonomic dysfunction, leading to severe and potentially fatal reactions, as in malignant hyperthermia induced during inhalation anesthesia by succinylcholine and perhaps other agents. Recently, reactions of comparable severity, associated with hyperpyrexia and rigidity, have been reported with the use of haloperidol and similar drugs (i.e., "neuroleptic

TABLE 53–10. Nonallergic Causes of Drug Fever

Mechanism	Examples
Endogenous release of bacterial pyrogen	Jarisch-Herxheimer reaction
Administration of exogenous pyrogen	Contaminated fluids or drugs
	Fever therapy; injection of endotoxin or typhoid vaccine
Release of endogenous pyrogen	Sterile inflammation after intramuscular drug injection
Secondary to another type of adverse reaction producing tissue injury	Hemolysis, hepatitis
Increased tissue metabolism	General anesthetics, succinylcholine (malignant hyperthermia)
	Neuroleptic malignant syndrome
Peripheral vasoconstriction and reduced heat loss	Norepinephrine effect
Central effect	Amphetamine intoxication
	Prostaglandins and prostaglandin-generating agents
Hormonal	Etiocholanolone fever

malignant syndrome") (Szabadi, 1984). Hyperpyrexia in children caused by certain psychotropic drugs has been recognized as an occasional problem for several years (Feigen and Shearer, 1976).

Prostaglandins are now used therapeutically and are frequently pyrogenic via a direct central effect. Alprostadil (PGE_1) should be of particular interest to pediatricians. It is used to help maintain patent ductus arterioses in infants with congenital heart disease, and 14 percent of these infants so treated develop hyperpyrexia. Human interferon often is pyrogenic. Until recently, this effect has been attributed to endotoxin or endogenous pyrogen contamination. However, human alpha interferon prepared by recombinant techniques, and thus free of such impurities, also is pyrogenic. The mechanism has recently been identified, and it is interferon-induced prostaglandin E_2 (PGE_2) generation in the hypothalamus (Dinarello et al., 1984).

Some other drugs probably are direct pyrogens, being commonly associated with fever, but the mechanisms are not known. Amphotericin B is the best known example; others are cimetidine, iron dextran, calcium disodium edetate, and dimercaprol. In children, *epinephrine as well as norepinephrine can cause fevers.* Atropine (even eye drops) and phenothiazine may inhibit sweating sufficiently to raise the body temperature above normal.

Perhaps the earliest description of allergic fever produced by a drug was reported by Jadassohn in 1896 (see Samter, 1969). He described a patient with contact dermatitis who subsequently swallowed a small amount of the offending chemical; several hours later, the patient developed fever and generalized erythroderma. Allergic fever can be part of drug-induced vasculitis, which may include manifestations similar to those of serum sickness. It may be the first sign of drug-induced hepatitis, or it may be the only physical manifestation. When allergic fever occurs alone, the patient may lack other symptoms associated with a febrile illness. This is a noteworthy feature to recognize when a fever due to an antimicrobial drug allergy appears after resolution of a fever caused by an infection. When treatment with the offending drug is stopped, the temperature almost always drops to normal within 48 hours. One exception is phenytoin. This drug has a high tissue affinity, and the temperature may not return to normal for several days after treatment is stopped.

Table 53–11 lists drugs that have been reported to cause allergic fevers without other allergic manifestations. The most commonly implicated are allopurinol, azathioprine, barbiturates, blood products, cephalosporins, hydroxyurea, iodides, methyldopa, penicillamine, penicillins, phenytoin, procainamide, and quinidine. Fever is relatively uncommon among all forms of adverse drug reactions in hospitalized patients but may make up as much as 25 percent of the total number of allergic reactions. In one study of 146 children with fevers of unknown origin, three had drug fevers (Feigin and Shearer, 1976).

The mechanism of allergic drug fever has not been established. Because the clinical features are consistent with allergy and because the fever has been produced in sensitized rabbits by a penicilloyl conjugate (Chusid and Atkins, 1972), there is general consensus that allergic drug fever is caused by the release of interleukin-1 during phagocytosis of complexes of antibody with drug-carrier conjugates.

Autoimmune Reactions

Systemic Lupus Erythematosus (SLE). First reported in patients receiving hydralazine treatment over 30 years ago, a syndrome similar to SLE has subsequently been associated with treatment with many other drugs. However, most cases have been caused by hydralazine or procainamide. The most frequent symptoms

TABLE 53–11. Drugs that can Cause Fever Without Other Signs of Allergy

Antimicrobials	Other Drugs
Aminosalicylic acid	Allopurinol
Cephalosporins	Antithymocyte globulin
Chloramphenicol	Blood products
Erythromycin	Heparin
Griseofulvin	Hydralazine
Isoniazid	Hydroxyurea
Kanamycin	Iodides
Nitrofurantoin	Mercurial diuretics
Penicillins	Methyldopa
Pyrazinamide	Penicillamine
Quinine	Phenobarbital
Streptomycin	Phenytoin
Sulfonamides	Pneumococcal vaccine
Tetracyclines	Procainamide
Trimethoprim	Propylthiouracil
	Quinidine

are malaise, fever, arthralgias, and pleuritic pain. A few patients also develop pericarditis, adenopathy, skin rash, and hepatosplenomegaly. Most develop mild anemia and leukopenia and demonstrate an elevated erythrocyte sedimentation rate. The lupus cell preparation and antinuclear antibody (ANA) titer become positive. In contrast to true SLE, central nervous system or renal involvement is unusual, serum complement remains normal, and antibodies to DNA are absent. Most patients with symptomatic drug-induced SLE have predominately antihistone antibodies, in contrast to patients with true SLE, in whom antibodies to multiple nuclear antigens usually are found, and in contrast to asymptomatic patients, in whom drug-induced ANAs are found (Epstein and Barland, 1985). The prevalence of positive ANA titers increases with the duration of treatment and the incidence of clinical manifestations may be dose related. The prevalence is so high (over 50 percent with positive ANAs from procainamide treatment and up to 12 percent with symptoms from hydralazine treatment) that the SLE syndrome is often considered toxic rather than allergic. Indeed, the reaction may be the outcome of a pharmacologic effect. Perhaps the drugs render native nucleoprotein antigenic. This is supported by experimental observations (Dubroff and Reid, 1980). There is no evidence that the drugs unmask latent SLE, and symptoms and ANA titers gradually diminish after drug treatment is stopped.

Other drugs that are documented causes of the SLE syndrome are chlorpromazine, isoniazid, penicillamine, phenytoin, and sulfasalazine. Acebutolol, a new beta-adrenergic blocking drug, has been associated with positive ANA titers and, less often, with symptoms (Anonymous, Medical Letter, 1985). At least a dozen more drugs have been implicated, but the evidence for a causal association is weak (VanArsdel, 1983).

Other Autoimmune Disorders. Penicillamine has been implicated in several immune complex disorders in addition to SLE. These include dermatomyositis, polymyositis, diffuse alveolitis, obliterative bronchiolitis, and myasthenia gravis. The last disorder is noteworthy because antiacetylcholine receptor antibodies and antistriated muscle antibodies have been identified in the sera of some patients being treated with D-penicillamine (Vincent et al., 1978). A syndrome similar to myasthenia gravis also has been reported during treatment with trimethadione and with quinidine.

Penicillin treatment has been associated with a clotting disorder caused by an autoantibody to Factor VIII (Parker, 1982). Drug-induced autoimmune hemolytic anemia is discussed in the next section.

Organ System Reactions

Hematologic

Eosinophilia. Eosinophilia usually accompanies other allergic manifestations of drug allergy, or it may be the first sign to appear. Although its appearance may serve as a warning of worse manifestations to come, this rarely is appreciated at the time. Furthermore, the appearance of eosinophilia alone is not a reason to terminate important therapy. Drugs that are commonly associated with eosinophilia are listed in Table 53–12. Only occasionally is eosinophilia the only manifestation of drug allergy. It is curious that eosinophilia alone is common during treatment with streptomycin (50 percent), kanamycin (10 percent), and digitalis, even though clinical allergy to the last is extremely rare.

The association between a drug and eosinophilia may not indicate cause and effect, particularly with antibiotic therapy. Eosinophilia is not an uncommon part of convalescence from infections, such as pneumococcal pneumonia.

Hemolytic Anemia. As indicated previously, it is useful to categorize drug-related cell destruction according to three types of mechanisms.

Haptene-Cell Type. In this type of reaction, the offending drug or its reactive intermediate binds to some portion of the red blood cell membrane. The immunogenicity of the drug

TABLE 53–12. Drugs Associated with Eosinophilia

Antimicrobials	Other Drugs
Aminosalicylic acid	Allopurinol
Cephalosporins	Carbamazepine
Erythromycin	Chloral hydrate
Isoniazid	Clonazepam
Kanamycin	Digitalis
Nalidixic acid	Ethosuximide
Nitrofurantoin	Papaverine
Penicillins	Penicillamine
Rifampin	Phenothiazines
Streptomycin	Probucol
Sulfonamides	Tricyclics
Tetracyclines	

may relate more to its serum protein binding than to its binding to that membrane. Accordingly, the effect of the reaction of antibody with the drug is more analogous to passive hemagglutination than to that of a reaction with a drug-membrane-protein carrier. Thus, the mechanism may be more appropriately termed "drug-adsorption" than "haptene-cell" (Petz, 1985). This reaction was first described with high-dose benzylpenicillin treatment in association with high-titered IgG antibody. The diagnosis is supported if the direct Coombs antiglobulin reaction is positive; the diagnosis is confirmed if the indirect test results, using normal drug-treated cells, also are positive (Van-Arsdel, 1970). A similar mechanism is responsible for the reaction to the antitumor drug, cisplatin. Cephalothin, commonly responsible for a positive Coombs test result, rarely causes hemolytic anemia. This positive test result is an artifact caused by nonspecific protein adsorption.

Immune Complex Type. When IgG or IgM antibody develops with specificity for an epitope on a drug or drug metabolite, the antibody forms a complex with the antigen (most likely bound to a macromolecular carrier) in the circulation. In susceptible individuals, this complex, after reacting with complement, develops a high affinity for red blood cells and attaches to them nonspecifically. After such an attachment, the antigen-antibody complex may remain on the cells only transiently, while the membrane attack complex of complement remains on the cell to produce injury. For this reason, the direct Coombs test result in drug-induced immune anemia may be positive only if a complement antiserum is used. This nonspecific binding to red blood cells or other formed blood elements, with subsequent cell damage, led Shulman (1964) to apply the term, "innocent bystanders" to these cells. More recently, however, receptors for immune complexes have been identified on red blood cells, suggesting that binding may not be so passive after all (Petz, 1985). Drugs in common use that can cause this kind of anemia are acetaminophen, phenacetin, chlorpromazine, insulin, isoniazid, quinidine, rifampin, sulfonamides, and sulindac.

The more severe reactions have been associated with evidence of intravascular hemolysis. An antidepressant drug, nomifensine, has been observed recently to produce these reactions in several patients. Although the drug is not used in the United States, investigation of

patients receiving it in Germany has provided further insight into the immune mechanism of drug hypersensitivity. Some complement-fixing IgG and IgM antibodies were found with drug specificity, but most antibodies were reactive with drug metabolites. The most consistent reactions were found using, as an antigen source, the urine from a normal person who had been given the drug. Most of the *"ex vivo"* reactive metabolites so obtained have not yet been identified (Salama and Mueller-Eckhardt, 1985).

Autoimmune. In this type of reaction, drug administration may lead to the production of an IgG autoantibody directed against an intrinsic red blood cell antigen. The direct Coombs antiglobulin test is strongly reactive, but the anticomplement test is not. The most commonly implicated drug, methyldopa, inhibits suppressor lymphocyte function, including those cells that prevent the unrestrained production of autoimmune antibodies (Kirtland et al.,1980). Ibuprofen, levodopa, mefenamic acid, and procainamide are others that may be responsible for this type of reaction.

Thrombocytopenia. An immune complex mechanism probably is responsible for most cases of drug-induced immune thrombocytopenia; although, as with anemia, the binding may be more active than previously thought. The sensitized patient will react within 30 minutes of receiving even a minute dose of the offending drug (e.g., quinine in tonic water) with chills, fever, petechiae, and mucous membrane bleeding as the platelet count drops precipitously. The antibody involved usually is an IgG immunoglobulin. In the laboratory, the suspected drug is incubated with the patient's serum and normal platelet-rich plasma. A positive reaction may be detected by complement fixation, platelet factor release, or serotonin uptake inhibition. Drugs now in common use that have been associated with immune thrombocytopenia are listed in Table 53–13. The most frequent offenders are cephalosporins, gold salts, hydantoins, isoniazid, procainamide, quinidine, quinine, rifampin, sulfonamides, and thiazide diuretics. In the case of acetaminophen, the responsible antigen was a sulfate metabolite (Eisner and Shahidi, 1972).

Granulocytopenia. Immune granulocytopenia is associated with the appearance of acute chills, fever, and arthralgias, accompanied by a rapid fall in the leukocyte count. By contrast, toxic or idiosyncratic leukopenia caused by bone marrow depression develops insidiously

TABLE 53–13. Drugs Causing Immune
Thrombocytopenia

Acetaminophen	Mefenamic acid
Acetazolamide	Meprobamate
Acetylsalicylic acid	Methyldopa
Aminosalicylic acid	Penicillamine
Carbamazepine	Phenacetin
Cephalothin	Phenylbutazone
Chloramphenicol	Procainamide
Chlorpheniramine	Quinidine
Desipramine	Quinine
Digitoxin	*Rauwolfia* alkaloids
Ethchlorvynol	Rifampin
Gold salts	Stibophen
Heparin	Sulfonamides
Hydantoins	Sulfonylureas
Isoniazid	Thiazide diuretics
Levodopa	Valproic acid

and becomes apparent if the patient is monitored with periodic blood counts or if an infection, such as stomatitis or pharyngitis, develops. Drugs' causing immune granulocytopenia are few in number compared with those causing predictable suppressive effects on bone marrow. Aminopyrine was the first drug reported to produce immune granulocytopenia; sensitivity was confirmed by demonstrating leukoagglutinating antibodies that transferred the sensitivity passively to normal recipients. Leukoagglutinins to other drugs have been identified inconsistently. The results may be inconsistent because granulocytes altered by drug-antibody complexes have short half-lives and remove the complexes when they are cleared from the circulation. Thus, any leukoagglutinin is present only transiently. A test based on the opsonization of normal neutrophils by sera of neutropenic patients' receiving various drugs appears to be more reliable than leukoagglutination (Weitzman et al., 1978). Immune granulocytopenia from any drug is rare. The more familiar drugs that are responsible occasionally are antidepressants, gold salts, methimazole, phenothiazines, phenylbutazone, semisynthetic penicillins, procainamide, quinidine, sulfonamides, and sulfonylureas.

HEPATIC

The liver, being a major site for drug metabolism, should be particularly susceptible to drug injury. Perhaps because the liver is such a vulnerable target, few drugs that are primarily hepatotoxic remain in use today. Occasionally, toxic dose–related reactions occur from acetaminophen or intravenous tetracycline; ne-

crosis and fibrosis are calculated risks in treatment with methotrexate or mercaptopurine. In children, idiosyncratic hepatotoxic reactions to aspirin may occur during the treatment of juvenile rheumatoid arthritis and allied diseases (Anderson, 1980). Most hepatic reactions have characteristics more consistent with allergy, although the evidence is based primarily on clinical clues such as the delay in the onset of symptoms or signs and the association with other signs of allergy.

The two main subclasses of hypersensitivity are *cholestatic* and *hepatocellular*. Drugs that may produce hepatic reactions are listed according to these two subclasses in Table 53–14. Jaundice usually is the first sign of a cholestatic reaction but may be preceded by the appearance of eosinophilia. Phenothiazines and erythromycin estolate have been more often responsible for the cholestatic reaction, although the latter is rarely used now because of this side effect. The clinical picture of hepatocellular reaction may be similar to that of viral hepatitis. Fever may be the first manifestation, or signs of obstructive jaundice may develop. The liver becomes enlarged and tender. A skin rash and arthralgias, eosinophilia, or both may develop. The reaction occurs frequently with pyrazinamide, rifampin, and aminosalicylic acid, and is the most frequent reaction in children treated with valproic acid. Rarely, the anesthetic agent halothane can produce an allergic hepatitis after repeated exposure, and some deaths have been reported. Patients with cholestatic hepati-

TABLE 53–14. Drugs Causing Hypersensitive
Hepatic Reactions

Primarily Cholestatic	
Aprindine	Gold salts
Chlorzoxazone	Griseofulvin
Erythromycin estolate	Halothane
Ethchlorvynol	Hydantoins
Haloperidol	Isoniazid
Imipramine	Ketoconazole
Nalidixic acid	Methyldopa
Nitrofurantoin	Monoamine oxidase
Papaverine	inhibitors
Phenothiazines	Nitrofurantoin
Sulindac	Oxyphenisatin
Sulfamethoxazole	Phenylbutazone
Sulfonylureas	Propylthiouracil
Troleandomycin	Pyrazinamide
Primarily Hepatocellular	Quinidine
	Rifampin
Aminosalicylic acid	Sulfonamides
Amphotericin B	Sulindac
Ethacrynic acid	Trimethadione
Furosemide	Valproic acid

tis always recover completely when drug treatment is stopped. Most with hepatocellular injury also recover, but the reaction may lead rarely to postnecrotic cirrhosis and can be fatal.

Granulomatous hepatitis has been associated with several drugs, but these associations may be coincidental. It has developed during allopurinol treatment along with other signs of vasculitis (see subsequent discussion), and a few cases of *chronic active hepatitis* have been reported following treatment with methyldopa, nitrofurantoin, and oxyphenisatin.

PULMONARY

Asthma. Asthma most often is a part of a generalized systemic reaction to an injected allergenic extract. It may occur occasionally as part of an anaphylactic drug reaction in a patient with an asthmatic diathesis. It rarely is the only manifestation of a systemic allergic reaction. Indeed, if asthma alone follows administration of some drug, it probably is a pharmacologic side effect of that drug. Such reactions are discussed elsewhere in this chapter. Inhaled agents such as antimicrobials and enzymes may provoke asthmatic reactions in sensitive individuals but are reported much more commonly from occupational exposure than from therapeutic use.

Infiltrative Reactions. These are acute reactions that usually develop 2 to 10 days after onset of treatment, with cough and dyspnea that are often associated with chills, fever, and malaise. A maculopapular rash may develop. The physical findings usually are limited to a few focal or basilar coarse rales. In contrast, the chest radiograph usually shows the following impressive changes: diffuse alveolar, reticulonodular, and focal migratory fluffy infiltrates. The reaction has been reported from inhaled drugs, even cromolyn, but is exceedingly rare. Reactions reported to be caused by systemic drug administration are listed in Table 53–15. *Eosinophilic pneumonitis* usually is associated with few symptoms or physical signs, but marked eosinophilia develops, followed by the radiographic appearance of nodular or fluffy infiltrates in the chest. In the *"other"* category are drugs that produce a diffuse interstitial infiltrate. Sometimes, patients develop symptoms and signs suggesting pulmonary edema, particularly with nitrofurantoin. This drug is the most common cause of acute reactions. Evidence that the acute reactions are allergic is mostly circumstantial. There are scattered reports of drug-in-

TABLE 53–15. Drugs Causing Infiltrative Pulmonary Reactions

Probably Allergic	Fibrotic
Eosinophilic pneumonitis	Bleomycin
Aminosalicylic acid	Busulfan
Carbamazepine	Methysergide
Chlorpropamide	Mitomycin
Gold salts	Nitrofurantoin
Naproxen	Nitrogen mustards
Penicillin	Nitrosoureas
Sulfonamides	
Other	
Gold salts	
Melphalan	
Methotrexate	
Nitrofurantoin	
Procarbazine	
Thiazide diuretics	

duced stimulation of a patient's lymphocytes in tissue culture, suggesting a cell-mediated hypersensitivity mechanism, but no consistent immune pattern has emerged.

Fibrotic Reactions. These are slowly developing reactions that are probably toxic-idiosyncratic. They are characterized by the gradual development of cough and dyspnea without any associated systemic symptoms. Responsible drugs are also listed in Table 53–15. Pulmonary toxicity of certain antineoplastic agents, particularly bleomycin, is a predictable, dose-related side effect. Fibrosis may continue to progress after drug treatment is terminated.

RENAL

Interstitial nephritis is the most common drug-induced hypersensitivity reaction. It is characterized by hematuria, proteinuria, pyuria, and varying degrees of azotemia. The reaction tends to be milder and of shorter duration in children than in adults. Most patients have other findings that suggest an allergic reaction, such as fever, skin rash, and eosinophilia of blood and urine. The renal biopsy specimen shows tubular degeneration and necrosis with infiltrates containing mononuclear cells, plasma cells, and eosinophils. The results of immunofluorescent studies have been variable and inconsistent. Methicillin has been the most common identified cause of interstitial nephritis. Other probable causes among drugs in common use are cimetidine, cephalosporins, diuretics (furosemide and thiazides), other penicillins, rifampin, and sulfonamides. Nonsteroidal anti-inflammatory drugs (NSAIDs) also can produce interstitial nephritis, but the symptoms and signs are those of nephrotic syndrome, and associated allergic features are rare. The predominant cells in the interstitial infiltrate are T lymphocytes. Allopurinol and phenytoin may produce interstitial nephritis, but usually reactions from these drugs are heterogeneous with vasculitis and variable glomerular involvement (Adler et al., 1985).

A patient with a drug-induced immune *glomerular injury* usually presents with nephrotic syndrome. Commonly, renal function is only mildly impaired. The biopsy findings are typical of membranous glomerulopathy, including the immunofluorescence findings of finely granular IgG and C3 deposits (Adler et al., 1985). Drugs that are most often implicated are captopril, gold salts, NSAIDs, and penicillamine.

Reactions with Inconsistent Drug Associations

Erythema Multiforme. This is an eruption characterized by concentric or "target"-shaped skin eruptions along with various combinations of macular, papular, urticarial, vesicular, and purpuric lesions. A severe form, called the *Stevens-Johnson syndrome,* is characterized by bullous skin lesions with mucous membrane and conjunctival involvement. It generally is preceded by fever, malaise, or other constitutional symptoms. Establishing or excluding a drug association usually is difficult, because the reaction can be associated with mycoplasma and other infections, neoplasms, connective tissue diseases, and even radiation therapy. As mentioned previously, a drug being used for treatment of a disease may be mistakenly blamed for a reaction that is actually a result of the disease itself. Nevertheless, hypersensitivity to the suspected drug has been proved in a few instances; the drug was inadvertently given again, and the skin eruption reappeared. Drugs so implicated in published cases are minoxidil, phenolphthalein, rifampin, sulfapyridine, and trimethoprim-sulfamethoxazole (VanArsdel, 1983). Commonly used drugs that have been implicated on circumstantial evidence alone are acetaminophen/phenacetin, carbamazepine, gold salts, hydralazine, penicillins, phenylbutazone, phenytoin, and sulfonylureas.

Exfoliative Dermatitis. This is a potentially fatal reaction that may begin as an apparently benign maculopapular eruption but progresses to a diffuse, highly pruritic desquamative erythroderma. If uncontrolled, it may become edematous and exudative and lead to severe fluid loss and secondary infection. About 10 percent of cases are thought to be drug induced; the remainder are associated with underlying diseases such as psoriasis, atopic dermatitis, and lymphocytic malignancies. There is only scanty evidence for an immune pathogenesis. The best evidence is clinical. Patients with known contact allergy to ethylenediamine may develop exfoliative erythroderma if treated with parenteral aminophylline (Petrozzi and Shore, 1976). Exfoliative dermatitis has been implicated as an unusual or rare adverse effect from treatment with the drugs listed in Table 53–16. Carbamazepine may be the most frequent offender (Kuokkanen, 1972). In children, exfoliative dermatitis may be a toxic reaction; it is one of several symptoms and signs of vitamin A poisoning.

Vasculitis. This reaction has other names, e.g., *allergic angiitis, hypersensitivity angiitis, and allergic purpura.* The patient presents with erythematous and maculopapular lesions that usually appear first on dependent areas. Frequently, purpuric lesions then appear. These are raised ("palpable purpura") and may become bullous and necrotic. Occasionally, urticaria and target lesions also are present. There may be systemic symptoms, such as fever, malaise, arthralgias, headache, and abdominal pain. A biopsy specimen of a typical skin lesion shows fibrinoid necrosis in walls of small venules and arterioles, endothelial swelling, hemorrhage, platelet thrombi, and disintegrating nuclei in the leukocyte infiltrate (*leukocytoclastic vasculitis*). Vasculitis is probably an immune complex disease, but most of the convincing laboratory evidence for this is found in patients with vasculitis that is not drug induced, i.e., vasculitis related to hepatitis B. In fact, most cases are not drug induced; only 4 of 39 cases reported recently were considered to be drug induced (Mackel and Jordon, 1982). Drugs in

TABLE 53–16. Drugs Implicated in Exfoliative Dermatitis

Allopurinol	Penicillin
Aminophylline (ethylenediamine)	Phenobarbital
Carbamazepine	Phenothiazines
Captopril	Phenytoin
Dapsone	Sulfonamides
Glutethimide	Trimethadione
Gold salts	Trimethoprim
Iodides	

common use that have been implicated are allopurinol, cimetidine, furosemide, hydantoins, penicillins, phenylbutazone, and sulfonamides. There is at least one report of vasculitis that reappeared when the offending drug (cimetidine) was taken again. The biopsy findings were positive both times (Mitchell et al., 1983).

Other. There is no evidence other than a small number of anecdotal reports that any drug causes either *erythema nodosum* or *Henoch-Schönlein purpura*.

Pseudoallergic Reactions

These reactions have been outlined previously (see Table 53–3) and discussed briefly. Three groups of drugs (NSAIDs, radiographic contrast media, and various additives) merit further discussion.

NSAIDs. One year after aspirin was first approved in 1909 by the Council on Pharmacy and Chemistry of the American Medical Association, a 40-year-old woman with a history of asthma developed acute difficulty in breathing after ingesting 5 grains of aspirin for a headache. Within a few years, aspirin reactions were thought to be among the most common examples of drug allergy. However, when similar reactions began to appear from anti-inflammatory drugs of significantly different chemical structure, it became clear that the commonality among these drugs was not immunochemical cross-reactivity, but pharmacologic similarity (VanArsdel, 1984). Starting with aspirin and indomethacin, this commonality now encompasses a substantial number of drugs — the NSAIDs — that share the property of inhibiting the enzyme cyclooxygenase and, thus, the generation of prostaglandins from arachidonic acid. The first reported patient is typical of patients who develop intolerance to aspirin and other NSAIDs. All such patients have a history of asthma, chronic rhinosinusitis, or both. Many have nasal polyps, and most have blood and tissue eosinophilia. Many do not have an atopic background, and most developed their first respiratory symptoms as adults. About 4 percent of unselected adult asthmatic patients give histories of symptoms provoked by NSAIDs, and as many more will show drops in ventilatory function after drug challenge. Up to 40 percent of patients with asthma, rhinosinusitis, and nasal polyps are intolerant or will become so. Some have the symptoms for several years before intolerance develops, although it is not uncommon for one with a history of rhinosinusitis to have the first asthma attack provoked by aspirin (Stevenson, 1984).

The NSAIDs produce or provoke both asthma and symptoms of rhinosinusitis in most intolerant patients; about 10 percent develop one or the other only. The degree of intolerance varies widely. Some patients may show nothing more than a 15 percent reduction in the forced expiratory volume in 1 second (FEV_1) and no symptoms when challenged with a full therapeutic dose; others may develop symptoms when challenged with a tenth that amount. Severe reactions can be anaphylactoid, leading to shock and death. Although most intolerant patients are adults, intolerance can develop in adolescents and in older children. Young atopic patients who have the misfortune to have asthma or allergic rhinitis complicated by chronic sinusitis and nasal polyps are at risk.

The mechanism of intolerance to NSAIDs is probably related in some way to their pharmacologic action. The most obvious explanation is that the inhibition of cyclooxygenase by these drugs increases arachidonic metabolism via the lipoxygenase pathway, thus increasing leukotriene generation. However, if the mechanism were this simple, NSAIDs should have an adverse effect on all asthmatic patients (VanArsdel, 1984).

Aspirin also aggravates symptoms of about one fourth of patients with chronic urticaria. The mechanism might be immune, but proof is lacking. Urticaria and other skin eruptions initiated by aspirin are rare.

Radiographic Contrast Media. Flushing, urticaria, wheezing, angioedema, and syncope with hypotension are occasional adverse reactions to the injection of iodine-containing radiopaque substances. The risk of these anaphylactoid reactions has been reported as high as 2.5 percent; most of the reported reactions occur in adults between 20 and 50 years of age (Erffmeyer et al., 1985). Contrary to some assertions, the risk of reaction is completely independent of any sensitivity to iodine, to iodides in the diet, or to shellfish. Reactions are much less frequent following arterial injections than intravenous ones. The incidence of reactions among those who had had previous reactions is 16 to 30 percent unless pretreatment is used (see subsequent discussion). Even though the symptoms may seem to be allergic, most reactions in fact are the results of the direct release or activation of mast cell–derived and complement-derived vasoactive mediators. A reaction is more likely if the material is hyperosmolar, a large amount is given, or is given rapidly. Individual differences in reactivity also may play roles. Recently, an increase in histamine levels was reported in the urine of all patients who were tested following the administration of radiographic contrast media. More important, the amount of histamine was significantly higher in the urine of those who had clinical reactions than in those who did not (Kaliner et al., 1984).

Sulfites and Other Food and Drug Additives. Sulfiting agents have been used for centuries to aid in food preservation. Sulfur dioxide, sodium sulfite, sodium and potassium bisulfite, and sodium and potassium metabisulfite are antioxidants and sanitary agents. They delay bacterial spoilage; minimize discoloration of various foodstuffs during processing, storage, and distribution; and inhibit undesirable microorganisms during wine making and other fermentation processes. Although the presence of metabisulfites in "salad bar" lettuce, processed potatoes, and shrimp has received the most publicity, sulfiting agents are found in a variety of other foods as well and are used in numerous drugs, including some bronchodilator solutions (see Settipane, 1984, for detailed tables listing foods and drugs that contain sulfites). Symptoms produced by sulfiting agents in susceptible individuals are flushing, urticaria and angioedema, laryngeal edema, asthmatic wheezing, and potentially fatal anaphylactoid shock. Some develop various gastrointestinal symptoms alone or in addition to the anaphylactoid symptoms. At least four deaths have been reported to the Food and Drug Administration (FDA). The prevalence of sulfite reactivity may be as high as 10 percent among asthmatic patients, and asthma has been provoked even by the small amount of sodium metabisulfite in the ophthalmic solution dipivefrin (Schwartz and Sher, 1985). Sulfite reactions most likely are mediated via irritant receptors in the upper airways through neural reflexes and vagal efferent pathways. In the recent past, about 80 percent of the sulfite reactions have occurred in restaurants. Through the efforts of the FDA, state regulatory agencies, and the National Restaurant Association, the use of sulfites in restaurants has been drastically curtailed.

Compared with sulfites, other additives produce rare or inadequately documented adverse reactions. Tartrazine (FD&C Yellow No. 5) has received the most attention because of reported reactions in some aspirin-sensitive asthmatic patients. However, such sensitivity rarely has been confirmed by proper placebo-controlled challenge testing. The evidence for intolerance to other food and drug coloring agents and to substances, such as sodium benzoate, is even less convincing. The role of food additives in the genesis of hyperactivity in children remains controversial; in general, the association has not been confirmed in properly controlled clinical studies (Lipton and Mayo, 1983).

MANAGEMENT

Prevention

Reducing Drug Exposure. The most effective way to prevent an adverse reaction to a drug is—don't use it! Hospital surveys have shown repeatedly that the number of adverse reactions is proportional to the number of drugs prescribed. The use of important drugs should be restricted to important conditions. For example, potentially life-saving antimicrobial drugs should not be prescribed for minor illnesses or for questionable indications. One or more earlier courses of treatment given for questionable indications may sensitize a patient to an important drug, making it difficult to use the drug safely later when it is really necessary.

Product Refinements. Improvements in the manufacturing methods and in the components of biologic products have reduced, but not eliminated, the sensitizing potential of many therapeutic agents. Examples are as follows:

- Reduction in the use of sensitizing preservatives, such as parabens and thimerosal.
- Elimination of impurities, including immunogenic polymers, from penicillin and its homologues.
- Development of purified insulin and manufacture of inexpensive human insulin by recombinant DNA technology.
- Substitution with synthetic polypeptides for pituitary polypeptide hormones of animal origin.
- Replacement of equine antitoxins with human antitoxins.
- Employment of purified gamma globulin instead of whole serum when an animal product must be used (e.g., antithymocyte serum).
- Development of vaccines free of egg and other animal proteins.

Importance of the History. Taking a careful history is the best possible action to minimize allergic drug reactions. However, a positive history must be interpreted carefully. For example, one that elicits a background of only atopic disease should not exert a significant influence on therapeutic decision making. It is of paramount importance, though, to document any previous drug reaction. The patient, or whoever is best informed about the patient's previous medical problems, should be asked not only the name of the drug, but also the kinds of symptoms, the severity of the adverse reaction, and the nature of the illness being treated at the time. The physician should be able to determine if any previous reaction was caused by a drug that is immunochemically or pharmacologically similar to the drug being considered for treatment. However, it is important to be careful in selecting and prescribing *any* drug for someone who gives a history of allergy to several different drugs.

Inevitably, some patients will be labeled as allergic who actually are not. By careful questioning alone, one may be able to correct the record. Symptoms of the previous reaction could be nonallergic (e.g., nausea, vomiting, and headache). The patient who gives a history of penicillin allergy may have been given ampicillin or some other homologue some time after the alleged penicillin reaction with no problem. As mentioned previously, ampicillin treatment may be associated with the development of a skin rash, but the patient may not be allergic to the drug. In a child, cutaneous and serum sickness–like reactions commonly accompany acute viral infections, and it is likely that a sick child will be given drugs of some sort, including antimicrobials. It is worth remembering that allergic drug reactions are uncommon in children, except for those who require repeated treatment, e.g., patients with cystic fibrosis.

As the promotion and distribution of nonorthodox medicines increase, so do adverse reactions to their various ingredients. In taking a thorough history, one should not forget to ask tactfully about the use of aberrant remedies. Herbal products may be "fortified" with glucocorticoids, NSAIDs, psychotropic agents, or thiazide diuretics. The herbal products themselves may contain a wide variety of plant allergens capable of aggravating asthma or even provoking anaphylaxis. Chamomile tea is prepared from flower heads that crossreact with ragweed. Ginseng can produce skin eruptions as well as toxic side effects. Alfalfa seeds may induce a reaction similar to systemic lupus erythematosus. "Bee pollen" causes severe anaphylactic reactions. "Cellular therapy," consisting of injections of various animal tissues,

has obvious and potentially severe risks. The many adverse effects of nonorthodox treatment schemes have been reviewed in detail recently by Vulto and Buurma (1984).

Routine Testing or Premedication. All patients should undergo skin tests for possible anaphylactic sensitivity before receiving any xenogenic protein or large polypeptide agent. A prick test is done with a 1 : 10 dilution of serum. If the reaction is negative in 10 minutes, this dilution is used again for an intradermal test reaction which, if negative, is followed by an intradermal test with the undiluted substance. A negative test reaction is one with a wheal diameter less than 5 mm 15 minutes after the test is placed. Skin testing for penicillin allergy is discussed subsequently. Suffice it to say that a recent multicenter study found that when all hospitalized patients about to receive penicillin were tested, allergy was identified in such a small number with no history of penicillin allergy that the potential benefit was not worth the effort expended!

Premedication of all patients about to be treated has not proved to be practicable. For example, premedication is no longer used routinely before administering a radiographic contrast agent. One exception is the premedication of a patient before chymopapain injection into a herniated intervertebral disc. The empiric use of diphenhydramine, cimetidine, and a glucocorticoid became a standard procedure before the efficacy of skin testing could be established.

The Patient with a Positive History

Frequently, a patient develops a problem in which it would be desirable to use a particular drug or diagnostic agent, but gives a history of suspected allergy or idiosyncrasy to that substance or a similar one. The decision pathways to use for such a patient are depicted in Figure 53–1 and are discussed next.

Alternative Drugs. If possible, a drug that is not known to crossreact with the suspect drug, but is equally effective, should be used. The risk of toxicity from the alternative drug, however, should not be overlooked. For example, vancomycin and aminoglycosides are alternatives to penicillins, but are substantially more toxic. It might be a better choice to prescribe one of the cephalosporins, even though there is some statistical probability of cross-reactivity; about 5 percent of patients with histories of penicillin allergy will react also to a cephalosporin. This is an acceptable risk unless the patient had an an-

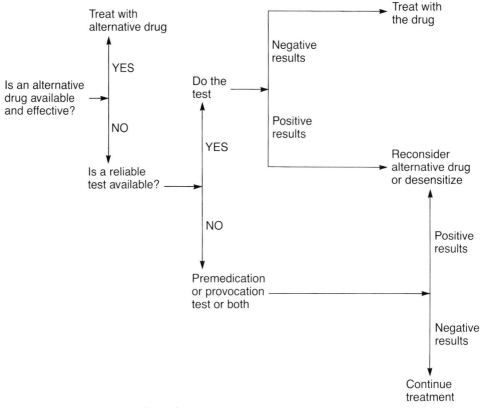

FIGURE 53–1. Decision pathway for assessing patients with positive histories of drug allergies.

aphylactic reaction to penicillin. Such patients should be tested for penicillin allergy (see subsequent discussion) or treated cautiously, beginning with small test doses. Aztreonam, one of a new class of beta-lactam antibiotics, the monobactams, shows no apparent cross-reactivity in penicillin-allergic subjects (Saxon et al., 1984).

Immunologic Testing. As discussed in the previous section, prick and intradermal skin testing are reliable for identifying IgE-mediated allergy to macromolecules, such as xenogenic sera and large polypeptides or polysaccharides. For most purposes, the skin test is sufficient to establish whether or not sensitivity is present. Serologic methods for measuring IgE antibodies, namely, the radioallergosorbent test (RAST) and the enzyme-linked immunosorbent assays (ELISAs), are available for testing to some agents but are more expensive, less sensitive, take longer, and add no further information than skin testing. Whereas routine skin testing to macromolecular agents can begin with a 1 : 10 dilution as described, it is prudent to start with a dilution of 1 : 1000, if the patient gives a history of a prior allergic reaction or is about to

receive an agent about which little clinical experience has been accumulated. If severe anaphylaxis was the previous reaction, the first test should be a prick test using a 10^{-5} dilution.

Before testing can be done for allergy to drugs of small molecular weight, the immunogenic metabolites and, ideally, the mode of their conjugation to macromolecular carriers should be identified. With the exception of penicillin, this goal has been achieved only rarely; a few isolated examples of metabolites responsible for hematologic reactions were previously cited. Testing for penicillin allergy has become a well-established procedure for screening patients who give histories of suspected previous reactions to one of the penicillins. One principal and immunogenic penicillin metabolite that forms a stable conjugate *in vitro* with protein or polypeptide carriers has been identified. It is commercially available as penicilloyl polylysine (PPL). Skin test reactions using this so-called *major determinant* reagent will be positive in most patients who are truly allergic. However, it will not detect sensitivity in some patients in whom reliable testing is needed the most: those at risk for anaphylactic reactions. Fortunately, almost all such individuals have positive skin reactions to penicillin G (PG) itself; a very small number have been found to react only to other metabolites, e.g., benzylpenicilloate, benzylpenilloate, and penicilloyl-n-propylamine. Collectively, PG and these metabolites are called *minor determinants*. A standardized mixture called the minor determinant mixture (MDM) has been tested extensively on hospitalized patients in eight medical centers around the United States and should be released for general use soon. In the meantime, the closest approximation to MDM that is generally available for testing is a fresh solution of PG. The standard procedure at the University of Washington Hospitals uses PPL, 6×10^{-5} M, and PG, $1000\ \mu/\text{ml}$. Any patient with a history of a severe, rapid-onset reaction should be tested first with $1:100$ dilutions of these reagents. Prick tests are done first; if these reactions are negative after 10 minutes, intracutaneous tests are then done, delivering not more than 0.02 ml into the skin. If the resulting wheal is less than 5 mm in diameter after 15 minutes, treatment probably is safe. Because of the rare allergic patient who is sensitive neither to PPL nor to PG, it is prudent to give the patients whose reactions are negative a small dose (1000 units or the equivalent) 30 minutes before the full therapeutic dose. Some consultants will perform skin tests also to the specific beta-lactam drug that is to be used. This seems reasonable, although evidence supporting the value of such testing is scanty.

In our study of hospitalized patients who underwent skin testing with PPL and MDM, approximately 85 percent of those who gave histories of penicillin allergy were no longer allergic by skin testing, and these findings were confirmed by subsequent uneventful treatment (VanArsdel et al., 1986). We did not attempt to treat any patients with positive test reactions with a penicillin because effective alternative drugs were available. In earlier studies, approximately two thirds of patients with positive skin test reactions had systemic allergic reactions when penicillin treatment was attempted (Levine and Zolov, 1969).

Systemic allergy to local anesthetics, whatever the chemical structure, is extremely rare. Skin testing is an effective way to rule out allergy. Each drug to be tested is obtained epinephrine free and is diluted $1:10$ and $1:100$. The patient first undergoes prick testing with the $1:100$ dilution. This is followed by intradermal tests to the $1:100$, $1:10$, and undiluted

drug 15 minutes apart. A test dose of 0.5 ml can then be given subcutaneously or into the area to be anesthetized as a final precaution. In over 100 patients tested at the University of Washington Hospital, we have yet to identify a patient who was allergic to a local anesthetic. Furthermore, we have not observed any reactions that were caused by sensitivity to parabens or any other additives.

Skin testing for allergy to other drugs of low molecular weight is not reliable. Serologic tests are no better, except for the tests used to confirm drug-induced hematologic reactions, and most of these are done reliably only in research laboratories. Since T cell–mediated allergy is suspected in a large proportion of drug reactions, several laboratories over the last two decades have tested suspected drugs for their possible blastogenic and lymphokine-producing effects on lymphocytes in tissue culture. Reports continue to appear of positive responses to a few drugs by lymphocytes from patients who have had recent allergic reactions. The most reliable reports have come from research laboratories interested in the immune mechanisms of the reactions (Knutsen et al., 1984). The *in vitro* lymphocyte response is a valuable research procedure, but its usefulness for diagnosing drug allergy, either prospectively or retrospectively, has yet to be established.

Provocative Testing. The only definitive test for drug sensitivity is to give the drug again under controlled conditions. The best example of a provocative test is the *patch test*. This is used to identify the cause of drug-induced allergic eczematous contact dermatitis. The drug or drugs in question are applied to the skin, in an appropriate vehicle, under an occlusive adhesive patch. Any positive reaction will develop within 48 (occasionally 72) hours as a pruritic, erythematous, and vesicular eruption similar to the original reaction but limited in severity and in scale. Other situations in which a provocation test may be advisable (i.e., when the offending drug is in doubt) are those in which the anticipated reaction is benign. Two common examples are the fixed-drug eruption and uncomplicated fever.

Whenever a drug is the probable cause of a reaction that is potentially serious, challenge rarely is justified. When the relationship is in doubt, the prior reaction was not a life-threatening one, and the suspected agent is clearly the best available one to use, then careful challenge testing will be necessary. This is done by giving a small dose at first, orally if possible. The starting dose can be 1 percent of the therapeutic dose unless the prior reaction was a severe one, in which case, the starting amount should be 100- or 1000-fold lower. Doses should be repeated in 10-fold increments every 15 to 60 minutes (depending on the route of administration). If any symptoms appear, the test either should be terminated or, if the need for the drug is sufficiently great, should evolve into a desensitization attempt. Properly maintained emergency resuscitative equipment must always be kept at hand whenever provocation testing, desensitization, or both are carried out.

Premedication. Various drugs have been used for several decades to suppress possible reactions from antituberculous drugs, transfusions of blood products, and allergen immunotherapy injections. Premedication usually includes some combination of glucocorticoids, NSAIDs, antihistamines, and adrenergic drugs. Such therapy may be applied routinely or initiated if and when allergic symptoms develop during provocation testing or desensitization. The best documented premedication program is the one for patients who have had previous reactions to radiographic contrast media. These patients are given oral prednisone, 50 mg every 6 hours for 3 doses before the procedure; diphenydramine, 50 mg intramuscularly, and ephedrine, 25 mg subcutaneously, are given 1 hour before. In one large series of patients, this pretreatment reduced the reaction rate to 3.1 percent, and none of those reactions was serious (Greenberger et al., 1984).

Desensitization. The strategies used in provocation testing and in premedication can be applied to desensitization as well. These strategies were used for many years to overcome sensitivity to antituberculosis drugs when alternative, first-line drugs were not available. Recent published reports have described the successful slow desensitization of patients to drugs, such as carbamazepine and sulfasalazine. *Desensitization to sulfasalazine* has become fairly common because no comparable alternative drug is available for treatment of inflammatory bowel disease (Purdy et al., 1984). The usual starting dose is 1 mg, doubled daily until the 2 gm therapeutic dose is achieved. The dose is reduced temporarily if a reaction occurs; medication for the reaction usually is not needed.

Desensitization to other agents is done more rapidly. The patient who is sensitive to *xenogenic serum* is given 0.1 ml subcutaneously of the smallest 10-fold dilution that gives a positive skin test reaction (see previous section,

Routine Testing or Premedication). The dose is doubled every 15 minutes until 1 ml of the undiluted serum has been given. This dose is then given intramuscularly, followed by the full therapeutic dose. Because the procedure is required only when there is an immediate and urgent need for the drug, *penicillin desensitization* also is done rapidly. The patient with a positive skin test reaction to one or more of the penicillin determinants can usually be desensitized in a few hours, and the skin test reaction becomes negative (for the duration of treatment, at least). Desensitization can be carried out successfully through oral or parenteral routes. The oral program begins with 100 units as a rule; it is safe and takes up to 5 hours to complete (Sullivan et al., 1982). The intravenous route should be used if the patient cannot take oral medication or if absorption from the gut is uncertain. Intravenous administration has an advantage over other routes because one can control both the concentration and the rate of administration. Furthermore, a reaction can be identified at the first hint of symptoms, and corrective action can be taken promptly. With emergency equipment and drugs at hand, a dilute solution of benzylpenicillin or a homologue is delivered intravenously according to the method given in Table 53–17. Each infusion is given slowly at first, then gradually more rapidly until warning symptoms such as pruritus and flush develop. If any symptoms develop, the flow rate is reduced and the patient is given an antihistamine and a glucocorticoid drug. The flow rate is increased again when the symptoms are gone. Thirty minutes should be sufficient to administer each dilution. A recent report of

TABLE 53–17. Intravenous Method for Penicillin Desensitization*

Bag No.	Concentration† μ/ml or μg/ml	Total Dose† μ or μg
1‡	0.01	0.5
2	0.1	5
3	1	50
4	10	500
5§	100	5000
6	1,000	50,000
7	10,000	500,000
8	Full dose	

*All solutions prepared in dextrose and water. 50-ml plastic bags for "piggyback" delivery.
† For simplicity of preparation, a unit of benzylpenicillin is equated with 1 μg rather than with the actual value of 0.6 μg.
‡ Starting point if prick test reaction is strongly positive.
§ Starting point if only the intradermal test reaction is positive.

children and young adults with cystic fibrosis, who were allergic to penicillin, described the successful use of intravenous desensitization in preparation for treatment with semisynthetic penicillins (Moss et al., 1984).

It also is customary to use *rapid desensitization for insulin allergy*, whether or not a sense of urgency exists. Insulin is a complete antigen, but systemic reactions to insulin are extremely rare unless there has been a lapse in treatment. Before desensitization is considered, one of the several alternative products should be tried, e.g., pork insulin, sulfated insulin, single peak insulin (partially purified), single component insulin (highly purified), and human insulin. The possibility of sensitivity to protamine or even zinc should not be overlooked. Patients who react even to human insulin are rare, but do exist (Grammer et al., 1985). Experience with human insulin desensitization is still limited. Conventional desensitization (using pork insulin) starts with the lowest concentration that gives a positive skin test reaction, proceeding with 10-fold increments given subcutaneously as often as every 15 minutes until a local reaction occurs. The next dose is lower, and the following doses are increased at smaller increments. For a recent review of insulin allergy in children see Ross (1984).

A few patients with rheumatoid arthritis and allied conditions who are intolerant to *aspirin* and other NSAIDs would benefit greatly if these drugs could be used. Desensitization is possible (Stevenson, 1984). Tolerance usually can be achieved (albeit with some risk of severe asthmatic reactions) by giving gradually increasing doses every 3 hours, beginning with an amount previously determined to be the threshhold for a reaction; it may be as little as 10 mg. Tolerance is maintained by taking the drug every day; it may lapse if the drug is not taken for more than 2 days. The use of desensitization to diminish the underlying respiratory symptoms of aspirin-sensitive patients remains experimental.

TREATMENT

Stopping the drug treatment may be sufficient to terminate relatively benign reactions, such as fever and nonpruritic fixed and generalized eruptions. Indeed, the presence of such reactions does not necessarily require that effective drug treatment be discontinued.

Urticaria and other pruritic skin eruptions can be treated with antihistaminic drugs with sedative or tranquilization properties. Hydroxyzine (25 to 100 mg, 2 to 3 times daily) usually is effective. Alternative drugs are diphenhydramine (25 to 100 mg, 4 times daily) and cyproheptadine, (4 to 8 mg, 4 times daily). Urticaria that develops rapidly after a drug is given should be treated in addition with epinephrine, 0.3 to 0.5 mg subcutaneously, in anticipation of a possible anaphylactic reaction. Anaphylaxis is discussed in detail in Chapter 51. Briefly, epinephrine is effective for most of the features of anaphylaxis. Other essentials of treatment are as follows:

- Prevent the absorption of the offending agent (if injected) with local infiltration of epinephrine and application of a tourniquet.
- Maintain plasma volume with ample amounts of intravenous fluids.
- Give drugs, including epinephrine intravenously (by slow drip), if the patient is hypotensive.
- Give oxygen and maintain patency of the upper airway; an intravenous antihistaminic may help.
- Watch for bronchospasm, and treat it.
- Monitor for cardiac dysrhythmias and cardiogenic shock.
- Consider glucocorticoid therapy to suppress a late reaction after the aforementioned have been done.

Pain of serum sickness, SLE syndrome, vasculitis, and some cases of urticaria may require analgesic therapy with a NSAID. Although aspirin may be adequate, indomethacin (25 to 50 mg every 8 hours for adults) may be more effective, particularly for vasculitis.

Systemic glucocorticoid therapy should be started without hesitation for treatment of severe urticaria, contact dermatitis, exfoliative dermatitis, and erythema multiforme. It may hasten recovery from pulmonary, hematologic, and hepatic reactions as well. The usual dosage range is 40 to 80 mg/day of prednisone or its equivalent, and the dose can be tapered rapidly as soon as the lesions begin to subside, usually within 3 days. Toxic epidermal necrolysis, vasculitis, and interstitial nephritis do not usually respond to glucocorticoid treatment, but a short trial may be appropriate. Topical glucocorticoids are ineffective in the treatment of urticaria and other pruritic dermatoses. Although they may be of some benefit in contact dermatitis, their systemic use is much more effective and just as safe over the usual short treatment period. Their use is most suited to severe, slowly resolving exfoliative dermatitis as an aid in tapering the dose of the systemic glucocorticoid.

REFERENCES

Ackroyd, J.F.: Fixed drug eruptions. Brit. Med. J. 290:1533, 1985.

Adler, S.G., Cohen, A.H., Border, W.A.: Hypersensitivity phenomena and the kidney: role of drugs and environmental agents. Am. J. Kidney Dis. 5:75, 1985.

AMA Drug Evaluations, 6th ed. Chicago, American Medical Association, 1986.

Anderson, J.A.: Drug allergies. In Bierman, C.W., Pearlman, D.S. (eds.); Allergic Diseases of Infancy, Childhood and Adolescence. Philadelphia, W.B. Saunders Co., 1980.

Anonymous: Acebutolol. The Medical Letter 27:60, 1985.

Bielory, L., Yancey, K.B., Young, N.S., Frank, M.M., Lawley, T.J.: Cutaneous manifestations of serum sickness in patients receiving antithymocyte globulin. J. Am. Acad. Derm. 13:411, 1985.

Bierman, C.W., VanArsdel, P.P., Jr.: Penicillin allergy in children. J. Allergy 43:267, 1969.

Bigby, M., Jick, S., Jick, H., Arndt, K.: Drug-induced cutaneous reactions: A report from the Boston collaborative drug surveillance program on 15,438 consecutive inpatients, 1975 to 1982. J.A.M.A. 256:3358, 1986.

Bryceson, A.D.M.: Clinical pathology of the Jarisch-Herxheimer reaction. J. Infect. Dis. 133:696, 1976.

Chusid, M.J., Atkins, E.: Studies on the mechanism of penicillin-induced fever. J. Exp. Med. 136:227, 1972.

Cluff, L.E., Caranasos, G.J., Stewart, R.B.: Clinical Problems with Drugs. Philadelphia, W.B. Saunders Co., 1975.

Cronin, E., Bandmann, H.J., Calnan, C.D., Fregert, S., Hjorth, N., Magnusson, B., Maibach, H.I., Malten, K., Meneghini, C.L., Pirilä, V., Wilkinson, D.S.: Contact dermatitis in the atopic. Acta Dermvenereol. 50:183, 1970.

Davies, D.M. (ed.): Textbook of Adverse Drug Reactions, 3rd ed. New York, Oxford University Press, 1985.

Derbes, V.J.: The fixed eruption. J.A.M.A. 190:765, 1964.

Dinarello, C.A., Bernheim, H.A., Duff, G.W., Hung, V.L., Nagabhushan, T.L., Hamilton, N.C., Coceani, F.: Mechanisms of fever induced by recombinant human interferon. J. Clin. Invest. 74:906, 1984.

Dubroff, L.M., Reid, R.J., Jr.: Hydralazine-pyrimidine interactions may explain hydralazine-induced lupus erythematosus. Science 208:404, 1980.

Dukes, M.N.G. (ed.): Meyler's Side Effects of Drugs, 10th ed. Amsterdam, Elsevier, Science Publishing Co. Inc., 1984.

Eisner, E.V., Shahidi, N.T.: Immunothrombocytopenia due to a drug metabolite. N. Engl. J. Med. 287:376, 1972.

Epstein, A., Barland, P.: The diagnostic value of antihistone antibodies in drug-induced lupus erythematosus. Arthr. Rheum. 28:158, 1985.

Erffmeyer, J.E., Siegle, R.L., Lieberman, P.: Anaphylactoid reactions to radiocontrast material. J. Allergy Clin. Immunol. 75:401, 1985.

Feigin, R.D., Shearer, W.T.: Fever of unknown origin in children. Curr. Prob. Pediatr. vol. 6, no. 10, 1976.

Gilman, A.G., Goodman, L.S., Rall, T.W., Murad, F. (eds.): Goodman and Gilman's The Pharmacological Basis of Therapeutics, 7th ed. New York, Macmillan Publishing Co. Inc., 1985.

Grammer, L.C., Roberts, M., Patterson, R.: IgE and IgG antibody against human (recombinant DNA) insulin in patients with systemic insulin allergy. J. Lab. Clin. Med. 105:108, 1985.

Greenberger, P.A., Patterson, R., Radin, R.C.: Two pretreatment regimens for high-risk patients receiving radiographic contrast media. J. Allergy Clin. Immunol. 74:540, 1984.

Horowitz, L., Parker, C.: Correspondence. N. Engl. J. Med. 292:1243, 1975.

Kaliner, M., Dyer, J., Merlin, S., Shelton, A., Greenhill, A., Treadwell, G., McKenna, W., Lieberman, P.: Increased urine histamine and contrast media reactions. Invest. Radiol. 19:116, 1984.

Kirtland, H.H., III, Mohler, D.N., Horwitz, D.A.: Methyldopa inhibition of suppressor-lymphocyte function. A proposed cause of autoimmune hemolytic anemia. N. Engl. J. Med. 302:825, 1980.

Knutsen, A.P., Anderson, J., Satayaviboon, S., Slavin, R.G.: Immunologic aspects of phenobarbital hypersensitivity. J. Pediatr. 105:558, 1984.

Kuokkanen, L.: Drug eruptions: a series of 464 cases in the Department of Dermatology, University of Turku, Finland, during 1966–1970. Acta Allergol. 27:407, 1972.

Lakin, J.D., Grace, W.R., Sell, K.W.: IgE antipolymyxin B antibody formation in a T cell–depleted bone marrow transplant patient. J. Allergy Clin. Immunol. 56:94, 1975.

Landsteiner, K., Jacobs, J.: Studies on the sensitization of animals with simple chemical compounds. J. Exp. Med. 61:643, 1935.

Levine, B.B.: Immunochemical mechanisms of drug allergy. Ann. Rev. Med. 17:23, 1966.

Levine, B.B., Zolov, D.M.: Prediction of penicillin allergy by immunological tests. J. Allergy 43:231, 1969.

Lipton, M.A., Mayo, J.P.: Diet and hyperkinesis—an update. J. Am. Diet. Assoc. 83:132, 1983.

Mackel, S.E., Jordon, R.E.: Leukocytoclastic vasculitis: a cutaneous expression of immune complex disease. Arch. Dermatol. 118:296, 1982.

Mackert, J.R., Fisher, A.A.: Hypersensitivity to mercury from dental amalgams. J. Am. Acad. Derm. 12:877, 1985.

Mandel, H.G., Cohn, W.H.: Fat-Soluble Vitamins: Vitamins A, K, and E. In Gilman, A.G., Goodman, L.S., Rall, T.W., Murad, F. (eds.); Goodman and Gilman's The Pharmacological Basis of Therapeutics, 7th ed. New York, MacMillian Publishing Co. Inc., 1985.

McKenzie, M.W., Marchall, G.L., Netzloff, M.L., Cluff, L.E.: Adverse drug reactions leading to hospitalization. J. Pediatr. 89:487, 1976.

Mitchell, G.G., Magnusson, A.R., Weiler, J.M.: Cimetidine-induced cutaneous vasculitis. Am. J. Med. 75:875, 1983.

Moss, R.B., Babin, S., Hsu, Y.P., Blessing-Moore, J., Lewiston, N.J.: Allergy to semisynthetic penicillins in cystic fibrosis. J. Pediatr. 104:460, 1984.

Parker, C.W.: Allergic reactions in man. Pharmacol. Rev. 34:85, 1982.

Pegram, P.S., Mountz, J.D., O'Bar, P.R.: Ethambutol-induced toxic epidermal necrolysis. Arch. Intern. Med. 141:1677, 1981.

Petrozzi, J.W., Shore, R.N.: Generalized exfoliative dermatitis from ethylenediamine. Arch. Dermatol. 112:525, 1976.

Petz, L.D.: Drug-induced immune hemolysis. N. Engl. J. Med. 313:510, 1985.

Purdy, B.H., Philips, D.M., Summers, R.W.: Desensitization for sulfasalazine skin rash. Ann. Intern. Med. 100:512, 1984.

Rocklin, R.E.: Clinical applications of *in vitro* lymphocyte tests. in Schwartz, R.S. (ed.), Progress in Clinical Immunology, Vol. 2. New York, Grune and Stratton, 1974.

Ross, J.M.: Allergy to insulin. Pediatr. Clin. N. Am. 31:675, 1984.

Rudolph, A.H., Price, E.V.: Penicillin reactions among patients in venereal disease clinics: a national survey. J.A.M.A. 223:499, 1973.

Salama, A., Mueller-Eckhardt, C.: The role of metabolite-specific antibodies in nomifesine-dependent immune hemolytic anemia. N. Engl. J. Med. 313:469, 1985.

Samter, M. (ed.): Excerpts from Classics in Allergy (see Jadassohn, J., page 27). Columbus, Ohio, Ross Laboratories, 1969.

Saxon, A., Hassner, A., Swabb, E.A., Wheeler, B., Adkinson, N.F., Jr.: Lack of cross-reactivity between aztreonam, a monobactam antibiotic, and penicillin in penicillin-allergic subjects. J. Infect. Dis. 149:16, 1984.

Schwartz, H.J., Sher, T.H.: Bisulfite intolerance manifests as bronchospasm following topical dipivefrin hydrochloride therapy for glaucoma. Arch. Ophthalmol. 103:14, 1985.

Settipane, G.A.: Adverse reactions to sulfites in drugs and foods. J. Am. Acad. Derm. 10:1077, 1984.

Shulman, N.R.: A mechanism of cell destruction in individuals sensitized to foreign antigens and its implications in autoimmunity: combined clinical staff conference at the National Institutes of Health. Ann. Intern. Med. 60:506, 1964.

Stevenson, D.D.: Diagnosis, prevention, and treatment of adverse reactions to aspirin and nonsteroidal anti-inflammatory drugs. J. Allergy Clin. Immunol. 74:617, 1984.

Sullivan, T.J., Yecies, L.D., Schatz, G.S., Parker, C.W., Wedner, H.J.: Desensitization of patients allergic to penicillin using orally administered beta-lactam antibiotics. J. Allergy Clin. Immunol. 69:275, 1982.

Szabadi, E.: Neuroleptic malignant syndrome. Brit. Med. J. 288:1399, 1984.

VanArsdel, P.P., Jr.: Serum Antibodies to Red Cell Conjugates in Penicillin Allergy. In Stewart, G.T., McGovern, J.P. (eds.), Penicillin Allergy. Springfield, Charles C Thomas, 1970.

VanArsdel, P.P., Jr.: Adverse Drug Reactions. In Middleton, E., Reed, C.E., Ellis, E.F. (eds.), Allergy: Principles and Practice, 2nd ed. St. Louis, C.V. Mosby Co., 1983.

VanArsdel, P.P., Jr.: Aspirin idiosyncracy and tolerance. J. Allergy Clin. Immunol. 73:431, 1984.

VanArsdel, P.P., Jr., Martonick, G.J., Johnson, L.E., Sprenger, J.D., Altman, L.C., Henderson, W.R., Jr.: The value of skin testing for penicillin allergy diagnosis. West. J. Med. 144:311, 1986.

Vincent, A., Newsom-Davis, J., Martin, V.: Anti-acetylcholine receptor antibodies in D-penicillamine–associated myasthenia gravis. Lancet 1:1254, 1978.

Vulto, A.G., Buurma, H.: Drugs used in non-orthodox medicine. In Dukes, M.N.G. (ed.), Meyler's Side Effects of Drugs, 10th ed. Amsterdam, Elsevier Science Publishing Co. Inc., 1984.

Weitzman, S.A., Stossel, T.P., Desmond, M.: Drug-induced immunological neutropenia. Lancet 1:1068, 1978.

Whyte, J., Greenan, E.: Drug usage and adverse drug reactions in paediatric patients. Acta Paediatr. Scand. 66:767, 1977.

Wilkin, J.K., Hammond, J.J., Kirkendall, W.M.: The captopril-induced eruption: a possible mechanism: cutaneous kinin potentiation. Arch. Dermatol. 116:902, 1980.

Woosley, R.L., Drayer, D.E., Reidenberg, M.M., Nies, A.S., Carr, K., Oates, J.A.: Effect of acetylator phenotype on the rate at which procainamide induces antinuclear antibodies and the lupus syndrome. N. Engl. J. Med. 298:1157, 1978.

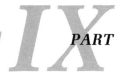
DIAGNOSTIC AND THERAPEUTIC DILEMMAS IN ALLERGIC PATIENTS

54

Chronic Cough

ROGER KATZ

Patients who have complaints of cough have many ways of presenting to the physician. If symptoms are recurrent or chronic, the diagnostic and therapeutic considerations can be confusing and frustrating for both patient and physician. Cough may be present from days to months before patients seek medical help. Patients often complain of upper or lower respiratory tract symptoms, but they also may have other symptoms, such as generalized fatigue, aches, pains, headaches, and weight loss. Frequently, patients are depressed, anxious, or otherwise concerned because the cough may disrupt their daily lives. Cough sufferers may seek medical attention only after experiencing an episode of syncope or an alarming episode of something unusual, such as expectoration with blood.

Cough can be of sudden onset, paroxysmal, or recurrent. It may be associated with swallowing, throat clearing, aphonia, and dysphonia; cough may or may not be accompanied by sputum production. The quality of cough, such as *brassy* (dry), *croupy, bovine, barking, hacking,* or *hawking* (throat clearing), may give clues concerning its cause and origin. For example, barking coughs tend to be laryngeal, whereas brassy coughs tend to be tracheal in origin. Cough is a symptom. The cause should be sought, and the underlying illness treated.

PATHOPHYSIOLOGY OF COUGH

Typically, cough is preceded by inspiration with opening of the glottis. The inflow of air increases lung volume and lengthens the bronchi. This phase is followed by a compression phase, with closing of the glottis and with rapid and forceful expulsion of air which also expels secretions or other materials from the respiratory tree.

The physiology of the cough reflex is not entirely defined. It is a complex response that involves the peripheral and central nervous systems, the irritant receptors in the lung and in other tissues, and the effector response. Cough receptors are located in upper, middle, and lower airways of cats and dogs and presumably also in humans. Those in the upper airways are situated in the paranasal sinuses, ear canals, tympanic membranes, nasal airways, and pharynx. In the middle airways, cough receptors are located in the larynx and trachea. Cough receptors in the lower airways are concentrated in the carina, in the bronchial bifurcations, and to a lesser extent in the peripheral airways (Widdicombe et al., 1962). Cough receptors also can be found in the pleura and diaphragm and, in nonpulmonary sites, the pericardium and stomach (Nadel, 1973).

Stimulation of cough receptors creates nerve impulses that travel through the afferent pathways to the medullary cough center, which in turn stimulates efferent nerve pathways (vagus, phrenic, and possibly spinal motor nerves) (Fig. 54–1). Sympathetic nerves involved in the cough reflex innervate the larynx, tracheobronchial tree, heart, and gastrointestinal tract (Dahlstrom et al., 1966). They apparently act to oppose the actions of parasympathetic nerves. In dogs, alpha-adrenergic constrictor pathways may not be important in airways (Cabezas, 1971); their importance in humans is unclear.

An alternative but less accepted concept of the physiology of cough postulates a direct reflex arc from the mucosa to the bronchial smooth muscles. According to this view, irritation of mucosal receptors initiates bronchospasm that in turn activates cough receptors in the lungs. Bronchoconstriction dynamically

COUGH REFLEX PATHWAYS

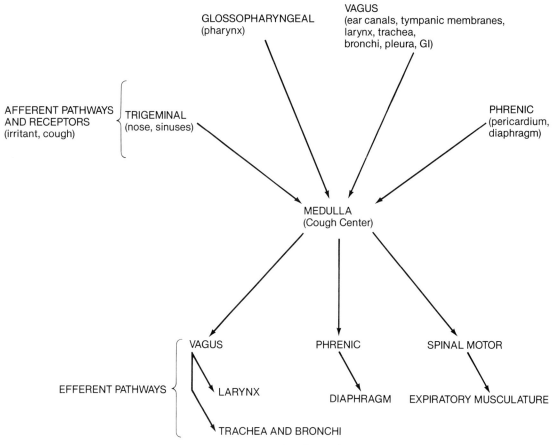

FIGURE 54–1. Cough reflex pathways.

compresses the tracheobronchial tree that in turn results in the forced expiratory phase of cough. This bronchoconstriction can be blocked by cutting the vagus nerve in animals and by atropine sulfate administration in humans, indicating that postganglionic cholinergic pathways are involved (Nadel et al., 1962).

COMMON CAUSES OF COUGH

Causes of cough are numerous and are listed in Table 54–1. The "allergic cough" may have several inciting factors, such as the action of inflammatory mediators released from mast cells, local inflammatory or irritant reactions to nasopharyngeal sections, and increased bronchial reactivity. Each may stimulate cough. Patients with asthma may present with only the symptom of cough (Corrao et al., 1979), and

TABLE 54–1. Causes of Cough

Allergy (all ages)
Irritants (all ages)
Physical factors (all ages)
  Cold
  Heat
  Humidity
Infection of the lower (and deeper?) respiratory tract
  Viral
    Respiratory syncytial virus, cytomegalovirus (infancy)
    Other viruses (preschool to adult)
  Mycoplasma (preschool to adult)
  Bacterial
    Specific: pertussis, *Chlamydia,* tuberculosis, histoplasmosis, coccidioidomycosis (all ages)
    Other bacteria (all ages)
  Cystic fibrosis (infancy to adolescence)
    Bacterial infections (especially *Pseudomonas, Staphylococcus, Streptococcus, Pneumococcus*)
Bronchospasm (all ages)
  Bronchial asthma
  Cystic fibrosis
  Associated with COPD, other diseases

TABLE 54–1. Causes of Cough (*Continued*)

Sinusitis
Inflammation or irritation of the tympanic membrane
Otitis externa
Nasopharyngitis (URIs)
Retropharyngeal and perifaucial infections
Epiglottitis and laryngitis
Tracheitis
Bronchitis and bronchiolitis
Interstitial lung disease
Gastrointestinal (intraluminal lesions)
CNS inflammation
Noninflammatory
  Upper airway
    Sinus and nasal polyps (school age to adult)
    Foreign body (infancy, preschool, school age)
    Elongated uvula, adenoidal and tonsillar hypertrophy
      (infancy to adolescence)
  Middle airway
    Epiglottic and laryngeal structural abnormalities (in-
      fancy to school age)
    Vocal cord paralysis (all ages); polyps and tumors (ado-
      lescence to adult)
    Foreign body (all ages)
    Tracheomalacia (infancy)
  Central airway
    Vascular ring (infancy)
    Tracheoesophageal fistula (infancy)
    Extraluminal compression from enlarged lymph nodes
      and tumor (all ages)
    Intraluminal obstruction from foreign body, mucus
      plugs, tumor (all ages)
    Bronchopulmonary dysplasia (infancy, early child-
      hood)
  Peripheral airway
    Congenital abnormalities (infancy)
    Sequestration and dysplasias (infancy)
    Cysts (all ages)
    Bronchiectasis (all ages)
    Atelectasis (all ages)
    Tumors
  Extrapulmonary
    Congenital heart disease (all ages)
    Congestive heart failure (all ages)
    Great vessel abnormalities (infancy)
    CNS disorders (edema, hysteria, paralysis, drug intoxi-
      cation) (all ages)
    Gastrointestinal (GER, hiatal hernia, esophagitis,
      tumor) (all ages)

cough may be the only symptom of exercise-induced asthma (Katz, 1970a).

Infectious rhinitis, chronic sinusitis, or both can cause profound coughing that is severe enough to interfere with sleep (Rachelefsky et al., 1982). Other physical or environmental factors, such as cold air, high humidity, and dry inhaled air, also stimulate irritant receptors and induce cough (Simonsson et al., 1967).

Cough associated with acute nasopharyngitis (the common cold) and sinusitis may be related in part to pharyngeal irritation from drainage. Other infections, such as pertussis and respiratory virus infections, induce coughing over a protracted postinfectious period by sensitizing epithelial cough receptors. Tuberculosis may cause cough by inflaming the airways or impinging upon the cough receptors of the middle and lower airways. Cough is a common feature of bronchiectasis and cystic fibrosis. Persistent atelectasis can induce chronic cough similar to that caused by a foreign body.

An extraluminal chest mass (e.g., mediastinal tumor) or intraluminal gastroesophageal lesion can induce a cough symptom complex, presumably through activation of a component of the cough reflex arc. Cough receptors in the large airway that may initiate a loud and brassy cough can be stimulated by such cardiovascular lesions as left atrial enlargement and aortic aneurysm. Other extrapulmonary lesions associated with cough include foreign bodies found in the upper or middle airways and in the esophagus.

Cough tic is associated frequently with psychologic problems and neurologic diseases. An important diagnostic point is that the cough tic usually disappears with sleep or other distractions. In such cases, psychologic intervention may be required to alleviate symptoms.

Gastroesophageal reflux should be considered when the patient's primary problem is at night or is associated with chest fullness, vomiting, or recurrent pneumonia. Cough and bronchospasm can occur in asthmatic children with gastroesophageal reflux or asthmatic adults with hiatal hernia, either due to the aspiration of gastric contents or the stimulation of vagal esophageal receptors (Euler et al., 1979).

COMPLICATIONS OF COUGH

Chronic cough can lead to potentially severe complications. One such complication is cough syncope. Paroxysmal coughing spasms induce facial congestion, turgidity, cyanosis, and syncope or a seizure-like episode, and unconsciousness that may last from seconds to several minutes. The syndrome occurs most frequently in asthmatics who have markedly decreased pulmonary compliance. The coughing spasm increases intrathoracic pressure, which results in decreased venous return, decreased cardiac output, and cerebral hypoxia due to diminished cranial blood flow (Katz, 1970b).

Painful muscle strain and even muscle rupture may complicate chronic cough. The Mallory-Weiss syndrome (esophageal bleeding due to tearing of the esophageal mucosa) may be caused by chronic coughing. Rib fractures due to cough along the lateral margins of the rib cage are frequent in adults but are rare in children. Pneumomediastinum, pneumothorax, and subcutaneous emphysema (examples of more severe complications), probably result from sharply increased intrathoracic pressure which causes rupturing of alveolar blebs or shearing of alveolar bases that permits air to enter perivascular spaces. Constitutional symptoms, such as fatigue, insomnia, anorexia, vomiting, weight loss, and headache, can be due to chronic cough.

DIAGNOSTIC EVALUATION

A meticulous history of present illness should focus on the onset, type, and timing of cough, aggravating factors (e.g., cold air, exercise, deep breathing, talking, eating, and drinking) as well as sputum production, associated pains, shortness of breath, wheezing, hoarseness, and dizziness. A family history of illness associated with coughing and a detailed environmental and occupational history may be helpful. A wide variety of diseases can manifest with chronic cough; knowledge of tissues or organs with cough receptors can aid in the evaluation of cough.

An abrupt onset of a harsh, barking, and irritative cough, associated with respiratory distress and dysphagia with or without wheezing, often is associated with a foreign body in the esophagus or lower respiratory tract; the sudden onset of a harsh, barking cough, and inspiratory stridor usually is associated with partial obstruction of the epiglottis, larynx, or trachea. Hyperinflation with dyspnea, wheezing, and recurrent coughing are associated more often with more peripheral airways obstruction, as in asthma and prolonged bronchiolitis. Chronic, hacking, day-and-night cough is most characteristic of upper airway disease, particularly of the sinuses. A loud, brassy, deep paroxysmal cough tends to be associated with the lower respiratory tract. Associated fever and green purulent sputum suggest infection of the middle to peripheral airway or sinuses. Infants should be evaluated for cough regardless of duration. Children should be evaluated for cough of 2 weeks duration or more, and adults, for cough of 2 months duration or more.

The history and physical examination will provide clues to the underlying cause of cough.

Specific laboratory tests may be used as indicated to help in establishing a diagnosis. These include blood tests (complete blood count, specific antibodies, sedimentation rate); sputum analysis; nasal or nasopharyngeal secretion smears for polymorphonuclear neutrophils (PMNs), eosinophils, and bacteria or yeast; audiometry and tympanograms; pulmonary functions tests; fiberoptic rhinoscopy, bronchoscopy, or both; and roentgenograms.

In the allergic child or adult, cough that persists both day and night should be evaluated for pulmonary and sinus involvement. Abnormal maxillary sinus radiographic findings can be seen in infants as young as 2 months (Rachelefsky et al., 1982); abnormal findings in maxillary and ethmoid sinuses can be seen in toddlers. In adolescents and adults, the maxillary and ethmoid sinuses are most commonly involved. In 90 percent of children and 80 percent of adults, a maxillary sinus film (Waters view) ordinarily is sufficient for diagnosis of sinus disease. In adults, tomograms occasionally are necessary to diagnose ethmoid sinus disease. Computed axial tomographic scans and magnetic resonance imaging rarely are needed, since ordinary roentgenograms usually are adequate. Additional radiographic examination of the pharyngeal regions and chest to establish the presence of pharyngeal lymphoid tissue and thymus gland may be important in the differential diagnosis of immune deficiency disease (see Chapter 3). The usefulness of echosinograms for evaluation of sinus disease is still controversial, since 30 to 40 percent of A-mode ultrasound patterns are falsely negative when evaluating maxillary sinusitis in adults (Rhor et al., 1986).

Headaches frequently are associated with sinus disease in adolescents and adults. They may be described as pressure like, aching, throbbing, painful, or migraine like. The location may be directly over the involved sinus or, more often, in the forehead and the glabella, retro-ocular, temporal, or parietal regions rather than in an area close to the involved sinus. Some headaches may be associated with negative pressure in the sinus due to resorption of air in a blocked sinus. In this case, the radiogram of the sinus is normal (see also Chapter 35 and Chapter 56).

Cough can be the sole manifestation of asthma; it may be due to bronchoconstriction or activation of cough receptors without bronchoconstriction. On the one hand, bronchodilators may ameliorate both cough and bronchospasm;

on the other hand, since bronchoconstriction may not necessarily be the entire cause of cough in an asthmatic, failure to alleviate cough with bronchodilators does not rule out this diagnosis. Exercise and exercise-induced asthma frequently manifest clinically as coughing. Respiratory water loss may be the mechanism of this effect (Banner et al., 1984) (see also Chapter 44).

Gastroesophageal reflux (GER) in both children and adults may be associated with cough, aspiration, and bronchospasm. These need not occur together. Studies to date are contradictory over the exact relationships among GER, esophagitis, and cough and bronchoconstriction. A reflex mechanism appears to be an important factor in some individuals, whereas aspiration may be a major factor in others. GER often can be determined by the cineesophagram or by the Tuttle test (Bernoken, 1978). In cases of chronic pulmonary lesions, tomography, bronchoscopy, and bronchography should be considered.

Evaluation of allergic disorders has been discussed in detail elsewhere. Pulmonary function testing may indicate obstructive and restrictive pulmonary lesions when the auscultatory examination findings are normal. Consider appropriate referrals for evaluation of congenital heart disease, GER, allergy, or foreign body removal.

TREATMENT

Successful therapy depends upon identification of the cause of cough. Treatment for specific disorders in which cough is a common symptom is discussed elsewhere in this text. Symptomatic treatment often is disappointing, especially in patients with severe coughs. Antitussives and expectorants used properly, however, may benefit some.

Cough preparations can be classified according to their site of action. Central cough suppressants act by depressing the medullary integrative cough center. Peripheral depressants appear to work chiefly on irritant receptors, either by anesthetizing them or otherwise decreasing their activity. Both narcotic and nonnarcotic antitussives are available. Codeine phosphate is the principal antitussive narcotic in clinical use. In the older child or adult, the oral dosage ranges from ½ to 1 grain up to four times a day; this should be reduced, if used at all in younger children. In general, there is little

experimental evidence for the effectiveness of non-narcotic antitussives, although dextromethorphan is claimed to be equally effective as codeine at comparable oral doses and clinical complications from excessive doses are less likely than with codeine. The use of these agents in children has not been studied extensively, however.

Anticholinergic agents, such as atropine sulfate and derivatives of atropine, may block the cough and irritant receptor responsiveness to acetylcholine. If given in large doses, they may induce such side effects as mouth dryness, blurred vision, and skin flushing. Recent evidence indicates that aerosolized atropine in doses of 0.5 to 2 mg may be beneficial in patients who have bronchospasm and cough.

Expectorants that include iodides and guaifenesin (glyceryl guaiacolate) are supposed to aid by thinning secretions. Evidence of their effectiveness is conflicting. Iodides as expectorants have adverse reactions that outweigh any possible benefits, at least in children (AAP Committe on Drugs, 1976). Side effects of iodides include parotid swelling, metallic taste, marked exacerbation of acne, skin rash, and goiter. Guaifenesin is made from wood distillate. It appears to act as a respiratory tract secretory gland irritant, but appropriate dosage (indeed, its effectiveness at all as an expectorant) is still in question. Daily dosage recommended ranges are from 100 to 400 mg, divided into 4 to 6 doses. Large dosages may cause platelet aggregation. In animal studies, ammonium chloride is effective as an expectorant, if given in large doses.

Mucolytic agents, such as acetylcysteine, pancreatic dornase, and streptokinase, are effective in reducing viscosity of secretions but must be delivered by aerosol. They are irritating, may induce severe bronchospasm, and are contraindicated in asthma. Adequate oral hydration to cause thinning of secretions is important, especially in acute asthma.

REFERENCES

American Academy of Pediatrics Committee on Drugs: Adverse reactions to iodide therapy of asthma and other pulmonary diseases. Pediatrics 57:272, 1976.

Banner, A.S., Green, J., O'Connor, M.: Relation of respiratory water loss to coughing after exercise. N. Engl. J. Med. 311:883, 1984.

Bernoken, I.L.: Asthma in adults. In Allergy, Vol. 2. Middleton, E., Jr., Reed, C.E., Ellis, E.F. (eds.), St. Louis, C.V. Mosby Co., 1978.

Berquist, W.E., Rachelefsky G.S., Kadden, M., Siegel S.C., et al.: Gastroesophageal reflux–associated recurrent pneumonia and chronic asthma in children. Pediatrics 68:29–35, 1981.

Cabezas, G.A., Graf, P.D., Nadel, J.A.: Sympathetic vs. parasympathetic nerve regulation of airway of dogs. J. Appl. Physiol. 31:651, 1971.

Corrao, W.M., Braman, S.S., Irwin, R.S.: Chronic cough as the sole presenting manifestation of bronchial asthma. N. Engl. J. Med. 300:633, 1979.

Dahlstrom, A., Fuxe, K., Hokfelt, T., Norberg, R.A.: Adrenergic innervation of bronchial muscles of cat. Acta Physiol. Scand. 66:507, 1966.

Euler, A.R., Byrne, W.J., Ament, M.E., Fondalsrud, E.W., Strobe, C.T., Siegel, S.C., Katz, R.M., Rachelefsky, G.S.: Recurrent pulmonary disease in children: A complication of gastroesophageal reflux. Pediatrics 63:47, 1979.

Katz, R.M.: Exercise-induced bronchospasm in childhood. Ann. Allergy 28:361, 1970a.

Katz, R.M.: Cough syncope in children with asthma. J. Pediatr. 77:48, 1970b.

Nadel, J.A.: In Asthma: Physiology, Immunopharmacology and Treatment. Austen, K.F., Lichtenstein, J.M. (eds.), New York, Academic Press, 1973.

Nadel, J.A., Widdicombe, J.G.: Reflex effects of upper airway irritation on total lung resistance and blood pressure. J. Appl. Physiol. 17:861, 1962.

Rachelefsky, G.S., Katz, R.M., Siegel, S.C.: Diseases of Paranasal Sinuses in Children. Current Problems in Pediatrics, Vol. 12, No. 5. 1982.

Rohr, A.S., Spector, S.L., Siegel, S.C., Katz, R.M., Rachelefsky, G.S.: Correlation between A-mode ultrasound and radiography in the diagnosis of maxillary sinusitis. J. Allergy Clin. Immunol. 78:58–61, 1986.

Simonsson, B.G., Jacobs, F.M., Nadel, J.A.: Role of autonomic nervous system and cough reflex in the increased responsiveness of airways in patients with obstructive airway disease. J. Clin. Invest. 46:1812, 1967.

Widdicombe, J.G., Kent, D.C., Nadel, J.A.: Mechanisms of bronchoconstriction during inhalation of dust. J. Appl. Physiol. 17:613, 1962.

55

Recurrent and Chronic Upper Respiratory Infections and Chronic Otitis Media

SHELDON C. SIEGEL, M.D.

Upper respiratory infections (URIs) of the ears, nose, and throat rank as the most frequent causes for patients of all ages to seek medical attention. They account for nearly two thirds of total illnesses in a community (Dingle et al., 1964) and are responsible for one third of school absences (Saliba et al., 1967). These illnesses also have a tremendous economic impact on society; the annual cost for laboratory tests, respiratory pharmaceuticals, and economic losses due to absenteeism and impaired work productivity alone in the United States has been estimated to run into billions of dollars. When these URIs become current and chronic in nature, they become challenging diagnostic problems.

Evidence has been presented suggesting that respiratory allergic disorders may predispose patients to primary (usually viral) or secondary (usually bacterial) respiratory infections. Furthermore, viral infections frequently precipitate asthmatic attacks. The similarity of the symptoms and signs of respiratory allergic diseases to those of respiratory illnesses adds an additional diagnostic dilemma for the physician. Moreover, the elderly, often compromised in their immune defense mechanisms, may display unusual clinical pictures of common URIs. In this chapter, possible etiologic and contributing factors (with special emphasis on the role of allergy) that may relate to the problem of chronic or recurrent upper respiratory or ear infections will be discussed along with practical diagnostic and therapeutic considerations.

What is a "recurrent" or "chronic" infection? These infections are extremely difficult to define precisely because of variations in frequency and severity of respiratory infections that occur in different anatomic sites (e.g., nose, sinus, pharynx, eyes) and because of different criteria in their classification. Physicians commonly diagnose all upper respiratory tract infections with the term "URIs." However, it is important for the physician to focus on the specific anatomic site that is initially or primarily involved and to consider the age of the patient. For example, a normal 3-year-old child attending nursery school, who has repeated exposures to respiratory viruses, might have as many as ten or more infections per year. It would be abnormal for an older child or adult to have so many respiratory infections. Consideration should also be given to increased susceptibility to infections, usually severe or prolonged infections, infections without symptom-free periods, unexpected manifestations or complications of infections, and infections with organisms of low pathogenicity.

FACTORS THAT CONTRIBUTE TO RECURRENT OR CHRONIC RESPIRATORY INFECTIONS

Numerous factors contribute to the number, severity, and chronicity of URIs (Table 55–1).

Etiologic Agents

Viruses cause the vast majority of respiratory infections. Over 150 different viruses have been isolated and are associated with respiratory infections. Although infectious agents seldom confine themselves to specific areas, URIs are classified commonly into clinical syndromes (e.g., common cold, pharyngitis, and laryngitis). Certain organisms tend to produce specific syndromes. Table 55–2 lists clinical upper respiratory syndromes and prinicipal viral and bacterial agents associated with their etiologies. The 120 or more serologically different rhinoviruses primarily infect the nose and are the major etiologic agents of common cold syndromes. These also are the most common causes of pharyngeal symptoms (sore, dry, or scratchy throat). The coronaviruses have also been implicated as etiologic agents in approximately 15 to 20 percent of the common cold

TABLE 55–1. Factors Contributing to Recurrent or Chronic Respiratory Infections

Etiologic agents
Viruses
Bacteria
Other organisms
Environmental factors
Exposure to infectious agents
At school
Family (related to size)
Baby sitters
Seasonal variations
Air pollution
Variations in host susceptibility
Age and sex
Genetic factors
Nutrition
Immunologic factors
Primary immune deficiencies
Secondary immunologic dysfunction
Microbial factors
Disorders leading to increased susceptibility to infections
Circulatory
Anatomic obstruction
Integument defects
Allergy

syndromes, but they account for only about 5 percent of pharyngitis symptoms. Less common causes of viral pharyngeal infections are herpes simplex virus, adenovirus, type A coxsackievirus, influenza virus, parainfluenza virus, cytomegalovirus, and Epstein-Barr virus. The last two viruses are important causes of infectious mononucleosis in adults as well as in children. Recently, the Epstein-Barr virus has been implicated as a cause of chronic recurring infections, suggesting some alteration in immunoregulation (see section Immune Factors).

Viruses are isolated infrequently from fluids obtained from middle ear infections despite the epidemiologic data suggesting that acute otitis media frequently is associated with upper respiratory tract viral infections. Respiratory syncytial viruses or influenza viruses account for most infections. Two types of bacteria, *Streptococcus pneumoniae* and *Haemophilus influenzae*, account for most secondary bacterial infections of the middle ear.

Acute laryngitis usually occurs with common cold and influenza syndromes; in children, however, parainfluenza viruses more commonly cause laryngotracheobronchitis (croup). Although the myxoviruses (respiratory syncytial, parainfluenza, and influenza viruses) cause URIs, they are the predominant pathogenic agents encountered in serious respiratory infections in infants, children, and the elderly. Respiratory syncytial viruses account for 75 percent of bronchiolitis in infants and children, whereas in older children and adults the infections usually are manifested as URIs. Following these infections in adults, airways hyperreactivity to cholinergic stimuli may occur for up to 8 weeks and may cause bronchopneumonia in the elderly (Hall et al., 1978). Influenza or viral infections are especially hazardous in elderly patients and in patients with chronic pulmonary, cardiac, metabolic, or other diseases; these infections frequently cause chest complications (e.g., tracheobronchitis and pneumonia). Whereas only 8 percent of children and

TABLE 55–2. Upper Respiratory Tract Clinical Syndromes and Their Principal Viral and Bacterial Etiology

Common Cold	Oropharyngitis	Otitis Media	Laryngeal Infections
VIRUSES			
Rhinovirus	Rhinovirus	Respiratory syncytial virus	Respiratory syncytial virus
Coronavirus	Coronavirus	Adenovirus	Adenovirus
	Herpesvirus	Influenza virus	Influenza and parainfluenza virus
			Rhinovirus
	Adenovirus		
	Coxsackievirus		
	Influenza and parainfluenza viruses		
	Epstein-Barr virus		
	Cytomegalic virus		
BACTERIA AND OTHER ORGANISMS			
	Streptococcus pyogenes (group A, B hemolytic)	*Haemophilus influenzae*	*H. influenzae* (epiglottitis)
		Streptococcus pneumoniae	*Streptococcus pyogenes*

adults under the age of 50 years have such complications, the incidence increases progressively after 60 years to more than 70 percent in those over 70 years of age. Although the classic illness produced by *Mycoplasma pneumoniae* is atypical pneumonia, this organism also may be the etiologic agent in upper respiratory disease and bullous myringitis. Thus, depending on the type of infecting viral agent, a wide spectrum of upper respiratory syndromes can be observed.

The role of *bacteria* and other organisms as causative factors in URI is more difficult to define. Bacteria that may cause unusually common, cold-like illnesses are *Coccidioides immitis, Histoplasma capsulatum, Bordetella pertussis, Chlamydia psittaci,* and *Coxiella burnetii* (Q fever). The only bacterial species commonly encountered as a cause of nasopharyngeal disease is the group A beta-hemolytic *Streptococcus.* In the past, diphtheria and tuberculosis occasionally were responsible for pharyngeal infections, and pertussis in its preparoxysmal catarrhal stage had to be differentiated from other common causes of URIs. Occasionally, in children under 3 years of age, *Haemophilus influenzae* may produce mild nasopharyngitis. This organism also is responsible for the distinctive clinical entity of acute epiglottitis, which can be fulminating and fatal if not recognized and treated promptly. On the one hand, there is little evidence that *Staphylococcus,* non-group A *Streptococcus,* or pneumococcus cause significant pharyngeal disease. On the other hand, chronic tonsillitis generally is due to streptococci. Once chronic scarring has occurred, the organism is difficult to eradicate with antibiotic therapy. Repeated attacks of nasopharyngitis also may be caused by chronic adenoiditis. Children with this infection generally have chronic rhinorrhea, repeated episodes of otitis media, and chronic mouth breathing. The diagnosis is established on physical examination by finding purulent postnasal drip or, with a gloved finger, by palpating and expressing pus from the enlarged adenoid mass. Antimicrobial therapy often is ineffectual, and removal of the hypertrophied tissue sometimes is necessary. Secondary bacterial infections, in general, account for many of the complications arising from the primary viral infections and undoubtedly contribute to the chronicity or recurrence of some infections seen in both children and adults. This will be discussed further under the section Differential Diagnosis and Complications.

Environmental Factors

Exposure to Infection. The frequency of respiratory infections in children increases sharply when they enter nursery school or kindergarten, because of exposures to a greater range of viruses. The infection rate in preschool children in a family also rises when an older sibling enters school. In general, the larger the family, the greater the individual "attack rate" for upper respiratory illnesses.

Seasonal Variations. Climatic, ecologic, epidemiologic, and other factors partially help to explain why some infections occur at certain times of the year. For most of the common URIs, the reasons for the seasonal cycles and increased incidences during the winter months remains unknown. Seasonal variations are found in areas of high mean temperatures in winter as well as in areas of colder climates. In the tropics, respiratory infections are more prevalent during the rainy season. However, there is no evidence that cold weather per se, chilling, wet feet, and drafts cause or increase susceptibility to URIs.

Knowledge of intraseasonal prevalences of viral respiratory illnesses, as well as pollinating seasons, can be helpful in narrowing the etiology of upper respiratory symptoms. In Figure 55–1, the peak prevalence periods of some of the more common respiratory infections and pollinating periods for the Midwest and Eastern areas in the United States are shown.

Air Pollution. The relationship of atmospheric air pollution to upper respiratory health has been controversial, and research has yielded disparate results. However, there is a significant correlation between increasing recurrent lower respiratory tract disease and increasing air pollution (Pierson et al., 1984; Goldstein et al., 1985; Spinaci et al., 1985). Air pollution, such as photochemical smog and sulfur dioxide, can cause increased bronchial hyperreactivity (especially during exercise), ciliary paralysis, mucous gland hypertrophy, excess secretions with airways obstruction, slow resolution of respiratory infections, and susceptibility to further infections. Evidence also suggests that parental smoking and indoor heating with woodburning stoves increases the incidence of respiratory infections in children (Kraemer et al., 1983; Honicky et al., 1985). Kraemer and associates (1983) reported that children exposed to passive cigarette smoke, with nasal congestion and atopy, were more than six times as likely to develop persistent middle ear effu-

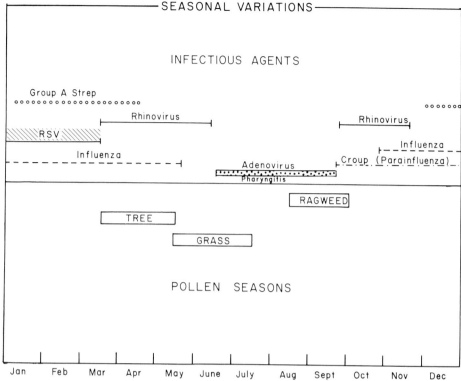

FIGURE 55–1. Pollen and seasonal variations for the Midwest and East in the United States.

sions compared to children whose histories did not include these characteristics.

Variations in Host Susceptibility

There are many host factors that can affect the incidence and severity of upper respiratory disease. These include age, sex, genetics, nutrition, immunity, microbial alterations of host susceptibility, and allergies, as well as various disorders that predispose patients to increased susceptibility to infections.

Age and Sex. URIs are more frequent in childhood, probably because of the increased number of viral pathogens capable of causing upper respiratory symptoms in this age group and because of accelerated transmission. Illness rates decline in older children and reach adult levels in adolescents. For reasons that are not clear, boys tend to have more URIs than girls until puberty. After adolescence, women have higher incidences, probably reflecting greater exposure to young children. The highest incidence of bacterial otitis media is between 6 and 24 months of age; the incidence then declines with age with the exception of another rise be-

tween 5 and 6 years of age, the time of school entry. Otitis media also is more frequent in young children than in adults, possibly because of anatomic changes, since children have less cartilage in the eustachian tubes as well as less efficient contraction of the tensor palatine muscles. Sinusitis is a common complication in both children and adults.

The elderly also are more susceptible to infection, possibly because of functional decline in cell-mediated immunity and decreased lung function.

Primary immunodeficiencies also are more common in males than in females. Under 5 years of age, approximately 80 percent of affected patients are males; in adults, the incidence in males is around 40 percent, as a greater late-onset common variable immunodeficiency exists in females.

Genetic factors. A relationship of genetic factors to susceptibility to infections has been appreciated for many years. Some racial groups (American Indians, Eskimos, and Australian aborigines) are at increased risk for high rates of infection and severe chronic middle ear diseases. Specific anthropometric differences in the middle ear cavity and differences in function of the eustachian tubes have been postulated for these racial differences. Other workers have implicated poverty, overcrowding, poor sanitation, and inadequate medical care.

Some individuals with hereditary disorders, such as cystic fibrosis, immotile cilia syndrome, and genetically associated immunodeficiencies, have increased susceptibilities to recurrent and chronic URIs, purulent otitis media, and sinusitis.

Nutrition. There is general agreement that nutritional deficiencies will reduce the host's defense mechanisms to infections (Katz and Stiehm, 1977). Severely undernourished children are especially vulnerable to life-threatening bacterial infections of the middle ears and lower respiratory tracts. A gradation in immune defects exists from the mild of malnutrition to the extreme of kwashiorkor. Humoral antibody response appears to be little affected, whereas cell-mediated immunity is profoundly affected in human malnutrition. Although all lymphoid tissue atrophies, the thymus gland is the most severely affected. It is of interest that, despite high levels of IgE in many malnourished children, allergy is uncommon. It has been postulated that the elevated IgE levels reflect diminished thymic inhibitory influence on IgE synthesis. Reyes and coworkers (1982) also found that intestinal parasitism was not a significant factor in the hyperimmunoglobulin E observed in moderately malnourished asthmatics. However, in patients predisposed to extrinsic asthma, moderate malnutrition did not impair the *in vitro* and *in vivo* expression of specific IgE.

Several mild defects of polymorphonuclear leukocyte function have been described in malnutrition, the most notable being diminished bactericidal and candidacidal activity. Complement components also decrease in proportion to the degree of malnutrition. Whether this has any practical consequences remains to be determined.

Obese patients are more susceptible to respiratory infections (Chandra and Newberne, 1977), perhaps because of local factors such as reduced vascularity of adipose tissue, restricted pulmonary function, or defective microbial activity of granulocytes.

Immune Factors. Both primary and secondary immunodeficiency diseases are associated with recurrent respiratory infection, recurrent diarrhea, and failure to thrive (Stiehm and Fulginiti, 1980). These disorders are discussed in detail in Chapter 3, and a few that are likely to be the causes of recurrent and chronic infections are considered briefly.

The most common of these disorders is selective deficiency of serum and secretory IgA. IgA deficiency may be associated with recurrent upper and lower respiratory infections, autoimmunity, gastrointestinal disorders, and increased risk of neoplasia; however, many individuals with this condition may be asymptomatic. The diagnosis is easily confirmed by demonstrating IgA serum levels less than 4 mg/dl, with usually normal levels of other immunoglobulins. However, a concomitant IgG$_2$ subclass deficiency has been reported in some cases. There is no specific treatment. Gamma globulin injections are contraindicated, since they may cause sensitization of the patient by the production of anti-IgA antibodies.

Primary and secondary hypogammaglobulinemias (e.g., common variable immunodeficiency, acquired agammaglobulinemia, and idiopathic late-onset immunoglobulin deficiency) also must be considered in patients predisposed to sinopulmonary infections. In both the congenital and common variable type, the diagnosis is established by quantification of serum immunoglobulins and antibody responses.

Although IgG subclass deficiency has been described in patients with well-defined immunodeficiency diseases (e.g., common variable immunodeficiency, IgA deficiency, ataxia-telangiectasia, and Wiskott-Aldrich syndrome), isolated selected deficiency of IgG$_2$ or IgG$_3$ subclass has been reported recently to be associated with recurrent sinopulmonary infections (Umetsu et al., 1985). The patients so affected have poor antibody responses to polysaccharide antigens, responses that reside predominantly within the IgG$_2$ subclass. Since IgG levels are generally elevated in children with recurrent infections, normal serum levels of IgG in association with chronic sinopulmonary disease may provide clues to this disorder. Establishment of the diagnosis is important in that the frequency of infections can be greatly reduced by antibiotic prophylaxis and gamma globulin replacement therapy.

The Wiskott-Aldrich syndrome, Buckley syndrome (Buckley et al., 1972), and ataxia-telangiectasia also are associated with frequent severe respiratory infections.

Microbial Alteration of Host Susceptibility. Microbial alteration of the host may also promote invasion by secondary pathogens (Machowiak, 1978). The diminished ability to resist these secondary invaders is brought about by alterations in the cellular or humoral immunity or by alterations in the anatomy of the host. Temporary suppression of cell-mediated immunity, phagocytosis, and macrophage function has been demonstrated in a wide variety of infections. The clinical significance of this effect is illustrated by the reports of reactivation and dissemination of tuberculosis during measles' epidemics. Acquired immune deficiency syndrome (AIDS) is the most striking example of how a viral infection (human immunodeficiency virus IV) can impair severely the host's T-cell immune resistance to opportunistic infections, which invariably are fatal.

Various microorganisms also predispose individuals to secondary infections by altering humoral immunity, inhibiting antibody production, stimulating production of sensitizing antibodies, or inducing blocking antibodies.

Recently, attention has been focused on the medical consequences of persistent viral infections (Southern and Oldstone, 1986). Chronic infectious mononucleosis is one of these chronic viral infections, which is likely to be encountered by the practicing physician. Some patients with chronic infectious mononucleosis complain of persistent symptoms for months and even years after an acute episode. Recently, Jones and associates (1985), in a study of 44 adults and children with one or more symptoms of fevers, recurrent tonsillitis, pharyngitis, anterior cervical or generalized lymphadenopathy, arthralgia, myalgia, fatigue, depressive symptoms, headaches, and paresthesias, found elevated Epstein-Barr viral antibody levels (antibodies to viral capsid antigen, early antigen, and nuclear antigen) highly suggestive of active infection for at least 1 year. None of the patients continued to have positive heterophil agglutinin. In other studies, women aged 25 to 40 years were more often infected, frequently had histories of allergy, and commonly had symptoms of chronic fatigue, low-grade fevers, and recurrent sore throats (Tobi et al., 1985). Caution should be exercised against overinterpretation of the serologic profile of Epstein-Barr viral antibodies, since many asymptomatic healthy persons have elevated early antigen and capsid antigen antibody titers. It has been postulated that a patient who develops this syndrome may have a selective cellular immune deficiency with an inability to recognize the K nuclear antigen of the virus. As with the acute disease, the treatment of this chronic disorder remains unsatisfactory. The therapeutic effectiveness of acyclovir and intravenous gamma globulin is currently under investigation.

Disorders Leading to Increased Susceptibility to Infection. In general, recurrent infections at one site, often with the same organism, should make one suspect a circulation disorder, a mechanical obstruction, or a skin function disorder. In contrast, infections due to a systemic immunodeficiency occur at multiple sites and frequently are caused by many different organisms. Examples of circulatory disorders that lead to recurrent infections include sickle cell anemia, diabetes, and nephrosis.

Mechanical obstruction frequently causes localized infection of the upper respiratory tract. Infants and children are especially prone to these infections. Because infants are obligatory nose breathers, nasal obstruction creates significant difficulties. For example, nasal mucosal edema in children with prominent lymphoid tissue and shorter, straighter, horizontal, less stiff eustachian tubes (compared with adults) predisposes them to obstruction and infection. Obstructions and dysfunctions of the eustachian tubes, obstructions of the ostia of the sinuses due to edema, and secretions due to allergy or polyps also frequently give rise to recurrent or chronic ear infections and sinusitis.

Micromechanical problems also have been recognized recently. Abnormalities of clearance mechanisms due to disorganized ciliary movement in cystic fibrosis and Kartagener syndrome (chronic sinusitis, situs inversus, and bronchiectasis) are examples (Eliasson et al., 1977). In the last decade it has been shown that the disease can occur without situs inversus, and the terms immotile cilia syndrome and primary ciliary dyskinesia were introduced (Mygind et al., 1983). The syndrome is an autosomal recessive inherited disease of the microtubules of ciliated cells and spermatozoa; it affects approximately 1 in 20,000 people. A variety of aberrations in the axonemal microtubular apparatus have been observed, the most common being a deficiency of the dynein arms. These defects cause abnormal mucociliary clearance, leading to chronic URIs and bronchiectasis, and sterility from immotile spermatozoa. Recently, three adult men with chronic sinopulmonary disease, nasal polyposis, and azoospermia with normal sweat chloride values and cilia structures were described (Schanker et al., 1985). These cases appear to represent a clinical entity distinct from cystic fibrosis and known immotile cilia disorders.

Skin defects, which alter the primary mechanical barrier to organisms, can also lead to increased susceptibility to infections. Such disorders include skull fractures, midline sinus tracts, burns, and eczema.

Allergy. A relationship between allergy and respiratory infection has long been recognized. URIs have been clearly associated with exacerbations of asthma in children (McIntosh et al., 1973); they are the single most common precipitating factors in this age group (Carlsen et al., 1984). In studies of adults with asthma, this association has been reported to be less striking (Halperin et al., 1985; Hudgel et al., 1979). However, even in normal adult subjects there is substantial evidence of an increase in bronchial hyperactivity lasting for several weeks following URIs (Stempel and Boucher, 1981). URIs also have been implicated in acute infectious exacerbations in patients with chronic bronchitis, a disorder that also frequently has a component of reversible bronchospasm. Specific pathogens responsible for causing wheezing episodes vary with age of the patient and season of the year. In children up to 5 years of age, respiratory syncytial virus, parainfluenza virus, and adenovirus are the most frequent causes; respiratory syncytial virus is the most common offender. In children between 5 and 15 years of age, *Mycoplasma*, parainfluenza virus, and respiratory syncytial virus have been identified as triggering wheezing, whereas in adults *Mycoplasma pneumoniae* and influenza virus are the organisms most frequently recovered. Asthmatic children also have been reported to have an increased number of URIs compared with their nonasthmatic siblings (Minor et al., 1974). It was postulated that the increased incidence of URIs (especially of rhinoviruses) might have been related to the increased time spent indoors or the increased inoculation due to nasal pruritus. Other investigators have found that viral infections occur with equal frequency in children with and without asthma or elevated levels of IgE (Welliver, 1983).

It is not clear how upper respiratory infections cause airways hyperreactivity. A single mechansim does not appear to explain virus-induced asthma (Busse, 1985). The most commonly postulated explanations include the following:

1. Upper respiratory infections cause inflammation of the larger airways which, in turn, produces an increased sensitivity of the cholinergic irritant receptors. Reflex bronchoconstriction then follows from stimulation of these receptors.

2. Certain metabolites produced by the virus-infected cell or the virus per se act to interfere with the beta-adrenergic tone in the airways of asthmatics. The beta receptor response is impaired not only in neurons but also in lymphocytes and polymorphonuclear cells. Thus, inflammation could be prolonged by interference with the normal catecholamine effects on the inflammatory leukocytes.

3. Release of mediators, which can sensitize the airway, is triggered by virus-specific IgE antibody (Welliver et al., 1981).

4. Respiratory viruses and products of virus-infected cells (e.g., interferon) enhance mediator release (Ida et al., 1977).

Other observations indicate that URIs (especially croup and bronchiolitis) in early childhood may play roles in the development of airways hyperreactivity and atopy (Weiss et al., 1985). The onset of allergic disease in children, in fact, has been linked specifically to URIs. Frick and coworkers (1979) found that 12 of 13 children had allergic sensitizations initiated by URIs; they developed increased IgE levels, positive radioallergosorbent tests (RASTs), leukocyte histamine release, and lymphocyte transformations following infection. Suggestive evidence exists that infections may cause an imbalance between suppressor and helper lymphocytes, resulting in an overproduction of IgE (Perelmutter and Potvin, 1980). Raised IgE levels in the early phase of infectious mononucleosis and increased incidences of seropositivity in the Epstein-Barr virus in atopic children also are compatible with the idea that this virus has a pathogenic role in the hyperproduction of IgE and in the development of atopic disease (Strannegard and Strannegard, 1981). It remains to be determined, however, whether the increased levels of airway responsiveness, atopy, or both, rather than being causally related to viral respiratory infections, simply predispose children to more severe illnesses.

The incidence of recurrent otitis media, chronic serous otitis media, and acute and chronic sinusitis may be greater in allergic individuals (Bierman and Furukawa, 1978; Fireman, 1985). Some investigators have contended that secretory otitis media can be a primary allergic response of the middle ear mucosa and contiguous tissues to a specific allergen. Most other investigators, however, believe that the mechanism by which allergy leads to otitis media with effusion is direct inflammation of the eustachian tube or of the nose and nasopharynx leading to abnormal eustachian tube function. Bernstein and his coworkers (1985) concluded that IgE-mediated reactions in the middle ear occurred in less than 10 percent of allergic children with recurrent otitis media with effusion; they postulated that the eustachian tube may have been the target organ in 30 percent of patients. Recent studies in human subjects and in monkeys strongly suggest a causal relationship between allergic reactions in the nasopharynx and obstruction of the eustachian tube, which, in turn, probably contributes to the development of otitis media with effusion (Fireman, 1985; Walker et al., 1985).

Frequently, both secretory otitis and chronic sinusitis coexist, suggesting a common etiology. One such factor may be underlying allergic respiratory disease (Howshaw and Nickman, 1974). Anecdotal data suggest that sinusitis occurs frequently in patients with allergic respiratory diseases and that, when present, it may be a precipitating factor in bronchial asthma. We studied 70 consecutive children referred for evaluations of allergies for the prevalence of sinus disease (see Chapter 35) (Rachelefsky et al., 1978). Abnormal sinus radiographic results compatible with disease were found in 37 subjects (53 percent), and 15 (21 percent) had complete opacification of one or more sinuses. Sinus disease appears to be extremely common in both allergic children and adults and often contributes to the chronicity of symptoms.

The role of sinusitis in precipitating asthma or bronchitis has been recognized for many years despite the fact the mechanisms by which paranasal sinus disease induces asthma and bronchitis are not fully understood. Certainly, sinusitis should be suspected in patients with chronic asthma that is difficult to control (Slavin, 1984; Rachelefsky et al., 1984).

Upper respiratory disease also is more frequent in allergic individuals. For example, in 304 subjects, the incidence of allergic disease was significantly higher in those who had five or more "colds" per year compared with those who had two or less "colds" per year (Siegel et al., 1952).

DIAGNOSIS AND TREATMENT

It is evident that there are numerous factors that can contribute to recurrent or chronic URIs. When a parent states "My child is sick all the time" or when an adolescent or adult patient inquires "Why am I having one cold after another?", how does the physician determine whether this is a variation of normal or is due to a more serious underlying disorder?

History

Foremost among helpful diagnostic procedures is a detailed history. Although emphasis should be placed on the respiratory system, the history should be complete, since symptoms involving other systems will provide clues to possible underlying disease processes.

Information regarding factors previously discussed that may contribute to the etiology of recurrent or chronic URIs should be obtained. It is particularly important to differentiate among *allergic rhinitis, vasomotor rhinitis, recurrent infectious rhinitis,* and *nonallergic eosinophilic rhinitis.* The salient features of each of these disorders are presented in Table 55–3. Often the diagnosis of each of these conditions can be established by history alone.

The development of specific therapeutic measures for some immune deficient disorders makes the early and accurate diagnosis of the immune incompetent patient more urgent. *The history often will provide the initial clues as to possible defects in host defense mechanisms and be sufficient to differentiate nonimmune problems.* Usually, immunologically compromised patients are constantly ill in contrast to normal individuals who are well between respiratory infections. Multiple sites of infections are the rule, whereas recurrent infections at one locale (such as otitis media) should suggest an anatomic defect. When infections involve the respiratory tract, allergy must be suspected. The type of organisms identified also may be of diagnostic significance. Gram-negative bacilli, such as *Pseudomonas aeruginosa,* are particularly likely to cause infection in patients with granulocytopenia and mucosal damage (and cystic fibrosis), whereas viruses, fungi, protozoa, or mycobacteria cause infection in patients with cellular deficiencies. *Streptococcus pneumoniae* and *Haemophilus influenzae* are frequent offenders in patients with humoral antibody deficiencies. A family history of early infant deaths, cancer, or allergic, collagen, or autoimmune diseases also may suggest heritable disorders of host immunity.

Physical Examination

The physical examination may suggest whether the patient's infections are "normal"

TABLE 55–3. Differential Diagnosis of Allergic, Infectious, Vasomotor, and Noneosinophilic Rhinitis

Findings	Allergic	Infectious	Vasomotor	Nonallergic Eosinophilic
HISTORY				
Usual age of onset	Childhood	Childhood	Adulthood but not uncommon in childhood	Older children and adults
Seasonal variations	Recurrent or perennial	Single attacks more frequent during winter months	Perennial	Perennial
Symptomatic between exacerbations	Often present	Asymptomatic	Persistent symptoms	Persistent symptoms
Nasal, ocular, or palatal pruritus	Marked	Absent	Absent	Occasional
Paroxysmal sneezing	Marked	Early in course only	Uncommon, mild sneezing	Occasional
Loss of taste or smell	Occasional	Rarely	Occasional	Occasional
Associated wheezing and coughing	Often	Coincidental	Occasional	Uncommon
Past history of atopic manifestations	Frequent	Coincidental	Coincidental	Coincidental
Etiologic allergens	Usual	Coincidental	Coincidental	Allergens not identifiable
Family history of allergy	Usual	Coincidental	Coincidental	Coincidental
Etiology	Allergens	Viruses	Unknown	Unknown
PHYSICAL EXAMINATION				
Appearance of mucosa	Usually pale	Hyperemic and red	Pale and edematous or erythematous	Pale and edematous
Turbinates	Moderately to markedly edematous	Mildly edematous	Edematous	Markedly edematous
Secretions	Watery or mucoid	Clear early, mucopurulent or purulent later	Watery or mucoid	Watery or mucoid
Nasal polyps*	Infrequent	Coincidental	Coincidental	Coincidental
Other manifestations of allergy	Often present	Coincidental	Occasional, nonallergic asthma	Coincidental
Allergic facies, shiners, nasal crease, gaping	Common	Usually absent	Usually absent	Uncommon
Allergic "salute"	Common	Absent	Usually absent	Uncommon
LABORATORY TESTS				
Nasal eosinophilia >10 percent	Positive	Negative	Negative	Positive
Peripheral eosinophilia	Usually positive	Negative†	Negative†	Occasional
Immediate skin tests	Usually positive	Negative†	Negative†	Negative
RAST results	Positive	Negative†	Negative†	Negative
Elevated IgE levels	Approximately 60 percent	Normal	Normal	Negative
RESPONSE TO THERAPY				
Environmental control	Improvement	No improvement	No improvement	No improvement
Antihistamines	Effective	Poor	Poor	Fair
Oral decongestants	Effective	Minimal effects	Poor	Fair
Topical cromolyn	Effective	Poor	Poor	Poor
Topical corticosteroids	Excellent	Poor	Fair	Excellent

* If present, cystic fibrosis and cilia immotile syndrome should be considered.
† Unless coincidental allergic disease also present.

or related to an underlying disorder. In addition to distinctive symptoms (especially nasal pruritus and paroxysmal sneezing), the nasal mucous membranes in a patient with allergic rhinitis often have a pale, bluish, moist, and glistening appearance (except when secondarily infected). However, the features of the nasal mucous membranes in vasomotor rhinitis and nonallergic eosinophilic rhinitis are similar, so that the diagnosis cannot be established by physical examination alone. Children with allergies also often exhibit a number of characteristic stigmata. "Allergic shiners," dark and often swollen circles of tissue below the eyes, are presumed to be caused by stasis of blood resulting from swollen nasal and paranasal mucous membranes compressing the veins that drain this area. (This sign is not confined to "allergy," however.) Chronic nasal pruritus often leads to a transverse crease, a horizontal or hypopigmented groove across the lower third of the nose. A gaping appearance also may be present due to long-standing nasal obstruction and associated mouth breathing. Evidence obtained by history or physical findings of other atopic manifestations in the patient or the family help to support the diagnosis of allergic rhinitis. If nasal polyps are present, the diagnosis of cystic fibrosis (in children) and cilia immotile syndrome (in all ages) must be ruled out.

The physical examination also may reveal important clues in immunodeficiency. Usually, immunodeficient children have poor growth, poor subcutaneous fat, and distended abdomens; they appear pale, irritable, and chronically ill. A robust, active child with normal growth is unlikely to have immunodeficiency disorder. Hepatosplenomegaly is common in both children and adults. Cervical nodes may be absent (despite a history of recurrent URIs) or may be unduly enlarged or suppurative. Lymphoid tissue often is absent or markedly diminished. Tympanic membranes are frequently scarred or perforated, and there may be purulent drainage. Thrush and mouth ulcers are common. Evidence of lower respiratory tract infection (deep cough, rales, or wheezing) frequently is found but should also suggest the possibility of asthma. Signs suggestive of bronchiectasis specifically may be present. Rashes, abscesses, purpura, pyoderma, petechiae, paronychia, alopecia, sparse hair, arthritis, or telangiectasia often are present.

Certain congenital immunodeficiency disorders are associated with characteristic physical findings. X-linked agammaglobulinemia is associated with recurrent bacterial sinopulmonary infections, otitis media, and diarrhea. Wiskott-Aldrich syndrome is characterized by severe eczema, thrombocytopenia, and recurrent infection with encapsulated bacteria. Ataxia-telangiectasia has the distinguishing characteristics of telangiectasia of the bulbar conjunctivae, nose, and ears, and ataxia and recurrent sinopulmonary infection. The DiGeorge syndrome can be diagnosed through the characteristic facial features (hypertelorism, ear anomalies), abnormalities of the aortic arch, and neonatal hypocalcemia.

Laboratory Studies

Laboratory tests that are helpful in differentiating allergic, infectious, vasomotor rhinitis, and nonallergic eosinophilic rhinitis are listed in Table 55 – 3. Microscopic examination of the type of cells in nasal secretions can be especially helpful. The presence of eosinophils (greater than 10 percent of the cells) is highly suggestive of allergic rhinitis, especially in children (Williams and Gwaltney, 1972). However, it must be kept in mind that nasal eosinophilia also occurs in nonallergic eosinophilic rhinitis, which is more prevalent in adults (Mullarkey, 1984). On the other hand, an absence or a small number of eosinophils in the quiescent periods of allergic disease or in the presence of secondary infection does not rule out either of these diagnoses. In addition, the ratio of eosinophils to neutrophils can be an important indicator of the role that infection may be playing in a patient with rhinitis.

Immediate type skin tests, RASTs, enzyme-linked immunosorbent assays (ELISA), or other serologic tests for IgE antibody, in conjunction with the history, may be of help not only in pinpointing specific etiologic allergens but also in determining whether the patient is allergic. However, elevation of IgE levels in the serum is of limited use in determining the presence or absence of allergy, since only about 60 percent of patients with allergic rhinitis have elevated serum IgE levels (Yunginger and Gleich, 1975).

It should be reemphasized that when nasal polyps are found in children, cystic fibrosis should be ruled out by a reliable sweat chloride determination. The possibility of immotile cilia syndrome can be evaluated by electron microscopic examination of either respiratory tract cilia or sperm flagella.

Although the precise diagnosis of an immunodeficiency requires special tests normally available only in specialized medical centers, a number of screening tests can be performed easily by the practitioner that help in resolving the dilemma of how to proceed with the patient presenting with recurrent or chronic infections (see Chapters 3 and 4).

Differential Diagnosis and Complications

Other disorders that need to be considered in the differential diagnosis (see Table 55–3) include rhinitis medicamentosa (due to persistent use of topical decongestants), structural derangements of the nose (deviated septum, enlarged adenoids, choanal atresia), nasal congestion due to drugs (*Rauwolfia* derivatives, aspirin, estrogens, cromolyn), endocrine disorders (hypothyroidism), foreign bodies, systemic immune disorders (immunodeficiency, Wegener granulomatosis, polyarteritis, sarcoid, Sjogren syndrome), and tumors (angiofibroma, teratoma, rhabdomyosarcoma, and others). In addition, some of the complications of allergic rhinitis or recurrent infectious rhinitis (Table 55–4) may contribute further to the chronicity of these infections and add to the therapeutic dilemmas when dealing with patients who "have one cold after another" or "are sick all the time." Although these conditions are discussed elsewhere, it should be emphasized that uncontrolled chronic rhinitis may lead to chronic sinusitis, recurrent acute or chronic otitis media, or facial deformities (Shapiro and Shapiro, 1984).

Treatment

Appropriate management of chronic and recurrent upper respiratory infection (RURI) requires recognition of the disorder as well as the

TABLE 55–4. Complications of Allergic Rhinitis and Recurrent Upper Respiratory Infections

Sinusitis
Bacterial infections
   Adenoiditis, tonsillitis, or both
   Pharyngitis
Lower respiratory infections
Triggering asthma
Otitis media

underlying contributing etiologic factors. In the young child with RURI due to unavoidable exposure in nursery school, it may be necessary to remove the child from the school temporarily. Antimicrobial therapy is not beneficial in shortening the duration of URIs nor in preventing secondary bacterial complications, with the possible exception of the prophylactic use of sulfisoxazole or an alternative antimicrobial agent (Schuller, 1983; Cotton et al., 1984; Medical Letter, 1984). Once a secondary bacterial infection such as otitis media or sinusitis has been identified, selection of an appropriate antimicrobial agent depends on the patient's age and clinical signs and symptoms and the physician's knowledge of the organisms most often involved and information regarding penetration of the the drug into the infected area (see Chapter 23).

In recurrent otitis media, *Staphylococcus aureus* and *Haemophilus influenzae* are more commonly isolated than *Streptococcus pneumoniae* and group A beta-hemolytic streptococci. If the organism is unknown, the preferred antibiotic for children is amoxicillin or cefaclor, and cloxacillin for adults and older children. The optimal therapy for chronically draining ears has not been established; therapy is best directed at the particular organism isolated. The most common isolates are *Staphylococcus aureus, S. epidermidis, Pseudomonas aeruginosa,* and occasionally proteus species. The presence of cholesteatoma, chronic mastoiditis, or both must also be considered in evaluating and treating patients with chronic otitis media. The predominant organisms in sinusitis usually are *H. influenzae* and *S. pneumoniae.* (In children, *Branhamella catarrhalis* is also isolated in about 20 percent of the patients.) Treatment with amoxicillin or cefaclor usually is effective, but therapy should be given for a minimum of 10 days because the antibiotic penetrates into the sinuses poorly. One should keep in mind that inadequate treatment with antimicrobial agents also may be a factor in contributing to chronic or recurrent infections.

Despite the wide usage of nasal and oral decongestants administered alone or in combination with antihistamines, their efficacy in the treatment of either acute or chronic secretory otitis media has not been demonstrated. Surgical management of persistent effusion of the middle ear includes the use of myringotomy, adenoidectomy, and placement of tympanotomy tubes (Cantekin et al., 1983; Schnore et al., 1986). The therapeutic value of myringotomy in acute otitis remains doubtful other than for relieving severe otalgia (Giebrink and Quie, 1978). Ventilation of the middle ear with tympanotomy tubes remains a debatable method of treatment. Recently, Paradise and Rogers (1986) have suggested that myringotomy and tympanotomy tube placement be deferred until middle ear effusions are unresponsive to adequate medical treatment over a period of 3 months. Similarly, the effectiveness of adenoidectomy or tonsillectomy for recurrent otitis media and throat infections has remained controversial (Paradise et al., 1980). Two recent reports of prospective controlled studies have suggested their benefit in selected cases (Maw, 1983; Paradise et al., 1984).

Numerous other remedies have been advocated for the prevention and management of RURI and chronic respiratory tract infections. These incude vitamins (especially vitamin C), antiseptic aerosols, ultraviolet irradiation, autogenous and stock bacterial vaccines, transfer factor, and levamisole. None have been proved to be of value, and some may be harmful. Although immunization in a few instances against specific viral and bacterial agents (e.g., influenza A and pneumococcus) has been successful, many major problems must be overcome before immunization for the vast majority of URIs can be successful. Chemoprophylaxis against viral infections is equally ineffective, with the possible exceptions of amantadine for influenza and intranasal interferon for the prevention of colds (Hayden et al., 1986).

The management of specific immune disorders is considered in Chapters 3 and 4. *The empirical and indiscriminate administration of serum immune globulin to a child with normal immune function (to prevent RURI or chronic respiratory tract infection) is without demonstrated value and may be harmful.*

When managing a child with recurrent or chronic respiratory tract infections, the physician should suspect a possible underlying allergic disorder. Appropriate measures should then be taken to treat the process, if it is present.

REFERENCES

Bernstein, J.M.: Recent advances in otitis media with infusion. Ann. Allergy 55:544, 1985.

Bierman, C.W., Furukawa, C.T.: Medical management of serous otitis in children. Pediatrics 61:768, 1978.

Buckley, R.H., Wray, B.B., Belmaker, W.E.: Extreme hyperimmunoglobulinemia E and undue susceptibility to infection. Pediatrics 49:59, 1972.

Busse, W.W.: The precipitation of asthma by upper respiratory infections. Chest 87:44, 1985.

Cantekin, E.I., Mandel, E.M., Bluestone, C.D., Rochette, H.E., Paradise, J.L., Stool, S.E., Fria, J.J., Rogers, K.D.: Lack of efficacy of a decongestant-antihistamine combination for otitis media with effusion ("secretory" otitis media) in children. N. Engl. J. Med. 308:297, 1983.

Carlsen, K.H., Ørstavik, I., Leegard, J., Høeg, H.: Respiratory virus infections and aeroallergens in acute bronchial asthma. Arch. Dis. Childh. 59:310, 1984.

Chandra, R.K., Newberne, P.M.: Nutrition, immunity and infection. In Mechanisms of Interactions. New York, Plenum Press, 1977.

Cotton, R.T., Bierman, C.W., Zalzal, G.H.: Serous otitis in children: Medical and surgical aspects, diagnosis and management. Clin. Rev. Allergy 2:329, 1984.

Dingle, J.H., Badger, G.F., Jordan, W.S.: Illness in the Home: A Study of 25,000 Illnesses in a Group of Cleveland Families. Cleveland, The Press of Western Reserve University, 1964.

Eliasson, R., Mossberg, B., Camner, P., Afzeluis, B.A.: The immotile-cilia syndrome, a congenital ciliary abnormality as an etiologic factor in chronic airway infections and male sterility. N. Engl. J. Med. 297:1, 1977.

Fireman, P.: Eustachian tube obstruction and allergy: A role in otitis media with effusion. J. Allergy Clin. Immunol. 76:137, 1985.

Frick, O.L., German, P.F., Mills, J.: Development of allergy in children. I. Association with virus infections. J. Allergy Clin. Immunol. 63:228, 1979.

Giebrink, G.S., Quie, P.G.: Otitis media: The spectrum of middle ear inflammation. Ann. Rev. Med. 29:285, 1978.

Goldstein, E., Hackney, J.D., Rokaw, S.N.: Photochemical air pollution. Parts I and II. West. J. Med. 142:369, 523, 1985.

Hall, W.J., Hall, C.B., Speers, D.M.: Respiratory syncytial virus infection in adults: Clinical virologic and serial pulmonary studies. Ann. Intern. Med. 88:203, 1978.

Halperin, S.A., Eggleston, P.A., Beasley, P., Suratt, P., Hendley, O., Groschel, M., Gwaltney, J.M., Jr.: Exacerbations of asthma in adults during experimental rhinovirus. Am. Rev. Respir. Dis. 132:976, 1985.

Hayden, F.G., Albrecht, J.K., Kaiser, D.I., Gwaltney, J.M., Jr.: Prevention of natural colds by contact prophylaxis with intranasal alpha-2-interferon. N. Engl. J. Med. 314:71, 1986.

Honicky, R.E., Osborne, J.S., III, Akpom, C.A.: Symptoms of respiratory illness in young children and the use of woodburning stoves for indoor heating. Pediatrics 75:587, 1985.

Howshaw, T.C., Nickman, N.J.: Sinusitis and otitis in children. Arch. Otolaryngol. 100:194, 1974.

Hudgel, D.W., Langston, L., Selner, J.C., McIntosh, K.: Viral and bacterial infections in adults with chronic asthma. Am. Rev. Respir. Dis. 120:393, 1979.

Ida, S., Hooks, J.J., Siraganiah, R.P., Notkins, A.L.: Enhancement of IgE-mediated histamine release from human basophils by viruses: role of interferon. J. Exp. Med. 145:892, 1977.

Jones, J.R., Ray, C.G., Minnich, L.L., Hicks, M.J., Kibler, R., Lucas, D.O.: Evidence for active Epstein-Barr virus infections in patients with persistent, unexplained illnesses: Elevated anti-early antigen antibodies. Ann. Intern. Med. 102:1, 1985.

Katz, M., Stiehm, E.R.: Host defense in malnutrition. Pediatrics 59:490, 1977.

Kraemer, M.J., Richardson, M.A., Weiss, N.S., Furukawa, C.T., Shapiro, G.G., Pierson, W.E., Bierman, C.W.: Risk factors for persistent middle-ear effusions: Otitis media, catarrh, cigarette smoke, exposure and atopy. J.A.M.A. 249:1022, 1983.

Machowiak, P.A.: Microbial synergism in human infections. Part I and Part II. N. Engl. J. Med. 298:21, 83, 1978.

Maw, A.R.: Chronic otitis media with effusion (glue ear) and adenotonsillectomy: prospective randomized controlled study. Brit. Med. J. 287:1586, 1983.

McIntosh, K., Ellis, E.F., Hoffman, L.S., Lybass, T.G., Eller, J.J., Fulginiti, V.A.: The association of viral and bacterial respiratory infections with exacerbation of wheezing in young asthmatic children. J. Pediatr. 82:578, 1973.

Medical Letter: Chemoprophylaxis for recurrent acute otitis media. 26:102, 1984.

Minor, T.E., Baker, J.W., Dick, E.C., DeMeo, A.N., Ouellette, J.J., Cohen, M., Reed, C.E.: Greater frequency of viral infection in asthmatic children as compared with their nonasthmatic siblings. J. Pediatr. 85:472, 1974.

Mullarkey, M.F.: Eosinophilic Nonallergic Rhinitis, A Review. In Settipane, G.A. (ed.), Rhinitis. Providence, Rhode Island, New England and Regional Allergy Proceedings, 1984.

Mygind, N. Pedersen, M., Nielsen, M.H.: Primary and secondary ciliary dyskinesia. Acta. Otolaryngol. 95:688, 1983.

Perelmutter, L., Potvin, L.: Studies on T gamma lymphocytes of atopics and nonatopics. J. Allergy Clin. Immunol. 65:223, 1980.

Pierson, W.E., Covert, D.S., Koenig, J.O.: Air pollutants, bronchial hyperreactivity and exercise. J. Allergy Clin. Immunol. 73:717, 1984.

Rachelefsky, G.S., Goldberg, M., Katz, R.M., Boris, G., Gyepes, M.I., Shapiro, M.J., Mickey, M.R., Finegold, S.M., Siegel, S.C.: Sinus disease in children with respiratory allergy. J. Allergy Clin. Immunol. 61:310, 1978.

Rachelefsky, G.S., Katz, R.M., Siegel, S.C.: Chronic sinus disease with associated airway disease in children. Pediatrics 73:526, 1984.

Reyes, M.A., Saravia, N.G., Watson, R.R., McMurray, D.N.: Effect of moderate malnutrition on immediate hypersensitivity and immunoglobulin E levels in asthmatic children. J. Allergy Clin. Immunol. 70:94, 1982.

Saliba, G.S., Glenzen, W.P., Chen, T.D.Y.: Etiologic studies of acute respiratory illness among children attending public schools. Am. Rev. Respir. Dis. 95:592, 1967.

Schanker, H.M., Jr., Rajfer, J., Saxon, A.: Recurrent respiratory diseases, azoospermia, and nasal polyposis. A syndrome that mimics cystic fibrosis and immotile cilia syndrome. Arch. Intern. Med. 145:2201, 1985.

Schnore, S.K., Sangster, J.F., Gerace, T.M.,Bass, M.J.: Are antihistamine-decongestants of value in the treatment of acute otitis media in children? J. Family Pract. 22:39, 1986.

Schuller, D.E.: Prophylaxis of otitis media in asthmatic children. Pediatr. Infect. Dis. 2:280, 1983.

Shapiro G.G., Shapiro P.A.: Nasal airway ostruction and facial development. Clin Rev in Allergy, 2(3):225–235, 1984.

Siegel, S.C., Goldstein, J.D., Sawyer, A., Glaser, J.: The incidence of allergy in persons who have many colds. Ann. Allergy, 10:24, 1952.

Slavin, R.G.: Sinus disease and asthma. Ear Nose Throat J. 63:45, 1984.

Southern, P., Oldstone, B.A.: Medical consequences of persistent viral infection. N. Engl. J. Med. 314:359, 1986.

Spinaci, S., Arossa, W., Bugiani, M., Natale, P., Bucca, C., deCandussio, G.: The effects of air pollution on the respiratory health of children. A cross-sectional study. Pediatr. Pulmon. 1:262, 1985.

Stempel, D.A., Boucher, R.C.: Respiratory infection and airway reactivity. Med. Clin. North Am. 65:1045, 1981.

Stiehm, E.R., Fulginiti, V.A.: Immunologic Disorders in Infants and Children. Philadelphia, W. B. Saunders Co., 1980.

Strannegard, I., Strannegard, O.: Epstein-Barr virus antibodies in children with atopic disease. Int. Arch. Allergy Appl. Immun. 64:314, 1981.

Tobi, M., Straus, S.E.: Chronic Epstein-Barr disease: A workshop held by the National Institutes of Allergy and Infectious Diseases. Ann. Intern. Med. 103:951, 1985.

Umetsu, D.T., Ambrosino, D.M., Fiunti, I., Siber, G.R., Geha, R.S.: Recurrent sinopulmonary infection and impaired antibody response to bacterial capsular polysaccharide antigen in children with selective IgG-subclass deficiency. N. Engl. J. Med. 313:1247, 1985.

Walker, S.B., Shapiro, G.G., Bierman, C.W., Morgan, M.S., Marshall, S.G., Furukawa, C.T., Pierson, W.I.: Induction of eustachian tube dysfunction with histamine nasal provocation. J. Allergy Clin. Immunol. 76:158, 1985.

Weiss, S.T., Tager, I.B., Munoz, A., Speizer, F.E.: The relationship of respiratory infections in early childhood to the occurrence of increased levels of bronchial responsiveness and atopy. Am. Rev. Respir. Dis. 131:573, 1985.

Welliver, R.C.: Pediatrics asthma: The role of infection. J. Resp. Dis. 4:46, 1983.

Welliver, R.C., Wong, D.T., Sun, M., Middleton, E., Jr., Vaughan, R.S., Ogra, P.L.: The development of respiratory syncytial virus specific IgE and the release of histamine in nasopharyngeal secretions after infection. N. Engl. J. Med. 305:841, 1981.

Williams, R.B., Gwaltney, G.J.: Allergic rhinitis or virus cold? Nasal smear for eosinophilia in differential diagnosis. Ann. Allergy 30:189, 1972.

Yunginger, J.W., Glieich, G.J.: The impact of the discovery of IgE on the practice of allergy. Pediatr. Clin. North Am. 22:3, 1975.

56

Headache

GILBERT A. FRIDAY, M.D.
D. LEE MILLER, M.D.
MICHAEL J. PAINTER, M.D.

Headache is not an uncommon complaint and is seen in a great variety of clinical conditions. Although it is difficult to assess the incidence of all types of headache, as many as 4 percent of school children appear to suffer from vascular headaches (Bille, 1962). Even before age 6, it is not unusual for a child to complain that his or her head hurts. Headache is common in adults. In most instances, headache in children and adults is not allergic in origin. Chronic headache may signal the presence of an underlying structural, physiologic, or psychologic disease process that warrants therapy, and all chronic and recurrent headaches demand painstaking consideration of their etiology. The determination of the cause of chronic headache requires careful and systematic history taking, thorough general physical and neurologic examinations, and selective laboratory studies. Rational therapy can best be accomplished after specific etiologic factors are found.

CLASSIFICATIONS OF HEADACHES

Classifications of headaches are necessarily inadequate, since the etiology and pathogenetic mechanisms in many instances are unknown. It is useful, however, to approach the diagnosis and treatment of headaches according to pathophysiologic processes of pain production, e.g., vascular, sustained muscle contraction, and traction-inflammatory.

Headaches of Vascular Origin.. Until recently, the preheadache phenomena in some vascular headaches was thought to be related to constriction of cerebral arteries, and the headache per se was due to sustained dilatation of cranial arteries (Bruyn, 1976; Dalessio, 1972a and 1974). Evidence, however, is now in doubt. The mechanisms for both may be related to

vasoconstriction and neuronal depression, including serotonergic neuronal depression (Olesen et al., 1980). Histamine, kinins, leukotrienes, 5-hydroxytryptamine, prostaglandins, tyramine, and phenylethylamine all have been implicated in migraine. In addition, adenosine triphosphate and its breakdown products, adenosine monophosphate and adenosine, may play a role in vasodilatation and pain that follow vasoconstriction induced by hypoxia (Burnstock, 1981).

Headaches Due to Sustained Muscle Contraction. A common factor in the production of headache is sustained contraction of head or neck musculature. Several important mechanisms for muscular spasm have been described. It must be remembered that not only can the pathologic process stimulate transmission of nerve impulses, which ultimately results in muscle contraction, but also the contracted muscle may send stimuli to the cord that augment the already existing spasm. Finally, muscular spasm is "perceived" by the cerebral cortex as painful.

Traction-Inflammatory Headaches. Another mechanism responsible for the production of head pain is direct traction, torsion, or inflammation of pain-sensitive structures of the scalp, skull, and intracranial contents. The principal intracranial pain-sensitive structures include the venous sinuses and their tributaries; parts of the dura in the vicinity of the large arteries of the brain, leading to and coming from the circle of Willis; and the arteries themselves. In addition, the anterior and middle meningeal arteries of the dura are pain sensitive. Extracranial structures that possess pain receptors include the periosteum of the skull, the skin of the scalp and its blood supply, and the nasal and paranasal appendages and muscles. Pain is conducted through the trigeminal, facial, vagus, glossopharyngeal, and second and third cervical nerves. The brain parenchyma, the pia mater, the ependyma lining the ventricles, and the choroid plexus are not pain sensitive.

CLINICAL SYNDROMES

Vascular headache syndromes include migraine, cluster, those caused by arteriovenous malformations, hypertension, and fever. *Sustained muscle contraction* is the basis of the common tension headache associated with spasm of scalp and neck musculature, pain in the temporomandibular joint area from malocclusion, and "ophthalmic headaches" from hyperopic refractive errors. Traction-inflammation headaches include head pain associated with meningitis, brain abscesses, and inflamed nasal and paranasal structures as well as traction on pain-sensitive structures by tumors, cysts, arteriovenous malformations, hematomas, hydrocephalus, periosteal elevation, and lumbar punctures (Friedman and Harms, 1967).

Migraine. Migraine headaches may be divided into classic and common types. Only about 10 percent of migraine headaches are of the classic variety, which consists of the three following phases: preheadache (prodrome), headache, and postheadache. During the preheadache phase, there may be pallor, scotomata, scintillations, tinnitus, and other sensations. This period lasts from minutes to hours. This prodromal phase gives way to a headache phase characterized by deep, aching, throbbing pain felt behind the eye on the affected side. The pain progresses to involve the ipsilateral hemicranium and, at times, the entire head. Photophobia, tearing, and blurred vision are frequent during this phase. Edema of the lid and face also is not unusual. The headache phase extends from hours to days; towards the end, vomiting may occur. This phase is associated with marked dilatation of the external carotid system, sometimes observable on the patient's forehead. With the ultimate dissipation of the headache, the third or postheadache phase occurs, which may be accompanied by dehydration produced by anorexia, vomiting, or both and feelings of euphoria or total apathy. Commonly, migraine may not be characterized by a prodromal stage or unilateral localization. "Migrainoid" syndromes may occur with or without headache, presenting as cyclic vomiting, abdominal pain, and paroxysmal vertigo.

Uncommon Vascular Headache Syndromes. Uncommon vascular headache syndromes include cluster headache, "malignant migraine," basilar artery migraine, head trauma, and vascular malformations. Cluster headaches, characteristically occurring nocturnally, consist of a series of closely spaced attacks followed by remission of months or years. "Malignant migraine" is characterized by extraocular muscle palsies, hemiplegia, hemiparesis, and confusional states. Basilar artery migraine

has been described as a type of migraine primarily in young women and in girls, often having a striking relation to menstruation and characterized by vertigo, ataxia, dysarthria, and paresthesias followed by severe, throbbing occipital headache with vomiting (Bickerstaff, 1961; Golden and French, 1975). Head trauma may precipitate vascular headaches. Vascular malformations can cause headache clinically indistinguishable from migraines; convulsions, focal signs outlasting the headache, and continuous cranial bruit are among the associated neurologic findings. Headache related to vascular malformations also can be due to subarachnoid hemorrhage. Hypertension is an occasional cause of vascular headache. Fever may produce head pain due to vasodilatation.

Muscle-Tension Syndrome. Muscle-tension headaches often are located in the bitemporal or occipital area and are characterized by band-like or constrictive pain of dull quality and moderate intensity. Historically, these headaches are often generated by anxiety-producing events. Disorders of the temporomandibular joint, regardless of the cause (e.g., malocclusion; arthritis; trauma; infection; and involuntary tension-relieving mechanisms, such as jaw clenching or bruxism), may produce muscle fatigue, subsequent spasm, and headache. The pain is dull, aching, constant, and centered in the ear or preauricular area and radiates to the temple, side of the neck, and angle of the jaw. The diagnosis is confirmed by tenderness of the temporomandibular joint, spasm of the mastication muscles, and restriction or deviation of the jaw opening (Guralnick et al., 1978).

Traction-Inflammatory Syndrome. Headaches caused by dural traction or meningeal inflammation, including meningitis, brain abscess, brain tumors, cysts, arteriovenous malformations, hematomas, and hydrocephalus, vary in quality and severity. Constant, severe, dull headache is the most consistent feature of brain abscess, whereas headache often is inconspicuous in hydrocephalus. Pain on eye movement can be a clue to the meningeal origin of headache. Head pain associated with increased intracranial pressure is dull and moderate in intensity, tending to be most severe early in the morning. Occasionally, the headache is localized adjacent to structural lesions because of dural traction but may be referred to a distant site.

Rhinocephalgia. The word rhinocephalgia has been coined to describe head pain originating from the nasal structures. Headaches, especially those associated with acute disease of the paranasal structures, often become clinically important components of upper respiratory problems. Allergic rhinitis with engorgement of the nasal turbinates may block the sinus ostia, resulting in sinusitis with subsequent inflammation of the pain-sensitive nasal structures leading to the so-called vacuum headache. Nasal engorgement per se usually does not produce head pain without inflammation or infection. Harold Wolff, through a series of careful experiments, identified the pain-sensitive structures in the nasal and paranasal areas (see Dalessio, 1972a). These areas are listed in Table 56–1. Stimulation of nasal turbinates may result in intense pain, depending upon the area stimulated. Stimulation of the ostia of the maxillary sinuses results in severe pain with referral to the nasopharynx, molars, zygoma, and temple. Stimulation of the duct of the frontal sinuses and the superior cavity also gives significant pain, which is felt locally as well as at the inner canthus of the eye, zygoma, temple, angle of the jaw, and molars. It is of interest to note that in such experiments, stimulation of the mucosa of the paranasal sinuses produced little discomfort. Stimulation of the cavity of the sphenoid sinus produces referred pain to the vertex of the skull. When the maxillary sinus is stimulated, discomfort can be felt about the eye,

angle of the jaw, and posterior molars (see Chapter 35).

Thus, inflammation of the sinuses involving the ostia, particularly the maxillary ostia, may result in "sinus headaches," whereas infection of the sinus per se may be painless. Pressure in the maxillary and frontal sinuses produces little or no discomfort. Wolff also found that headaches originating in paranasal sinuses are uncommon. When headaches did occur, they were usually deep, dull, aching, and nonpulsating. Sinus headaches rarely cause nausea or vomiting and seldom rival migraine headaches in intensity. In acute sinus disease, headaches are more intense than in chronic sinus inflammation.

ROLE OF INGESTANTS IN HEADACHE PRODUCTION

It has been claimed that migraine headaches may be caused by food hypersensitivity (Egger et al., 1983; Monroe et al., 1984; Page et al., in press). The relationship between food ingestion and migraine may be based in part on IgE-specific food allergy in some patients, as shown in double-blind food challenges with a rise in plasma histamine levels (Mansfield et al., 1985).

Certain foods and substances, such as alco-

TABLE 56–1. Experimental Study of Pain from Nasal and Paranasal Structures*

Structures Stimulated	Sites of Pain	Intensity (1 to 10+)
Pharynx and posterior nasopharynx	Local, deep throat	1–2+
Tonsil	Local, behind ear	1–2+
Nasal floor	Local	1–2+
Nasal septum		
Middle	Zygoma to ear	1–2+
Upper	Inner and outer canthus of eye	1–2+
Turbinates		
Upper	Local, inner canthus, forehead, lateral wall of nose	4–6+
Middle	Local, zygoma, to ear and temple	4–6+
Lower	Local, upper teeth, under eye, zygoma to ear	4–6+
Ostium of maxillary sinus	Local, nasopharynx, back teeth, zygoma, temple	5–8+
Nasofrontal duct	Inner canthus, zygoma, temple, angle of jaw, upper back teeth	5–7+
Sinuses		
Frontal	Local, bridge of nose	1–2+
Sphenoid	Vertex of skull	1–2+
Maxillary	Eye, jaw, back teeth	1–2+
Superior nasal cavity		
Anterior	Over eye, upper canthus, teeth	6+
Posterior	Teeth, outer canthus	5–6+
(Vicinity of ethmoidal sinuses)		

*Data obtained after Wolff (see Dalessio, 1972a). Structures were stimulated by pressure from a probe and by faradic current. Pain was described as 1+, 2+, and so forth. The magnitude of the current used for stimulation was based on a scale in which a 1+ pain was the lower limit of pain perception by the tip of the tongue.

hol, do precipitate migraine headaches in some susceptible individuals (Dalessio, 1972b). Patients with cluster headaches are sensitive to small amounts of alcohol. Food containing vasoactive amines, such as tyramine-rich aged cheeses, pickled herrings, chicken livers, and canned figs, may set off migraine by some biochemical alteration of vascular tone. Chocolate contains phenylethylamine, a vasoactive amine found also in certain cheeses, which may cause migraine headaches in some individuals sensitive to the tiny amount found after the conche manufacturing process. Hypoglycemia has been known to trigger migraine, possibly through a reflex vasodilatation of vascular structures. Another example of a vasoactive substance precipitating headache is unusual sensitivity to the sodium nitrite used in cured meats, such as hot dogs, bacon, ham, and salami. Large amounts of ingested monosodium glutamate may produce generalized vasomotor reactions that include headache ("Chinese restaurant syndrome").

PRACTICAL CONSIDERATIONS IN THE EVALUATION OF HEADACHE

A careful history should include the location, duration, intensity, quality, and time of head pain. Sustained contraction headache is usually occipital or bitemporal in location, moderate in severity, and constrictive or band-like in quality. A vascular headache is a severe "pounding or throbbing" headache that is associated frequently with vomiting. The headache usually is unilateral, but may alternate sides, and may be bilateral. A pounding headache that occurs on the same side and is associated with focal neurologic deficit should raise the suspicion of an underlying structural abnormality (e.g., arteriovenous malformation). Dull constant headaches, which are primarily in the morning, should raise the suspicion of elevated intracranial pressure.

A careful dietary history is of value in eliciting inciting agents. As mentioned, in some patients subject to migraine, headaches may be precipitated by chocolate (phenylethylamine), alcohol, or foods with a high content of tyramine or other vasoactive substances. Systemic steroids, including the endogenous hormones (e.g., those of the menstrual cycle) and those of the oral contraceptives, commonly precipitate vascular headaches.

General physical examination including determination of blood pressure should be performed. Neurologic evaluation must include auscultation of the skull and neck; visual field evaluation by confrontation; funduscopic examination; and evaluation of sensation, gait, and reflexes. Soft systolic bruits are heard on auscultation of the skull in many children between the ages of 3 and 15 years. However, detection of a loud, continuous cranial bruit is an indication for more extensive neurodiagnostic procedures. It must be recognized, however, that angiography is undertaken with particular care in the evaluation of individuals with vascular headaches, since there is an increased risk of complications, including stroke. An electroencephalogram and a computerized axial tomographic scan should be considered in a patient with a focal neurologic deficit, a headache at a consistent location, a scalp or periosteal tenderness, and a refractory headache. However, it should be recognized that a significant number of migraine sufferers may have abnormal electroencephalogram patterns that do not reflect epilepsy or underlying structural disease. Positive emission tomography and nuclear magnetic resonance also may be considered. In the presence of fever and meningeal signs, lumbar puncture is indicated. However, if there is a significant possibility that a space-occupying intracranial lesion such as a tumor or an abscess is present, lumbar puncture is to be avoided as an initial diagnostic procedure.

Head pain consistent with rhinocephalgia may require radiographic examination of the paranasal sinuses, evaluation of allergy, and possibly further study of immunologic factors. Pale engorgement of the nasal turbinates suggests allergy or vasomotor rhinitis. In chronic purulent rhinitis, abnormalities of the humoral, cell mediated, or phagocytic limb of the immune system must be considered.

TREATMENT OF HEADACHES

Intelligent therapy of headache rests upon proper diagnosis. Headaches of inflammatory origin or those due to intracranial space-occupying lesions and arteriovenous malformations are beyond the scope of this text and will not be further considered. Muscle contraction headache usually responds to analgesics. In evaluating patients with muscle tension headaches, however, signs of depression should be sought and, if present, psychiatric evaluation obtained. Cluster headache is considered a migraine variant but may be responsive to corticosteroid and lithium carbonate therapy (Medina et al., 1980).

Various drugs have been advocated for the treatment of migraine. Ergot alkaloids, because of their constrictive effect on cerebral vasculature, should be used judiciously in migraine. A drug combination containing isometheptene mucate, a sympathomimetic amine, acts by constriction of dilated cranial and cerebral arterioles and may be helpful in treating mild migraine. Anticonvulsants, such as phenobarbital and phenytoin, have been used in children for treatment of migraine. However, hirsutism, gingival hyperplasia, changes in collagen structure, and other side effects are associated with the use of phenytoin, and this drug should be avoided in the treatment of childhood migraine.

Propranolol can be an effective prophylactic agent in migraine (Ludvigesson, 1974). Since it must be employed on a daily basis therapy is inconvenient. If the headache is of sufficient severity and frequency to warrant daily prophylaxis, propranolol would appear to be the most efficacious agent but should be avoided in patients with asthma, since it can precipitate or intensify bronchospasm. Tricyclic antidepressants (Couch et al., 1976); cyproheptadine, especially in children; and calcium channel blockers are alternative forms of therapy in patients with migraine and asthma. Calcium channel blockers, such as verapamil, offer another alternative for the prophylaxis of migraine (Markley et al., 1984). Before embarking on a therapeutic regimen of daily prophylaxis utilizing potent pharmacologic agents, the response of an individual patient with headache to less potent agents, such as acetaminophen and aspirin, should be evaluated.

Management of allergic factors and of sinusitus are discussed in detail elsewhere in this text.

REFERENCES

Bickerstaff, E.R.: Basilar artery migraine. Lancet 1:15, 1961.

Bille, B.: Migraine in school children. Acta Paediatr. Scand. 5:136, 1962.

Bruyn, G.W.: Biochemical Basis of Migraine: A critique. In Klawans, J.R. (ed.), Clinical Neuropharmacology. New York, Raven Press, 1976.

Burnstock, G.: Pathophysiology of migraine: A new hypothesis. Lancet 1:1397, 1981.

Couch J.R., Ziegler, D.K., Hassanein, K.: Amitryptyline in the prophylaxis of migraine. Neurology 26:121, 1976.

Dalessio, D.J.: Wolff's Headache and Other Head Pain, 3rd ed. New York, Oxford University Press, 1972a.

Dalessio, D.J.: Mechanisms and biochemistry of headache. Postgrad. Med 56:55, 1974.

Egger, J., Carter, C.M., Wilson, J., Turner, M.W., Soothill, J.F.: Is migraine food allergy? Lancet 2:865, 1983.

Friedman, A.T., Harms, E.: Headaches in Children. Springfield Ill., Charles C Thomas, 1967.

Golden, G.S., French, J.D.: Basilar artery migraine in young children. Pediatrics 56:722, 1975.

Guralnick, W., Kaban, L.B., Merrill, R.G.: Temporomandibular joint afflictions. N. Engl. J. Med. 313:123, 1978.

Ludvigesson, J.: Propranolol used in prophylaxis of migraine in children. Acta Neurol. Scand. 50:109, 1974.

Mansfield, L.E., Vaughan, T.R., Walker, S.F., Haverly, R.W., Ting, S.: Food allergy and adult migraine. Double-blind and mediator confirmation of an allergic etiology. Ann. Allergy 55:126, 1985.

Markley, H.G., Cheronis, J.C., Piepho, R.W.: Verapamil in prophylactic therapy of migraine. Neurology 34:973, 1984.

Medina, J.L., Fareed, J., Diamond, S.: Lithium carbonate therapy for cluster headache, changes in number of platelets, and serotonin and histamine levels. Arch. Neurol. 33:559, 1980.

Monroe, J., Cavin, C., Brustoff, J.: Migraine is a food allergic disease. Lancet 2:719, 1984.

Olesen, J., Larsen, B., Lauvitzen, M.D.: Focal hyperemia followed by spreading oligemia and impaired activation of r CBF and classic migraine. Ann. Neurol. 9:344, 1980.

Page, R.A., Fireman, P., Wolfson, S.K., Painter, M.J.: Food-induced cerebral blood flow and migraine headaches. (In press.)

57

Controversial Concepts and Practices in Allergy

JAMES G. EASTON, M.D.
MICHAEL S. KAPLAN, M.D.

Allergic diseases of various types, especially in the pediatric age group, are responsible for a significant amount of morbidity, school or work absence, and financial expenditure. Primary physicians and allergists are not able to provide definitive cures for many of these long-term problems. Consequently, as occurs with many chronic disease states, multiple alternative and controversial concepts and techniques have been promulgated for the management of allergic problems.

Some of the controversy related to these concepts and techniques appears to be semantic in nature, but some is related to the nature and amount of scientific investigation considered necessary for a hypothesis to be reasonably accepted as "fact" and, therefore, clinically applicable. Allergy usually is defined as "an altered state of immune reactivity, usually denoting hypersensitivity" (Stites et al., 1984). This definition implies involvement of immune mechanisms, and the term allergy is probably best not applied if such a mechanism has not been demonstrated. In several circumstances to be discussed, the term "food intolerance" would be preferable to "food allergy," since immune mechanisms have not been implicated. Furthermore, patient response to suggestion, placebo administration, or both is a well-recognized occurrence in clinical medicine, and the incidence of this type of response has been reported to be as high as 30 percent in allergic patients. Therefore, data from carefully conducted double-blind clinical studies should be essential to the acceptance of new concepts or techniques. Unfortunately, these studies are not always done. Van Metre (1983) has discussed this problem, and the reader is referred to his critique for further insights.

BEHAVIORAL DISTURBANCES

A variety of behavioral disturbances, especially irritability and hyperkinesis, have been attributed to ingestion of foods or food additives, and the disturbances frequently are labeled "food allergies." In many instances, these behavioral patterns have been described in patients with coexisting classic allergic diseases, such as rhinitis and asthma, and under these circumstances it is important to consider that behavioral or personality changes may be a result of the chronic illness itself or a side effect of the medications used in treatment. An example of such a situation might be one of a child with inadequately controlled asthma who has frequent sleep interruptions, resulting in fatigue and irritability leading to underachievement at school. Additionally, side effects of medication, such as theophylline, may cause hyperactivity, abdominal pain, and headache. It is easy to understand that these sleep and behavioral disturbances could have profound impacts on family interrelationships, resulting in further aggravation of behavioral problems.

Hyperkinetic Behavior Syndrome

The hyperkinetic behavior syndrome is a term generally used to describe a child who displays hyperactive and impulsive behavior, who has unusual distractibility, and who generally receives poor grades in school. This syndrome is estimated to occur in 5 to 10 percent of school-age children and is felt to have multiple etiologies. In 1975, Ben Feingold, M.D., (now deceased) published the book, *Why Your Child Is Hyperactive*, in which he proposed that this syndrome was frequently the result of ingestion of food additives and that often these children could be treated effectively with an additive-free diet. Since Dr. Feingold was an allergist, this concept was interpreted by many to imply an allergy to these additives, although this was never specifically stated in his writings and no immune mechanism was proposed.

Feingold's results were anecdotal in nature, with no attempt at confirmation using double-blind controlled trials. The concept was accepted by many physicians, however, and the

735

Feingold or Kaiser-Permanente* diet became popular in the management of hyperkinetic behavior. Because of the far-reaching implications associated both with the implementation of this rather strict diet and the possibility of control of hyperactive behavior, appropriate studies were considered critical and were performed by others. These studies are summarized in the proceedings of the Consensus Development Panel on *Defined Diets in Childhood Hyperactivity* sponsored by the National Institutes of Health (National Institutes of Health, 1982). An additional concise review of this subject was published in 1983 (Lipton and Mayo, 1983). The results strongly suggest that additive-free diets at best benefit only a very small percentage of children with hyperkinetic behavior (no greater than 2 percent), and evidence for immune reactions to these substances as a pathogenetic mechanism is lacking.

"Sugar Allergy"

More recently, similar behavior patterns of hyperactivity, aggressiveness, and poor school achievement have been attributed to diets high in sugar, perhaps associated with an abnormality of sugar metabolism, and have been referred to as "sugar allergy" (Crook, 1980). Hypoglycemia itself and the associated compensatory mechanisms, such as epinephrine release, may produce symptoms of restlessness, confusion, and irritability, but these are physiologic in nature with no immune basis. Thus, the term sugar allergy is not appropriate. Two recent well-controlled studies suggest that this syndrome, if it exists at all, is exceedingly rare (Rappaport, 1982/83; Mahan et al., 1985).

"Allergic Tension-Fatigue Syndrome"

Symptoms of the "allergic tension-fatigue syndrome" were originally described in 1922 by Shannon. Periods of anxiety, hyperactivity, and poor sleep alternating with periods of listlessness and fatigue are the primary manifestations often associated with headache, abdominal pain, infraorbital discoloration of the skin (so-called allergic shiners), and leg aches. The syndrome has been attributed primarily to food allergies, with milk, corn, wheat, and chocolate implicated most frequently. In some patients respiratory allergic symptoms coexist. Symptoms are said to resolve when the offending foods are removed from the diet.

That some or all of these symptoms may exist in patients with allergic disease is accepted by most authorities. Infraorbital discoloration occurs commonly in children with allergic rhinitis, and abdominal pain may occur as a manifestation of gastrointestinal allergy. Other symptoms may be nonspecific manifestations of chronic disease, side effects of medication, as discussed earlier, or both. However, no evidence exists that this syndrome is primarily the result of food allergy or, as has been suggested, is a primary allergic disorder of the central nervous system (Crook, 1973). Double-blind placebo-controlled studies investigating the effects of removal and reintroduction of suspect foods have not been performed. Crook (1975) attributes symptoms to "nonreaginic allergy" mediated by sensitized lymphocytes, but no investigational evidence exists to substantiate this theory.

Megavitamin therapy has been proposed as treatment in hyperactive behavior syndromes and therefore by implication in certain allergic states. There are no controlled studies investigating this type of treatment; with the known side effects of large doses of certain vitamins, this type of therapy cannot be recommended.

ENURESIS

Enuresis has been reported to be associated with allergic disease, especially food allergies (Breneman, 1965; Crook, 1974). Milk, corn, chocolate, cola, citrus fruits, and food coloring have been implicated most frequently. It is theorized that urinary bladder smooth muscle acts as an allergic target organ, much as airways smooth muscle does in asthma, with spasm causing decreased bladder capacity and enuresis. Success with elimination diets has been reported, but adequately designed placebo-controlled studies have not been done. When one considers the social and emotional impact that a problem such as enuresis may have on a child and on family relationships, control for a placebo effect in evaluating any therapeutic intervention is essential.

---

*Named after the Kaiser-Permanente Medical Center in California where Dr. Feingold practiced.

HEADACHE

Headache is a frequent complaint in the general population, although less common in children than in adults. It may occur more frequently in persons with respiratory allergies. Head pain as the result of disturbances in the nasal cavities and paranasal sinuses, so-called rhinocephalgia, is a well-recognized entity. Allergic rhinitis with nasal obstruction as the result of mucosal edema, often with obstruction of sinus ostia, is a common cause of this type of headache (see Chapter 56). Headaches may also occur as side effects of drugs (e.g., theophylline, sympathomimetics) given for the control of allergic diseases, and tension headaches may occur in association with any chronic disease, including allergy.

The association of food allergies and migraine headache (allergic migraine) is less certain. Earlier studies suggesting this association were entirely anecdotal in nature. However, in 1983, Egger and colleagues reported an investigation of 88 children with migraine, 77 of whom became symptom free on a strict elimination diet. The offending foods were then identified by careful dietary reintroduction. Forty of the 77 responders were tested with double-blind challenges to the identified food, and 26 reacted with headaches. No evaluation of allergy in the participants was done, so that evidence for or against an allergic mechanism is not available from this study. Mansfield and coworkers (1985) studied 43 adult patients with classic recurrent migraine headaches. Sixteen had at least one positive immediate skin test reaction to a large battery of commercial food extracts, and 13 of these 16 showed at least a 66 percent reduction in headache frequency when the food was eliminated from their diet. Only seven of the 16 were available for double-blind food challenges, but in five, at least one food provoked the headache. Thus, it seems possible that food ingestion may be the precipitating factor for migraine headache in some patients, and headache can be a manifestation of an immediate-type immune reaction.

"CANDIDIASIS HYPERSENSITIVITY SYNDROME"

The most recently proposed controversial concept is the "candidiasis hypersensitivity syndrome" or "the yeast connection." The strongest advocate of this concept is Crook (1984) who has espoused it in a book entitled, *The Yeast Connection —A Medical Breakthrough.* He refers to the recognition and management of this syndrome as "the coming revolution in medicine." Symptoms said to occur as the result of this problem are varied, involve multiple organ systems, and in general are rather nonspecific. The symptoms include fatigue, depression, various skin disorders, gastrointestinal and respiratory symptoms, aching muscles and joints, and hyperactivity.

Crook lists 15 sets of circumstances under which this syndrome should be especially suspect as follows:

1. Feeling bad "all over," yet the cause can't be identified and treatment of many kinds hasn't helped.

2. Prolonged courses of broad-spectrum antibiotics.

3. Consumption of large amounts of yeast and sugar.

4. Craving for sweets.

5. Craving for other carbohydrates, especially breads and pizza.

6. Ingestion of sweets worsening symptoms or causing a "pickup" followed by a "let down."

7. Symptoms of "hypoglycemia" but tests fail to confirm this diagnosis.

8. Craving for alcohol.

9. Use of birth control pills or corticosteroids.

10. Multiple pregnancies.

11. Recurrent problems related to reproductive organs, such as abdominal pain, premenstrual tension, and impotence.

12. Persistent or recurrent digestive or nervous system symptoms or both.

13. Persistent or recurrent athlete's foot or "jock itch."

14. Feeling bad on damp days or in moldy places.

15. Ill feelings when exposed to perfumes, tobacco smoke, and some chemicals.

Most of the preceding symptoms and circumstances are, of course, nonspecific and highly subjective and may be experienced at one time or another in a significant percentage of the general population. Dr. Crook also points out that these symptoms may be caused by medical problems other than "*Candida* hypersensitivity" and that a thorough evaluation by the patient's physician is advisable when such symptoms are present. He further indicates that the diagnosis must be suspected from a history of the aforementioned complaints and is then confirmed by the response to treatment. Laboratory tests are said to be of little if any value, even though dysfunction of the immune system is said to be present (see following section).

The basis for this syndrome, as described in Dr. Crook's book, is as follows:

1. Antibiotics, especially broad-spectrum types, kill "friendly germs" at the same time they kill "enemies."

2. Killing "friendly germs" allows "yeast germs" *(Candida albicans)*, normally present in the body in small numbers, to multiply. Diets rich in carbohydrates and the use of birth control pills, corticosteroids, and "other drugs" also stimulate yeast growth.

3. Large numbers of yeasts produce sufficient toxins to weaken the immune system. This alteration in the immune system, not further defined, is then responsible for the multiplicity of symptoms.

4. As the result of the weakened immune system additional infections occur, which are treated with antibiotics allowing additional yeast growth, toxin production, and so forth.
It is further suggested that fatigue, depression, allergies, and possibly cancer and acquired immune deficiency syndrome (AIDS) may result from this type of weakening of the immune system.

The proposed treatment of candidiasis hypersensitivity includes (1) avoiding consumption of foods that promote yeast growth (although the specifics of such a diet are not entirely clear), (2) avoiding birth control pills, antibiotics, and environmental mold sources, (3) initiating steps to improve general health, and (4) in some cases injections with *Candida* extracts and the use of antifungal agents.

Dr. Crook's book contains much testimonial evidence and anecdotal data regarding the prevalence of this syndrome and the response to treatment. However, it offers no scientific evidence in the form of controlled studies to substantiate *Candida albicans* as the cause or that the proposed management, including treatment with antifungal agents, permits improvement. Furthermore, no data on abnormal functioning of the immune system allegedly caused by *Candida* "toxins" in these patients are presented. It is important that this syndrome not be confused with chronic mucocutaneous candidiasis which is associated with documented immune dysfunction.

INTRACUTANEOUS TITRATION FOR INHALANT ALLERGENS

In 1926, Phillips popularized the use of intracutaneous titration with aqueous allergens to determine a safe starting dose for coseasonal injection therapy with inhalant allergens. The end point was a wheal "the size of the palm" (Phillips, 1926). Hansel (1941) outlined a specific protocol for determining starting dose and stepwise coseasonal treatment.

Rinkel modified the technique in 1949 and again in 1962 by using five-fold dilutions to determine the end point. The end point was the dilution that produced a wheal greater than 7 mm in diameter, initiated progressive wheals with higher concentrations, and was 2 mm larger in diameter than the preceding test. He used nine dilutions of a basic 1:20 pollen or mold mix (1:20–1:4,000,000). The optimal treatment dose was that volume of the end point dilution that resulted in clinical improvement within 4 hours after the injection and lasted up to a week or more (Rinkel, 1949 and 1962). Since 1949, other practitioners have applied their own interpretations of the "end point" (Greico, 1982). The end point is variable in any given patient on any given day. Reasons for the variation and reasons for the treatment failure with the Rinkel technique are listed in Table 57–1.

As Greico (1982) has pointed out, most of Rinkel's patients had an "optimal dose" that would be equivalent to 40 to 1000 protein nitrogen unit (PNU) per ml, a low treatment dose by conventional standards. Double-blind studies comparing the Rinkel technique with conventional immunotherapy confirm that low dosages are used in the Rinkel technique (i.e., 0.001 to 0.006 μg protein median dose). Conventional immunotherapy was more effective in reducing symptom and medication scores compared with the Rinkel technique or placebo; in these studies, the Rinkel technique was no more effective than placebo (VanMetre, et al., 1980; Hirsch et al., 1981).

Skin test end point titration is a useful guide to determine a safe starting dose of injection therapy, but controlled studies have not shown this technique to be useful for optimal treatment of pollenosis. The technique tends to overestimate the sensitivity of the patient, providing a wide margin of safety for starting injections. It has been our experience that patients can tolerate higher antigen doses subcutane-

TABLE 57–1. Rinkel Technique Pitfalls*

Variability of Endpoint	Treatment Failure
Modified by prior therapy	Suboptimal treatment dose
Modified by pollen inhalation	Unidentified antigens
Prior overdose and suboptimal dose	Concomitant food allergy
Dose provokes systemic reaction	Inaccurate endpoint determination
Infection or fever	Reduced antigen temperature
Ambient air temperature	Alternate injection site†

* Adapted from Golbert, T.M.: A review of controversial diagnostic and therapeutic techniques employed in allergy. J. Allergy Clin. Immunol. 56:170–190, 1975.
† Some have observed that the same antigen concentration injected into a different site in the same patient produces a different reaction.

ously than are indicated by their sensitivities to intracutaneous injections of the same antigens. This finding may be due to a sparser population of reactive cells in the subcutaneous tissues compared with the layers of the dermis.

INTRACUTANEOUS AND SUBCUTANEOUS PROVOCATION

An extension of the Rinkel technique was designed to treat patients who have chronic symptoms that are not limited to classic allergic symptoms. The technique introduced by Lee in 1961 and expanded by Rinkel in 1964 attempts to provoke then to neutralize specific symptoms by subcutaneous and intracutaneous injections mainly of food antigens. Proponents point out the advantages of a double end point, involving both wheals (objective) and symptoms (subjective), and an ability to provide rapid symptom relief. An algorithm of the diagnostic and treatment techniques is presented in Figure 57–1.

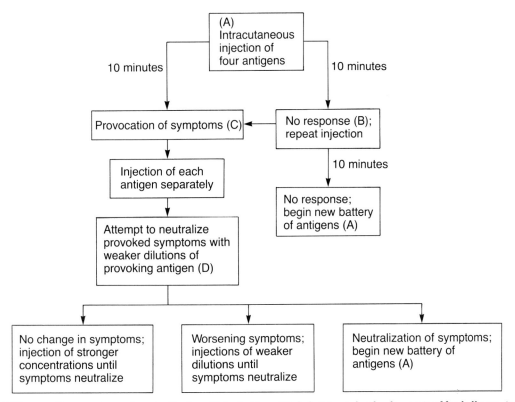

FIGURE 57–1. Provocation and neutralization. (Adapted from Rinkel, H.J., et al.: The diagnosis of food allergy. Arch. Otolaryngol. *79:* 71–76, 1964.)

Rinkel pointed out that neutralization fails when the dose is too strong or too weak; the practitioner often has to reverse the direction of progressive doses, using either more concentrated or more dilute extract. The neutralizing dose is usually injected by the patient twice weekly, or, in some cases, daily, to allow tolerance to the ingestion of offending foods (Miller, 1972).

It has been suggested that intracutaneous administration of antigen allows substances such as proteoses and peptones to bypass the gastrointestinal tract and to directly interact with lymphocytes. Lymphocytes are thought to be necessary to continue the reaction. Neutralization is thought to be achieved by subanaphylactic doses of systemically administered antigen given frequently enough to maintain the lymphocytes in a "desensitized state" (Morris, 1969).

Most practitioners employing this technique allow their patients to self administer the neutralizing doses at home. However, doses in the range usually used have been reported to cause serious, even fatal reactions when food extracts (especially fish, nuts, and seeds) have been administered in conventional intradermal skin testing (Hale, 1960). On the one hand, the practice of intradermal skin testing to food extracts in concentrations stronger than 1:1000 has largely been abandoned by conventional allergists. On the other hand, Willoughby (1965) reported no fatal anaphylactic reactions after 200,000 provocation tests.

In 1977, Miller reported results of a double-blind crossover study of eight patients successfully treated with provocation and neutralization. During the study period, patients adhered to individualized diets that included foods for which neutralization solutions were being given. The study covered four consecutive 20-day periods of alternating active and placebo injections. An elaborate symptom improvement score was used to evaluate the patients, i.e., from 0 (no change) to 4+ (complete relief of symptoms). Symptom changes were recorded during and at the end of the four 20-day courses but not daily. Symptoms included migraine headaches, nausea, vomiting, emotional lability, hyperactivity and other behavior problems, aphthous stomatitis, vertigo, enuresis, skin rashes, and nasal symptoms. It is unclear from the report whether the physician or the patient recorded the symptoms. The placebo was mushroom extract. Each patient was first given an open trial with the "neutralizing" solution to test the adequacy of the "neutralizing dose" and the ability of the patient to adhere to the individual diet. Therefore, each of the eight patients knew beforehand the appearance of the active solution, which may have influenced symptom reporting. As a group, the active treatment was stated to produce a statistically significant improvement compared with the placebo. However, two patients in the active group had little improvement over those in the placebo group, and three other patients had only modest improvement (less than the mean for the group).

Kailin and Collier (1971), in a double-blind trial, found no difference in symptom relief among patients using sublingual or intracutaneous "neutralizing" solutions versus saline. They allowed five physicians with at least 7 years experience with provocation and neutralization procedures to choose the patients and the food antigens based on previous provocation responses. Interestingly, 23 of 34 provocation trials with antigen resulted in relief of symptoms (71 percent), but 28 of 40 trials with saline also resulted in symptom relief (70 percent). Rinkel reported no discrepancy in results between provocative skin tests and oral food challenges. However, no individual data were presented, and the data were aggregated by food (Rinkel et al., 1964). Draper (1972) compared 193 positive intracutaneous provocation test results with oral food challenge results with the same antigen. Of the oral challenge results, 120 were positive (62 percent); in other words, there were falsely positive "provocative" skin tests in 38 percent. The rate of positive correlation for the two tests is less than that reported for conventional skin tests and for end-organ provocation for inhalant allergens (Hosen, 1965).

The American College of Allergists studied 70 patients in a double-blind crossover fashion for responses to subcutaneous food antigen provocation. Although some foods did provoke symptoms, results were not reproducible. Moreover, skin test results did not correlate with oral food challenge results (Caplin, 1973). A double-blind study by the American Academy of Allergy also found the subcutaneous food provocation test to be a poor predictor of food sensitivity (Crawford et al., 1976).

An assessment by the National Center for Health Care Technology in 1981 concluded that the clinical effectiveness of intracutaneous or subcutaneous food neutralization has not been conclusively demonstrated, citing the aforementioned studies and drawing from the communication of the American Academy of Allergy that provocation cannot be explained on the basis of any known sequence of immune events (Heyse, 1981).

SUBLINGUAL PROVOCATION AND NEUTRALIZATION

In 1964, Dickey and Pfeifer expanded Hansel's suggestion of sublingual administration of antigen. Diluted food extracts are administered by dropper sublingually. If symptoms appear within 20 minutes, a more dilute solution of the same antigen is applied sublingually to "neutralize" the symptoms. The "neutralizing" dose then is used regularly when an offending food cannot be avoided. As with subcutaneous provocation, the proponents of sublingual provocation claim that it allows systemic absorption of intact food allergens by bypassing the gastrointestinal tract where it would otherwise be transported and altered. The systemically absorbed food extract theoretically stimulates lymphocytes with small doses of antigen to "desensitize" them. Self administration of diluted food extracts sublingually, avoiding injection, is more acceptable to patients, and adverse reactions are reported to be rare.

Despite several anecdotal reports on the successful use of sublingual provocation, there are no convincing studies of its safety or efficacy. Kailin and Collier (1971) reported that 70 percent of 40 patients experienced relief using saline drops in a double-blind controlled study. The Food Allergy Committee of the American College of Allergists found approximately 30 percent positive reactions using food extracts of various concentrations but concluded that the tests did not discriminate between reactions to control solutions and food extracts (Breneman et al., 1974). Lehman (1980a) also did not find significant differences between placebo and food extracts in the provocation of symptoms.

Subanaphylactic doses of antigen administered systemically may desensitize lymphocytes and basophils to antigen *in vitro* (Gatien et al., 1975; Mendoza, 1982), but there is no evidence that mast cells or basophils can be desensitized by sublingual administration of antigen. Drawing on penicillin desensitization as a model for allergen tolerance, the state of such tolerance is a delicate balance, requiring more or less continuous antigen exposure. One would expect neither rapidly induced nor sustained tolerance by the intermittent sublingual administration of food extracts as described previously.

LEUKOCYTOTOXIC TESTING

The leukopenic index, described initially in the 1930's, measures the fall in total white blood cell count and polymorphonuclear neutrophils (PMNs) compared with baseline levels after ingestion or inhalation of antigen. Squire and Lee (1947) reported that ragweed antigen added to sensitized leukocytes *in vitro* results in lysis of these cells, although this could not be substantiated by Franklin and Lowell (1949). These observations were the basis for Black's leukocytotoxic test for the diagnosis of allergy (Black, 1956). The technique involves mixing cells from the buffy coat layer of the patient's blood with the patient's plasma or serum on a glass slide and adding a small amount of food extract or control solution. After appropriate incubation, the slide is examined for cytolytic changes, which are graded from negative to severe, as depicted in Figure 57–2. Theoretically, the cytotoxic effect on the polymorphonuclear leukocytes is triggered by antigen-antibody complexes, containing the reactive food, or by a direct toxic effect of that food. Black used the test to "diagnose" ten patients for whom no clinical correlates were offered. Bryan and Bryan (1960) applied Black's technique for food antigens in 107 pediatric and adult patients and reported subjective improvement of symptoms in 80 percent after elimination of the reacting food. Chambers et al., (1958) could not duplicate Black's results using the same method. Thirteen children with well-documented sensitivities to pollen, dander, or food were tested. Only 1 of 24 known sensitivities was identified.

Ulett and Perry (1975) found *in vivo* leukocytosis after ingestion of a sensitizing food and reported a perfect correlation with *in vitro* leukocytotoxicity, especially when the leukocytotoxic test was done at the peak of leukocytosis. In a controlled, blinded clinical trial, 45 adult and pediatric patients were divided into three groups as follows: 20 nonatopic, 15 atopic with well-documented and reproducible reactions to ingested foods, and 10 with suspected but unconfirmed reactions to foods (fatigue, nonurticarial rash, rhinitis, diarrhea, and shortness of breath). In the atopic group, the test failed to detect 73 percent of known sensitivities and 80 percent of suspected sensitivities. All atopic

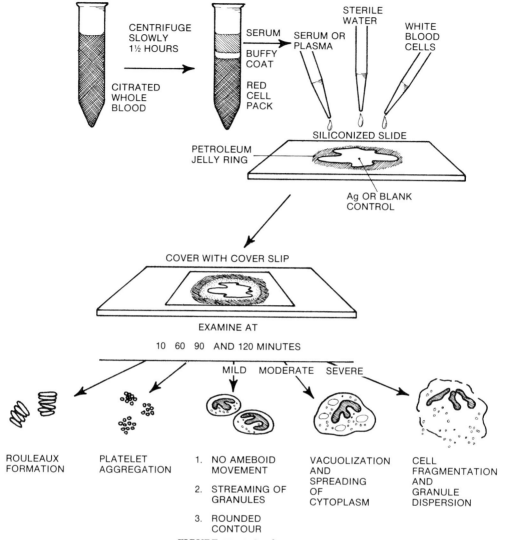

FIGURE 57–2. Leukocyte test.

subjects had false-positive test results to at least three foods, and 44 of 45 patients had false-positive test results to an average of 5.5 foods. When duplicate tests were examined in a blinded fashion, there was a lack of reproducible interpretation of cytotoxic changes (Lieberman et al., 1975). Lehman (1980b) did not find the results of cytotoxic tests reproducible from day to day, even when controlled for possible interference from elimination diets and sublingual food drop therapy. This result contrasts with another study in which an 80 percent intraobserver agreement was reached on 3 consecutive days when technicians were properly trained and supervised (Holopainen et al., 1980).

The problems of interpretation notwithstanding, Benson and Arkins (1976) were able to achieve reproducible *in vitro* test results in nine atopic and five control patients, using six replicate samples that were reviewed by one examiner in a blinded fashion. However, the atopic group had 70 percent and the control group had 57 percent false positive test results. The investigators did not look for reproducibility of results on subsequent days. They concluded that cytotoxic tests offered no reliable help in the diagnosis of food allergy.

It appears that the leukocytotoxic test requires well-trained and well-supervised technicians to achieve reproducibility. It is time-consuming and tedious work. Moreover, the test results do not correlate with clinical food sensitivity. In March of 1985, the Food and Drug Administration (FDA) ruled that *in vitro* leukocytotoxic testing is an "unproven diagnostic procedure" and ruled against the marketing and use of cytotoxic testing kits (FDA Compliance Guide, March 1985).

URINE AUTOINJECTION

In 1930, Oriel and Barber described increased proteoses in the urine of allergic individuals, especially during acute allergy attacks. They believed that the proteoses contained antigens to which patients were sensitive. Subsequently, proteoses were found not only in the urine of atopic individuals between attacks but also in the urine of nonatopic individuals. Oriel (1932) and Conybeare and Oriel (1931) reported positive intradermal skin reactions in sensitive patients using the patients' urine. They reported that urine from a nonatopic individual did not give a positive skin test result and that urine from a sensitive individual gave a positive test result only in another individual with similar sensitivities. Freeman (1932) was not able to duplicate these results, however, and concluded that the reaction was nonspecific and toxic in nature.

Cornblect and Kaplan (1933) dialyzed away the toxic substance and eliminated the erythema produced by skin testing with the native urine. Upon identifying a patient with a positive skin test reaction to their own urine, the urine was injected into the patient to "desensitize" against the antigen or proteose. Urine was prepared by treating it with a "little" chloroform and acidifying it with H_2SO_4, followed by ether extraction, alcohol precipitation, centrifugation, and drying. The preparation was then resuspended in dilute NaOH and diluted in buffer. Injection schedules were either arbitrary or based on skin test titration reactions (Libman, and Biglony, 1937). The early proponents of urine proteose injections reported significant cures for allergic skin disease, asthma, hayfever, rheumatoid arthritis, and epilepsy (Oriel and Barber 1930; Oriel, 1932; Yoeman et al., 1932; Burgess, 1933; Eichenlaub, 1933; Darley and Whitehead, 1931). Almost immediately, however, reports appeared denying any therapeutic benefits from urinary proteose injections for these same disorders (Freeman, 1932; Minchin and Haviland, 1932; Cormia, 1934; Templeton, 1934; Trashoff and Meranze, 1932).

The use of autogenous urine injections resurfaced in 1947 when Plesch reported success in treating 12 patients. The evidence for relief of allergic and constitutional symptoms was entirely anecdotal. He sterilized the urine by boiling or filtration then injected it intramuscularly in doses of 0.25 to 5.0 ml. Since then, there have been only further anecdotal reports of "cures" for a variety of allergic disorders. As of 1981, the American Academy of Allergy was not able to find a published report to support the use of this modality (Reisman, 1981). Autogenous urine injection therapy should be considered experimental and potentially dangerous. Autogenous injections can induce autoimmune nephritis in rabbits due to glomerular basement membrane antigens excreted in the urine (Hawkins and Cochran, 1965). Humans also excrete protein immunologically related to glomerular basement membrane (McPhaul and Dixon, 1969).

FOOD IMMUNE COMPLEX ASSAY

Anaphylactic sensitivity to food causes rapid, recognizable symptoms, which usually can be confirmed by skin tests, serologic tests for IgE antibody, or both. Delayed reactions to foods are claimed to occur hours to days after the ingestion of implicated food or combination of foods and are not classic anaphylactic reactions. Patients are purported to present with headaches, abdominal cramps, muscle cramps, fatigue, and mood changes. Tests to confirm this type of reaction, however, have not been validated. It has been postulated that these reactions are mediated by non-IgE antibodies that form immune complexes, a belief that is fostered by the detection of such antibodies in the sera of some patients who give histories of food sensitivities (Parish, 1971; Goodwin, 1983; Necessary et al., 1984).

Assays for food immune complexes are available through some commercial clinical immunology laboratories. The proponents of these assays state that they offer the advantages of (1) diagnosing of delayed reactions to foods when routine allergy test reactions are negative, (2) not requiring a discontination of medications, (3) mailing of serum samples, (4) automated testing not requiring subjective interpretation. Although the idea for such a relatively simple test for diagnosing "hidden" food allergy is attractive and is fueled by the frustration that many practitioners and their patients have in attempting to evaluate the causes of a myriad of vague complaints, there is no scientific documentation of the validity of this test for diagnosing any clinical problem.

Circulating immune complexes are thought to play a role in a variety of diseases but are found in healthy individuals as well and in individuals with physiologic conditions such as pregnancy (Paganelli et al., 1981) (Table 57–2). Using extremely sensitive radioimmunoassays, IgG antibodies to bovine gamma globulin can be detected in 70 percent of normal individuals, and precipitating antibodies to ingested food antigens can be found in virtually all IgA deficient patients, even in the absence of symptoms (Foucard et al., 1975). Circulating immune complexes reflect antigenic stimulation; individuals with decreased gastrointestinal mucosal barriers for any reason are more likely to absorb antigens and produce serum antibodies in moderate to high titers, therefore, predisposing them to the development of immune complexes. These complexes peak after a meal, clear rapidly, and, in the vast majority of patients, do not appear to cause disease. Atopic individuals may differ from nonatopic individuals to some extent in the biologic properties of immune complexes involving milk antigen after an oral milk challenge. However, Paganelli and coworkers (1983) were unable to correlate any immediate or delayed reactions in eczematous children with the different types of immune complexes generated.

Inflammatory changes consistent with immune complex disease either have been absent or have not been looked for in studies attempting to correlate the detection of these complexes with clinical findings (Parish, 1970 and 1971; Dannaeus et al., 1977; Brostoff et al., 1979). Serum sickness type reactions have not been reported in such patients. Brostoff and colleagues (1979) suggested that the pathologic changes in eczema are consistent with the changes induced by the injection of immune complexes in the skin of experimental animals, but immune complexes have not been demonstrated in the lesions of naturally occurring human eczema.

In addition to the biologic activities of the particular immunoglobulin involved, differences in size and binding capacities of various immunoglobulins and of complexes formed also influence the biologic effects of the complexes. These could result either in a variety of disease syndromes not limited to an Arthus type reaction or in no disease at all (Lambert et al., 1978).

Three different assays have been used to identify food immune complexes as follows: polyethylene glycol precipitation, inhibition of rheumatoid factor agglutination, and two-site radioimmunosorbent assay. Circulating immune complexes of all immunoglobulin classes can be precipitated in polyethylene glycol. The precipitate can then be disassociated in an acid pH and the antigen adsorbed onto polystyrene tubes. The antigen is detected by radiolabeled, affinity purified specific antibody. Enzyme linked immunosorbent assay (ELISA) can be used instead of the radiolabeled antibody (Paganelli et al., 1981). Using this method, Paganelli and coworkers found circulating immune complexes containing beta-lactoglobulin and bovine serum albumin in a majority of healthy individuals. Peak levels occurred at 1 hour and at 3 to 5 hours after milk challenge. Patients with eczema had higher levels of immune complexes, with peaks occurring in the same time sequence as normal individuals (Paganelli et al., 1981). Another assay indirectly reflects the presence of food antigens in circulating IgG immune complexes by inhibiting rheumatoid factor agglutination of IgG-coated latex particles. Addition of food antigens identical to those in the complex causes antigen excess and a dissociation of the immune complex, resulting in an inhibition of agglutination (Lurhuma et al., 1976). These assays are time consuming and technically difficult. Leary and Halsey (1984) developed an assay that is antigen and isotype specific. Antigen conjugated paper discs are exposed to rabbit antibody that is specific for the food antigen. The same or cross-reacting antigen in the patient's serum (presumably complexed to circulating antibody) will fix to the rabbit antibody on the disc. This new complex, consisting of disc food, antigen food–specific rabbit IgG and food antigen-antibody complex, is then reacted with I[125] horse or goat antihuman immunoglobulin purified for specificity

TABLE 57–2. Clinical States in Which Food Immune Complexes are Detected*

No Disease Association	Possible Disease Association
Young infants†	Inflammatory bowel disease†‡
Healthy individuals	Eczema†
Pregnancy	Selective IgA deficiency†

* Adapted from Johannson et al., 1984.
† States in which there is increased gastrointestinal absorption of antigen
‡ During remission antibodies to foods decrease or disappear.

against a given human immunoglobulin isotype. A control disc with normal rabbit IgG allows measurement of nonspecific binding of IgE in a patient with serum IgE concentrations over 1000 IU/ml. These assays are limited by the availability of specific antisera, not only to native food but also to new antigens generated by the digestive products of the native foods (Haddad et al., 1979; Schwartz et al., 1980).

Brostoff and associates (1979) looked at the time course of food entry via the gastrointestinal tract and the production of immune complexes in atopic and nonatopic individuals. Five nonatopic patients showed rises in either IgG or IgA complexes after ingestion of 2 pints of milk. There was either a single early peak or an early and 3 to 5 hour delayed peak. The level of IgG containing circulating immune complexes remained within the normal range while the peak level of IgA complexes exceeded the normal range. The patients did not develop symptoms. In egg sensitive patients, there were reciprocal relationships between monomeric IgE and IgE immune complexes. Within 30 minutes after ingestion of egg, a rapid disappearance of monomeric IgE occurred with a return at 3 hours and another decline at 7 hours, which roughly corresponds to apparent clinical symptomatology. Unfortunately, no pathologic correlates were obtained and no chemical mediators were measured. The IgE complexes cleared rapidly. In this same study, oral cromolyn inhibited the late fall in monomeric IgE as well as the early and late rise in IgE containing immune complexes. One might postulate that cromolyn, by inhibiting anaphylactic mediator release, prevents further absorption of antigen and subsequent antigen stimulation that result in the formation of complexing antibody.

Necessary and colleagues (1984) used a two-site radioimmunoassay to identify IgE and IgG complexes of food allergic patients. Of 45 patients whose history suggested food sensitivity, 25 had immune complexes to milk and 10 had positive RAST reactions to milk. All 15 patients with acute allergic symptoms, including urticaria and eczema, had IgG complexes. Only two patients had IgE complexes. The incidence of IgG complexes in patients with more vague symptoms was lower and was absent in controls. Claims by commercial laboratories that assays of this type can be used to diagnose hidden (clinically inapparent) food allergy or the cause of a multitude of symptoms, including headache, abdominal pain, fatigue, muscle ache, and tension are not substantiated by this study, nor is there other literature to support the association of food immune complexes with the type of symptoms mentioned. May and colleagues (1977) could not find any correlation in older children between high levels of nonIgE antibodies to milk protein and ovalbumin and intolerance to these food substances.

Food immune complexes appear to be normal physiologic mechanisms for antigen elimination. Rather than cause disease, IgG food immune complexes may be tolerogenic by interacting with T cells, B cells, and macrophages to hinder the synthesis of further specific antibody, as well as the production and release of lymphokines (Delire, 1979). Thus, a relationship between food immune complexes and clinical disease remains to be proved.

REFERENCES

Benson, T.E., Arkins, J.A.: Cytotoxic testing for food allergy: Evaluation of reproducibility and correlation. J. Allergy Clin. Immunol. 58:471–476, 1976.

Black, A.P.: A new diagnostic method in allergic disease. Pediatrics 17:716–724, 1956.

Breneman, J.C.: Nocturnal enuresis, a treatment regimen for general use. Ann. Allergy 23:185, 1965.

Breneman, J.C., Hurst, A., Heiner, D., Leney, F.L., Morris, D., Josephson, B.M.: Final report of the Food Allergy Committee of the American College of Allergists on the clinical evaluation of sublingual provocation testing method for the diagnosis of food allergy. Ann. Allergy 33:164–166, 1974.

Brostoff, J., Carini, C., Wraith, D.A., Paganelli, R.: Immune Complexes in Atopy. In Pepys, J., Edwards, A.M. (eds.), The Mast Cell. Pitman, London, 1979.

Bryan, W.T., Bryan, M.P.: The application of *in vitro* cytotoxic reactions to the clinical diagnosis of food allergy. Laryngoscope 70:810–824, 1960.

Burgess, N.: Experiences with proteoses in treatment of diseases of skin. Brit Med. J. 1:914, 1933.

Caplin, I.: Report of the committee on provocative food testing. Ann. Allergy 31:375–381, 1973.

Chambers, V.V., Hudson, B.H., Glaser, J.A.: A study of the reactions of human PMNs to various antigens. J. Allergy 29:93–102, 1958.

Conybaere, E.T., Oriel, G.H.: Some experiments on pollen sensitization in asthma. Guys Hosp. Report 81:458, 1931.

Cormia, F.E.: Urinary proteose: Allergic dermatoses and eczema-asthma-hayfever complex. Arch. Derm. Syph. 28:346, 1934.

Cornblect, T., Kaplan, M.A.: Urinary proteose in eczema. Arch. Derm. Syph. 29:497, 1933.

Crawford, L.V., Lieberman, P., Harfi, H.A., Hale, R., Nelsen, H., Selner, J., Wittig, H., Postman, M., Zietz, A.: Double blind study of subcutaneous food testing (Food Committee of the American Academy of Allergy). J. Allergy Clin. Immunol. 57:236, 1976.

Crook, W.G.: Your Allergic Child. New York, Medcom Press, 1973.

Crook, W.G.: Genitourinary allergy. In Speer,F., Dockhorn,

R.J. (eds.), Allergy and Immunology in Childhood. Springfield, Illinois, Charles C Thomas, 1974.

Crook, W.G.: Food allergy-the great masquerader. Pediatr. Clin. N. Am. 22:227, 1975.

Crook, W.G.: Can what a child eats make him dull, stupid or hyperactive? J. Learning Disabil. 13:281, 1980.

Crook, W.G.: The Yeast Connection; A Medical Breakthrough, 2nd ed. Jackson, Tennessee, Professional Books, 1984.

Dannaeus, A., Johannson, S.G.O., Foucard, T., Ohmen, S.: Clinical and immunological aspects of food allergy in childhood. Acta Pediatr. Scand. 66:31, 1977.

Darley, W., Whitehead, R.: Studies on urinary proteose: Skin reactions and therapeutic response to injections. Proc. Soc. Exp. Biol. New York 28:668, 1931.

Delire, M.: Detection of circulating immune complexes in infants fed cow's milk. In Pepys, J., Edwards, A.M. (eds.), The Mast Cell. Pitman, London, 1979.

Dickey, L.D., Pfeiffer, G.: Sublingual therapy in allergy. Trans. Am. Soc. Ophth. Otolaryngol. Allergy 5:37, 1964.

Draper, L.W.: Food testing in allergy: Intradermal provocative vs. deliberate feeding. Arch. Otolaryngol. 95:196, 1972.

Egger, J., Wilson, J., Carter, C.M., Turner, M.W., Soothill, J.F.: Is migraine food allergy: A double-blind controlled trial of oligoantigenic diet treatment. Lancet 2:865–868, 1983.

Eichenlaub, F.J.: Urinary proteoses in dermatoses. Arch. Derm. Syph. 27:316, 1933.

FDA Compliance Policy Guide 7124.27 – Chapter 24. Devices. March, 1985.

Feingold, B.F.: Why Your Child Is Hyperactive. New York, Random House, 1975.

Foucard, T., Bennich, H., Johannson, S.G.O., Lundkvist, V.: Human antibodies to bovine gammaglobulin: Occurrence in immunological disorders and influence on allergy radioimmunoassays. Int. Arch. Allergy Appl. Immunol. 48:812, 1975.

Franklin W., Lowell, F.C.: Failure of ragweed pollen extract to destroy white cells from ragweed sensitive patients. J. Allergy 20:375, 1949.

Freeman, J.: Specificity of proteose intradermal reactions. Lancet 1:561, 1932.

Gatien, J.G., Merler, E., Colten, H.: Allergy to ragweed antigen E: Effect of specific immunotherapy on human T lymphocytes in vitro. Clin. Immunol. Immunopath. 4:32–37, 1975.

Golbert, T.M.: A review of controversial diagnostic and therapeutic techniques employed in allergy. J. Allergy Clin. Immunol. 56:170–190, 1975.

Goodwin, B.F.J.: Nonreaginic anaphylactic antibodies in man. Clin. Rev. Allergy 1:249, 1983.

Grieco, M.H.: Controversial practices in allergy. J.A.M.A. 247:3106–3111, 1982.

Haddad, Z.H., Kalra, V., Verma, S.: Antibody to peptic and peptic-trypsin digests of beta-lactoglobulin. Ann. Allergy 42:368, 1979.

Hale, R.: Seeds as a source of food testing material. Ann. Allergy 18:270, 1960.

Hansel, F.K.: Coseasonal treatment of hayfever. J. Allergy 12:457–461, 1941.

Hawkins, D., Cochran, C.G.: Glomerular basement membrane damage in immunologically induced glomerulonephritis. Immunology 14:665, 1965.

Heyse, H.P.: Intracutaneous and subcutaneous provocation and neutralization testing and neutralization therapy

for food allergies. U.S. Dept. Health Human Serv. Vol. 1, No. 10, 1981.

Hirsch, S.R., Kalbfleish, J.H., Golbert, T.M., Josephson, B.M., McConnell, L.H., Scanlon, R., Knicker, W.R., Fink, J.N., Murphee, J.J., Cohen, S.H.: Rinkel method: A multicenter controlled study. J. Allergy Clin. Immunol. 68:133–155, 1981.

Holopainen, E., Palva, T., Stenberg, P.T. Backman, A.: Cytotoxic leukocyte reaction. Acta Otolaryngol. 89:222–226, 1980.

Hosen, H.: Provocative nasal tests for the diagnosis of inhalant allergens. Ann. Allergy 23:497, 1965.

Johannson, S.G.O., Dannaeus, A., Lilja, G.: The relevance of antifood antibodies for the diagnosis of food allergy. Ann. Allergy 53:665, 1984.

Kailin, E.W., Collier, R: Relieving therapy for antigen exposure. J.A.M.A. 217:78, 1971.

Lambert, P.H., Dixon, F.J., Zubler, R.H., Agnello, V., et al.: A WHO collaborative study for the evaluation of eighteen methods for detecting immune complexes in serum. J. Clin. Lab. Immunol. 1:1, 1978.

Leary, H.L., Jr., Halsey, J.F.: An assay to measure antigen specific immune complexes in food allergy patients. J. Allergy Clin. Immunol. 74:190, 1984.

Lee, C.H.: A new test for the diagnosis and treatment of food allergies. Buchanan Co. Med. Bull. 25:9–12, 1961.

Lehman, C.W.: A double blind study of sublingual provocative food testing: A study of its efficacy. Ann. Allergy 45:144, 1980a.

Lehman, C.W.: The cytotoxic food allergy test: A study of reliability and reproducibility. Ann. Allergy 45:150, 1980b.

Libman, J., Biglang, A.D.: Autogenous urine proteins in asthma and other allergic diseases. Brit. Med. J. 1:62, 1937.

Lieberman, P., Crawford, L., Bjelland, J., Connell, B., Rice, M.: Controlled study of the cytotoxic food test. J.A.M.A. 231:728–730, 1975.

Lipton, M.A., Mayo, J.P.: Diet and hyperkinesis — an update. J. Am. Diet. Assn. 83:132, 1983.

Lurhuma, A.Z., Cambiaso, C.L., Masson, P.L., Heremans, J.F.: Detection of CICs by inhibition of rheumatoid factor agglutination of IgG coated latex articles. Clin. Exp. Immunol. 25:212, 1976.

Mahan, K., Chase, M., Furukawa, C., Shapiro, G., Pierson, W., Bierman, C.W.: Sugar "allergy" and children's behavior. (Abstract.) J. Allergy Clin. Immunol. 75:177 (Part 2), 1985.

Mansfield, L.E., Vaughn, T.R., Waller, S.F., Haverly, R.W., Ting, S.: Food allergy and adult migraine — double-blind and mediator confirmation of an allergic etiology. Ann. Allergy 55:126–129, 1985.

May, C.D., Remigio, L., Feldman, J., Bock, S.A., Carr, R.I.: A study of serum antibodies to isolated milk proteins and ovalbumin in infants. Clin. Allergy 7:583, 1977.

McPhaul, J.J., Dixon, F.J.: Basement membrane antigens in serum and urine. Transpl. Proc. 1:964, 1969.

Mendoza, G.: Subthreshold and suboptimal densitization of basophils. Intern. Arch. Allergy Appl. Immunol. 69:282, 1982.

Miller, J.B.: Food Allergy: Provocative Testing and Injection Therapy. Springfield, Illinois, Charles C Thomas, 1972.

Miller, J.B.: A double blind study of food extract injection therapy: A preliminary report. Ann. Allergy 38:185–191, 1977.

Minchin, R.L., Haviland, D.: Significance of urinary proteose in idiopathic epilepsy. Brit. Med. J. 2:97, 1932.

Morris, D.L.: Use of sublingual antigen in the diagnosis and treatment of food allergy. Ann. Allergy 27:289–294, 1969.

National Institutes of Health Consensus Development Panel: Defined Diets in Childhood Hyperactivity. Bethesda, Maryland, Office of Medical Applications of Research, N.I.H. Bldg. No. 1, 1982.

Necessary, P.C., Leary, L., Dockhorn, R.J., Halsey, J.F.: Allergen specific immune complexes in food sensitive patients. Ann. Allergy 52:232, 1984.

Oriel, G.H.: Letter to the editor. Lancet 2:1304, 1932.

Oriel, G.H., and Barber, H.W.: Proteoses in urine, excreted in anaphylactic and allergic conditions. Lancet 2:1304, 1930.

Paganelli, R., Levinsky, R.J., Atherton, D.J.: Detection of specific antigen within circulating immune complexes: Healthy and food allergic patients. Clin. Exp. Immunol. 46:44, 1981.

Parish, W.E.: Short term anaphylactic IgG antibodies in human sera. Lancet 2:591, 1970.

Parish, W.E.: Detection of reaginic and short term sensitizing anaphylactic antibodies to milk in sera of allergic and normal persons. Clin. Allergy 1:369, 1971.

Phillips, E.W.: Relief of hayfever by intradermal injections of pollen extract. J.A.M.A. 86:182–186, 1926.

Plesch, J.: Urine therapy. Med. Press 218:128, 1947.

Rappaport, J.L.: Effects of dietary substances in children. J. Psychiatr. Res. 17:187, 1982/83.

Reisman, R.E.: American Academy of Allergy position statement—controversial techniques. J. Allergy Clin. Immunol. 67:333, 1981.

Rinkel, H.J.: The whealing response of the skin to serial dilution testing. Ann. Allergy 7:625–630, 1949.

Rinkel, H.J.: Management of clinical allergy: General considerations. Arch. Otolaryngol. 76:491–499, 1962.

Rinkel, H.J., Lee, C.H., Brown, D.W., Jr., Willoughby, J.W., Williams, J.M.: The diagnosis of food allergy. Arch. Otolaryngol. 79:71–76, 1964.

Schwartz, H.R., Nevurkar, L., Spies, J.R., Scanlon, R.T., Bellanti, J.A.: Milk hypersensitivity: RAST studies using new antigens generated by pepsin hydrolysis of beta-lactoglobulin. J. Allergy Clin. Immunol. 65:212, 1980.

Shannon, W.R.: Neuropathic manifestations in infants and children as a result of anaphylactic reactions to foods contained in their diet. Am. J. Dis. Childh. 24:89, 1922.

Squire, T.L., Lee, H.J.: Lysis *in vitro* of sensitized leukocytes by ragweed. J. Allergy 18:156–163, 1947.

Stites, D.P., Stobo, J.D., Fudenberg, H.H., Wells, J.V. (eds.): Basic and Clinical Immunology. Palo Alto, California, Lahge Medical Publications, 1984.

Templeton, H.J.: Letter to the editor. Arch. Derm. Syph. 28:346, 1934.

Trashoff, A., Meranze, D.R.: Urinary proteoses in bronchial asthma. J. Allergy 4:136, 1932–1933.

Ulett, G.A., Perry, S.G.: Cytotoxic testing and leukocyte increase: An index of food sensitivity. II. Coffee and tobacco. Ann. Allergy 34:150–160, 1975.

VanMetre, T.E., Jr.: Critique of controversial and unproven procedures for diagnosis and therapy of allergic disorders. Pediatr. Clin. N. Am. 30:807, 1983.

VanMetre, T.E., Jr., Adkinson, N.F., Jr., Amodeo, F.J., Lichtenstein, L.M., Mardiney, M.R., Norman, P.S., Rosenberg, G.L., Sabotka, A.K., Valentine, M.D.: A comparison of the effectiveness of the Rinkel method and the current standard method of immunotherapy for ragweed pollen hayfever. J. Allergy Clin. Immunol. 66:500–509, 1980.

VanMetre, T.E., Jr., Adkinson, N.F., Jr., Lichtenstein, L.M., Mardiney, M.R., Norman, P.S., Rosenberg, G.L., Sabotka, A.K., Valentine, M.D.: A controlled study of the effectiveness of the Rinkel method of immunotherapy for ragweed pollen hayfever. J. Allergy Clin. Immunol. 65:288–298, 1980.

Willoughby, J.W.: Provocative food test technique. Ann. Allergy 23:543, 1965.

Yoeman, W., Miller, S., Rutherford, R.P.J., Wesley-Smith, J.L.: Letter to the editor. Lancet 2:1303, 1932.

58

Surgery in Allergic Patients

DENNIS L. FUNG, M.D.
MICHAEL SCHATZ, M.D.

Asthma and drug allergy constitute the majority of allergic conditions that are encountered in the perioperative period. In the general population, risk of mortality from anesthesia is believed to be approximately 1 per 10,000. Mortality from anesthesia is higher in pediatric cases (approximately 5 per 10,000). In a recent review of 27 deaths due to anesthetics, only one death involved asthma; none was due to an allergic drug reaction (Keenan and Boyan, 1985). There are no recent statistics on the perioperative morbidity and mortality due to asthma. The incidence of severe anaphylactoid reactions during anesthesia is estimated to be between 1 per 5000 and 1 per 20,000, with 4 percent mortality (Fisher and Baldo, 1984). Although these figures suggest a low risk of mortality from anesthesia, administration of anesthesia in allergic patients, in fact, is of special concern because of the potential suddenness and severity of reaction, such as bronchospasm and anaphylactic shock. Each would require immediate and appropriate action if a fatal outcome is to be averted. Recent reviews of these topics have appeared in the anesthesiology-related literature (Kingston and Hirshman, 1984; Stoelting, 1983; Sage, 1985).

Little has been written concerning the management during anesthesia of patients with other allergic conditions. Anesthesia for patients with more uncommon allergic states must be determined by the existing or potential clinical manifestations. In such cases, the anesthetist is often dependent upon the patient's primary care physician for insight (Table 58–1).

ASTHMA

Preoperative Assessment and Preparation

Preoperative assessment includes a consideration of the following: the severity of asthma and the adequacy of therapy, and whether complications have occurred from asthma or from its treatment. Severe bronchial hyperreactivity is suspected when the history reveals frequent asthma episodes, steroid therapy, multiple changes in medication or dose adjustments, theophylline toxicity, hospitalization, and intubation for respiratory failure. A review of the patient's experience with prior anesthetic agents is important. Although previously encountered problems do not necessarily recur, parental or patient anxiety concerning anesthesia is to be expected if complications have been experienced, and this anxiety should be discussed. Known triggering factors may have implications for anesthetic management. For example, a patient who is sensitive to cold air should receive warmed humidified anesthetic gases. Some patients suffer extreme anxiety related to face masks or physical restraints; this anxiety should be recognized and dealt with sympathetically.

Physical examination may reveal a hyperexpanded chest, the use of accessory respiratory muscles, secretions, and wheezing. These are the findings in a patient with already compromised ventilatory reserve and impaired ability to clear secretions. The addition of general anesthesia may be sufficient to cause hypoventilation, atelectasis, and hypoxemia. When this possibility is likely and the surgery cannot be postponed, the patient or the patient's parent should be prepared for the possibility of postoperative intubation and ventilator support.

Ideally, the patient should be asymptomatic, free of wheezing and bronchospasm, and free of secretions prior to surgery. When clinical abnormalities are present, considerable related expertise may be required to decide how much evaluation is needed before proceeding and whether further therapy is required. Preoperative indications for procedures, such as chest x-ray, pulmonary function testing, and arterial blood gas analysis, have not been established for asthmatics, but when an asthmatic presents

TABLE 58–1. Contributions of Primary Care Physicians to Perioperative Care

Comparison of the patient's preoperative condition to his or her usual status.

Assessment of the limitations and benefits of outpatient versus inpatient management when the patient's condition has been difficult to control.

Advice to the surgical team on ways to avoid exacerbations.

Advice to the surgical team on options for managing intraoperative exacerbations.

Participation in the preoperative and postoperative management of the patient's disease and alerting the surgical team to potential or actual conflicts in therapy so that solutions can be agreed upon.

Communication to the patient and family, if appropriate, of adjustments that may have to be made during the perioperative period.

TABLE 58–2. American Society of Anesthesiologist (ASA) Classification of Physical Status*

Class 1

The patient has no organic, physiologic, biochemical, or psychiatric disturbance. The pathologic process for which operation is to be performed is localized and does not entail a systemic disturbance.

Class 2

Mild to moderate systemic disturbance caused either by the condition to be treated surgically or by other pathophysiologic processes.

Class 3

Severe systemic disturbance or disease from whatever cause, even though it may not be possible to define the degree of disability with finality.

Class 4

Severe systemic disorders that are already life threatening, not always correctable by operation.

Class 5

The moribund patient who has little chance of survival but is submitted to operation in desperation.

EMERGENCY OPERATION (E)

Any patient in one of the classes listed previously who undergoes operation on an emergency basis is considered to be in poorer physical condition. The letter E is placed beside the numerical classification.

* Adapted from Dripps, R.D.: Introduction to Anesthesia. Philadelphia, W.B. Saunders Co., 1982.

with wheezing, secretions, and cough, the adequacy of therapy must be questioned. Under these circumstances, physiologic measurements and a review of the clinical history will be needed to establish that no further improvement can be achieved. In adults and children, measurements of expiratory flow rates before and after bronchodilators are useful in determining whether additional bronchodilators would be beneficial. Greater than 15 percent improvement following a bronchodilator has been recommended as an indication for further therapy (Kingston and Hirshman, 1984).

The patient's preoperative condition is summarized by the anesthesiologist according to the classification of the American Society of Anesthesiologists (ASA) (Table 58–2). The ASA classification includes assessment of concomitant medical conditions, but several important factors that may contribute to overall risk are not included (Table 58–3). Procedures involving the airways and lungs, such as laryngoscopy, intubation, bronchoscopy, tracheal suctioning, and thoracotomy can be expected to increase the risk of perioperative asthmatic complications. Surgical incisions in the chest or upper abdomen cause postoperative splinting and impaired cough. Although attention frequently focuses on assessing the severity and control of asthma, it is too easily overlooked that hospitalization, examinations, testing, and discussions with parents or staff overheard by the patient may have an adverse effect on the child or adult, especially the child. Consequently, close attention should be given to the child's and the adult's emotional adjustment during the preoperative phase.

Preparation for surgery should be individualized, according to the patient and the antici-

pated surgical stress. Bronchodilator therapy may be interrupted inadvertently or deliberately. When appropriate, preoperative instructions should be given to continue therapy. In patients on theophylline who are still symptomatic, theophylline plasma concentrations will need to be determined. When there is strong evidence (e.g., low plasma theophylline concentrations, poor compliance with medications, recent respiratory infections, and seasonal al-

TABLE 58–3. Additional Risk Factors in Asthmatics

Surgery

Operations involving the airway, chest, and upper abdomen are more often associated with pulmonary complications. In adults, operations lasting more than 3 hours have a higher risk of pulmonary complications.

Patient

Poor cooperation and interaction with staff may lead to unsafe compromises.

Staff

Lack of experience and skill in dealing with asthmatic patients may lead to errors.

lergies) that control can be improved, elective surgery should be postponed until optimal control is achieved. In most cases, preoperative asthma preparation can be completed without hospitalization. Preoperative admission for the management of asthma is a consideration if outpatient control has been inadequate or if surgery cannot be postponed. In such a case, there is a risk of theophylline toxicity during dose adjustment; moreover, intensive pulmonary care for secretions may be needed. Hospitalization also can facilitate joint assessment by the physicians who will be involved with the care of a difficult to manage patient.

Preoperative Medications

There are two frequently cited indications for the preoperative administration of corticosteroids in asthmatics. When a corticosteroid has been recently used in the treatment of asthma, and adrenal suppression is suspected, 100 mg hydrocortisone hemisuccinate or equivalent intravenously every 8 hours for 24 hours is recommended as coverage to prevent perioperative adrenal insufficiency. There is uncertainty as to which patients actually require such coverage. In an adult, a 5-day course of high dose steroid can cause at least transient adrenal suppression (Streck and Lockwood, 1979); it is reported that in some instances evidence of suppression may persist for up to 1 year (Livanou et al., 1967). Although there is no consensus, liberal use of perioperative steroids has been advocated in order to eliminate adrenal insufficiency as a cause of perioperative hypotension. The second indication advanced for perioperative corticosteroid treatment in asthmatics is prophylaxis against bronchospasm. This treatment is believed to offer an extra measure of protection, although there has been no controlled clinical trial to demonstrate added protection. Again, no consensus exists for this indication, and as with steroid coverage liberal application is based upon an apparent lack of adverse effects from brief high dose steroid therapy.

Premedication with sedative-hypnotics, narcotics, or both also is controversial. Practice varies widely, ranging from no premedication to heavy sedation. Personal preference and experience have a large influence on this decision. In addition, there is no assurance that premedication schedules that work well in one case will be successful in another. The need, efficacy, and safety of premedication depend on factors that are difficult to describe or measure. The patient's understanding and anxiety and the degree of respiratory impairment must receive prime consideration. The usefulness of anticholinergic drugs also is debated. On the one hand, atropine has the beneficial effect of antagonizing reflex bronchoconstriction and bradycardia; on the other hand, it may lead to tenacious secretions and exaggeration of beta adrenegic–induced tachycardia.

Because specific guidelines for preoperative corticosteroid and preanesthetic medication differ, they are a potential source of misunderstanding among physicians. It is important to recognize that the crucial issue is the question of prophylaxis versus the risk of unnecessary prophylaxis. When information is lacking to permit a clear decision, such a question is frequently resolved on the basis of personal experience and temperament.

Selection of Anesthetic Technique

When improvement appears unlikely in a symptomatic patient, local infiltration anesthesia should at least be considered. In many children, minor procedures can be undertaken successfully with local anesthesia and sedation. Although local anesthesia does not preclude the possibility of severe intraoperative bronchospasm, airway manipulation and general anesthesia usually can be avoided. Occasionally, local anesthesia will fail, and general anesthesia will be needed anyway. In other words, local anesthesia is not a completely satisfactory alternative to adequate preoperative control, but it may be a satisfactory alternative to general anesthesia. Similar considerations apply to the use of regional anesthesia, such as spinal subarachnoid block, brachial plexus block, and epidural block. For adult asthmatics who require lower abdominal or extremity surgery, there are strong arguments for the use of regional anesthesia. Uncomplicated regional anesthesia also circumvents the need for airway manipulation and avoids the respiratory impairment of general anesthesia. However, with few exceptions (Esther, 1975), regional anesthesia has not been extensively applied in children, and anesthesiologists who are experienced in regional anesthesia in children are not available in every hospital. Even when regional anesthesia is practical in infants and children, some additional hazards must be considered as follows: poor cooperation; inadequate emotional preparation; inadequate sedation; oversedation; and inadequate block, with the necessity of inducing anesthesia and managing the airways in those who already have been draped and who are less accessible because of their small size. General anesthesia usually is selected for pediatric patients.

Risks of General Anesthesia

There are numerous potential complications from general anesthesia in asthmatic patients. Airway manipulation can lead to bronchospasm and respiratory failure. Airway and pulmonary complications can be misdiagnosed as asthma, resulting in delayed or inappropriate management. Retained secretions can progress to postoperative atelectasis and pneumonia. Drug interactions between anesthetics and bronchodilators can cause cardiac dysrhythmias or seizures. Some anesthetic drugs cause histamine release (Table 58–4).

The hazards of induction in asthmatic patients are threefold as follows: an emotionally stressful induction can precipitate bronchospasm, endotracheal intubation can trigger severe bronchospasm, and interaction can occur between the induction agent and bronchodilators.

General anesthesia invariably jeopardizes

TABLE 58–4. Anesthetic Drugs that Cause Histamine Release*

Drugs	Estimated Frequency (percent)
INDUCTION AGENTS	
Thiopental	90
Methohexital	75
NEUROMUSCULAR BLOCKING AGENTS	
d-Tubocurarine	70
Pancuronium	15
Succinylcholine	40
OPIATES	
Alfentanil	10
Fentanyl	20–25
Morphine	100
OTHER	
Atropine	20

* Adapted from Doenicke et al., 1985.

the upper airway. For some operations, endotracheal intubation is not required; when intubation is required, the risk of bronchospasm is increased (Shnider and Papper, 1961). Whenever possible, intubation of a lightly anesthetized or awake asthmatic patient is avoided. Three measures are employed to reduce the risk of bronchospasm from intubation as follows: (1) establishment of deep anesthesia before intubations; (2) employment of intravenous agents, such as atropine and lidocaine, to block reflex bronchoconstriction; and (3) application of topical anesthetic spray on the trachea. Tracheal spray is probably the least effective and may even stimulate bronchospasm.

In the patient with pulmonary secretions, anesthesia will inhibit their natural removal by mucociliary action and coughing. The retention of secretions and the drying effect of inhaled gases through an endotracheal tube can result in atelectasis and hypoxemia. For lengthy procedures, it is essential that inspired gases be humidified and warmed. In addition, the patient's airway must be accessible under the drapes for suctioning. Potential adverse effects from anesthetic drugs are summarized in Table 58–5.

Selection of Anesthetic Agents and Ventilation Techniques

In a cooperative, calm patient, inhalation induction proceeds smoothly, without airway stimulation and with gradual control of ventilation until the patient is anesthetized deeply enough to tolerate intubation without coughing. On the one hand, halothane is widely used for inhalation induction in asthmatics because of its bronchodilating effect; it also is less irritating to breathe than either enflurane or isoflurane. On the other hand, halothane has the disadvantage of potentiating catecholamine-induced ventricular dysrhythmias to a greater extent than the others. Consequently, in a patient who is on theophylline or any of the beta-adrenergic bronchodilators, isoflurane may be preferred. Contraindications to induction with a potent inhalation anesthetic include elevated intracranial pressure, risk of malignant hyperthermia, and cardiac failure. Emergency inhalation induction may be impractical (i.e., too slow) in a patient with severe respiratory failure because the speed of induction depends upon alveolar ventilation.

In the child who will not accept an inhalation

TABLE 58-5. Potential Adverse Effects from Anesthetic Agents in Asthmatic Patients

Anesthetic Agent	Adverse Effect
INDUCTION AGENTS	
Thiopental	Histamine release.
Ketamine	Seizures in patients who are receiving aminophylline/theophylline.
INHALATION ANESTHETICS	
Nitrous oxide	Hypoxemia if an increased inspired oxygen concentration is needed.
Halothane, enflurane, and isoflurane	Ventricular dysrhythmia in the presence of catecholamines or theophylline. Risk may be negligible with isoflurane.
NEUROMUSCULAR BLOCKING AGENTS	
d-Tubocurarine	Histamine release.
Pancuronium	One case reported of sudden tachycardia during status asthmaticus.
OPIATES	
Morphine	Histamine release.
OTHER	
Atropine	Possible inspissation of secretions.
Neostigmine	Bronchoconstriction.

induction or who cannot be given a potent inhalation anesthetic, an alternative is intravenous induction with thiopental, diazepam, or ketamine. The severely asthmatic child usually will have an intravenous catheter in place before coming to the operating room. Ketamine is a bronchodilator and in isolated cases has been reported to be more effective than halothane (Corssen et al., 1972). Intramuscular ketamine induction can be used when an intravenous catheter is not available, but it is potentially hazardous to undertake induction of a severely asthmatic child without intravenous access. In adults who are on theophylline, ketamine induction may induce a transient seizure (Hirshman et al., 1982); combination with thiopental should reduce this hazard. As with the inhalational agents, there are contraindications to the use of ketamine as follows: elevated intracranial pressure; open eye injuries; and, possibly, seizure disorders.

During general anesthesia, severe bronchoconstriction can lead to hypoventilation, CO_2 retention, and hypoxemia. Exhalation is impaired by the effects of anesthesia and paralysis on expiratory muscle activity. The combination of positive pressure ventilation and impaired exhalation leads to progressive air trapping and hypoventilation. Bronchoconstriction also leads to a decrease in ventilation to perfusion ratios and hypoxemia. Under these conditions, a high concentration of nitrous oxide may increase the risk of hypoxemia, both by reducing the inspired oxygen concentration and possibly by expanding the volume of trapped air. An effect of nitrous oxide on gas trapping has not been demonstrated but is theoretically plausible.

Because the ventilatory responses to hypercarbia and hypoxemia are blunted or absent during general anesthesia, ventilation usually will be controlled by the anesthesiologist. Manual ventilation rather than mechanical ventilation may be preferable, since changes in pulmonary compliance and resistance are more readily detected and compensated for during manual ventilation. If mechanical ventilation is required, a volume limited ventilator should be used, and peak airway pressures should be monitored for changes in airway mechanics. For long cases, the adequacy of gas exchange should be monitored, but access to the patient may be limited by surgical drapes. Arterial blood gas analyses may not be readily available for small children. If so, venous blood samples may be used to estimate arterial values for pH and P_{CO_2}, and pulse oximetry or a transcutaneous oxygen electrode can be used to monitor oxygenation. During bronchospasm, end tidal CO_2 analysis may be an unreliable indicator of arterial P_{CO_2} because of variations in the end tidal to arterial difference. Breath sounds should be auscultated continuously for secretions, wheezing, and degree of air exchange.

Intraoperative Bronchospasm

In an asthmatic patient, bronchospasm is the most likely cause of increased airway pressure and wheezing. However, in the presence of surgical draping, other conditions can mimic bronchospasm, and limited access to the patient significantly increases the risk of misdiagnosis or delayed diagnosis by the anesthesiologist. Endotracheal tube obstruction by mucus or tension pneumothorax can cause resistance to ventilation and wheezing, and both conditions are rapidly fatal if mistaken for asthma and not corrected. Bronchospasm during anesthesia usually has a cause: Airway stimulation under light anesthesia, lapse in bronchodilator therapy, and drug-induced histamine release are causes to be considered, and they should be avoided or corrected. Because the inhalational anesthetics are bronchodilators and because light anesthesia is not an uncommon cause of wheezing, many anesthetists deepen the anesthetic and increase the inspired oxygen concentration as first steps in managing bronchospasm. Intravenous lidocaine, ketamine, aminophylline, isoproterenol, and hydrocortisone; subcutaneous terbutaline; and inhalation of isoetharine, metaproterenol, and albuterol have been used with success during anesthesia to reduce or eliminate bronchospasm (Table 58–6).

Beta-adrenergic drugs and aminophylline expose the patient to the hazard of ventricular dysrhythmia, but the risk is probably reduced if isoflurane instead of halothane is used as the anesthetic. The effect of anesthesia on the pharmacokinetics of theophylline has been studied in dogs. The early distribution phase appears to be unaffected by both halothane and enflurane, but the elimination phase is prolonged by thiopental plus halothane, enflurane, or isoflurane. There are currently insufficient data to indicate how the loading dose and infusion rate should be adjusted during anesthesia. A cautious approach might be to reduce both by half. Because there are no data on the dosage adjustments of bronchodilators in subjects during anesthesia, the recommended dosages in Table 58–6 are for conscious subjects. The efficacy of passively inhaled bronchodilator aerosol administration during anesthesia versus intravenous administration has not been studied. During severe bronchospasm, the intravenous route may be more effective.

Postoperative Analgesia

Inadequate postoperative analgesia is frequent in pediatric patients in particular. The usual reasons given by clinicians are fear of side effects, respiratory failure, and airway obstruction. These concerns also are heightened in the case of the patient who has symptomatic asthma. The price of inadequate analgesia may be poor patient cooperation, loss of intravenous catheters, and even premature extubation. Postoperative care in an intensive care unit will decrease the hazards of providing adequate analgesia. When the risk of postoperative pulmo-

TABLE 58–6. Drug Therapy for Intraoperative Bronchospasm

Inhalational Anesthetics	
Halothane Isoflurane	} Inhalation to effect or to side effect.
Intravenous Anesthetics	**Dose in Conscious Patients**
Lidocaine	1 mg/kg IV
Ketamine	1 to 2 mg/kg IV
Intravenous Bronchodilators	
Aminophylline	Loading dose of 3 mg/kg over 15 minutes. Infusion of 0.5 mg/kg/hr
Terbutaline	5 μg/kg
Albuterol	1 μg/kg over 5 minutes
Hydrocortisone	7 mg/kg
Inhalational Bronchodilators	
Isoetharine Metaproterenol Albuterol Terbutaline	} Periodic inhalation of 1 or 2 breaths to effect or to side effect.

nary complications is particularly high, it may be preferable to plan on postoperative sedation, analgesia, and intubation for the first 24 hours. Epidural narcotics and caudal analgesia have been used with success and low morbidity in children, but their current availability is limited.

DRUG ALLERGY REACTIONS DURING GENERAL ANESTHESIA

Preoperative Assessment

The most reliable sources of information in a patient with a history of a prior allergic reaction are a letter from the attending physician who managed the reaction and a Medic-Alert bracelet, the medical record, anesthetic record, recovery room record, or postanesthesia notes. Even when documentation is available, the offending drug frequently cannot be identified unequivocally. Suggestive characteristics of an allergic reaction include a history of atopic phenomena, multiple drug sensitivities, occurrence of the reaction during induction, and implication of a drug that is known to be associated with anaphylactic reactions.

Allergic reactions to anesthetic drugs are uncommon in the pediatric patient. This finding may be due to the widespread use of inhalational rather than injectable agents in children and also due to the low rate of drug exposure.

Many instances of "allergic reactions" are actually dose-related side effects. Young patients usually are unable to provide details, and their parents and even adult patients themselves may not recall or may erroneously recall the nature or cause of previous adverse reactions.

Table 58–7 lists the anesthetic drugs that have been associated with possible allergic reactions. Most reports concern adult patients, and the most common offending agents are intravenous induction agents, such as thiopental, and neuromuscular blocking drugs, such as succinylcholine. In the clinical setting, anaphylactic reactions are usually indistinguishable from severe anaphylactoid reactions (see Table 58–4). Since nearly all anesthetic-related allergic reactions are due to injectable drugs, drug inhalation induction and maintenance of anesthesia usually will be satisfactory alternatives. However, when inhalation induction and maintenance of anesthesia are not possible, as in patients who are at risk for malignant hyperthermia, safe intravenous agents must be identified. Since induction agents differ significantly in chemical structure, it usually is possible to find a noncrossreacting alternative to an induction agent suspected of causing a prior reaction. Neuromuscular blocking agents present a potentially greater problem because of their common quaternary ammonium group. When anesthetic management is unduly re-

TABLE 58–7. Anesthetic Agents that may Produce Anaphylactic or Anaphylactoid Reactions

Anesthetic Agents	Comments
INDUCTION AGENTS	
Sodium thiopental	1:30,000 incidence
Sodium methohexital	1:43,000 incidence
Ketamine	One case reported of generalized rash
Diazepam	
Althesin (alflaxalone/alphadolone)	1:1000 incidence
INHALATION AGENTS	
Halothane	One case of urticaria
Enflurane	One case of delayed bronchospasm
NEUROMUSCULAR BLOCKING AGENTS	
d-Tubocurarine	Histamine release
Metocurine	
Gallamine	Five cases in Australian women
Pancuronium	One case report of bronchospasm
Succinylcholine	Contains methylparaben
OPIATES	
Morphine	Histamine release
Meperidine	One case of anaphylaxis

stricted because of suspected or substantiated drug allergy, testing is advisable.

Testing for Anesthetic Allergy

Systematic evaluation includes a complete history of the reaction and, if possible, identification of the offending drug. The significance of positive skin tests for induction and neuromuscular blocking drugs in the immediate preoperative period is unclear. For example, Lavery and colleagues (1985) found that the response to intradermal injection of *d*-tubocurarine, atracurium, or vecuronium did not correlate with the flushing or hypotensive response to subsequent intravenous administration of these agents. Similarly, Wood and colleagues (in press) performed preoperative prick and intradermal skin tests to atracurium or *d*-tubocurarine in 22 patients who had no prior exposures to either of these drugs. Although positive intradermal skin test reactions were found to one or the other of these drugs in 17 of 22 patients, no obvious adverse clinical responses were observed in any of their 22 patients after clinical exposure to either drug 24 hours later. Consequently, direct incremental challenge with appropriate precautions may be more informative in the high risk patient. Unless the allergic reaction is of the delayed type, incremental challenge can be performed prior to anesthetic induction while the patient is monitored, with means for resuscitation at hand.

Preoperative Preparation

Once a history of allergic drug reaction is obtained, it must be clearly noted on the patient's chart. This is particularly important in a child who cannot be relied upon to communicate this information. In addition, many procedures are done at outpatient facilities where the person obtaining and evaluating the allergic history may not be the one who subsequently gives the anesthetic.

In patients who are at risk for drug reactions, premedication with antihistamines, such as diphenhydramine (0.5 to 1.0 mg/kg) and cimetidine (4 to 6 mg/kg), may have a protective effect. Doenicke and associates (1985) recommend slow (2-minute) intravenous administration of H_1-receptor and H_2-receptor antagonists. Oral corticosteroids have also been sug-

gested. However, to date, there are no data available on the efficacy of pretreatment in the prevention of reactions during general anesthesia in patients with prior histories of such reactions.

Selection of Anesthetic Agents

In the practice of anesthesia, many drugs are almost routinely given, sometimes for prophylactic reasons. Thus, the anesthetic plan should include a careful review of drugs that will be used. The use of those with potential for causing reaction is discouraged (see Table 58–4 and Table 58–7). The number of drugs used should be minimized in order to reduce the risk of a new reaction. To facilitate identification of an offending agent if a new reaction occurs, simultaneous administration of drugs should be avoided. Intravenous drugs should be given slowly. One may argue that a small test dose will permit discrimination between an anaphylactic or an anaphylactoid reaction and the circulatory depressant effect of some anesthetics. Should a reaction occur to the test dose, resuscitation may be easier in the absence of circulatory depression. There is no evidence that anesthesia suppresses the mechanism of anaphylaxis.

Inhalation induction is probably the safest technique. Hepatic necrosis following halothane has some of the features of an allergic reaction, but the evidence is not strongly supportive of this hypothesis and there are many "anomalous" observations that cannot be explained by an allergic mechanism (Walton, 1981). Halothane-associated hepatitis is probably an idiosyncratic reaction due to toxic metabolites of halothane. Interestingly, halothane-associated hepatitis is uncommon in children, even after multiple administrations.

When more rapid induction is needed, ketamine, fentanyl, or sufentanil is a reasonable alternative. Anaphylactoid reactions to intravenous opiates, such as meperidine, codeine, and morphine, seem to consist of localized urticaria, usually without systemic effects. In the case of morphine, the transient circulatory response to histamine release can be reduced by a combination of H_1- and H_2-receptor antagonists.

There are many reports of induction reactions to thiopental and alflaxalone/alphadolone (Althesin) see Table 58–7; Althesin was withdrawn from the market in March, 1984. Since anaphylactic shock has not been reported with either diazepam or ketamine, and has been reported rarely for etomidate, these agents would probably be preferable to other intravenous induction agents in patients with histories of prior adverse reactions during general anesthesia. Similarly, no anaphylactic or anaphylactoid reactions have been reported for the newer neuromuscular blocking drug, vecuronium, and only one case has been reported for pancuronium. A low potential for histamine release has also been estimated for these drugs, particularly for vecuronium (Lavery et al., 1985). Therefore, vecuronium or pancuronium may be useful in a high risk patient (Watkins, 1985).

Intraoperative Diagnosis and Management

Routine anesthetic monitoring of blood pressure, heart rate, and breath sounds will detect the signs of anaphylaxis. In addition, the anesthetist should be able to observe the patient's skin and face. Most reactions will occur within minutes after injection of an offending drug. Sudden hypotension during induction usually is due to a relative overdose of the induction agent and will almost always respond to administration of fluid and vasopressors. When hypotension is not immediately corrected by these measures, other signs of anaphylaxis, such as wheezing, urticaria, and generalized flushing, should be sought. Wheezing after induction and intubation usually is due to light anesthesia and will not be accompanied by hypotension unless the patient is hypovolemic or severely hypoxic. The combination of wheezing and hypotension must be treated initially as anaphylaxis until another etiology is determined.

The emergency management of an allergic drug reaction during anesthesia differs from the office management of anaphylaxis. Intravenous epinephrine (5 μg/kg over 2 minutes), rapid crystalloid infusion, and endotracheal intubation are standard. However, during inhalation anesthesia, especially with halothane, epinephrine may cause ventricular dysrhythmia, and treatment for ventricular irritability must be available. Intravenous infusions that might still contain the suspected drug should be stopped and replaced with warmed crystalloid solution. Nitrous oxide should be discontinued and 100-percent oxygen given to compensate for the hypoxemia associated with anaphylaxis. Corticosteroids and antihistamines may be helpful and can be given after initial resuscita-

tion has been accomplished. If surgery has not begun and is elective, the procedure should be cancelled in order to devote full attention to the management of the life-threatening complication. Continuation of anesthesia exposes patients to further hazards from anesthetic drug reactions.

Postanesthetic Management

Since manifestations of anaphylaxis can reappear after initial resuscitation, continued monitoring is required postoperatively. The endotracheal tube may have to remain in place if hypotension, severe bronchospasm, hypoxemia, or glottic edema is present. When upper airway edema has occurred, premature extubation can be catastrophic, even though equipment and personnel for reestablishing the airway are available.

A description of the drug reaction should be carefully detailed in the patient's record. Although the mechanism and responsible drug may be unknown until studies are performed, the parent or patient must be informed of the event. A brief written account, including the date, name of the hospital, and medical record number, can be provided for future reference. The written account should also list drugs that were used, probable offending drug, confirmatory tests that were done, and recommendations for prevention. Skin tests to determine the mechanism and etiology of the reaction should be considered. On the one hand, most patients will not experience frequent exposures to anesthetic agents. On the other hand, a distinction between anaphylactic and anaphylactoid reactions has important implications for future drug exposures. Even when a drug seems to be clearly implicated, testing is advisable, since reactions can be due to a preservative, such as methylparaben, rather than to the anesthetic. The highest priority should be given to identifying and documenting allergic reactions to drugs that are frequently used in emergency anesthesia, such as thiopental and succinylcholine. Fisher (1984) has suggested that positive skin test reactions at dilutions of 1 : 100 for induction agents, 1 : 10,000 for d-tubocurarine, and 1 : 1000 for other muscle relaxing agents do not occur in nonsensitive controls, and thus positive skin test reactions at these dilutions should be considered significant. Although suspected drugs that elicit positive skin test reactions should be avoided during subsequent surgical procedures, a negative skin test reaction has not been validated as indicating the safety of an induction or muscle relaxing agent upon subsequent exposure.

DRUG ALLERGY REACTIONS DURING LOCAL ANESTHESIA

General Considerations

True allergic reactions to local anesthetics (LA) are rare and probably account for less than 1 percent of all adverse reactions during local anesthesia. More common are reactions associated with the operative procedures (e.g., hyperventilation, vasovagal syncope, endogenous or exogenous sympathetic stimulation, operative trauma) but not due to LA and reactions associated with the toxic effects of LA (most commonly local, central nervous system, and cardiovascular). Urticaria, bronchospasm, or distant angioedema within 1 hour of local anesthetic injection suggest true IgE-mediated reactivity. Local swelling, dyspnea, hypotension, lightheadedness or syncope could be IgE-mediated but could also be mediated by the other mechanisms described previously. There are currently no immunologic tests that conclusively confirm or exclude the diagnosis of an IgE-mediated anaphylactic local anesthetic reaction.

Patients who exhibit symptoms and signs suggestive of IgE-mediated reactions during local anesthesia should receive standard antianaphylaxis therapy (see Chapter 51). The treatment of other types of adverse local anesthetic reactions is largely supportive. The major challenge is the approach to the patient with a history of a prior adverse local anesthetic reaction who requires subsequent local anesthesia.

Preoperative Assessment of Patients with Prior Local Anesthetic Reactions

The first step is to obtain as much information as possible about the prior reaction as follows: when it occurred, the specific drug involved, the preservative or stabilizer content of the drug, the vasoconstrictor content, the time of the reaction after exposure, and the specific symptoms and signs. Medical records describing the prior reaction should be reviewed if possible. A history of possible contact sensitivity to agents containing LA or parabens should be identified.

The next step is to discuss with the patient and the patient's parents, if appropriate, the significance of the prior reaction and the alternative approaches available for the upcoming surgery as follows: no anesthesia, general anesthesia, and skin testing and incremental challenge to local anesthetic not expected to cross react with the prior incriminated drug (see next section). Most patients will choose the last procedure after considering the benefits, risks, and alternatives.

Local Anesthetic Skin Testing and Incremental Challenge

The first step in the process of local anesthetic skin testing and incremental challenge is the choice of a drug. LA have been divided into two main groups based on their chemical structure as follows: group I consisting of benzoic acid esters (e.g., benzocaine, procaine, tetracaine, hexylcaine), and group II consisting of others (e.g., lidocaine, mepivacaine, prilocaine, bupivacaine, etidocaine). On the basis of the data available, group I drugs are considered to frequently crossreact immunologically with each other, whereas group II drugs are considered not to crossreact with each other or with group I drugs. If the drug that caused the prior reaction is known, a noncrossreacting alternative drug should be chosen for the current procedure; if the drug that caused the prior reaction is unknown, a group II drug, usually lidocaine, should be chosen. Although the preparation for skin testing should not contain a vasoconstrictor, the data in the related literature would support the use of a local anesthetic containing epinephrine or levonordefrin for incremental challenge and subsequent clinical use (Schatz and Fung, 1986). Finally, since parabens have been incriminated as the causes of some local anesthetic reactions (Schatz, 1984), and since local anesthetic preparations without parabens are becoming increasingly available, we recommend that local anesthetic preparations without parabens be utilized for skin testing, incremental challenge, and subsequent clinical use in patients with histories of prior adverse local anesthetic reactions.

Various skin testing and incremental challenge protocols have been utilized to identify a local anesthetic that will be safely tolerated in a patient with a history of a prior adverse local anesthetic reaction. Although there is no published data documenting the superiority of any one protocol, we recommend the one described in Table 58–8, which was derived from a re-

TABLE 58-8. Skin Testing and Incremental Challenge in Subjects with Histories of Prior Adverse Reactions to Local Anesthetic Agents*

Step†	Route	Volume (ml)	Dilution
1	Puncture	—	1:100
2	Puncture	—	Undiluted‡
3	Intradermal	0.02	1:100
	INCREMENTAL CHALLENGE		
1	Subcutaneous	0.1	1:100
2	Subcutaneous	0.1	1:10
3	Subcutaneous	0.1	Undiluted
4	Subcutaneous	0.5	Undiluted
5	Subcutaneous	1.0	Undiluted

* Reprinted with permission from Schatz, M., Fung, D. L.: Anaphylactic and anaphylactoid reactions due to anesthetic agents. Clin. Rev. Allergy 4:215–227, 1986.
† Administer at 20-minute intervals. See text for approach in subjects with histories of delayed adverse reactions.
‡ The concentration of local anesthetic (usually 1 to 2 percent) to be used for the procedure.

view of published data regarding skin testing and incremental challenge in the evaluation of local anesthetic allergy (Schatz, 1984). If the skin test reaction is negative (< 5 mm wheal), one may proceed to the incremental challenge part of the protocol. In patients who report prior adverse reactions beginning 12 to 24 hours after local anesthetic injection, negative skin test reactions at 24 to 48 hours must be confirmed before proceeding to incremental challenge. Although a positive skin test result may be falsely positive, it would generally be prudent to start over with a potentially noncrossreacting drug in a patient with a definitely positive skin test result.

Although false-negative skin test reactions have been documented only rarely (Schatz, 1984), their possible occurrence dictates that negative skin test reactions be confirmed by a negative incremental challenge before clinical use of that local anesthetic is recommended. As for skin testing, the clinical use of a local anesthetic tolerated during incremental challenge should be delayed until no adverse reactivity within the ensuing 24 to 48 hours can be assured in patients with histories of delayed prior reactions. Although reported reactions during subcutaneous incremental challenge procedures have been rare, mild, and not usually suggestive of IgE-mediated mechanisms, incremental challenge must be performed under careful observation with appropriate medical personnel and facilities immediately available to treat a patient with a potentially severe adverse reaction.

Patients are usually referred to either an allergist or an anesthesiologist for evaluation of a local anesthetic reaction. After a local anesthetic has been tolerated during incremental challenge, the referring dentist or physician should be informed in writing of the following: (1) the specific drug used, (2) the drug's vasoconstrictor, preservative, and stabilizer content, and (3) the final dose given. It is important that the local anesthetic administered clinically be identical to the one tolerated during incremental challenge, including its vasoconstrictor, preservative, and stabilizer content. Finally, the referring dentist or physician should be advised that the patient is at no increased risk for experiencing an IgE-mediated reaction to subsequent administration of the local anesthetic that was tolerated during incremental challenge.

REFERENCES

Corssen, G., Gutierrez, J., Reves, J.G., Huber, F.C., Jr.: Ketamine in the anesthetic management of asthmatic patients. Anesth. Analg. 51:588, 1972.

Doenicke, A., Ennis, M., Lorenz, W.: Histamine release in anesthesia and surgery: A systematic approach to risk in the perioperative period. Intern. Anesth. Clin. 23:41, 1985.

Esther, K.: Regional anesthesia for infants and children. Intern. Anesth. Clin. 12:19, 1975.

Fisher, M.: Intradermal testing after anaphylactoid reaction to anesthetic drugs: Practical aspects of performance and interpretation. Anesth. Intens. Care 12:115, 1984.

Fisher, M.M., Baldo, B.A.: Anaphylactoid reactions during anaesthesia. Clin. Anaesth. 2:677, 1984.

Hirshman, C.A., Krieger, W., Littlejohn, G., Lee, R., Julien, R.: Ketamine aminophylline–induced decrease in seizure threshold. Anesthesiology 56:464, 1982.

Keenan, R.L., Boyan, C.P.: Cardiac arrest due to anesthesia. J.A.M.A. 253:2373, 1985.

Kingston, H.G.G., Hirshman, C.A.: Perioperative management of the patient with asthma. Anesth. Analg. 63:844, 1984.

Lavery, G.G., Clarke, R.S.J., Watkins, J.: Histaminoid responses to atracurium, vecuronium and tubocurarine. Ann. Fr. Anesth. Reanim. 4:180, 1985.

Livanou, T., Ferriman, D., James, V: Recovery of hypothalamopituitary-adrenal function after corticosteroid therapy. Lancet 2:856, 1967.

Sage, D.J. (ed.): Anaphylactoid reactions in anesthesia. Intern. Anesth. Clin. 23: no. 3, 1985.

Schatz, M.: Skin testing and incremental challenges in the evaluation of adverse reactions to local anesthetics. J. Allergy Clin. Immunol. 74:606, 1984.

Schatz, M., Fung, D.: Anaphylactic and anaphylactoid reactions due to anesthetic agents. Clin. Rev. Allergy 4:215–227, 1986.

Shnider, S.M., Papper, E.M.: Anesthesia for the asthmatic patient. Anesthesiology 22:886, 1961.

Stoelting, R.K.: Allergic reactions during anesthesia. Anesth. Analg. 62:341, 1983.

Streck, W.F., Lockwood, D.H.: Pituitary adrenal recovery following short-term suppression with corticosteroids. Am. J. Med. 66:910, 1979.

Walton, B.: Immunological Aspects of Adverse Reactions to Inhalational Anaesthetic Agents. In Thornton, J.A. (ed.), Adverse Reactions to Anaesthetic Drugs. New York, Excerpta Medica/Elsevier North-Holland Biomedical Press, 1981.

Watkins, J.: Adverse anesthetic reactions. Anesthesiology 45:797, 1985.

Wood, M., Watkins, J., Wild, G., Levy, C.J., Harrington, C.: Skin testing in the investigation of reactions to intravenous drugs: A prospective trial of atracurium and tubocurarine. Ann. Fr. Anesth. Reanim. 4:176–179, 1985.

DISORDERS THAT MAY INCLUDE IMMUNE MECHANISMS

59

Overview of Autoimmune and Immune Mechanisms

LEONARD C. ALTMAN, M.D.

DISORDERS OF BLOOD CELLS

Immune Anemias. Autoimmune hemolytic anemias are a group of disorders in which antibodies develop against antigens on red blood cells. These disorders are characterized by reduced erythrocyte survival and hemolysis. The traditional and most helpful way to categorize autoimmune anemias is by the class of antibody responsible for hemolysis. Specifically, these anemias can be divided into those mediated by IgM antibodies, often referred to as cold hemagglutinin disease because the antibodies are active at low temperature, and IgG antibodies, often referred to as warm hemolytic anemia because these antibodies are maximally active at 37°C. IgM erythrocyte antibodies generally are agglutinating and active in complement fixation, whereas IgG antibodies are nonagglutinating and less active in complement fixation (Kaplan, 1985; Rosse, 1985).

IgG Antibody–Induced Autoimmune Anemia. In IgG antibody–induced anemia, the antibody is directed at either a protein of the Rh system or a sialoglycoprotein. Antibodies reacting with an Rh protein are noncomplement fixing, whereas sialoglycoprotein-reacting IgG antibodies are complement fixing. In about 60 percent of IgG antibody–induced hemolytic anemias, the conditions are idiopathic or primary; the remainder are secondary to any of a

variety of underlying disorders, such as chronic lymphocytic leukemia (CLL), other lymphoproliferative diseases, ovarian teratoma, systemic lupus erythematosus, and other collagen vascular diseases. The most common association is with CLL. The other diseases are less commonly associated. The mechanism of red blood cell destruction in IgG antibody–induced anemia generally involves immune adherence and sequestration of red blood cells, particularly in the spleen. This occurs because IgG antibodies, particularly antibodies of the IgG1 and IgG3 subclasses, are effective promoters of immune adherence. If complement also is activated, C3B and C4B can bind to the erythrocytes and promote adherence and phagocytosis by the splenic and hepatic macrophages, thus hastening erythrocyte destruction (Fig. 59–1). Frequently, red blood cells are only partially phagocytosed, and the portion remaining in the circulation becomes a spherocyte. These damaged erythrocytes have a shortened life span, because they are poorly deformable and are generally filtered out by the spleen.

The symptoms of IgG antibody–induced anemia are highly variable depending on the rate of red blood cell destruction, the degree of anemia, and the presence or absence of an underlying disease. If the hemolysis is rapid, the patient may be weak, pale, and dizzy and experience dyspnea on exertion. If the anemia develops slowly, the patient may be relatively asymptomatic. Physical findings include mild jaundice and splenomegaly.

IgM Antibody–Induced Autoimmune Anemia. IgM antierythrocyte antibodies react with red blood cell membranes at low temperatures and produce clinical hemolysis only if they retain immune reactivity up to temperatures about 30 to 32°C; these temperatures can occur naturally *in vivo*. The temperature range over which antibodies retain biologic activity is termed thermal amplitude. IgM antierythrocyte antibodies often develop a few weeks after cer-

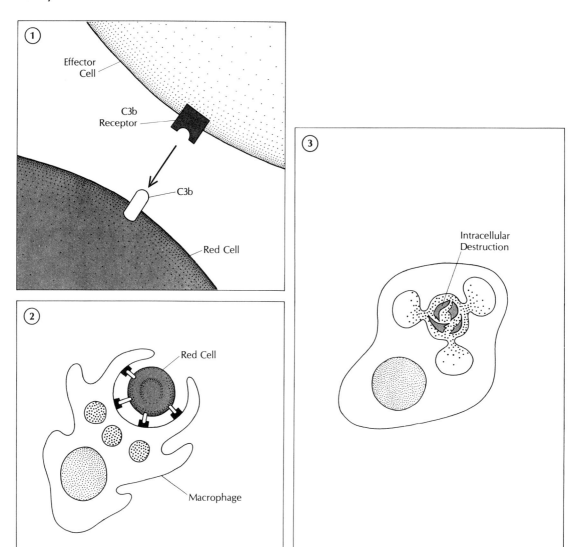

FIGURE 59–1. Immune adherence and removal of red cells. (From Rosse, W.: Autoimmune hemolytic anemia. Hosp. Pract: *20*:105–119, 1985.

tain infections, notably of *Mycoplasma*, Epstein-Barr virus, cytomegalovirus, and some protozoa (trypanosomiasis, malaria). These antibodies usually are polyclonal and of insufficient titer to produce hemolysis. Cold agglutinins can develop in patients with lymphoproliferative disorders in which case they are monoclonal often in amounts detectable by serum protein electrophoresis. Cold agglutinins also develop without an underlying cause, notably in elderly patients. These antibodies usually are monoclonal kappa IgM. This disorder is termed idiopathic cold agglutinin disease. IgM red blood cell antibodies generally are

directed against complex membrane polysaccharide antigens known as "I" antigen, which is strongly expressed on adult red blood cells, and "i" antigen, which is expressed on fetal red blood cells. IgM antired blood cell antibodies are efficient complement activators and produce hemolysis, since red blood cells bearing the complement fragments C3B and C4B are readily removed from the circulation and destroyed by splenic and hepatic macrophages.

Idiopathic and lymphoma associated cold hemolytic anemia are worse in winter, and patients so affected can present with painful acrocyanosis. Patients usually are jaundiced. Cold agglutinins associated with infections rarely cause hemolysis.

Laboratory Tests. Agglutination tests are used to detect IgM antierythrocyte antibodies. Results usually are expressed as the dilution of the patient's plasma capable of agglutinating human red blood cells in the cold. The antiglobulin or direct Coombs test detects IgG or C3B molecules on red blood cells. This test uses heterologous (often rabbit) antiserum against human IgG or C3 to detect these immune reactants bound to red blood cells. If the test result is positive with polyspecific antiserum, the precise class of immunoglobulin, complement fragment, or both bound to the red blood cells can be identified with monospecific antisera. Approximately 95 percent of patients with autoimmune anemias have positive direct antiglobulin test results. The indirect antiglobulin test detects antibodies in the sera of patients that have the potential for attaching to red blood cells. In this assay, the test serum is incubated with a panel of defined erythrocytes and the binding of an antibody to the cells is detected by the antiglobulin reaction.

Treatment. In many cases of IgG and IgM antibody–induced autoimmune anemias, the process is mild or self limited and requires no treatment. In more severe IgG antibody associated disease, corticosteroid therapy, in the range of 40 to 120 mg of prednisone a day, generally is effective. Corticosteroids appear to work by decreasing IgG production and interfering with macrophage IgG and C3B receptor function. Approximately 80 percent of patients have initial responses to steroid therapy, but only 20 to 30 percent have sustained responses when steroid therapy is stopped. Once a response is achieved, tapering of steroids should be gradual, and alternate day therapy may be effective. If the response to steroids is inadequate (when hemolysis or anemia fails to improve within 2 weeks or when a dosage greater than 20 mg/day is required to maintain improvement), other treatment is required. Other drugs that have been used are azathioprine (50 to 200 mg a day) or cyclophosphamide (50 to150 mg a day). Responses are variable but may permit steroid reduction. Splenectomy often is effective in a patient with shortened red blood cell survival and a predominance of red blood cell sequestration in the spleen. Before surgery is performed, ^{51}Cr red blood cell survival and sequestration studies should be done to verify the shortened red blood cell half-life and the predominant role of the spleen. Trans-

fusion may be necessary in severely anemic patients but can be hazardous because of donor to patient incompatibility, and specialized blood bank tests are indicated.

Treatment of IgM antibody–induced hemolytic anemia includes avoidance of low temperatures (i.e., moving to a warm climate if severe and poorly controlled hemolysis is a problem). Corticosteroids and splenectomy generally do not benefit the IgM antibody–induced form of disease, but chlorambucil, 2 to 4 mg, may benefit the idiopathic cold agglutinin syndrome (Schreiber, 1985).

Immune Leukopenias. Leukopenia is defined as a reduction in total blood leukocyte count to less than 4000 cells/dl. Since neutrophils and polymorphonuclear leukocytes (PMNs) are the majority of leukocytes in the blood, leukopenia usually is a reflection of neutropenia. Neutropenia can occur as an isolated problem or may be accompanied by lymphopenia; by reduction in monocytes, eosinophils, or basophils; or by both; most often in the setting of aplastic anemia. Neutropenia can result from four mechanisms as follows: (1) decreased size of the marrow production pool, (2) ineffective marrow production, (3) abnormal distribution between the circulating and marginated pools known as pseudoneutropenia, and (4) accelerated cell destruction. Neutropenia can be congenital, drug induced, or the result of other diseases, notably leukemias, Felty syndrome, and vitamin B_{12} and folate deficiencies. Autoimmune neutropenia usually occurs in association with other diseases (Table 59–1) or with the use of certain drugs (Table 59–2) (Boggs, 1985; Dale, 1985).

Clinical Features. Infections and oral ulcers are the usual findings in neutropenic patients. The locations of infections in neutropenic patients generally are the lungs, the oral cavities, and the perianal areas. Infections may be more virulent and rapidly progressive than in normal patients because they are not contained by the

TABLE 59–1. Autoimmune Diseases and Other Disorders Associated with Antineutrophil Antibodies and Neutropenia

---

Felty syndrome (rheumatoid arthritis and neutropenia)
Systemic lupus erythematosus
Idiopathic thrombocytopenic purpura
Coombs positive hemolytic anemia
Lymphoproliferative disease
Chronic hepatitis
Hashimoto thyroiditis

TABLE 59-2. Drugs Associated with Antineutrophil Antibodies and Neutropenia

Penicillins
Cephalosporins
Sulfonamides
Quinidine
Procainamide
Phenytoin (Dilantin)

actions of PMNs. In particular, local infection may spread rapidly to the circulation, and septicemia may develop without an apparent site of entry, especially in a neutropenic cancer patient undergoing chemotherapy.

Pathogenesis. Autoimmune neutropenia is caused by circulating antineutrophil antibodies that bind to neutrophils, increasing their rate of loss from the circulation beyond the capacity of the marrow to compensate. In the case of drug-induced neutropenia, the drug may act as a hapten to promote the production of antineutrophil antibodies or the antibody may be directed against the drug, which can attach to the neutrophil that is then destroyed as an "innocent bystander." Neutropenias associated with other diseases also are caused by antineutrophil antibodies. Felty syndrome, the best studied example, is characterized by circulating immune complexes, neutrophils with membrane-bound immunoglobulins, and circulating antineutrophil antibodies.

Laboratory Tests. The total blood leukocyte count, differential leukocyte count, and absolute neutrophil count should be measured and followed serially. A bone marrow aspirate or biopsy often is necessary to help determine the cause of neutropenia and to establish if the problem is due to reduced production or increased utilization. Assays for antineutrophil antibodies can be either direct, measuring antibody on the patient's own cells, or indirect, determining if the patient's serum has antibodies that attach to normal cells. Furthermore, assays for antineutrophil antibodies can be either immunochemical or functional. Immunochemical assays include a leukoagglutinin and an antiglobulin consumption test; a radioassay using ^{125}I-labeled staphylococcal protein A, which binds to the Fc portion of IgG bound to neutrophils; and a similar assay using fluorescein labeled protein A. Functional assays are difficult to perform and usually require specialized research support. Examples of functional tests are the antibody-dependent, lymphocyte-mediated granulocytotoxicity assay and the rate of reduction of nitroblue tetrazolium.

Treatment. The need for therapy generally is determined by the neutrophil count. Patients with levels around 1000 cells/μl rarely require therapy; those with levels in the range of 100 to 500 require close attention for signs of infection or fever; those with levels below 100 require urgent treatment. Corticosteroids generally are the first approach to therapy. Usually, a short burst of 60 to 100 mg/day of prednisone in adults is employed, followed by alternate day therapy at 20 to 30 mg. Other agents that have been tried on a limited basis are androgens, lithium, cyclophosphamide, azathioprine, and vincristine. Splenectomy sometimes is employed for patients with severe Felty syndrome manifested as splenomegaly, very low neutrophil counts, and recurrent infections. In about 60 to 75 percent of cases, the neutrophil count rises after splenectomy.

Immune Thrombocytopenias. Platelets are cytoplasmic fragments derived from bone marrow megakaryocytes. These cells are 2 to 3 microns in diameter and circulate for about 10 days. Approximately 70 percent of platelets are in the circulation, and 30 percent are sequestered in the spleen. The production and release of platelets are under the control of soluble factors known as thrombopoietins, of which there may be two as follows: one regulates the number of committed megakaryocyte stem cells and the other controls the maturation of megakaryocytes. The normal platelet count is 150,000 to 400,000/mm³. Thrombocytopenia ordinarily is defined by values below 150,000 mm³. Thrombocytopenias result from the following four basic mechanisms: (1) decreased or ineffective production of platelets, (2) increased destruction of circulating platelets, (3) sequestration of platelets in the spleen, and (4) dilution of circulating platelets. Immune thrombocytopenias are caused by the second of these mechanisms, i.e., increased platelet destruction, and may be either drug induced or idiopathic in etiology. Drugs also may cause thrombocytopenia directly by damaging the bone marrow or nonimmunologically by damaging the circulating platelets. Table 59-3 is a list of some of the drugs and chemicals known to produce thrombocytopenia (Marcus, 1985).

Clinical Features. In general, patients with platelet disorders present with cutaneous, mucous membrane, and, more rarely, central nervous system hemorrhage. Petechiae and purpura are common, while hemarthroses are rare. Bleeding in patients with platelet disorders usually occurs immediately following trauma and is of short duration. In contrast, bleeding due to coagulation deficits is often in joints, visceral organs, or intramuscular sites. It can be spontaneous or follow only mild trauma and may be delayed with persistent oozing.

In drug-induced thrombocytopenia, petechiae and purpura are common and most often in dependent areas, although the palms and soles rarely are affected. Of significance is the fact that petechiae are nonpruritic and are not painful in contrast to those observed in vasculitic conditions. Hemorrhagic bullae in the oral cavity also may occur as may hemorrhage in the urinary and gastrointestinal tracts. Since many drugs and chemicals can produce immune thrombocytopenia, a detailed history is required. It also is important to recognize that medications can be used for long periods without difficulty prior to the development of thrombocytopenia.

Idiopathic thrombocytopenic purpura (ITP) is a disorder associated with low platelet counts and shortened platelet survival time in the absence of splenomegaly or drug or chemical exposure, with normal or increased megakaryocytes in the marrow. There are two forms of ITP; acute ITP usually is a disease of childhood, occuring most commonly between ages 2 and 6 and affecting both sexes equally. This disease usually occurs 1 to 3 weeks after an upper respiratory viral illness. Petechiae, purpura, oral hemorrhagic bullae, and gastrointestinal and urinary tract bleeding are characteristic. Platelet counts often are below 20,000 mm³, which places patients at risk for central nervous system hemorrhages. In 80 percent of cases, the disease spontaneously remits in 2 to 3 weeks. However, when adults are affected the likelihood of recovery is less. Chronic ITP usually occurs in adults between the ages 20 and 40 years and affects females three times more commonly than males. The onset of chronic ITP usually is gradual and without an antecedent history of a viral respiratory infection. Patients generally develop mild and episodic petechiae and tend to bleed excessively after trauma or minor surgical procedures; women may develop hemorrhagia. Chronic ITP is characterized by repeated relapses and remissions over long periods of time, and severe bleeding is rare. Some patients with chronic ITP also develop other autoimmune disorders, such as autoimmune hemolytic anemia, systemic lupus erythematosus, and lymphoproliferative disorders. The platelet count in most patients ranges between 30,000 and 80,000 mm³.

Pathogenesis. Drug-induced immune thrombocytopenia occurs when the drug, acting as a haptene, along with a plasma protein, serving as a carrier, stimulates the production of circulating antidrug antibodies. The newly formed antibodies then bind the drug, and the formed immune complexes bind nonspecifically to platelets. Thus, the platelets act simply as "innocent bystanders." Once coated, platelets are removed by fixed macrophages of the spleen and liver.

ITP is caused by IgG autoantibodies against platelet glycoproteins. These antibodies, of the IgG1 and IgG3 subclasses, are species specific and can fix complement. In some cases of ITP, the autoantibodies are formed against functionally important glycoproteins on the platelets, specifically IIb and IIIa, which are important in platelet aggregation, and Ib, which is important in platelet adhesion. These occur in 5 to 10 percent of ITP patients. These individuals are at more serious risk of severe and frequent bleeding because their platelets not only are sequestered and destroyed, but also are functionally impaired. Such patients may bleed, therefore, with platelet counts of 50,000 to 100,000 mm³. Following viral illness and vaccination, particularly with pneumococcal vaccine, a patient with previously stable, chronic ITP may have a severe exacerbation. Although the precise mechanism is unknown, it is thought possibly to reflect polyclonal activation of B cells, thus nonspecifically increasing the production of antiplatelet antibodies. Additionally, these insults may increase splenic reticuloendothelial function, thereby increasing platelet destruction.

Laboratory Tests. The essential test required for the diagnosis of any thrombocytopenic disorder is a quantitative platelet count. The bleeding time, usually performed by the modified Ivy method, remains the most valuable functional test of platelet function. The test is performed by making a 1-cm long, 1-mm deep incision on the volar aspect of the forearm while a blood pressure cuff is inflated on the upper arm to 40 mm Hg. Prolongation of the bleeding time beyond 9 minutes reflects thrombocytopenia, abnormal platelet adhesion, or aggregation. In drug-induced immune thrombocytopenia, no *in vitro* tests are routinely available for identifying circulating or cell bound antibodies. Removal of the suspected drug remains the best diagnostic test; afterwards, clearing of the purpura within a few days and resolution of the thrombocytopenia within 2 weeks should occur. If this is not the case, alternative diagnoses should be considered. In ITP, again, no single standard diagnostic laboratory test exists.

TABLE 59–3. Drugs and Chemicals Known to Produce
Thrombocytopenia

Direct Marrow Suppressants

GENERALIZED MARROW HYPOPLASIA OR APLASIA

Antimetabolites
Antimitotic agents
Antitumor antibiotics
Benzene and derivatives
Ionizing radiation
Nitrogen mustard and congeners

OCCASIONAL ASSOCIATION WITH MARROW HYPOPLASIA OR APLASIA

Chloramphenicol
Gold compounds
Methylphenylethylhydantoin (Mesantoin), trimethadione (Tridione)
Phenylbutazone
Quinacrine

SELECTIVE SUPPRESSION OF MEGAKARYOCYTES

Chlorothiazides
Estrogenic hormones
Ethanol
Tolbutamide

Production of Thrombocytopenia by an Immune Mechanism

Acetazolamide (Diamox)
Carbamazepine
Chlorothiazides
Chlorpropamide
Desipramine
Digitoxin
Gold salts
Hydroxychloroquine
Methyldopa
p-aminosalicylic acid (PAS)
Phenytoin (Dilantin)
Quinidine
Quinine
Rifampin
Stibophen (Fouadin)
Sulfamethazine
Sulfathiazole

Direct Damage to Circulating Platelets

Heparin
Ristocetin

Probable Immune Mechanism; Antibodies Not Always Demonstrated

Acetaminophen
Aminopyrine
Aspirin and sodium salicylate
Barbiturates
Bismuth
Carbutamide
Cephalothin
Chloroquine
Chlorpheniramine maleate
Chlorpromazine
Codeine
Dextroamphetamine sulfate
Diazoxide
Digitalis and digoxin
Disulfiram (Antabuse)
Ergot
Erythromycin
Insecticides

TABLE 59–3. Drugs and Chemicals Known to Produce
Thrombocytopenia *(Continued)*

Ipanoic acid (Telepaque)
Isoniazid
Meperidine
Meprobamate
Mercurial diuretics
Organic hair dyes
Nitroglycerin
Paramethadione
Penicillin
Phenacetin
Phenylbutazone
Potassium iodide
Prednisone
Prochlorperazine
Promethazine
Propylthiouracil
Pyrazinamide
Reserpine
Spironolactone
Streptomycin
Sulfonamides (sulfadiazine, sulfadimetine, sulfamerazine,
    sulfamethoxazole, sulfisoxazole)
Tetracycline
Tetraethylammonium
Thiourea
Trimethadione
Turpentine

There are, however, about 30 different assays available to measure platelet associated IgG. Some of the more commonly used tests are the antiglobulin consumption assay, the competitive binding radioimmunoassay, and the fluorescent anti-IgG assay. In general, normal subjects have less than 0.3 pg/platelet of IgG, whereas patients with ITP have 0.5 to 3.4 pg/platelet. Tests to measure platelet bound C3 also are available. Binding of this protein usually is proportional to the amount of platelet bound IgG. Tests of platelet bound IgG or C3 are more helpful than measurements of antiplatelet antibodies in serum.

Treatment. Drug-induced immune thrombocytopenia usually requires no treatment other than to stop the offending drug. If the bleeding or purpura is severe or if the platelet count is below 30,000 mm^3, corticosteroids should be administered. In life-threatening situations, platelet transfusions and exchange transfusions can be used. The latter therapy is effective because it removes antidrug antibody and lowers the plasma level of the drug. Further use of the offending agent obviously is contraindicated.

The treatment of chronic ITP involves corticosteroids, splenectomy, and immunosuppressive agents. First, however, it is necessary to determine which patients require treatment. Since platelet function determines the likelihood of bleeding, the most important determinant of who to treat is the bleeding time. If bleeding time is normal, treatment usually is not necessary even with platelet counts as low as 30,000 mm^3. If treatment is required, prednisone at 1 mg/kg/day is indicated. This therapy usually shortens the bleeding time within 2 to 3 days and elevates the platelet count within 5 to 10 days. After approximately 4 to 6 weeks, the dose of corticosteroid should be tapered, using the patient's bleeding time, platelet count, and bleeding tendency as indices of responsiveness. Seventy to 90 percent of patients respond to corticosteroids; after one course of prednisone, approximately 10 percent of patients will have permanent remissions or can be maintained subsequently on sufficiently low doses, such as 5 mg every other day, so that side effects are minimal. The mechanism of action of corticosteroids is uncertain but likely therapeutic effects include an increase in platelet production, a suppression of macrophage phagocytic activity, an inhibition of platelet and antibody interaction, and a reduction of capillary fragility. For a patient who relapses upon reduction of steroid dosage splenectomy is indicated. In approximately 70 percent of patients who undergo this procedure, adequate hemostasis is achieved. However, approximately 5 to 20 percent of patients fail to respond to both corticosteroids and splenectomy. In such patients, vincristine may be effective and is the immunosuppressive agent of choice, since it does not suppress bone marrow production of platelets and may have an antiphagocytic effect. Cyclophosphamide and azathioprine also have proved beneficial in difficult cases after failure of corticosteroids. Two new treatments for very refractory patients are danazol and intravenous gammaglobulin; the gammaglobulin acts by saturating macrophage receptors, thus blocking their ability to clear sensitized platelets (Karpatkin and Karpatkin, 1985).

IMMUNE DISORDERS OF THE KIDNEY

Most immune kidney diseases are associated with the glomerular disposition of IgG and complement. For many years immune renal diseases were classified into two categories, depending upon whether the pattern of IgG and complement deposition was linear or granular. A linear pattern was thought to be diagnostic of an antiglomerular basement membrane nephritis, and a granular pattern was thought to be the result of trapping of circulating immune complexes in the glomeruli. This schema now is

considered to be an oversimplification. Rather, it is believed that immune renal disease is more accurately categorized according to the immune reactants found in subepithelial, subendothelial, and mesangial locations. Figure 59–2 is a diagram of glomeruli, showing these various patterns of immune reactant deposition (Adler and Couser, 1985).

Renal diseases associated with subepithelial deposits usually are characterized by large increases in glomerular permeability and nephrotic syndrome. Renal function in these diseases generally is good, and histologic changes in glomeruli are minimal. Diseases in which subepithelial deposits usually are found include poststreptococcal glomerulonephritis; the membranous form of systemic lupus nephritis; and drug-induced, idiopathic, tumor associated and other types of membranous nephritis. Tissue injury in subepithelial immune nephritis appears to be due to the direct effect of complement deposition without the involement of inflammatory cells. It is thought that terminal components of complement attack structures in the subepithelial capillary wall, resulting in loss of glomerular barrier function. The principal reason for the formation of immune deposits in the subepithelial space is an interaction between negatively charged anions in the glomerulus and positively charged antigens or antibodies.

Intramembranous immune complex formation results from the *in situ* binding of autoantibodies to antigens in the glomerular basement

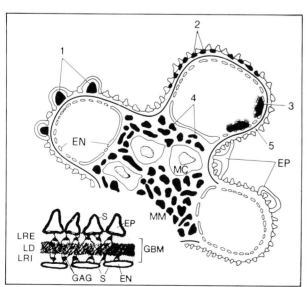

FIGURE 59–2. Schematic representation of three glomerular capillary loops showing the sites of glomerular immune complex deposition or formation along the subepithelial surface of the capillary wall as the "humps" of poststreptococcal glomerulonephritis (1) or the diffuse, finely granular deposits of membranous nephropathy (2). Subendothelial deposits (3) are seen in SLE and type I membranoproliferative glomerulonephritis, and deposits in the mesangial matrix *(MM)* (4) are characteristic of SLE, IgA nephropathy, Henoch-Schönlein purpura with nephritis, and other diseases. The deposits in mesangial matrix surround mesangial cells *(MC)*. Anti-GBM antibody deposits are in a linear pattern within the capillary wall itself (5). The inset illustrates the three layers of the normal glomerular capillary wall, endothelial cells *(EN)*, GBM, and epithelial cells *(EP)*. The negative charge on the capillary wall results from the sialoglycoprotein (S) coating endothelial and epithelial cell surfaces and the heparan sulfate containing glycosaminoglycans *(GAG)* which are distributed discontinuously in the lamina rara interna *(LRI)* and externa *(LRE)* of the *GBM*. (From Adler, S., and Couser, W.: Review: Immunologic mechanisms of renal disease. Am. J. Medical Sci. *289*:55–57, 1985.)

membrane. The physical nature of these deposits gives a linear appearance when visualized with an immunofluorescence microscope. Since alveolar basement membrane of the lung has antigens that crossreact with renal basement membrane, many patients with antiglomerular basement membrane disease develop pulmonary hemorrhage as well as nephritis, a disease known as Goodpasture syndrome. In these patients, radioimmunoassays can detect circulatory antiglomerular basement membrane antibodies in 95 percent. Experimental evidence suggests that the mechanism of renal damage in this form of nephritis is complex, involving direct antibody effects, direct complement effects, and complement stimulated neutrophil accumulations with subsequent release of neutrophil generated toxic oxygen species.

Subendothelial immune deposits are seen commonly in severe lupus nephritis, type 1 membranoproliferative glomerulonephritis (MPGN), and other immune complex diseases that affect the kidney. Subendothelial deposits may form *in situ* through cationic antigens binding to anionic sites on endothelial cells or through passive trapping of preformed immune complexes. Subendothelial deposits generally are associated with poor renal function, severe disease, and poor prognosis. The glomeruli usually show an inflammatory and proliferative response, and heavy protein loss is characteristic. Tissue injury in subendothelial immune renal disease is due primarily to the activity of neutrophils recruited through complement activation or through binding to immune deposits.

Mesangial immune deposits are seen in many immune renal diseases, including all forms of lupus nephritis, type 1 MPGN, IgA nephropathy, and Henoch-Schönlein purpura with nephritis. The mesangium is a major site for clearance of macromolecules from the glomerulus, and it is likely that the mesangium is a site of immune complex deposition in most diseases characterized by sigificant levels of circulating immune complexes. The mechanism of immune complex deposition in the mesangium is uncertain. Possibilities include antibody reacting with intrinsic mesangial antigens, antibody reacting with previously trapped exogenous antigens, or passive trapping of preformed immune complexes. In IgA nephropathy and Henoch-Schönlein purpura, there is evidence for trapping of circulating IgA complexes. Lastly, it has been shown that mesangial cells can produce proteolytic enzymes, reactive oxygen radicals, arachidonic acid metabolites, and interleukin-1 (IL-1); therefore, these cells may be partially responsible for the damage produced.

With the foregoing information as a background, the diagnosis and treatment of selected immune renal diseases is discussed. Table 59–4

TABLE 59–4. Immune Nephritic Diseases*

| Entity | Typical Features | |
	IMMUNOLOGIC	PATHOLOGIC[†]
Idiopathic hematuria	Uncertain mechanism	FPGN, rare deposits
Berger nephropathy	IgA, IgG complexes	Mesangial, FPGN, rarely crescentic GN
Henoch-Schönlein nephritis	IgA excess, vasculitis	Similar to Berger nephropathy
Membranoproliferative glomerulo-nephritis	Low complement, C3NeF	MPGN types 1, 2, 3; rarely crescentic GN
Rapidly progressive glomerulone-phritis	Type 1, anti-GBM Type 2, immune complex Type 3, no deposits	Crescentic GN
Systemic vasculitis	Uncertain mechanism	Glomerular ischemia, FPGN, DPGN, crescentic GN
Wegener granulomatosis	Uncertain mechanism	Focal necrotizing GN, crescentic GN
Systemic lupus erythematosus	ANA, anti-DNA, low complement, immune complexes	Mesangial, FPGN, DPGN, MPGN, membranous GN
Poststreptococcal nephritis	Latent phase with rise in antibody titer, low complement	DPGN, subepithelial hump deposits
Other postinfectious nephropathies (endocarditis; shunt disease)	Hyperglobulinemia, rheumatoid factor, low complement	FPGN, rarely DPGN, MPGN, membranous GN

* From Austin, III, H.A., Balow, J.E.: Immunologically mediated nephritic renal diseases. In Lichtenstein, L.M., Fauci, A.S. (eds.). *Current Therapy in Allergy, Immunology and Rheumatology.* Burlington, Ontario, Decher, 1985.
† FPGN = focal proliferative glomerulonephritis; GN = glomerulonephritis; DPGN = diffuse proliferative glomerulonephritis; MPGN = membranoproliferative glomerulonephritis; RPGN = rapidly progressive glomerulonephritis; C3NeF = C3 nephritic factor.

lists all immunologically mediated nephritic disease; Table 59–5 lists the primary renal and systemic diseases capable of causing nephrotic syndrome.

IgA Nephropathy (Berger Disease). This is a recently recognized form of glomerulonephritis that is diagnosed by demonstration of mesangial IgA deposits in the absence of other systemic diseases capable of producing the same lesion. IgA nephropathy causes 20 percent of acute glomerulonephritis in the United States and is more common in Europe. The history is usually one of macroscopic hematuria following a recent upper respiratory infection. However, the same disease can occur after pneumonia, osteomyelitis, gastroenteritis, vaccinations, minor surgery, and trauma. The disease is regarded as a monosymptomatic form of Henoch-Schönlein purpura, with the kidneys being the only organs affected. The characteristic histologic lesion is focal and segmental proliferative glomerulonephritis. IgA nephropathy is more common in males than females, and most cases occur before the age of 35 years. Laboratory test results show impaired renal function, with an increased creatinine level in 25 percent of patients; proteinuria usually of less than 1 gm/day; gross and microscopic hematuria; normal serum complement values; and absence of antistreptococcal antibodies.

TABLE 59–5. Diseases that Cause Nephrotic Syndrome*

	Approximate Relative Incidence	
	Adults (percent)	Children (percent)
PRIMARY GLOMERULAR DISEASE	(75)	(90)
Membranous nephropathy	30	
Minimal change (lipoid) nephrosis	15	80–90
Focal glomerular sclerosis	15	
Membranoproliferative GN, including dense deposit disease[†]	7	
Mesangial proliferative GN, including IgA nephropathy	5	
Rapidly progressive GN	3	
Acute poststreptococcal GN	—	
SYSTEMIC CONDITIONS	25	

RELATIVELY COMMON

Diabetes mellitus
Systemic lupus erythematosus (SLE)
Amyloid, including multiple myeloma

LESS COMMON CAUSES

Other immune disease (in addition to SLE)
    Polyarteritis (small vessel form), Wegener granulomatosis, scleroderma, Takayasu disease, Sjögren disease, Henoch Schönlein purpura, serum sickness, transplant rejection, sarcoid, mixed cryoglobulinemia

ASSOCIATED WITH MALIGNANCY

Hodgkin lymphoma, usually minimal change
Other tumors, usually membranous

HEAVY METALS, DRUGS, ALLERGENS

Gold, mercury, probenecid, penicillamine, paramethadione, trimethadione, "street" heroin, nonsteroidal anti-inflammatory drugs

INFECTIONS

Bacterial endocarditis and shunt infections, malaria, hepatitis, secondary and congenital syphilis, schistosomiasis

CONGENITAL OR FAMILIAL

Fabry, Alport, nail patella

PREGNANCY ASSOCIATED

* From Dale, D.C.: Autoimmune leukopenia. In Lichtenstein, L.M., Fauci, A.S. (eds.). *Current Therapy in Allergy, Immunology and Rheumatology.* Burlington, Ontario, Decher, 1985.
† GN = glomerulonephritis.

Circulating IgA immune complexes are elevated intermittently; serum IgA levels are elevated in about 50 percent of patients but do not correlate with clinical manifestations. IgA nephropathy leads to renal failure in 15 to 20 percent of patients in 6 months. In general, the prognosis is worse for males who develop hypertension or proteinuria values exceeding 3 gm/day. No specific therapy exists for IgA nephropathy except careful management of hypertension, intercurrent infections, and hemodialysis or renal transplantation.

Postinfectious Glomerulonephritis. Acute glomerulonephritis can occur following many bacterial, viral, and parasitic infections. Group A beta-streptococcal infection of the nephritogenic type M is the prototype of such diseases. However, a similar nephritis can occur in subacute bacterial endocarditis, infected ventriculoatrial shunts, pyogenic visceral abscesses, syphilis, leprosy, malaria, and toxoplasmosis. Poststreptococcal glomerulonephritis can follow pharyngeal infection, in which case the average latency is 10 days. The disease only occurs in about 5 percent of those with streptococcal pharyngitis and is more common in males. Glomerulonephritis also can follow streptococcal pyoderma, in which case the attack rate generally is 25 to 50 percent, the latency is approximately 20 days, and the male to female ratio is equal. The pathologic finding of this disease is a diffuse proliferative glomerulitis with hypercellularity, including neutrophil and monocyte accumulation. Epithelial cell proliferation and crescent formation can occur and reflect a poorer prognosis. Subepithelial and mesangial deposits of IgG and C3 in a lumpy distribution are seen on electron microscopy. The disease is most common in children between 3 and 12 years. The typical presentation is abrupt onset of hematuria, oliguria, malaise, gastrointestinal symptoms, headache, periorbital edema, and hypertension. Proteinuria is common with 20 percent experiencing loss of greater than 3 gm/day, and 50 percent demonstrating impaired renal function.

Over 90 percent of patients with poststreptococcal glomerulonephritis make complete recoveries with spontaneous diuresis. About 5 percent of patients have oliguria lasting more than 9 days, and many of these patients have glomerular crescents on biopsy findings. About half these patients recover spontaneously. Some others have only partial or minimal recoveries characterized by impaired renal function, persistant proteinuria, and progressive renal failure. The remainder experience partial recoveries and may be left with mild hypertension, slightly reduced renal clearance, and mild proteinuria for many years. Laboratory diagnosis of poststreptococcal glomerulonephritis is made employing a urinalysis showing red blood cells, white blood cells, casts, and protein; a low serum complement level; and antibodies to streptococcal exoenzymes. Specifically, the complement profile suggests alternative pathway activation with normal values for Clq and C4. Streptococcal serology frequently is studied with a streptozyme test, which measures antibodies to five antigens and is sensitive and specific. Treatment of poststreptococcal glomerulonephritis usually is not necessary, since spontaneous recovery is expected. Antibiotics are indicated if the streptococcal infection still is present but do not alter the course. Sodium restriction, diuretics, and antihypertensives may be necessary. Dialysis may be required transiently for some patients. For those who fail to recover, pulsed steroid administration or plasma exchange may be considered.

Goodpasture Syndrome. Goodpasture syndrome is a disorder resulting from the deposition of antibasement membrane antibodies in the lung and kidney. It is one of the causes of rapidly progressive glomerulonephritis and accounts for about 20 percent of cases (Bolton, 1985). In about two thirds of cases in which antiglomerular basement membrane antibodies are produced, there is accompanying pulmonary disease or typical Goodpasture syndrome. In the remaining one third of patients antiglomerular basement membrane nephritis develops without pulmonary involvement. The histologic lesion in Goodpasture syndrome is a focal proliferative and necrotizing glomerulonephritis that progresses to become diffuse with crescent formation. There also is a characteristic linear immune complex deposition of IgG and C3. The disease is one of young males, with a 6:1 male to female ratio. The first signs and symptoms are usually hemoptysis, dyspnea, and pulmonary infiltrates followed in a few days to weeks by hematuria, proteinuria, and rapid renal failure. A recent preceding flulike illness or exposure to possible pulmonary toxins is common. The diagnosis can be confirmed in over 95 percent of patients by radioimmunoassays, which detect circulating antiglomerular basement membrane antibodies. HLA typing may be useful, since there is a strong association with the HLA-DRw2 haplotype.

Treatment has improved significantly in recent years with the overall survival rate increasing from 10–15 to 50 percent. Rapid diagnosis and confirmation by renal biopsy are essential so that treatment can be initiated promptly. The treatment of choice is plasma exchange combined with prednisone (1 mg/kg/day) and cyclophosphamide (2 to 3 mg/kg/day). Plasma exchange is continued daily or every other day until antiglomerular basement membrane antibody is no longer detectable (Austin and Balo, 1985).

Rapidly Progressive Glomerulonephritis. The term rapidly progressive glomerulonephritis (RPGN) is used to define the loss of 50 percent of renal function in a 3-month period associated with extensive crescent formation in the glomeruli. In about 40 percent of cases, the disease is associated with granular glomerular immune complexes; in 20 percent, antiglomerular basement membrane antibodies are involved; and in the remainder, there are no associated immune deposits (Couser, 1985). Table 59–6 lists the many conditions that are associated

with RPGN. Since Goodpasture syndrome was discussed previously, this section addresses RPGN of idiopathic cause.

Idiopathic RPGN is not associated with immune complex deposition. Glomerular crescent formation is characteristic and usually involves 50 to 100 percent of glomeruli. Idiopathic RPGN is a disease of older adults, with a slight male predominance, and often has a prodrome characterized by myalgias, arthralgias, generalized pain, and fever. Idiopathic RPGN presents with acute onset of hematuria, proteinuria, and rapid renal failure often without hypertension or edema. There are no specific laboratory findings. The diagnosis is made through clinical presentation and biopsy findings in the absence of data supportive of any known disease responsible for causing RPGN. Until recently, the treatment of patients with idiopathic RPGN was poor, and 75 percent died or required dialysis within 2 years. Currently, intravenous pulse corticosteroid therapy and intensive plasma exchange are used and are effective in improving renal function in up to 75 percent of patients.

TABLE 59–6. Classification of Rapidly Progressive Glomerulonephritis (RPGN)*

Type of RPGN	Frequency
ANTI-GBM ANTIBODY MEDIATED RPGN	20 percent
Goodpasture syndrome	
Idiopathic anti-GBM nephritis	
Membranous nephropathy with crescents	
RPGN ASSOCIATED WITH GRANULAR IMMUNE DEPOSITS	40 percent
Postinfectious	
Poststreptococcal glomerulonephritis	
Bacterial endocarditis	
"Shunt" nephritis	
Visceral abscesses, other nonstreptococcal infections	
Noninfectious	
Systemic lupus erythematosus	
Henoch-Schönlein syndrome	
Mixed cryoglobulinemia	
Solid tumors	
Primary Renal Disease	
Membranoproliferative glomerulonephritis	
IgG-IgA nephropathy	
Idiopathic "immune complex" nephritis	
RPGN WITHOUT GLOMERULAR IMMUNE DEPOSITS	40 percent
Vasculitis	
Polyarteritis	
Wegener granulomatosis	
Idiopathic RPGN	

* From Couser, W.B.: Glomerular disorders. In Wyngaarden J.B., Smith, L.H. (eds.) *Cecil Textbook of Medicine.* Philadelphia, W.B. Saunders Co., 1985.

Neither form of treatment has been tested in a prospective controlled fashion (Austin and Balo, 1985).

Membranoproliferative Glomerulonephritis. The term membranoproliferative glomerulonephritis (MPGN) refers to a disorder primarily seen in young adults characterized by idiopathic nephrotic syndrome, hypocomplementemia, and a histologic renal lesion of basement membrane thickening and cellular proliferation. There are two types of MPGN as follows: type 1 in which there are subendothelial immune deposits and type 2 in which there are dense deposits. Type 1 MPGN is twice as common as type 2 disease. Type 1 MPGN is an immune complex disease with granular deposits of IgG and C3 in subendothelial and mesangial locations, evidence of classic complement pathway activation, and presence of cryoglobulins and circulating immune complexes. Type 2 MPGN does not appear to be an immune deposit disease, and its etiology remains unknown. The pathology of MPGN shows a proliferative lesion with thickened capillary walls and increased mesangial cellularity and matrix. Crescent formation is more frequent in type 2 disease. The clinical presentations of types 1 and 2 MPGN are similar. Onset usually is between ages 5 and 30 years, and sex distribution is equal. Nephrotic syndrome is the presenting manifestation in 50 percent of patients. Up to 20 percent may have nephritis, which is more common in type 2 disease. Hematuria is common. Hypertension occurs in one third; reduced glomerular filtration rate occurs in one fourth on initial presentation. One third of patients develop chronic renal failure in 6 to 10 years, one third have persistent nephrotic syndrome, and one third have persistent hematuria and non-nephrotic levels of protein loss. Type 2 MPGN has a poorer prognosis and a more rapid progression to renal failure. Circulating immune complexes are present in about one half of patients, and depression of complement components also is characteristic. In type 1 disease the classic and alternative pathways are activated, whereas in type 2 only the alternative pathway is activated. Also, in type 2 disease, most patients have circulating IgG autoantibody termed C3 nephritic factor, which is directed against the C3 convertase of the alternative pathway. There is no standard method for treating MPGN, and no therapeutic distinctions have been made for type 1 and type 2 disease. Alternate-day steroid therapy appears to be effective (Couser, 1985; Austin and Balo, 1985).

DISORDERS OF THE NERVOUS SYSTEM

Multiple Sclerosis. Multiple sclerosis is a demyelinating disease of the central nervous system that is diagnosed by findings of two or more central nervous system lesions that are present at two points in time, usually with at least a month's interval between symptoms. The disease onset usually is between ages 20 and 40 years. Its course characteristically is one of recurrent exacerbations and remissions. Multiple sclerosis has a prevalence of 60 per 100,000 in North America and Northern Europe. The disease is rare in black Africans and in Orientals. The incidence varies dramatically in different parts of the world, being greatest at the higher latitudes on both sides of the equator (Ellison, 1984). Localized outbreaks also have been reported.

Clinical Features. Because the pathologic lesions are diverse and random in distribution, the clinical presentation of multiple sclerosis is variable. Common signs and symptoms include weakness; incoordination; paresthesias; vertigo; and urinary symptoms, such as incontinence, frequency, and retention. Sensory symptoms may include the previously mentioned parethesias, pain, and loss of vibration and position senses. Findings in regard to vision include blurring, loss of sight, nystagmus, and diplopia. In approximately 70 percent of patients, the disease is characterized by recurrent exacerbations and remissions, whereas in the remainder, the disease progresses without apparent remissions. The average period from disease onset to death is 35 years (Silberberg, 1985).

Pathogenesis. Although multiple sclerosis remains a disease of unknown cause, a great deal of evidence supports the concept that it is an autoimmune disease possibly triggered by an infectious agent. Pathologically, macrophages, T lymphocytes, and plasma cells are found in and around affected tissue. Also, multiple sclerosis is a disease that is strongly limited to individuals of certain HLA haplotypes. The particular haplotype varies in different population groups; in North America the association is with HLA-Dw2. Experimental studies have shown that peripheral suppressor cell function is low in patients with multiple sclerosis during attacks and often normal during remissions. Other studies have found reduced suppressor T cell numbers, as determined with an OKT5 monoclonal antibody, during active stages of multiple sclerosis, although this finding is controversial (Arnason et al., 1984). The B lymphocyte system also is abnormal in multiple sclerosis as evidenced by increased cerebrospinal fluid (CSF) IgG levels that are oligoclonal in nature in virtually all patients with multiple sclerosis; furthermore, the IgG is synthesized in the brain, and some of the IgG is directed against measles virus. The antigenic specificity of most of the CSF IgG and of the major oligoclonal bands is not known, however, suggesting that no presently identified single agent causes the disease and drives the B cell immunoglobulin synthesis. Other immune aberrations in these patients include increased killer cell functions during the acute episodes and reduced interferon production by the lymphocytes in about one third (Ellison, et al., 1984). Although multiple immune abnormalities exist in multiple sclerosis, it is not known if these are primary events or secondary phenomena (Waksman, 1984; Waksman and Reynolds, 1984).

Many studies have attempted to isolate a specific infectious agent as the cause of multiple sclerosis. Agents have been isolated from cultures of materials from some patients, but in most cases, these probably represent contaminants or coincidental rather than causal agents. Perhaps the most suggestive evidence for an infectious cause of multiple sclerosis is work with DNA probes, which suggest that measles virus may be an etiologic factor (Haase et al., 1981). Serologic studies of IgG in the CSF of multiple sclerosis patients, while often showing elevated antimeasles virus titers, have been inconclusive with regard to the role of measles virus in the disease because the specificity of most of the IgG remains unknown.

Laboratory Tests. As indicated previously, IgG levels in CSF from most patients is elevated, and the distribution is oligoclonal in about 90 percent of cases. The CSF also contains mononuclear cells, usually 5 to 15/mm², and during disease activity myelin basic protein also can be detected. Electrophysiologic measurements usually are slowed owing to demyelination. This effect is measured by the appearance of an evoked potential after an appropriate stimulus. Most commonly, the visual evoked

response is measured. Also, computed tomographic scans and nuclear magnetic resonance imaging can be used to detect the so-called hypodense demyelination lesions in the white matter.

Treatment. Acute episodes are treated usually with ACTH, 40 to 80 units/day, or prednisone, 40 to 60 mg/day for 2 to 4 weeks. There is no evidence that this modifies the long-term course of the disease, but the length of acute exacerbations often is shortened. Baclofen or diazepam may help spasticity. Bacterial suppressant therapy can help reduce infectious complications in patients with bladder dysfunctions. Physical, occupational, and psychologic therapy are important.

Guillain-Barré Syndrome. Guillain-Barré syndrome is an acute inflammatory demyelinating polyradiculoneuropathy in which the patient presents with a rapidly evolving paralytic illness. Other related but rare neuropathies include chronic inflammatory polyneuropathy and acute sensory neuropathy. Guillain-Barré syndrome occurs at a rate of 1.7 per 100,000 and is the most common cause of acute paralysis in young adults.

Clinical Features. Guillain-Barré syndrome is a rapidly progressive, symmetric, largely reversible motor neuropathy. It causes hyporeflexia and symmetric and progressive weakness and generally begins in the lower extremities and ascends proximally. Weakness commonly involves the face and the bulbar muscles and may appear as dysphagia, dysarthria, and rarely ophthalmoparesis. Many patients have histories of preceding viral or mycoplasma infections of which Epstein-Barr virus, viral hepatitis, and infectious mononucleosis are most common. Other less common antecedent factors include immunization, surgery, pregnancy, and lymphoma. Patients with Guillain-Barré syndrome usually are afebrile and have no constitutional symptoms. Central nervous system involvement does not occur. Sensory symptoms, such as paresthesias and neuropathic or radicular pain, may occur but are not progressive or persistent. Autonomic dysfunction also may develop, appearing as orthostatic hypotension or hypertension and bladder and bowel dysfunctions. The clinical features of Guillain-Barré syndrome are summarized in Table 59–7 (Miller, 1985; Schaumburg, 1985).

Course and Prognosis. The disorder progresses rapidly with maximal paralysis in 50 percent of the patients in 1 week and in 90

TABLE 59–7. Clinical and Laboratory Features of Guillian-Barré Syndrome*

Progressive ascending weakness over days to a few weeks
Relative symmetry
Mild sensory signs and symptoms
Cranial nerve involvement
Onset of recovery 2 to 4 weeks after cessation of new symptoms
Autonomic dysfunction
Initial lack of fever or constitutional symptoms
Elevated CSF protein
Abnormal electrophysiologic study results

---

* From Miller R.G.: Guillain-Barré syndrome: current methods of diagnosis and treatment. Postgrad. Med. 77(7):57–64, 1985.

percent, in 1 month. Recovery usually starts about 2 to 4 weeks after the cessation of new symptoms. Most patients notice good recoveries, although these usually are gradual, with greater than 80 percent of patients being ambulatory in six months. Approximately 50 percent of those affected have some permanent nervous system damage, 15 percent remain seriously incapacitated, and 5 percent die.

Pathogenesis. Pathologic studies of spinal nerves from autopsy findings of Guillain-Barré syndrome patients have shown edema and swelling of myelin sheaths and axis cylinders and macrophage and lymphocyte infiltration (Haymaker and Kernohan, 1949). Subsequent work has shown that demyelination occurs only at sites of inflammatory cell infiltration and that destruction is directed at the part of the Schwann cell that forms the myelin sheath and not at the remainder of the plasma membrane of the body of the Schwann cell (Prineas, 1981). Experimental studies have demonstrated that lymphocytes from Guillain-Barré patients react to peripheral nerve myelin with increased proliferation and macrophage inhibitory factor synthesis. Other experiments have indicated increased circulating immune complexes and decreased suppressor T cell activity in this disease. Sera from patients with Guillain-Barré syndrome have been reported to demyelinate cultured peripheral nerves in experimental systems (Iqbal et al., 1981). In addition, many studies have documented that sera from Guillain-Barré patients contain complement-fixing antineural antibodies with significantly more frequency than sera from patients with other neurologic diseases or from healthy controls (Cook and Dowling, 1981).

Laboratory Tests. The CSF initially is normal, but after 1 week the protein level rises. CSF leukocytes are rare, and more than 10/mm³ mononuclear cells is unusual. Electrophysiologic studies are helpful, and 80 to 90 percent of patients exhibit distinctive changes of an acquired demyelinating neuropathy.

Treatment. Most patients require intensive therapeutic care. For those who develop respiratory failure (20 percent), mechanical ventilation is indicated. Meticulous nursing care, physical and psychologic therapy, and nutritional support by nasogastric tube usually are necessary. Corticosteroid therapy has been shown to be of no benefit, but plasma exchange, although controversial, appears to be of benefit when performed at specialized medical centers.

IMMUNE THYROID DISEASES

Graves Disease. Graves disease is a syndrome that includes diffuse thyromegaly, hypermetabolism, exophthalmos, and pretibial myxedema. While thyroid disease is the usual manifestation, the diagnosis can be made when only one of the three major manifestations (thyroid, cutaneous, and ocular) is present. The disease is relatively common, affecting up to 2 percent of females and 0.2 percent of males. Graves disease occurs most frequently in the fourth and fifth decades of life and has a strong familial component. Pathologically, the thyroid gland is hypercellular with lymphocytic infiltration. Orbital pathology, which is found only in severe cases, shows extraocular muscle edema and lymphocyte and polymorphonuclear neutrophil infiltration. The pretibial myxedema is characterized by a mucopolysaccharide infiltrate of the subcutaneous tissues (Larsen, 1985).

Pathogenesis. The thyroid abnormalities in Graves disease are caused by the actions of a 7S gammaglobulin, which appears to bind to the thyrotropin receptors (TSH) of the thyroid cells. In so doing, these immunoglobulins apparently activate the adenylate cyclase of the thyroid cell and thereby promote thyroid growth, increased vascularity, and hypersecretion of hormone. The terminology for the immunoglobulin capable of stimulating thyroid gland activity is complex and depends on the assay used for its detection. Long-acting thyroid stimulator (LATS) was the first described factor based on an activity found in the sera of about 50 percent of patients with Graves disease. Detection of LATS was classically performed using a mouse bioassay. Another assay uses human thyroid cell membrane fractions and measures whether the sera of patients can block LATS binding to these fractions. The IgG responsible for this activity is called LATS-protector, and it is detectable in the sera of nearly 90 percent of patients with active Graves disease. The tests currently in common use in Graves disease detection are radioreceptor techniques employed to demonstrate that the pathologic IgG in these patients is capable of inhibiting the binding of ^{125}I-labeled bovine TSH to the binding sites on human or porcine thyroid membranes. This immunoglobulin is called TSH-displacing antibody or TSH-binding inhibitory immunoglobulin. This activity is present in the sera of more than 90 percent of patients with active Graves disease. Thus, there is a heterogeneous group of antithyroid antibodies present in patients with Graves disease, some of which produce functional stimulation of the gland and are thereby responsible for the clinical syndrome of thyrotoxicosis. In contrast, the pathogenesis of the ophthalmopathy and dermopathy are essentially unknown (Volpe, 1984; Weetman and McGregor, 1984).

Clinical Features. The clinical features of hyperthyroidism of all causes, including Graves disease, are nervousness, anxiousness, palpitations, heat intolerance, weight loss, increased bowel frequency, and emotional lability. In females, amenorrhea or oligomenorrhea is common; males may develop gynecomastia. In older patients, the usual signs of hypermetabolism may be lacking, and the so-called apathetic hyperthyroidism may be the clinical presentation. These patients often have new onsets of atrial fibrillation and congestive heart failure.

Eye symptoms are lid lag, stare, easy tearing, a foreign body "feeling," and rarely severe irritation and inflammation. In the rare patient who develops pretibial myxedema, orange colored plaques occur on the lower legs. Common physical findings include tachycardia, systolic hypertension, fine tremor, thyromegaly, proximal muscle weakness, exophthalmos, and rarely impairment of eye movement.

Laboratory Tests. The free T4 index is elevated in virtually all patients with Graves disease. Patients seriously ill for any reason or individuals receiving propranolol, large doses of glucocorticoids, or a few other drugs may have impaired ability to convert T4 to T3, thus producing an elevated free T4 without hyperthyroidism. In these patients and in those with normal free T4 indices in which the suspicion of

Graves disease is high, the serum T3 should be determined. In Graves disease, the ratio of T3 to T4 is increased. Some Graves disease patients have an elevation of T3 only; this occurs in about 5 percent of patients and is known as T3 thyrotoxicosis. In rare situations, a thyrotropin-releasing hormone (TRH) infusion test may be necessary. This measures pituitary TSH reserve and is reduced in patients with hyperthyroidism. As mentioned previously, antithyroid antibody tests also may be very helpful.

Treatment. Propylthiouracil (PTU) and methimazole inhibit organic processing of iodine and thereby suppress thyroid hormone synthesis. Methimazole is about 15 fold more potent than PTU. Initial treatment with PTU usually is 300 to 450 mg/day (or the equivalent of methimazole) in three divided doses. Later in treatment with PTU, the dosage often is reduced to 100 to 300 mg/day. Patients should be monitored with clinical evaluations and with measurements of free T3 and T4 values. Skin rash, liver damage, and agranulocytosis are potential complications of PTU. In patients with severe symptoms of hyperthyroidism, propranolol, 20 to 40 mg every 4 to 6 hours, may produce rapid symptomatic improvement.

Following the initial control of the symptoms of hyperthyroidism with antithyroid drugs, long-term therapy must be initiated. Three choices are available as follows: continued use of antithyroid drugs, surgery and administration of radioiodine. If continued antithyroid drugs are used, it should be realized that treatment may be necessary for 6 to 18 months while waiting for spontaneous remission. Signs of remission are shrinkage of the thyroid gland and reduction of the necessary dosage of the antithyroid agent. Thyroid function should be monitored with free T3 and T4 serum values. T3 determination is especially helpful, since it often becomes elevated before the T4 when a relapse occurs. Surgery to remove a portion of the thyroid gland is another effective treatment in hyperthyroidism. The major problem with this therapy is that 50 to 80 percent of patients eventually become hypothyroid. Prior to surgery, a saturated solution of potassium iodide is given to reduce the vascularity of the thyroid gland. Treatment with ^{131}I also is effective. Its major complication also is hypothyroidism, occurring in about 10 percent of patients in the first year and another 5 percent/year thereafter. The average dose is 5 mCi or 80 to 90 μCi/gm of estimated gland weight. This produces effective control of hyperthyroidism in about 80 percent of patients in 6 months. Long-standing follow-ups for patients treated with radioiodine are necessary in order to diagnose and treat delayed hypothyroidism, which occurs eventually in 80 to 90 percent.

Hashimoto Thyroiditis. Hashimoto thyroiditis is an autoimmune disorder that is closely related to Graves disease. Patients with this condition have serum antibodies to various thyroid antigens, including thyroglobulins, thyroid microsomes, and colloid antigens. Furthermore, the lymphocytes of patients with this disease respond *in vitro* to thyroid antigens with the production of the lymphokine migration inhibitory factor. In experimental animals, a similar clinical condition can be produced by injection of thyroid tissue and transferred passively to other animals with transfused lymphocytes. These findings suggest that a cell-mediated mechanism underlies Hashimoto thyroiditis.

A patient with this disorder has an increased prevalence of other autoimmune diseases, including systemic lupus erythematosus, idiopathic thrombocytopenic purpura (ITP), Sjögren syndrome, and pernicious anemia. The pathologic findings in Hashimoto thyroiditis are fibrosis and lymphocyte and plasma cell infiltration.

Clinical Features. Two clinical presentations are seen as follows: an atrophic form of the disease in which the patient has a small thyroid gland and a form in which the patient has thyroid gland enlargement and goiter. In the last form, the thyroid gland usually is firm and diffusely enlarged. Both forms have characteristic signs and symptoms of hypothyroidism, including hoarseness of the voice; constipation; and swelling of the hands and feet. Women are affected with Hashimoto thyroiditis four to five times more frequently than men.

Laboratory Tests. The free serum T4 level is reduced and the TSH level is elevated in nearly all patients. Antimicrosomal antibodies are present in about 95 percent of patients, and a thyroid scan usually shows heterogeneous update.

Treatment. Treatment can be effected with desiccated thyroid, L-thyroxine (T4), L-triiodothyronine (T3), or products that combine T3 and T4. Evaluation of therapy requires measurement of the free serum T4 and TSH levels. Dosage should be increased until these values are normal. Patients in otherwise good general health can have therapy initiated at half their estimated replacement dose and advanced to full levels in 1 month. In elderly patients and those with coronary disease, treatment usually is initiated at lower doses and advanced more slowly.

IMMUNE ASPECTS OF FEVER

Fever is an elevation of body temperature that accompanies infections; traumatic injuries; many neoplastic diseases; some hematopoietic disorders, such as hemolysis; serious vascular accidents, such as myocardial, cerebral, and cardiac infarctions; most immune diseases; and certain metabolic disorders. Certain systemic signs and symptoms may accompany fevers, such as chills, delirium, convulsions, and herpes labialis or the so-called fever blisters, which result from activation of latent herpes simplex virus.

The mechanism of fever has been investigated extensively, using endotoxin-induced fever as a model. Approximately 25 years ago, this investigation showed that endotoxin-induced fever was mediated by a heat labile, host-derived substance termed either endogenous or leukocyte pyrogen. This substance is not preformed in leukocytes; following exogenous stimulation with endotoxin, leukocytes release pyrogen in 2 to 3 hours. Synthesis can be blocked with inhibitors of protein synthesis, such as actinomycin D and puromycin, but not by cyclooxygenase inhibitors, indicating that the suppressive effect of aspirin on fever is not due to inhibition of leukocyte pyrogen synthesis. Leukocyte pyrogen is produced by blood monocytes and macrophages. Prior reports showing that it was a polymorphonuclear neutrophil (PMN) product were incorrect, most likely because of monocyte contamination in the PMN preparations. Physicochemical characterization of leukocyte pyrogen has demonstrated that it is a protein of an apparent molecular weight of 15,000 daltons, with multiple isoelectric points. The mechanism by which leukocyte pyrogen produces fever appears to be stimulation of prostaglandin E synthesis in cells of the preoptic area of the hypothalmus, which is the primary area of thermosensitive neurons in the brain (Dinarello, 1983).

The relationship of leukocyte pyrogen to the immune system recently has been defined in studies which indicate that leukocyte pyrogen, interleukin-1 and epidermal thymocyte–

activating factor (ETAF) are identical. Interleukin-1, previously known as lymphocyte activating factor, is a hormone-like soluble helper factor required for maturation and amplification of T cell responses. It is a product of monocytes and macrophages. In the skin, it appears that keratinocytes produce a functionally and physicochemically identical factor. This fact has been substantiated by studies which show that an antibody to leukocyte pyrogen will block the activities of ETAF (Sauder, 1983). Leukocyte pyrogen, interleukin-1, and ETAF are chemotactic for PMNs (Sauder et al., 1984). Hence, leukocyte pyrogen appears to be important not only in promoting fever but can also induce proliferation of thymocytes and promote the directed migration of PMNs.

REFERENCES

Adler, S., Couser, W.: Review: Immunologic mechanisms of renal disease. Am. J. Medical Sci. 289(2):55-57, 1985.

Arnason, B.G., Antel, J.P., Reder, A.T.: Immunoregulation in Multiple Sclerosis. In Scheinberg, L., Raine, C.S. (eds.), Multiple Sclerosis: Experimental and Clinical Aspects, Vol. 436. New York, New York Academy of Sciences, 1984.

Austin, H.A., III, Balo, J.E.: Immunologically Mediated Nephritic Renal Diseases. In Lichtenstein, L.M., Fauci, A.S. (eds.), Current Therapy in Allergy, Immunology and Rheumatology. St. Louis, C.V. Mosby Co., 1985.

Boggs, D.R.: The Leukopenic State. In Wyngaarden, J.B., Smith, L.H. (eds.), Cecil Textbook of Medicine. Philadelphia, W.B. Saunders Co., 1985.

Bolton, W.K.: Goodpasture's Syndrome and Rapidly Progressive Glomerulonephritis. In Lichtenstein, L.M., Fauci, A.S. (eds.), Current Therapy in Allergy, Immunology and Rheumatology. St. Louis, C.V. Mosby Co., 1985.

Cook, S.D., Dowling, P.C.: The role of autoantibody and immune complexes in the pathogenesis of Guillain-Barré syndrome. Ann. Neurol. 9:70–79, 1981.

Couser, W.G.: Glomerular Disorders. In Wyngaarden, J.B., Smith, L.H. (eds.), Cecil Textbook of Medicine. Philadelphia, W.B. Saunders, Co., 1985.

Dale, D.C.: Autoimmune Leukopenia. In Lichtenstein, L.M., Fauci, A.S. (eds.), Current Therapy in Allergy, Immunology and Rheumatology, St. Louis, C.V. Mosby Co., 1985.

Dinarello, C.A.: Molecular mechanisms in endotoxin fever. Agents. Actions. 13:470–486, 1983.

Ellison, G.W. (moderator): Multiple sclerosis. Ann. Intern. Med. 101:514–526, 1984.

Hasse, A.T., Ventura, P., Gibbs, C.J., Jr., et al.: Measles virus nucleotide sequences: detection by hybridization *in situ*. Science 212:672–675, 1981.

Haymaker, W., Kernohan, J.W.: The Landry-Guillain-Barré syndrome. A clinicopathologic report of fifty fatal cases and a critique of the literature. Medicine 28:59–141, 1949.

Iqbal A., Oger J.J-F., Arnason, B.G.W.: Cell-mediated immunity in idiopathic polyneuritis. Ann. Neurol. 9:65–69, 1981.

Kaplan, M.E.: Acquired Hemolytic Disorders. In Wyngaarden, J.B., Smith, L.H. (eds.), Cecil Textbook of Medicine. Philadelphia, W.B. Saunders Co., 1985.

Karpatkin, S., Karpatkin, M.B.: Autoimmune Thrombocytopenic Purpura in Adults and Children. In Lichtenstein, L.M., Fauci, A.S. (eds.), Current Therapy in Allergy, Immunology and Rheumatology. St. Louis, C.V. Mosby Co., 1985.

Larsen, P.R.: The Thyroid. In Wyngaarden, J.B., Smith, L.H. (eds.), Cecil Textbook of Medicine, Philadelphia, W.B. Saunders Co., 1985.

Marcus, A.J.: Hemorrhagic Disorders: Abnormalities of Platelet and Vascular Function. In Wyngaarden, J.B., Smith, L.H. (eds.), Cecil Textbook of Medicine, Philadelphia, W.B. Saunders Co., 1985.

Miller, R.G.: Guillain-Barré syndrome: current methods of diagnosis and treatment. Postgrad. Med. 77:57–64, 1985.

Prineas, J.W.: Pathology of the Guillain-Barré syndrome. Ann. Neurol. 9:6–19, 1981.

Rosse, W.F.: Autoimmune hemolytic anemia. Hosp. Pract. 20:105–119, 1985.

Sauder, D.N.: Immunology of the epidermis: changing perspectives. (Editorial.) J. Invest. Derm. 81:185–186, 1983.

Sauder, D.N., Mounessa, N.L., Katz, S.I., Dinarello, C.A., Gallin, J.I.: Chemotactic cytokines: the role of leukocytic pyrogen and epidermal cell thymocyte–activating factor in neutrophil chemotaxis. J. Immunol. 132:828–832, 1984.

Schaumberg, H.H.: Inflammatory Polyneuropathy (Guillain-Barré Syndrome and Related Disorders). In Wyngaarden, J.B., Smith, L.H.(eds.), Cecil Textbook of Medicine. Philadelphia, W.B. Saunders Co., 1985.

Schreiber, A.D.: Autoimmune Hemolytic Anemia. In Lichtenstein, L.M., Fauci, A.S. (eds.), Current Therapy in Allergy, Immunology and Rheumatology. St. Louis, C.V. Mosby Co., 1985.

Silberberg, D.H.: The Demyelinating Diseases. In Wyngaarden, J.B., Smith, L.H. (eds.), Cecil Textbook of Medicine. Philadelphia, W.B. Saunders Co., 1985.

Volpe, R.: Autoimmune thyroid disease. Hosp. Prac. 19:141–158, 1984.

Waksman, B.H.: Pathogenetic mechanisms in multiple sclerosis: a summary. Ann. N.Y. Acad. Sci. 436:125–132, 1984.

Waksman, B.H., Reynolds, W.E.: Multiple sclerosis as a disease of immune regulation. Proc. Soc. Exp. Biol. Med. 175:282–294, 1984.

Weetman, A.P., McGregor, A.M.: Autoimmune thyroid disease: developments in our understanding. Endo. Rev. 5:309–345, 1984.

60

Collagen Vascular Disease

ROGER HOLLISTER, M.D.

Collagen vascular diseases are listed frequently in the differential diagnoses of patients with intermittent and confusing symptoms. Patients and physicians often consult with allergists to obtain diagnoses and to identify extrinsic agents for illnesses that currently are understood to be autoimmune or rheumatic in origin. In this chapter, the description of these diseases will focus on symptoms, often respiratory, which may mimic allergic disease. The laboratory will be considered as a tool in differentiating autoimmune and allergic disease.

SYSTEMIC LUPUS ERYTHEMATOSUS

Although not the most common collagen vascular disease, systemic lupus erythematosus (SLE), with its multiorgan symptomatology and intermittent episodes, may appear the most "allergic" in origin. SLE is a disease with an 8 : 1 female predominance. It is rare under the age of 10 years and occurs throughout life, even in the elderly. The prevalence may be as high as 1 in 2000 women of childbearing age. Although the prognosis has improved greatly in the past three decades, a significant mortality remains. A correct diagnosis is therefore demanded as soon as possible.

Symptoms and signs of SLE are protean with skin rashes, respiratory symptoms, and obscure swellings of an intermittent nature, often suggesting allergic origins. Table 60–1 lists the precentage of SLE patients with various symptoms and findings during the course of the illness. Although these symptoms may not be present at disease onset, the majority of patients soon develop manifestations of multisystem disease. Particular attention should be paid to a history of intermittent arthritis (swelling within joints as opposed to angioedema), for this

symptom is present in 85 percent of patients with SLE. Also of note is the fact that only about a third of patients with SLE are sun sensitive (see Table 60–1), although this feature may trigger severe systemic disease in those who demonstrate it. Skin manifestations may include any rash and distribution with a vasculitic appearance as well as the classic malar rash. Disease onset may include urticaria or angioedema, but this is rare.

Respiratory symptoms most frequently include dyspnea and pleurisy (Hauft et al., 1981). Pleural effusions are the most common radiographic findings (Fig. 60–1), but interstitial lung disease also has been found, similar to other collagen vascular syndromes. Wheezing or productive cough is a distinctly unusual manifestation. In the febrile toxic patient, thoracocentesis is indicated to rule out an infectious etiology. Complement levels are reduced, and there is a moderate pleocytosis in pleural effusions of SLE origin.

Laboratory tests are very important in the diagnosis of SLE. Over 95 percent of SLE patients have positive antinuclear antibody (ANA) results, usually in high titers (greater than 1 : 160) when the disease is active. A negative ANA result essentially excludes the diagnosis of SLE, therefore. The fluorescent ANA test is a sensitive diagnostic one, but low titer, false-positive results are significant problems. Repetition of the test and testing for antibodies to native DNA frequently resolves these problems, however. The issue of SLE should not be raised to the patient until unequivocal test results diagnostic of SLE are obtained, since this diagnosis produces considerable anxiety.

The ANA profile has been a significant addition to the laboratory assessment. Two of the following antibodies are found only in SLE patients: anti-DNA and anti-SM, but only in 60 percent and 20 percent, respectively, of all SLE patients. Other antibody specificities have been helpful in diseases such as mixed connective tissue disease, Sjögren syndrome, and scleroderma. Elevated levels of anti-DNA antibodies and depressed levels of complement (CH50 or C3) are associated with active disease and will return to normal with successful treatment. "Lupus anticoagulant" and anticardiolipin antibody are two new additions to the SLE autoimmune profile, and their presence correlates with an increased risk of thrombosis and central

779

TABLE 60–1. Frequency (Percentage) of Signs and Symptoms in Systemic Lupus Erythematosus

Sign or Symptom	Percentage
Butterfly rash	64
Alopecia	43
Photosensitivity	37
Chronic discoid SLE	17
Oral ulceration	15
Raynaud phenomenon	20
Nondeforming arthritis	84
Pleurisy or pericarditis	60
Profuse proteinuria	20
Urinary casts	48
Convulsions or psychosis	20
False-positive VDRL	17
Hemolytic anemia, leukopenia, or thrombocytopenia	40
Positive ANA	95

nervous system (CNS) disease, respectively. The detection of other autoantibodies, such as in a positive Coombs test and a ("false-positive") Venereal Disease Research Laboratory (VDRL) is consistent but not diagnostic of SLE.

Routine urinalysis is the best indicator of active lupus nephritis. Since renal involvement is still a leading cause of death in SLE patients, hematuria, proteinuria, and especially the presence of casts suggest the necessity of renal biopsy to establish a morphologic diagnosis and

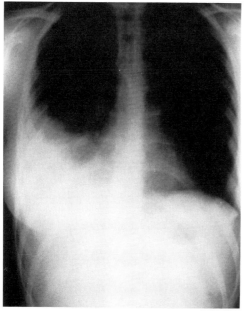

FIGURE 60–1. Systemic lupus erythematosus (SLE) patient with large right-sided pleural effusion obscuring the diaphragm, which cleared completely with high-dose steroid therapy.

a prognosis. If diffuse proliferative glomerulonephritis is seen on the renal biopsy specimen, aggressive treatment is needed to control the disease.

In summary, the laboratory data can eliminate SLE as a diagnosis and can give support to SLE as a positive diagnosis. However, it cannot be used to make a diagnosis of SLE in the absence of the appropriate multisystem disease presentation.

Treatment of SLE has changed the prognosis in this illness from a 15 percent survival at 5 years to an 85 percent survival at 10 years in the most recent series. Part of this increased survival has been due to more judicious use of hazardous medications. For instance, nonsteroidal drugs and the antimalarial drug hydroxy cholorquine sulfate (Plaquenil) have been used successfully in the treatment of patients with arthritis and skin disease. High-dose steroid therapy (1 to 2 mg/kg/day) should be reserved for patients with life-threatening renal or central nervous system (CNS) involvement. Alternate day steroid management frequently is possible after the acute stage of the disease is controlled. Immunosuppressive therapy has added a measure of control for refractory cases. Pulse cyclophosphamide therapy appears to have advantages over other regimens. Plasmapheresis and total lymph node irradiation are considered experimental therapies at this time.

A rare complication in SLE is massive pulmonary hemorrhage. Hemoptysis, dyspnea, and the rapid development of anemia are the clinical signs. Although pulmonary vasculitis seems a logical cause, pathogenesis has been difficult to prove. Treatment with large doses of steroids and plasma exchange may be needed to reverse this life-threatening event.

HENOCH-SCHÖNLEIN PURPURA

Henoch-Schönlein purpura (HSP), or anaphylactoid purpura, is one of the better defined forms of vasculitis which may present as an allergic phenomenon. The definitive clinical finding is a purpuric rash, primarily of the lower extremities or of the buttocks (Fig. 60–2), but it can be seen on other parts of the body. Before the rash becomes purpuric, it may appear urticarial or petechial, or it may appear as angioedema. Other symptoms, such as arthritis, abdominal pain, and hematuria, may precede the purpuris rash and suggest the vasculitic nature of this disorder. A unique inciting agent has not been found.

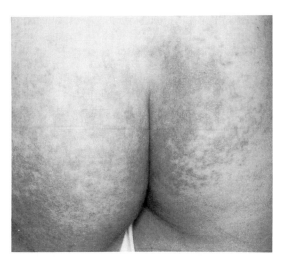

FIGURE 60-2. Characteristic lower extremity and buttock rash in patient with Henoch-Schölein purpura.

There are no specific laboratory tests for patients with HSP, but tests of an exclusionary nature, such as negative ANA results, are important. An elevated serum IgA level is a frequent finding. Should a patient require a skin or renal biopsy, HSP is unique in that IgA is the predominant immunoglobulin deposit found with fluorescent microscopy. Microscopic hematuria, proteinuria, and heme-positive stools indicate vasculitis of kidneys and bowel.

The prognosis for HSP varies considerably between adults and children. In children 3 to 5 years old, the prognoses are excellent with recovery in 7 to 10 days unless nephritis is severe enough to cause azotemia. In the adolescent population, the illness may last several months, and recurrences are not unusual. In the adult, significant renal disease frequently is found, and the response to treatment is disappointing.

The treatment of HSP depends on the organ system involved. In children, prednisone, 1 mg/kg/day, may be necessary if abdominal pain, melena, or the threat of intussusception is present. The rash rarely requires treatment, and nonsteroidal agents can adequately treat arthritic symptoms. Steroids and immunosuppressive agents have been used in the IgA nephropathy of HSP, but the response has been unimpressive.

WEGENER GRANULOMATOSIS

This disease masquerades frequently as chronic sinus disease, recurrent otitis media, or persistent pulmonary disease (Fauci et al., 1983). Incidence figures are not available, but it is an uncommon disease. The cause is unknown. Since its original description as "lethal midline granuloma," Wegener granulomatosis has been found to involve several organ systems, with giant cell vasculitis. The disease is rare in children; however, the diagnosis should be considered early in the work-up of patients with persistent upper respiratory symptoms. A history of nasal septal perforation, hemoptysis, pleurisy, fever, weight loss, or hematuria should alert the physician to consider Wegener granulomatosis in a patient with chronic upper respiratory symptoms. A purpuric skin rash occurs in 50 percent of patients.

The laboratory data show evidence of systemic inflammation, but there are no definitive tests. The anemia of chronic inflammation, leukocytosis, elevated sedimentation rate, and polyclonal hypergammaglobulinemia are frequent. Test results for autoantibodies usually are negative. Microscopic hematuria suggests renal imvolvement. Sinus radiographs may demonstrate bony erosion. Pulmonary infiltrates are the most common findings on chest radiographs; these abnormalities may suggest the proper tissue to biopsy to establish definitively the diagnosis.

The diagnosis of Wegener granulomatosis does not carry the lethal prognosis of a generation ago. With cyclophosphamide and steroid treatment, long-term remissions that may become cures are now possible.

OTHER VASCULITIS SYNDROMES

Depending on the classification, there are many other vasculitic syndromes (Fauci et al., 1976), but for consideration of diseases that may be confused with allergic diseases, polyarteritis nodosa and Kawasaki disease deserve mention.

Polyarteritis nodosa, when it involves the lung and appears as asthma, is known as Churg-Strauss syndrome (allergic granulomatosis). Other involved organ systems are the skin, kidney, and peripheral nervous system. Patients are constitutionally ill with fever, weight loss, myalgia, hypertension, and abdominal pain. Symptoms of mononeuritis multiplex suggest peripheral nervous system vasculitis. The symptoms of asthma may exist for years before other organ system manifestations. The cause of this vasculitis is unknown, and the disease is rare. Multisystem symptomatology should alert the clinician, but there are little epidemiologic data on how often vasculitis appears in the asthmatic population.

In allergic granulomatosis, eosinophilia may reach striking proportions, but hypertension is not common. Conversely, patients with polyarteritis nodosa experience more hypertension and demonstrate less eosinophilia. In polyarteritis nodosa patients, 20-70 percent may have hepatitis B antigenemia detected; in Churg-Strauss patients, an offending agent is identified less frequently. Both conditions produce a medium sized arteritis with subsequent aneurysm formation. In biopsy material, a neutrophilic necrotizing arteritis is found in polyarteritis nodosa, whereas in Churg-Strauss a perivascular, eosinophilic granulomata is found.

In the asthma patient whose clinical picture appears to be evolving into a multisystem disorder, the work-up should include electromyelography (EMG) of suspicious peripheral nerves, ultrasonography or angiography to detect aneurysm formation, and biopsy of suspicious skin lesions or sural nerve (Lanham et al., 1984). Blind biopsies, such as testicular biopsies, are no longer recommended because they are so frequently normal.

Treatment of affected patients relies on high dose steroid therapy, with immunosuppressive trials in patients with resistant cases. The prognosis is variable and must remain guarded until the initial response to therapy can be assessed.

RHEUMATOID ARTHRITIS

The chronic, deforming joint disease of rheumatoid arthritis is not likely to pose problems in diagnosis to the allergist or pulmonologist, but lung involvement may produce several clinical patterns (Petty and Wilkins, 1966). The cause of this systemic autoimmune disease remains unknown. Many aspects of the local, chronic inflammatory cycle have been delineated and include immune complex formation, complement fixation, and subsequent tissue injury by enzymes released from invading neutrophils, macrophages, and lymphocytes. However, no single pathogenetic sequence appears to explain the multiplicity of lung disease.

In children and adults alike, the most common symptoms of lung involvement are pleural inflammation and subsequent effusion. Patients present with dyspnea, tachypnea, and chest pain. Inflammation usually is unilateral but may be bilateral. It occurs in the clinical setting of active joint disease in adults or active systemic disease in children. Fever is absent or low grade, and cough is neither prominent nor productive.

Radiographs demonstrate pleural effusion or pleural thickening. Lateral decubitus films are helpful to demonstrate fluid for diagnostic thoracocentesis. Infections and metastatic effusions are the critical differential diagnoses to eliminate. In rheumatic pleural effusions, an inflammatory exudate is found with cell counts of 5000 to 20,000/mm^3, a neutrophil predominance, a high protein level, and a gram-negative stain. A low peural fluid glucose level is characteristic of both rheumatic and infectious effusions. The pleural fluid complement level will be low relative to the serum level in rheumatoid arthritis, and normal or high in infection. Of the various lung manifestations, pleural effusions seem most likely to derive from local immune complex deposits. Other laboratory parameters, such as leukocytosis, elevated sedimentation rate, positive rheumatoid factor test result (80 percent in adults; 5 to 10 percent in children), are not helpful in distinguishing the cause of the effusion.

Treatment with prednisone (1 mg/kg/day) brings prompt symptomatic relief, and the majority of patients have prompt resolution of radiologic abnormalities. Residual pleural thickening may occur, and brief episodes of pleuritic chest pain may occur without a new effusion for months afterward. Rarely is there a residual abnormality of lung function.

Interstitial lung disease is the next most common pattern in rheumatoid arthritis and is also associated with SLE, scleroderma, and dermatomyositis (Fig. 60-3). It appears to be a common pathway for many of the autoimmune diseases (Hunninghake and Fauci, 1979). Symptoms are insidious at onset with slow progression to exercise intolerance, shortness of breath, and nonproductive cough. Radiographs may be quite unremarkable initially but eventually demonstrate interstitial infiltrates diffusely. Pulmonary function test results show restrictive not obstructive patterns and a decreased diffusing capacity for carbon monoxide (DL$_{co}$) may be the earliest indication of disease. Serum immune complexes can be found frequently, but the antigen or provocative agent is unknown (Dreisin et al., 1978). Bronchoalveolar lavage and open lung biopsy are used to stage the lung disease, with a range from inflammatory to fibrotic. Patients in the inflammatory stage appear to respond better to corticosteroids. High

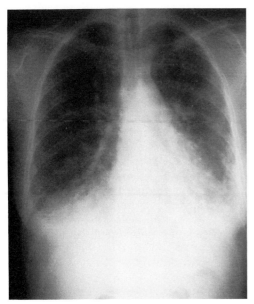

FIGURE 60-3. Diffuse granular interstitial infiltrates in a patient with rheumatoid arthritis.

dose therapy should be used for several months to reverse the process. Other treatments beyond steroids, such as immunosuppressive agents and plasmapheresis, may be tried in individual patients, although there are no large series data on which to predict success.

Bronchiolitis obliterans and Caplan syndrome (Fig. 60-4) are rarer manifestations of rheumatoid lung disease. In the former, an obstructive pattern with wheezing begins the symptomatology that progresses to hypoxia. In Caplan syndrome, pneumoconiosis is superimposed on the autoimmune background of rheumatoid arthritis. Cavitary granulomas are

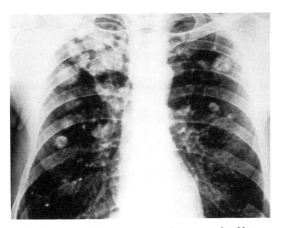

FIGURE 60-4. Widespread granulomata and infiltrates in a patient with Caplan syndrome.

found on chest radiographs. A solitary parenchymal coin lesion can represent a rheumatoid nodule, but biopsy of the mass may be required to distinguish it from neoplastic disease.

SPONDYLOARTHROPATHY

The so-called rheumatoid variants compose a group of disorders that share a common immunogenetic background (the B27 antigen) and often have epidemic environmental triggers (Reiter syndrome, *Yersinia enterocolitica*). The arthritic involvement is primarily of the lower extremities and spine. Sacroiliitis is the hallmark of these diseases (ankylosing spondylitis, Reiter syndrome, and psoriatic arthritis). Acute iritis distinguishes these disorders from juvenile rheumatoid arthritis with chronic uveitis. There is a marked male predominance of approximately 8:1 compared with rheumatoid arthritis, which has a female predominance of 3:1.

Upper lobe fibrotic involvement is a unique pulmonary feature of these diseases (Campbell, 1965). In advanced disease, a productive cough and hemoptysis signal progression of the disease to cyst formation with occasional *Aspergillus* superinfection. This clinical constellation is similar to pulmonary tuberculosis from which it must be distinguished. The cause is not understood, and there is no effective treatment. In a patient with arthritis of the back and no lung involvement, respiratory muscle exercise can maintain vital capacity and function.

DERMATOPOLYMYOSITIS

Autoimmune inflammation of muscles and skin is an acquired and treatable cause of muscle weakness. Five different subtypes of dermatopolymyositis have been proposed, but the most important considerations applicable to possible allergic or pulmonary disease apply across subtypes. In dermatomyositis, the skin rash demonstrates a unique distribution that distinguishes it from eczema (Fig. 60-5). Although the rash of dermatomyositis includes hyperkeratosis, itching, and eventual atrophy, it occurs on extensor surfaces including the knuckles. Eczema, however, is a condition affecting mainly flexor surfaces. The association between inflammatory muscle disease and occult malignancy is real but applies only to those patients over age 40 years. The muscle weakness of dermatopolymyositis is proximal in dis-

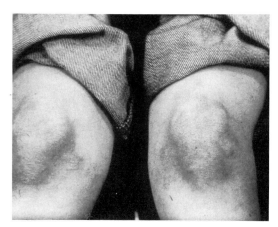

FIGURE 60–5. Erythematous, scaling, raised lesions on the elbows of a patient with dermatomyositis.

tribution, and pelvic girdle weakness is more common than shoulder girdle weakness. Distal muscles are not affected until late in the disease, and deep tendon reflexes are maintained until much later. Sensitized T lymphocytes may be more important to the pathogenesis of this disease than autoantibodies. The childhood form of dermatopolymyositis is a vasculitis that may have widespread visceral involvement.

There are three patterns of respiratory involvement in dermatopolymyositis. Interstitial pulmonary fibrosis, as described in other collagen vascular diseases, may be subclinial and found on DL$_{CO}$ testing (Duncan et al., 1974). A more urgent and obvious pathology in some patients is weakness with palatal muscle involvement, predisposing them to aspiration

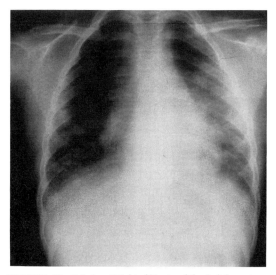

FIGURE 60–6. Interstitial infiltrate of the left lung in a patient with mixed connective tissue disease (MCTD).

often of unanticipated, catastrophic proportions. Extraordinary doses of steroids may be needed to reverse this muscle involvement. Lastly, profoundly weak patients with myositis may have diaphragmatic or intercostal involvement with decreased vital capacity to the point of respiratory failure requiring ventilation. This obviously ominous situation may still be quite reversible. The treatment for dermatopolymyositis is high dose steroid therapy (60 mg/m^2/day or 2 mg/kg/day). In resistant cases, immunosuppressive agents, especially methotrexate, have produced improvement and decreased steroid requirements. In a child, the disease may run a single inflammatory cycle with subsequent permanent remission, but many adults and children have chronic persistent symptoms.

SCLERODERMA AND MIXED CONNECTIVE TISSUE DISEASE

The spectrum of scleroderma has been widened in recent years to include patients with overlapping symptoms who may be responsive to steroids as well as patients with better prognoses. Systemic sclerosis (scleroderma) can involve many organs with a destructive fibrotic process associated with high mortality, or it may be limited to the skin where the process produces the characteristic hidebound appearance, with atrophy of underlying tissue. The pathogenesis of this disorder remains obscure. Immune mechanisms implicated in other autoimmune diseases do not appear to play a role. The extraordinary incidence of Raynaud phenomena in patients with scleroderma may point to a primary vasculopathy. Medical treatment remains inadequate.

Pulmonary involvement in scleroderma is of the interstitial fibrotic pattern. If combined with sclerodermatous involvement of the heart or with hypertension due to renal involvement, the prognosis is grim. There is no convincing evidence that steroids or immunosuppressive agents can reverse these manifestations. The newer antihypertensive agents, such as captopril and minoxidil, may improve the renal complications temporarily.

Mixed connective tissue disease is an overlapping syndrome with elements of scleroderma, arthritis, myositis, and rash resembling SLE. The diagnosis requires a positive antinuclear antibody test result specific for ribonucleoprotein, which usually is present in very high titer. When originally reported, this overlapping syndrome was thought to be a more steroid-responsive form of scleroderma. However, longer follow-up has shown cause for a more guarded prognosis. In children, in particular, interstitial fibrosis may be progressive and poorly responsive to treatment (Fig. 60–6).

The second scleroderma variant is named CREST for the involvement of calcinosis, Raynaud disease, esophageal dysmotility, sclerodactyly, and telangiectasia. The prognoses for this group of patients are believed to be better than for the group of patients with systemic sclerosis who have more lethal renal involvement. The antibody to SCL-70 antigen serves to identify these patients. CREST patients may present with pulmonary hypertension but no other evidence of parenchymal lung involvement (Stupi et al., 1986).

KAWASAKI DISEASE

Kawasaki disease or mucocutaneous lymph node syndrome is a multisystem disease described in 1974 by Kawasaki and associates. Since then it has been reported to occur in epidemic proportions in children. Symptoms include prolonged fever, conjunctivitis, lymphadenopathy, oral mucosal lesions, and desquamating skin rash. There is a small but significant mortality from cardiac complications with aneurysm formation. Pathology is that of diffuse vasculitis indistinguishable from infantile polyarteritis. Involvement of nearly every organ system has been reported. It would not be unexpected to see patients with pulmonary involvement.

GOODPASTURE SYNDROME

This disease, first described by Ernest Goodpasture in 1919, is the prototype of autoimmune disease in which complement-fixing, tissue-specific antibody produces tissue damage. Clinical hemoptysis and dyspnea and pathologic crescentic glomerulonephritis in the presence of antiglomerular basement antibody constitute the syndrome. The antibody crossreacts with the basement membrane of the pulmonary vasculature. Although the two-organ system manifestations of the disease coincide in 70 percent of patients, up to 3 months may separate the two manifestations. Immunofluorescent techniques demonstrate pathogenetic antibody in a linear distribution along the basement membrane.

The syndrome carries a poor prognosis. Although high dose steroid therapy appears to control the hemoptysis, the renal disease rapidly progresses to renal failure. A series of patients has been described in which plasmapheresis has removed the putative antibody in combination with steroid and immunosuppressive therapy, stabilizing or reversing the life-threatening kidney disease (Simpson et al., 1982).

RHEUMATIC FEVER

The Jones criteria have withstood the test of time for diagnosis of rheumatic fever. However, endocarditis and migratory polyarthritis following streptococcal infection are the keystones of diagnosis. Erythema marginatum, chorea, and rheumatic nodules seldom are seen for unknown reasons. Inflammation of the lung with an alveolar infiltration (rheumatic pneumonia) has been reported. Differentiation from congestive heart failure is important but may be difficult. Steroids are indicated for carditis that is severe enough to produce heart failure, but there is no proof that steroids reduce the incidence of residual rheumatic heart disease. Penicillin G (Bicillin) injections remain the most effective prophylactic treatment; they should be given every 3 weeks if exposure rate is high, such as in a day care center (Markowitz, 1985).

THE CLINICAL IMMUNOLOGY LABORATORY

The immunology laboratory can assist the clinician but rarely provides a diagnosis that was not suggested on clinical grounds. Table 60–2 summarizes specific tests and their relationships to various collagen vascular diseases.

A few general comments apply to these tests. A negative ANA test result is most helpful in excluding the diagnosis of SLE, since over 95 percent of active SLE patients have high titer positive test results. Similar to the other autoantibody tests, the techniques involve "sticky" proteins, and low titer "false-positive" results are seen. Many "false-positive" test results occur in the setting of a reactive phenomenon due to a virus, some other infection, or an inflammatory process. In such cases, the ANA usually will be absent on repetition. With all

TABLE 60-2. Laboratory Tests in Collagen Vascular Disease

	Rheumatoid Arthritis	SLE	Scleroderma	Acute Rheumatic Fever	Vasculitis	Spondyloarthropathy
Rheumatoid factors	+++	+/−	−	−	+/−	−
Complement	−	++	−	−	+/−	−
aDNA	−	++++	−	−	−	−
ANA*	+/−	++++	+	−	+/−	−
Streptozyme, ASO	−	−	−	++++	+/−	−
Histocompatibility tests (B27 and DR4)†	+	−	−	−	−	++
Immune complex assays	+	+	−	+	+	−
D_{LCO}‡	+	+	+	−	+	+

+ = positive.
++ =
+++ = } frequently positive.
++++ = always positive.
+/− = occasionally positive.
− = negative.
* ANA profile specificities especially helpful in scleroderma and mixed connective tissue disease.
† Carriage higher in disease population than in normal population.
‡ Most sensitive test of interstitial lung disease.

autoantibody tests, a high titer has a much greater significance than one that is positive only at the screening dilution.

If one had to choose a single test to distinguish collagen vascular disorders from others, the erythrocyte sedimentation rate is useful. Rheumatic diseases are chronic conditions that stimulate the production of acute phase reactants, many of which elevate the sedimentation rate. Conversely, allergic, viral, and metabolic diseases infrequently do so. Even in the perplexing situation of a fever of unknown origin, an elevated sedimentation rate serves to separate chronic systemic diseases from those that are self limited and resolve spontaneously.

The rheumatoid factor test result can be positive in any individual undergoing prolonged antigen stimulation. Subacute bacterial endocarditis is a classic example, but a wide variety of chronic or parasitic diseases also are associated with positive test results. The presence of rheumatoid factors, therefore, is not disease specific but suggests the need for other tests to identify specific antigens.

Newer assays of complement activation rather than simply total complement activity (CH50) are on the horizon. Some of these appear very sensitive and yet do not require special handling. Antibodies to native DNA are highly specific for SLE, but they occur in only 60 percent of SLE patients.

Histocompatibility testing, such as the B27 antigen or the B cell antigen DR4, is useful in patients with spondyloarthropathy or rheumatoid arthritis. The results connote a susceptibility to the disease but are in no way diagnostic.

The D_{LCO} is reduced in patients with interstitial lung disease regardless of the associated collagen vascular disease. Of the panoply of pulmonary manifestations in patients with autoimmune diseases, interstitial lung disease occurs in all the disorders from rheumatoid arthritis to dermatomyositis and even scleroderma. Although it lacks disease specificity, the D_{LCO} is sensitive to this kind of lung involvement, even in patients with normal chest radiographs.

REFERENCES

Campbell, A.H.: Upper lobe fibrosis associated with ankylosing spondylitis. Brit. J. Dis. Chest 59: 90, 1965.

Crystal, R.G.,, Bitterman, P.B., Rennard, S.I., et al.: Interstitial lung diseases of unknown cause. N. Eng. J. Med. 310: 154, 235, 1984.

Dreisin, R.B., Schwartz, M.I., Theofilopoulos, A.N., et al.: Circulating immune complexes in the idiopathic interstitial pneumonias. N. Eng. J. Med. 298: 553, 1978.

Duncan, P.E., Griffin, J.P., Garcia, A.: Fibrosing alveolitis in polymyositis. Am. J. Med. 57: 621, 1974.

Fan, P.T., Davis, J.A., Somer, T., Kaplan, L., et al.: A clinical approach to systemic vasculitis. Semin. Arthr. Rheum. 9: 248, 1980.

Fauci, A.S., Haynes, B.T., Kate, P.: The spectrum of vasculitis: clinical, pathologic, immunologic and therapeutic considerations. Ann. Int. Med. 89: 660, 1976.

Fauci, A.S., Haynes, B.F., Kate, P., et al.: Wegener's granulomatosis: prospective clinical and therapeutic experience with 85 patients for 21 years. Ann. Int. Med. 98: 76, 1983.

Haupt, H.M., Moore, G.W., Hutchins, G.M.: The lung in systemic lupus erythematosus. Am. J. Med. 71: 791, 1981.

Hunninghake, G.W., Fuci, A.S.: Pulmonary involvement in the collagen vascular diseases. Am. Rev. Resp. Dis. 119: 471, 1979.

Kawasaki, T., Kosaki, F., Okawa, S., et al.: A new infantile febrile mucocutaneous lymph node syndrome (MLNS) prevailing in Japan. Pediatrics 54: 271, 1974.

Lanham, J.G., Elkon, K.B., Pesey, C.D., et al.: Systemic vasculitis with asthma and eosinophilia: A clinical approach to the Churg-Strauss syndrome. Medicine (Baltimore) 63: 65, 1984.

Markowitz, M.: The decline of rheumatic fever: role of medical intervention. J. Peds. 106: 545, 1985.

Petty, T.I. Wilkins, M.: The five manifestations of rheumatoid lung. Dis. Chest 49 :75, 1966.

Simpson, I.J., Doak, P.B., Williams, L.C., et al.: Plasma exchange in Goodpasture's syndrome. Am. J. Nephrol. 2: 301, 1982.

Stupi, A.M., Steen, V.D., Owens, G.R., et al.: Pulmonary hypertension in the CREST syndrome variant of systemic sclerosis. Arth. Rheum. 29: 515, 1986.

INDEX

Note: Numbers in italics *refer to figures; numbers followed by (t) refer to tables.*